BERRY AND KOHN'S INTRODUCTION TO OPERATING ROOM TECHNIQUE

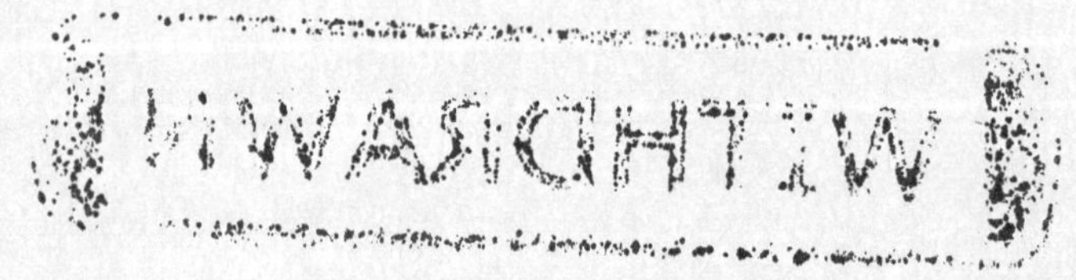

BERRY AND KOHN'S INTRODUCTION TO OPERATING ROOM TECHNIQUE

SIXTH EDITION

Lucy Jo Atkinson, B.S.N., R.N., M.S.

Director of Educational Services, Ethicon, Inc.
Formerly Assistant Director of Nursing
for Operating Rooms and Recovery Room,
Cedars of Lebanon Hospital, Los Angeles

Mary Louise Kohn, A.B., R.N., M.N.

Formerly Instructor in Operating Room Technique
Frances Payne Bolton School of Nursing
Case Western Reserve University, Cleveland

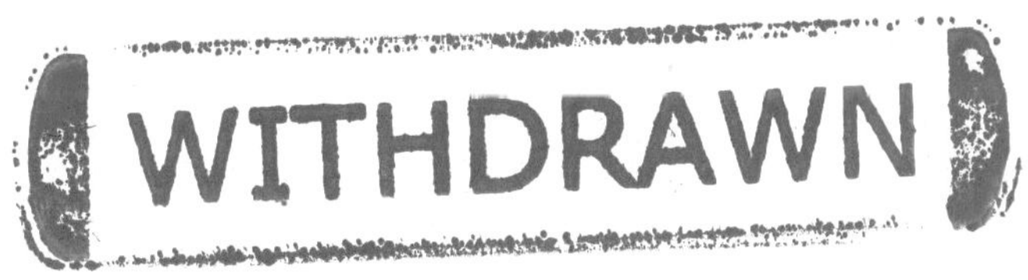

McGRAW-HILL BOOK COMPANY

New York St. Louis San Francisco Auckland Bogotá
Hamburg Johannesburg London Madrid Mexico Montreal New Delhi
Panama Paris São Paulo Singapore Sydney Tokyo Toronto

This book was set in Times Roman by University Graphics, Inc. (ECU).
The editor was Sally J. Barhydt;
the production supervisor was Leroy A. Young;
the cover was designed by Laura Stover.
Cover photograph by UPI/Bettmann Newsphotos.
Project supervision was done by The Total Book.
Semline, Inc., was printer and binder.

Notice

As new medical and nursing research and clinical experience broaden our knowledge, changes in treatment and drug therapy are required. The editors and the publisher of this work have made every effort to ensure that the drug dosage schedules herein are accurate and in accord with the standards accepted at the time of publication. Readers are advised, however, to check the product information sheet included in the package of each drug they plan to administer to be certain that changes have not been made in the recommended dose or in the contraindications for administration. This recommendation is of particular importance in regard to new or infrequently used drugs.

BERRY AND KOHN'S INTRODUCTION TO OPERATING ROOM TECHNIQUE

1 2 3 4 5 6 7 8 9 0 SEMSEM 8 9 8 7 6 5

ISBN 0-07-002541-X

Library of Congress Cataloging in Publication Data

Berry, Edna Cornelia.
Berry & Kohn's Introduction to operating room technique.

Bibliography: p.
Includes index.
1. Operating room nursing. I. Kohn, Mary Louise.
II. Atkinson, Lucy Jo. III. Title. IV. Title:
Berry and Kohn's Introduction to operating room
technique. V. Title: Introduction to operating
room technique. [DNLM: 1. Operating Room Nursing.
2. Operating Room Technicians. WY 162 B534i]
RD32.3.B4 1986 617'.91 85-9634
ISBN 0-07-002541-X

To the memory of Edna Cornelia Berry,
whose devotion to teaching was surpassed
only by her devotion to the
care of surgical patients in the operating room.

CONTENTS

PREFACE TO THE SIXTH EDITION

The sixth edition of this internationally established text is sincerely dedicated to the memory of Edna Cornelia Berry, the original senior author. To the many students and operating room nurses who were privileged to work with her and to know her personally, she was a positive role model and mentor. To thousands of others, she was a teacher through four editions of this text. Miss Berry passed away in 1983 at the age of 86. Her professional life was devoted to the care of her patients and to the nurturing of all practitioners of operating room nursing.

The current authors have maintained the fundamental purposes of this text: to develop an understanding of the principles of sterile and aseptic techniques and the necessity for their application in all operative procedures; and to develop an understanding of the physiological and psychological impact of surgical intervention on the surgical patient as a unique individual.

Following publication of the fifth edition, Miss Berry commented, "This text is now more than an introduction to operating room technique." Although the authors have retained this title, indeed the content was expanded and has been updated in this edition to include current technology and trends in operating room nursing practice.

As technology has become more complex, many operative procedures not envisioned when this text was originally published in 1955 are frequently on the daily schedule of operations. Likewise, specialization within surgical practice has fostered specialization in nursing practice in many operating room suites. *The focus on teamwork remains unchanged,* however. A new chapter is added to this edition describing the multidisciplinary team approach specifically to head and neck surgery.

The practice setting has changed for many operating room nurses and surgical technologists. Because of the increasing trend toward postoperative recovery in the home rather than hospital setting, a chapter is devoted to ambulatory care. This includes consideration of the pre-, intra-, and postoperative care of surgical patients operated in an ambulatory care facility.

Whether in a hospital or ambulatory care setting, the concept of perioperative nursing extends the role of the nurse. A new chapter delineating this professional role emphasizes the nursing process as the mechanism for care of all surgical patients. Although this role is conceptually valid, it is difficult to implement in some clinical settings. Perioperative nursing is a worthy objective of professional operating room nurses, however. Inclusion of the chapter devoted to this concept will help learners and practitioners understand the correlation between theory and practice.

The technical component of patient care in the operating room cannot be overlooked and, therefore, is emphasized throughout this text. This edition retains the general format and accepted principles and practices of previous editions. Although it is assumed the reader has a foundation in the basic sciences, some microbiology, anatomy and physiology, and behavioral science concepts are included for reference and clarification. The material has been resequenced to reflect current emphasis on the need to understand use and care of sophisticated instrumentation to ensure patient safety and quality care, to minimize risks of legal liability in rendering care, and to effect cost containment ultimately for the patient. Some chapters have been divided to more accurately reflect current surgical specialization and practices, e.g., thoracic and vascular surgery, patient monitoring for many specialties.

This text is addressed to all learners of operating room technology, be they students in formal basic or postgraduate educational programs or graduate nurses or surgical technologists developing skills in a new or different area of specialization. To give encouragement to those entering the field of operating room nursing, in whatever capacity, the new last chapter of this edition presents some of the challenges and realities of practice.

Everyone who works in an operating room is responsible and accountable to self, to employer, but primarily to the patient. The authors hope this text will continue to serve as a reference resource for all who are involved in the intraoperative phase of the surgical patient's care. Knowledge is the basis on which skills are developed. References cited in bibliography were current at the time of preparation of this edition. But it is incumbent on every practitioner to keep up with current literature on a regular basis.

The authors sincerely appreciated the recommendations offered by Beverly Baker, C.S.T., Gerald B. Goethals, B.S.N., and Carol Tyler, B.S., C.N.O.R., who reviewed the previous edition, and Edgar Montgomery, C.S.T., who reviewed both the fifth edition and part of the manuscript for this edition. We gratefully acknowledge and give sincere appreciation to the professors/instructors who reviewed the entire manuscript for the sixth edition: Joyce Borndahl, R.N., Moraine Park Technical Institute, Fond du Lac, Wisconsin, Betty Fitzgerald, B.A., C.N.O.R., University of South Alabama, Mobile, and Claire Olson, M.S., C.N.O.R., Nassau Community College, Garden City, New York.

Other reviewers to whom we are indebted for reading specific portions are Frederick S. Cross, M.D., Ph.D., David E. Klein, M.D., Howard D. Kohn, M.D., and Lawrence E. Lohman, M.D., St. Luke's Hospital and the faculty of the School of Medicine, Case Western Reserve University, Cleveland; Ellen V. Mausser, M.D., and Alan M. Oliver, D.O., St. Luke's Hospital, Cleveland; Barbara Daly, M.S.N., C.C.R.N., F.A.A.N., Marcia R. Kohn, B.S.N., C.I.C. and W. Budd Wentz, M.D., University Hospitals of Cleveland; Ira L. Eisenstein, D.M.D., Somerset Medical Center, Somerville, New Jersey; Dwight C. Hanna, M.D., Western Pennsylvania Hospital, Pittsburgh; Mary Senna, R.N., Westfield Orthopaedic Group, Westfield, New Jersey; and Virginia R. Thompson, R.N., B.A., St. Luke's Hospital, San Francisco.

The authors also wish to acknowledge Anita Rogoff, illustrator for previous editions, and Maura Wright for illustrations added to this edition. Appreciation is extended to Grace M. Plumbo, Carole A. Loboda, and Joan A. Bozoklian for assistance with typing of the manuscript.

Lucy Jo Atkinson

Mary Louise Kohn

PREFACE TO THE FIRST EDITION

The material in this text is the outgrowth of the coauthors' experience in the operating room—one as instructor of students, the other as head nurse with some responsibility for instructing and guiding students. It is an adaptation of the instructor's teaching outline for which there have been many requests.

The aim of the book is to facilitate the nurse's study of aseptic technique and care of the patient in the operating room. Although this text is intended primarily for the student, the authors hope it may prove useful to the graduate nurse as well.

Since it is assumed that the student has studied pathological conditions necessitating surgical treatment, these conditions are not discussed. When applicable, and as a matter of emphasis, there is a reiteration of principles of sterile technique and safety factors for the patient. It is hoped this will aid in fixing the principles as patterns of thought and work.

While operative routines vary in different hospitals, underlying principles are the same. Consequently, basic principles are stressed and the authors have endeavored to keep the material as general as possible. Principles must be adapted to suit the situations found in individual hospitals. Specific linen, equipment, and procedures are mentioned merely to serve as a framework upon which to demonstrate principles or as samples for points of departure. However, the specific examples mentioned are workable procedures that have evolved. They are kept as uncomplicated as possible for student teaching and for use in the practical situation.

Instruments for operations are not listed and few are mentioned, because each hospital has its instrument lists, standardized for each case, to which students can refer.

Emphasis is placed upon meeting the psychological as well as the physical needs of the surgical patient. An endeavor is made where possible to correlate briefly the preoperative and postoperative care with the operative procedure, to give the student a complete concept of patient care.

The frequent use of the imperative mood is for the purpose of brevity, organization, and emphasis. Questions and assignments in each chapter are to aid the student in reviewing the material, in recalling pertinent facts, and in applying the principles to her specific situation.

Obviously, if the student starts scrubbing for cases with an older nurse after her first day or two in the operating room and if her operating-room theory is given concurrently with the practice, much of the material in this book will have been covered by individual instruction before class discussion.

The authors have attempted to maintain simplicity and brevity, and to present a concise outline for preliminary study. They suggest that the student supplement this material by reference reading.

The authors wish to express their grateful appreciation and thanks to those persons who by their interest and cooperation supported them:

To Miss Edythe Angell, Supervisor of the Operating Rooms at University Hospitals of Cleveland, for helpful suggestions during the preparation of the manuscript and for reading, critically, the entire manuscript. We are gratefully indebted to her because we have learned from her much of what appears in this text.

To Miss Janet McMahon, Educational Director, School of Anesthesia, University Hospitals of Cleveland, for valuable assistance in preparing Chapter 21. Also, to Dr. Edward Depp, Anesthesiologist, Euclid-Glenville Hospital, Cleveland, who offered suggestions on this chapter and reviewed it.

To Dr. C. C. Roe Jackson, of the faculty of Western Reserve University School of Medicine, for constructive criticism in reviewing Chapter 17. To Dr. Howard D. Kohn, also of the faculty, who has been most helpful in reading the manuscript and offering suggestions.

To Mrs. Geraldine Mink, Librarian, for her assistance; to Mrs. Leona Peck for her patience in typing the manuscript and for her helpful suggestions; to Miss Ruth Elmenthaler and Miss Margaret Sanderson of the operating-room staff for their assistance in making the photographs; and to Mrs. Anita Rogoff for drawing the illustrations.

Edna Cornelia Berry

Mary Louise Kohn

CHAPTER **1**

INTRODUCTION FOR THE LEARNER

MODERN SURGERY

Health is a personal and economic asset. Needs are altered in proportion to one's ability to function normally. *Optimal health* has been defined as the best an individual can feel and function in the particular circumstances or with a disease process. *Disease* is a failure of the adaptive mechanisms to adequately counteract stimuli or stresses, resulting in disturbance in function or structure of any part, organ, or system of the body. *Illness* is often a composite of many reactions or diseases.

Since time immemorial, human beings have searched for the causes of illnesses and ways to relieve suffering. To participate as a health care worker increases one's awareness of some basic facts of life:

1 No one is immune to suffering, but to alleviate it is worth the effort and cost, for life is priceless.

2 One should not try to face suffering alone; let others help.

3 Vulnerability is an important component of life. Anne Morrow Lindberg's insight is most applicable. "Suffering is always individual . . . to suffer is to be alone. . . . To suffering must be added mourning, understanding, patience, love, openness, and the willingness to remain vulnerable."*

*AM Lindberg, *Hour of Gold, Hour of Lead: Diaries and Letters of Anne Morrow Lindberg 1929–1932,* New York: Harcourt Brace Jovanovich, 1973, p. 212.

Fifty years ago only a small percentage of hospitalized patients were admitted for operations. Today, surgical intervention, one step in the total process of restoring or maintaining health, offers hope to a population of all ages with conditions that can be treated surgically. The number of operations performed and anesthetics administered increases annually. This is due to the population explosion, the increased incidence of congenital abnormalities, the ever-increasing number of aged persons, and the rapid progress in all facets of medicine. Many former contraindications to surgery have changed. Because of better diagnostic and supportive services and drug therapies, many persons are now considered candidates for surgery.

The word *surgery* designates the branch of medicine that encompasses preoperative care, intraoperative judgment and management, and postoperative care of patients. Surgery as a discipline is total care of illness with an extra modality of treatment, the *operation,* for correction of deformities and defects, repair of injuries, diagnosis and cure of disease processes, relief of suffering, and prolongation of life. At the time of operation, pathologic conditions are documented and treated. Surgical intervention encompasses more than technical performance of an operative procedure. In fact, the operation may constitute a minor part of the total therapy for surgical patients.

Surgical science has progressed far beyond what was envisioned years ago. Modern surgery is safer and surer than ever before. Reliable diagnostic techniques and equipment enable physicians to more precisely measure the effects of illness and injury and to more accurately make diagnoses and predict surgical outcomes. Surgeons and equipment manufacturers consult together constantly to develop and perfect instrumentation. Improvement in the knowledge and management of the surgical patient's nutritional and physiological condition, plus the many complex, precise skills of the surgeon are also beneficial to the effectiveness and safety of surgical care. Specialization in all areas of medicine, and increasingly in nursing too, brings to patient care a vast augmentation of available consultative services for helping to determine what is wrong, what needs to be done, and how best to do it. Some of the greatest gains have been in methods of preparing patients for operation, and of caring for them postoperatively in the rehabilitation period. These new methods of patient care are based on the premise that each patient is a unique individual requiring individualized care. Exceptionally rapid advances have been made in the development of safe anesthesia, which is so vital to a favorable surgical outcome.

Patients come to the operating room for a variety of reasons, including:

1 To preserve life, e.g., relief of intestinal obstruction or decompression of a skull fracture
2 To maintain dynamic bodily equilibrium, e.g., removal of a diseased kidney
3 To undergo diagnostic procedures, e.g., breast biopsy, bronchoscopy
4 To prevent infection and to promote healing, e.g., burn debridement
5 To obtain comfort and to ensure the ability to earn a living, e.g., elective herniorrhaphy

Most, but not all, operations are performed in hospitals. Many are performed in surgeons' offices or in independent, nonhospital-based, free-standing surgical facilities if they are not complex enough to require hospitalization of the patients. Not all patients operated on in a hospital-contained operating room unit are admitted to the hospital. Surgeons view postoperative activity as beneficial rather than hazardous for surgical patients. Consequently, operation on an ambulatory care or an outpatient basis is feasible and safe for carefully selected patients. Ambulatory surgery is discussed in more detail in Chapter 5. Although reference will be made throughout this text to *hospital,* the practices and procedures described are applicable in all surgical care settings.

The types of operations performed in a hospital or other facility vary according to the expertise of the surgeons on the staff, the community in which the facility is located, and the equipment available. The daily schedule of operations is as variable as the type of facility and the types of operations performed. Regardless of the circumstances that bring patients to the operating room (OR), the intraoperative phase of care becomes an integral part of nursing service, filling a need that cannot be met by the individual patient or his or her family. In the operating room you must accept the challenge of this critical phase of nursing care upon which the patient's ultimate recovery is so dependent. Nursing care of patients undergoing surgical intervention as the therapeutic modality of choice is carried out at two levels: professional and technical.

PROFESSIONAL NURSING

Characteristics of a Profession

The characteristics of a profession are that:

1 It defines its own rules and code of ethics.
2 It sets its own standards and conducts its own affairs and self-regulation.
3 It identifies and develops its own body of knowledge unique to its role, through research.
4 It engages in periodic self-evaluation and peer review to control and alter its practices and behaviors.

The members of a profession must act responsibly in accord with their commitment to public trust and service. However, professional conduct is not synonymous with ritualism, detachment, or denial of feeling. Simply stated the word *profession* implies a combination and coordination of knowledge, skills, and ideals that are communicated through a highly specialized educational discipline. In this way education sets the standards for practice.

Professional Nursing

Professional nursing is dedicated to the promotion of optimal health for all human beings in their various environments. In addition to performing many other roles including teaching health-seeking behaviors, promoting preventive medicine, taking part in patient rehabilitation, and participating in nursing research, the professional nurse in the acute-care setting performs functions that are primarily curative and restorative in nature. The professional nurse practitioner's role, as reflected in the *Standards of Nursing Practice* developed by the American Nurses' Association (ANA), includes nursing diagnosis as a basis for planning, providing, directing, collaborating in, and evaluating direct patient care.

As a helping profession, nursing's ideal characteristics include the ability and commitment to respond with compassion to human needs and society's expectations for health care services. If we deny humanity to others, we dehumanize ourselves as well. Professional nurses are committed to life, health, and death with dignity. In practice, they help each client/patient to attain his or her highest possible level of general health. Nurses are morally responsible and legally accountable for the quality of their practice.

Professional and legal standards extend the nurse's responsibility and accountability beyond procedural steps. Their purpose is to fulfill the profession's obligation to provide and improve practice. Standards and recommended practices have been established by professional organizations, federal and state governments, the Joint Commission on the Accreditation of Hospitals (JCAH), and other voluntary agencies. Definitions, standards, and recommended practices give guidance to nursing service and nursing education. They have been progressively elevated and are continually assessed, maintained, and improved.

Data have shown that care tends to move to the lowest level of preparation of personnel. Therefore, the better prepared the staff, the higher the quality of care given. Professional education should be built upon a solid base of general education in liberal arts, humanities, and natural and behavioral sciences. The nurse, educated to assess the total patient, is an indispensable member of the OR professional team. A person with quality education approaches challenges creatively and with confidence that solutions can be found. As changes occur with surprising rapidity, and nursing develops as a profession in its own right, its responsibilities to the patient, to itself, and to its correlated professions increase as well. The source of professional authority is an understanding of the role functions of the professional.

Operating Room Nursing

New developments are constantly taking place in the field of surgery. As diagnostic and supportive services have become increasingly complex, so have operative procedures. Intricate procedures have become part of daily operating room routine. It is therefore essential that nurses have extensive specialized technological knowledge and skills. They also must have the theory-based critical judgment and intellectual skills needed to apply a humanistic approach to their responsibilities as patient advocates. Concurrently, the role of the OR nurse is expanding as nurses relinquish non-nursing activities in order to accept newer nursing responsibilities. Nursing care of surgical patients extends behind and beyond the doors of the operating room.

Professional nursing in the operating room has been defined as "the identification of the physiological, psychological and sociological needs of the patient, and the implementation of an individualized program of nursing care that coordinates the nursing actions, based on a knowledge of the natural and behavioral sciences, in order to restore, or maintain, the health and welfare of the patient before, during, and after surgical intervention."*

The professional operating room nurse practitioner, a duly licensed registered nurse, is legally responsible for the nature and quality of the nursing care patients receive during surgical intervention, i.e., the operation itself. The scope of operating room nursing practice encompasses those nursing activities that assist the individual surgical patient in a conscious or unconscious state. These activities are directed toward providing continuity of care through preoperative assessment and planning, intraoperative intervention, and postoperative evaluation. The program for nursing care prescribes:

1. What nursing actions are to be performed
2. How the nursing actions are to be done
3. When these actions are to be performed
4. Where these actions are to be performed
5. Who is to perform the nursing actions†

Nursing actions, the functions of professional nursing, provide the foundation of the nursing

*AORN Statement Committee: Definition and objective for clinical practice of professional operating room nursing, AORN J 10(5):48, Nov 1969.

†Association of Operating Room Nurses and American Nurses' Association Division on Medical-Surgical Nursing Practice: *Standards of Perioperative Nursing Practice,* Kansas City, Missouri: American Nurses' Association, 1981. Reprinted with permission of ANA.

process used in assessing, planning, implementing, and evaluating patient care. These actions are:

1 Application and execution of the physician's legal orders
2 Observation of the patient's symptoms and reactions
3 Supervision of the patient
4 Supervision of others who contribute to the care of the patient
5 Reporting and recording
6 Application and execution of nursing procedures and techniques
7 Promotion of the patient's physical and emotional health by directing and teaching

The first action is dependent upon the physician, and the other six are independently taken by the nurse. The activities of professional nurses are supplemented and complemented by the services of allied technical health care personnel who function as assistants to nurses.

The concepts of total patient care and continuity of nursing care encompass the *perioperative role* of the OR nurse. This role has both technical and professional components in carrying out the nursing process preoperatively, intraoperatively, and postoperatively. The preoperative phase of a surgical patient's care extends to the time the patient is moved onto the operating table. The intraoperative phase begins at this time and ends when the patient is admitted to the recovery room. Postoperative care continues through the immediate recovery period to complete rehabilitation. The scope of nursing activities the OR nurse assumes in the perioperative role is contingent upon his or her personal knowledge, skills, and experience, and upon the expectations delineated in the job description of the nurse's position. The perioperative role is discussed in detail in Chapter 4.

OR nursing is an intellectually and physically demanding yet rewarding acute care specialty of clinical nursing practice. The OR is a dynamic, ever-changing critical care setting where the care given is a decisive factor in postoperative outcome. Since no two days are alike, OR nursing is always challenging, never tedious.

A wise physician once said that the physician's role is to cure sometimes, to relieve often, to comfort always. The same can be said for the OR nurse who embodies all the word *nurse* has traditionally meant to a patient—provider of safety and comfort, supporter and confidante—no less so because the practice environment within the OR suite is geographically separated from most of the hospital complex to reduce traffic, noise, and sources of microbial contamination. The professional OR nurse holds a unique position. Patients' safety and welfare are entrusted to the nurse from the moment of their arrival in the operating room until their departure, and until the transfer of responsibility for their care has been made to another professional health care team member. The primary emphasis of the nurse's responsibility is that of total nursing care. He or she is accountable to patients and responsible for the scope of nursing practice whether it is accomplished personally or by qualified assisting personnel. The patient relies on the nurse:

1 To provide competent, skilled, trustworthy care during the operation
2 To mitigate anxiety and pain
3 To meet aggregate needs for which the nurse is qualified through extensive, in-depth education and experience

The nurse fulfills a vital function in the continuity of care of the surgical patient as he or she pursues goals to enable persons to experience ever more healthy, productive lives.

TECHNICAL NURSING/ALLIED TECHNOLOGY

The activities of registered professional nurses are supplemented and complemented by the services of allied technical health care personnel who function as assistants to nurses. *Technical nursing practice* has been defined as the carrying out of delegated techniques with a high degree of skill through the use of principles learned through didactic education and clinical experience. Technical nursing practice is unlimited in depth, but limited in scope.

Broadly, the term *allied health care personnel* refers to individuals trained in a health care related science with responsibility for the delivery of health care related services, but who are not graduates of schools of medicine, osteopathy, dentistry, podiatry, or nursing.* About two-thirds of the health care work force is designated as allied health professionals. Educational preparation may be offered in colleges, vocational-technical schools, hospital-based programs, or military service schools. Technologists, technicians, and ther-

*Adapted from definition recognized by the National Commission on Allied Health Education in 1980.

apists in over 130 occupational categories work collaboratively with medicine, nursing, or other health-related professions.

The *surgical technologist* (ST), sometimes still referred to as an *operating room technician* (ORT), works with the surgeon, anesthesiologist or anesthetist, and professional registered nurse as a member of the direct patient-care team during surgical intervention. This team is referred to as the *OR team.* The surgical technologist assists by preparing and handling supplies and equipment to maintain a safe and therapeutic environment through a system of specific techniques and practices designed to exclude all pathogenic microorganisms from the operative wound.

A surgical technologist completes a nine-month to two-year intensive educational program. This includes courses in biology, chemistry, anatomy and physiology, and microbiology as prerequisites to courses involving theory and application of the dynamics of operating room technology to operative procedures and the operating room environment. Other courses in the curriculum, such as pathology and pharmacology, help explain the underlying basis for technical tasks to be mastered. Courses in psychology and interpersonal communication are fundamental to an appreciation of the humanities. These generic courses are beyond the scope of this text, which focuses on the essentials of operating room technique that all nursing personnel, professional and technical, must master.

Because they are administratively responsible to nursing service, and considered part of the nursing staff complement in the OR, *surgical technologists will be included in reference to nursing personnel throughout this text.*

CORRELATION OF THEORY AND PRACTICE

Knowledge and technology advance so rapidly that physicians, nurses, and allied health care personnel must remain learners throughout their professional or vocational careers or face obsolescence in five to ten years. The types of learners in any setting are as varied as their backgrounds, personalities, experiences, and abilities to learn.

Some learning of OR technique can take place in the classroom setting or the self-study laboratory. Lecture and demonstration may be given to learners who then practice the procedure, which, in turn, is followed by the instructor's evaluation of their work. Books, journals, films, slides, and videotapes may supplement the lecture approach. Many audiovisual materials are self-contained units for self-study. A bibliography in a text such as this provides reference leads to add to and broaden the learner's theoretical knowledge. The amount of literature is almost without limit. Each instructor plans classes or self-study units according to available materials and learner needs.

Reading the literature and using audiovisual teaching aids are only part of providing adequate preparation for clinical practice. Skills are gained by active participation. Theory becomes meaningful and of value only when it is put to practical use. Some learning will be accomplished through observation, but skills will be learned through actual experience in applying the theory learned in the classroom or self-study laboratory.

In the operating room you will see living anatomy, its alteration by congenital deformities, disease, or injury, and its restoration or reconstruction. You will see the important part operative procedures play in the care of life-threatening emergencies. You will learn to function in these situations for the patient's welfare.

Your practice in the operating room will give you opportunity to apply your knowledge of the basic sciences. Much theory is translated into practice and can be observed, such as the effect of a tourniquet in creating a dry operative site, the effect of warm tapes in restoring circulation to a strangulated bowel, the gangrene that results from prolonged strangulation, the dark appearance of blood not properly oxygenated, the expansion of the lungs, the movement of the diaphragm.

Operating room nursing is an invaluable experience in preparing one to be a more understanding, observing, and efficient person. In close teamwork with surgeons and anesthesiologists, the nurse participates in vital resuscitative measures, and learns to evaluate their effectiveness and to care for anesthetized, unconscious, and/or critically ill patients. In addition, the learner discovers that such emergencies as cardiac arrest are more easily prevented than treated. He or she gains valuable experience applicable to any nursing situation by learning:

1 To fully realize what surgical intervention in all its aspects means to a patient. When one is familiar with operative procedures, the *whys* of postoperative pain, complications, and care are clearly apparent.

2 To realize the importance of optimal physical and emotional preoperative preparation for all patients and the need for constant patient observation intraoperatively. One deficiency can have a snowballing effect. For example, if an adequate blood volume is not maintained, cardiac output is reduced, the blood pressure then falls, and renal function is impaired; retained body wastes then further disturb delicate acid-base, potassium-sodium balances. The heat-regulating mechanism is also upset. Fluid and electrolyte maintenance is important to prevent dehydration and acid-base imbalance in blood and tissues.

3 To differentiate between innocuous occurrences and situations that, if unrecognized and allowed to progress, will lead to disaster.

4 To cope with any eventuality in a calm, efficient manner; to think clearly and act quickly in crisis situations.

5 To attend to every pertinent detail, to keenly observe, and to anticipate the needs of the patient and of colleagues.

6 To know the need for and to comprehensively practice aseptic and sterile techniques.

Above all, operating room experience teaches that *no operation is minor!* The only predictable element in the operating room is the potential for the unpredictable occurrence. Operations may be classified as major or minor by hospitals for practical use but in reality no such distinction exists. An operation has a deep personal meaning for each patient, and the possibility of death cannot be ruled out completely. Every operative procedure carries an element of inherent risk. A supposedly relatively safe procedure can rapidly become a catastrophic one, even a fatal one, if the patient is allergic to medication or anesthetic drug, develops uncontrollable bleeding, irreversible shock, overwhelming postoperative infection, or experiences a cardiac arrest on the operating table. While every precaution is taken to foresee and prevent adverse reactions, such reactions do occur on occasion. No matter how simple a procedure, an experienced OR team member has indelibly inscribed in memory such occurrences and gives undivided attention to the patient at *all* times.

During your experience, you may participate in or observe the preparation of operating room supplies and learn their use. You will gain an appreciation of the precision with which surgical instruments and equipment are made for particular functions. Also, in helping to carry out a daily schedule of operations, you will become aware of the interdependence of the various departments of the hospital, and how they work together for the well-being of the patient. One of the most valuable learning experiences in the OR is the opportunity to see and become a part of real teamwork in action. This will be discussed in Chapter 2.

THE LEARNER

The beginning learner in the OR may be either a student nurse or surgical technologist enrolled in a formalized educational program or a registered nurse, who was recently graduated or who is reentering the profession, learning first-level basic competencies in perioperative nursing.

All learners in the OR environment are adults. Therefore, regardless of level of learning, advanced or beginning, the general characteristics of the adult learner apply.

1 As a person matures, time perspective changes from one of postponed application of knowledge to immediacy of application. Accordingly, learning shifts from a subject-centered orientation to a problem-solving approach. Adults will learn what they need to know to solve problems, i.e., to function effectively.

2 An ego involvement in self-concept moves an adult from a dependent personality toward that of a self-directing individual who wants to be responsible for one's own behavior.

3 The readiness to learn becomes oriented to the need to increase developmental skills.

4 As experience accumulates, the resources for learning enhance individual participation and involvement in the learning process, i.e., practical application of developing skills through an expanded knowledge base.

Each hospital has its learner level of work more or less defined. In most hospitals, beginning learners are not used to fill staff positions. Learners actually help prepare for, assist during, and clean up following operations. Novices will not be expected to assume responsibilities for which they are not fully prepared. Only through continued study and experience can individuals qualify as team members during the most complex operations.

The learner is usually taught the scrub role functions early in the OR experience. These functions are discussed in detail throughout this text. At first, an experienced instructor or staff member scrubs with the new person, gradually permitting the learner to take over more of the work in the sterile field until the learner is able to function without help. The types of operations to which the novice may be assigned vary from hospital to hospital, depending upon many factors peculiar to each. However, rarely does the beginning learner scrub on operations of the heart, lung, or brain.

Since one of the objectives of learning is to gain a thorough knowledge of sterile technique, repetition of the scrub functions serves a valuable purpose by impressing it indelibly in the mind of the learner. It is better to learn the fundamentals thoroughly than to try to observe many complicated operations and retain little. Knowing how to do a procedure is not enough. All OR procedures must be practiced. You will sense greater satisfaction when you gain skill in performing them. To make the experience as profitable as possible, the learner should assist the circulating nurse as well as scrub. This necessitates constant supervision and help from the instructor or another experienced RN. Contribution to the accomplishment of the work of the entire team becomes real and is a necessary part of the learning process.

The learner is not the only one who benefits from this learning process. The OR team gains from each learner contact. The surgeons actively participate in the learning experience by acquainting the learner with patients' situations, by explaining why operations are being performed, and by answering questions.

Learning as many procedures as the course of study permits can benefit in the following ways:

1 You will have a more complete understanding of the implications that surgical interventions have on the health status of patients.

2 You will appreciate the proper care of expensive instruments and the need for economy in the use of all supplies.

3 You will know how to do the work in order to assist others. In helping others, you will be stimulated to increased effort and will feel more a part of the department.

4 You will be better able to evaluate and compare other methods for the purpose of improvement, if you know the methods in use.

5 You will be better qualified to supervise others and to evaluate their performance if you know the time and labor involved in their work.

OBJECTIVES FOR LEARNING

Education for first-level entry into professional practice prepares nurses to be knowledgeable generalists capable of working with and through others in all clinical settings. The operating room can be used as a clinical laboratory for learning generalist nursing behaviors by focusing on what happens to the patient during surgical intervention. Some schools of nursing offer a course in perioperative nursing either in the core curriculum or as a student elective. After graduation from any generalist program, the nurse needs further preparation in the clinical area of specialization. This may take place in a postbasic perioperative nursing course, or it may be provided through a well-planned and well-taught on-the-job inservice educational program, plus self-study. The purpose of a formalized postgraduate program is to meet the nurse's needs for theoretical and technical knowledge and to provide supervised clinical experience. The RN in the OR must have full knowledge and experience in all the roles that are tangentially connected and interdependent with the care of the surgical patient.

The operation itself is the focal point of surgical intervention for the patient. Management of this critical act requires a team whose members understand the dynamics of the problems presented, the methods to solve them, and the gravity of the situation for the patient. All team members must have theoretical scientific knowledge of the principles of technique, referred to as *aseptic and sterile techniques,* in order to provide an environment free from pathogenic microorganisms. These principles must be thoroughly learned by nurses and technologists who work in the operating room. They are applicable, in various measures, to nursing in other clinical settings. For example, the principles learned in the OR apply to procedures requiring isolation or a sterile field to prevent hospital or self-acquired infection. However, the need for understanding and applying aseptic and sterile techniques is greatly intensified and emphasized in the OR. Surgeons are able to maximize their skills effectively through strict adherence to these techniques by all team members. Therefore, the concepts to be learned and the objectives to be met for all beginning learners of operating room technology must include the following:

1 To demonstrate ability to apply principles of sterilization, disinfection, aseptic and sterile techniques in preparation and use of all supplies and equipment under all conditions and circumstances imperative to prevent the potential eventuality of an environmentally acquired infection.

2 To increase and clarify knowledge of anatomy and physiology in normal structure and function, and in patterns altered by disease processes. This knowledge will be demonstrated by ability to correctly position patients on the operating table and to select appropriate instrumentation, equipment, and supplies.

3 To demonstrate an understanding of the more common operations by anticipating the needs of members of the OR team and by organizing work efficiently in the best interests of patient safety and welfare.

4 To understand the action and use of anesthetic agents, fluids, and electrolytes and patient responses to them by having appropriate supplies available in the event of adverse reactions.

5 To recognize the trauma inflicted, and consequent legal implications involved, on each patient undergoing surgical intervention and to carry out the care required to ensure patient safety.

6 To identify the potential environmental dangers to the patient through an understanding of the function and care of surgical instruments, supplies, and equipment, so as to prevent hazards to patient safety and subsequent incidents of negligence.

7 To identify the members of the OR team and the legal responsibility of each member for the care of the conscious or the unconscious patient as a basis for establishing and maintaining inter- and intradepartmental functions that ensure continuity of surgical patient care.

8 To participate in making collaborative decisions that demonstrate willingness to cooperate with members of the OR team on behalf of the patient.

9 To function as a team member by showing consideration for and cooperation with others within the OR and by communicating with the interdependent departments of the hospital that work together for the well-being of the patient.

10 To develop flexibility, adaptability, and self-reliance as a team member by acquiring a working knowledge of all aspects of the operating room environment and the functions of all personnel.

11 To develop manual dexterity and the ability to manage personal anxiety by learning basic techniques so well that correct activity response is quickly carried out in life-threatening emergency or stressful situations as well as in normal circumstances.

12 To identify factors that create stress and the coping mechanisms exhibited by members of the OR team in their cooperative effort as a basis for evaluating and modifying your own behavior in order to enhance your personal participation in the team effort on behalf of the patient.

13 To exert a conscientious effort to carry out all duties accurately and with integrity, in compliance with hospital policies and recognized standards of practice, and thus to develop pride in performance consistent with personal, professional, and vocational ethical and moral values.

14 To help control patient and hospital costs through the correct, safe, and economical use of supplies and equipment and personal efficiency in time and motion.

THE CLINICAL INSTRUCTOR

Experience in the OR clinical setting must be planned and supervised. A designated resource person, either a faculty member or nursing staff member employed by the hospital, is available to guide and assist you in competently applying newly acquired knowledge. *The term* instructor *will be used throughout this text to refer to the resource person responsible for planning, implementing, and evaluating learners' experiences, both in the classroom or self-study laboratory and in the clinical setting.* The instructor who is a faculty member employed by a teaching institution may not be a member of the hospital staff. Hospitals offering the clinical setting for educational and training programs have their own policies and procedures that must be adapted and adhered to by both the instructor and the learner. During clinical experience, the instructor supervises learner activities.

The instructor must objectively assess your skills and knowledge. When your deficiencies are identified, you must be provided with learning experience to enable you to reach your highest potential. You must be involved in the teaching/learning process too. Effective education develops from the needs of the learner. It is essential for the instructor to discover what the learner wants to know as well as what will be required for the learner to know.

The instructor must determine in what areas the learner is knowledgeable and in what areas additional experience is needed. A written knowledge and skills inventory checklist can assist in identifying learning needs. This involves rating the actual skills and knowledge of the learner against a standardized listing of the skills and knowledge required for optimum performance. This framework provides a means for the learner to identify his or her own learning needs as well as to request new learning experiences.

The instructor must use a variety of approaches with learners to achieve the desired results, such as formulation of clear-cut explicit behavioral objectives; use of skill in questioning and encouraging learners to make discoveries and correlations; employment of written guidelines and assignment for feedback to assure that learning has taken place. Learner conferences should be held on a regular basis to discuss procedures as well as problems.

The instructor must work closely with the *OR nursing supervisor* (ORS). Classroom hours and clinical experience assignments are worked out together. The supervisor offers suggestions and criticism for the benefit of the learner. The instructor offers suggestions to the supervisor for the experiences of the learner. The ORS is aware of the planned program for the learner. An effort is made to confer and to coordinate any changes in the program. This fosters a friendly and cooperative relationship. The ORS is advised of each learner's progress.

The instructor must also acquaint the entire operating room staff with the proposed learning experiences. All staff members should assist in teaching the learners. Everyone should be familiar with the level of the learners, the learning goals, and the roles that staff members will be expected to assume with respect to teaching. Learner performance objectives should be prepared to specifically describe:

1 The condition under which the task is to be performed

2 The specific action or performance to be demonstrated

3 The standard of acceptable performance as a basis for evaluating learner's competency and achievement

EXPECTED BEHAVIOR OF O.R. PERSONNEL

Nurses are expected to be both human and humane, as well as competent. The standard for the behavior of all OR nursing personnel is no less high. The ability to successfully discharge duties contributes to efficient teamwork, but more importantly, to patients' sense of security. Perceived behavior makes a lasting impression that patients associate with their experiences in the operating room. It reveals self-confidence (or lack of it), interest (or indifference), proficiency and authority (or ineptitude). In addition to possessing special technical expertise, OR nursing personnel must have personal attributes that inspire confidence, trust, and honesty in patients and team members. OR nursing personnel must be:

1 *Empathic.* Feeling persons can put themselves in another's place. As allies of patients, they convey compassion and a sense of personal worth. They understand and are sensitive to feelings, values, points of view, and actions. Yet they do not let emotions indiscriminately obscure or override professional judgment and rationale, or interfere with care. Caring can be painful, so caring persons are vulnerable. However, in order to insulate or steel against anxiety, suffering, or even death, nursing personnel sometimes lose their ability to interact with patients or colleagues.

The sedated patient is not totally unaware of the OR milieu. Soft-spoken, reassuring words are another valuable way to express concern. Never be reticent to communicate your empathy to a patient.

2 *Conscientious.* These persons will not compromise or sacrifice principles of self-accountability, to ensure quality in practice.

3 *Efficient and well-organized.* Persons who develop organized work habits know, and know that they know, that patients are properly prepared and the OR is ready for their operations with the required equipment in working order. They anticipate needs of patients and team members to save time and energy. They are prepared for the unexpected. Efficiency provides reassurance and comfort to patients and surgeons alike.

4 *Flexible and adaptable.* Team members react quickly to changing circumstances in a calm manner and rearrange routine. Discriminating judgment prepares adaptable people to cope with all situations with professional decorum.

5 *Sensitive and perceptive.* Nursing personnel are responsive at all times to areas of need and to problems that must be solved. Perceptive persons exhibit genuine interest and kindness in caring for patients, and in looking after them and letting them know that they mean something to them. OR nurses are sensitive to the special kind of caring that their patients need.

6 *Understanding, reassuring, and supportive.* In a kind and emotionally controlled way, team members allow others to express their feelings. This conveys to patients the team's ability to relieve physical and emotional discomfort.

7 *Skilled listeners, keen observers, and able communicators.* People who watch, look, and listen will act effectively. Aware personnel will not underestimate the importance of communications in their relations with patients and colleagues.

8 *Considerate.* These individuals respect other people's concepts and do not automatically reject those different from their own. Consideration extends to all interpersonal relationships.

9 *Informative and sincere.* Nursing personnel should answer questions and share pertinent information for the mutual benefit of patients, families or significant others, and colleagues. All health care team members must have the same information to deal honestly and factually with patients and their families. Shared information and forewarning can avoid problems. Nurses should explain procedures before touching patients and give the rationale for them. Patients must never be permitted to feel lost, confined, or abandoned. Control and trust are enhanced by knowledge. Patients have greater confidence when an open, facilitating approach is used. Nurses should reinforce the physicians' explanations.

10 *Aware of individuality.* All personnel convey to patients and colleagues an interest in them as unique persons and act accordingly.

11 *Manually and intellectually dextrous.* These people have quick hands, sharp minds, and keen eyes. Manual dexterity, inherent in most OR team members, is perfected with experience.

12 *Objective.* Such individuals assemble factual data before making a judgment. They view situations from all sides before taking action. Objectivity requires experience and self-discipline. This attribute does not exclude concern but is combined with empathy. Nurses should remain sensitive to problems while acknowledging their own feelings. However, fear must never be obvious to patients, whom it would affect adversely.

13 *Impartial, nonjudgmental, open-minded.* These individuals set value judgments aside when making decisions and do not permit their own values and attitudes to distort observations. Accept others as they are without attaching conditions to acceptance.

14 *Versatile.* These persons have a comprehensive knowledge of an extensive amount of instrumentation and equipment. They are familiar with numerous operative procedures and care required for many diverse patients.

15 *Analytical.* These persons are competent in analyzing and correlating significant data. *They know the* why *as well as the* how *of surgical intervention.* Patients depend on their judgment.

16 *Creative.* These individuals are innovative in devising effective methods of approach to meeting individual needs and helping patients and colleagues to utilize available resources.

17 *Humanistic.* OR team members act in a humane way toward others. They consider the patient as a person as opposed to someone hooked up to technology.

18 *Sense of humor.* These are the people who can maintain a balance for their own mental health through their perception of the ironies in life situations.

19 *Enduring.* Personnel with endurance maximize their physical and emotional capacities and stamina. OR personnel interact in a critical setting under stress, often for prolonged periods of time. Continual demands are made on them for keen observation, rapid judgment, and fast action. All personnel must be disaster-prepared and work rapidly, often under pressure, without sacrificing competency.

20 *Intellectually eager and curious.* Nurses and technologists have a legal responsibility to keep current in their knowledge, to be present-oriented and informed. Documented proof of continuing education and demonstrated competence in performing functions are of value in litigation. Educational development is a dynamic, ongoing process. Continuing education is a shared responsibility of the hospital, the nursing service, and the individual. The instructional environment should be individually designed. Learning is not just subject-centered, but more problem-centered. Participating in research improves nursing practice and patient care.

21 *Ethical.* These persons use ethical principles, moral values, and professional codes as the basis for making decisions and solving problems. Personal values do influence behavior, but they should not violate legal or ethical rights of patients or the hospital. Always be honest; tell the truth. Respect the equality of human rights and the dignity of others as human beings, but also "to thine own self be true." You will encounter ethical dilemmas that must be resolved in the best interests of all involved. (Refer to Chapter 37.)

NECESSITY FOR STANDARDIZED PROCEDURES AND TECHNIQUES

Standardized procedures and techniques are essential. While there are different ways of arriving at the same ends, it is necessary that one method in each hospital be established and practiced. This prevents chaos for learners and other new personnel. When you are expected to follow accepted procedures, you may sometimes feel that you are being regimented, but that is not the case. Standardized procedures are a great aid in the development of skill and efficiency because:

1 They have as their chief aim the safety and welfare of the patient.

2 It is easier for the instructor or nursing staff member to teach the learners if there is a clearly defined method of work.

3 Learning is easier if everyone does the procedures in the same way.

4 When procedures are kept up-to-date, they set a high standard of work performance.

5 Deviations show a need for evaluation of the procedures and the staff. Do the procedures need revision? Or have staff members become careless?

6 They provide an efficient check during the preparation for any operation. They supplement the memory of the OR staff.

7 One person can take over for another at any time during the operation, if necessary, and know exactly where to find instruments and supplies.

8 Routine procedures establish patterns of habit that increase speed in thought and action. These habits act as motives for doing work in a certain way, which means a high level of proficiency when keyed to high standards of performance.

All personnel involved in the care of surgical patients during the critical intraoperative phase must be thoroughly familiar not only with setups, policies, and procedures, but also with equipment and surgeons' routines. OR nursing personnel must be able to cope with all situations in order to provide patients with the utmost in skill, knowledge, and abilities. The enhancement of each individual's potential will provide the best guarantee of high quality patient care.

Inasmuch as details vary from hospital to hospital, discussion of specific equipment has been minimized in this text. However, certain items and techniques for handling are basic. Comparable if not identical equipment is in use in all hospitals. Efficiency is increased by knowledge of equipment and its use. Many items are a part of the operation only. Others are returned to units with patients, and their use carries over to the nursing care and safety of patients there. You must have a broad scope of general knowledge concerning OR procedures and equipment and you must be able to bring it into immediate use as the need arises.

The following is a list of *reference sources* and *learning aids* that all personnel will find useful in mastering and carrying out accepted procedures and techniques:

Hospital Policy Manual. This book contains written basic and general administrative and patient care policies that apply to all hospital personnel. A copy is retained on each nursing unit and in all departments of the hospital.

Operating Room Policy Manual. This book, usually a hardcover ringed binder, contains the policies pertaining solely to the administration and operation of the OR department. A copy is available for reference either in the supervisor's office or at the control desk or both.

Operating Room Procedure Manual. Procedure manuals are assembled for the OR department, as for other hospital departments, to ensure the optimum safety of patients. The primary purpose of the OR procedure manual is to detail how procedures should be specifically performed within the OR suite. It includes those procedures involving direct patient care and supportive procedures.

Instrument Book. The instruments for each operation may be listed in a separate book, which is kept in the instrument room or processing area. Photographs or catalog illustrations help learners identify the vast number of instruments used.

Surgeon Preference Cards. A preference card is maintained for each operation that each surgeon performs. A set of cards is kept in a central file under the surgeon's name. The file is kept where it is readily available. Each day the cards are pulled for operations scheduled and taken to the appropriate OR. The nurses and technologists consult them, along with the procedure book, as they prepare for each operation. The surgeon's specific preference and any variance from the procedures in the procedure book are noted on the card. It is inexcusable for nurses and technologists to fail to prepare the equipment and supplies that a surgeon routinely uses.

These cards are revised as necessary as procedures and personal preferences for new technology change. These cards permit surgeons to maintain their individuality. Figure 1-1 is a sample surgeon preference card.

Directories. Alphabetical listings of the location of supplies and equipment are maintained for the instrument room, general workroom, sterile supply room, and general operating room suite storage areas. Regardless of where the storage areas are located, personnel must know the location of supplies and equipment. Directories save valuable time in trying to locate items.

Checklist for learners. The instructor provides a checklist of work assignments for the learners. Learners check off their assignment as they observe or complete it. New assignments are made each day from this list, according to the experience needs of each learner. Learners should avail themselves of every opportunity to learn by observation and practice to enhance their competency.

Checklist of operations. The instructor maintains a record sheet for operations on which learners have scrubbed or circulated. It contains a list of operations for each surgical service. Learners check off their daily experience. This enables the supervisor to see at a glance the experience needed by each learner when making out assignments.

Library and literature file. Books and current periodicals are available for learner reference in the department library. These may be found in the supervisor's office, the nursing staff lounge, or the classroom or conference room if there is one within the OR suite. In addition to books and periodicals, educational literature is available from surgical supply and instrument manufacturers. The literature that accompanies new equipment is of inestimable value to all the staff as well as to learners. This is filed and kept available as part of the inservice educational program.

NOTE. 1. The *Cumulative Index to Nursing and Allied Health Health Literature* is the most widely used index for nursing and allied health. In addition to the printed version, the on-line computer version (CINAHL) is available through data base vendors DIALOG and BRS. The 30,000 record data base includes indexing by subject headings from virtually all English language nursing journals and allied health literature from January 1983, with bimonthly updates. CINAHL also indexes pertinent articles from the medical literature, and lists nursing and allied health books.

2. Medical Literature Analysis and Retrieval System On-Line (MEDLINE) is a computer-

SURGEON:	PROCEDURE:
GLOVE SIZE: ________	POSITION OF PATIENT: ________
SKIN PREP:	DRAPES:
SUTURES AND NEEDLES	**INSTRUMENTS AND EQUIPMENT**
TIES:	BASIC:
PERITONEUM:	
FASCIA:	SPECIAL:
SUB-CU:	
SKIN:	
RETENTION:	
OTHER:	
DRESSINGS:	

FIGURE 1-1
Surgeon preference card. (*Reproduced by permission of Ethicon, Inc.*)

based reference system available at over 800 libraries in institutions and government agencies in the United States and Canada. Over 3000 biomedical journals, including 200 nursing journals, are referenced.

3. Audiovisual aids have become increasingly important in teaching and continuing education. The National Library of Medicine has established Audiovisuals On-Line (AVLINE), a data base of references to audiovisual aids in the health sciences. AVLINE is available through the same on-line network as MEDLINE.

Self-help aids. Habit patterns are formed early in one's learning. Carry in your pocket a memorandum book and pencil. After the completion of an operation, as a reminder, write down in a notebook any questions concerning the patient, or the operation and duties regarding it, and discuss them with the instructor before going off duty. Whenever in doubt, ask for clarification and direction. Always complete an assignment thoroughly and neatly. Ask for help or consult the procedure book when in doubt. Report any assignment as finished or unfinished and ask to have it checked. Seek new experiences. This demonstrates your interest. Remember your purpose: to learn about the nursing care of patients during surgical intervention, the critical phase of surgical patient care, so that you can be a functional member of the operating room team.

CREDENTIALING

Credentialing refers to the processes of accreditation, licensure, and certification of institutions, agencies, and individuals. These processes establish quality, identity, protection, and control for competency-based education and performance of professional and allied technical health care personnel.

Accreditation

An accrediting body of a voluntary organization evaluates and sanctions an educational program or an institution as meeting predetermined standards and/or essential criteria. The National League for Nursing accredits schools of nursing. The Committee on Allied Health Education and Accreditation of the American Medical Association accredits surgical technology programs. The Joint Commission on Accreditation of Hospitals (JCAH) accredits hospitals.

Licensure

A license to practice is granted to professionals by a governmental agency, such as the state board of nursing or medicine. Upon completion of formal academic education, nurses and doctors who successfully pass a state examination receive a license to practice in that state. To maintain this license, they must register with the state as required by law, hence the term *registered nurse* (RN). Practical/vocational nurses also are licensed (LPN/LVN). Some states require evidence of continuing professional education for renewal of a license.

Most states grant a license by reciprocity to applicants who move into their state to practice, but who took the examination in another state.

Some states require licensure for some categories of allied health occupations, however, surgical technologists are not currently licensed in any state.

Certification

A nongovernmental, private organization can award a credential that attests to the competence or excellence of an individual who meets predetermined qualifications. Certification is voluntary, as opposed to licensure, which is mandatory.

Doctors, nurses, and allied health care personnel may be certified by their specialty association as competent in knowledge and skills to practice. Applicants must take an examination that tests basic knowledge in the area of specialization. Surgical technologists who successfully pass an examination attesting to their theoretical knowledge are certified by the Association of Surgical Technologists, Inc. These individuals are *certified surgical technologists* (CST). Similarly, a nurse anesthetist becomes a *certified registered nurse anesthetist* (CRNA) by passing the examination of the American Association of Nurse Anesthetists.

Some nursing associations grant recognition of professional achievement and excellence in current practice. In addition to an examination, applicants must demonstrate actual performance competence. This must be validated by peer review. Operating room nurses who successfully complete the process are certified by the Association of Operating Room Nurses National Certification Board, Inc. Each is recognized as a *certified nurse operating room* (CNOR).

Certification is usually granted for a limited time period. To retain this credential, the individual must complete the recertification process established by the certifying body.

CHAPTER **2**

THE HEALTH CARE TEAM

TEAM CONCEPT

This text is directed to the health care personnel who care for the surgical patient primarily during the most critical phase of intervention—the operative procedure. When the patient is reconciled to and has given consent for surgical intervention, the patient is dependent on the health care team. A *team* is a group of two or more persons who recognize common goals and coordinate their efforts to achieve them. Broadly defined, the *health care team* includes all personnel relating to the patient, those in direct patient contact as well as those who are not but whose services are essential and contribute indirectly to patient care.

The team's approach to patient care must be harmonious. Members must employ ethical practices that foster trust and confidence. Unethical discussions or conduct, carelessness, or forgetfulness makes a negative impression on a patient or other team members.

Pride in one's work and in the team as a whole leads to personal satisfaction. High morale is facilitated by adequate staff orientation, staff participation in departmental decision making and problem solving, receipt of deserved praise, opportunity for continuing education, and motivation to reach and practice at one's highest potential.

The team's common goal is the efficient and effective delivery of care to the individual patient for the relief of suffering, the restoration of bodily structure and function, and a favorable postoperative outcome contributing to the patient's optimal health and return to society, or death with dignity.

TOTAL DEPENDENCE OF THE PATIENT ON THE O.R. TEAM

At no other time during the hospital experience will the patient be so well attended as during the operation. The patient is surrounded by a surgeon and one or two assistants, a scrub nurse or technologist, an anesthesiologist or anesthetist, and a circulating nurse. These individuals, each with specific functions to perform, comprise the operating team. *Reference will be made throughout this text to this direct patient care team as the OR team.* This team literally has the patient's life in its hands. The OR team is like a symphony orchestra; each person is an integral entity in unison and harmony with his or her colleagues for the total accomplishment of a successful outcome.

Persons who function in stressful situations, such as those who work in acute and critical care units, are among the most qualified of professionals and allied technical personnel. They are motivated to maintain high standards. There is no place for mediocrity in the OR! For the welfare and safety of the patient, all persons need to work rapidly and efficiently as a functioning single unit of *one,* often under tension in a critical setting. They must be thoroughly familiar with procedures, setups, equipment, and policies, and must be able to cope with the unpredictable. They must have high morale, mutual understanding, trust, cooperation, and consideration. Anyone who cannot function wholeheartedly as a qualified team member, practicing at his or her optimum level at all times, has no place in the OR! This team works to promote the best interests of the patient every single minute.

O.R. Team

The OR team is subdivided according to the functions of its members:

1 The *scrubbed sterile* team
- **a** Operating surgeon
- **b** Assistants to the surgeon
- **c** Scrub nurse or technologist

These team members scrub (wash) their hands and arms, don sterile gown and gloves (see Chap. 9), and enter the sterile field. The *sterile field* is the area of the operating room that immediately surrounds and is especially prepared for the patient. To establish the sterile field, all items needed for the operation are *sterilized,* which are the processes by which all microorganisms are killed (see Chap. 8). Thereafter, the scrubbed, sterile team members function within this limited area and handle only sterile items (see Chaps. 7 and 10).

2 The *unscrubbed unsterile* team
- **a** Anesthesiologist or anesthetist
- **b** Circulating nurse
- **c** Others: In complicated, critical operations such as those in which the chest is opened for procedures on the heart or lungs, the OR team is enlarged to include biomedical engineers or technicians who may be needed to set up and operate the heart-lung machine, monitoring devices, and other instruments that safeguard patient welfare during the operation.

These team members do not enter the sterile field. They function outside and around it. They must assume responsibility for maintaining sterile technique during the operation, but they handle supplies and equipment not considered sterile. Using the principles of aseptic technique, they keep the sterile team supplied, give direct patient care, and handle other requirements that may arise during the operation.

STERILE TEAM MEMBERS

Operating Surgeon

The surgeon must have the knowledge, skill, and judgment required to successfully perform the intended operation and any deviation in procedure necessitated by unforeseen difficulties. The American College of Surgeons (ACS) has stated principles of patient care that dictate ethical surgical practice. Protection of the patient and quality care are preeminent in these principles. The surgeon's responsibilities include preoperative diagnosis and care, selection and performance of the operation, and postoperative management of care. The care of many surgical patients is so complex that considerably more than technical skill is required of a surgeon. Advance prediction of simple and uncomplicated operations is uncertain. A surgeon must be prepared for the unexpected with a knowledge of the fundamentals of the basic sciences and the ability to apply them to the diagnosis and management of the patient before, during, and after surgical intervention.

The surgeon assumes full responsibility for all medical acts of judgment and for the management of the surgical patient. The surgeon is a licensed physician (MD), osteopath (DO), oral surgeon (DDS or DMD), or podiatrist (DPM) especially trained and qualified by knowledge and experience to perform operative procedures.

Most surgeons, by virtue of their postgraduate surgical education, engage in practice within a specific surgical specialty. Qualification for surgical practice, although not a rigid requirement, is certification by an American surgical specialty board approved by the American Board of Medical Specialists or fellowship in the American College of Surgeons. Ten American Specialty Boards grant certification for surgical practice or include surgery. Highly trained and qualified surgeons limit themselves to their specialty except perhaps in emergency situations.

Operations may also be performed by physicians who do not meet these criteria. These physicians include: a physician who received the MD degree prior to 1968 and who has had surgical privileges for over five years in a hospital approved by the Joint Commission on Accreditation of Hospitals where most of his or her surgical practice is conducted; a physician who renders surgical care in an emergency or in an area of limited population where a surgical specialist is not available; or a physician who by reason of education, training, and experience is eligible but who has not yet obtained certification or fellowship.

The surgeon must become a member of the medical staff and be granted surgical privileges by each hospital in which he or she wishes to practice. Standards for admission to staff membership, and retention of that membership, are clearly delineated in the bylaws formulated by the medical staff and approved by the governing body of the hospital. The credentials committee has the primary responsibility for investigating thoroughly not only the training of an applicant but also the surgeon's integrity, technical competence, and professional judgment. In making its recommendations, the committee sets any limitations it sees fit on the surgeon's privileges. The fact that the hospital has assigned privileges does not mean that the surgeon has a free hand. Each hospital sets specific rules, which must be strictly adhered to by each member of the medical staff.

Patients are entitled to the protection and assurance of knowing that surgical privileges are limited to those for which the surgeon has been educated and in which his or her competence has been demonstrated. The patient's choice of and confidence in a surgeon, as well as adherence to directions and advice, are potent factors in the outcome of surgical intervention. A discerning patient will check the qualifications of a surgeon preoperatively.

A competent surgeon has been described as one who realistically appreciates his or her own cognitive skills and personal characteristics to effectively intervene in a patient's particular illness or injury. This surgeon accepts responsibility based on competence, humanistic concern, and accountability to choose a course of action that will not harm the patient.

Assistants to the Surgeon

Under the operating surgeon's direction, one or two assistants hold retractors in the wound to expose the operative site, place clamps on blood vessels, and assist in suturing during the operation. Ideally, another competent surgeon should back up the operating surgeon during every operation in the event of an unanticipated incident to the latter. Such sudden incapacities are, however, rare. For many simple procedures it is clearly not feasible to have a second surgeon, or even another physician as assistant, on the operating team. It would be superfluous to insist upon a physician as assistant at all operations. The degree of hazard of an operation is not so much in the nature of the procedure itself as in the condition of the patient. The operating surgeon must evaluate all individual patient factors to determine the needs for adequate assistance during the operation. The surgeon must be prepared to defend his or her decision before the medical staff and the governing body of the hospital.

In most medical staff bylaws, a section reads, "A qualified physician shall assist during all major operations." The surgical staff of some hospitals maintains a listing of operations by classification as major or minor. If policy stipulates that a physician must assist on all major operations, the surgeon should not be allowed to operate unless a qualified MD assistant is present. Differentiation of major versus minor begs the question. The technical procedure itself may be relatively minor, but performing it without complications sometimes is not. In any operation with unusual hazard to life, a qualified physician must be present and scrubbed as first assistant. Determination of what constitutes unusual hazard rests with the conscience of the operating surgeon and is part of his or her responsibility to the patient.

First Assistant to the Surgeon The first assistant should be capable of assuming the responsibility of the operating surgeon in case of an emergency. A qualified assistant is an individual acknowledged by the credentials committee of the medical staff as having sufficient knowledge, skill, and experience to properly and adequately assist and act for the benefit of the patient.

When the magnitude of the situation warrants, the surgeon may employ another surgeon to first assist. This may be an associate with whom surgical practice is shared and to whom part of the care of the patient may be delegated.

A referring staff physician who is not a surgeon by education and training, but who has a contractual relationship with the patient, may assist the surgeon if granted this privilege by the medical staff. These physicians are usually engaged in general or family practice and have had some training in basic operative principles and techniques. Specially trained nonmedical personnel such as oral surgeons and podiatrists perform or assist with operative procedures in a hospital only under the authority of the medical staff and the surgeon responsible for the surgical service.

In hospitals with accredited postgraduate surgical residency training programs, the surgical resident in the third or more year usually acts as first assistant. The resident is given sufficient responsibility under supervision at the operating table to acquire skill and judgment. This experience is progressively graded so that on completion of training the resident is able to assume individual responsibility for operations.

All ten boards governing the surgical specialties require at least three years of approved formal residency training, and most set the minimum at four or five years. Any physician who aspires to become a board certified surgeon must meet these requirements while assuming increasing responsibility in the care of surgical patients and learning operative techniques under supervision.

The responsible staff surgeon may delegate the performance of part of an operation to a resident assistant, provided the surgeon is an active participant throughout the essential part of the operation. If a senior resident is to operate on and take care of the patient under the general supervision of an attending surgeon who will not participate actively but who is readily available, the patient should be so informed and give consent prior to operation.

The medical staff may approve privileges for a nonphysician allied health practitioner who is qualified by academic and clinical training to perform designated procedures in the operating room and in other areas of surgical patient care. *Physician assistant (PA)* is a generic term with two subcategories: the *assistant to the primary care physician (PCA)* and the *surgeon's assistant (SA)*. The PCA must have additional surgical training to first assist at the operating table. Authorization by the medical staff is based upon the individual's training, experience, and demonstrated competency. Eligibility for appointment as an allied health nonphysician assistant for specified services is determined by the following critieria:

1 Exercising judgment within areas of competence, with the physician member of the medical staff having the ultimate responsibility for patient care

2 Participating directly in the management of patients under the supervision or direction of a member of the medical staff

3 Recording reports and progress notes on patients' records and writing orders to the extent established by the medical staff

4 Performing services in conformity with the applicable provisions of the medical staff bylaws

A member of an allied health profession is individually assigned to an appropriate clinical department as a staff affiliate to carry out activities subject to departmental policies and procedures. The surgeon's assistant must perform duties under the direct supervision of the surgeon. The assistant may help take care of patients in any setting for which the surgeon assumes responsibility and may perform tasks delegated by the surgeon. The ultimate role of the surgeon's assistant cannot be rigidly defined because of variations in practice requirements due to geographic, economic, and sociological factors. The high degree of responsibility an assistant may assume requires that at the conclusion of formal education he or she will possess the knowledge, skills, and abilities necessary to provide those services appropriate to the surgical setting, which may include those of first assistant at the operating table. After completion of a formal academic program, the PAC and SA must pass a standardized certification examination.

The surgeon's assistant may become highly skilled and specialized in the area in which the immediate supervisor has interest, or may remain a generalist for a wide variety of procedures such as those performed by a family practitioner in a community hospital. The frequency of performance of certain duties will in part determine the degree of special expertise such an individual acquires. A surgeon's assistant usually is employed by the surgeon, not the hospital, but must receive approval from the medical staff. The medical staff bylaws delineate the assistant's practice privileges within the hospital.

The functions of the surgeon's assistant are not an extension of the role of the registered nurse or surgical technologist in the OR. In the absence of a qualified MD or SA, the RN who has acquired additional knowledge, technical skills, and judgment through specialized instruction and supervised practice may serve as the first assistant under direct supervision of the surgeon. The assigned nurse should function solely as the first assistant and not try to also fulfill the scrub nurse functions. Similarly, a surgical technologist trained to perform the necessary skills may act as the first assistant in the absence of more qualified individuals.

A nurse may not be compelled to perform an action outside the scope of competence or the legal limits of nursing practice. He or she is free to refuse to act as first assistant, out of concern both for the well-being of the patient and for one's own professional accountability. Before any nurse or surgical technologist acts as a first assistant at the operating table, he or she should check to be certain that a written hospital policy permits this action. *If RNs and/or surgical technologists are expected to act as first assistants, this function should be part of their written job descriptions and inservice education.* Moreover, the individual must be familiar with state statutes and regulations relevant to this role, particularly nurse and medical practice acts. Several states have determined that acting as first assistant at the operating table is not within the scope of nursing practice.

Regardless of whether the employer is the surgeon or the hospital, practice privileges for surgical residents and nonphysician first assistants must be based on verifiable credentials that attest to essential knowledge and skills.

Second Assistant to the Surgeon Qualified nurses and technologists may be utilized as second or third assistants during operations requiring a physician first assistant, or a first assistant as delineated above, in which the surgeon deems their assistance is adequate and *for which they have been trained.*

Prior to entering postgraduate programs in the surgical specialties, physicians complete at least one year of general surgical residency immediately following graduation from medical school. Medical students also receive some exposure to the operating room during surgical clerkship. These first year general surgical residents and medical students usually function as second assistants at the operating table in teaching centers.

Scrub Nurse

Scrub nurse is a term used to designate the nursing member of the sterile team who actually may or may not be a nurse. The role of scrub nurse may be filled by a registered nurse, a licensed practical/vocational nurse, or a surgical technologist. The scrub nurse may also be called the scrub assistant, sterile nurse, instrument nurse, or suture nurse. *The term* scrub nurse *will be used throughout this text to designate this role and to elaborate the specific functions of the individual performing in this capacity.*

The scrub nurse is responsible for maintaining the integrity, safety, and efficiency of the sterile field throughout the operation. Knowledge of and experience with aseptic and sterile techniques qualify the scrub nurse to prepare and arrange instruments and supplies, and to assist the surgeon and assistants throughout the operation by providing the sterile instruments and supplies required. *This demands that the scrub nurse anticipate, plan for, and respond to the needs of the surgeon and other members of the team by constantly watching the sterile field.* Manual dexterity, along with physical stamina, is required. A stable temperament and ability to work under pressure are also important assets of the scrub nurse, as well as a keen sense of responsibility and concern for accuracy in performing all duties.

During extremely complicated or hazardous operations or in teaching situations, two scrub nurses may join the team. One may pass instruments and supplies to the surgeon while the other prepares supplies. An experienced nurse often joins the team to teach, guide, and assist the learner to function in the scrub nurse role. When unexpected, unusual, or emergency situations arise, specific instructions and guidance are received from the surgeon or registered nurse. The surgical technologist provides services under the supervision and responsibility of a qualified registered nurse at all times.

Some hospitals permit nurses or surgical technologists employed by surgeons to come into the OR to perform the scrub role for their employers. These *private scrub nurses* must adhere to all hospital policies and procedures and to approved written guidelines for the functions they may fulfill.

UNSCRUBBED TEAM MEMBERS

Anesthesiologist or Anesthetist

An *anesthesiologist* is an MD, preferably certified by the American Board of Anesthesiology, or a DO who specializes in the art and science of administering anesthetics to produce the various states of anesthesia. An *anesthetist* is a qualified nurse, dentist, physician, or anesthesia assistant who administers anesthetics. When a drug or gas is administered by an anesthetist, this individual works under the direct supervision of an anesthesiologist or the surgeon. The majority of anesthetists are nurses who have a background in OR nursing. Graduates of an accredited nurse anesthesia program, which is a minimum of two years in length, must pass the certification examination of the American Association of Nurse Anesthetists to become certified registered nurse anesthetists (CRNA). They must be recertified every two years.

It has been said that no anesthetic agent is safer than its worst administrator. *Throughout this text the term* anesthesiologist *will be used to refer to the person responsible for inducing anesthesia, maintaining anesthesia at the required levels, and managing untoward reactions to anesthesia throughout the operation.* Recognizing that anesthesiology is a practice of medicine, the value of well-trained anesthetists is also acknowledged. Medically delegated functions of an anesthetic nature are performed under the overall supervision of a responsible physician or in accordance with individual written guidelines approved within the health care facility.*

Anesthesia and surgery are inseparable; they are the two parts of one. These parts must not go their independent ways, but must go together and remain together. Adequate communication between the surgeon and the anesthesiologist is the greatest safeguard the patient has. The anesthesiologist is an indispensable member of the OR team (see Chaps. 3, 13, and 14). Functioning as guardian of the patient, the anesthesiologist must also observe the principles of aseptic technique (see Chap. 7).

Modern anesthesia is vastly superior to anesthesia of previous years. A continuing increase in the number of anesthetic agents available and refinements of administration techniques have broadened its scope. Improvement in understanding of the pharmacologic action of anesthetic drugs has led to safer anesthesia. The choice and application of appropriate agents and suitable techniques of administration, monitoring of physiologic functions, maintenance of fluid and electrolyte balance, and blood replacement are all essential parts of anesthesiologists' responsibilities. They also share responsibility for minimizing the hazards of shock, electrocution, and fire. Appropriate precautions must be taken to ensure the safe administration of anesthetic agents. They must be able to use and interpret correctly a wide variety of monitoring devices (see Chap. 14).

Anesthesiologists are not confined to the operating room, although this is their primary arena. In addition to providing relief from pain for patients and optimal conditions for surgeons during operation, they oversee the recovery room to provide resuscitative care until each patient has regained control of vital functions. They also participate in the hospital's program of cardiopulmonary resuscitation as teachers and team members. They act as consultants or managers for problems of acute and chronic respiratory insufficiency requiring inhalation therapy, and for a variety of other fluid, electrolyte, and metabolic disturbances. Their advice may be sought in the total care of unconscious, critically ill, or injured patients with acute circulatory disorders or neurologic deficits in the intensive care unit or emergency department. Anesthesiologists also are integral staff members of pain therapy clinics.

Some anesthesiologists prefer to specialize in one area, such as cardiothoracic or obstetric anesthesia. The latter involves care of two lives simultaneously. In some settings, they participate in teaching and research as well as in clinical practice.

Circulating Nurse

The *circulating nurse* plays a role that is vital to the smooth flow of events before, during, and after the operation. Patients undergoing surgical intervention experience physical and psychosocial trauma. They enter an alien environment removed from the personal contact of family and friends. Physical and psychological needs reach ultimate proportions. Because most patients are unconscious, they are powerless and unable to make decisions concerning their welfare. At this critical time, patients need the professional judgment of others who must function on their behalf. These advocates must be within close physical and social proximity. The surgeon is in charge at the operating table, but he or she relies upon the circulating nurse to take care of the activities of the room outside the sterile field and to manage the nursing care required for each patient. To some extent, the circulating nurse controls both the physical and

*American Association of Nurse Anesthetists Guidelines for the Practice of the Certified Registered Nurse Anesthetist, copyright © 1983.

emotional atmosphere in the room. The role of the OR nurse as the patient's advocate, protector, guardian angel, and provider cannot be stressed enough. Therefore, the circulating nurse must always be a registered nurse. Surgical technologists may assist in circulating duties under direct supervision of a qualified RN.

The role of the circulating nurse is vital to the provision of that care that includes but is not limited to:

1 Application of the nursing process in directing and coordinating all nursing activities related to the care and support of the patient within the OR to meet individualized patient needs. Nursing judgment and decision-making skill are requisites to assessing, planning, implementing, and evaluating nursing care before, during, and after surgical intervention. This is the professional role of the circulating nurse (see Chap. 4).

2 Creation and maintenance of a safe and comfortable environment for the patient through implementing the principles of asepsis (see Chap. 7). The circulating nurse must see the OR as a whole and be so "technique conscious" that any break or near-break on the part of anyone in the room is evident instantly. Although sterile technique is the responsibility of everyone in the room, the circulating nurse must be on the alert to catch any breaks that others may not have seen. Standing farther away from the sterile field than others, the circulating nurse is better able to observe the entire field.

3 Provision of assistance to any member of the OR team in any manner in which the circulating nurse is qualified. This requires current knowledge of the legal implications of surgical intervention. The circulating nurse must know the organization of the work and the relative importance of factors involved in accomplishing it. The effective circulating nurse will know the fine points of performance as a scrub nurse to be able to anticipate the needs of the scrubbed team. He or she must be alert to these needs and see that the team is supplied with every item necessary to perform the operation efficiently. The circulating nurse must know all supplies, instruments, and equipment, be able to get them quickly, and guard against inadvertent hazards in their use and care. He or she must direct the scrub nurse and stay close to assist with unfamiliar equipment.

4 Identification of any potential environmental dangers or stressful situations involving the patient and/or other team members. This requires constant flexibility to meet the unexpected and to act in an efficient, rational manner in emergency situations.

5 Maintenance of the communication link between events and team members at the sterile field and persons not in the OR but concerned with the outcome of the operation. The latter includes the patient's family or significant other, and other personnel in the OR suite and in other departments of the hospital. The ability to recognize and effectively communicate situations involving the patient and/or other team members is a vital link in the continuity of patient care.

6 Direction of the activities of all learners. The circulating nurse must have supervisory capability and the teaching skills needed to ensure maintenance of a safe and therapeutic environment for the patient. Assistance kindly given builds up the learner's confidence. In this capacity the circulating nurse acts as supervisor, advisor, and teacher.

DIRECT PATIENT CARE TEAM IS PART OF TOTAL DEPARTMENT

The OR team, as described, immediately surrounds the patient throughout the operation. This direct patient care team functions within the physical confines of a specific room, *the operating room* (OR). This room is one part of the physical facilities that comprise the total *operating room suite*. Similarly, this team makes up only one part of the human activity directed toward the care of the surgical patient. Many other people function in an indirect relationship with the patient, contributing vital supporting services toward the common goal of ensuring a safe, comfortable, and effective environment for the safety and welfare of the patient within the OR suite. All of the nursing personnel assigned to work in the operating room suite are collectively referred to as *the operating room nursing staff of the OR department*. The relationship and duties of those staff members within the OR department will vary from hospital to hospital depending on the size and extent of the physical facilities and the number of personnel employed. No one's job is small! Each staff member fits into the general scheme of the department. Each has important functions to perform and is responsible for assuming a part of the total workload.

Job Descriptions

Each OR staff member must understand his or her own functions and responsibilities. A *job description* provides a written summary of the job to be done, lists the duties and requirements of the job as it must be performed in order to fulfill the department's requirements, and states to whom the employee is accountable.

The staffing plan must delineate those functions for which nursing service is responsible, and indicate all positions to carry out these functions. Job descriptions delineate the functions, responsibilities, and desired qualifications of each classification of professional, allied technical, and ancillary personnel. They serve as a guide for individual employees as well as for the supervisor; give order to individual work assignments and orderly, intelligent direction to the activities of the department; and prevent duplication of effort or neglect of duties.

Job descriptions must be written by each hospital for its own OR department staff to plan and coordinate work, and to establish methods of accomplishing it. An employee is not required to assume responsibility not specified in the job description. Work satisfaction is promoted by giving members of the staff basic duties and fixed responsibilities. Because the job description spells out each job requirement, it provides the supervisor with a means of checking that the employee understands the assignments and carries them out.

Performance Standards

Performance standards complement job descriptions. They are precise criteria for evaluating what an employee must do under present working conditions to perform a specific duty in a manner that is completely satisfactory. They are the measurements by which the employee's performance is judged in terms of quality, quantity, and manner. Standards of acceptable practice in the OR department are based on sound principles of the natural and behavioral sciences.

A standard developed by a profession or regulatory body is an authoritative statement of the range of acceptable variation from a norm or criterion by which quality can be judged. Standards of nursing practice are a means of determining the quality of nursing care that a patient receives regardless of whether such care is provided solely by professional nurses or by nurses in conjunction with allied technical and/or ancillary assistants. For the individual practitioner, standards provide a yardstick for the day-to-day evaluation of patient care. Since the professional nurse is primarily accountable to the patient, the standards focus on the nursing process and reflect a systematic approach to nursing practice. They are intended to provide safe individualized patient care, detect inadequacy of care, prevent legal implications resulting from alleged nursing malpractice or negligence, and improve the integrated nursing care program offered each patient.

NURSING ADMINISTRATIVE PERSONNEL

The *operating room supervisor* is responsible for the administration and supervision of nursing service in the OR department. This title is not used universally in all hospitals; neither is it always representative of the position's major functions. In large hospitals, the title *director of operating rooms* or *assistant director of nursing service* may more appropriately reflect the extent and complexity of the administrative responsibilities. Actual supervision of personnel is then delegated to an assistant or assistants who may be titled *supervisor* or *coordinator.* In smaller hospitals, where the volume of administrative and supervisory work is limited, the operating room supervisor often approaches the level of head nurse and may hold this title. In other situations, one nursing supervisor may be responsible for managing more than one clinical service such as OR, central services, recovery room, and/or emergency departments.

The title should indicate the scope of the responsibilities of the nurse who is accountable for coordination of all nursing care given and all related supporting services of the OR department and its staff. *The title* operating room supervisor (ORS) *will be used throughout this text to designate this position.*

Operating Room Supervisor

An operating room supervisor must have thorough knowledge of general nursing theory and practice and specialized knowledge of operating room technique and management. The ORS must be an RN in order to supervise and direct all nursing care given to patients, both directly and indirectly by nursing service personnel within the OR department, according to nursing principles and standards. The main function of the ORS is that of leadership—of promoting cooperative effort. To be a leader requires an additional set of skills and knowledge. These concern functions of management that include planning, organizing, staffing, directing, and controlling, plus the connecting processes of decision making, coordinating, and communicating.

The ORS is responsible for the allocation and completion of work, but does not do it all or make all of the decisions. Capable personnel are employed and given increasing responsibility as they develop competence in their work under the guidance of the ORS. He or she develops the will and desire among all staff members to cooperate with one another. The ORS creates an organization that can function well in his or her absence.

Personnel must know the direction of the entire organizational effort as a prerequisite for their successful functioning. The ORS interprets the hospital and departmental philosophy, objectives, policies, and procedures to the OR staff.

Philosophy Statement of beliefs regarding patient care and the nature of perioperative nursing that clarifies the overall responsibilities to be fulfilled.

Objectives Statements of specific goals to be accomplished during the course of action and definitions of criteria for acceptable performance.

Policies Specific authoritative statements of governing principles or actions, within the context of the philosophy and objectives, that assist in decision making by providing guidelines for action to be taken or, in some situations, for what is not to be done.

- **Basic Policies** Statements of the principles of administration and its approach to functioning.
- **General Policies** Guidelines of the principles dealing with everyday situations that affect all personnel within the hospital.
- **Departmental Policies** Guidelines structured to meet the needs of a specific work unit, i.e., OR policies.

Procedures Statements of actions to be taken in the implementation of policies.

The ORS must implement and enforce these hospital and departmental policies and procedures. He or she also analyzes and evaluates continuously all nursing services rendered and, through participation in research, seeks to improve the quality of patient care given. The ORS retains accountability for all nursing care given, all related activities in the OR department, and all aspects of environmental control in the OR suite. Areas of this accountability include:

1 Assistance to surgeons in operations through provision of adequately prepared OR team members
2 Delegation of responsibilities and duties to professional, allied technical, and ancillary personnel
3 Responsibility for performance evaluation of all department personnel
4 Provision of educational opportunities to increase knowledge of all personnel
5 Coordination of administrative duties to ensure proper functioning of the staff
6 Provision and control of materials, supplies, and equipment
7 Coordination of activities within the OR suite with other departments of the hospital

Assistant Operating Room Supervisor

The *assistant operating room supervisor* (AORS) aids in the administration and supervision of nursing service in the OR department and is directly responsible to the OR supervisor. This person acts as the administrative head in the absence of the supervisor. The position usually does not exist in small hospitals. In large hospitals, one or more *patient care coordinators* or *clinical coordinators* supervise nursing activities.

Head Nurse

The *head nurse* functions in a middle management position as liaison between staff members and administrative personnel. In some hospitals, the title of head nurse is given to the person whose position is comparable to an AORS. In other hospitals, usually smaller ones, the ORS functions more or less in the capacity of head nurse.

In large hospitals with many surgical specialty services, a head nurse may be responsible for the administration and direct supervision of nursing service in a designated room or rooms within the OR suite assigned to a particular specialty service, such as ophthalmology, neurosurgery, cardiovascular surgery, urology. With this structure, there will be several head nurses in the department. These head nurses should have the technical proficiency required for the specialty service for which they are responsible and should have sufficient management ability to plan for and administer effectively the nursing service activities.

The duties of the head nurse will include, but are not limited to:

1 Planning for and supervising the nursing activities within the entire OR suite or specific room(s) to which assigned

2 Coordinating nursing activities with those of the surgeons and anesthesiologists to provide for the care of patients

3 Maintaining adequate supplies and equipment and providing for their economical use

4 Observing the performance of all staff members pertaining to nursing activities

5 Interpreting to personnel the procedures and policies adopted by the department and hospital administration

6 Informing the ORS of needs and problems arising in the department

7 Assisting with orientation of new staff members

Functions vary in different hospitals, but the position of head nurse, with its direct and continuous responsibility for both patients and staff, is an important one.

O.R. Inservice Education Coordinator

Planned educational experiences are provided in the job setting to help staff members perform effectively and knowledgeably. Most hospitals have a nursing staff development department or committee to plan, coordinate, and conduct educational and training programs.

A program is planned to ensure a thorough orientation for each new nursing service employee. Many hospitals have established a hiring policy so that all new employees begin their first day of employment on designated days of each month, i.e., the first and third Monday. For at least the first week or two of employment, all employees attend the orientation classes. All new personnel must become familiar with the philosophy, objectives, policies and procedures of the hospital and nursing service. This general orientation program assists the new employee to adjust to the organization and environment. It is coordinated with an orientation to the duties in the unit to which the employee is assigned.

The *OR inservice coordinator* may be a member of the staff development department and/or a member of the OR administrative staff. This person is responsible for planning, scheduling, and coordinating the orientation of new OR staff. This includes review of policies and procedures, personnel duties, and performance standards specific to the OR. Based on an individual skills assessment, the new employee is given guidance and supervision for a period of weeks to months until basic competencies are adequate to function independently. (Refer to Chapter 37 for basic competencies in OR nursing.) Head nurses, preceptors, and other experienced staff members assist with the orientation of new personnel.

An inservice educational program must also be planned to keep the nursing staff up-to-date on new techniques, equipment, and concepts of nursing care. Programs focusing on fire prevention, electrical hazards, security measures, and resuscitation training are important to ensure personnel and patient safety. Professional and technical programs designed to develop specialized job knowledge, skills and/or attitudes affecting patient care are planned and presented for the appropriate segment of the nursing service department and the OR staff. The OR inservice coordinator is responsible for planning, scheduling, and coordinating these inservice programs. This individual may conduct some of the sessions.

Staff development programs, on a continuing basis, enhance performance by maintaining job knowledge and clinical competence. Inservice programs, presented in the hospital, may be supplemented by attending other appropriate continuing educational offerings held outside the hospital.

O.R. Unit Manager

To relieve the OR supervisor of nonnursing duties, some hospitals employ an *OR unit manager.* This manager may report to the ORS or directly to the hospital administrator. Lines of authority and responsibility between the unit manager and the ORS must be clearly defined regardless of the organizational structure. The OR unit manager directs the management of the nonnursing and nondirect patient care functions in the OR suite, while the OR nursing supervisor and other administrative nursing personnel direct and supervise patient care and the professional and allied technical nursing personnel.

In addition to directing and supervising all nursing care given to patients within the OR, administrative duties must include maintaining a clean, orderly, safe environment within the OR suite for patients and personnel. This entails more than removing visible dust and dirt. A safe environment is one that is free of contamination, free of electrical and fire hazards, and free of negligence. Formulation of procedures is necessary. Personnel must be trained. But inspection and followup are equally important. The OR unit manager coordinates these efforts with the supporting service departments: housekeeping, maintenance, central services, laundry, central storeroom, and purchasing. The unit manager may prepare and administrate the department budget. This may include maintaining inventories and evaluating supplies and equipment. If the hospital does not employ an OR unit manager, the ORS must assume responsibility for these duties.

Clinician

Within any organization a formal structure of authority and responsibility exists. However, the evolution of nursing as a profession has changed the focus of functions for many nurses within the hospital organization. With experience and advanced study, a nurse can become recognized as being capable of organizing and providing complex care, and of using initiative and independent judgment. Specific job titles vary considerably from one locale and one hospital to another. This clinician may hold the title of *team leader, senior clinical nurse, nurse clinician,* or *clinical nurse specialist.* Although the *term* clinician *will be used to describe any or all of these roles,* differentiation is made within the profession on the basis of formal academic educational preparation.

In general, minimal preparation for this role is a baccalaureate degree in nursing. The *clinical nurse specialist,* however, has been defined as a graduate of a master's program in nursing, with a major in a clinical specialty, who enhances the quality of nursing care directly with patients and indirectly through guidance and planning of care with other nursing personnel. The clinical nurse specialist serves as a role model by teaching patients and personnel, and by demonstrating the highest level of interpersonal skills and promoting collegial relationships. These skills can be utilized as effectively in the OR as in any nursing unit.

The clinician is capable of exercising a high degree of discriminative judgment in planning, executing, and evaluating nursing care based upon the assessed needs of patients having one or more common clinical manifestations. A clinician may develop the nursing care plan for a group of orthopaedic patients, for example. This plan is coordinated for each patient with the surgeon, other professional nurses, and allied technical personnel who assist in the performance of functions related to the nursing care plan.

Clinical nursing is not necessarily performed by the clinician. This nurse decides what needs to be done, then determines which nursing functions can be done by others and which he or she must do. These decisions are based upon personal interaction with each patient and a knowledge of the clinical condition. The clinician exercises a degree of autonomy and independence within the clinical setting and serves as the patient's advocate.

Since a clinician has extensive academic preparation in theoretical knowledge and clinical experience in a particular clinical nursing setting, and is an expert in nursing situations in that setting, qualified OR supervisors may function as clinicians. In this role, they assist in planning a program of total nursing care for each surgical patient, coordinating nursing and supportive services, participating in the orientation, development, and evaluation of nursing personnel assigned to direct patient care functions in the OR, and conducting research studies to evaluate nursing interventions. Supervisors who also assess individual patient needs through personal patient interviews and who plan for individualized nursing care in the OR truly function as clinicians. They have the title of *OR nurse clinician* or *OR clinical specialist* in some hospitals. These supervisors make decisions relative to the direct and indirect nursing care of the patient in the OR setting, utilizing specialized judgments and skills. Decision making is the heart of professional management and professional leadership.

The OR clinician, whatever the organizational title may be, may not be the nurse charged with the overall management and leadership functions in the OR department. OR nurses may be assigned to work solely or primarily with the surgeons in a specific surgical specialty. This concept of nursing specialization coincides with the specialization of surgeons. With practice and formal or informal study, nurses develop expertise in planning and implementing nursing care for patients with similar surgical problems. Skills and knowledge become highly specialized, and the surgeons in that particular specialty rely on such nurses to supervise the nursing care of their patients and to direct less-experienced nursing personnel on the OR team. Clinicians may fulfill the circulating nurse duties in one OR or serve as consultant-coordinators for several rooms in which patients are being operated on by surgeons within a given surgical specialty. The job title for the nurse and the assignment structure will vary with the size of the hospital and the manner in which it is organized. With either type of assignment, these nurses are clinicians of very narrow scope unless they visit patients preoperatively to assess their individual needs, plan nursing care on the basis of need assessment, and evaluate the quality of nursing care postoperatively through direct patient interaction. Then they are clinicians in the broader context of perioperative nursing (see Chap. 4).

STAFF NURSING PERSONNEL

General Duty Registered Nurse

Under the immediate supervision of the head nurse and/or OR supervisor, *general duty professional staff nurses* provide direct care to patients utilizing the nursing process and discriminative judgment in making independent nursing decisions. They work in a collaborative relationship with surgeons and anesthesiologists to determine the needs of patients during the operation and assume responsibility for planning nursing care. Preoperatively they help alleviate patient anxiety and identify nursing care problems (see Chap. 4).

Staff nurses perform either scrub or circulating functions. In general, the more experienced nurse functions as the circulating nurse to supervise the management of all nursing activities during the operation. If staffing does not permit an RN staff nurse in both positions, the RN must circulate.

As part of their professional practice in the OR, staff nurses assess the effectiveness of nursing actions taken, identify and carry out systematic investigations of clinical problems, and engage in periodic review of their own contributions to nursing care and those of their professional peers. To assure a safe environment for patients, they assist other nursing staff members through teaching and supervising aseptic and sterile techniques and other procedures. They also assist in the control and maintenance of drugs, supplies, equipment, and records. Staff nurses assist all members of the OR team. They work cooperatively with members of the nursing staff and other departments to promote continuity of patient care.

By actively participating in the operation, scrubbing or circulating, teaching, and directing, the OR staff nurse maintains nursing skills, extends area of competence, and keeps abreast of current developments in patient care and treatment. OR nursing is a specialty of clinical nursing practice.

Those professional OR nurses who are certified nurses operating room (CNOR) serve as role models for others to emulate. Since they influence others by their nursing practice, behavior, and appearance, their conduct must be exemplary. Demeanor should express dignity, self-confidence, and genuine concern for patients and team members.

Licensed Practical/Vocational Nurses

Licensed practical/vocational nurses (LPN/LVNs) who are qualified by training, experience, and demonstrated ability may be utilized to give nursing care that does not require the skill and judgment of a registered nurse. With specialized training in surgical technology, these nurses may be permitted to serve as scrub nurses at the operating table. LPN/LVNs are not permitted to function independently as circulating nurses in the OR. They may assist in implementing the nursing care plan by working with a qualified registered nurse. *Throughout this text the functions of the LPN/LVN on the OR staff will be considered the same as those of surgical technologists.*

Surgical Technologist/O.R. Technician

Surgical technologists, referred to as *operating room technicians* (ORTs) in some hospitals, are responsible for their own acts, but must function under the supervision of a registered nurse at all times. They assist with the nursing care of patients in the OR by performing routine and delegated duties according to the standards of practice and the policies of the hospital and department. They are restricted from administering medications, completing patient records, or carrying out direct physician orders regarding treatment of patients. They are permitted to serve as scrub nurses, but they are not permitted to function as circulating nurses in the OR. They may be permitted to second assist the surgeon at the operating table or second assist the RN circulating nurse.

Routine duties of surgical technologists also include stocking, replenishing, preparing, and/or selecting supplies and equipment for storage or for immediate use during operations. They also assist with housekeeping duties to maintain cleanliness in the OR suite in order to ensure a safe patient environment.

Ancillary Personnel

Ancillary personnel are lay workers trained through an inservice educational program.

Clerical Personnel One or more ancillary workers may perform clerical duties associated with activities within the OR suite. These duties may include assisting with preparation of the schedule of operations, ordering supplies, and maintaining records and reports.

A control desk is usually located at the entrance to the OR suite where a clerk-receptionist can see and check all visitors and personnel. Unauthorized persons can be intercepted.

Clerical personnel serve as vital communication links between the OR department and other departments. They receive and send messages by telephone, intercommunication system, and mail.

The hospital telephone exchange operators frequently relay messages for surgeons while they are operating. The clerk in the OR suite must be aware of the arrival and departure of the surgeons in order to be certain that they receive their messages without being disturbed during operations.

Most hospitals have an intercommunication system between the OR and other areas in the OR suite. Clerical personnel coordinate messages through this system. They can arrange for transportation of patients to and from the OR, obtain supplies or additional personnel for the OR team if needed, etc.

Many hospitals have a pneumatic-tube system that provides a quick means for the delivery of written communications and small, nonbreakable supplies to all parts of the hospital. The clerk operates this system.

Clerical personnel relieve nurses of much paper work by doing the departmental record keeping.

Nursing Assistants Ancillary personnel are employed to perform certain indirect nursing care activities. A *nursing assistant* may be male or female. Most OR departments have both. Their duties include, but are not limited to:

1 Assisting with transporting, moving, and positioning of patients

2 Performing errands to other departments as needed

3 Cleaning, processing, and storing instruments and supplies

4 Maintaining assigned work area in a clean and orderly condition

A male assistant, sometimes titled an *orderly,* may be asked to do the heavier work in the department, such as lifting patients and moving or setting up large pieces of equipment.

INTERDEPARTMENTAL RELATIONSHIPS

The operating room is one of many departments within the total hospital organization, just as the operation is one phase of total surgical patient care. To provide continuity in total patient care, the staffs of many departments must cooperate. Their efforts are coordinated through the administration of the formal organizational structure of the hospital.

Every hospital has a *governing body* that appoints a chief executive officer, usually titled the *hospital administrator,* to provide appropriate physical resources and personnel to meet the needs of patients. Administrative lines of authority, responsibility, and accountability are defined to establish the working relationships between departments and personnel.

The *director of nursing service* reports to the hospital administrator. The OR supervisor will report to the director of nursing if the OR department is structured as a unit within nursing service. In some hospitals, the OR is considered an independent department separate from nursing service. This OR supervisor then reports directly to the hospital administrator or an assistant administrator, or to the chief of the department of surgery. Through either channel of administration, many activities in the OR department must be coordinated with other nursing units and hospital departments.

Nursing Units

Patients come to the OR directly from the emergency department, inpatient nursing units, or outpatient ambulatory care area. It is vital that channels of communication be kept open between OR personnel and nursing personnel in these other nursing units in order to coordinate preoperative preparation and transportation of patients. Many hospitals use a checklist to assure adequate preparation of surgical patients. An RN or LPN/LVN signs or initials for each item accomplished. By the time the patient leaves for the OR suite, all the preparations have been completed.

Emergency Department

Victims of trauma and acutely ill patients often are initially seen in the hospital emergency department (ED). Cardiopulmonary resuscitative and other equipment are available to initiate prompt triage and treatment. Minor injuries usually can be treated in the ED. Some patients must be scheduled for an emergency operation, however. These patients may arrive in the OR before the results of all diagnostic tests are confirmed. Therefore, communication between OR, ED, laboratory, and x-ray personnel is vital to the success of surgical intervention. OR personnel must be advised of the nature of the injury or illness to prepare all needed equipment and obtain supplies for the emergency operation.

Labor and Delivery Room

The obstetrical unit is divided into three separate areas: labor and delivery, postpartum care, and newborn nursery. Some labor and delivery areas have an operating room for delivery by cesarean (C) section. However, patients scheduled either for an elective or emergency C-section are brought to the operating room suite in other hospitals. In addition to the supplies needed for the operation, adequate resuscitative equipment must be available for the newborn (see Chap. 22).

Recovery Room/Postanesthesia Care Unit

The inestimable value of a good postanesthesia care unit to provide maximal safety for patients immediately following their operation is undisputed. Recovery rooms evolved to meet a need for trained personnel to constantly observe patients within facilities equipped for specialized care until recovery from anesthesia is stabilized sufficiently for safe transfer to their rooms elsewhere in the hospital. Because this is the purpose, the *recovery room* (RR) is referred to as the *postanesthesia room* (PAR) in some hospitals.

The recovery room is usually physically adjacent to the OR suite. Included in the RR may be partitioned isolation areas for patients with known infectious organisms or who are highly susceptible to infection, such as burn patients, or patients with radioactive implants. These patients need the same postoperative care as others do. They should be sent to the RR unless they can receive the same care in an isolation room on the nursing unit. Hospital policy should determine this. If the RR does not have a partitioned isolation area, patients may be placed at the end of the room, separated from others by screens or curtains. Extra care must be used in handling bedding and equipment. Hand washing is essential after each patient contact to prevent cross contamination.

In large hospitals, the recovery room may be open 24 hours a day. In other hospitals, especially if most of the operations are performed in the morning hours, the RR may be open only during the day. The extent of utilization of the operating rooms will determine the routine hours of available recovery room care. Special arrangements for constant observation must be made for patients during hours in which the recovery room is closed. These arrangements are established by hospital policy.

The recovery room is under the supervision of an anesthesiologist in coordination with a nursing supervisor. This supervisor may be the OR supervisor who has a head nurse assigned to the recovery room to directly supervise the activities in this specialized area.

The recovery room is staffed by specially trained registered nurses and other nursing personnel. The patients are under their constant observation. Respiratory and circulatory depressions are at once detected and corrected. Monitoring and emergency resuscitation equipment is always at hand. An intercommunication system or emergency call system connects the recovery room personnel with the OR suite so that additional personnel are readily available in situations that are life-threatening to patients.

The goal of postanesthesia nursing care is "to assist the patient in returning to a safe physiological level after an anesthetic."* The application of physiologic and psychosocial knowledge, principles of asepsis, and technical knowledge and skills are necessary to promote, restore, and maintain the patient's physiological processes in a safe, comfortable, and effective environment, and to fa-

*American Society of Post Anesthesia Nurses Guidelines for Standards of Care and Management in the Post Anesthesia Care Unit, copyright © 1984.

cilitate the patient's adaptation to the surgical experience.

Patients remain in the recovery room until they have reacted from anesthesia and their vital signs have stabilized. Clinical evaluation of patients by listening, watching, and feeling is augmented by electronic devices to monitor respiratory and cardiac functions. These monitors aid personnel in keeping a careful check on patients during the critical postoperative period.

Family members are notified when the patient is admitted to the recovery room so that they will know when the operation is over. This helps relieve their anxiety during the hours of waiting. The period of time spent in the recovery room postpones visits with family and friends until the patient is better able to see them. However, by policy, some hospitals permit visitors in the recovery room.

Intensive Care Units

As surgery has become more specialized and operations of great magnitude have been developed and perfected, specialized facilities where concentrated treatment can bring the patient to a satisfactory recovery have become a necessity. This care is provided in an *intensive care unit* (ICU) open 24 hours a day, 7 days a week. It is staffed by highly trained and specialized registered nurses. Critically ill patients who need constant care for several days are admitted directly from the operating room, recovery room, emergency department, or other nursing unit. Each bedside is equipped with therapeutic and monitoring equipment.

Depending on the size of the hospital and its specialty services, more than one specially designed and equipped intensive care unit may be provided. One ICU may admit only cardiovascular surgical patients, another burn patients, another only pediatric patients, another transplant patients. In addition to surgical intensive care units, most hospitals also have a *coronary care unit* (CCU) and/or a unit for nonsurgical (medical) patients. The increased efficiency these units afford serves the best interests of both the hospital and the patient. They create the most effective utilization of personnel and equipment, and lower morbidity and mortality rates.

Movements of patients to and from the surgical intensive care units must be closely coordinated with the operating room schedule, the OR team, and the recovery room personnel. If the surgeon anticipates that a patient will need intensive care postoperatively, a bed in the ICU must be reserved before the patient is scheduled for operation. Sometimes the patient must wait in the OR or recovery room for another patient to be transferred out of the ICU when the former's condition warrants intensive care that was unanticipated.

Many surgeons prefer to transfer their patients directly from the operating room to the intensive care unit, thus bypassing the recovery room. This facilitates immediate initiation of treatment that will be prolonged in the postoperative period and eliminates the stress that additional movement causes patients.

Radiology and Nuclear Medicine Departments

Frequently, personnel from the radiology (x-ray) and nuclear medicine (radiation therapy) departments assist with diagnostic or therapeutic procedures in the OR. For some procedures it may be necessary for OR nursing personnel to go to the x-ray department to assist the surgeon during a procedure requiring sterile technique. Whenever a diagnostic procedure or operation is scheduled that will require use of x-ray or a radioactive implant, all departments must be notified at least the day before. This is not only common courtesy, but facilitates the scheduling of personnel and the workload in all departments.

Pharmacy

Many drugs are routinely stocked in the OR suite for the anesthesiologists' use and some for use by the surgeons during operations. These are obtained by requisition from the pharmacy. When received, narcotics are always kept under lock, and each dosage is recorded as dispensed.

The pharmacy is not an isolated department but an integral part of the hospital. Pharmacists are resource persons who convey drug information to physicians and nurses. They cooperate with physicians in obtaining new, unusual, or special drugs for patients, and in providing information about actions and interactions. They also recommend new or improved products or forms of packaging drugs. Pharmacists should be responsible for the preparation of all admixtures and for the quality control of associated drug product services throughout the hospital.

Blood Bank

If the surgeon anticipates in advance of the operation that blood loss replacement may be necessary, a sample of the patient's blood is sent to the blood bank for type and cross match. In emergency situations this may be sent from the emergency department or the OR. The units of blood products ordered by the surgeon are prepared and labeled with patient's name and blood data.

Blood products for transfusion are kept in a refrigerator at a constant temperature between 36 and 43°F (2 and 6°C), verified by a recording thermometer. Blood banks usually dispense whole blood, plasma, or packed cells only as they are needed (see Chap. 10, p. 173).

Pathology Department

The *pathologist,* an MD who specializes in the cause and effect of disease, may be on call at a few minutes' notice to examine tissue while the patient is under anesthesia. This enables the surgeon to proceed immediately with a definitive operation, if malignant tumor cells are found, without subjecting the patient to a second operation at a later time. A small laboratory may be located within the OR suite with equipment for microscopic tissue examination. This laboratory may be used for other tests and/or for taking photographs of tissue specimens removed from patients.

All tissue removed during operations ultimately is sent to the pathology department for routine examination. These tissues may be stored in a refrigerator in the laboratory or some other location within the OR suite until they are taken to the pathology department at the end of or at intervals during each day's schedule of operations.

Bacteriology Laboratory

Biological testing of the OR environment and sterile supplies is done periodically according to hospital routine and always when a problem of contamination is suspected. The *bacteriologist,* who specializes in the study of microorganisms, may come into the OR suite to collect samples for testing, or samples may be collected and sent to the laboratory by OR personnel. The results provide a method for evaluating the effectiveness of procedures and the degree of adherence to environmental standards.

Medical Records

Clinical records must be complete. They include the admitting diagnosis, the patient's chief complaint, complete history and physical examination, the records of laboratory examinations, and the physicians' and nurses' care plans. Records must state therapy employed including operations, and include progress notes, consultation remarks, condition on discharge or observations in case of death. A summary of the hospitalization experience must be complete. These records are signed by all physicians and nurses attending the patient.

The anesthesia record completed during the operation by the anesthesiologist also becomes part of the patient's record. Nursing care must also be documented on the patient's chart. Therefore, the circulating nurse should write pertinent remarks pertaining to nursing care rendered in the OR and the patient's response to care on the nurses' note sheet or the progress notes. *Documentation is a responsibility of all professional team members implementing direct patient care.*

Notes about the operation must be explicit, dictated promptly after the operation, and incorporated into the record of each surgical patient. For the surgeons' convenience, many hospitals have dictating machines or a phone hookup with the medical records department installed within the OR suite, usually located in the dressing room or lounge. Details of the pre- and postoperative diagnosis and the operation itself may have medical and legal significance. It is the responsibility of the medical records department to accurately transcribe the surgeon's dictation and maintain the patient's chart after his or her discharge from the hospital. The patient's chart may be put on microfilm for storage.

Environmental Services/Housekeeping Department

Housekeeping functions are recognized as important preventive measures to eliminate microorganisms from the hospital environment. Each hospital establishes a routine for its particular needs. Usually environmental services/housekeeping department personnel and nursing personnel share the housekeeping duties in the OR suite. The amount of cleaning done by the OR personnel varies from one hospital to another. In many, the members of the housekeeping department clean all furniture, flat surfaces, lights, and floors once a day at the end of the operating schedule. In others, they also clean the furniture and floors before the schedule starts and between each operation throughout the day. Whatever plan they follow, housekeeping personnel must have a storage area within the OR suite in which to keep their equipment and supplies. Equipment used for cleaning in the OR is not taken outside the suite.

The *director of environmental/housekeeping services* and the OR supervisor or unit manager plan the division of work. Personnel in each department must understand their responsibilities. The OR supervisor or unit manager checks the work of housekeeping personnel and keeps in touch with the director concerning their performance.

The director must have a thorough knowledge of the job. He or she evaluates and chooses the proper solutions for effective cleaning, sets up a program and standard of performance for employees, and sees that they are properly oriented and taught the procedures and standards. Using a checklist helps to cover all areas to be cleaned and inspected on a routine basis, whether it is daily, weekly, or monthly. A weekly or monthly cleaning routine is set up that includes walls and ceilings, in addition to the daily cleaning schedule within the OR suite (see Chap. 10).

The director impresses upon the personnel the importance of the work and the important part they play in enabling the OR personnel to carry out aseptic technique. The housekeeping personnel do indeed function as members of the OR team when working with the scrub and circulating nurses between operations.

Engineering and Maintenance Department

The engineering and maintenance department personnel work in close cooperation with the OR department by providing a continuous preventive maintenance program. This includes routine monitoring of ventilation and heating, electrical and lighting systems, emergency warning systems, and water supply. Humidity is recorded every hour in the maintenance department. All electrical equipment is checked monthly by maintenance department personnel. In addition, they regularly test the autonomous emergency power source and maintain a written record of inspection and performance.

The hospital water supply system should not be connected with other piping systems, or with fixtures that could allow contamination of the water supply. The hot water supply and steam lines have temperature control devices regulated by the maintenance department personnel. They are cleaned on a routine schedule, usually weekly, to prevent accumulation of mineral deposits.

Conductive flooring is a means of electrically connecting people and objects to prevent the accumulation of electrical charges and to equalize potentials in anesthetizing locations where flammable agents are used. The maintenance department checks the conductivity of the flooring and furniture in these locations at least once a month and keeps a permanent record of the levels.

Competent technical personnel must be available to every area of the hospital to ensure the safe operation of equipment. Nearly every operation uses some form of powered instrumentation. Because of the variety and complexity of the instrumentation currently in use, most hospitals have a clinical engineer and/or biomedical equipment technician on staff or available. This technical support group assists OR personnel in evaluating and selecting new equipment, in installing and operating it, and in maintaining it. The *clinical engineer* is systems and applications oriented. This individual can compare different models and manufacturers' specifications and provide recommendations for purchase. The *biomedical equipment technician* is knowledgeable about the theory of operation, the underlying physiological principles, and the practical, safe clinical applications of biomedical instrumentation. This individual can test, install, calibrate, inspect, service, and repair equipment. Every preventive service or repair is recorded in an instrument history file.

Central Services/Materiels Management

One area of the hospital is designed specifically for processing, storing, and distributing supplies and equipment used in patient care. This department may be referred to as central services, central supply, central processing, sterile processing, or materiels management depending on the services provided. *References to* central services *will be used throughout this text as the all inclusive term for this area.* The functional design and work flow patterns provide for separation of soiled and contaminated supplies from clean and sterile items.

A myriad of sterile supplies are used in the OR. Many of these are commercially prepackaged, presterilized, disposable, one-time use products.

Some are prepared in the OR suite. Other items used in the OR are processed for reuse by central services department personnel. These items are decontaminated, cleaned, packaged, and sterilized. Central services personnel may package and sterilize linen packs unless this is done in the laundry or unless disposable packs are used. In many hospitals, central services personnel replenish supplies on the nursing units daily, according to standard inventories. A similar system may be established for the OR suite or supplies may be requisitioned as needed.

Many hospitals built or renovated after the mid-1960s utilize a surgery case cart system. Personnel in central services prepare individual carts with the required supplies for each scheduled operative procedure. These are transported to the appropriate operating rooms. After each operation, the cart with the soiled supplies is returned to the decontamination areas of central services. The decontaminating and reprocessing of OR instruments and equipment usually are done in areas separated from the rest of the department. This prevents mixing surgical instruments with those supplied to other units. The personnel assigned to the surgery case cart areas must be familiar with the supplies needed for each operation: how they are used, and how they are processed.

Laundry

Many hospitals use disposable nonwoven fabrics. In others, the laundry processes the linens used in the OR. These are either sterilized in the laundry, central services, or in the OR suite, depending on where the sterilizing equipment is located. Even if the use of disposables negates this need, some linen is processed for the OR suite. Hospitals that do not have laundry facilities as part of their physical plant use a commercial laundry. Linen supplies are usually requisitioned on a daily basis to maintain inventory level. The *laundry manager* may assist in determining appropriate inventories.

Central Storeroom and Purchasing

A limited stock of supplies is kept in the OR suite. However, storage is generally a problem in every OR suite. Therefore, bulk inventories of many supplies are stocked in the central storeroom for requisition as needed. Usually these supplies are requisitioned on a weekly basis.

Items that are too expensive to stock in large quantities or that are used infrequently are ordered through the purchasing department as needed. In some hospitals this department is referred to as materiels management. As the central storeroom is a part of this department, the purchasing director determines the supplies to be stocked for requisition and those for direct purchase as needed.

Personnel Department

Even though the availability of supplies and equipment and the physical facilities are important, these are secondary to the functioning of the OR department. The efficiency of any department depends on the persons employed in it. Therefore, the careful selection of capable, highly motivated people contributes to the efficiency and effectiveness of interdepartmental relationships. The personnel department helps screen applicants. Those seen with potential for available positions are referred to the appropriate department head. If the OR supervisor reports through nursing service, potential employees may be processed through nursing service before an interview with the OR supervisor is scheduled. Or, the OR supervisor may be contacted directly by the personnel department to arrange an interview with an applicant. In either situation, the personnel department assists in the hiring and terminating of all employees.

COORDINATION THROUGH COMMITTEES

Operating Room Committee

The OR committee is a committee of the medical staff. One surgeon is appointed chief or director of the department of surgery. In teaching hospitals, a director is appointed chief of each specialty service, e.g., chief of orthopaedics. The anesthesia department also designates a director of this department. These individuals are responsible for professional practice and administrative activities within their respective departments. They must maintain continuing surveillance of the professional performance of all members of the medical staff granted privileges in their specialty. They also serve as liaison representatives between the medical staff and hospital administration.

Vital to the management of the OR suite is an active OR committee. The chief of surgery, the chiefs or representatives of the specialty services, the chief of the anesthesia department, the OR nursing supervisor, the assistant ORS and/or the OR unit manager meet at regular intervals to review and formulate policies and procedures concerning OR suite activities. The hospital administrator and director of nursing service may also be members of this committee or may be invited to attend meetings relevant to their concerns.

The OR committee must consider policies and procedures pertaining to utilization of facilities, schedule of operations, maintenance of a safe environment, evaluation of techniques, and selection of new products. This may require the review of reports from other departments or committees in addition to those prepared by OR personnel.

Since this committee determines policy and procedures for efficient functioning within the OR suite, persistent problems are brought before the committee where recommendations for corrective action are made. For example, if temperature and humidity controls are not being effectively monitored or maintained, the committee may recommend to the hospital administration that procedures be reviewed and revised by the maintenance department or that new equipment be installed. If surgeons are repeatedly late in arriving, thus delaying the OR schedule, stronger policy may be indicated for the control and better utilization of facilities. If a new product is purchased, a new procedure may need to be written to specify its use and care.

Through utilization of the problem-solving approach to decision making, the OR committee seeks to improve the working relationships of all members of the OR team and the supportive services concerned with activities within the OR suite.

Operating room activities related to procedures and techniques are supervised indirectly by the OR committee, which is responsible for enunciating policy. Policies and associated directives formulated and approved by the committee serve as guides for governing the actions of surgeons, anesthesiologists, and the OR nursing staff while in the OR suite. The ORS shares with the OR committee, hospital administration, and nursing service the responsibility for clarification, implementation, and day-by-day enforcement of approved policies and procedures.

Infection Control Committee

The infection control committee investigates hospital-acquired infections and seeks to prevent or control them. Membership may vary in different hospitals, but generally includes representatives of the medical staff, resident staff, hospital administration and nursing service, and the epidemiologist or infection surveillance coordinator, bacteriologist and/or pathologist. Representatives from other departments may be invited to attend meetings when the agenda is relevant to their particular concerns.

The committee meets at least once every two months. Members form a defense against hospital-acquired infections by reviewing environmental factors and by determining if the hospital is providing a safe environment for patient care. They review all infection reports and investigate nosocomial infections. Committee members also review the procedures and scrutinize the entire chain of asepsis in an effort to determine and then eliminate possible sources of infection.

This committee has the authority to carry out any changes necessary and to enforce strict rules to eliminate any hazardous practices. Included in its jurisdiction is the education of personnel so that they can provide a high standard of patient care. *The hospital has a moral duty to provide a safe environment for its patients.* The infection control committee aids the hospital in fulfilling this duty. Surveillance personnel assist in directing infection control policies, procedures, and practices.

Nursing Supervisors

The supervisors of all the nursing units usually meet weekly, or at least monthly, to discuss problem situations. This is an excellent mechanism for resolving conflicts between the units and for working out procedures that are mutually beneficial. The OR supervisor should attend these meetings to stay aware of staffing problems on other units, and breakdowns in communication between the OR department and the units, if these exist. Only through the identification of problems can solutions be sought, and decisions made.

Quality Assurance Committee

The membership of the quality assurance committee includes representatives of both clinical and administrative personnel. This committee monitors routine activities, audits incident reports, and conducts problem-focused studies in an effort to change practices deemed substandard or in violation of hospital policy. A productive and efficient committee will implement actions designed to eliminate identified real or potential problems, to improve patient care, and to reduce financial loss. Because of the emphasis on cost containment, review of utilization of facilities and risk management also may be concerns of this committee. Some hospitals employ a *quality assurance coordinator* and/or a *risk manager* to assure implementation of committee decisions.

Hospital Safety Committee

Representatives from administration, nursing service, medical staff, the engineering and maintenance department, housekeeping and dietary departments, and the safety director form the nucleus of the hospital safety committee. This group writes policies and procedures designed to enhance safety within the hospital and on hospital grounds. They exchange information with the infection control and quality assurance committees and conduct hazard surveillance programs. They meet at least monthly to investigate and evaluate reported incidents. Action is taken when a hazardous condition exists that could result in personal injury or damage to equipment or facilities.

Disaster Planning Committee

Hospitals have an organized plan for caring for many casualties if a mass disaster occurs within the community. Planning by the intrahospital committee includes consultation with local civil authorities and representatives of other medical agencies to establish an effective chain of command and to make appropriate jurisdictional provisions. This planning results in disaster-site triage to separate and distribute patients in order to ensure the most efficient use of available facilities and services.

Disaster drills are held at least twice a year to try out the plan developed by the committee, to seek to improve it, and to acquaint personnel with it. Disaster plans include:

1 An information center at the hospital to facilitate a unified medical command and the movement of patients.

2 A receiving area for the severely wounded. Casualties are given emergency care according to their needs and are sent at once to the OR or to other units as indicated, or transferred to another facility.

3 Arrangements for sending ambulatory patients to a special area. These patients are treated in the emergency department for slight injuries and are sent home, or are admitted to the hospital as indicated.

4 Special disaster medical records or tags accompany patients at all times.

5 A plan of organization of personnel. As soon as word of disaster comes to a hospital, if it is during the evening or night, several key persons are called. These in turn phone others previously assigned to them, and these call still others, until the full staff has been notified. If the disaster occurs during the day, the full staff is usually on duty, although any off-duty personnel may be called.

Other departments are alerted and come on duty as needed; these include personnel for the blood bank, central services department, pharmacy, central storeroom, x-ray, and the various nursing units. If disposable linen packs are not in use, it may be necessary to alert some laundry personnel. Some key maintenance personnel must be available, especially electricians.

Personnel are periodically given drills so that each member knows where to report, what to do, and where extra supplies are kept in case of an emergency. Extra supplies are stored in reserve in sufficient quantities to fill possible needs for a minimum of one week.

TEAMWORK TO MEET OBJECTIVES

Several factors contribute to the restoration of optimal patient health:

1 Interdisciplinary communication, mutual cooperation, consideration, and smooth, efficient collaboration are essential.
   - **a** Unit, emergency department, operating room, recovery room, and intensive care unit nurses and physicians share pertinent information concerning patients. Collected data are documented by accurate recording, thereby protecting the patient, the medical personnel, and the health care institution.
   - **b** Personnel work together in a congenial atmosphere of equality with knowledge of and respect and appreciation for each other's unique skills and contribution to patient safety and well-being. Team members benefit from the expertise of each other. Team nursing is at its finest in the OR. In some hospi-

tals, a multidisciplinary team meets regularly to share information and exchange ideas. This enables each member to support the goals of other team members.

c Personnel are considerate of each other as well as of the patient. For example:

1 Surgeons inform their teammates ahead of time of any anticipated potential deviation from their regular routine or the scheduled procedure. They respond to questions courteously, and show appreciation for thoughtful preparation and assistance.

2 Nurses do all in their power to provide the best possible atmosphere to ensure the surgeon's uninterrupted concentration. The surgeon is not to be interrupted with messages that are not of immediate urgency. Neither should loud, irrelevant messages come over the intercom system to startle the surgeon. If the surgeon becomes tense, he or she may develop a tremor or cause inadvertent tissue trauma. It is always a risk to interrupt an ongoing team's concerted effort during any procedure.

3 The anesthesiologist and circulating nurse assist each other with certain procedures, such as starting and checking intravenous infusions. The circulating nurse stands beside the patient during induction to be ready to assist as necessary. The anesthesiologist, while concentrating on physiologic modalities, must watch the progression of the procedure. For example, there are appropriate and inappropriate times to inflate a blood pressure cuff.

NOTE. Adequate preparation and familiarity with the operation and the surgeon's individual preferences are fundamental. If the nurses are unfamiliar with the routine and equipment, it distracts the surgeon's train of thought. The dedicated surgeon's plea is for nursing personnel and other assistants who are knowledgeable and caring. Only then can the surgeon, who needs their expertise and cooperation, help the patient. Surgeons want to work in collegial relationships with their team members. By not being properly oriented, assigned, prepared (both patient and the OR), or attentive (to patient and team), one puts both the patient and the surgeon's skill in jeopardy. An adequately experienced and skilled OR team is mandatory!

2 Assignment of adequately oriented and competent personnel avoids delays and keeps anesthesia time to a minimum. The potential for complications increases proportionately with the length of anesthesia time and the operation. Calm, experienced personnel greatly reduce all hazards, especially in critical situations. Lack of knowledge, personnel shortage, and inadequate rest pose a serious threat to the patient and to the expected outcome of the operation. Both patient and surgeon are entitled to an adequate number of qualified nurses and technologists in the OR. Everyone must care about what happens to their patient. The need for communication and cooperation cannot be overemphasized!

3 Attention to the patient's welfare must be constant. The patient on the operating table has an unconditional right to the team's complete concentration and attention at all times. The members of the team must be concerned with meeting that patient's needs, regarding him or her as a unique individual completely dependent on them for survival. The patient is, however, also a planner and participant in decision making regarding his or her own health care.

While the ideological differences of personnel may at times be a source of conflict, teamwork and the task at hand must overcome any disparities. Also problems in the OR suite due to many complex procedures, heavy operating schedules, or shortages of personnel or available staff must not interfere with the delivery of efficient, individualized patient care.

The remainder of this text details the many procedures OR nurses and technologists perform in implementing nursing care. Applicable standards of care and recommended practices are incorporated in these procedures (see sources in Chap. 12).

CHAPTER 3

THE PATIENT: THE REASON FOR YOUR EXISTENCE

PATIENT-CENTERED CARE

Hippocrates (b. 460 B.C.) advocated, "To cure the human body you must have knowledge of the whole thing." His concept is still valid. The human body is a miraculously complex creation that functions as a coordinated unit, an organized entity, and as a person who interacts with family and society.

A person facing an impaired health status strives for wholeness that acts as a catalyst to healing. As a patient, this person looks to the hospital staff to fulfill his or her multiplicity of diversified needs, which are not presented in an orderly, categorized manner. Specialization tends to separate the body into systems and parts, to fragment and categorize care. A *patient-centered approach* to total surgical care involves meeting all the patient's basic needs during the preoperative, intraoperative, and postoperative phases. As noted in Chapter 2, many persons contribute to this care. Each has specific functions in the continuity of care process. The health care team is dedicated to maintaining optimal health and/or restoring it when altered by disease, injury, or deformity. Although the team members may vary with the situation and the patient, the goal is for a favorable outcome from surgical intervention.

In viewing the team in its broadest scope, one can consider the patient as the central part or hub of a wheel with many persons and departments as the supporting framework (see Fig. 3-1). All focus their efforts at the hub, meaning that the patient is the center of attention always, not only when under the OR spotlight. The ultimate beneficiary of teamwork is the patient. Imperfection in any one part of the wheel imperils the performance and security of all. Each team member makes a unique contribution in reaching the goals. The patient is your reason for existence as a health care team member.

THE PATIENT

A *patient* may be defined as an individual seeking medical care. To effectively meet the patient's requirements and wants, personnel must have knowledge of his or her needs, understanding of individuality, and realization of what an operation means to a patient.

Certain beliefs exist concerning a human being. In our society, human beings:

1 Are worthwhile and unique singular beings.

2 Respond psychosocially to their environment.

3 Have the capacity to adapt to both their internal and external environments.

4 Have certain basic needs that must be met in order to maintain homeostasis.

Homeostasis may be defined as the maintenance of steady or stable states in the organism by coordinated physiologic processes. The body strives to maintain equilibrium within normal limits. This stability depends partly on the intactness of

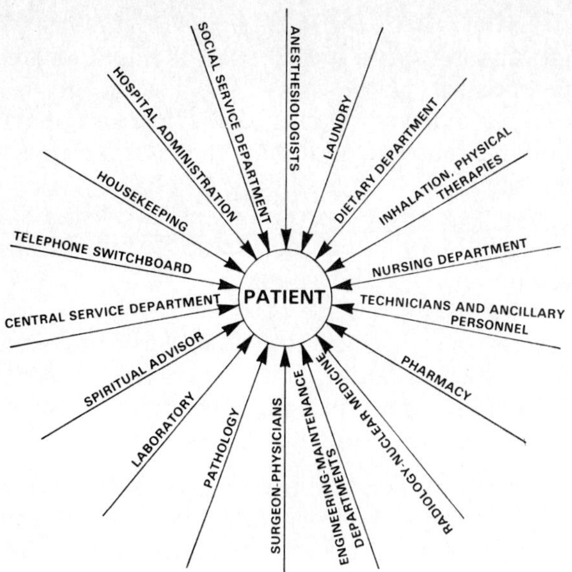

FIGURE 3-1
The patient is the focus of attention of the entire health care team.

the body, the consistency of its functions, and its surroundings. Change requires adjustment.

THE PATIENT'S BASIC NEEDS

Needs are factors that must be controlled or redirected to restore altered function. Nursing judgments are based on knowledge of patient needs. It is therefore essential to understand basic human needs of all persons (well or ill), because fulfilling them is an integral part of the nursing process. The surgical patient faces a grave threat to the basic needs classified as physical, emotional or psychosocial, and spiritual.

Physical Needs

Physical needs are the life-sustaining necessities such as food, water, oxygen, sleep, warmth. In illness, the patient becomes acutely aware of these needs. However, patient care does not focus entirely on bodily needs.

Psychosocial Needs

Concern for the patient's emotional well-being should be as intense as it is for his or her physical health for the two are inseparably intertwined. The society the patient lives in is an integral factor in developing feelings of identity, self-worth, and satisfaction. Thwarted feelings can lead to a state of helplessness or inferiority. Development of self-actualization, what the patient can be and the best he or she is capable of, is the highest level of human development. Examples of *psychosocial* needs that also require fulfillment are:

1 *Security.* People need to be secure, feel safe, and trust those around them. They also need to feel comforted, reassured, protected, and cared about.

2 *Belonging, inclusion, affection.* Individuals need to receive empathetic understanding and response to the self-expression of their feelings and attitudes, both negative as well as positive.

3 *Recognition.* People need to be accepted as worthy individuals.

4 *Self-esteem, identity, control.* People need to be productive, make their own choices and decisions, and control their behavior and environment. They also need their confidentiality respected.

People are social beings who need to establish satisfying meaningful interpersonal relationships, mutual trust and respect, and to know that someone cares. Risk is involved in sharing feelings with others, however. Emotional stress develops if individuals do not feel secure. If they are treated with love and kindness they feel worthy and can respond to others in the same way. Human beings also need a sense of order in their lives, as well as recreational diversion.

Spiritual Needs

Spiritual needs include support of a person's religious views or belief in a supreme being(s), whose guidance influences life. People have an inherent drive for spirituality, a desire to achieve a sense of oneness with the total universe. Especially in times of stress and fear, a person reaches out or turns to religious convictions for spiritual sustenance, since fear of death has a spiritual as well as a physical dimension. Uncertainty about one's relationship with one's God can enhance patient anxiety as the operative procedure draws near. The inner strength derived from a strong religious faith can be a bulwark of hope for the patient facing an operation.

The hospital chaplain, available to patients of all faiths, or the patient's personal cleric provides the anxious, suffering patient with a human element of comfort, warmth, and strength. The giving of sacraments to the ill does not necessarily mean that the patient is dying. Rather, through an understanding of life's subjective aspects, the clergy can be a source of great support, giving courage as patients feel free to share their fears. The spiritual advisor, available as the patient needs him or her, fulfills a basic need by utilizing the reassuring symbols of the patient's religious experiences.

Hierarchy of Needs

Using Maslow's concept of a hierarchy of needs to set priorities for care (see Fig. 4-2, p. 63), basic lower-level or physiologic needs—those essential for survival—must be met first. Then satisfaction of the higher-level needs for safety, security, belonging and love, esteem, and self-actualization can be met. Health care personnel must be concerned with a total picture of the patient's needs and consider all of them. In illness, factors such as location of pathology, type of operation, and effectiveness of therapy can influence needs. Also, priorities may change with changing situations. Preoperatively, anxiety and nutritional status are two factors that must be dealt with. Intraoperatively, the team must concentrate on basic physiological needs such as oxygenation, circulation, and prevention of shock and infection. Postoperatively, team members must prevent complications and encourage patient self-actualization. If one's needs are not satisfactorily met, undesirable consequences can occur.

PATIENT REACTIONS TO ILLNESS

To meet patient needs, the health care team must be sensitive to patients' feelings about their illnesses. Patients' reactions influence their behaviors and the staff's behavioral responses to them.

Behavior

Health and human behavior are interdependent. Individuals with physiological problems, regardless of age, experience some emotional change that influences behavior. Patients react to a new interpersonal environment according to their learned behavioral patterns. The following are facts about behavior.

1 Perception of interaction within the environment creates individualized differences in personality, behavior, and needs.

2 A person's physical and psychosocial behavior is a response to stimuli in an attempt to maintain homeostasis.

3 Behavior is complex. Behavioral acts have multiple causes in addition to a major precipitating one.

4 A person functions on many levels simultaneously. Many factors determine an individual's reaction in a given situation.

5 Behavior must be evaluated in light of the person's specific situation and of pertinent social forces such as family, culture, and environment. To understand the meaning of behavior, one must know about the individual.

Patients respond to crises or personal threats in different ways. Some persons face suffering and surgical intervention with extreme courage, dignity, and fortitude. Others may revert to extreme fear or helplessness when faced by even a relatively safe procedure. Overt behavior is not necessarily consistent with one's feelings but often reflects them most accurately. Patients often express frustration and fear behaviorally in an effort to cope with stimuli.

Adaptation

Any deviation from a person's normal daily pattern of living necessitates adaptation through innate or acquired defenses. Adaptation may involve physiological or psychological changes.

Personality includes a patient's characteristic responses to anxiety (either calm acceptance or disorganization, depression, and resistance) as well as to self-image. *Self-image,* an individual's concept or ideas about self and personal philosophy of life, is often affected by other people's reactions. It may also involve constantly changing and evolving perceptions of self. These perceptions may be on both the conscious and unconscious levels. Interpersonal relationships in early childhood are among the most important social determinants of personality formation. A person's adaptive and defensive mechanisms are a basic part of personality and heredity. Therefore, individuals vary in their adaptive abilities, as demonstrated by varied behavioral responses to illness.

Illness disrupts normal living and equilibrium. It also alters self-image. One may worry about what others think, especially if the illness involves disfigurement as from severe burns or a communicable disease such as syphilis. A patient's initial reaction to illness may be irrational, impulsive behavior requiring patience and understanding from others. He or she may have difficulty thinking clearly, concentrating, or making intelligent, rational decisions. Both mind and body must adapt successfully in order for the patient to recover. Adaptation requires energy, ingenuity, and persistence.

The coping mechanism that creates physiological or psychological changes constitutes an attempt to counteract stimuli by limiting site, lessening impact, or neutralizing effects so the individual can continue to function. If adaptation is interfered with, the effects can be detrimental. Adaptation to illness includes the following three stages:

1 Transition from health: development of symptoms
2 Acceptance: coping and making decisions
3 Convalescence or resolution

Adaptation may be rapid or slow depending on the nature of the stimuli, the individual's heredity, learned responses, and developmental needs. Adaptations may be sensory, motor, or sensorimotor. The extent of adjustment required is contingent on the type of illness, the magnitude of disability, and the patient's personality.

Stress

Stress can be defined as a physical, chemical, or emotional factor that causes tension. It may be a factor in disease causation. It is the result of threat perception, and is manifested by changes in physiological and psychosocial behavior. Tolerance of stress depends on the individual and on the intensity of stress, its duration, and type—either localized or generalized, as pain.

Inescapable in the process of daily living, a certain degree of stress can be beneficial if it motivates an individual to increased productivity. Conversely, it can be harmful if increased or simultaneous stresses occur, straining the individual's coping ability. If the individual's adaptive powers are inadequate or malfunctioning, the stress may become overwhelming. In the latter situation, new secondary stresses more incapacitating than the initial one develop, creating a continuous stress-adaptation cycle. Adaptive reserve may become depleted as a result.

Stressful factors can originate from within the individual or from the external environment. *Intrinsic factors,* those originating from within, that affect a patient include:

1 Hereditary or genetic factors, such as hormonic or enzymic system competency.
2 Nature of the illness or disease process. This may be influenced by nutritional status.
3 Severity of the illness or presence of a stigma.
4 Previous personal experiences with illnesses. Chronic illness has a disruptive effect on life-style.
5 Age. Children feel threatened. Adolescents resent an interruption of activities and are painfully aware of body changes. Older people think about infirmity and death.
6 Intellectual capacity.
7 Disturbed sensorium. Hearing or sight loss intensifies a stressful experience.
8 General state of personal well-being.

Extrinsic factors originating from external sources include those dependent on:

1 Environment. The physical and social environment of the hospital is not the same as that of the home.
2 Family role and status. Expectations and authoritative relationships affect life-style, modesty, attitudes.
3 Economic, financial situation.
4 Religion. Beliefs influence attitudes and values toward life, illness, and death. For example, Jehovah's Witnesses will not permit transfusion of whole blood or blood components. Orthodox Jews must follow dietary laws in any environment. The fatalistic attitudes derived from some religious beliefs give a person little control over his or her environment; they can render a patient passive and apathetic.
5 Cultural background, education, and social class. These are closely related to the patient's emotional response and living habits. Significant elements such as food habits, daily living patterns, hygiene, family organization, child care, orientation to past, present, and future time should be analyzed in relationship to culture. An ethnic community is really a larger family. Roles taught by a cultural group influence mores, beliefs, and social interactions of individuals. Also, responses to pain may vary according to one's cultural or ethnic background. Some groups commonly show an exaggerated emotional response; in others it is more appropriate to conceal suffering.

Social factors, such as a breakdown in the role and closeness of the family and the emphasis on isolationism and independence, increase one's need for reassurance and for a sense of being cared about. The nurse must not, however, assume or make specific predictions in regard to cultural or social influences.

Disability, illness, and hospitalization accentuate feelings of vulnerability and are stress-producing, stress-exaggerating experiences that threaten a person's security and stability. They may create a crisis state that diminishes defenses and increases an emotional response to threats. The individual patient's needs, strengths, and innate defense mechanisms create unique responses to these threats. The severity of the reaction may be unrelated to the seriousness of the illness. It is often not the problem itself that is devastating, but one's perception of it. Also, the same illness may hold different meanings for different individuals. For many persons hospitalization and surgical intervention represent a critical life experience.

To decrease the traumatic consequences of an operation, health care personnel must realize that stress and pain are both physical and psychological. These components of illness become inseparable parts of the total patient experience. Stress can affect appetite and bodily functions such as digestion, metabolism, and fluid and electrolyte balance. However, during times of markedly increased stress one's emotional needs come to the fore. In facing personal threat, a person tends to mobilize defense mechanisms for flight or fight. One's ability to adapt depends in part on the support one receives. Effective nursing intervention at any stage of the adaptation process can alter the exigencies of illness and direct the patient's emotional reactions. This will facilitate therapy and recovery through behavior modification.

Coping with Stress Reactions

Each individual patient's natural inclination toward health or illness influences preoperative response and contributes to postoperative recovery. Psychologic reactions are significant factors affecting the outcome of surgical intervention. To give adequate support in the patient's periods of crisis, the health care team must assess the patient's ability to cope with stress. Psychological preparation is as important as physical preparation but it is all too often overlooked. Crisis intervention includes comprehensive nursing care of the patient under stress through interactions with patient, family or significant other, and staff, directed toward controlling crisis behavior in reaction to stress.

Persons assessing the patient must ascertain his or her needs and share this information with others. All patients' reactions to preoperative stress should be documented, discussed with attending physicians, and reduced by appropriate interventions. Severe or prolonged reactions require psychiatric consultation. Some stress and anxiety are a natural part of surgical patient experience. Specific reactions to the stresses of surgical intervention are described in detail in Chapter 4.

PATIENT'S RIGHTS

Hospital services are a commodity that the patient as a consumer purchases to fulfill health care needs. The patient is entitled to certain rights. Access to quality care is recognized as a right, not a privilege, for every human being.

In the interest of "more effective patient care and greater satisfaction for the patient, his physician, and the hospital organization," the American Hospital Association adopted a Patient's Bill of Rights as a national policy statement and distributed it to its member hospitals. Intended to be supported by the hospital on behalf of its patients, these rights, in summary, are:

1 The patient has the right to considerate and respectful care.

2 The patient has the right to obtain from the physician complete and current information concerning diagnosis, treatment, and prognosis in terms the patient can be reasonably expected to understand.

3 The patient has the right to receive from the physician information necessary to give informed consent prior to the start of any procedure and/or treatment. Except in emergencies, such information for informed consent should include but not necessarily be limited to the specific procedure and/or treatment, the medically significant risks involved, and the probable duration of incapacitation.

4 The patient has the right to refuse treatment to the extent permitted by law, and to be informed of the medical consequences of his action.

5 The patient has the right to every consideration of his privacy concerning his own medical care program.

6 The patient has the right to expect that all communications and records pertaining to his care should be treated as confidential.

7 The patient has the right to expect that within its capacity a hospital must make reasonable response to the request of a patient for services.

8 The patient has the right to obtain information as to any relationship of his hospital to other health care and educational institutions insofar as his care is concerned.

9 The patient has the right to be advised if the hospital proposes to engage in or perform human experimentation affecting his care or treatment. The patient has the right to refuse to participate in such research projects.

10 The patient has the right to expect reasonable continuity of care.

11 The patient has the right to examine and receive an explanation of his bill regardless of source of payment.

12 The patient has the right to know what hospital rules and regulations apply to his conduct as a patient.

Further, the American Hospital Association statement concludes that no bill of rights:

> can guarantee for the patient the kind of treatment he has a right to expect. A hospital has many functions to perform, including the prevention and treatment of disease, the education of both health professionals and patients, and the conduct of clinical research. All these activities must be conducted with an overriding concern for the patient, and, above all, the recognition of his dignity as a human being. Success in achieving this recognition assures success in the defense of the rights of the patient.*

This document gives patients the right to know what is being done to, for, and about them and their illnesses. For those patients not wishing to know the details during a crisis, their wish for only capsule explanations or essential information should be respected. The duty of disclosure is not absolute.

PATIENT-PHYSICIAN RELATIONSHIP

The attending physician must adequately explain, in clear, simple language, the nature, purpose, extent, potential hazards, and expected outcome of the procedure proposed, as well as other available options of therapy. The patient usually wants to know about anticipated duration of hospitalization, absence from work, and cost of operation. Physicians, both surgeons and anesthesiologists, must inform the patient, and not delegate this responsibility to a nurse or assistant.

> NOTE. Adequate translation must be provided for patients with a language barrier and interpretation for deaf patients.

The physician-patient relationship is a contractual one. However, the physician is under no legal obligation to accept any person as a patient. The potential for litigation may influence the surgeon since positive guarantee of a favorable outcome of surgical intervention can never be fully given. Patients want and deserve reassurance, but the key to all medical discussion is the risk versus benefit ratio. Everyone wants a black and white answer. This is not possible in medicine.

If the physician or patient has doubts as to the necessity for an operation, the American College of Surgeons recommends that another opinion be secured from a qualified specialist in the appropriate field of surgery. A second opinion may be particularly indicated if the procedure involves extended disability, such as amputation of an extremity or removal of an eye. Special consultation or consent may be required by hospital policy for procedures to terminate reproductive capability through sterilization and/or therapeutic abortion. Consultation is a common and desirable part of good surgical practice.

The surgeon is responsible for informing the patient about a proposed operation, and its inherent risks and complications. The explanation should reasonably include discussion of removal of parts, disfigurement, disability, and what the patient may expect in the postoperative period. It should be meaningful without creating unnecessary anxiety over very rare or insignificant hazards. Preoperative discussion also should include advice to the patient regarding diet, bathing, smoking, and other factors that might affect the outcome.

The anesthesiologist also has a responsibility to inform the patient of any unfavorable reactions to a medication or anesthetic agent that may be given during the operation. The risks of anesthesia must be explained, but without causing the patient undue stress.

*American Hospital Association Statement: A Patient's Bill of Rights, copyright © 1975. Reprinted with permission.

Explanations are given prior to the time the patient or legal guardian signs a written, informed consent document. Written, *informed consent* is necessary for any procedure that may possibly be injurious to the patient. The surgeon is responsible for making certain that the patient or legal guardian is adequately prepared to sign this document.

It is valuable to have a family member or significant other present during the physician's explanation to the patient, especially if the patient is elderly. Persons facing a proposed operation are under stress. They often do not listen to or comprehend the physician's explicit information, even if it is repeated. Also, they may misconstrue what is said. Some patients go to the OR still not clear about the operative procedure to be performed in spite of a careful discussion beforehand. For this reason, many physicians will again, in a nonstressful manner, simply repeat the basic facts on a second occasion preoperatively. For legal protection, physicians should record a brief progress note covering the explanatory conversation and the patient's reaction. Failure to provide full disclosure of the risks of the procedure and alternative modes of therapy has led to successful negligence suits. The physician is liable for misrepresentations, whether by affirmative statement or nondisclosure. To prevent legal liability, some surgeons tape record their conversations with patients about the planned operations.

Immediately after the operation, the surgeon speaks to the patient's family and discusses with them the procedure performed, patient's tolerance, and prognosis. On the rare occasion when a patient expires during an operation, the attending physician is responsible for informing the family or next of kin. The surgeon has the ultimate responsibility of facing the patient and the family whether the outcome of surgical intervention is satisfactory or unsatisfactory.

Postoperatively, the surgeon follows the patient's progress until discharge from his or her care, or return to a referring physician is indicated.

ACCEPTANCE OF OPERATION

The patient must reconcile the need or weigh the advantages and disadvantages for surgical intervention. Every patient is entitled to receive sufficient information upon which to intelligently base a decision. The patient has the right to decide what will or will not be done to him or her. Only after making this decision is the patient asked to sign a written consent for operation.

Written Consent

A written consent is not an infallible legal protection for the surgeon and hospital, but it does have legal value for all concerned with patient care. Consent documents vary from hospital to hospital and state to state.

General Consent Most hospitals ask the patient or legal guardian to sign a *general consent* form upon admission, usually in the hospital admitting office. This form authorizes the physician in charge and hospital staff to render such treatment or perform such procedures as the physician deems advisable. This general consent is relied on only for routine duties carried out in the hospital. Physicians and nurses must be knowledgeable about the statement on the form used in their hospital. A signed consent is legally regarded as valid for a period of about six months.

Operative Permit A consent document specifically relating to any procedure possibly injurious to the patient also should be signed before procedure is performed. Often referred to as an *operative permit,* the patient's consent is generally required for:

1 Each operation performed, including secondary procedures such as incision and drainage

2 Any procedure for which general anesthesia is administered, such as the examination of a child under anesthesia

3 Procedures involving entrance into a body cavity, such as endoscopy

4 Any hazardous therapy, such as radiation or chemotherapy

Purposes of Informed Consent An informed consent provides a mechanism to protect a patient's right to self-determination regarding surgical intervention. It also serves:

1 To protect patient from unratified and unwanted procedures

2 To protect surgeon and hospital or facility from claims of an unauthorized operation or other invasive procedures

Validity of Consent The document must contain the patient's name in full (a married woman's given name), surgeon's name, procedure to be performed, patient's and authorized witness(es)' signatures, and date of signatures.

The patient giving consent must be of legal age, mentally alert, and competent. The patient must sign before premedication is given and prior to going to the OR or other treatment area, except in life-threatening, emergency situations. Before elective operation, the patient should be asked to sign at least one day preoperatively. This may be done in the surgeon's office, hospital admitting office, or on the nursing unit, but *it must be an informed consent freely given without coercion.* If the patient is:

1 A minor, a parent or legal guardian must sign.

2 An emancipated minor, married or independently earning a living, he or she may sign or a spouse of legal age may sign.

3 An illiterate, he or she may sign with an *X*, after which the witness writes *"patient's mark."*

4 Unconscious or inebriated, a responsible relative or guardian signs.

5 Mentally incompetent, the legal guardian who may be either an individual or an agency must sign. A court of competent jurisdiction may legalize the procedure in the absence of the legal guardian.

6 A child of an unwed minor parent, consent is signed by the next of kin to the unwed parent.

Witnessing a Consent The patient's or guardian's signature must be witnessed by one or more authorized persons. They may be physicians, nurses, or other hospital employees as established by policy. By his or her signature the witness signing a consent document attests to:

1 Identification of patient or legal substitute
2 Fact that the signing was voluntary

Consent in Emergency Situations In a life-threatening emergency, consent is desired but not essential. While every effort should be made to contact the family, the patient's perilous physical condition takes precedence over operative permit. The patient's condition usually prevents his or her signing. Permit for operation, especially on a minor, may be accepted from a legal guardian or responsible relative by telephone, telegram, or written communication. If by phone, two nurses monitor the call and sign the form, which is signed by the parent or guardian on arrival at the hospital. In lieu of the aforementioned methods, a written consultation by two physicians other than the surgeon will suffice until a relative can sign a consent.

Responsibility for Permit The ultimate responsibility for obtaining consent is the surgeon's. The consent document becomes a permanent part of the patient's medical record and accompanies him or her to the OR. It is the duty of the circulating nurse (RN or charge nurse) and the anesthesiologist when checking the patient's identity and chart on arrival in the OR to be certain that:

1 Consent is on the chart and properly signed.
2 Information on the form is correct.

NOTE. Checking a form does *not* ensure that it is an informed consent, however.

The attending surgeon should also check the consent before an anesthetic is administered. If the surgeon intends or wants to perform a procedure not specified on the consent form, the OR nurse has a responsibility to inform the surgeon and/or a proper administrative authority of the discrepancy.

Right to Refuse Operation

The patient has a right to withdraw written consent prior to operation if his or her determination to do so is reached in a rational state. The surgeon is notified and the patient is not taken to the OR. The operation is postponed until the patient is willing. The patient makes the final decision on what treatment is acceptable.

The surgeon or referring physician should explain to the patient the medical consequences of refusing the operation. If therapeutically valid, alternative methods of medical management should be offered.

The physician should inform hospital administration of the patient's refusal to consent to treatment if the consequences will be adverse and substantial. The physician should also obtain a written refusal from the patient, parent, or legal guardian to absolve him or her and the hospital from liability for failure to perform the recommended operation or other treatment.

Some states by law have placed restrictions on the right of a patient, or someone on his or her behalf, to refuse surgical or medical treatments.

Hospital personnel need to be familiar with these laws in their state.

PATIENTS WITH SPECIAL NEEDS

In general, the healthy body can tolerate the trauma of a surgical procedure without serious sequelae. However, the debilitated, chronically ill, or age-extreme patient has increased difficulty combating the stress of trauma to tissues and alteration of physiology from anesthetic agents. An added hazard is the patient's possible concealment from the surgeon of pertinent facts or conditions that, if uncorrected, may predispose to intra- and/or postoperative complications.

The importance of sending each patient to the operating room in the best possible physical and emotional condition must be emphasized. Adequate rest and balanced nutrition are essential factors. Diagnostic and laboratory studies assist in establishing diagnoses and pinpoint areas of deficiencies. Surgical intervention is often postponed until a cardiovascular situation is optimized, for example, by lowering hypertension or correcting cardiac arrhythmias. Preoperative therapy may be indicated to control diabetes, reduce obesity, or treat infection in order to decrease risk of anesthesia and postoperative complications.

Patients of various ages and stages of development have different needs. Ways of meeting those needs will vary. A family-centered approach to care is valuable. Particularly with aged patients, family cooperation is essential for communication with, interpretation to, and assistance with the patient.

Many patients have special needs, but space precludes mention of them all. The more common secondary problems associated with surgical intervention will be discussed. These may be encountered in patients coming to the OR for all types of operations.

Nutritional Needs

Nutrition refers to the sum of the processes concerned in the growth, maintenance, and repair of the body as a whole or its constituent parts. Decreased intake and increased metabolic demands create nutritional problems in surgical patients.

Perhaps as many as 50 percent of hospitalized patients are malnourished to some degree. *Malnutrition* in the surgical patient is due to inadequate intake or utilization of calories and protein pre- and/or postoperatively. This creates a state of impaired functional ability and structural integrity because of a discrepancy between the intake of essential nutrients and the body's demand for them. As a result of malnutrition, the surgical patient may have:

1 Poor tolerance of anesthetic agents
   a Decreased metabolism of agents by the liver
   b Inadequate excretion of toxin by the kidneys
2 Failure of blood clotting mechanisms
3 Negative nitrogen balance with a serum albumin of less than 3.5 gram (g)/100 millimeter (ml)
4 Decreased wound healing potential from a decrease in protein synthesis
5 Immunologic incompetence from a total lymphocyte count of less than 1800/millimeter (mm) that increases susceptibility to infection
6 Increased risk of morbidity and mortality

Metabolism is the phenomenon of synthesizing foodstuffs into complex elements and complex substances into simple ones in the production of energy. It involves two opposing phases:

1 *Anabolism,* or constructive metabolism, the conversion of nutritive material into complex living matter—tissue construction

2 *Catabolism,* or destructive metabolism, concerned with the breaking down or dissolution by the body of complex compounds, often with the release of energy

Metabolic disorders can complicate the outcome of surgical intervention. Dietary deficiencies disturb the body's nutritional homeostasis and may markedly alter a patient's nutritional status and needs. Hormonal response to physical stress involves both anabolic and catabolic effects on the body with catabolism predominant. The degree of metabolic reaction may depend greatly on the body's reserve of labile protein. The type and extent of the operative procedure, the preoperative nutritional state, and the effect of the operation on the patient's ability to digest and absorb nutrients affect immediate postoperative metabolism.

Biochemical changes accompany surgical intervention. One of the major ones is *protein catabolism.* Limited food intake preoperatively, catharsis, and adrenocortical response to crisis augment a catabolic response. Trauma and blood loss also have a contributory effect. Metabolic disease, dehydration, and fever increase one's need for calories and nutritional substances. This is also true in patients with severe burns, infection, or toxemia where essential nutrients such as nitrogen are lost. Abnormalities of the gastrointestinal tract and digestive organs may produce malnutrition through incomplete digestion, absorption, or excretion of nutrients. Digestion and absorption are also affected by deviations in digestive secretions, timing of passage through gastrointestinal tract, and stomach capacity.

Biochemical tests monitor nutritional status. These include proteins, albumin/globulin determination and ratio, and blood urea nitrogen level. Body weight is significant also. If calorie intake is inadequate, protein is converted into carbohydrate for energy. Protein synthesis then suffers.

The average adult patient needs about 1500 calories daily to spare body protein. Hypermetabolic states can double that requirement to 3000 calories and 18 to 19 gram (g) of nitrogen for nitrogen retention, if liver function is normal. Depleted reserves of essential elements must be replenished to replace tissue loss and expedite wound healing. Protein deficiency impairs collagen formation, thereby delaying the healing process. Vitamins K and C are also important (see Chap. 17). The application of principles of aseptic technique, gentle handling of tissues, and physiological support are preeminent in modern surgery but they are not enough for patients with *protein calorie malnutrition.* The surgeon is justifiably concerned about the patient's nutritional status, since malnutrition lowers host resistance by impairing lymphocyte and neutrophilic functioning. A definite relationship has been demonstrated between hypoproteinemia and terminal postoperative infection.

Electrolyte and metabolic disturbances other than protein catabolism may accompany surgical intervention and lead to imbalance. These disturbances can result from:

1 Cell destruction leading to potassium depletion.

2 Changes in blood lipids; calcium and magnesium are depleted by poor absorption.

3 Stress; diminishes glucose tolerance.

4 Gastric drainage; chlorides are lost.

5 Fluid loss from drainage tubes, diaphoresis, vomiting, or diarrhea.

6 Maxillofacial injury; inhibits oral intake.

7 Radiation enteritis.

8 Disease of bowel, liver, or biliary tract, intestinal tract obstruction, or gastrointestinal fistula.

9 Drugs; adverse affect on metabolic balance. Broad-spectrum antibiotics, while limiting a disease process can, in association with dietary inadequacy, cause vitamin K deficiency in aged patients by inhibiting the intestinal bacteria that produce that vitamin. Drug detoxification and/or excretion may be altered in patients with kidney or liver damage, leading to possible drug overdosage. Metabolism is altered by immunosuppressive drugs and antimetabolites that interfere with nutritional function. Corticosteroids may increase susceptibility to infection and loss of muscle protein.

10 Loss of muscle tissue; leads to increased nitrogen loss.

11 Inadequate oxygen/carbon dioxide exchange; disrupts acid-base balance.

Nutritional Supplements Changes in fluid and electrolyte balance affect kidney function, cellular metabolism, and oxygen concentration in circulation. Tissue hydration and distribution of body electrolytes are essential. Adequate essential nutrients at the cellular level are crucial. Therefore, by dietary management, physicians aim to correct metabolic and nutritional abnormalities prior to the operative procedure. In some patients, special nutritional supplements are indicated to build up or compensate for a permanent metabolic handicap. Successful therapy is indicated by weight gain, a rise in plasma albumin, and a positive nitrogen balance. A chemically defined elemental diet may be administered via:

1 Oral intake.

2 Nasogastric tube.

3 Gastrostomy tube, with or without constant infusion pump.

4 Intravenous (IV) infusion through a peripheral vein. Isotonic fat emulsions can be administered via this route, but only about 2000 calories per day can be provided.

5 Central venous cannulation for hyperalimentation.

Hyperalimentation [Total Parenteral Nutrition (TPN)] *Parenteral hyperalimentation* is another method of fulfilling nutritional requirements. Essential nutrients are delivered directly into the bloodstream intravenously via an indwelling catheter. This mode of therapy is used for patients with nutritional defects not amenable to oral therapy or nasogastric intubation, or who fail to gain weight by other means. Intravenous infusion by peripheral vein is precluded in some patients because the amount of fluid necessary to supply the adequate calories and nitrogen would exceed the body's fluid tolerance, leading to pulmonary edema and congestive heart failure. For these select patients and for those requiring long-term intravenous therapy, hyperalimentation provides the daily nutrition necessary for protein synthesis.

Hyperalimentation is coordinated with other therapy to establish adequate nutrition, fluid, and electrolyte balance. Increasing protein nourishment in the pre- and postoperative periods lessens protein loss and destruction of cell nuclei, muscle, and connective tissue. It also counteracts the increased catabolism resulting from the stress of surgical intervention. The therapy is beneficial to select patients but is not without danger or complications.

Basic Solution To provide 2500 to 3000 calories daily in small volume, a concentrated hypertonic solution is administered. It usually consists of 25% glucose with amino acids to provide 1000 calories and 6 g nitrogen per liter for protein synthesis. The physician orders the solution contents for each patient. Specific serum electrolyte needs determine the essential elements, vitamins, and minerals to be included.

Solutions are prepared in the pharmacy with strict aseptic technique under a laminar airflow hood (see Chap. 7). The solution is a medium for bacterial and fungal growth, so it must be stored at 4°C (39°F) until used. It is warmed to room temperature before administration and may hang for no more than 12 hours if it is a casein protein hydrolysate solution; no longer than 24 hours if an essential amino acid solution.

> NOTE. 1. Commercial solutions are available. If used, they are modified to meet individual needs. Mixing of additives poses a risk of sepsis.
>
> 2. Each flask should be inspected and the expiration date noted before use. Also, a cloudy solution with floating particles should not be used as it may be contaminated.

Central Venous Cannulation A large-diameter vein in a region of high blood flow must be selected to instantly dilute the irritating hypertonic solution, which has high osmolarity, in order to prevent thrombus or vein occlusion at the introduction site. A Broviac or Hickman catheter is inserted through the cephalic, external or internal jugular, or subclavian vein into the superior vena cava or the right atrium of the heart. (Refer to Chapter 35 for further discussion of these catheters, their placement and uses.)

Central venous catheter insertion should be performed in a controlled environment; an area with an air-filtering system where microbial levels are acceptable. Because strict aseptic technique is required, catheter insertion may be done in the OR by a scrubbed sterile team.

Cyclical variations in intracaval venous pressure occurs because the superior vena cava is situated within the thorax, contiguous to the right atrium. This pressure becomes negative during atrial filling and during respiratory inspiration. Therefore, any leaks in the external portion of the tubing can permit the sucking of air into the system during negative venous pressure. Precautionary measures must be taken against inadvertent introduction of air into the system, which can result in air embolus. Leakage in the line must be prevented. All connections in the parenteral hyperalimentation setup should be taped to prevent accidental separation. The patient is instructed not to touch the insertion site, but to report any discomfort.

During catheter insertion and subsequent tubing changes, the patient may be requested to bear down with mouth closed. Forced expiration against a closed glottis (Valsalva maneuver) produces a positive phase in the central venous pressure.

Infusion Rate A constant infusion rate of the prescribed solution is calculated on the basis of the amount of fluids ordered for a 24-hour period. Slow administration is necessary because bypassing the regulatory mechanism in the gastrointestinal tract and liver places an increased burden of elimination on the cells and kidneys. The flow rate must be maintained as ordered. An overload of hypertonic solution can cause massive dehydration of body cells. The solution should not be infused more rapidly than it can be metabolized or hyperglycemia can result. Insulin may then be prescribed. Hypoglycemia may develop from too slow an infusion rate. A decreased flow rate may result from a plugged filter or change in body position. *Constant monitoring is necessary.* The flow rate and patency of the infusion system should be checked every 30 minutes.

Precautions Strict asepsis for catheter insertion, maintenance, and infusion is mandatory. Sepsis is a serious complication. Maintenance of a closed intravenous system with minimal catheter manipulation is important. The technique itself introduces a foreign body and exposes the circulation to a potentially dangerous external environment at a time when the patient can least afford complications. Possibility of sepsis is the greatest deterrent to hyperalimentation therapy. Conscientious care is obligatory.

NOTE. Every time the line is entered there is risk of contamination. Therefore, the parenteral alimentation line should be used *only* for the delivery of nutrition. It should not be used for piggyback intravenous setups as for administration of blood constituents, medications, central venous pressure monitoring, or blood drawing for laboratory analysis.

Hyperalimentation therapy is discontinued gradually to permit adjustment to a lowered glucose level. Rebound hypoglycemia must be guarded against.

Other Considerations Hyperalimentation therapy is not a contraindication to ambulation. Long-term parenteral hyperalimentation, although hazardous, can be accomplished at home with adequate professional instruction, supervision, assistance, and unyielding observance of strict aseptic technique.

Diabetic Patients

Diabetes mellitus is an endocrine disease that increases the risk for morbidity and mortality. The stress of an operation is reflected in all body systems in relatively healthy patients. For the labile diabetic patient who vacillates from the precipice of insulin shock to ketoacidosis, the hazards are even greater. Surgical intervention upsets normal regimen of caloric intake and insulin or oral hypoglycemic agents. Anesthesia and reduced activity postoperatively also have disruptive effects on the diabetic. These factors can increase blood glucose and free fatty acids and decrease serum insulin level.

The stress of physical and emotional trauma, infection, or fever present additional problems of metabolic regulation. All three raise the blood sugar level. Stress stimulates the pituitary and adrenal glands. The former secretes an *adrenocorticotropic hormone* (ACTH), which stimulates the production of glucocorticoids. These in turn increase *gluconeogenesis,* the formation of glucose by the liver from noncarbohydrate sources. The resulting extra glucose enters the bloodstream. Coincidentally, the adrenals secrete epinephrine, which accelerates the conversion of glycogen in the liver to glucose, also raising the blood sugar. More insulin is needed. The primary goal of diabetes control is to maintain a stable internal environment thereby averting a metabolic crisis. Extreme care must be taken to *prevent:*

1 Hyperglycemia and its accompanying severe fluid loss, causing dehydration.
   a Some medications increase blood sugar level, e.g., cortisone.
2 Ketoacidosis and acetonuria.
   a These are due to insulin insufficiency from natural cause, or reduced or omitted insulin dosage.
   b They may result in coma if allowed to progress untreated.
3 Hypoglycemia and hypoglycemic shock.
   a These are due to too much insulin.
   b They are of faster onset than ketoacidosis.
   c Hypoglycemia is especially dangerous. It can occur during major procedures because of omission or delay of oral intake.
   d These can cause brain damage and stress on the cardiovascular system.

Prevention of these states is dependent on:

1 Physician's treatment of choice of diabetes
2 Severity of the disease
3 Type of onset, i.e., juvenile or adult
4 Existence of complicating conditions and type of operation

Preoperative preparation includes careful laboratory testing, including fasting and postprandial blood sugar determinations, urinalysis for sugar and acetone, complete blood count, blood urea nitrogen, and serum electrolyte determinations. A chest x-ray and electrocardiogram are also advisable.

Common Complications of Diabetes Persons with a mild form of the disease usually withstand surgical intervention without crisis. Intraoperative metabolic control is more difficult in patients with juvenile onset, who have marked unpredictability and greater extremes in blood sugar levels, as well as in severe diabetics. Lengthy major procedures with extensive tissue trauma present the greatest challenge to regulation. Diabetic patients are prone to:

1 Dehydration and electrolyte imbalance.
2 Infection.
3 Inadequate circulation from premature vas-

cular disease, causing deficient tissue perfusion. Hyperlipemia affects both coronary and peripheral arteries.

4 Delayed wound healing, due to increased protein breakdown. Glycogenolysis diverts protein from tissue regeneration.

5 Neuropathy; any nervous system disorder causing motor and sensory dysfunctions.

6 Nephropathy; small blood vessels in the kidney are affected.

7 Diabetic retinopathy and blindness; small vessels in the eye are affected.

8 Biliary and pancreatic diseases.

Postoperative blood glucose control may be a problem, especially if the patient remains under stress from a diagnosis necessitating changes in life-style or body image, for example, amputation of a gangrenous extremity.

Special Considerations To minimize the potential risks, special precautions need to be taken in the care of the diabetic surgical patient.

1 Blood for fasting serum glucose and urine for glucose and acetone tests should be obtained preoperatively prior to induction of anesthesia. The results provide baseline data to assess postoperative control.

2 Preoperative insulin dose may be reduced or eliminated to guard against hypoglycemia or insulin shock during operation.

3 Preoperative medication may be reduced by 25 to 50 percent of a normal dosage. Narcotics may cause vomiting, which predisposes to fluid and electrolyte imbalance. This can precipitate a hypoglycemic reaction from a decreased need for insulin. Adequate glucose is essential to central nervous system function.

4 Continuous intravenous access is vital throughout the operation in case of a metabolic problem. An infusion of dextrose in water may be started to begin administration of daily carbohydrate requirement before the patient comes to the operating room.

- **a** Optional methods of management for insulin-dependent patients are determined by the severity of the disease, preoperative control regimen, and type of operation. Insulin may be added to the infusion or administered by subcutaneous injection. Amounts are determined by serum glucose levels.
- **b** Adequate hydration must be maintained because a rising blood glucose level upsets osmotic equilibrium. Electrolytes may be added to the infusion to maintain metabolic status.

5 Metabolic crisis in an unconscious patient is difficult to detect. Therefore, during long operations blood glucose levels are monitored for hyper- or hypoglycemia, plus fractional urine specimens for ketones, in order to ascertain requirements for insulin and/or glucose.

6 Nasogastric suction may cause acidosis, dehydration, or electrolyte imbalance.

7 Antiembolic stockings usually are worn by the patient during the operation and postoperatively as a precaution against thrombophlebitis and thromboembolism.

8 Skin integrity must be guarded to avoid sepsis.

- **a** Strict aseptic and sterile techniques are extremely important to the infection-prone diabetic patient.
- **b** Air or water mattress should be placed on the operating table for operations expected to take more than three hours, to protect bony prominences.
- **c** Hyposensitive tape is used to affix dressings.

Obese Patients

Obesity is prevalent in our society. It may be of:

1 Endocrine origin; usually associated with biliary, hepatic, or endocrine disease.

2 Nonendocrine origin; usually associated with excessive caloric intake, is referred to as *morbid obesity* when weight exceeds 100 lb (220 kg) over the ideal weight for one's height.

Common Complications of Obesity Surgical patients who are ten percent or more overweight have an increased incidence of morbidity and mortality due to concomitant systemic diseases and physical problems. The degree of morbidity varies with the severity of the obese condition. Obesity predisposes to:

1 Increased demand on the cardiac system. Pulse rate, cardiac output, stroke volume, and blood volume increase to meet the metabolic demands of the adipose tissue (fat). Eventually this overload leads to myocardial hypertrophy (enlargement of the heart). Congestive heart failure may ensue.

2 Hypertension (high blood pressure). The vascular changes in the kidneys, associated with hypertension, affect elimination of protein wastes and maintenance of fluid and electrolyte balance.

3 Varicose veins and edema in the lower extremities. These conditions are due to poor venous return as a result of pressure on pelvic veins and the vena cava. Venous stasis can ultimately contribute to thrombophlebitis and thromboembolism.

4 Pulmonary function abnormalities. Hypoxemia may be associated with decreased tidal volume or poor gaseous exchange due to excessive weight on the thoracic cavity. These patients are susceptible to pulmonary infection and pulmonary embolism postoperatively.

5 Diseases of the digestive system, such as liver or gall bladder disease.

6 Osteoarthritis. This may limit mobility of spine.

7 Diabetes mellitus.

8 Malnutrition. Even though the patient is overweight, the obese patient may have a protein deficiency or other metabolic disturbance.

Special Considerations The marked increase in the physical size of obese persons presents problems for the OR and RR teams. Safety precautions against injury, falls, and burns must be emphasized. Problems include the following:

1 Transporting and lifting the patient. Mechanical patient lifters are desirable (see Chap. 10). If these are not available, extra persons are needed to ensure safety in lifting.
  - **a** Tables and stretchers must be stabilized.
  - **b** In moving from stretcher to operating table, suggest that the patient feel for the far side of the table, so that he or she does not move too far and fall.

2 Obese patients are frequently self-conscious; keep exposure to a minimum.

3 Induction, intubation, and maintenance of anesthesia.
  - **a** Venous cutdown may be necessary to establish an IV line if peripheral veins are invisible.
  - **b** Mobility of the cervical spine to hyperextend the neck for intubation may be limited.
  - **c** Inefficient respiratory muscles, poor lung/chest wall compliance, and/or increased intraabdominal pressure in supine position reduce ventilation capability.
  - **d** Lower concentrations of gases entering the lungs, due to inefficient ventilation, prolongs induction time.
  - **e** Continuous uptake by adipose tissue requires higher concentrations of anesthetic agents to maintain anesthesia.
  - **f** Recovery period may be prolonged because adipose tissue retains fat soluble agents and the poor blood supply in this tissue eliminates all agents slowly.

4 Positioning on the operating table.
  - **a** Extra personnel may be necessary to assist.
  - **b** Massive tissue and pressure areas must be protected. Protuberances must be padded to prevent bruising.
  - **c** Ventilation and circulation must be assured.
  - **d** The electrosurgical unit patient ground must not be surrounded by overlapping skin folds; the tissue could be burned.

5 Mechanics of operation lengthen operating time.
  - **a** Accessibility of deep organs, such as the gall bladder, may be a problem.
  - **b** Large instrumentation may contribute to operative trauma and postoperative pain.

6 Thromboembolic complications may occur due to venous stasis, erythrocytosis which increases the viscosity of the blood, and a decrease in fibrinolytic activity. Anticoagulants may be given prophylactically.

7 Healing may be delayed because of poor vascularity of adipose tissue. Obese patients have an increased incidence of postoperative wound infection and disruption (see Chap. 17).
  - **a** A sterile closed drainage system is often used to drain accumulated fluid, thereby facilitating healing.
  - **b** It is harder to eliminate "dead space" in wound closure.

Hematologic Disorders

All patients have a complete blood count, SMA-18, and urinalysis done prior to operation. The results of these laboratory tests may reveal or confirm the presence of an abnormal or pathologic condition affecting the blood. Some of these hematologic disorders or blood dyscrasias demand special consideration during perioperative care.

Anemia Anemia is a symptom of a deficiency in either the quantity or quality of red blood cells (erythrocytes). *Red cell count* (RBC) is normally

5.4 ± 0.8 million/cubic millimeter (cu mm) of blood in males, 4.8 ± 0.6 in females, and 4.5 to 5.1 in children. Normal *hematocrit,* the volume of red blood cells expressed as a percentage of volume of whole blood, is 47% ± 7 in males and 42% ± 5 in females. *Hemoglobin,* the chief component of these cells, delivers oxygen to the tissues. Normal hemoglobin values are 16.0 ± 2 g/100 ml of blood in males, 14.0 ± 2 g/100 ml in females, and 11.2 to 16.5 g/100 ml in children. These values are decreased in anemic patients. Thus anemia may result in tissue hypoxia. The various types of this disorder may be caused by:

1 Blood loss from massive bleeding, as from a traumatic injury, or chronic blood loss, as from a gastric or intestinal ulcer. This blood loss can be replaced by transfusion of blood products.

2 Dietary deficiency of sufficient iron, protein, vitamins, and minerals to form red blood cells or produce hemoglobin. Dietary supplements are given to correct the deficiency.

3 Diseases or drugs that inhibit the bone marrow from producing blood cells, such as tumors or chronic renal disease. The cause must be diagnosed and treated.

4 Destruction of red blood cells by an overactive reticuloendothelial system in the spleen or liver. A splenectomy may be indicated for hypersplenism or hereditary spherocytosis, for example.

5 Destruction of red blood cells by foreign substances entering the circulatory system, such as an incompatible blood transfusion. Treatment may necessitate an exchange transfusion.

6 Abnormal blood cells produced by the bone marrow, usually by genetic or hereditary factors. Precautions can be taken to minimize risks of surgical intervention.

The average normal life span of red blood cells is 120 days. In patients with any one of the many forms of *hemolytic anemia,* red blood cells have a shortened life span. Hemolytic anemias may be acquired or inherited. All must be adequately assessed preoperatively.

Sickle Cell Hemoglobinopathies A severe chronic inherited hemolytic disorder, *sickle cell anemia* is most prevalent among blacks of African descent. It may be found in other ethnic groups, particularly people of Mediterranean, north African, and south Asian descent. Due to the pairing of identical abnormal recessive genes, the substitution of a single amino acid for glutamic acid in the polypeptide chain alters the hemoglobin. These abnormal cells, known as *hemoglobin S,* become distorted in shape when exposed to low oxygen tension in the venous circulation. Dehydration, cold, infection, and physical or emotional stress may precipitate crisis periods that vary in duration and intensity when sickling occurs. A crisis also may occur spontaneously without apparent cause. The resultant sickle-shaped red blood cells occlude the microcirculation through the capillaries, arterioles, and venules. This produces blood stasis, hypoxia, vasospasm, ischemia, and necrosis that causes pain and ultimately permanent damage to tissues and organs. Osteomyelitis, stasis ulcers, ischemic bone, and joint lesions are common complications that may require surgical intervention. Elective operations are performed when the patient is not in crisis, but these patients are always at risk of crisis.

Sickle cell trait is present when one abnormal gene is inherited. The red blood cells have both hemoglobin A (normal) and hemoglobin S (sickle cell). Persons with this trait usually are asymptomatic and tolerate routine anesthesia and surgical intervention well. But when stressed by hypothermia, acidosis, or hypoxemia, local or regional sickling can occur during operation.

Sickle cells have a life span of 15 to 30 days. The severity of the hemolytic process is proportional to the amount of hemoglobin S in the blood. Hemoglobin in patients with sickle cell anemia usually ranges from 6 to 9 g with a hematocrit of 25 to 30 percent. All blacks and other susceptible persons who do not have a sickle cell test recorded on their chart must be tested preoperatively. Electrophoresis is the standard laboratory test for hemoglobin S. Consideration then must be given to the following in the perioperative management of patients with sickle cell anemia or sickle cell trait:

1 Transfusion of whole blood, packed cells, or low molecular dextran is essential preoperatively if the patient's hemoglobin is 5 g or less.
2 Urea may be given orally or by IV prophylactically to prevent a sickle cell crisis. It may also be used to reverse a crisis.
3 Systemic antibiotics are initiated preoperatively because these patients are susceptible to postoperative infection.
4 Normal body temperature must be maintained. Any lowering increases oxygen requirement.

The patient must be kept warm to avoid hypothermia.

a Add extra blankets during transport to OR suite.
b Avoid drafts from air-conditioning system in the holding area, OR, and recovery room.
c Raise temperature in the operating room to 80 to 85°F (27 to 29°C).
d Place patient on a hyperthermia blanket on the operating table.
e Monitor the patient's temperature throughout the operation with an electronic probe.
f Put warm blankets over patient before transfer to the recovery room.

5 Oxygen is administered during induction of anesthesia, during operation, and following extubation to prevent deoxygenation of the sickle cells.

6 Blood gases are monitored to avoid hypoxia, acidosis, hypotension, and hypovolemia.

7 Fluid and blood replacement during operation reduce the risk of crisis from dehydration. Scheduling elective operation early in the morning minimizes dehydration following period of nothing by mouth (NPO).

Hemorrhagic Disorders Patients with a disorder in the mechanism of blood coagulation (see Chap. 17) have abnormal bleeding tendencies. These may be related to:

1 Hemorrhagic diseases, such as a type of *purpura* in which spontaneous bleeding occurs under the skin, through mucous membranes, or in the gastrointestinal tract that is idiopathic (cause unknown) or secondary to a systemic or an infectious disease or to exposure to chemical agents.

2 Platelet deficiency in the blood, such as *thrombocytopenia* as a result of decreased production of platelets by bone marrow or excessive destruction of platelets in the peripheral circulation.

3 Abnormal blood clotting factors, such as in hemophilia and von Willebrand's disease which are inherited genetic disorders.

Preoperatively, a complete blood count including platelets, plasma clotting time, bleeding time, prothrombin time, and partial thromboplastin time must be established. Adequate blood replacement of the deficient factors must be available during operation and postoperatively.

Hemophilia The term hemophilia refers to a group of genetic bleeding disorders characterized by abnormal blood clotting factors.

Hemophilia A, the classic disorder, is due to a deficiency of functional Factor VIII, the antihemophilic globulin in plasma. *Hemophilia B,* also known as Christmas disease, is due to a lack of functional Factor IX, the plasma thromboplastic cofactor. A carrier mother transmits to her son this sex-linked recessive trait of the specific clotting factor. Hemophilia occurs most commonly in males of the Jewish faith of Russian descent. The sons of hemophiliacs are normal, but their daughters are carriers, unless the mother is also a carrier as in a consanguineous relationship.

Severity of the disorder depends on the percentage of functional versus nonfunctional factor in the blood. Partial thromboplastin times or thromboplastin generation times are the standard tests for this determination. These patients have normal vasculature and platelets (150,000 to 400,000/cu mm of blood), so bleeding time (1 to 3 minutes by Duke method) and prothrombin time (9.6 to 11.8 seconds) tests are normal.

Severely affected hemophiliacs will have spontaneous bleeding episodes into the skin, muscles, and joints, those most commonly being the ankles, knees, wrists, and elbows. If untreated, joint deformities can result. Bleeding will be excessive from even a minor wound, such as a bruise or cut.

For hemostasis after a severe bleeding episode, trauma or during operation, replacement therapy must be initiated to bring the clotting factor up to 30 percent or more. This is started preoperatively for elective surgery. Concentrates available for replacement therapy are:

1 Factor VIII
a Fresh frozen plasma, stored at −4°F (−20°C).
b Cryoprecipitate, stored at 68°F (20°C).
c Courtland VIII lyophilized cryoprecipitate reconstituted with 30 ml of sterile water, stored at 35 to 77°F (2 to 25°C).
d Hemophil VIII concentrate reconstituted with sterile water, stored at 35 to 46°F (2 to 8°C).

2 Factor IX
a Fresh frozen plasma, stored at −4°F (−20°C).
b Konyne prothrombin complex reconstituted with sterile water.

Dosage for the factor deficiency is calculated on the basis of plasma volume, half-life of the factor, and percentage of deficit. Care must be taken in administration of these blood products to avoid hypovolemia and hemolytic anemia.

NOTE. Because they may receive many blood transfusions and/or infusions of clotting factor concentrates, hemophiliacs are susceptible to acquired immune deficiency syndrome. (See Chapter 7 for description of AIDS.)

Pediatric Patients

Pediatric patients react differently than adults. Infants, especially the premature, and young children are especially susceptible to the trauma of operative procedures, physically and emotionally. Responses that are supportive and nurturing can reduce trauma and prevent complications. Accurate information with explanations geared to how the child looks at things, previews of procedures through play techniques, and as much individual care as possible during critical periods pre- and postoperatively are the desired protocol.

Modern pediatric surgery has opened new horizons. For example, a newborn infant with a congenital defect, who formerly lived only a few days or spent a life of restricted activity, now may live a normal, active life. Chapter 33 details the special needs of infants and children.

Geriatric Patients

Surgery for the over-65 age group once was considered out of the reach of surgeons' skills because the risks were too high. Now, many of these persons are successfully operated on for pathologic conditions prevalent within this increasing population.

Persons are not ill simply because they are old. But chronic illness and multiple pathology often are companions of the aged due to a gradual deterioration in physiologic functions. Geriatric patients are prone to have hypoproteinemia and cardiovascular, renal, digestive, or pulmonary problems. Coronary artery and cerebrovascular diseases are prevalent. Chronic bleeding may decrease blood volume and oxygenation of tissues. Decreased vital capacity, oxygen intake, and carbon dioxide removal reduce cardiac reserve. General debilitative changes, such as atherosclerosis, deteriorated skin and muscular integrity, and weakened sensorium (hearing, sight, and feelings that includes sensation of pressure or temperature), develop gradually over the years and present additional problems.

Assessment of older persons differs somewhat from that of younger people. Because of loss of cognition, the elderly usually function best mentally and physically in a familiar setting. Therefore, home visits and supportive health services are particularly helpful. For emotional health, the aged need to be involved and to retain control over their lives. A loss of physical and financial security and life-long friends can be devastating. Aged patients gain comfort from familiarity. During hospitalization, having a personal possession, such as a clock, calendar, or photograph, assists in orienting the elderly to new surroundings. Good lighting is also helpful. Many persons are past- rather than present-oriented, so always introduce yourself to expedite their adjustment. Also give special attention to individual living patterns and idiosyncrasies, and indulge them within limits of safety. Drugs, altered sleeping and eating patterns, an unfamiliar environment, and the physical changes of aging all contribute to mental confusion.

Treating geriatric patients in a respectful manner is not only commendable but expected, and serves to preserve their self-esteem. Special precautions and patience are always indicated in caring for these patients. The following factors should be taken into account:

1 Slow adaptation, reduced cardiac reserve, and diminished blood flow throughout the body with inadequate perfusion result in an inability to respond rapidly to sudden change in position.

2 Older people do not tolerate fluid and blood loss well. Hypovolemia can rapidly progress to a crisis situation.

3 Slow circulation or hypotension predispose the elderly to thrombus formation. Antiembolic stockings, leg exercises, and early ambulation are precautionary measures. Bruising is common.

4 The aged must be well supported during diagnostic procedures as dizziness and weakness can result from slow cardiac compensation. Also, it is difficult for an orthopneic cardiac patient to lie flat as some tests require. These persons need extra pillows. Do not lay them flat until necessary. Older people also tire easily.

5 Geriatric patients are especially susceptible to infection because of immunologic changes and decreased immunoglobulin production. They may have hidden infection with masked symptoms and muted febrile reactions.

6 Pulmonary complications, such as atelectasis or pneumonia, often follow operations on patients with chronic pulmonary diseases, e.g., emphysema. They also are susceptible to hypoxia. These patients must be kept warm.

7 Arthritis is a common affliction. Support a stiff knee or spine curvatures with pillows.

8 Drug tolerance may be poor and detoxification slow due to slow blood flow to the liver or impaired hepatic function. Usually narcotics and sedatives are given only with extreme caution; the normal dosage is reduced; the patient is observed closely for untoward reaction. Sometimes medications are administered early because of slow absorption. All drugs interact with anesthetic agents and affect physiologic functioning. Therefore, a minimum number of medications is desirable. Characteristically, the aged have a high pain threshold. Anesthetic agents are myocardial and respiratory depressants; they must be thoughtfully selected and the patient carefully monitored (see Chap. 14).

9 Acute renal problems preclude operation. Impaired renal function or dehydration may cause renal failure.

10 Most aged patients require special attention to nutrition. Edentia or poor teeth, inadequate eating habits, and limited finances may contribute to malnutrition.

11 Aged persons have a diminution in respiratory tract reflexes, such as cough. They have difficulty swallowing due to loss of secretions, reduced esophageal peristalsis, and neuromuscular changes. They must be watched for, often silent, aspiration.

12 All of the responses of older people are slower than normal; for this reason the utmost patience is required. Do not rush them or confuse them with a multiplicity of instructions. Give them time to respond without loss of dignity.

13 Provide for sensory deficiencies and do not distract the patient from the situation at point; at best, concentration is difficult.

14 Motivate the patient toward recovery by encouraging self-help.

In summary, geriatric patients require thorough preoperative assessment, an experienced anesthesiologist, and careful postoperative management.

Catastrophic Illnesses

Although OR nursing personnel are most frequently involved with patients who have favorable prognoses, they also care for those of all ages with terminal illnesses who are operated on to relieve a specific problem. Maximum patient comfort and relief of physiological disturbances are the primary concerns. Included in this category are some of the patients with malignancies. Those who have metastatic disease are often severely debilitated. All require highly individualized care.

The manner in which patients are told the diagnosis and prognosis naturally has a great impact on their hope of recovery. Significantly, patients who have been judiciously and thoughtfully informed are easier to talk to, accept therapy more readily, and have greater trust in and communicate more openly with the hospital staff. The suspense of uncertainty is frequently harmful. Each patient handles in his or her own way the pain of and the living with the diagnosis. Although not always so, many persons consider the diagnosis of cancer a death warrant and react accordingly. The nurse must emphasize the present, focusing on the patient's strengths and attributes, and how these can best be utilized. It is difficult to find hope when one faces a radical procedure such as a laryngectomy or radical neck dissection. The discerning nurse will offer a philosophy of hope, but not focus on the positive without acknowledging the negative.

Listening to these patients is particularly important. Be completely supportive. It is wise not to be ultracheerful. Patients are not deceived. To be effective, the nurse should mentally review the stages of dying: denial, isolation, anger, bargaining, depression, acceptance. These stages do not always occur in this sequence, however.

Persons caring for patients with a terminal or catastrophic illness must remember that they are interacting with people who have different priorities and values. These patients are present-oriented, for many have little future. They review their existing sense of values and the quality of their lives in hopes of living each day to the fullest, since such a diagnosis alters one's perspective. They rearrange their ultimate goals for existence. Some persons appreciate living each day. Others are anxious to end their suffering.

The chronically ill patient feels especially threatened, for disability requires a reorientation of self-image. Another problem is that chronic illness often creates an emotional and financial burden on the family. Consequently, family members may have ambivalent feelings toward the patient because of the necessary changes in their lives that the illness precipitates.

A few of the special problems these conditions give rise to are as follows:

1 The common therapies, e.g., radiation, chemotherapy, and steroids, frequently cause gastrointestinal disturbances and severe hematological depressions, such as leukopenia or lymphopenia (see Chap. 35).

2 Inhibition of blood supply and nourishment can result in necrotic tissue. Prolonged confinement in bed increases one's susceptibility to decubitus ulcers.

3 Inactivity promotes catabolism and muscle wasting.

4 Preoperative preparation must be intensive for patients whose surgical intervention is palliative rather than curative.

5 Many operations are long and complex radical procedures, such as hemipelvectomy.

PREPARATION OF ALL PATIENTS FOR OPERATION

Emotional Preparation

By fulfilling spiritual and psychosocial needs, the hospital staff should furnish the preoperative patient with as much peace of mind as is possible. Understandably, as the time for operation approaches, the patient's tension level rises.

If the patient has not seen his or her cleric or the hospital chaplain before coming to the OR and makes such a request, the OR nurse should make every effort to get in touch with that person before anesthesia induction.

Physical Preparation

Preoperative physical preparation is designed to help the patient overcome the stresses of anesthesia, fluid and blood loss, immobilization, and tissue trauma. Preparation often begins before the patient's hospital admission, with the institution of nutritional or drug therapy and a special bathing regimen (see Chap. 16). Physical preparation on the unit is as follows.

On Admission A history is taken and a physical examination performed routinely. A chest x-ray and laboratory tests may be required by hospital policy or medically indicated. Usually a complete blood count, SMA-18 multichemistry profile, and urinalysis are ordered. If the patient is over 35 years old, or has a special problem such as a cardiac disease, then an electrocardiogram is taken. If transfusion is anticipated, the patient's blood is typed and cross-matched. Special diagnostic procedures are performed when specifically indicated. An attempt is made to bring all patients to their best possible physical status preoperatively. Appropriate consultations are sought when necessary.

Evening Before an Elective Operation The surgeon writes specific orders for the appropriate preoperative preparation that may include:

1 Hair removal and/or skin cleansing of the operative site. This is done according to hospital policy (see Chap. 16).

2 Special procedures, for example a douche or enema. "Enemas till clear" are usually ordered when it is advantageous to have the bowel and rectum empty as for gastrointestinal procedures, such as bowel resection or colonoscopy, and operations in the pelvic, perineal, or perianal areas.

3 Bedtime sedative for sleep.

4 Nothing by mouth (NPO) for six to eight hours preceding the operation, to prevent regurgitation or emesis and aspiration of gastric contents. NPO time usually is reduced for infants and small children.

> NOTE. Some oral medications may be taken with a minimal fluid intake preoperatively. However, the nurse should remind the physician to order essential medications normally taken orally, if they must be given or substituted by another route.

Nail polish may be removed from fingers and toes, by hospital policy or at discretion of the anesthesiologist, to permit observation of nail bed color during operation, one indication of oxygenation and circulation.

Ideally, both the OR nurse and anesthesiologist visit the patient. (Refer to preoperative visits by OR nurses in Chapter 4.)

Preoperative Visit by Anesthesiologist The anesthesiologist is knowledgeable in the pathophysiology of disease as it pertains to anesthetic agents. Participation in the patient's preoperative preparation can reduce intraoperative complications as well as postoperative morbidity and mortality. The anesthesiologist assesses patients scheduled for anesthesia, usually the evening before operation.

Judgment and skill are important in selection of agents and administration of anesthesia, but firsthand knowledge of the patient is extremely valuable. The anesthesiologist visits the patient seeking information, but also to establish rapport, inspire confidence and trust, and alleviate fear. Preparation for anesthesia begins with this visit.

Before meeting the patient, the anesthesiologist reviews the patient's past and present hospital records and charts. If recent laboratory or other test reports are not in the chart, due sometimes to late admissions, decisions and the operation are delayed until all essential information is available. The administration of anesthesia requires no compromise with quality. Special attention is given to past operations and any disease or complicating processes, especially those involving vital organs.

After introduction to the patient, the anesthesiologist:

1 Takes a history pertinent to administration of anesthetic agents by questioning patient in regard to past anesthetic experiences, allergies, adverse reactions to drugs, and habitual drug usage. Tranquilizers, cortisone, reserpine, alcohol, and recreational drugs, for example, influence the course of anesthesia. Smoking habits, genetic and metabolic problems, and reactions to previous blood transfusions also influence the choice of anesthesia.
2 Evaluates the patient's physical, mental, and emotional status to determine type and amount of anesthesia most appropriate.
   a Examines patient as necessary to obtain information desired, with particular interest in heart and lungs.
   b Palpates needle insertion site and observes for skin infection if regional block anesthesia is contemplated.
   c Assesses subjectively the patient's mental state and cognitive ability, and observes for signs of anxiety.
3 Investigates patient's cardiac reserve, and observes signs of dyspnea or claudication during a short exercise tolerance test, if indicated.
4 Asks about teeth. If indicated, explains that dental work may be damaged inadvertently during airway insertion.
5 Evaluates patient's physique for technical difficulties in administration of anesthesia:
   a A short, stout neck may cause respiratory problems or difficult intubation.
   b Active athletic persons and obese persons require more anesthesia than inactive persons.
6 Explains preference of anesthetic, pending the surgeon's approval, and informs the patient what to expect concerning anesthesia. The patient's wishes are taken into consideration, if expressed.
7 Tells patient about restricted or prohibited oral intake before anesthesia and gives reasons for this. IV therapy is explained.
8 Discusses preoperative sedation in relation to time operation is scheduled to begin.
9 Reassures patient that constant observation will be given during the operation and in the immediate postoperative period. Also the methods of monitoring vital functions are explained.
10 Explains risks of anesthesia, but without causing the patient undue stress.

Following visit with patient, the anesthesiologist:

1 Estimates effect of the necessary position during operation on patient's physiologic processes.
2 Records preliminary data on anesthesia chart.
3 Writes preanesthesia orders, including times for medication administration.
4 Writes a summary of the visit and the proposed anesthetic management of the patient on the physicians' progress note. This has medicolegal value if a problem subsequently develops.
5 Assigns the patient a physical status category, for the purpose of anesthesia, as per the classification adopted by the American Society of Anesthesiologists (ASA):
   a Class I theoretically includes relatively healthy patients with localized pathologic processes. Emergency operation, designated E, signifies additional risk. For example, a hernia that becomes incarcerated changes the patient's status to Class I-E.
   b Class II includes patients with mild systemic disease, for example, diabetes mellitus controlled by oral hypoglycemic agents or diet.
   c Class III includes patients with severe systemic disease that limits activity, but is not totally incapacitating, for example, chronic obstructive pulmonary disease or severe hypertension.
   d Class IV includes patients with an incapacitating disease that is a constant threat to life, for example, cardiovascular and renal diseases.
   e Class V includes moribund patients who are not expected to survive 24 hours with or

without operation. They are operated on in an attempt to save life; the operation is a resuscitative measure, as for a massive pulmonary embolus.

6 Consults with surgeon and other physicians, for example a cardiologist, about patient assigned a Class III, IV, or V status. Consideration is given to the critical nature of the operation in relation to the anesthesia risks.

a In elective situations, the operation is postponed until anesthesia will be less hazardous, for example, following acute respiratory infection or cardiac decompensation.

b In emergency situations, ideal practices may be altered or disregarded to meet the exigencies of the situation. For example, if a patient is hemorrhaging, there is no time to wait to restore a low red blood count. A multiple trauma victim with a full stomach may need a nasogastric tube inserted and suction applied, endotracheal intubation while awake or spinal anesthesia as applicable, and be operated on in spite of food ingestion.

The role of the anesthesiologist as a member of the OR team was referred to in Chapter 2. Specific functions related to the administration of anesthetic agents will be discussed in Chapter 13. In addition to preoperative assessment of the patient and administration and maintenance of intraoperative anesthesia, the anesthesiologist may see the patient postoperatively. *He or she has a responsibility to inform the patient of any unfavorable reaction to a medication or agent given* so the patient will be forewarned in the future and report these reactions to other physicians and anesthesiologists.

Before Leaving for the OR At this time, the patient's physical and emotional status and vital signs should be assessed and recorded by the unit nurse. Any untoward symptoms or extreme apprehension must be reported to the surgeon as they could affect the patient's intraoperative course. The following preparations are made:

1 Bed linens are changed and the patient puts on a clean hospital gown.

2 All jewelry is removed for safekeeping. If a wedding ring is not removed, it must be loosely taped or tied securely to prevent loss.

3 Dentures and removable bridges are removed, unless otherwise ordered, prior to general anesthesia to safeguard them and prevent obstruction to respiration under anesthesia. Dentures may be permitted during local anesthesia, especially if the patient can breathe more easily with them in place.

4 Prostheses, such as eye, extremity and breast, contact lenses, eyeglasses, and hearing aids are removed for safekeeping.

NOTE. In some instances of marked impairment in visual or hearing acuity, the patient may be permitted to wear eyeglasses or hearing aid to the OR. The circulating nurse must safeguard them.

5 Long hair is braided. Wigs are removed. Hairpins are removed to prevent scalp injury.

6 Antiembolic stockings or an elastic bandage may be ordered applied to the lower extremities to prevent embolic phenomena. This is often done prior to abdominal or pelvic procedures, and for patients who have varicosities, are prone to thrombus formation, or have a history of embolus, and some geriatric patients.

7 The patient voids to prevent overdistention of the bladder or incontinence during unconsciousness. This is especially important for abdominal or pelvic procedures where a large bladder may interfere with adequate exposure of abdominal contents or may be traumatized. Time of voiding is recorded.

NOTE: Indwelling catheter insertion, when indicated, is usually done in the OR after the patient is anesthetized (see Chap. 16).

8 Preanesthesia medications are given as ordered. Their purpose is to eliminate apprehension by making the patient calm, drowsy, and comfortable. Patients receiving preanesthesia medication should be cautioned to remain in bed and not to smoke. Many of the drugs cause drowsiness, vertigo, or postural hypotension. Therefore, the siderails should be raised on the bed.

9 The patient, bed, and chart are accurately identified and identifications fastened securely in place.

A preoperative checklist will help the unit nurse to assure that the patient has been properly prepared and that all essential records are accompanying him or her to the operating room. If preparation is inadequate, operation may be canceled.

Transportation to the OR Suite

Patients usually are taken to the OR suite about 45 minutes before scheduled procedure time. For safety, they are transported via stretcher. Elevators should be designated "For OR use only." This ensures privacy and minimizes microbial contamination. The patient must be comfortable, warm, and safe during transport. Siderails are raised and restraint straps applied. Intravenous solution bags hung on poles or standards during transportation must be attached securely to minimize danger of injury to the patient if the container should fall. Gentle handling is indicated to prevent dislodging intravenous needles or indwelling catheters. A unit nurse or nursing assistant should stay with the patient until relieved by an operating room nurse or anesthesiologist, to whom the patient's chart is given. If the patient has a language barrier, an interpreter may accompany him or her to the OR and stay until anesthesia induction.

Admission to the OR Suite

Exchange and Holding Areas Patients are brought through the outer corridor to the holding area by outside personnel. OR personnel may transfer patient to an OR stretcher where he or she remains until taken into the operating room. The patient goes to the recovery room and from there to the unit on this stretcher. It is then brought back to a stretcher-cleaning room where the entire stretcher, including the wheels, is decontaminated before being brought into the OR suite.

This procedure is ideal from the standpoint of contamination control. But some conditions justify bringing patients to the OR suite in their beds. These include patients in traction, on Stryker frames, or cardiac patients who must not be moved until transferred to the operating table.

A patient on a Stryker or similar frame should have broad muslin bands across the body and legs while being transported. These should be left in place until the patient is moved onto the operating table. Some patients may be operated on while on the frame. The surgeon chooses the course that best benefits the individual patient. The bed or frame can be decontaminated in the exchange area and made up with clean linen before being brought into the room after the operation.

Beds, stretchers, frames, and tables must be stabilized by locking the wheels and by personnel when a patient is moving from one to the other. The patient should be instructed and assisted to prevent a fall or injury. Once transferred to a stretcher or the operating table, the patient is not left unattended.

Some hospitals have individual anesthesia induction rooms where the patient waits and is administered an anesthetic before being taken into the operating room.

A quiet, restful atmosphere enables the patient to gain full advantage of premedication. Some holding areas and operating rooms have piped-in recorded music. Music diverts attention from the many other sounds in the environment, especially for patients under local anesthesia. Music with a soft, slow, easy rhythm and low volume is most conducive to relaxation. Familiar music is more pleasing and relaxing because the patient can associate it with pleasant past experiences. Some hospitals provide earphones or headsets so patients can listen to the type of music each prefers. These also muffle extraneous noises and conversations. Ideally the patient should have a choice in the selection of music or no music at all; this is the advantage of providing individual headsets rather than piped-in systems.

Immediate Preanesthesia Preparation A line-up of stretchers with each patient gowned alike is not conducive to preserving a patient's personal identity. Nowhere may a patient feel more alone than in a holding area. By introducing themselves and pleasantly greeting patients by name, circulating nurses can do much to dispel apprehensions and assure patients they are not alone nor among disinterested people.

Patients appreciate seeing a familiar face. It is advantageous if the nurse has made a preoperative visit (see Chap. 4). A compassionate expression in the eyes and voice, a reassuring touch of the hand, and a positive statement such as, "You look rested and comfortable; is there anything I can do for you?" can convey concern and expectance of the patient's arrival. Respect and genuine warmth rather than superficially endearing words inspire confidence. An anxious patient looks to this nurse for comfort, reassurance, and personal attention. He or she must know that the nurse will be constantly there. Also, because of lethargy, a medicated patient needs and wants direction.

If the patient is drowsy, unnecessary conversation should be avoided. However, the nurse should answer questions and see to the patient's comfort. Keep the patient warm or turn down the cover if he or she is too warm. Place an extra pillow under the patient's head or under an arthritic knee. Moisten dry lips, if requested. Any delay or unusual circumstances should be explained.

The circulating nurse has a number of important duties to fulfill in a short period of time.

1 Check identity of the patient, stretcher or bed, and chart.
  a When patient comes to the hospital, an identifying wristband is put on in the admitting office. The unit nurse checks the band before the patient leaves for the OR. The circulating nurse compares the information on the wristband with information on the chart, and with the information on the operative schedule: name, anticipated procedure, time, surgeon.
  b Identification on the stretcher or bed assures the patient's return to the same one following operation if this is the procedure. If the patient is an infant or child, the identification tag on the crib should be out of reach.
2 Put an OR cap on patient to protect hair if vomiting occurs and for purpose of asepsis.
3 Check siderails, restraining straps, intravenous infusions, and indwelling catheters.
4 Observe patient for reaction to medication.
5 Observe patient's anxiety level.
6 Check physical exam, medical history, laboratory tests, x-ray reports, and operative consent form in the patient's chart.
  a Pay particular attention to allergies and any previous unfavorable reactions to anesthesia or blood transfusion.
7 Review orders and nursing care plan.

Usually for physical and psychological comfort, the patient is not transferred to the operating table until time for anesthesia induction. Ideally, the main preparations for the procedure will have been completed before the patient is taken into the OR so that the circulating nurse can then devote undivided attention to the patient. If the nurse is more intent on equipment than on the patient, the patient may feel abandoned.

The anesthesiologist also has immediate preanesthesia duties. He or she must:

1 Check and assemble equipment before patient enters the room. Airways, endotracheal tubes, laryngoscope, suction catheters, labeled prefilled medication syringes, etc., are arranged on a cart or table. (Refer to Chapter 13 for discussion of anesthesia equipment.)

2 Review the preoperative physical examination, history, and laboratory reports in the chart.

3 Make certain the patient is comfortable and secure on the operating table. (Refer to Chapter 15 for discussion of safety measures.)

4 Check for denture removal or any loose teeth. The latter may be secured with thread taped to the patient's cheek to prevent possible aspiration.

5 Ask patient when last took anything by mouth.

6 Check pulse, respiration and blood pressure to serve as a baseline for subsequent vital signs under anesthesia.

7 Listen to heart and lungs, then connect monitor leads (see Chap. 14).

8 Start intravenous infusion. This may be done in the holding area or an induction room. Some patients arrive with an infusion line in place.

9 Prepare for and explain induction procedure to patient. If properly premedicated, patient should be able to respond to simple instructions.

TEAMWORK

A discussion of the patient would not be complete without another mention of teamwork. A team approach is necessary for patient-centered care. Consideration must be given to each patient's basic and special needs, both physiological and psychosocial. Surgeons, other attending physicians, anesthesiologist or anesthetist, the nursing staff and supporting services must coordinate their efforts to ensure successful outcome from surgical intervention. Comprehensive care includes adequate preoperative preparation and postoperative rehabilitation.

CHAPTER **4**

PERIOPERATIVE NURSING

Surgery today, as defined in Chapter 1, encompasses all elements in the scientific care of surgical patients. The operation is the focal point for these patients. It is imperative that the patient comes to the OR optimally prepared physically and emotionally before performance of an operative procedure. The persons concerned with and/or contributing to surgical patient care are many, as discussed in Chapter 2. This chapter focuses specifically on the operating room nurse who fulfills the patient's needs by carrying out the perioperative role. *The term* perioperative nurse *used in this chapter refers to the professional OR nurse who performs functions encompassing the full scope of perioperative nursing practice.*

PERIOPERATIVE ROLE

The perioperative role has been delineated to consist of "nursing activities performed by the professional operating room nurse during the *preoperative, intraoperative* and *postoperative phases* of the patient's surgical experience."* *Perioperative,* therefore, is an encompassing term that incorporates the patient's total experience when surgical intervention is accepted as the treatment of choice. *Role* refers to the expected behavior patterns and clinical activities the OR nurse performs during the three phases of surgical patient care. Knowledge, judgment, and skill to fulfill the perioperative role are based on principles of biological, physiological, behavioral, and social sciences. The operating room nurse functioning in this role makes decisions about patient's needs, and assists and supports the patient to meet these needs.

*Operating room nursing: Perioperative role, *AORN J 27* (6): 1165, May 1978.

Patient-Nurse Relationship

Perioperative nursing involves patient-nurse interaction through direct patient contact and care; consequently, it is a discipline in nursing. It is not purely technical nor procedure-oriented. Both nurses and technologists work, in different capacities, toward the common goal of the safest possible care of the patient and of a favorable surgical outcome. While technical assistants provide a very real contribution to surgical patient care, nowhere in the hospital are the qualities of the professional nurse more needed or better utilized than in the OR as the RN implements a personalized, patient-oriented approach to care through his or her understanding, judgment, and skills. Therefore, the perioperative role incorporates both professional and technical components of nursing practice.

The professional nurse shares a special experience with the patient at a time of great stress and need in his or her life. Their relationship encompasses feelings, attitudes, and behavioral approaches. It must be humanized in structure.

The nurse's first goal is to promote and establish a meaningful, therapeutic relationship so that individualized care can be given. It is not the length of time the nurse spends with the patient that is so important, but the quality of the association. Mutual trust and understanding are the vital components. Effective interaction involves concern for the personhood of both patient and nurse. Then patient goals can be formulated together and decisively achieved.

As the nurse and patient begin to know each other, their identities and roles become apparent, and they develop feelings for each other. To achieve a viable cooperative relationship, the patient must know that the nurse unconditionally cares about his or her life both within and outside of the hospital. The nurse is aware that personal interaction is often predicated on attitudes and past experiences. Knowledge of the patient and the impact of surgical intervention on his or her life situation is therefore indispensable.

Objectives of Perioperative Nursing

A basic understanding of operating room technique and intraoperative procedures is essential for the total care of the surgical patient. To plan and manage the preoperative, intraoperative, or postoperative nursing care regimen of the surgical patient in order to meet individualized needs, the professional nurse must have a knowledge of the operative site and procedure, the effects of operative trauma and anesthesia on the body, and the problems of recovery and rehabilitation. Participation in perioperative nursing can help the nurse:

1 To apply nursing process to nursing actions in the OR so they correlate the operative procedure with other aspects of patient care.

2 To promote an understanding of the patient's total surgical experience by demonstrating the ability to assess physiological, psychological, and sociological patient needs and prepare a nursing care plan.

3 To reinforce basic knowledge of anatomy and physiology and to gain knowledge of the total patient experience as a basis for management of preoperative patient anxiety related to body image and postoperative pain related to site of incision and intraoperative procedure.

4 To assist patients with the management of anxiety by assessing their needs for psychological support preoperatively and by anticipating their psychological and physiological needs in the postoperative recovery period through an understanding of the total surgical experience.

5 To recognize the effects of preoperative medication, anesthesia, positioning on the operating table, site of incision, and operative procedure as the basis for planning the patient's postoperative recovery and rehabilitation.

6 To develop an appreciation of the meaning of the surgical experience for patients and their families as a basis for correlating the intraoperative phase with establishment of priorities for teaching and planning all aspects of surgical patient care to promote continuity of care.

7 To become an effective communicator with patients through pre- and postoperative teaching based on knowledge of the intraoperative procedure as it relates to each individual patient.

The overall objective of perioperative nursing is to improve the intraoperative care rendered to surgical patients by the OR team and the patients' outcomes of surgical intervention.

Communication with, for, and about Patient

Communication is the basis for the continuum of patient care and for teamwork among the staff. Relationships between people are established through communication. Therefore, the nurse must know general principles specifically applicable to the perioperative role.

Communication has been defined as a process by which meanings are exchanged between individuals; everything that one mind can use to affect another. It is an effort by one person to get close to another. In therapeutic communication, the goals are patient-directed, patient-centered. Communication is effective only when the patient, physician, and nurse understand one another. A capacity for feeling is the most effective constituent of communication.

Importance of Communication

1 Communication is necessary for successful interpersonal relations.

2 Patients need support in adjusting to health-related problems and hospital environment.

3 We fallaciously assume that others know what we mean; communication serves to clarify our meaning.

Communication is facilitated by using the acronym EARS—listen:

1 Earnestly—look into the speaker's eyes
2 Actively—give the speaker your attention

3 Receptively—acknowledge what message the speaker is conveying

4 Sensitively—interpret the speaker's message

Briefly, some principles are as follows:

1 Communication incorporates:
  a A sender (speaker, encoder).
  b A message sent via a transmission channel.
  c A receiver (listener, decoder).

2 The sender puts thoughts into words or some other channel of communication, then transmits an idea in the form of a message to the receiver who attempts to understand the thought.

3 Goals are to inform, to obtain information, to release tension, to explore problems.

4 Channels of communication are:
  a Verbal—audio-aural language and word symbols.
  b Nonverbal—(kinesthetic) facial expression, tone of voice, gesture, posture, body movements.

5 The setting for communication and the attitudes of those involved influence the degree of effectiveness. One's emotional state affects listening. An anxious patient may not hear, may misunderstand, or may draw erroneous conclusions.

6 The use of unqualified statements is avoided.

7 Communication should be source-centered rather than message-centered.

8 Prerequisites are to know what you're going to say and to say what you mean. As the speaker, verify or paraphrase until you are convinced that the receiver has the message.

9 Shadings of meanings a message can have are:
  a What the speaker means to say—what the speaker actually says.
  b What the receiver hears—what the receiver thinks he or she hears.
  c What the speaker says—what the receiver thinks the speaker said.

NOTE. 1. Two people must have mutual understanding about the meaning of a word. Language should convey meaning.

2. The mind seems to decode messages in relationship to its own background of experiences, prejudices, moods. A person can hear and repeat what you said without believing a word of it.

3. Don't evaluate the receiver's comprehension totally on the basis of language.

10 For accurate interpretation of communication one should know the other's level of intellect.

11 Barriers to communication can be:
  a Verbal—changing the subject, having a judgmental attitude (stating one's own opinion about a patient or situation), offering false or inappropriate reassurance, jumping to conclusions or taking things for granted, using medical facts or nursing knowledge inappropriately.
  b Nonverbal—showing a lack of trust or feeling, disinterest, revulsion.

Criteria for Determining the Success of Communication

1 Feedback. Letting the sender know how you perceived the message so the sender can discover if it was understood as intended. There is a breakdown in communication when the idea of the receiver doesn't match the idea of the sender.

2 Appropriateness of reply.

3 Efficiency. Is the sender overloading the listener?

4 Flexibility. Is there no control versus too much control?

5 Specific results. Behavioral changes indicate that the goal is reached.

Through communication the nurse can influence individual behavior to encourage the patient to express feelings or redirect them toward more beneficial behavior.

Verbal communication is directed toward patient care in conference, study of patient problems, teaching, providing interdisciplinary liaison, and safeguarding the patient. It is the keynote of care planning among all personnel. *Nonverbal communication* provides clues to feeling and attitude in one's interpretation of them as signals. We often communicate through nonverbal channels without realizing it, and those forms of expression sometimes speak louder than words. When the patient is feeling sad, lonely, or isolated, touch is a most effective means of communicating empathy.

Patients can indicate their needs by what they say or do not say. Physicians and nurses must verify that their transmissions are being internalized by the patient. They must repeatedly affirm to the patient how much he or she means to them. Patients under stress have a deep need to communicate and establish a positive relationship with their physicians and nurses.

NURSING PROCESS

The patient-nurse relationship is an ongoing one. Perioperative nursing care requires meticulous preplanning with goals developed through the nursing process. This process, the dominant nursing modality, provides systematic nursing care planning and delivery. A *process* is the act of proceeding through a series of actions that contribute to an end. It provides a framework for cyclic problem solving in a logical, interrelated sequence of steps. All these steps are recorded for documentation and sharing among health care team members. These steps comprise a rational method of determining patient problems, formulating a plan for solving them, implementing the plan, and evaluating its effectiveness in resolving the problems identified.

A *problem* may be defined as any condition or situation in which the patient requires help to maintain or regain physical, emotional, or social equilibrium. The scientific process of problem solving furnishes an organized approach to nursing care and a mode of determining patient outcomes resulting from that care, while adhering to the philosophies of nursing. An *independent nursing function* is the selection of priority needs in a given situation. Rationale for the selection and the patient's viewpoint are needed.

The systematic approach to nursing practice utilizing problem solving techniques has four major components:

1 Assessment
2 Planning
3 Implementation
4 Evaluation

NOTE: The nursing process can be described as A PIE for the patient, the four parts of which make a whole.

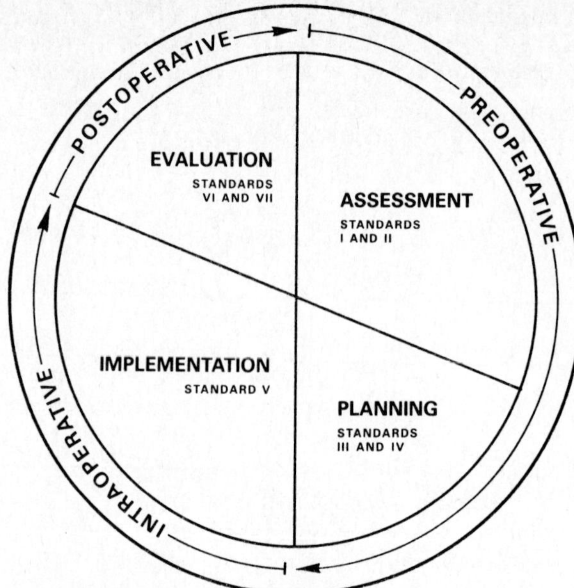

FIGURE 4-1
Nursing Process: A PIE for the patient. The three phases of perioperative nursing incorporate the four components of nursing process and the seven standards of perioperative nursing practice.

Integration of Nursing Process into Phases of Perioperative Role

The four components of the nursing process are integrated into the three phases of the perioperative role (see Fig. 4-1).

Preoperative The preoperative phase of the patient's surgical experience begins when the decision is made to undergo surgical intervention. This phase ends when the patient is transferred to the operating table. During this phase, the perioperative nurse performs the assessment and planning components of the nursing process. The nurse identifies the patient's physiological, psychosocial, and spiritual needs and existing or potential problems. Then the nurse plans the nursing actions necessary to achieve the determined goals for patient outcomes following surgical intervention.

Intraoperative Beginning with transfer of the patient to the operating table, the intraoperative phase of care extends to the time the patient is admitted to the recovery area. The implementation component of nursing process is completed during this phase. The perioperative nurse either personally carries out the plan or supervises others in carrying out the plan of nursing actions with skill, safety, efficiency, and effectiveness.

Postoperative The postoperative phase begins with admission of the patient to the recovery area, which may be a recovery room or an intensive care unit as described in Chapter 2. Unless the operation is performed as an ambulatory care procedure (refer to Chapter 5), the patient will transfer from the immediate postoperative recovery area to progressive stages of self-care on a surgical unit prior to discharge from the hospital. The postoperative phase ends when the surgeon discontinues follow-up care. Evaluation, the fourth component of nursing process, takes place during this phase. The perioperative nurse appraises the quality of nursing care rendered during the preoperative and intraoperative phases of care. Evaluation determines whether or not the assessment, planning, and implementation processes were effective in terms of the patient's achievement of the predetermined goals/outcomes.

STANDARDS OF PERIOPERATIVE NURSING PRACTICE

A standard is an authoritative statement established and published by a profession by which the quality of practice can be measured. The setting of standards for nursing practice is a means of assuring the quality of the services nurses offer, *provided nurses implement the standards.*

Standards of Perioperative Nursing Practice was published in 1981 by the American Nurses' Association following approval by the Executive Committee of the ANA Division on Medical-Surgical Nursing Practice and the Board of Directors of the Association of Operating Room Nurses. The seven basic *standard statements* reflect the nursing process and state the activities to be performed. The *interpretive statements* that accompany each standard provide definitions of terms and actions, and provide guidelines to achieve the standards. *Criteria* for achievement of each standard also are enunciated. These are written in behavioral terms so nurses can measure to what degree each standard has been met.

The nursing activities inherent in each standard are incorporated in the nursing process during the three phases of the surgical patient's experience (see Fig. 4-1). The seven standards* will be presented under the four major headings of the nursing process, *A PIE* for the patient.

PREOPERATIVE ASSESSMENT

A purposeful patient-nurse interaction that continues through all phases of the nursing process begins by the nurse getting to know the patient and what is happening to him or her. *Assessment* consists of appraising the patient and his or her existing and potential nursing care needs. This is the basis for individualized care planning and establishment of nursing goals related to the patient's problems. From specific data collected and analyzed, the nurse constructs a data base, a composite picture of the patient's condition, to serve as a basis for comparison with subsequent observations and postoperative status. The data collected through interview and observation become the *nursing history.* The nursing history includes subjective material (what the patient states he or she is experiencing such as pain or anxiety) and objective material (that which can be validated by another person such as the unit nurse, family member, social worker).

From the nursing history, the perioperative nurse determines the appropriate nursing diagnoses that are consistent with accepted nursing interventions during the preoperative and intraoperative phases of patient care. A *nursing diagnosis* includes a concise, descriptive statement of the patient's existing or potential health problem and its etiology as related to the signs and symptoms, i.e., observable cues or defining characteristics, leading to identification of the problem. For example, a sensory perceptual alteration may be related to etiology of a visual or hearing problem. Nursing diagnoses are developed after the patient is assessed.

Maslow's hierarchy of basic needs can be used as a basis for developing the nursing history and nursing diagnoses (see Chap. 3 and Fig. 4-2). The

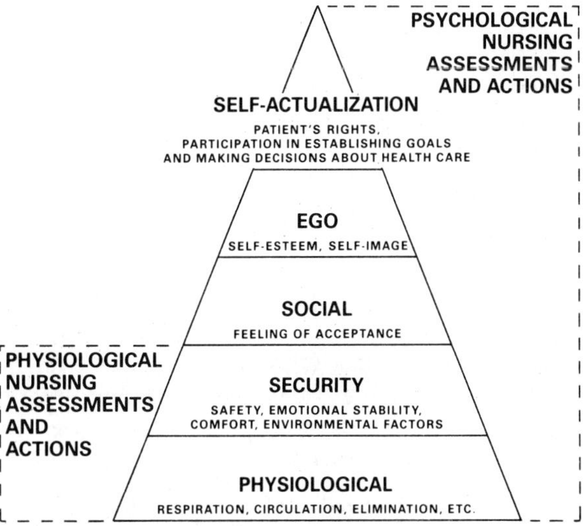

FIGURE 4-2
Maslow's hierarchy of basic needs related to a surgical patient's needs during perioperative care.

*American Nurses' Association Division on Medical-Surgical Nursing Practice and Association of OperatingRoom Nurses: *Standards of Perioperative Nursing Practice,*American Nurses' Association, Kansas City, Missouri, 1981.Reprinted with permission of ANA.

National Group for Classification of Nursing Diagnosis has attempted to standardize nursing diagnoses to facilitate interpretation of patient needs and problems.

Standard I

The collection of data about the health status of the individual is systematic and continuous. The data are retrievable and communicated to appropriate persons.

Data may be collected in the preoperative holding area in the OR suite, on the surgical unit, or in the clinic or home. It can be obtained from the patient's chart, by consultation with other members of the health care team (unit nurses, surgeon, anesthesiologist, etc.), through interview with the patient and/or family or significant others, and by observation and physical assessment of the patient. Data collection is a progressive and orderly process to gather meaningful information pertinent to the planned surgical intervention. This includes, but is not limited to, the following:

1 Current medical diagnosis and therapy
2 Diagnostic studies and laboratory tests results
3 Physical status and physiological responses including allergies, sensory, or physical deficits
4 Psychosocial status
5 Spiritual needs and cultural background
6 Previous responses to illness, hospitalization, and surgery
7 Patient's understanding, perceptions, and expectations of the operative procedure

Pertinent data collected through physiological and psychosocial assessment must be recorded, and problems communicated to other team members. These data become the nursing history.

Physiological Assessment

Fulfilling basic life-sustaining needs are of the highest priority during surgical intervention. Therefore, in addition to the physician's physical examination, the perioperative nurse can make a physical assessment of the patient. Techniques include inspection/observation, palpation, percussion, and auscultation. Physiological manifestations of anxiety may be identified (refer to following discussion of anxiety). Assessment of the major body systems provides a basis for planning appropriate preoperative and intraoperative nursing actions. It also provides baseline data for evaluation in the postoperative phase.

The perioperative nurse must also be familiar with laboratory norms so that critical deviations are identified in all phases of surgical intervention.

Psychosocial Assessment

Individuals vary in their ability to cope with illness and stress situations. Coping mechanisms are normal and natural to some extent, but their exaggeration or overuse is cause for concern. Illness produces heightened self-awareness. Stress initiates an exaggerated response of the normal defense mechanisms for self-protection. Surgical patients are in a psychologically perilous situation. They are threatened by loss of life, body parts, or function, and by unfamiliar social relationships. The strangeness of the OR itself, its noise, odors, and equipment, represents to the patient a potential hazard. Stress, perceived by the patient as *distress,* may be expressed in one or many ways.

Anxiety (Tension) Anxiety is a painful, apprehensive uneasiness, a feeling of uncertainty, or a solicitous concern stemming from anticipation of a real or imagined threat. It incites the body's defenses. All patients experience anxieties preoperatively whether they verbalize them or not. Physiologic manifestations of anxiety may be rapid pulse usually associated with palpitation, rapid respiration, diaphoresis, dry mouth, dilated pupils, clammy skin, and, if very severe, even paralysis. The patient may become so anxious that physiologic manifestation becomes exaggerated. For example, a controlled hypertensive patient may suddenly experience increased blood pressure and electrocardiogram changes that may cause postponement of the operation. Other indications of increasing tension are stuttering, word blockage, confusion, and distortion of events. Anxiety impairs intellectual functioning. Perception, concentration, feeling of security, and self-image are also disturbed.

Anxiety from stress is experienced on both physical and emotional levels. *Psychophysiological reaction* refers to anxiety reactions in which the symptoms center around one organ system, such as the cardiovascular. Psychosomatic illness results from a combination of physiologic and emotional factors that can cause structural change, such as ulcerative colitis, which may necessitate bowel resection. A person's emotional strength influences the ability to view him- or herself objectively. The intensity of feelings is multiform. Sharing a feeling with another often reduces the intensity.

Varying degrees of anxiety are to be expected. Normally patients are worried to some extent about what will happen during the operation and consequently may be restless and unable to sleep. However, patients are accessible to meaningful communication and will ask questions, desiring to know the facts. These patients are not likely to develop significant emotional disturbances.

Highly anxious patients exhibit hyperactive behavior and dwell on the dangers of the operation, apparently overwhelmed by them. They may not hear what you say or be able to accept reassurance against their magnified fears. You can help these patients only if you can calm them. Research has shown the highly anxious patient to be a high-risk patient. Extreme preoperative apprehension predisposes this patient to a more difficult anesthesia induction and intraoperative period, as well as to more postoperative discomfort and complications. As poorer surgical risks, these patients are prone to shock, laryngeal spasm, or cardiac arrest. A patient's unresolved severe anxiety or premonition of death will usually alert the surgeon to delay the operation until a more favorable time.

Alteration of time perception is not an unusual aspect of anxiety. To a waiting patient a minute may seem like an hour. The patient's disability strikes at his or her sense of security. In addition, the anxious patient experiences a feeling of alienation. Surrounded by strange people and equipment in an alien environment, separated from loved ones, the patient is expected to conform to an unfamiliar routine. He or she may feel helpless and alone. For surgical patients, alterations of the body produce tremendous anxiety associated not only with the procedure but also with its potential outcomes. The independent, secure individual can cope more easily than the insecure, inferior-feeling person who may disguise underlying concern with false gaiety and independence. Anxieties originating from reality sources can have a cumulative effect and add fuel to other emotional problems. For example, a young mother facing an operation, with no responsible person to care for her family and home, has enhanced feelings of dread. Similar anxiety-inducing factors are:

1 Confusion about present and future activity: "Will I be able to do all the things I did before?"

2 Worry by the family provider: "Will we have to go into debt?"

3 Concern for unfinished projects: "Will I be able to make up my exam?" or "Will I be able to keep my new job?"

Relieving contributory stresses helps the patient to cope with the main stress—his or her illness. The individual's specific concerns depend greatly on how illness frustrates his or her specific needs.

Fear An emotion marked by dread, apprehension, and alarm, fear is caused by anticipation or awareness of danger. Visceral manifestations of anxiety may occur when a person is afraid. As the patient realizes that he or she is vulnerable, the body prepares to physiologically cope with crisis. Many childhood fears remain with a person in various forms throughout life. In illness, anxiety causes repressed fears to resurface from the subconscious and become magnified. The patient may imagine and dread something more frightening than the actual experience. Anticipatory fears are many and varied and include:

1 *Fear of the unknown.* Research has shown feelings of uncertainty and suspense to be the most common and virulent type of the psychologic reactions. The expected is less traumatic than the unexpected. One can more easily deal with feelings when the factors causing them are known and recognized. Fear of what might be discovered in an exploratory operation augments the patient's anxiety. Advance warning and explanations of stress-producing situations are important for all patients, but especially for those with a low degree of predanger anxiety.

2 *Fear of death.* In many instances this is a very valid fear. The patient who fears death in the operating room runs a greater risk of cardiac arrest on the operating table than patients with known cardiac disease. This fear must be dealt with preoperatively to determine its source.

3 *Fear of anesthesia.* Some patients fear loss of consciousness. This is closely aligned with fear of death. The patient who asks, "Will I survive the operation?" or "Who will care for my family if I die?" may really be asking, "Will I wake up?" General anesthesia invokes complete dependency on the OR team for survival.

4 *Fear of impending procedure and resultant prognosis.* An operation may be a new experience for the patient. "Will the operation be successful and help me?" "What will the surgeon find?" "Do

I have cancer?" This is a universal fear. Or fear may be caused by the trauma of a previously unpleasant surgical experience.

5 *Fear of disfigurement, mutilation, or loss of a valued body part.* Patients facing amputation of an extremity or breast, the loss of an eye, or other disfigurement abhor the thought of an incomplete body. "Will my family and society accept me or be revolted by my altered condition?" An operation on the reproductive organs also may affect self-image. This fear provokes real suffering.

6 *Fear of isolation, rejection, neglect, abandonment.* Separation anxiety is common in the elderly, children, immature persons, and those without a family. A sense of being alone and alienated from others, identified as the single most consistent fear, accentuates the realization that everyone truly lives life alone. Loved ones can't protect us from pain, suffering, or death. No one can face uncertainties or adversity for us. Everyone must experience stress and pain personally but, in so doing, may turn to the hospital staff for protection, comfort, and warmth. A threat to one's security reawakens earlier fears of separation or abandonment. Loss of functions and fear of death may be symbolically related to separation.

7 *Fear of incompetency of medical personnel.* The patient may express such a fear by asking questions such as, "Do they know what they are doing?" "Am I being experimented on or victimized?" "Will they remove all of the cancer?"

8 *Fear of depersonalization and loss of self-control.* In the complexity of the hospital organization, the patient fears impersonal treatment and dependence on others. Health care personnel strip the individual of identity and a sense of worth by taking away personal possessions, such as clothes, and by invading the patient's body. As a result, the patient may feel insignificant and depersonalized.

9 *Fear of invasion of privacy.* Patients must answer personal questions about their bodies and affairs; give information about their families; expose bodies to pain, instrumentation, and examination by strangers; accept help with bodily functions; and be subjected to other indignities. Adolescents and aged persons are especially self-conscious about bodily exposure. Invasive procedures, representing a bodily assault to a patient, must be carried out with minimal embarrassment.

10 *Fear of outcomes regarding goals and expectations.* Vain persons, for example, grieve when radiation therapy causes permanent skin discoloration or chemotherapy causes loss of hair.

11 *Fear of loss of livelihood.* Illness can precipitate financial crisis, especially during chronic illness or prolonged rehabilitation.

12 *Fear of burdening others.* Patients experience this fear especially during the course of a severely debilitating condition.

13 *Fear of reliance on a mechanical object or a transplanted organ.*

14 *Fear of restriction of movement or activity.*

15 *Fear of pain and discomfort.* Many patients dread pain more than the operation itself. Pain can be produced by overwhelming fear rather than a sensation. This is sometimes indistinguishable from actual physical pain. Both are physically tiring and deleterious to bodily defenses. While neurological factors and the brain play a part in perception, the psychological component is well recognized. Alteration of pain perception can be achieved by attention to psychological needs. Perception can also be influenced by circumstance and by one's attitude toward a wound or degree of disability. For example, many war casualty amputees needed only minimal analgesic medication and were in high spirits because of their dismissal from active duty and its concomitant threat of death. In contrast, paraplegic patients required considerably more medication, support, and attention because of their prolonged severe depression and, on the part of some, a desire not to survive their disability.

Questioning Anxious patients seek a reason for their illness. They ask the question, "Why me?" Others will acknowledge, "I neglected my health for other things."

Suspicion Suspicious patients lack complete trust. They do not wholly accept what they are told or believe they have not been told everything. These patients take time to adapt because of their "on guard" reaction. Hard-of-hearing patients excluded from communication may be suspicious.

Guilt, Shame, Punishment The patient may feel ashamed of an illness or may think it is a form of punishment for prior behavior or imagined wrongdoing. Invasive procedures involving body orifices may evoke fantasies that reactivate childhood fears of multilation, deprivation, or punishment that threaten self-image. Consciously, this may be experienced as pain or may precede depression.

Depression Illness fosters introspection that can depress the patient who wishes to escape an intolerable situation. Depression may be manifested by agitated signs of despair, hopelessness, disinterest, or desolation. Passive depression is characterized by a sad, frowning face or one with little expression, lassitude, somatic complaints, impaired thinking and memory, retarded movement and body processes, anorexia, withdrawal from others, and neglect of appearance and body hygiene. Rather than being passive and inert, the agitated depressed person is hyperactive and talkative. Excessive depression may be detrimental to recovery and rehabilitation. This is cause for concern and requires understanding on the part of the nurse to motivate the patient to accept illness.

Denial To protect their egos, patients may reject reality and danger, thereby reducing anxiety, maintaining stability, and deterring panic. By denying concern or joking inappropriately, they repel overwhelming threats and make their difficulties more bearable. Such patients divert meaningful conversation and are superoptimistic. They are high-risk patients because they are not prepared to cope postoperatively. Often restless and difficult in the recovery room, tolerance for even normal discomfort is poor.

Denial should not be mistaken for courage. This reaction can be dangerous if the patient refuses to recognize a serious illness and to accept appropriate therapy.

Withdrawal The patient may withdraw from others and from communication. This is a reaction to feeling that one's physical and emotional privacy has been violated. Withdrawal may accompany depression. Apathetic, detached, evasive, and silent, the patient may ignore the presence of others by feigning sleep or by turning to face the wall. The patient's actions may reveal what cannot be verbalized as a result of mistrusting staff members or of believing they lack interest. In turn, lack of feedback creates a nursing problem.

Dependency Illness forces the patient to be dependent on others. Many patients feel inadequate because others are making decisions for them. They must be reassured that a normal degree of dependency can be beneficial in providing needed rest. Hospitalization, however, may provide an overly dependent person with desired mothering as early conflicts and childhood fears resurface. The nurse may be viewed as a mother-substitute. The enforced dependency of the handicapped, for example blind persons, does not fall in this category, however. Emotionally dependent patients center attention on themselves and the present moment. They are overly concerned about body functions. They interpret others' behavior in terms of rejection or acceptance. These patients lack motivation to help themselves. They find peace of mind and security when relieved of making decisions or choices, but they need explanations related to their care.

Regression Regression is a path of least resistance that leads to inertia. It may accompany dependency. Patients may regress to less mature levels of behavior. They may view the staff with ambivalence, i.e., affection and resentment.

Anger, Hostility Independent self-image is damaged by the passivity caused by illness. Emotional stress may be expressed verbally through open criticism of authority figures, such as physicians and nurses, or nonverbally through physical expressions, such as clenched fists or pursed lips. Patients respond to their feelings of insecurity and dependency by being aggressive and demanding in an attempt to control their environment. They are defensive in an effort to protect themselves. They may be reacting to a feeling of being assaulted, rebelling against enforcement of rules, or emerging from apathy.

Shock Shock provokes a sense of unreality that acts as protective insulation. The patient may respond in an automatic manner without thought or feeling, or may be unable to answer questions or function coherently. This is a common reaction when a malignancy is first revealed. The immediate need is for understanding and support to face reality.

Grieving and Mourning Feelings of loneliness, loss, and unhappiness are common with the loss of something valued or with any body disfigurement, be it from severe burns, amputation of a part, or an alteration in body structure. The patient mourns the change or may grieve over impending death due to advanced malignancy. This reaction occurs especially in "-ostomy," or "-ectomy" patients. The intensity of reactions, i.e., fatigue, depression, anxiety, altered sensorium, anger, and/or loneliness, depends on the extent and significance of the loss. Interest in life and living is regained as one's dependence on the lost object decreases. Visits by others who have lived through the same travail help patients in the period of adjustment by indicating that they are not separated from the rest of humanity.

NOTE. The patient's level of anxiety and fear must be assessed preoperatively. Every effort is made through supportive measures to minimize the potential hazards of adverse psychosocial distress.

Preoperative Visits

While the primary area of the OR nurse's practice is within the OR suite, the broadened scope of the perioperative role encompasses phases of pre- and postoperative care that contribute to the continuity of total patient care. Preoperative visits to patients are made by perioperative nurses skilled in interviewing, a technique for the development of the patient-nurse relationship. These interviews afford nurses an opportunity to learn about the patients and to establish rapport prior to the time they are brought to the operating room.

Before the inception of preoperative visits, the OR nurse had only minimal time to see and get to know the unanesthetized patient. A preoperative visit to collect data at the patient's bedside, or in the clinic or home, gives the perioperative nurse the time to learn about the patient, to observe patient behavior directly, and to plan appropriately before assuming responsibility for that patient's care. Since knowledge about the patient and how he or she views the impending operation are prerequisites for effective nursing intervention, the visit also fosters quality patient care by providing the perioperative nurse with a basis for implementing the nursing process and developing an ongoing relationship with the patient. The nurse is, therefore, included in all aspects of care, not just in the intraoperative phase when the patient is medicated and possibly unconscious.

Pros of Preoperative Visits The *advantages* of visits with patients are self-evident. They include:

1 As an expert, the OR nurse is well qualified to discuss a patient's OR experience, to orient and prepare patient and family for it and for the postoperative period.

2 The OR nurse can review critical data before the procedure and access the patient before planning nursing care.

3 Visits improve and individualize intraoperative care and efficiency; avoid needless delays in the OR.

4 Visits prolong OR nurse-patient contact. Some patients are reluctant to reveal their feelings and needs to someone in a short-term relationship.

5 Visits reduce the isolation of OR nursing from other clinical specialities.

6 Visits make intraoperative observations more meaningful.

7 Visits contribute to patient cooperation and involvement.

8 Visits facilitate all communications.

9 Visits enhance the positive self-image of the OR nurse and contribute to job satisfaction, which in turn reduces job turnover, a benefit to the hospital. Because of increased patient contact, visits make OR nursing more attractive to those who enjoy patient proximity and teaching.

Cons of Preoperative Vistis The *problems* associated with preoperative visits include:

1 Visits require additional time, energy, training, and often staffing.
2 Late patient admissions and heavy OR schedules make timing of visits difficult.
3 Visits may produce friction among different team factions if the program is not well planned and executed.
4 Repetitious interviewing may lead to a stereotyped manner and a lack of enthusiasm and spontaneity on the part of nurse-interviewers.
5 If skill is not employed, patients may feel their privacy is being invaded.
6 Barriers to visits may arise from the nurse's inability to
  a Verbalize.
  b Handle or accept dying.
  c Handle emotionally upset or angry persons.
  d Function efficiently outside of his or her customary environment.

Nurse-Interviewers Preoperative interviewing should be done by professional nurses with operating room orientation, experience, and complete knowledge of operative procedures, as well as pre- and postoperative care. Ideally, the circulating nurse who will be with the patient during the operation makes the visit, but this is not feasible in all situations due to staffing and time factors. Patient interviewing requires training and special skills in data collection, physical assessment, and observation. OR nurses who have learned and are adept at these skills will be comfortable visiting patients.

In some hospitals, a *visiting-nurse team,* working an afternoon-evening shift of duty, visits patients scheduled for operation, fills out forms, and prepares the written individualized care plans. The circulating nurses review these plans before the operative procedures and implement the plans. The visiting team may be comprised of staff nurses, clinicians, or an OR and a recovery room nurse. The two-nurse team approach provides nurse orientation (role model concept) and feedback when a less-experienced interviewer accompanies an experienced one. For group instruction, teams of nurses representing the operating room, recovery room, and intensive care unit are effective.

Interviewing Skills Interviewing, a form of verbal interaction, is a valuable tool for obtaining information. There is a great range of interviewing techniques. The interview can be *directive,* structured with predetermined questions in a fixed order that limit responses, or *nondirective,* in which the patient is given more latitude in responding. An example of a directive question is: "Have you had an operation before?" An example of a nondirective question is: "Tell me about your previous operation." The choice of technique depends on the information desired.

A structured form of interview is valuable in learning about an individual's health and work history. The unstructured type gives one a portrait of the patient's emotional reactions, concerns, and personality. An effective preoperative interview usually includes questions about both facts and feelings with informal observation an essential component. All questions should be relevant. The setting should be conducive to communication. The interviewer must be able to handle the situation with spontaneity, judgment, and tact. The interview must be meaningful to both the patient and the nurse.

Steps to Successful Preoperative Visits

1 Carefully review the patient's chart and records so that you can quickly focus on critical issues. These data reveal medical and nursing histories, diagnosis, and operation to be performed. Collect any information relevant to planning care in the OR. Discuss the patient and the nursing care plan with the unit nurses if possible prior to visiting the patient. Find out all you can about the patient. The nursing history, taken on admission by the unit nurse, includes the following pertinent information:

- **a** Biographical information: name, age, ethnic background, educational level, patterns of living, previous hospitalization and operations, religion.
- **b** Physical findings: vital signs, height, weight, skin integrity, allergies, presence of pain, drainage, bleeding, state of consciousness and orientation, sensory or physical deficits.
- **c** Special therapy: tracheostomy, inhalation therapy, hyperalimentation.
- **d** Emotional status: understanding, expectations, and specific problems concerning comfort, safety, language barrier, etc.

These parameters are essential for accurate intra- and postoperative assessment.

2 Greet the patient by introducing yourself and explaining purpose of visit. Tell the patient that your visit is a routine part of his or her total care, so the patient does not feel singled out because of his or her medical diagnosis.

- **a** Put the patient at ease. *Sit* close so the patient can easily see and hear you. Choose an optimal time without interruptions. Early evening is usually best, after supper and before visitors, or during the morning or afternoon of the day before the operation if the patient is in the hospital. Do *not* conduct your interview the morning of the operation! If the patient is in acute physical distress, consider rescheduling the visit.
- **b** Allow adequate time for the interview. This is usually 10 to 20 minutes, unless the patient has special needs, and thus requires more time. Give the patient time to think and express himself or herself.
- **c** Except in the case of children, persons needing an interpreter, or the mentally handicapped, it is advisable to first speak with the patient alone. Then, if the patient is willing, the family may be invited to participate and ask questions. This affords the patient privacy so he or she may feel free to talk. The family should be present during teaching to learn how to assist the patient.

d Allow the patient to maintain his or her self-respect.

e Instill confidence in the patient by your appearance and attitude. Establish rapport by demonstrating warmth and genuine interest. Avoid an authoritative manner.

f Use language at the patient's level of development, understanding, and education.

3 Obtain information by asking about the patient's understanding of the operative procedure.

a Assess information the patient has and check its accuracy to ascertain what further instructions are needed. Ask a question such as, "What has your surgeon told you about the operation?" Clarify any misconceptions about the procedure as appropriate within the scope of nursing.

b Permit the patient to talk. Your objective is to gather data that will assist the OR staff in providing care.

c Direct questions must be used with caution and are not suitable for collecting all objective data. Word questions to elicit more information than one-word answers.

d *Listen attentively.* To preserve self-esteem, the patient may tell you what he or she thinks you want to hear.

e A patient's statement that ends in a question may be either a request for more information or an expression of a feeling or attitude about the nurse's competence.

4 Orient the patient to the OR suite environment and interpret hospital policies and routines.

a Tell the patient the time operation is scheduled, approximately how long it will take, and how long the stay will probably be in the recovery room. Explain that the patient will be taken to the preoperative holding area before the operation, if this is the routine procedure.

b Ask the patient who will be at the hospital during the operation, i.e., family members or friend(s). They should be informed how early to be there to see the patient before sedation is given. Tell the patient and family where the waiting room is located.

c Tell the patient the family will be informed when he or she arrives in recovery room and returns to unit, if this is hospital policy.

5 Review the preoperative preparations the patient will experience and provide information about what to expect postoperatively.

a Familiarize the patient with whom and what will be seen in the OR and RR. If you will not be in the OR, tell the patient a colleague will be there to greet and take care of him or her.

NOTE. Many OR nurses wear OR attire and laboratory coat with name tag when they visit patients. This familiarizes the patient with the way they will see personnel the next day. Attire must be changed if the nurse reenters the OR suite after the visit.

b Use your discretion as to how much the patient should know and *wants to know.* Use well-chosen words that do not connote an anxiety-inducing situation. Do not use words with unpleasant associations such as knife, needle, or nausea.

c Postoperative recovery begins with preoperative teaching, but keep explanations short and simple. Excessive detail can increase patient anxiety, which itself reduces the attention span. (Preoperative teaching will be discussed in more detail later in this chapter.)

d Give practical information about what the patient should expect such as withholding fluids, the drowsiness and/or dry mouth from preoperative medications, transportation to the OR, the holding area, and where he will be taken after the operation. Instruct him not to hesitate to ask for assistance at any time. Give any other relevant special precautions.

e Give reasons for procedures and regulations; this reduces patient anxiety. With children and the elderly, one often needs to repeat information.

f Be realistic about what you can accomplish. Explain only the procedures of which the patient will be aware.

6 Tell the patient that the anesthesiologist will visit him to discuss specific questions relative to anesthesia, if this is routine. (See discussion of anesthesiologist's visit in Chapter 3.)

7 Answer the patient's questions about the operative procedure in general terms. Refer specific questions to the surgeon.

a Be honest and responsible in your communications about a proposed diagnostic or operative procedure. Complement, but do not overlap, the surgeon's area of responsibility. Do not be unrealistic, falsify truth, or give false reassurance to patient or family.

b Be extremely cautious about spelling out specific details of treatment, procedure, and postoperative care unless you have been thoroughly briefed by the surgeon in charge. Surgeons' care plans are also individual and tailored to their own techniques as well as to the patients' problems. Forms of therapy may be controversial. Continual interdisciplinary communication is mandatory.

8 Encourage the patient and family to discuss feelings or anxieties regarding the operation and anticipated results.

a Motivate and assist the patient and family to gain perspective, objectivity, awareness, and insight. A skilled professional nurse will know how to discourage wishful thinking for miraculous cures while at the same time communicating understanding of their fears and wishes for an easy, fast recovery.

b Observe emotional reactions.

c As an interviewer, be emotionally objective yourself about pain, mutilative surgery, death, sexuality. Listen to what the patient is asking without feeling threatened if you have to talk about painful aspects or don't know the answers to questions such as "Why me?" Show that you care. Patients scheduled for spinal or local anesthesia and/or for operations on the face or genitalia often experience great anxiety.

d Acknowledge the impact of the procedure on the patient's sexuality, if appropriate.

e Try to help the patient solve own problems when possible. Ask questions that help explore a subject or feelings but do not probe to elicit responses. Do not destroy his or her coping mechanism. Encourage an appropriate one. The visit is not a structured psychiatric counseling session!

f Listen to anxieties in a realistic time frame and get others to follow through as necessary. Don't attempt too full an agenda. Sort out what is legitimate. You can't solve all problems in 20 minutes. For example, say "I'll share this information with the doctor or unit nurse so someone else can help you with this problem." Use colleagues' expertise to assist you or to make proper referral.

g Comfort the patient if indicated; convey a sense of security. Touch as appropriate. A perceptive nurse can tell when the patient resents touch; respect feelings. Patients with decreased visual acuity appreciate the assurance that a touch can give, but always speak first to avoid startling the patient. Reassure the patient that he or she will not be alone, but will be *constantly* attended by competent staff.

h Alert the family as to what they will see in the intensive care unit, such as monitors and machines, if the patient will be there.

i Ask the patient, "Do you have any concerns about tomorrow?" Never bring a patient's feelings into the open and then cut him off. Allow time to deal with problems. Try to increase the patient's trust in the team.

9 Use audiovisual materials—pamphlets, notebooks, photographs, drawings, etc.—to supplement the interview, if available and appropriate.

a These materials are especially useful for explaining complicated procedures such as total joint replacement.

10 Note information which will improve nursing care in the operating room, i.e., physical problems which might affect positioning or require special setups.

a The preoperative visit is a time for discovery and planning for problem prevention. The nursing care plan will include preparation for extra tall, obese, paralyzed, or left-handed patients to guard against a traumatic experience. For example, an intravenous infusion should be started in the right arm of a left-handed person, to minimize limitation of manual dexterity.

b Observe physical limitations such as pain on moving, loss of an extremity, or sensory loss. These tell the nurse how much cooperation to expect from the patient. A pad and pencil may be needed to communicate with a patient who is unable to speak or is deaf.

c Ask if the patient wears any type of prosthetic devices. Explain, per accepted hospital policy, that these must be removed prior to operation either at the bedside or in the OR.

d While talking to the patient, assess special needs. It is important for the OR nurse to know about the presence of an implanted pacemaker, for example. Electrosurgery could cause it to malfunction, and so would

be contraindicated. Preexisting medical conditions alter how the patient should be managed in the OR. (See Chapter 3: Patients with Special Needs.)
  e Know the patient's special requests.

11 Let the patient ask questions.
  a If you are unable or unprepared to answer a legitimate question, tell the patient that you will find out the answer. For example, say, "I don't know, but I'll get that information for you."
  b *Don't:* interrupt the patient; avoid eye contact; interrogate or belittle an expressed fear; avoid answering questions; introduce irrelevant topics; argue; use hospital jargon; conduct the visit out of curiosity; relate your own experiences in detail; moralize; joke inappropriately; contradict; offer false reassurance; avoid an uncomfortable situation—face it and resolve it.

12 Offer reassurance when possible. Maintain an attitude of hope.
  a Help both yourself and the patient turn negative feelings into positive useful responses.
  b Offer realistic hope but do not minimize the seriousness of the operative procedure.

Preoperative Teaching The overall nursing care plan includes directives for educating the patient and family about the illness and their part in managing it. *Teaching,* a function of nursing practice, is a process of action embracing perception, thought, feeling, and performance. During the preoperative visit, the perioperative nurse supplements instruction by other nursing team members and gives information unique to the patient's specific operation. The nurse teaches patients how to assist and encourages them to participate in their own postoperative recovery. He or she teaches patients:

1 How they will feel and the nursing actions that will provide comfort.

2 What will happen postoperatively.

3 What is expected of them. The aim of using specific measures is to prevent a health crisis or postoperative complication.

4 What they can do to make their own postoperative period easier and hasten recovery. The nurse makes patients aware that actions can be taken that are effective.

Effective Teaching Patient teaching involves emotional energy on the part of the nurse. It can produce behavioral changes in patients, however, as they become involved in the learning experience. By learning, patients can participate in their care and be better prepared physically and emotionally for the operation. They also learn how to utilize the health care system. Learning self-help has a positive effect on the patient. Another advantage is that the patient knows what to expect and where to go for help after discharge, if needed, such as to an -ostomy or -ectomy club.

Patient teaching may be conducted in an informal, individual manner or in a formal group teaching setting adapted for patients with similar problems such as laryngectomy, colostomy, or mastectomy. The nurse-instructor should first formulate, in conjunction with other team members, attainable objectives with patient input and determine the patient's emotional receptivity and mental capacity. The nurse also assesses the patient's acceptance of his or her problem, developmental level, sight, hearing, etc. Also, before beginning an explanation, the nurse should ascertain what the patient already understands about the condition and the topic to be taught. Verify what the patient knows, needs to know, and wants to know. Identify, by observation and what the patient says, where problems exist. An understanding relationship with the patient facilitates teaching.

Teaching should be slanted to family members' particular circumstances to help these persons cope with the problem to the extent of their ability. Success or failure of treatment is often contingent on what happens after the patient leaves the hospital. The family's knowledge, ability to cope, and help are important factors. Other points to consider:

1 Arrange conditions so that learning can occur; an undisturbed environment and proper timing are important and conducive to it.

2 Language is the fundamental tool for education. Use understandable terminology and be knowledgeable. Do not equate intelligence level with educational level. The nurse is accountable for what is taught.

3 Set priorities and teach what is significant and appropriate to patient's particular problems.
  a Break down instruction into manageable steps; for example, instruct patient to deep breathe, then cough.
  b Put content in sequence of activities to facilitate learning.
  c Give reasons and benefits; for example, movement of legs and toes postoperatively,

unless contraindicated, aids circulation and prevents venous stasis.

d Adapt teaching method to the specific situation. The patient may reject teaching not relevant to immediate present. For example, a patient about to be operated for a heart valve replacement may listen, but may actually be concentrating on the fact that his or her heart is going to be incised.

e Don't overburden the patient with a multitude of facts.

4 Recognition of need, not pressure, should be the motivating factor in learning.

5 To evaluate understanding, ask patient to repeat in own words what you explained.

6 Written instructions are helpful for review. Go over material with the patient. Test comprehension by asking questions, since pain, anxiety, and medication can hinder understanding.

7 As resource person, be consistent, concise, and organized. Repeat instructions to help patient retain them.

Patients who receive preoperative instruction from and interact with the perioperative nurse may suffer less apprehension, tolerate the procedure better, and seem more secure and comfortable postoperatively. Usually they remember what they are taught and react more positively to their surgical experience than other patients not given the benefit of this interaction with the perioperative nurse.

At the end of the preoperative assessment and teaching session, the perioperative nurse should not depart from the patient abruptly, but should leave an entree for the return postoperative visit (to be discussed later in this chapter).

From the data obtained, the perioperative nurse records the nursing history. The acronym SOAP is helpful to incorporate the basic elements of a nursing history.

S Subjective response: Patient's perceptions and expectations of surgical intervention and problems the patient has identified.

O Objective perception: Nurse's impressions of the patient and his or her problems as determined from chart data and observation of patient during preoperative visit.

A Analysis: Determination of basic needs, as outlined in Maslow's hierarchy (see Fig. 4-2) and defining characteristics of patient's existing or potential health problems.

P Plan: The data collected must be organized, analyzed, and interpreted to formulate the nursing diagnoses.

Documentation

Immediately after leaving the patient's bedside the nurse writes a summary of the visit on the nurses' note or progress sheet in the patient's chart to convey pertinent information to the unit nurses and surgeon. Written documentation is necessary also to correlate the visit with the nursing audit, a part of the evaluation phase of the nursing process. This information includes the teaching given as well as the patient's needs for further pre- and postoperative information and instruction. Identified family attitudes and needs are also included. This becomes a permanent part of the patient's record.

Assessment guidelines or nursing interview forms specifically designed for the perioperative nurse are valuable tools to organize and record data gleaned during preoperative visits. However, it is inappropriate for patients to see nurses writing during an interview. They may become uncomfortable and less communicative. Nurses should concentrate on remembering pertinent data, unusual observations, and teaching to record the appropriate information after the visit.

Standard II

Nursing diagnoses are derived from health status data.

Nursing diagnoses are conclusions the perioperative nurse makes based on analysis and interpretation of data collected. These are concise written statements about the patient's health status deviations and problems amenable to nursing intervention. Current scientific knowledge supports the nursing diagnoses, which should be congruent with diagnoses of other health care professionals.

Nursing diagnoses are synonymous with specific patient problems as determined by the patient's responses during physiological and psychosocial assessment. The format of nursing interview forms or assessment guides vary from hospital to hospital, but all elicit essentially the same information as a basis for writing nursing diagnoses and preparing written nursing care plans.

PREOPERATIVE PLANNING

From the nursing diagnoses the nurse structures a flexible, individualized nursing care plan designed to seek ways to achieve solutions to the patient's problems. This plan designates specific, necessary actions and possible nursing interventions to meet each problem listed, indicating priority of each goal and expected outcome. Plans to assist the family in helping the patient orient to reality as well as supportive, therapeutic, palliative, preventive, and rehabilitative measures to assist the patient are included. The nursing diagnoses and rationale are written into the nursing care plan.

The nurse's plan is only as good as the data, the information known about the patient. The nurse's actions are never better than the plan. All factors that influence subsequent actions, utilizing the total care concept, are included. Consultation with other health professionals while planning helps ascertain how best to meet the patient's needs. In formulating a care plan, the nurse utilizes analysis, application of knowledge, interpretation, and decision making.

NOTE. The acronym SOAP also applies in developing a nursing care plan. It means Subjective/Objective Analysis and Planning. It incorporates the first two components of nursing process and the first four standards of perioperative nursing practice.

Standard III

The plan of nursing care includes goals derived from the nursing diagnoses.

Goals are the *desired patient outcomes* following surgical intervention within specified time frames and with specific criteria for evaluation. They direct the nursing actions to modify or maintain the patient's present or potential physical capabilities and behavioral patterns. The patient's rights and preferences are considered. Goals should be realistic, attainable through available human and material resources, and consistent with medical regimen and the patient outcome standards for perioperative nursing.

In formulating goals as written statements of outcomes, the perioperative nurse should consider, but not be limited to, the following:

1 Absence of infection.
2 Maintenance of skin integrity.
3 Absence of adverse effects through proper application of safety measures related to positioning, chemical, physical, and electrical hazards.
4 Maintenance of fluid and electrolyte balance.
5 Knowledge and understanding the patient and family or significant others have of the potential physiological and psychological responses to surgical intervention and their participation in the rehabilitative process.

These goals are prioritized to maximize the therapeutic effect of the nursing actions. Immediate, actual problems must be resolved first by the safest, most efficient approach. Then highly probable, followed by potential problems, are addressed.

Standard IV

The plan for nursing care prescribes the nursing actions to achieve the goals.

The perioperative nurse asks creative questions such as, "In what ways can I assure the safety and welfare of this patient?" "What specific or unusual problems does this patient have?" "What are this patient's needs?" Based on the nursing history, nursing diagnoses, and goals, the perioperative nurse devises a plan for intraoperative care to fulfill needs and expedite the operation safely for the patient. The plan also should include provision for preoperative supportive and comfort measures and postoperative evaluation of outcomes specifically related to the intraoperative phase of nursing care. Points to consider in planning perioperative nursing care are:

1 Medical diagnosis and impact of surgical intervention on body systems
2 Location of operative site
3 Calculated risks of the proposed procedure on other physical needs
4 Psychosocial and spiritual needs
5 Environmental safety

Standardized nursing care plans may be developed for the common, expected problems of patient populations undergoing similar procedures, e.g., abdominal operations, open heart surgery, intracranial surgery. These written care plans can be organized to include the usual, predictable problems/nursing diagnoses and expected outcomes/goals. Space must be provided for the unusual, not routine, problems that must be considered for individualized patient care. Alternative options or interventions are a necessary part of the plan. They permit modification at any phase of the process as necessary. Regardless of format, the nursing care plan specifies the following:

1 Nursing actions necessary to achieve goals
2 Priorities for nursing actions
3 Logical sequencing of nursing actions

4 How the nursing actions are to be performed
5 When the nursing actions are to be performed
6 Where the nursing actions are to be performed
7 Who is to perform the nursing actions

Human and material resources must be available to implement the plan. Therefore, the planning phase of nursing process also includes assurance that appropriate and properly prepared and functioning supplies and equipment will be available. Methods for monitoring environmental safety should be delineated, as well as those for psychological and physiological monitoring of the patient. Communication of the plan to all personnel involved in providing care to the patient is essential for continuity of care. It should also be communicated to the patient and family or significant others, as appropriate.

Documentation

The JCAH standards for nursing services state: "The plan of care must be documented and should reflect current standards of nursing practice. The plan shall include nursing measures that will facilitate the medical care prescribed and that will restore, maintain or promote the patient's well-being."*

Perioperative nurses have a responsibility to plan as well as give care. If the planned and performed nursing activities are not documented, legally it can be assumed that the care did not take place.

PRE- AND INTRAOPERATIVE IMPLEMENTATION

Implementation, the third component of the nursing process, begins when the written nursing care plan is put into action in the OR suite during the preoperative phase of the patient's experience and continues throughout the intraoperative phase. All actions focus on the patient and are directed to the goals. Nursing actions directly affect patient outcomes.

The perioperative nurse who wrote the plan personally carries it out or communicates it to others to assure that the identified patient's goals are achieved. The patient's responses are monitored during performance of the planned nursing actions. Hopefully, the nursing interventions, which are the execution of the nursing regimen, will be therapeutically effective.

Being a surgical patient oneself is perhaps the only way of gaining insight into knowing what it feels like to be on the receiving side of perioperative care. Riding horizontally in an elevator on a stretcher is an extremely different sensation from moving vertically. Although premedication dulls the senses, when the circulating nurse asks and assists the patient to move onto the operating table, the patient is jolted from a sedated calm state by the realization that "This is it—the moment I've dreaded is now actually here." The starkness of the operating room is completely obvious (see Fig. 4-3). The patient looks to the nurse as mentor. It is then that the patient-nurse relationship, the basis of nursing, is revealed. A fundamental element in this relationship is effective communication, both with and for the patient.

Professional education prepares the perioperative nurse for fundamental functions as a clinical nursing practitioner-leader, a coprofessional with physicians in giving and promoting continuous

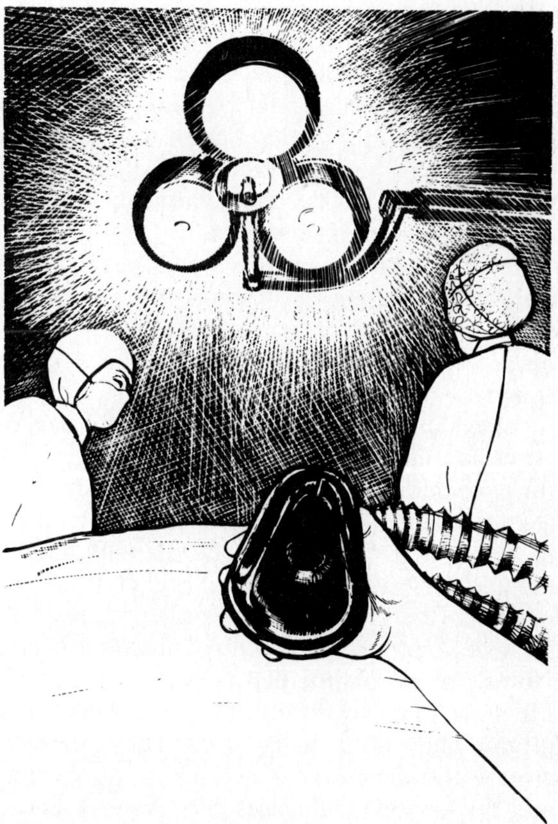

FIGURE 4-3
The operating room from the patient's perspective.

*Joint Commission on Accreditation of Hospitals: *Accreditation Manual for Hospitals,* Chicago: Joint Commission on Accreditation of Hospitals, 1984 edition.

care of surgical patients. In the OR, the surgeon is in charge of the operation, but the RN circulating nurse is the organizer, coordinator, stabilizer, and manager of the OR to which assigned. The surgeon relies on the circulating nurse to prepare for and keep the operation running smoothly as a result of meticulous planning and experiential expertise. The nurse coordinates and implements the nursing care plan with and through team members.

Standard V

The plan for nursing care is implemented.

Scientific principles provide the basis for nursing actions. These actions are consistent with the plan to foster continuity of nursing care in the preoperative, intraoperative, and postoperative phases. They must be performed with safety, skill, efficiency, and effectiveness.

The patient's welfare and individual needs are paramount in every facet of activity within the OR suite. They must not be compromised. Seemingly routine details have significant importance. For example, taking a defective instrument out of circulation may prevent injury to the patient. Checking the operating light helps to assure the surgeon of clear vision in the operative site. All preoperative preparations within the operating room must provide for the physical safety of the patient in an aseptic, controlled environment. The OR nurse also provides emotional support to the patient prior to transfer to the operating table and during induction of anesthesia.

Even though preoperative and postoperative visits are made, nurses' contacts with patients are limited and less than those of the unit nurses. OR nurses have a relatively short time in which to gain patients' trust and to reassure them. The risks involved in the operation are reduced when patients have hope, confidence, and are reconciled to the need or desire for the procedure. The nurse, as a central figure in patient care, can do much to relieve fear and provide security. Patients look to the OR nurse as a knowledgeable expert. In times of crisis, they want the physical presence of a trusted, competent, compassionate person. Human beings are interdependent. Patients expect the nurse to be cognizant of their problems, conditions, and willing to help them. They interpret a nurse's attitude as one of acceptance or rejection, and this concept influences effectiveness. Behavior is related to expectation. Consequently, the nurse's behavior affects the patient in either a positive or negative way. Positive actions include spending time with and staying close to the patient as distance may be interpreted as disapproval; giving concerned attention to the patient's needs and discomfort; looking directly at the patient when he or she speaks; touching the patient with kindliness; appearing poised and confident in a professional manner. Negative actions include frowning; ignoring the patient; failing to respond to patients' feelings or needs. The way in which something is said and done is equally as important as what is said and done. Sometimes inaction is indicated. The perceptive nurse can determine such instances.

Human beings react through their senses. Research has documented the positive effects of *touch* as a helpful nonverbal communication in establishing nurse-patient rapport within a short time. Touch says that someone is there and cares. Gentle touch can bridge a language barrier through the establishment of human contact. Warmly holding a patient's hand or laying a hand on an arm during induction of anesthesia or a painful procedure can do much to alleviate that patient's anxiety and elicit trust. A smile has been called the universal language. Above one's mask one's eyes can convey a smile or hope. Likewise, they can reveal fear, anger, or hostility. Physiognomy, the ancient Chinese art of discovering qualities of the mind and temperament from the expression of facial features, still has relevance. Facial expressions, eye contacts, and body movements have a positive or negative effect on the patient. Warmth and solicitude can be conveyed by a pleasant manner and the expression of the eyes.

Although formal routines for care, procedures, and teaching have been set up, each patient, as a frightened human being, deserves personalized care in the face of a disruptive life experience. The patient must not be treated as an inanimate object or anonymous person beneath the drapes, or categorized by disease or operative procedure. The patient is a living, feeling person, not "Dr. Brown's hysterectomy," "the cardiac in Room 4," "the arthritic I need help in moving," or "the case we just sent to recovery." Medical jargon such as this is depersonalizing, demoralizing, and totally unacceptable, as well as offensive to the patient. The goal of OR nursing is to combine *efficiency with caring.* The nurse must never become insensitive to patients because of depersonalized hospital routines or own prejudices.

Protection of modesty, dignity, and privacy whether the patient is conscious or unconscious is essential. Unnecessary exposure must be avoided. The gown and cotton blanket protect modesty in addition to keeping the patient warm. Also, the operating room door should be kept closed for privacy; this is a point in aseptic technique as well. Operations may be viewed only by authorized persons with a definite function and all privileged information is kept confidential.

Patients are unnerved by perceptible harmful stimuli such as strange odors; disturbing sights such as a used but uncleaned operating room, soiled linen, instruments, equipment, unconscious patients, bright lights; isolation or detachment from others or the group; hustle and bustle type of activity or unpreparedness; embarrassment from body exposure; loud noises such as voices, inappropriate conversation or whistling, staff disagreements, patient's moaning, instruments clattering, sterilizer noises.

Anxiety and preoperative sedation tend to alter the patient's ability to interpret events objectively. The patient may relate everything heard to self, although he or she may not actually be the subject of conversation. Lack of consideration can destroy the patient's confidence in the team. An overheard, thoughtless comment can produce a lasting traumatic memory and fear that the patient may pass on to others. Negative recall can become anxiety-inducing in similar future experiences. Think before speaking and do not converse near the patient while excluding him or her from the conversation. Sedation does not imply exclusion. The patient may be aware of conversation although appearing to be asleep! Out of the patient's hearing, conversation should pertain only to the work at hand, for the OR is not the place for social discourse. The patient may misinterpret or react unfavorably because hearing is the last sense lost as a person becomes unconscious, as in general anesthesia. It is not known at precisely what moment a person can no longer hear and interpret what is said.

Time is of the essence to keep anesthesia and procedure time to a minimum, a protective factor for patients to provide as little disturbance to physiologic homeostasis as possible. However, *efficiency and safety must not be sacrificed for speed.* Circulating nurses are responsible for patient and employee safety. *Safety is the prime concern.* The OR suite is generally considered the most critical area of the hospital in relation to safety. It imposes a high degree of vulnerability on patients and the entire professional, allied technical, and ancillary staff. Patients lack the power to defend and protect themselves during surgical intervention. Therefore, nurses are advocates, representatives, and protectors. They give supportive care and safeguard patients from emotional or physical harm by constant vigilance. Circulating nurses can minimize potential hazards by:

1 Never leaving a sedated patient unguarded. In addition to causing mental anguish from a feeling of abandonment, if left unattended the patient may fall or be injured on equipment.

2 Using good body mechanics and adequate restraints. Injury can occur to personnel during positioning or alignment of a patient due to faulty body mechanics. Or, the patient can fall due to inadequate assistance, restraints, or stabilization during transport or transfer to the operating table.

3 Correctly identifying patients, operative sites, drugs, or medications. An incorrect operation on a patient or error in medication is usually the result of inadequate identification.

4 Creating, maintaining, and controlling an optimally therapeutic environment in the OR. This involves control of the physical environment, such as temperature and humidity, and personnel. Traffic flow in and out of the room should be kept to a minimum. The more movement and talking, the greater the room's microbial count. Once the patient is in the OR, it should be kept quiet so that the effects of sedation are not counteracted. A tranquil, relaxed atmosphere is conducive to team concentration and orderly functioning so all can go well. Standards of ethical conduct should be strictly enforced.

5 Assuring that mandatory aseptic principles are adhered to by the entire team at all times. There is no compromise with sterility. Proper sterilization and housekeeping practices must be followed without deviation.

6 Preventing a foreign body from remaining in the wound of the patient. All needles, sponges, and instruments are counted. Sharp items must be protected before disposal to prevent injury to personnel.

7 Careful handling and accurate labeling of all specimens and cultures. An error could cause an inaccurate diagnosis, improper therapy, or reoperation.

8 Respecting equipment. Proper care and handling assure efficient functioning, a protection for both patient and team members, and an economic benefit for the hospital. Faulty electrical or anesthesia equipment or their improper usage can cause burns, electrocution, or explosion.

Documentation

All nursing interventions, both routine and complicated, observations of patient responses and resultant outcomes delineated in the care plan are documented as evidence of the care given. This written documentation becomes a part of the patient's permanent record. The RN accountable for the patient's care is responsible for the documentation. Nursing actions contributing to patient comfort and safety must be identified. Also activities other than direct nursing care not recorded elsewhere that may affect patient outcomes are included, for example, disposition of tissue specimens.

Writing nurses' notes or progress notes on the patient's chart or completing an intraoperative observation checklist provides a profile of what has happened to the patient. Records and forms must be accurate and specific (see Chap. 12). State what happened and why. Besides having legal value, records are of value to the postoperative care team in their assessment and interpretation of altered physiological status, i.e., pain or drainage from the trauma to living tissue occurring during operation.

INTRA- AND POSTOPERATIVE EVALUATION

Evaluation is a comparison of actual results with expected outcomes. The evaluation component of nursing process begins after the planned nursing actions are carried out or, by unanticipated circumstances, during implementation of the plan in the intraoperative phase of care. The effectiveness and appropriateness of goals, plans, and actions are measured by the interpretation of the patient's responses to and outcomes from nursing interventions.

Tools used for evaluation include outcome audit of charts, records, and care plans or intraoperative process audit (see Chap. 12), peer review (see Chap. 12), and/or postoperative visits with patients. The purposes of evaluation are:

1 To provide feedback to providers about the surgical patient's total care.

2 To influence policy making and procedures. New methods are devised from evaluation and research.

3 To reveal areas where inservice education is needed for nursing personnel.

4 To formulate and revise the hospital's quality assurance program. Evaluation provides an objective means for upgrading nursing care.

5 To provide data for self-evaluation. Every nurse is accountable for his or her own actions and those of personnel under the nurse's supervision.

Standard VI

The plan for nursing care is evaluated.

Determination of patient responses and degree of goal realization can be verified by direct observation of the patient and/or conversation with the patient. In the narrowest scope of the perioperative role, the OR nurse observes the patient's responses to nursing actions during the immediate preoperative and intraoperative phases of care in the OR suite. Or the OR nurse may accompany the patient to the recovery room to compare and communicate results of nursing actions with desired goals to the extent that they can be evaluated in the immediate postoperative period.

Ideally, the perioperative nurse visits the patient a day or two postoperatively, or phones an ambulatory care patient at home. In the broadest scope of the role, the perioperative nurse may see the patient after discharge in the clinic or home for follow-up evaluation of outcomes of surgical intervention.

Postoperative Visit

A postoperative visit is one made to the patient, at the bedside on the surgical unit, by the perioperative nurse for the purpose of evaluating preoperative preparation and intraoperative nursing care. Preferably, the perioperative nurse who assessed the patient preoperatively and who then prepared and implemented the nursing care plan will visit the patient postoperatively. This visit provides a means for evaluating the goals and determining the degree of their attainment. It discloses omission in the effectiveness of the nursing process as well as errors of commission such as injury, complications, and infection.

During the postoperative visit, the patient tells the perioperative nurse how preoperative and intraoperative care was perceived. The patient is asked to focus on physical and emotional needs, safety, environment, and teaching in preparation for postoperative rehabilitation. In addition to judicious examination of nursing management of the patient in comparison with actual patient outcomes, the preoperative visit and nursing care plan are evaluated in terms of objective achievement of the goals. The perioperative nurse needs to determine what factors influenced goal achievement or lack of it.

1 Was the preoperative visit helpful to the patient?
2 Was the patient's preparation for operation adequate physically, emotionally, and spiritually?
3 What could have been improved?
4 Were all patient needs identified?
5 Did planned care meet the identified needs?
6 Was the plan instructive, practical, adaptable?
7 Did the preoperative visit and care plan contribute to a positive surgical experience?
8 Was the preoperative teaching utilized, helpful, adequate?
9 Did the preoperative visit effect change in the patient postoperatively? Did it effect change on a long term basis?

The postoperative visit terminates the direct perioperative patient-nurse relationship. However, many hospitals give patients an evaluation form to be filled out objectively. This provides additional feedback for all of the hospital staff. An effective evaluation program and positive patient experiences promote good public relations. The pre- and postoperative visits by perioperative nurses present a friendly, caring hospital image to the public it serves.

To be successful, a visiting program requires the cooperative effort of and input from unit, RR, ICU, and perioperative nurses, surgeons, anesthesiologists, and hospital administrators. They should participate in structuring the program at its inception to avoid duplication of action and feelings of resentment. The program should be reviewed periodically and revised as necessary. The perioperative nurse also confers with the rest of the nursing team and the physicians to evaluate patient care and make recommendations for improvement in it and in interpersonal relationships. An interdisiciplinary conference is an effective medium for the accomplishment of these goals. Excellent intraoperative management of the patient can be nullified by inadequate pre- and/or postoperative care.

Standard VII

Reassessment of the individual, reconsideration of nursing diagnosis, resetting of goals, and modification and implementation of the nursing care plan are a continuous process.

Evaluation is a continual process of reassessing patient needs, modifying goals and priorities, and revising plans when expected outcomes are not achieved or the patient's condition or adaptive levels change. In the OR one deals continually with anxiety and stress. A sense of tension more or less prevails from the team's constant need to accommodate to a variety of intense situations within a short period of time. The OR team is always on the alert and prepared to respond to any eventuality. Therefore, the four components of the nursing process are taken concurrently and recurrently during the intraoperative phase as changes occur in the patient's internal and external environment.

The patient is observed during the operation and evaluated for responses to nursing actions and medical interventions. Changing conditions may require reassessment for new data and identification of new problems, revision of goals, implementation of alternative actions, or other modification of the initial nursing care plan.

Documentation

The patient's permanent record should reflect the evaluation of perioperative nursing care and its outcomes. Documentation provides legal evidence of results of planned nursing actions and revisions of the plan based on reassessment of the patient's needs.

QUALITY ASSURANCE

A discussion of perioperative nursing would not be complete without mention of quality assurance, since the patient is the focus of concern for perioperative nursing care.

Each patient deserves the best possible care. Without the structure the nursing process provides, health care services would be fragmented and accountability for the quality of services rendered made difficult. Society demands accountability of those who provide services. Patients are protected by laws, standards, and recommended practices.

Nursing practices must comply with established policies and procedures of the hospital or ambulatory care facility and with professional standards of practice. Nurses can be held legally responsible for unethical, illegal, or unsafe practices if they fail to exercise judgment that is considered standard nursing practice. They are responsible for their own acts in the patient-physician-nurse relationship and are required to exercise skilled judgment in making decisions. Nurses must see that all nursing procedures and techniques are correctly executed, always keeping patient outcomes in mind.

Quality assurance programs (see Chaps. 2 and 12) provide a means for determining the quality of care received by a patient in a particular health care setting. Nursing care in the OR can be evaluated in the context of the total nursing process: assessment, planning, implementation, evaluation. Quality is determined by identifying observable characteristics, judged according to standards, for an optimum achievable degree of excellence of care. For example, postoperatively the patient should be free from infection, skin breakdown, and injury related to positioning, instrumentation, or chemical agents. Quality assurance is important for professionalism, accountability, and cost containment. A program includes:

1 Determining standards and criteria.
2 Implementing and achieving standards.
3 Evaluating the results. Did the program succeed? What changes need to be made to improve practice and action?

Health care professionals continually aim to improve the health/wellness outcomes for patients; alteration in health status is the end result of care. A provocative thought: The essence of quality care is in the utilization of the therapeutic potential present in each interaction in which the nurse practitioner is involved. Nurses may improve the quality of patient care by:

1 Comprehending nursing problems, providing specialized nursing interventions, and meeting the patient's physiological and psychological needs based on observation and assessment of the patient's responses
2 Helping the patient and family adapt to what happens in the OR in relation to their perceptions and expectations through teaching
3 Delivering and supervising clinical patient care with skilled planned nursing intervention and interdisciplinary collaboration
4 Coordinating all activities in the OR by planning, preparing for, and expediting the operative procedure, keeping in mind individual patient, surgeon, and team needs

To summarize, productive care and improved patient outcome result from better directed efforts as indicated by evaluation, the fourth component in the nursing process.

CHAPTER **5**

AMBULATORY SURGERY

AMBULATORY SURGICAL CARE FACILITY

Many operative procedures minimally curtail physiologic functions and are anatomically superficial in nature. These are amenable to operation in an ambulatory care facility. *Ambulatory surgery* refers to a method of delivering surgical care whereby patients enter the facility, are operated on, and are cared for postoperatively in anticipation of being discharged to return home the same day.

Various terms are used to describe ambulatory care facilities including outpatient surgery, same day surgical unit, one day surgery, or ambulatory surgery center. Irrespective of its name or location, an ambulatory care facility must provide an admitting room, area for patients to change clothes, preoperative holding area, operating room(s) with appropriate areas for preparation and storage of supplies, recovery room with patient lavatory, and family waiting room.

In addition to obtaining a state license and certificate of approval, an ambulatory care facility must meet standards set by various accreditation agencies. The facility may be a hospital-based unit, a hospital-affiliated satellite unit, or an independent freestanding ambulatory surgery center. The latter must have a patient transfer/admission agreement with a nearby hospital. If complications develop, such as adverse reactions to anesthesia or postoperative bleeding, or if an unexpected finding of a malignancy or other diagnosis necessitates further surgery, the patient may need to be admitted to a hospital.

Studies have shown that up to 45 percent of all operative procedures can be safely performed on an ambulatory basis without compromising the quality of care. However, some facilities limit utilization to only those procedures that can be performed with local or regional block anesthesia. Other facilities allow surgeons to perform operations under general anesthesia. Although procedures performed in an ambulatory care facility usually are of short duration, 15 to 90 minutes, appropriate selection and evaluation of patients are essential. Nursing care and anesthesia management also are crucial factors in the ambulatory surgical patient's experience.

THE AMBULATORY SURGICAL PATIENT

Many persons prefer to recuperate after operation in their home environment, rather than be hospitalized. These patients may be candidates for ambulatory surgery, depending on the nature and extent of operation, and on the ability to follow instructions for care at home.

Patient Selection

Patients eligible for ambulatory surgery are carefully selected. Criteria considered include:

1 General health status. Acceptable patients are in Class I or II of the American Society of Anesthesiologists' physical status classification (see Chap 3, p. 55). Patients are evaluated physically and emotionally to determine the possibility of complications occurring during or after operation.

2 Results of preoperative tests.
   a Laboratory tests usually include a complete blood count and urinalysis for all patients.
   b Multichemistry profile and chest x-ray may be required for adults scheduled for general anesthesia.
   c Electrocardiogram (ECG) may be required prior to general anesthesia for patients over age 35.

   NOTE. 1. Patients may have tests upon admission the morning of operation, but preferably they are performed before the scheduled date of operation so the results can be evaluated preadmission. This avoids cancellation on the day operation is scheduled if unsatisfactory results so warrant. The results must be on the chart that accompanies the patient to the OR.

   2. If the surgeon documents that the patient has had a normal chest x-ray and/or ECG within the past six months, these requirements may be waived.

   3. Requirements may be waived by written policy for specific minor procedures or based on age. However, JCAH standards state, "When surgical services are provided in an ambulatory care setting, the policies and procedures shall be consistent with those applicable to inpatient surgery, anesthesia, and postoperative recovery."

3 Willingness of the patient. The patient must be willing and able to recuperate at home. Some persons will feel more secure in a hospital or lack adequate home care. Each patient must be individually assessed. Provision must be made for competent care at home for all ambulatory care patients.

4 Recovery period. The surgeon should anticipate minimal or no postoperative complications. Patients in whom a prolonged period of nausea and vomiting is anticipated, or in whom pain will not be relieved by oral analgesics are not ideal candidates for ambulatory surgery.

Patient Instructions

Written instructions are given to the patient by the surgeon during an office visit or by the nurse during a preadmission visit to the ambulatory care facility. These describe the operative, admission, recovery, and discharge procedures. To protect the physicians and the facility, the patient should sign for receipt of these instructions as well as sign a consent form for operation. Instructions include:

1 Preoperative preparations
   a Make appointment for preadmission testing and teaching session, unless these instructions are given at this time.
   b Take nothing by mouth after midnight, or other specified hour, before admission.
   c Arrive at facility by ____ A.M./P.M. (Time will depend on time operation is scheduled.)
   d Notify surgeon immediately of a change in physical condition, such as a cold or fever.
   e Wear comfortable casual clothing, and leave jewelry and valuables at home.

2 Postoperative discharge
   a Arrange for a responsible adult to accompany you home. You will not be permitted to drive or leave unattended.
   b Do not ingest alcoholic beverages, drive a car, or operate complex machinery for 24 hours.
   c Delay important decision making until a full recovery is made.
   d Take medications only as prescribed and maintain as regular a diet as tolerated.
   e Shower or bathe daily unless instructed otherwise. This helps relieve muscle tension or discomfort, and keeps the wound clean.
   f Call surgeon if postoperative problems arise.
   g Keep follow-up appointment with surgeon.

The patient's level of understanding of these instructions and concept of what is to happen must be assessed preoperatively. The consent form signed by the patient prior to premedication or anesthesia may include the statements: I have been NPO since ____ o'clock; my physical condition has not changed; I understand that admission overnight may be necessary.

PATIENT-NURSE RELATIONSHIP

Good patient-nurse rapport is essential in an ambulatory care facility. Patients are alert and often anxious as preoperative medication is kept to a minimum. Personnel with warm people-oriented personalities are essential. The need to provide continual reassurance throughout procedures demands qualified personnel with maturity, proficiency, and an ability to convey empathy. Staff, more than environment, contribute to the warm caring atmosphere essential in dealing with alert patients and their families.

The patient-nurse relationship begins with the preoperative interview. Patients are questioned about past medical/surgical history; if they see a physician or take medication on a regular basis; and if they wear glasses, contact lenses, false teeth, or prosthesis of any kind. Particular attention is given to medications. Many patients are vague regarding what they take and what allergic responses they have to drugs. If comprehension of the questions is doubtful or a language barrier exists, access to a family member, friend, or interpreter is essential.

Following the interview, the patient changes from street clothes into a patient gown. The nurse escorts the patient into the preoperative holding area where the patient is prepared as necessary for the specific operation. Unless sedation is given, the patient may walk from this area into the operating room. This helps minimize the patient's feeling of dependency. Conversation with the nurse reinforces the patient-nurse relationship.

Following the procedure, the patient receives specific discharge instructions in writing and the nurse verbally reinforces them. If problems occur after discharge, patients are encouraged to contact their surgeon. However, many patients feel more comfortable using the nursing staff of ambulatory care facilities as resource agents. This is encouraged as the units provide an ongoing environment for patient education.

INTRAOPERATIVE CARE

Anesthesia management is rarely difficult if careful selection of patients, preoperative evaluation, and instructions are adhered to. Premedication, if given, is minimal. Local anesthesia or regional block is preferable if appropriate. Spinal anesthesia seldom is used.

Patients who receive general anesthesia are scheduled early in the day to allow maximum recovery time. Rapidly dissipating agents are administered. Intravenous agents associated with prolonged recovery are avoided unless there is specific indication for their use. Doses of intravenous agents, such as narcotics and barbiturates, may be reduced to avoid delayed recovery. Indications for endotracheal intubation are the same as for inpatients. (Refer to Chapter 13 for indepth discussion of all anesthetic agents and their administration.)

Intraoperatively the same precautions are observed by all team members as for any operative procedure. These include strict adherence to the principles of aseptic and sterile techniques (see Chap. 7) and other operating room routines.

The patient is monitored continuously for reaction to drugs, and for behavioral and physiologic changes (see Chap. 14). If an anesthesiologist is not in attendance, the circulating nurse takes and records vital signs before the injection of a local or regional block anesthetic agent or analgesic and every 15 minutes thereafter, monitors physiologic status according to written policy and procedure, and institutes emergency measures if an adverse reaction occurs. Therefore, the circulating nurse must have a basic knowledge of the function and use of monitoring equipment that includes attaching electrocardiograph leads and identifying and reporting abnormal ECG readings. Additional functions upon request of the surgeon, as permitted by policy, may include starting oxygen therapy when clinically indicated, administering intravenous therapy, or giving medications. Cardiopulmonary resuscitation equipment must be available. All pertinent data and therapy must be documented.

The awake and alert patient must receive physical and emotional comfort throughout the operation. This patient should be told what is about to take place, for example, "You will feel a needle sting"; what to expect, for example, "You will have a burning sensation"; and what is expected of him or her, for example, "Tell us if you feel pain." The patient's questions should be answered truthfully and realistically. Conversation by team members must be appropriate and kept to a minimum. Hand signals between surgeon and scrub nurse are more useful than a verbal request for instruments. However, the surgeon may request a number 10 or 15 rather than a knife, a Kay or Converse rather than a scissor. Strange noises should be explained to the patient, for example, suction to remove irrigating solution or the sound of electrosurgical unit. Background music *of the patient's choice* may help relax and distract the patient.

RECOVERY, DISCHARGE, AND FOLLOW-UP

Postoperatively, management of pain, nausea, and vomiting, plus monitoring of vital signs are responsibilities of the recovery room nurse. Medications usually are given intravenously in small dosages, as oral medications on an empty stomach tend to increase nausea and vomiting. Routine orders may be established by policy for these analgesics and antiemetics.

Consciousness, rational behavior, and ambulation do not imply full recovery. Blood pressure and pulse rate may return to normal range while residual myocardial depression continues. Patients may lapse back into sleep or drowsiness as drugs are metabolized. Discharge to home must be contingent on patient safety in all respects.

Patients are discharged on written order of the anesthesiologist and/or surgeon as per policy, in the company of a responsible adult, when all discharge criteria are met. These criteria include:

1 Stable vital signs
2 Able to swallow and cough; gag reflex present
3 Able to ambulate, per developmental age, or per physical limitations
4 No or minimal dizziness, nausea, or vomiting
5 No respiratory distress, hoarseness, or croupy cough following endotracheal intubation
6 Alert and oriented
7 No bleeding and no or minimal drainage on dressings
8 Able to tolerate fluids and has voided
9 No excessive pain that will not be alleviated with oral medications at home.

Ideally the day following, or at least within three days of discharge, a nurse from the ambulatory care facility phones to check on the patient's progress and to reiterate postoperative instructions. The nurse reminds the patient of his or her follow-up appointment with the surgeon. Since many patients return to work within a day or two, they may not be home to receive the nurse's call.

Supplemental questionnaires are sent to surgeons and/or patients to determine if postoperative infection has occurred. These assist in infection control surveillance.

ADVANTAGES OF AMBULATORY SURGERY

The development of rapid-acting anesthetics that have minimal prolonged side effects, and the availability of short-acting narcotics to control pain and antiemetics to reduce nausea allow the surgeon to perform many operative procedures in an ambulatory care facility. The advantages are that ambulatory surgery:

1 Lowers cost for the patient.
2 Returns patient immediately to familiar surroundings that are less stressful than a hospital environment.
3 Reduces period of patient's dependency and disability.
4 Eliminates psychological trauma of hospitalization and separation from parents for infants and children.
5 Frees hospital bed space for patients who require more extensive care without increasing hospital bed capacity.
6 Frees hospital staff and resources for patients with more serious problems.
7 Reduces risk of nosocomial infection that is inherent in hospitalization (see Chap. 7).
8 Offers immediate and personalized patient care.

The concept of ambulatory health care services is expanding to community emergency care centers, rather than hospital-based emergency departments, for treatment of minor trauma and illness. Many surgeons perform minor operative procedures in their offices.

CHAPTER **6**

PHYSICAL FACILITIES

PHYSICAL LAYOUT OF THE O.R. SUITE

Utilization of the physical facilities is important; however, it is secondary to the functioning of the people within a department. The design of an OR suite offers a challenge to the planning team to optimize efficiency by creating realistic traffic and work flow patterns for patients, personnel, and supplies. Design should also allow for flexibility and for future expansion. Architects consult surgeons and OR nursing administrative personnel before allocating space.

No one plan suits all hospitals; each is designed on an individual basis to meet projected, specific future needs.The number of rooms required is a function of:

1 The number and length of operations to be performed
2 The type and distribution by specialties of the surgical staff
3 The proportion of elective inpatient and ambulatory patients to emergency operations
4 The scheduling policies related to the number of hours per day and days per week the suite will be in use
5 The systems and procedures established for the flow of patients, personnel, and supplies

Location

The OR suite is usually located in an area accessible to the critical care surgical patient areas and the supporting service departments, i.e., central service department, pathology, and radiology. The size of the hospital is a determining factor as it is impossible to locate every desirable unit or department immediately adjacent to the OR suite. A terminal location is necessary to prevent unrelated traffic from passing through the suite. A location on a top floor is not necessary for microbial control since all air is filtered to control dust. Traffic noises may be less evident above the ground floor. Artificial lighting is controllable so that outside daylight is not a factor; in fact, it may be a distraction. Many OR suites are underground or have solid walls without windows.

Principles in Design

The universal problem of environmental control to prevent wound infection exerts a great influence upon the design of the OR suite. As much as the floor plan will permit, clean and contaminated areas are differentiated. Architects follow two principles in planning the physical layout of an OR suite:

1 Exclusion of contamination from outside the suite with sensible traffic patterns within the suite
2 Separation of clean from contaminated areas within the suite

Physical planning of an OR suite, which separates clean from contaminated areas, makes it easier to carry out good aseptic technique. The clean area is often referred to as the *restricted area.*

Type of Design

The hospital where you are working probably was constructed according to a variation of one of four basic designs:

1 A central corridor, or hotel plan
2 A double central corridor, or clean core plan
3 A peripheral corridor, or race track plan
4 A grouping, or cluster plan

Each design has its advantages and disadvantages. Efficiency is affected if corridor distances are too long in proportion to other space, if illogical relationships exist between space and function, or if inadequate consideration was given to storage space, materiel handling, and personnel areas.

Space Allocation

Space is allocated within the OR suite to provide for the work to be done, with consideration of the efficiency with which it can be accomplished. The OR suite should be large enough to allow for correct technique yet small enough to minimize the movement of patients, personnel, and supplies. Provision must be made for traffic control. The type of design will predetermine traffic patterns. All persons, i.e., staff, patients, and visitors, should follow the delineated patterns in appropriate attire. The OR suite is divided into three areas.

Unrestricted Street clothes are permitted. A corridor on the periphery handles traffic from outside, including patients. This area is isolated by doors from the main hospital corridor or elevators and from other areas of the OR suite. It serves as an outside to inside access area.

Semirestricted OR attire is required (see Chap. 9, p. 145). This area includes peripheral support areas and access corridors to the operating rooms. The patient may be transferred to a clean "inside" stretcher or wheel base upon entry to this area.

Restricted Masks are required to supplement OR attire. Sterile procedures are carried out in these rooms.

EXCHANGE AREAS

Both patients and personnel enter the semi- and restricted areas of the OR suite through an exchange area.

Preoperative Holding Area

A designated room or area should be available for patients to wait in the OR suite that shields them from potentially distressing sights and sounds. The corridor outside the OR is the least desirable area. The area should provide privacy. Individual cubicles are preferable to curtains. Hair removal, insertion of intravenous lines, indwelling urinary catheters, and/or gastric tubes may be done here.

Dressing Rooms and Lounges

Clothes-changing area must be provided for both men and women. Access is from an unrestricted area to change from street clothes to OR attire before entering the semirestricted area, and vice versa. Lockers are usually provided. Doors separate this area from lavatory facilities and adjacent lounges. Walls in lounge areas should have an aesthetically pleasing color or combination of colors to foster a restful atmosphere. Dictating equipment and telephones should be available for the surgeons in the lounges or an adjacent semirestricted area.

PERIPHERAL SUPPORT AREAS

Central Administrative Control

At a central control point, traffic in and out of the suite is observed. This area may be within the unrestricted or semirestricted area. Offices for administrative personnel are best located where they have access to both areas, as these persons frequently need to confer with persons outside as well as to be informed of activities within the suite.

The clerk-receptionist is located at the control desk in the best position to coordinate communications. A pass-through window may be used to stop unauthorized persons, receive drugs, blood, and various small supplies, or to schedule operations with a surgeon.

Computers may be located in the control area. Automated information systems and computerization assist in financial management, statistical recording and analysis, scheduling of patients and personnel, materiels management, patient data retrieval, and other functions to integrate utilization of facilities with patient care outcomes.

Conference Room

Some hospitals have a conference room within the semirestricted area. This is used for nursing staff inservice educational programs and by surgical staff for teaching. Closed circuit television (see p. 93) and/or videocassettes may be available for self-study.

Work and Storage Areas

Clean and sterile supplies and equipment must be separated from soiled items and trash. If the suite has a clean core area, soiled materials are not taken into this area. They go to the decontamination area for processing, then storage, or to the disposal area.

Conveyors or monorails may move bags of soiled linen and trash out of the suite. Conveyors may also connect the OR suite with a central processing area on another floor of the hospital. If efficient materiel flow can be accomplished, support functions can be removed from the OR suite. Effective communications and a reliable transportation system must be established, however. Some hospitals send all their instruments and supplies to the central service department for cleaning, packaging, sterilizing, and storing. This system eliminates the need for work and storage areas within the OR suite.

Processing of Supplies

Utility Room Some hospitals use a closed-cart system and take contaminated instruments to a central area outside the OR suite for cleanup. Some do their cleanup procedures in the substerile room. Many, by virtue of the limitations of the physical facilities, bring the instruments to a utility room. This room contains washer-sterilizer, sinks, cabinets, and all necessary aids to cleaning. If the washer-sterilizer is a pass-through one, it opens also into the general workroom. This eliminates the task of physically moving instruments from one room to another.

General Workroom The general work area should be as centrally located in the OR suite as possible to keep contamination to a minimum. The work area may be divided into a cleaning area and a preparation area. If instruments and equipment from the utility room are received from the pass-through washer-sterilizer into this room, an ultrasonic cleaner should be available here for cleaning instruments that the washer-sterilizer has not adequately cleaned. Otherwise, the ultrasonic cleaner may be in the utility room.

Instrument sets, basin sets, trays, and other supplies are wrapped for sterilization here. The preparation of instrument trays and sets in a central room ensures better control.

This room also contains the stock supply of other items that are packaged for sterilization. The sterilizers that are used in this room may open also into the next room—the sterile supply room. This helps to eliminate the possibility of mixing sterile and nonsterile items.

Storage

Sterile Supply Room Most hospitals keep a stock supply of sterile linen, sponges, gloves, and other sterile items ready for use in a sterile supply room within the OR suite. As many shelves as possible should be freestanding from the walls, which permit supplies to be put into one side and removed from the other; thus, older packages are always used first.

The use of disposable products may necessitate a change in physical facilities. Less space is needed for cleaning equipment, wrapping packages, etc. The need for sterilization equipment may ultimately be reduced. More sterile storage space may be needed. These factors influence the design of new hospitals or the renovation of old ones for greater efficiency.

Instrument Room Most hospitals have a separate room, or section of the general workroom, for storing nonsterile instruments. The instrument room contains cupboards in which all clean instruments are stored when not in use. Instruments usually are segregated on shelves according to surgical specialty services.

Sets of basic instruments are usually cleaned, assembled, and sterilized after each use. However, special instruments designed for specific use, such as intestinal clamps, kidney forceps, bone instruments, may be stored after cleaning. Sets are then made up according to each day's schedule of operations.

Storage Room Some large, portable equipment must also be stored within the OR suite, readily accessible for use. A storage room for this equipment, such as the orthopaedic table that may not be used daily, keeps equipment out of corridors when not in use.

Architects sometimes plan for extra space to be used presently for storage but later for expansion. Rapidly changing needs, and increased efficiency in meeting them, will call for new equipment. Operating rooms become outdated due to the problem of keeping up-to-date with technological advancements. Many large pieces of sophisticated equipment are used for patients operated on because of trauma or diseases that yield to surgical intervention with the current technologies (see Chap. 19).

Scrub Room

Enclosed area for surgical scrubbing of hands and arms must be provided adjacent to each operating room (see Chap. 9, p. 149). Water that spills on the floor is particularly hazardous if the scrub area is in a traffic corridor.

THE OPERATING ROOM ITSELF

Size

The size of individual operating rooms vary. In the interest of economy and operational flexibility, it is desirable to have all operating rooms the same size, so that they can be used interchangeably to accommodate elective and emergency operations. Adequate size for multipurposes is 20 by 20 by 10 or 400 square feet (ft^2) or approximately 37 square meters (m^2) of floor space; the maximum beyond which efficiency is lost is 20 by 30 by 10 or 600 ft^2 (approximately 60 m^2). Specialized rooms, such as those equipped for cardiopulmonary bypass, may require as much as 600 ft^2 (approximately 60 m^2) of useful space.

Substerile Room

A group of two, three, or four operating rooms may be located around a central scrub area and a small substerile room. *Only if this latter room is immediately adjacent to the OR and separated from the scrub area will it be considered the* substerile room *throughout this text.*

A substerile room adjacent to the OR contains a sink, autoclave, and/or washer-sterilizer. Although some hospitals centralize their cleaning and sterilizing facilities, either inside or outside of the OR suite, a substerile room with this equipment offers the following advantages:

1 It saves time and steps. Emergency cleaning and flash sterilization of items can be done here by the circulating nurse. This reduces waiting time for the surgeon, anesthesia time for the patient, and saves steps for the circulating nurse. The circulating nurse, or scrub nurse if necessary, can lift sterile articles directly from the autoclave onto the sterile instrument table without transporting them through a hallway or another area.

2 It reduces the need for a messenger service to obtain sterile instruments and allows the circulating nurse to stay within the room.

3 It allows for better care of instruments and equipment that require special handling. Certain delicate or sensitive instruments, or perhaps a surgeon's personally owned set, usually are not sent out of the OR suite. They are handled only by the personnel directly responsible for their use and care, i.e., the circulating and scrub nurses. These nurses can clean up within the confines of the OR and this adjacent room. (See Chapters 10 and 11 for precautions.)

The substerile room also usually contains a combination blanket and solution warmer, cabinets for storage, and perhaps a refrigerator for blood and medications. Specimen containers with labels may be conveniently stored in this room. Slips for charges or other records may be kept here. Individual hospitals may find it convenient to keep other items in this room to save the time of the circulating nurse and to allow him or her to remain in or immediately adjacent to the OR during the operation.

Doors

Ideally, sliding doors should be used in the OR. They eliminate the air currents caused by swinging doors. Microorganisms that have previously settled in the room are disturbed with each swing of the door. The microbial count is usually at its peak at the time of the skin incision because this follows disturbance of air by gowning, draping, movement of personnel, and doors. During the operation, the microbial count rises every time doors swing open from either direction. Also, swinging doors may touch a sterile table or person.

Sliding doors should not recede into the wall but should be of the surface-sliding type. Fire regulations require that sliding doors for ORs be of the type that can be swung open if necessary. *Doors do not remain open either during or between operations.*

Ventilation

The ventilation system in the OR must ensure a controlled filtered-air supply. Air changes and circulation provide fresh air and prevent accumulation of anesthetic gases in the room. The concentration of gases is dependent solely on the proportion of pure air entering the air system to air recirculated through the system. Twenty-five air exchanges per hour is recommended. The microbial filters in the ducts do not remove anesthetic waste gases. They do filter the air to practically eliminate dust particles.

Architectural codes permit up to 80 percent recirculation of air. If air is recirculated, a gas scavenger system is mandatory to avoid buildup of waste anesthetic gases which are hazardous health risks for team members. Various types of scavengers are used (see Chap. 13, p. 240).

Some hospitals have installed laminar airflow. This high-flow unidirectional air-blowing system is housed in an enclosure within the OR. The air is filtered through high-efficiency particulate air (HEPA) filters. The value of this system is inconclusive (see Chap. 7, p. 109). Other types of filtered air-delivery systems that have a high rate of airflow are as effective in controlling airborne contamination. The ventilating system in the OR suite is separate from the hospital's general system.

Positive air pressure in each OR is greater than that outside in corridors, scrub areas, and substerile rooms. Positive pressure forces air out of the room. The inlet is at the ceiling. Air leaves through the outlets at floor level. If the reverse is true, air is drawn into the room around the doors and through open doors. Microorganisms in the air can enter the room unless positive pressure is maintained.

An air-conditioning system is ideal and valuable. It controls humidity to help reduce the possibility of explosion. High relative humidity (weight of water vapor present) should be maintained; 60 percent is preferable. Not less than 50 percent is mandatory in flammable anesthetizing locations. Moisture provides a relatively conductive medium, allowing static charge to leak to earth as fast as it is generated. Sparks form more readily with low humidity.

Room temperature is maintained within a range of 68 to 80°F (20 to 26°C). Even with controls of humidity and temperature, air-conditioning units may be a source of microorganisms that come through the filters. These must be changed at regular intervals. Ducts must be cleaned regularly.

Floors

Floors should be conductive enough to dissipate static from equipment and personnel, but not conductive enough to endanger personnel from shock. To prevent the accumulation of electrostatic charges in locations where flammable anesthetic agents are used, conductive flooring must be installed. Conductive floors are available in many materials including asphalt tile, linoleum, and terrazzo. The electrical resistance of these materials may change with age and cleaning. The resistance of conductive floors is measured monthly and must fulfill the provisions of the National Fire Protection Association Standard 56A (see Chap. 11, p. 204). The surface of the floor shall provide a path of moderate electrical conductivity between all persons and equipment making contact with the floor.

Flooring in nonflammable anesthetizing locations does not have to be conductive. A variety of hard plastic, seamless materials are used for nonconductive floors. The surface of all floors must not be porous, but suitably hard for cleaning by the flooding, wet-vacuuming technique.

Walls and Ceiling

Requisites of all surface materials are that they be hard, nonporous, fire resistant, waterproof, stainproof, seamless, and easy to clean. In addition, walls should be free from glare. The ceiling may be acoustical (sound-proof) tiles.

Wall paneling of hard vinyl materials, such as Formica, is easily cleaned and maintained. The seams can be sealed by a plastic filler. Laminated polyester or smooth, painted plaster provides a seamless wall. Epoxy paint has a tendency to flake or chip, however. Tiled walls collect dust and microorganisms between the tiles. The mortar between them is not smooth, and most grout lines are porous enough to harbor microorganisms even after cleaning. Tiles can crack and break. A material able to withstand considerable impact without affecting the surface also may have some value in noise control. Stainless steel cuffs at collision corners help avoid damage.

The walls and ceiling often are used to mount devices, utilities, and equipment in an effort to reduce clutter on the floor. In addition to the overhead operating light, the ceiling may be used for mounting an anesthesia service core, operating microscope, cyrosurgery device, x-ray tube and image intensifier, electronic monitor, closed-circuit television, and a variety of hooks, poles, and tubes. Demands for ceiling-mounted equipment are diversified. However, suspended track mounts are not recommended because they engender fallout of dust-carrying microorganisms each time they are moved. If movable or track-ceiling devices are installed, they should not be mounted directly over the operating table, but away from the center of the room and preferably recessed into the ceiling to minimize the possibility of dust accumulation and fallout.

Piped-In and Electrical Systems

Vacuum, compressed air, oxygen, and/or nitrous oxide may be piped into the OR. The outlets may be located on the wall, on the ceiling, or suspended from the ceiling. As a protection to other rooms, the supply of oxygen and nitrous oxide in any room can be shut off at panels for that purpose in the corridor should trouble occur in a particular line. A panel light comes on. A buzzer rings in the room and in the maintenance department. The buzzer can be turned off but the "abnormal" panel light stays on until the problem is corrected. The anesthesiologist can switch to the tanks of gases on the anesthesia machine.

Because flammable gases and vapors are heavier than air and settle to the floor when released, electrical outlets and fixtures located less than 5 ft (1.5 m) above the floor must meet rigid, explosion-proof code requirements. Explosion-proof electrical plugs are widely used. An alternative is to install grounded plugs above the 5-ft (1.5-m) level and to lead cords down the wall and across the floor to the equipment. Electrical cords on the floor are hazardous to personnel. Straight or curved ceiling-mounted tracks are satisfactory for bringing piped-in gases, vacuum, and electrical outlets close to the operating table. They eliminate the hazard of tripping over cords, but they can also produce a hazard. Insulation materials around electrical power sources from mobile, ceiling mounted tracks must be protected from repeated flexing when moved along the tracks to prevent cracks and damage to wires. Rigid or retractable ceiling service columns eliminate these hazards.

Multiple electrical outlets should be available from separate circuits. This minimizes the possibility of a blown fuse or a faulty circuit shutting off all electricity at a critical moment.

All personnel must be aware that the use of electricity introduces the hazards of electric shock, power failure, and fire. Faulty electrical equipment may cause a short circuit or the electrocution of patients or personnel (see Chap. 11 for detailed discussion). This hazard can be prevented by:

1 Using only electrical equipment designed for use in the OR. Equipment must have cords of adequate length and adequate current-carrying capacity to avoid overloading.

2 Testing portable equipment immediately before use and grounding correctly.

3 Discontinuing use immediately and reporting any faulty electrical equipment.

Should *fire* ever occur in a room during an operation, the burning article must be moved immediately from proximity to the oxygen source and the anesthesia machine or outlet of piped-in gases to prevent explosion. The fire should be extinguished in the room, if possible, but the patient must be immediately removed from any danger area. Fire safety systems are installed throughout the hospital. *All personnel must know the fire rules.* They must be familiar with the location of the alarm box and the use of fire extinguishers.

Lighting

General illumination is furnished by ceiling lights. Most room lights are white fluorescent, but may be incandescent. Recessed lights do not collect dust. Lighting should be evenly distributed throughout the room. The anesthesiologist must have sufficient light, at least 200 footcandles, to adequately evaluate the patient's color.

To minimize eye fatigue, the ratio of intensity of general room lighting to that at the operative site should not exceed one to five, preferably one to three. This contrast should be maintained in corridors and scrub areas as well as the room itself, so the surgeon becomes accustomed to the light before entering the sterile field. Color and hue of the lights also should be consistent.

Illumination of the operative site is dependent upon the quality of light from an overhead source and the reflection from the drapes and tissues. White, glistening tissues need less light than dull, dark tissues. Light must be of such quality that the pathologic conditions are recognizable. The overhead operating light must:

1 Make an intense light, within a range of 1000 to 9000 footcandles, into the incision without glare on the surface. It must give contrast to the depth and relationship of all anatomic structures. The light may be equipped with an intensity control. The surgeon will ask for more light when needed. A reserve of light should be available.

2 Provide the diameter light pattern and focus appropriate for the size of the incision. These are adjusted with controls mounted on the fixture. The focal point should avoid a dark center at the operative site. A 10 to 12 in. (25 to 30 cm) depth of focus allows the intensity to be relatively equal at the surface and depth of the incision. To avoid glare, a circular field of 10 in. (25 cm) in diameter provides a 2 in. (5 cm) zone of maximum intensity in the center of the field with one-fifth intensity at the periphery.

3 Be shadowless. Multiple sources and/or reflectors achieve reduction of shadows. In some units the relationship is fixed; others have separately maneuverable sources to direct light beams from converging angles.

4 Be near the blue/white color of daylight. Color quality of normal or diseased tissues is maintained within a spectral energy range of 1800 to 6500 Kelvin (K). Most surgeons prefer a color temperature about 5000K, which approximates the white light of a cloudless sky at noon.

5 Be freely adjustable to any position or angle. The downward movement is limited, however, to 5 ft (1.5 m) above the floor if flammable anesthetic agents are used. When only nonflammable agents are administered, the fixture can be lowered as desired. Most overhead operating lights are ceiling-mounted on mobile fixtures. Some have dual lights or dual tracks with sources on each track. These are designed for both lights to be used together to provide adequate intensity and minimize shadows in a single incision. Many fixtures are adapted so the surgeon can direct the beam by manipulation of sterile handles. Fixtures should be repositioned as little as possible to minimize dispersion of dust over the sterile field.

6 Produce a minimum of heat to prevent injury to exposed tissues, to ensure the comfort of the sterile team, and to minimize airborne microorganisms. As the lights heat up, convection currents tend to disturb settled microorganisms and cause them to become airborne. Heat produced from some fixtures is discharged by fans to outside the room. Most overhead lights dissipate heat into the room where it is cooled by the air-conditioning system. Halogen lights generate less heat than other types.

7 Produce less than 25,000 microwatts per square centimeter of radiant energy. If multiple light sources are used, collectively they must not exceed this limit at a single site. Beyond this range, the radiant energy produced by infrared rays changes to heat at or near the surface of exposed tissues. Some infrared and heat waves are absorbed by the filter globe over the light bulb.

8 Be easily cleaned. Tracks recessed within the ceiling virtually eliminate dust accumulation. Suspension-mounted tracks or a centrally mounted fixture must have smooth surfaces easily accessible for cleaning.

9 Adhere to electrical safety regulations for anesthetizing locations.

An auxillary light may be needed for a secondary operative site. Some hospitals have portable explosion-proof lights. Others have satellite units that are part of the overhead lighting fixture. These should only be used for secondary sites unless the manufacturer states the additional intensity is within safe radiant energy levels when used in conjunction with the main light source.

A source of light from a circuit separate from the usual supply must be available for use in case of power failure. This may require a separate emergency spotlight. It is best if the operating light is equipped so that an automatic switch can be made to the emergency source of lighting when the usual power fails.

Some surgeons prefer to work in a darkened room with only stark illumination of the operative site. This is particularly true of surgeons working with endoscopic instruments and the operating microscope. (This equipment is discussed in Chapter 19.) If the room has windows, light-proof shades may be drawn to darken the room when this equipment is in use. Because of the hazard of dust fallout from shades, hospitals have painted the windows in rooms where this equipment is used. Even though the surgeon prefers the room darkened, the circulating nurse or anesthesiologist must be able to see adequately to observe the patient's color and to monitor his or her condition. If only nonflammable anesthetic agents are used, a grazing light over the floor can be installed.

Some surgeons wear a headlight designed to focus a light beam on a specific small area, usually in a recessed body cavity such as the nasopharynx. Fiberoptic headlights produce a cool light and reduce shadows. Both the surgeon and first assistant may wear a headlight. Or, a light source that is an integral part of a sterile instrument such as a lighted retractor or fiberoptic cable may be used to illuminate deep cavities or tissues difficult to see with only the overhead operating light.

X-Ray Viewing Boxes

X-ray viewing boxes must be installed on the wall 5 ft (1.5 m) above the floor unless they are explosion-proof. The viewing surface should accommodate standard-size films. The best location is in the line of vision of the surgeon standing at the operating table. Lights for x-ray viewers should be of high intensity.

Clock with a Second Hand

A time-elapsed clock, which incorporates a warning signal, is useful for indicating that one or more predetermined periods of time have passed. This may be used during operations for total arterial occlusion, when using perfusion techniques or a pneumatic tourniquet, or during cardiac arrest.

Cabinets or Carts

Each OR is supplied with cabinets unless a cart system is used. Supplies for the types of operations done in that room are stocked, or every OR may be stocked with a standard number and type of supplies. These supplies save steps for the circulating nurse and help eliminate traffic in and out of the OR. Glass shelves and sliding doors provide ease in finding and taking out items. Many cabinets are stainless steel, however. Wire shelving minimizes dust accumulation. One cabinet in the room may have a pegboard at the back to hang items, such as table appliances.

Pass-through cabinets, that circulate clean air through them while maintaining positive air room pressure, allow transfer of supplies from outside to inside the OR. They help assure rotation of supplies in storage, or can be used only for passing supplies as needed from a clean center core.

In lieu of or as an adjunct to cabinets, some hospitals stock carts with special sutures, instruments, drugs, etc., for some or all of the surgical specialties. The appropriate cart is brought to the room for a specific operation.

Other hospitals stock an individual cart with those items necessary for each operation. This cart usually is prepared in the central service department and is sent to the operating room suite by clean dumbwaiter or an overhead monorail system. The cart is covered or enclosed during transport. With the monorail system, the wheels of the cart never touch the floor until ejected into the clean corridor of the OR suite. From the delivery point, the cart may be taken into the OR or substerile room, or remain in the clean corridor until needed.

With the individual cart system, each cart is adequate in size to hold the supplies, both sterile and nonsterile, for one operation. These are selected according to standard routines and the individual surgeon's preferences. Some carts are designed for both storage of supplies needed throughout the operation and to serve as the instrument table during the operation.

Furniture and Other Equipment

All furniture and equipment, permanent or portable, should contact a conductive floor by means of conductive materials. Dry graphite or graphited oil is preferred as lubricant for conductive rubber or metal caster wheels. Conductive rubber is used on feet of furniture without wheels. Furniture and equipment should be metal or some equally conductive material. Shelves and top surfaces of furniture also should be conductive. Stainless steel furniture is plain, durable, and easily cleaned. Each OR is equipped with:

1 Operating table with a mattress covered with conductive rubber, attachments for positioning patient (see Chap. 15), and armboards.

2 Instrument tables.

3 Mayo stand. The *Mayo stand* is a frame, with a removable rectangular stainless steel tray, that slides under the operating table. It is placed just above and across the patient, below the operative field. It serves to bring near the operative field a supply of instruments in constant use during the operation.

4 Small tables for gowns and gloves and/or patient's preparation equipment.

5 Ring stand for basin(s).

6 Anesthesia machine and table for anesthesiologist's equipment.

7 Sitting stools and standing platforms.

8 Standards or hangers for intravenous solution bags.

9 Suction bottle and tubing, either wall mounted or portable in a low-wheeled base.

10 Linen hamper frame.

11 Kick buckets in wheeled bases.

12 Wastebasket.

13 Writing surface. This may be a wall-mounted, stainless steel desk or an area built into a cabinet for the circulating nurse to keep and write records.

Communication Systems

A communication system is a vital link to summon routine or emergency assistance or to relay information to and from the OR team. Many OR suites are equipped with either monodirectional or bidirectional voice communication systems connecting each room with the clerk-receptionist's desk, the OR supervisor's office, pathology and radiology departments, blood bank, and recovery room. These systems make possible instantaneous consultation through direct communication. They are useful devices for the OR team, but are potentially hazardous for the patient.

Sounds are distorted by the patient in the early stages of general anesthesia. Incoming calls over a voice intercommunication (intercom) system should not be permitted to disturb the patient at this time. Also, an awake patient should not receive traumatic information about a pathologic diagnosis, for example, from a strange voice coming through an intercom speaker box after a biopsy has been performed. Installation of any type of intercom equipment in either the adjacent substerile room or scrub area, rather than in the OR, helps eliminate disturbance for both the patient and the surgeon.

In addition to or instead of a voice system, a call-light system can summon assistance from the anesthesia staff, ORS, pathologist, nursing assistant, and/or housekeeping personnel. Activated in the OR by a foot switch or hand switches, a light alerts personnel at a central point in the suite or displays varied needs at several receiving points simultaneously.

Closed-Circuit Television

Television surveillance provides an easy method for the ORS to keep abreast of activities in each OR. By means of a black-and-white television camera with a wide-angle lens mounted high in the corner of each OR, the ORS may make rounds simply by switching from one room to another by means of push buttons at his or her desk and a screen in the office.

More commonly, television serves a number of useful purposes for the surgeon in the OR. It is widely used for teaching operative techniques. This keeps visitors out of the OR, which, in the interest of sterile technique, is advantageous. In addition, television provides a better view for more persons to see the operation from a remote area, or through a microscope or endoscope. It can also provide record keeping and documentation for legal purposes for the surgeon.

As an aid to diagnosis, an audiovideo hookup between the OR and the x-ray department permits x-rays to be viewed on the television screen in the OR without transporting the films into the OR and mounting them on viewing boxes. With an audiovideo connection between the OR and x-ray department, the surgeon gains the advantage of remote interpretive consultation when it is desired.

A two-way audiovideo system between the frozen-section laboratory and the OR enables the surgeon to examine the microscopic slide by video in consultation with the pathologist without leaving the operating table. The pathologist can view the site of the pathologic lesion without entering the OR.

For these purposes, the color television camera may be mounted over the operating table in one of a number of ways. Usually it is attached to the stem of the operating light and outfitted with detachable sterilizable handles. An operating light with a television camera mounted in the center is available.

Video screens usually are adapted television sets and may be wall-mounted or placed on floor stands that can be moved readily. All pieces of television equipment must be labeled to indicate that they comply with applicable electrical safety regulations for use in the OR. They also must be encased in nonporous materials that can be easily cleaned.

Monitoring Equipment

Monitors and computers are designed to keep the OR team aware of the physiologic functions of the patient throughout the operation and to record patient data. The anesthesiologist uses monitoring devices as an added means to ensure safety for the patient during the operation (see Chap. 14).

In some hospitals a central room may be set up to monitor all patients undergoing operations. More frequently, the monitors are housed in a room immediately adjacent to the OR, separated by a glass partition. These rooms are staffed by well-trained personnel familiar with the types of monitoring or computerized equipment in use.

CHAPTER **7**

ASEPSIS, INFECTION CONTROL, AND PRINCIPLES OF STERILE TECHNIQUE

HISTORICAL INTRODUCTION

Early concepts of infection and the crude methods used to combat it seem strange indeed in the light of modern scientific knowledge, yet they were devised by the ablest minds of the times. Those minds, working on the three basic techniques—elimination of infection, control of hemorrhage, and anesthesia—have made possible the progress of modern surgery.

In ancient times, demons and evil spirits were thought to be the cause of pestilence and infection. Weird methods to drive them away were replaced by purification with fire.

In the pre-Christian era, Hippocrates (b. 460 B.C.) foreshadowed asepsis when he advocated irrigating wounds with wine or boiled water.

Galen (A.D. 131–200), the Greek physician and founder of experimental physiology, was the most distinguished physician of antiquity after Hippocrates. He practiced in Rome and upheld high standards of technique for his time. There is some evidence he boiled instruments used in caring for wounded gladiators. His anatomical investigations were unrivaled for their accuracy and fullness. His writings, and those of Hippocrates, were the established authority for medicine for many centuries.

Andreas Vesalius, born in Brussels in the early sixteenth century, was impressed by Galen's *De anatomicis administrandis.* After obtaining an MD degree, Vesalius and an artist collaborated to publish six very large plates—the *Tabulae anatomicae sex,* which became a landmark in the history of anatomical nomenclature. The plates were based on the physiology theorized by Galen. Modern anatomical nomenclature is an adaptation of that of Vesalius.

Early records are extant with descriptions of epidemics, purulence, fumigation, and wound management. Sporadically, light began to be shed after the Middle Ages on methods to improve operative technique. Although a few surgeons from the twelfth to the nineteenth centuries felt that wounds need not suppurate, even the learned Vesalius believed and taught that "laudable pus" was an essential part of the healing process. This universally accepted thought persisted in spite of the fact that some pioneering surgeons found that ventilation, sanitation, and heat-treated bed linens reduced patient infection rate. But acceptance of scientific inquiry was slow and the inquirer subject to condemnation, even death.

The concept of contamination by air or fomites did not surface until Girolama Francastoro, an Italian physician, in 1546 held that contagion was due to the passage of minute bodies, capable of self-multiplication, from the infector to the infected. He was the first to describe typhus fever, a prevalent disease of the times. His theory opened the way to the modern concept of infection and communicable diseases of epidemic proportions.

By the seventeenth century the world had barely begun to discard superstitions. Science was just beginning to emerge. Into such a world, Antony Leeuwenhoek was born in Holland. He heard that if one very carefully ground very small lenses out of clear glass, one could see objects much larger than they appeared to the unaided eye. His invention of the microscope was the precursor of many great discoveries. His painstaking work with minutia was challenged by his contemporaries. By the middle of the century, European rebels stated they would trust only perpetually repeated observations from their own experiments.

Leeuwenhoek's follower was Lazarro Spallanzani, a young Italian, who experimented on the multiplication of microbes and their "spontaneous generation." He proved that microbes may live without air. Humanity owes much to these bold, persistent explorers and fighters of death.

Europe was not the only seat of interest in disease and infection in the eighteenth century. America was struggling with epidemics as it battled to survive as a new nation. Diseases that are controlled today by inoculations and antibiotics ravaged the Revolutionary Army. Dr. Zabdiel Boylston of Boston introduced inoculation for smallpox in 1721. Some of Washington's troops were inoculated, but many uninoculated soldiers died. Diseases that plagued the losing side frequently tipped the scales of history and were often dreaded more than the enemy.

The field of medicine interested Noah Webster throughout his long life. The pestilence of the Revolutionary War camps was embedded in his memory. In 1799, he wrote the first American work of any real worth on general epidemiology.

Dr. Oliver Wendell Holmes, the renowned nineteenth-century Harvard physician and poet, wrote in 1843 of the contagious nature of puerperal fever ("childbed fever"). He expressed the belief that it was carried from patient to patient by nurses and doctors. However, many physicians still believed infection occurred by an act of Providence.

The true pioneer was Ignaz Semmelweis (1818–1865), an Austrian who established the etiology of puerperal fever, then a major cause of maternal mortality. He required doctors and medical students on his wards to wash their hands in a chlorinated-lime solution before examining patients. In a year's time Semmelweis reduced the mortality rate to one-twelfth of its previous level. However, his ideas were not understood and created controversy. The great value of his discovery was not recognized by other doctors of his time. Presumably because of this, he was committed to a hospital for the insane, and met with an early death.

It was Louis Pasteur, the French chemist and microbiologist, who established the validity of the germ theory of disease. He discovered that fermentation of wine is the result of minute organisms. All previous explanations had been without experimental foundation. He found that heat could halt the organisms' growth. By experimentation in the pure air of the high Alps, he destroyed the theory of spontaneous generation of organisms, proving that they came from similar organisms with which ordinary air was impregnated. His discoveries led to his studies of infection and putrefaction in living tissue. He isolated the bacillus of anthrax and developed the Pasteur vaccine for rabies. His greatest contribution was laying the foundation for bacteriology as a science and teaching the role of bacteria in causing disease.

The German physician Robert Koch was also a founder of bacteriology and won a Nobel prize for isolating the tubercle bacillus. Every modern student of bacteriology learns Koch's postulates:

1 A specific organism must be seen in all cases of an infectious disease.

2 This organism must be obtained in pure culture.

3 Organisms from pure cultures must reproduce the disease in experimental animals.

4 The organism must be recoverable from the experimental animals.

These postulates served as guides to discovery of etiologic agents in many of the most important diseases of man, animals, and plants. Koch traveled extensively studying the prevalent infectious diseases. His advocacy of use of bichloride of mercury as an antiseptic was the forerunner of interest in antisepsis.

Before and during the mid-nineteenth century, wounds or injury to an extremity invariably resulted in gangrene. Amputation was routinely performed in an attempt to prevent *septicemia,* a significant invasion of microorganisms into the bloodstream.

Surgical technique has advanced markedly since the nineteenth century, when the surgeon of that time operated in a Prince Albert coat and used the same blood- and pus-absorbing sponges for every patient he treated. During an operation, he often held the scalpel between his teeth, to protect the blade. The nineteenth-century surgeon unwound sutures from a nonsterile spool and hung them in a buttonhole of his Prince Albert. He kept a household pincushion nearby for his needles. Some instruments had beautifully carved ivory or bone handles, filled not only with bacteria but with dirt.

Joseph Lister, an English surgeon, is known as the father of modern surgery. Of all the persons who heard of Pasteur's work at the time, Lister was the one to see the value of the germ theory in relation to surgery, and to pursue its course. Since the relationship between bacteria and infection was known, he searched for a chemical to combat the bacteria and surgical infections. He first used a carbolic solution on dressings that somewhat reduced the mortality rate of his patients. Lister believed infections were airborne and his principle was to kill them in the wound and the surrounding area. In 1865, he started to use carbolic spray in the operating room. Then he used it in the wound, on articles in contact with the wound, and on the hands of the operating team. The result was a notable decrease in mortality rate. However, the carbolic solution caused wound necrosis and skin irritation in both patients and operators, and was said to "favour hemorrhage," making hemostasis difficult. Although unable to decide whether putrefaction was "germinal or chemical," some surgeons were convinced of the value of antiseptics. However, Lister's principle of antiseptic surgery, which initiated the modern era of surgery, was derided by other surgeons of the day. It was not until 1879 at a medical meeting in Amsterdam that Lister's antiseptic principle of surgery was truly accepted by the medical profession.

Developments in nursing accompanied advances in medicine. During the mid-nineteenth century, Florence Nightingale advocated the use of pure air, pure water, efficient drainage, cleanliness, and light for health. Her nursing experience during the Crimean War proved the efficacy of these practices. In 1876, Dr. Henry Bigelow of Massachusetts General Hospital took student nurses from the Boston Training School to the operating room for clinical instruction. In 1889, Johns Hopkins University opened its hospital. It included operating room nurse specialization.

Progress in sterile technique was slow, no doubt hindered by tradition, but with the advent of sterilization, continual progress was made. German surgeons assisted the transition from antisepsis to asepsis. Gustav Neuber was resolute about requiring complete cleanliness of the operating room, advocating scrubbing the furniture with disinfectant solution, and requiring the wearing of gowns and caps. He eventually sterilized everything in contact with wounds.

"Sterilization" by boiling was introduced in the 1880s. Everything used during an operation, including linens, dressings, and gowns, was boiled, although some surgeons still believed Lister's method to be adequate.

In 1876, heat-resistant bacteria were demonstrated. About 1886, Ernst von Bergmann and his associates introduced the steam sterilizer, a great improvement over von Bergmann's previous method of soaking surgical supplies in bichloride of mercury. However, surgeons soon learned that steam in itself is inadequate for sterilization. Steam must be under pressure to raise the temperature sufficiently to kill heat-resistant microorganisms. Pressure steam sterilizers were developed to kill resistant spores. Vacuum-type pressure sterilizers and hot air sterilizers followed.

Used as a fumigant for insects in the early twentieth century, ethylene oxide was recognized as an antibacterial agent around 1929, when it was used to sterilize imported spices. It has been employed as a sterilizing agent in industry and hospitals since the 1940s. Sterilization by irradiation developed thereafter. It is used for commercial sterilization of surgical supplies.

Coincidental with the development of sterilization, other factors in aseptic technique evolved. These include refinement of operative technique by William Halsted (see Chap. 17, p. 324), use of controlled environment, modern OR attire, and precise housekeeping methods. Surgeons learned that all things that come in contact with a wound should be free from microorganisms and spores, i.e., sterile.

SURGICAL CONSCIENCE

The key words of operating room practice are caring, conscience, discipline, and technique. Optimal patient care requires an inherent surgical conscience, self-discipline, and the application of principles of asepsis and sterile technique. All are inseparably related.

A surgical conscience may simply be stated as a surgical Golden Rule, i.e., do unto the patient as you would have others do unto you. One must consider each patient as oneself, or as a loved one. An individual develops a surgical conscience that remains inherent thereafter. In the last century, Florence Nightingale well summarized what is, in essence, its meaning. She said, "The nurse must keep a high sense of duty in her own mind, must aim at perfection in her care, and must be consistent always in herself." Surgical conscience involves a concept of self-inspection coupled with moral obligation. Involving both scientific and intellectual honesty, it is self-regulation in practice according to a deep personal commitment to the highest values. It incorporates one's own values and attitudes at a conscious level and monitors one's own behavior and decision making in relation to those values. In short, a surgical conscience is one's inner voice for the conscientious practice of asepsis and sterile technique *at all times.* This conscientiousness applies to every activity and intervention, as well as to personal hygiene.

Correct practice of asepsis provides a foundation for development of a mature conscience—mastery of personal integrity and discipline. Development of this conscience incorporates knowledge of aseptic principles, perpetual attention to detail, and experience. All are facets of responsibility, which involve trust. A surgical conscience does not permit a person to excuse an error but rather to readily admit and rectify one. It becomes so much an automatic part of the person that he or she can see at a glance or instinctively know if a break in technique or violation of a principle occurs. *Conscience dictates that appropriate action be taken, whether the person is with others or alone and unobserved.* A surgical conscience therefore is the foundation for the practice of strict aseptic and sterile techniques. Practice according to that conscience results in pride in self and in accomplishment, as well as an inner confidence that one is giving quality care.

A very important aspect in assisting the development of a surgical conscience in others is communication skill. Do not castigate a person for an error but praise that person instead for admitting it, and help him or her correct the violation. Fear of criticism is the primary deterrent in admission of fault. No one should be reluctant to admit a frank or questionable break in technique. However, any individual unmotivated to carry out aseptic practices as closely to perfection as possible has no place in the operating room suite.

DEFINITIONS

To understand infection, infection control, the principles of aseptic and sterile techniques, and the application of these principles in the operating room, you will need to know the meaning of the following terms.

Aerobe Microorganism that requires air or presence of oxygen for maintenance of life. Adj., *aerobic.*

Anaerobe Microorganism that grows best in oxygen-free environment or one that cannot tolerate oxygen, e.g., *Clostridium* species that causes gas gangrene. Adj., *anaerobic.*

Antibiotics Substances, both natural or synthetic, that inhibit growth of or destroy microorganisms. Used as therapeutic agents against infectious diseases, some are selective for a specific organism; some are broad-spectrum.

Antisepsis Prevention of sepsis by the exclusion, destruction, or inhibition of growth or multiplication of microorganisms from body tissues and fluids.

Antiseptics Organic or inorganic chemical compounds that combat sepsis by inhibiting growth of microorganisms without necessarily killing them. Used on skin and tissue to arrest growth of endogenous (resident flora) microorganisms, they must not destroy tissue.

Asepsis Absence of microorganisms that cause disease; freedom from infection; exclusion of microorganisms. Adj., *aseptic;* without infection.

Aseptic Technique Methods by which contamination with microorganisms is prevented. Alternate term: *aseptic practice,* to maintain asepsis.

Bactericide Agent that destroys bacteria. Adj., *bactericidal.*

Bacteriostasis Inhibition of growth of bacteria. Bacteria are undamaged to extent that they will grow if placed in a favorable medium, away from action of chemicals. Adj., *bacteriostatic.* Most antiseptics are bacteriostatic because they do not kill bacteria.

Bioburden Degree of microbial contamination on a device or object prior to sterilization.

Carrier Apparently healthy person who harbors and can transmit a pathogenic microorganism.

Contaminated Soiled or infected by microorganisms.

Cross Contamination Transmission of microorganisms from patient to patient and from inanimate objects to patients and vice versa.

Cross Infection Infection contracted by a patient from another patient or staff member, and/or contracted by a staff member from a patient.

Disease Specific entity that is the sum total of numerous expressions of one or more pathological processes; failure of the body's adaptive mechanisms to counteract adequately the stress to which it is subjected, resulting in disturbance in function or structure of any part, organ, or system of the body.

Disinfectants Agents that kill all growing or vegetative forms of microorganisms, thus completely eliminating them from inanimate objects. Syn., *germicide.* The suffix *-cide* means to kill; adj., *-cidal.* Reference is made frequently to the specific action of the following disinfectants:

Bactericide Kills gram-negative and gram-positive bacteria unless specifically stated to the contrary. Action against a specific species of bacteria may be elaborated; i.e., pseudomonacide kills *Pseudomonas aeruginosa,* tuberculocide kills tubercle bacillus.

Fungicide Kills fungi.

Sporicide Kills spores.

Virucide Kills viruses.

Disinfection Chemical or physical process of destroying all pathogenic microorganisms except spore-bearing ones; used for inanimate objects, but not on tissue. Degree of disinfection depends primarily on strength of agent and nature of contamination.

Droplet Minute particle of moisture, as expelled from respiratory tract by talking, sneezing, or coughing, which carries microorganisms.

Droplet Infection Infection transmitted from one person to another by airborne droplets.

Epidemiology Study of occurrence and distribution of disease; the sum of all factors controlling presence or absence of a disease.

Flora Bacteria and fungi normally inhabiting the body, often delineated as *resident* or *transient.*

Fomite Inanimate object that may be contaminated with infectious organisms and serves to transmit disease.

Gram's Stain Bacteriologic test to classify species of bacteria. Bacteria are stained with solutions of crystal violet and iodine, followed by exposure to alcohol, and then counterstained. Bacteria that retain blue color are *gram-positive;* those that remain pink are *gram-negative.*

Infection Invasion of the body by pathogenic microorganisms, and the reaction of tissues to their presence and to toxins generated by the organisms. Adj., *infectious.*

Microaerophilic Pertaining to microorganisms that require free oxygen for growth but thrive best when oxygen is less in amount than that in the atmosphere.

Microorganisms Living organisms, invisible to the naked eye, including: bacteria, fungi, viruses, yeasts, and molds. Syn., *microbe;* adj., *microbial.*

Opportunists Microorganisms that do not normally invade the tissue, but are capable of causing infection or disease if introduced mechanically into the body through injury. The tetanus bacillus is an example.

Pathogenic Producing or capable of producing disease.

Pathogenic Microorganisms Those microorganisms that cause infectious disease. They can invade healthy tissue through some power of their own, or can injure tissue by a toxin they produce.

Sepsis Severe toxic febrile state resulting from infection with pyrogenic microorganisms, with or without associated septicemia.

Septicemia Clinical syndrome characterized by significant invasion of microorganisms from a focus of infection in tissues into the bloodstream. Microorganisms may multiply in the blood. Infection of bacterial origin carried through the bloodstream is sometimes referred to as *bacteremia.*

Spores Inactive but viable state of microorganisms in the environment. Certain bacteria and fungi sustain themselves in this form until environment is favorable for vegetative growth. The spore stage is highly resistant to heat, toxic chemicals, and other methods of destruction.

Sterile Free of microorganisms, including all spores.

Sterile Field Area around the site of incision into tissue or introduction of any instrumentation into a body orifice that has been prepared for use of sterile supplies and equipment. This area includes all furniture covered with sterile drapes and personnel who are properly attired.

Sterile Technique Methods by which contamination with microorganisms is prevented to maintain sterility throughout the operative procedure.

Sterilization Processes by which all pathogenic and nonpathogenic microorganisms, including spores, are killed. This term refers *only* to a process capable of destroying *all* forms of microbial life, including spores.

Sterilizer Chamber or equipment used to attain either physical or chemical sterilization. Agent used must be capable of killing all forms of microorganisms.

Superinfection Secondary subsequent infection caused by a different microorganism as seen following antibiotic therapy.

Surgically Clean Mechanically cleansed but unsterile. Items are rendered surgically clean by the use of chemical, physical, or mechanical means that markedly reduce the number of microorganisms on them.

Terminal Sterilization and Disinfection Procedures carried out for the destruction of pathogens at end of operative procedure in the OR or in other areas of patient contact, i.e., recovery room, ICU, nursing unit.

Unsterile Inanimate object that has not been subjected to a sterilization process; outside wrapping of package containing sterile item; or person who has not prepared to enter sterile field. Syn., *nonsterile.*

To understand the principles of sterile technique (pages 116 through 120), their purpose and application, one must comprehend infection—the process, causes, and types, especially wound infection.

INFECTION

Careful attention is given to preoperative preparation of the patient and to creation and maintenance of a therapeutic environment. All possible measures are utilized to prevent complications. Postoperative infection is very serious and potentially fatal complication that may result from a single break in technique. Therefore, knowledge of causative agents and their control as well as meticulous practice of aseptic and sterile techniques are the basis of prevention.

The development of passive and active immunization, sterile and aseptic techniques, and antibiotic therapy have had revolutionary effects on surgical practice. Nevertheless, the ideal state of infection-free operative procedures is not always a reality. Wound and systemic infections continue to occur because all the facts are not understood, and individual discipline in carrying out techniques is sometimes lacking. The worldwide problem of infection persists to plague patient and physician alike. Infection is a health hazard of great expense and significance, affecting the final outcome of operative treatment. The quality of life, both physical and psychological, can be drastically altered, sometimes permanently, by infection and the associated "d's": *delayed healing, discomfort, distress, dependency,* and *dollars.* Not infrequently, *disability, deformity,* and *disaster* with ultimate *death* are the result of infection. A mild infection is potentially a severe one.

Clinically, infection is the product of entrance, growth, metabolic activities, and pathophysiological effects of microorganisms in living tissue. It can develop in the surgical patient as a preoperative complication following an injury, or as a postoperative complication of cross contamination or cross infection.

Process of Infection

Sepsis involves three stages: invasion, localization, and resolution leading to recovery. However, the progress toward recovery may revert back to extension of the infection. The characteristics, invasive qualities, and sources of the etiologic microorganism are important in prevention and treatment. Prompt identification of the infecting agent and sensitivity testing are essential so that appropriate antibiotic therapy can be instituted.

Acute bacterial infection is the most common sepsis in surgical patients. Infection usually develops as a diffuse, inflammatory process, known as *cellulitis,* characterized by pain, redness, and swelling. This inflammatory response is the body's initial defense directed toward localization and containment of the infecting agent. Red blood cells, leukocytes, and macrophages infiltrate the cells, with abscess formation (suppuration) often following. An *abscess* is the result of tissue liquefaction with pus formation, supported by bacterial proteolytic enzymes that break down protein and aid in the spread of infection. Fibrolysin, for example, an enzyme produced by hemolytic Streptococcus, may dissolve fibrin and delay localization of a streptococcal infection. However, the body attempts to wall off an abscess by means of a membrane that produces surrounding induration (hardened tissue) and heat. Localized pus should be promptly drained.

If localization is inadequate and does not contain the infectious process, spreading and extension occur, causing regional infection. Microorganisms and their metabolic products are carried from the primary invasion site into the lymphatic system, spreading along anatomic planes, causing lymphangitis. Failure of the lymph nodes to hold the infection results in uncontrolled cellulitis. Subsequently, regional and/or systemic infection may develop, characterized by chills, fever, and signs of toxicity. Septic emboli may enter the circulatory system from septic thrombophlebitis of from the primary invasion site into the lymphatic tions. These emboli and pathogenic microorganisms in the blood seed invasive infection and abscess formation in remote tissues.

Sepsis elevates the patient's metabolic rate 30 to 40 percent above average, imposing additional stress on the vital systems. For example, cardiac output is about 60 percent above normal resting value. The body's defenses and ability to meet the stress govern whether the infectious process progresses to septic shock (see Chap. 36) with grave prognosis, or whether resolution and recovery are the outcome. Multiple infection sites, the presence of shock, and inappropriate antibiotic therapy result in poor prognosis.

The ultimate resolution of infection depends on immunological and inflammatory responses capable of overcoming the infectious process. This is associated with drainage and removal of foreign material, including debris of bacteria and cells, lysis (disintegration) of microorganisms, resorption of pus, and sloughing of necrotic tissue. Healing then ensues.

Classification of Infections

Surgical infections may be classified in various ways: by source or base, by anatomic location and pathophysiological changes, or by etiology.

Classification by Source This broad classification includes the following types of infections:

1 *Community-acquired infections.* These are natural disease processes that develop or were incubating before a patient's admission to the hospital. *Spontaneous* infections requiring operative diagnosis and/or treatment for management, or as adjuvants to medical therapy, include acute appendicitis, cholecystitis, or bowel perforation with peritonitis. Therapy consists of identification of infection site, etiology, excision or drainage, prevention of further contamination, and augmentation of host resistance.

2 *Nosocomial infections.* Infections in hospitalized patients that were not present or incubating when patient was admitted are *hospital-associated.* They may occur as complications of operative or other procedures performed on uninfected patients. The term also refers to complicating infections in organs unrelated to the operative procedure, occurring with or as a result of postoperative care. About 70 percent of all nosocomial infections develop in surgical patients. The majority are related to instrumentation of the urinary and respiratory tracts. Wound infection is the second most common infection. Examples of various nosocomial infections are:
   - **a** Urinary tract or respiratory tract infection, infected decubiti
   - **b** Cellulitis or abscess formation, related to operative procedure, such as intraabdominal abscess following gastrointestinal procedure
   - **c** Thrombophlebitis or peritonitis, regional extensions of postoperative or posttraumatic infections
   - **d** Liver, lung, or visceral abscess following operation often performed for penetrating injuries or malignant metastases
   - **e** Bacteremia or septicemia, postoperative systemic infection resulting from dissemination of microorganisms into the bloodstream from a distributing focus

Hospital-associated infections may be *exogenous,* from sources outside the body such as personnel or environment, or *endogenous,* from sources within the body. Most postoperative wound infections result from seeding by endogenous microorganisms. Disruption of balance between potentially pathogenic organisms and host defenses permits invasion of microorganisms for which the patient is the primary reservoir. For example, abdominal sepsis may result from enteric flora if the intestine is perforated or transected. However, cross contamination occurs when organisms are transferred to the patient from another individual.

Classification by Etiology This classification of infections includes:

1 *Bacterial infections.* Infections caused by aerobic bacteria, microaerophilic bacteria, anaerobic bacteria, or mixed infections (aerobic and anaerobic, gram-positive and gram-negative, synergistic microorganisms).

2 *Nonbacterial infections.* Infections caused by fungi or by viruses. Specific organisms are discussed later in this chapter.

Factors Affecting Infection Rates

Incidence and types of infections that occur in surgical patients are affected by the following adjuvant factors, which substantially increase the risk.

1 Malnutrition. Whether primary or secondary to catabolic disease, malnutrition is a major factor influencing response to all types of infections since a number of factors, such as inflammatory response, are altered in the malnourished host. Protein deficiency is especially significant in extensive burn or multiple injury patients with greatly raised caloric requirements.

2 Age. Premature or newborn infants, and geriatric patients are especially prone to infection.

3 Obesity. Avascular subcutaneous fatty tissues are especially susceptible.

4 Chronic disease. Fibrocystic disease, diabetes, alcoholism, and malignancies upset normal physiology.

5 Remote focus of infection, especially in the respiratory or urinary tracts. Remote infection is a contraindication for any elective operation as it increases threefold the chance of wound infection.

6 Impaired defense mechanisms. Immunologic response is deficient because of disease, drug therapy such as steroids and immunosuppressive agents, or radiation. Patients of this status, referred to as *immunosuppressed* or *compromised hosts,* are often victims of infection caused by endogenous microbial flora, which are normal but potentially pathogenic flora within their own bodies. Lack of integrity of the immune system, such as leukopenia or defective immunoglobulin synthesis, can be life-threatening.

7 Cardiovascular or respiratory determi-

nants. Examples are tissue perfusion or structural bronchopulmonary disease.

8 Duration of preoperative hospitalization. Some organisms maintain virulence by passing from patient to patient. The hospital environment is a concentrated reservoir of microorganisms that can colonize patients, especially those who have received antibiotics. The organisms are rapidly and easily transferred between people and equipment. A noncarrier may become a carrier of an organism that eventually causes an infection of endogenous origin. Studies show short preoperative stays are associated with low wound infection rates. Risk of infection increases with length of hospitalization.

9 Certain types of operations. Many procedures involve the genitourinary or gastrointestinal tracts. Some contamination occurs whenever these tracts are opened. Extent of contamination at operation is an important factor.

10 Duration of operation. The longer the procedure, the greater the chance of contamination and infection.

11 Operative technique. Injured ischemic tissues, denuded bone, implanted foreign bodies or prosthetic devices have a propensity for microbial invasion. A wound heals faster if tissues are gently handled because fewer cells are destroyed. Necrotic tissue is microbial media. All invasive techniques are potential contaminants.

12 Catheters and drains. Closed drainage systems are preferred to minimize microbial migration.

13 Indiscriminate use of antibiotics (see p. 114). Suppression of normal flora of the skin, bowel, and pharynx, which may play a protective role in defense against pathogenic organisms, may predispose the patient to infection. Antibiotics suppress normal flora.

14 Breakdown of isolation procedures (see p. 111). This may be due to lack of knowledge on the part of hospital personnel regarding epidemiology.

In summary, many factors influence incidence of infection. Exposure of an increasingly high number of high-risk patients to the hospital environment, inhabited by virulent antibiotic-resistant organisms, contributes to infection. High-risk patients increasingly undergo complex and/or prolonged diagnostic and operative procedures under anesthesia. The accompanying instrumentation and use of medical devices open more portals for microbial entry. Complex therapeutic or supportive procedures, such as invasive monitoring by means of indwelling intraarterial or intravenous catheters, may provide microorganisms with an entry to the bloodstream. Continuous urinary catheterization increases the prevalence of urinary tract infection. The concomitant administration of drugs that reduce bodily resistance is a significant factor that favors development of nosocomial infection.

Factors Contributing to Infection

Infection results from interaction of three elements: organisms, tissues, and host defenses. Stated as an equation, infection equals number of organisms multiplied by virulence and divided by host resistance. Surgery reduces resistance.

1 *Pathogenic microorganisms* must be introduced or already present, then survive and propagate in wound or other body tissue. Severity of infection depends in part on size and virulence of inoculum (microbe-containing substance). The infecting agent must reach the host.

2 *Local factors* such as location of operative or invasive site and condition of tissues therein are significant. Necrotic, devitalized avascular tissue, or presence of foreign bodies or accumulated blood, enhance infection by providing excellent media for microbial growth. Various body tissues have different powers of resistance. The abdomen, thigh, calf, and buttocks are especially susceptible. The face, scalp, and chest are more resistant. Severe traumatic injuries and debilitating chronic diseases can make all tissues susceptible to infection.

3 *Host defense mechanisms* are extremely important. Biologic relationships between host defense, trauma of operation, and antibiotic therapy are complex. Body responses vary with the type of infecting microorganism, immune response of the patient, severity of infection, and effectiveness of treatment. The general health of patient influences resistance to microbial invasion.

Etiologic Microorganisms

Infections may be caused by one or several types of organisms. Types are numerous and vary in regard to incidence and significance of infection produced. Reader is referred to a standard textbook of microbiology for details.

Bacteria are classified as gram-positive or -negative and by the environment that sustains their life. The most common *pathogens* are:

1 Aerobic bacteria (require oxygen)
   a Gram-positive cocci, such as *Staphylococcus aureus, Staphylococcus epidermidis, Streptococcus Group B, Streptococcus Group D*
   b Gram-negative cocci, such as *Neisseria gonorrhoeae*
   c Gram-positive bacilli, such as *Bacillus* species, *Mycobacterium* species
   d Gram-negative bacilli, such as *Escherichia coli, Klebsiella* species, *Pseudomonas aeruginosa, Pseudomonas cepacia, Proteus* species, Providence species, *Serratia marcescens, Citrobacter* species, *Salmonella* species, *Alcaligenes faecalis, Hemophilus influenzae, Enterobacter aerogenes, Enterobacter cloacae*
2 Microaerophilic bacteria (require oxygen less than in atmosphere)
   a Gram-positive cocci, such as hemolytic and nonhemolytic streptococci
3 Anaerobic bacteria (grow in absence of oxygen)
   a Gram-positive cocci, such as peptostreptococcus, peptococcus
   b Gram-positive bacilli, such as *Clostridium tetani* and *Clostridium welchii*
   c Gram-negative bacilli, such as *Bacteroides* species, *Bacteroides fragilis*
4 Nonbacterial microorganisms
   a Viruses, such as *Herpesvirus,* hepatitis virus
   b Fungi, such as *Candida albicans, Histoplasmosis capsulatum, Phycomycosis* species.

NOTE. This list is incomplete but includes *the organisms that most frequently cause nosocomial infections.* Some organisms are primary invaders; others are opportunists that secondarily invade or superimpose upon an already infected host with inhibited resistance. Identification of causative organisms will direct investigation, e.g., streptococcus or *Staphylococcus aureus* from personnel, mycobacterium from inanimate objects. Epidemics caused by gram-negative microorganisms may be spread from environmental sources. Every microorganism is a potential pathogen given dense enough contamination and a crippled enough host.

Viability of Organisms Organisms need moisture, food, proper temperature, and time to reproduce. When they are transferred from one place to another, they pass through a dormant or lag phase of about five hours. Then each organism divides itself every 20 minutes. Air or objects containing live microorganisms contaminate on contact. Viable microorganisms are killed by the processes of sterilization (see Chap. 8).

Toxins of Microbial Origin Pathogenic microorganisms produce substances that adversely affect the host locally and/or systemically upon invasion. Toxic substances affecting tissues, cells, and possibly enzyme systems diffuse from the microbial cells. The cellular substance of a wide variety of organisms is toxic also. In addition, harmful effects may be produced indirectly by activation of tissue enzymes by bacteria. Such toxic substances include:

1 *Exotoxins,* classic bacterial toxins, are most potent toxins known. As little as 7 oz (200 cc) of crystalline botulism type A toxin is said to be able to kill the world's entire population. Exotoxins appear to be proteins, are denatured by heat, and are destroyed by proteolytic enzymes which break down protein. The formation of exotoxins is relatively uncommon but their actions are multiple.
2 *Endotoxins* are contained within the cell wall of bacteria. They are heat stable and are not digested by proteolytic enzymes. On parenteral inoculation they cause a rise in body temperature and are known as *bacterial pyrogens.* They increase capillary permeability with resultant production of local hemorrhage. Although causing injury to body cells at site of infection, endotoxins more importantly cause serious, often lethal, effects by dissemination and widespread injury to many tissues throughout the body. Endotoxic shock may occur in bacteremia due to gram-negative bacteria.
3 Microorganisms also form a variety of other heterogeneous toxic substances, often enzymatic in nature, which may contribute to the disease process directly or facilitate the establishment of foci of infection. Toxins, which diffuse from the intact microbial cell, have the following various effects:
   a *Cytotoxic effect* affects red and white blood cells, e.g., causing leukopenia (reduction of leukocytes below normal).
   b *Clotting effect* interferes with the clotting mechanism of blood.
   c *Enzyme effect* causes bacterial hemolysins to dissolve red blood cells or fibrin, thereby in-

hibiting clot formation. *Coagulase,* a substance of bacterial origin, is causally related to thrombus formation. Coagulase-positive staphylococcus, *B. subtilis, E. coli, S. marcescens,* accelerate clotting of blood and induce intravascular clotting.

4 Toxic substances are also associated with viruses.

5 Some bacteria are encapsulated, a defense mechanism against phagocytic activity of leukocytes. These bacteria may be ingested by white blood cells, but instead of being killed and digested they remain within the phagocyte for a time, then are extruded in a viable condition. The presence of a capsule is associated with virulence among pathogenic bacteria.

Wound Infections

Wound infections warrant special attention because many occur in clean wounds as a result of microorganisms introduced into the wound at time of operation. Secondary contamination is uncommon because fibrin seals the wound within hours after operation. However, wound healing can be interrupted by infection at almost any phase (see Chap. 17). Infection results from introduction of virulent microorganisms into the receptive wound of a susceptible host. Moisture and warmth in wound creates an environment conducive to bacterial growth.

Operative wound infection may be related to the incisional wound or to deep structures that were entered or exposed. The nature and severity vary because of local, systemic, technical, or environmental factors. Each factor is important; all are interrelated in clinical infection. Usually an infection is localized and does not progress to a major complication, but severe local or systemic reaction is possible. The specific pathogen and site of infection largely determine its gravity. Infection involving an implanted foreign body or gross necrotic tissue is prone to serious sequellae. Gram-negative bacteria and *Staphylococcus aureus* are the most frequent pathogens isolated from operative wounds.

Classification of Operative Wounds Classification provides standardization and a resource for comparison of wound infection rates. The circulating nurse should ask the surgeon to classify the wound at end of operation. This classification should be recorded in the patient's record and OR log. The information is used to compute the hospital's infection rate. Reduction in infection can be attributed to surveillance for infection, informing surgeons of their infection rates, and implementation of other infection control measures. The OR staff should be cognizant of wound infection statistics. Operative wounds may be specifically classified by:

1 Clinical significance
   a *Uninfected.* Heal without discharge.
   b *Possibly infected.* Inflamed, with no discharge or culture-positive serous fluid.
   c *Infected.* Suppuration present.
2 Contamination-infection risk
   a *Clean.* Alimentary, respiratory, genitourinary tracts or oropharyngeal cavity not entered; no inflammation present. No break in technique occurred. Elective procedure with wound made under ideal OR conditions. Primary closure usually not drained. Example: herniorrhaphy. Expected infection rate: 1 to 3 percent.
   b *Clean-contaminated.* Alimentary, respiratory, or genitourinary tracts or oropharyngeal cavity entered under controlled conditions without significant spillage or unusual contamination. No inflammation or infection. Minor break in technique occurred. Wound drained. Example: hysterectomy, cholecystectomy. Infection rate: 8 to 11 percent.
   c *Contaminated.* Gross spillage/contamination from gastrointestinal tract. Major break in technique occurred. Open fresh traumatic wounds of less than four hours. Acute nonpurulent inflammation encountered. Entrance into genitourinary or biliary tracts with infected urine or bile present. Example: inflamed but unruptured gallbladder, cystitis. Infection rate: 15 to 20 percent.
   d *Dirty and infected.* Existing clinical infection; acute bacterial inflammation with or without purulence encountered; abscess. Perforated viscus. Old traumatic wounds of over four hours duration from dirty source or with retained necrotic tissue, foreign body, or fecal contamination. Organisms present in operative field before procedure. Example: abdominal gunshot wound with perforated viscus. Infection rate: 27 to 40 percent.

The critical issue is elimination of infection in clean wounds, for overt tissue destruction can result. The aim should be for a clean wound infection rate of one percent or less. Infection rates vary by surgical specialty, type of procedure, and individual surgeon, but reflect the intraoperative care in an institution. Wound sepsis remains one of the prime problems in the surgeon's daily practice (see Chaps. 17 and 36).

SOURCES OF CONTAMINATION

In spite of many variables associated with sepsis, people remain the major source of microorganisms in the environment. Everything on or around a human being is contaminated by him or her in some way. Additionally, the action and interaction of personnel and patients contribute to prevalence of organisms.

Operating room personnel are primarily concerned with protecting the operating room suite environment. Operative procedures should be performed under optimal conditions within the limits of professional capability. The three most critical areas for the introduction and spread of microorganisms are:

1 Unrestricted interchange area, open to personnel generally

2 Semirestricted intermediate zone, open to properly attired authorized personnel

3 Restricted sterile work area or inner zone, occupied by the operating teams and patients, including the operating rooms, scrub rooms, and induction areas (see Chap.6).

Many sources contaminate the OR environment.

Skin

Skin of patients, operating team members, and visitors constitutes a hazard. Hair follicles, sebaceous and sweat glands (sudoriferous) contain abundant resident microbial flora. An estimated 4000 to 10,000 viable particles are shed by an average individual's skin per minute. Some people disperse up to 30,000 particles per minute. *Shedders* are persons who present an additional hazard. They are densely populated with virulent organisms that they shed with skin cells into the environment. These organisms usually are *Staphylococcus aureus.* Shedders have a much higher incidence of wound infection. True shedders are estimated to be 1 in 50 persons. Cosmetic detritus is also laden with skin bacteria. Major areas of microbial population on all persons are the head, neck, axilla, hands, groin, perineum, legs, and feet. Microbial shedding is contained most effectively by maximum skin coverage (see Chaps. 9 and 16).

Hair

Hair is a gross contaminant and major source of staphylococcus. The microbial population attracted to and shed from hair is directly related to length and cleanliness. Hair follicles and filaments harbor resident and transient flora.

Nasopharynx

Organisms forcibly expelled by talking, coughing, or sneezing give rise to bacteria-laden dust and lint as droplets settle on surfaces and skin. Persons known as *carriers* harbor many organisms, notably *Group A Streptococcus* and *Staphylococcus aureus,* which may be carried pharyngeally or rectally. They usually are transmitted by direct contact. More surgeons and anesthesiologists are carriers than nurses because of intimate contact with patients' respiratory tracts. Carriers do not usually present a real threat in absence of an overt lesion. However, when clusters of infection break out postoperatively, shedders and carriers who disseminate organisms and whose organism matches that of infected patients are sought.

Fomites

Contaminated particles are present on inanimate objects such as furniture, operating room surfaces (walls, floors, cabinet shelves), equipment, supplies, linens. Stringent measures, to be discussed, are used to control contact contamination from such sources. Covert contamination may result, however, from improper handling of equipment such as anesthesia apparatus, or intravenous lines and fluids. Contamination may result from the administration of unsterile medications or use of unsterile water to rinse sterile items.

Air

Thousands of submicron size particles per cubic foot of air are present in the OR. During a long operative procedure, particle count can rise to over a million particles per cubic foot. Air and dust are vehicles for transporting microorganism-laden particles. Air movement and thermal currents entrain dust and microbial particulates that remain airborne and can then settle onto open wounds, burns, or other susceptible tissue. Since airborne contamination is generated by personnel, every movement increases potential for wound infection. Microorganisms have an affinity for horizontal surfaces, the largest of which is the floor. From it, they are projected into the air.

Endogenous, as well as exogenous, microbial flora is significant. The patient's skin, oropharynx, tracheobronchial tree, and gastrointestinal tract support growth of innumerable organisms, which reflects the amount and kind of infection in the hospital population. Microorganisms from infected patients or carriers settle on equipment and flat surfaces, then become airborne.

An effective ventilation system is essential to avoid patients and staff breathing contaminated air that predisposes them to respiratory infection and that increases the incidence of microbial carriers among OR personnel. It is generally believed that objects, not air, are the major vehicles for the transmission of pathogens and that person-to-person contact remains the most frequent means by which infection is spread.

Human Error

Human error is an exogenous source of contamination not be be underestimated. Lives are at stake, no less so if breaks in technique occur through lack of knowledge or lack of adherence to principles of technique and their applications. Errors must be readily admitted and corrected.

INFECTION CONTROL

Infection control translates knowledge into action. It incorporates development and maintenance of an attitude of awareness of infection with acceptance of individual and collective responsibility to prevent infection. Although the scope of infection control encompasses the entire hospital, the focus of this text is infection control in the surgical patient, primarily control of wound infection that can obviate the benefits of surgical intervention. Infection control concerns keeping number of microorganisms to an irreducible minimum.

The purposes of infection control are to:

1 Minimize infection, and hopefully to eventually obliterate it
2 Improve wound healing
3 Minimize disability, morbidity, and mortality
4 Reduce the cost of hospital care

The many aspects of infection control include:

1 Establishment and utilization of an effective infection control program
2 Recognition of hazards and consistent adherence to established control practices
3 Provision of maximum protection to patients by means of physical barriers to microorganisms and functional measures of control
4 Limitation of the use of antibiotics to reduce resistant strains of microorganisms

Infection Control Program

An effective infection control program aims to reduce the incidence of infections and to control sources. Information collected through surveillance serves as a basis for corrective action. This information includes written records and reports of known or potential infections among patients and personnel.

Guidelines and standards for a comprehensive infection control program and surveillance are published by the Joint Commission on the Accreditation of Hospitals (JCAH) in the *Accreditation Manual for Hospitals.* In general, these standards and guidelines include:

1 Establishment of an effective hospital infection control program monitored by a multidisciplinary infection control committee
2 Development of specific written infection control policies and procedures for all services throughout the hospital
3 Preventive surveillance and control procedures relating to the hospital environment
4 Provision for essential laboratory support
5 Written policies defining indications for isolation and necessary provisions for it
6 Definitions of nosocomial infections for surveillance purposes to provide early uniform identification and reporting of infections
7 Determination of hospital infection rates
8 Coordination with the medical staff on action regarding findings from the staff's review of clinical use of antibiotics
9 Ongoing review and evaluation of all aseptic, isolation, and environmental control techniques of the hospital
10 Orientation of new employees regarding

personal hygiene and importance of infection control while caring for patients

11 Input into content and scope of employee health service

12 Reporting, evaluating, and maintaining records of infections occurring in patients and personnel

Infection Control Coordinator

An infection control program utilizes the services of a key person and agent of the infection control committee, the *infection control coordinator.* Since this person is often a registered nurse with special training in epidemiology, microbiology, statistics; and research methodology, he or she may be referred to as an *infection control nurse (ICN)* or *nurse epidemiologist.* The infection control coordinator keeps a finger on the pulse of the infection situation in the hospital by monitoring the hospital environment for infections. While in close collaboration with the infection control committee, the ICNs duties include all aspects of control activities such as:

1 Prompt investigation of outbreaks of disease or infection above expected levels.

2 Prompt identification of origin and etiology of outbreaks by epidemiologic study.

3 Acquisition, correlation, analysis, and evaluation of surveillance data and bacterial colony counts for infection control. This includes gathering information to compute and classify specific wound infection rates for all operations. Rates should be entered in infection control committee record, and be available to the department of surgery.

4 Tracing factors that contribute to infection problems.

5 Consultation with directors of critical areas, such as OR. In the case of clusters of wound infections, ICN confers with the ORS and reviews OR log to see if infected patients had same procedure, same operating team, or operative problem.

6 Conduction of educational programs for personnel who influence infection control. The ICN is a consultant to all hospital personnel and a liaison officer in dissemination of information on infection control.

7 Assistance in employee health programs in regard to screening, immunizing, and monitoring personal health of OR personnel.

8 Assistance in development and implementation of improved patient care procedures.

9 Comparison of monthly statistics. There is cause for concern if the monthly reported operative wound infection rate rises significantly. Reports and data can help improve aseptic technique, if brought to attention of personnel.

10 Supervision of reporting appropriate diseases to public health authorities.

11 Comparison of products for effectiveness.

12 Obtaining information about evidence of infection after discharge from ambulatory surgery facility or conducting retrospective study after inpatient discharge, per hospital policy.

In short, the infection control coordinator identifies problems, collects data to find the causes, investigates solutions, and makes recommendations for determining hospital policies and procedures relative to infection control. In evaluating infection problems, the ICN attempts to find a common denominator. This often leads to the source of the problem. For example, an outbreak of postoperative respiratory infections would lead to investigation of cleaning and sterilizing anesthesia equipment and respirators. If a patient develops signs and symptoms of infection within the immediate postoperative period, a causative factor in the OR is suspect. A ratio of one coordinator for every 250 hospital beds is recommended. Success of the control program depends in part on the information provided by a conscientious coordinator.

Surveillance

The Centers for Disease Control (CDC) in Atlanta is an agency of the Department of Health and Human Services, and is the third largest section of the United States Public Health Service. Functioning on both national and international levels, its activities are multifaceted. It carries out a national surveillance of disease incidence and a broad national program against disease, including health education, especially in regard to communicable diseases. Through liaison with state and local health departments, assistance and consultation from the CDC are available to local hospitals for specific problem solving, analysis of surveillance data, or on-site investigation of a serious infection outbreak. As part of its commitment to the prevention of nosocomial infections, the CDC furnishes to hospitals information on how to structure an infection control program. In addition, CDC renders aid to local or state health departments in times of epidemics.

Utilization of the Centers' facilities is optimized in the training course that CDC sponsors for nurses who wish to work in infection control. This course includes basic microbiology, principles and methodology of epidemiology, role of the infection control nurse, and guidance in setting up a hospital infection control program. Follow-up support is given trainees in their subsequent work situations, as needed.

The CDC provides worldwide service as a valuable resource for information. Its many publications include: *Outline for Surveillance and Control of Nosocomial Infections; Guideline for Isolation Precautions in Hospitals; Morbidity and Mortality Weekly Report;* and *Guidelines for Prevention of TB Transmission in Hospitals.* In conjunction with continuous research, CDC establishes guidelines for prevention of wound infections, for intravenous therapy, respiratory therapy, urinary catheterization, and other at-risk procedures, and for isolation techniques (see p. 111).

Effective action results from adequate background information. An important aspect of infection control, *surveillance* involves input or data collection, analysis, and action or regulatory activities. Quality control, establishment of and conformance to standards, is a prerequisite for rational infection control. The value of a surveillance program is the establishment of a statistical data base that can be subsequently correlated with testing to locate a problem or pinpoint changes in infection rates over a period of time. This is accomplished by a comprehensive culturing program or careful periodic checks on the effectiveness of essential equipment, such as sterilizers and anesthesia equipment. However, extensive random bacteriologic sampling of personnel and environment when no problem exists is not recommended by the CDC. Effective surveillance, predicated on an understanding of epidemiology, requires:

1 Investigation of every instance where a patient becomes infected to ascertain if infection is nosocomial or community-acquired.

2 Prompt reporting of infection in any patient to define incidence and type of infection in the hospital.

3 Monitoring of hospital patients, personnel, and environment according to written standards.

4 Identification of factors that place a patient at risk.

5 Clear definitions of infections, an infection control coordinator, computerized records. Storage and programming provide comparisons.

6 Monitoring of wound infection rate to alert staff to deviations from normal and to assess need for changes in procedures because of technological developments.

7 Protection of the patient from reasonable risk for which reasonable control is available. Alerting the surgeon to symptoms of an infection. These measures help to avoid litigation.

Surveillance data are studied to ascertain trends of infection, high rates associated with specific surgical services or operative procedures, or clustering in certain areas. Microbiological surveys are important in evaluating procedures. For example, sampling of floors indicates if the cleaning procedure is effective. Surveys help to answer the question, "What is the problem?" Surveillance provides a basis for improving conditions, procedures, and quality of patient care.

Microbiological Sampling

Routine culturing of air and equipment has not been found to be beneficial. Results are not cost effective. Microbiological sampling, to be purposeful:

1 Investigates an outbreak of nosocomial infection; type of problem directs type of culturing needed for personnel and/or environment.

2 Determines effectiveness of cleaning methods and products.

3 Monitors steam and gas sterilizers (see Chap. 8, p. 137).

4 Audits an increase in postoperative clean wound infection rate.

ENVIRONMENTAL CONTROL

Control of the *operating room environment* is a necessary part of an overall infection control program. The inanimate, as well as animate, environment in the OR suite presents a risk for transmission of infection and disease. The aim of a microbiologically controlled environment is to keep contamination to an irreducible minimum and to maintain balance in favor of the patient, not the microorganisms.

OR suites are designed with optimal function

and safety in mind, and to protect patients from sources of contamination. The suite includes specific areas for traffic, support systems, administration, communication, and storage. Clean and soiled activities, areas, and personnel, as well as sterile and unsterile supplies, should be distinctly separated. Traffic patterns are designed to flow smoothly and to prevent backtrack or cross-over traffic (see Chap. 6).

Barriers

Contact contamination plays a major role in bacterial spread. Therefore, barriers are established to create a safe environment. They protect sterile zones, isolate operative wounds from infectious contaminants, and keep number of microorganisms to a minimum. To retard or prevent transfer of organisms, barriers must be impervious to their passage under ordinary operating conditions posed by team members, a major source of microbial contamination in the OR. Procedures are established to provide barriers against migration of microorganisms from:

1 Skin
- **a** Preoperative skin preparation of patient (see Chap. 16) and operating team (see Chap. 9).
- **b** Special OR attire worn only within the OR suite (see Chap. 9).
- **c** Sterile drapes to cover patient and sterile field (see Chap. 16).
- **d** Occlusion of incised skin edges from the operative wound (see Chap. 16).

2 Nasopharyngeal flora and hair
- **a** Masks worn to cover nose and mouth, changed between patients (see Chap. 9).
- **b** Caps or hoods worn by personnel, part of attire, and by patient to cover hair.
- **c** Removal of hair from operative site (see Chap. 16).
- **d** Exclusion of personnel with acute infection or skin lesion from OR.
- **e** Anesthesia screen to separate anesthesia area from sterile field.

3 Fomites
- **a** Proper packaging of supplies and sterilizing procedures (see Chap. 8).
- **b** Dust covers placed over cool, dry, sterile items in storage.
- **c** Disinfection of OR surfaces, although no residual environmental disinfectant exists.
- **d** Clean, preoperative bed linen.

4 Airborne contamination
- **a** *Conventional air-conditioning systems,* when properly designed, installed, and maintained, effectively reduce the number of airborne bacteria by removing dust and aerosol particles. As fresh clean outside air is supplied, lint- and dust-contaminated air is removed. Recirculation of filtered air at a rate of no less than 25 air volume exchanges per hour is considered safe and economical. Using high-efficiency particulate air (HEPA) filters, the system reduces organisms to 1 to 3 per cubic foot. The dilution principle is used. Air enters from the ceiling, is diluted, and passes out through the lower portion of the room. Filters should be located downstream of air-processing equipment so microorganisms will not be drawn into the room. Warming and cooling fresh air to totally resupply the OR air is expensive. All air, recirculated or fresh, should be filtered before entering the OR.
- **b** *Laminar airflow* is a special air-handling system for the filtration, dilution, and distribution of air. It may be used during operative placement of implants, such as total hip replacement, or other high-risk procedures. Laminar airflow is a controlled unidirectional, positive pressure stream of air that moves either horizontally or vertically across the operative area and room. The controlled airstream entrains particulate matter and microorganisms to prevent their drifting with uncontrolled movement; it sweeps up dormant particles as well. The flow returns to the system and passes through a prefilter to remove gross particles. It then passes through a HEPA filter in each module that traps and eliminates over 99 percent of all particles larger than 0.3 micron. This includes virtually all bacteria and most viruses. A rate of 100 to 400 air changes per hour is possible; most systems deliver about 240 an hour. While the system provides microbial-free air (0 to 1 organism per cubic foot) with minimal air turbulence, *it is not a substitute for meticulous aseptic technique.* No substantial evidence indicates the decrease in particle count results in a significantly reduced rate of operative wound infection.

  The system, available in horizontal or vertical flow, comes with a vacuum hose inlet for use with multiple negative pressure masks and gowns. This bodysuit and hood vacuum system, resembling a spacesuit, prevents bacteria shed by team from reaching the patient. The entire body is covered. Air, piped into the headpiece, is removed through filtered tubes. The hood or helmet is equipped for hearing and speaking. Negative pressure gowns are impervious to moisture and microorganisms. No mask is needed with the helmet. The system provides body cooling of the wearer.

Unidirectional clean-air systems are a valuable adjunct to controlling airborne contamination. They reliably reduce bacterial contamination at the wound site.

NOTE. A bioclean room, a special enclosure within an OR, referred to as a *greenhouse,* may be installed in conjunction with laminar airflow.

c *Doors* to and in the OR should be kept closed except as needed for passage of patient and personnel or supplies and equipment. Disrupted pressurization mixes inside OR air with corridor air of higher bacterial count. Cabinet doors should remain closed.

d *Traffic* in and out of the OR must be kept to a minimum. Persons within OR during preparation and operation should be restricted to OR team and authorized technologists to reduce fallout from bacterial shedding.

e *Activity* increases air turbulence which carries bacteria to wound. Movement in OR must be reduced to minimum.

f *Textile lubricant* added to final rinse during laundering minimizes lint resulting from friction of fibers against each other. Disintegrated paper from disposable products is a source of lint on fabrics. Paper products should not be discarded with soiled linen.

Environmental Services/Housekeeping

Housekeeping practices using the most effective supplies, techniques, and equipment available are a most important aspect of infection control. *Housekeeping* procedures include cleaning and disinfecting the operating rooms and suite, handling soiled laundry, and disposing of solid wastes. They are carried out according to established practices, policies, and schedules. These procedures are performed by environmental service personnel under supervision. Good housekeeping cleaning techniques should reduce microbial flora by about 90 percent. *Detergent-disinfectants alone are no substitute for thorough mechanical cleansing,* the proverbial "elbow grease." Locations that by design or construction are difficult to clean and areas that may be touched by patients or personnel are of primary concern.

Any equipment or procedure requiring water in its operation presents a hazard, especially if water is not continually changed or sinks cleaned. Unsterile water, the universal solvent and transporter, can support, maintain, and protect almost every contaminant produced by human beings. The numbers, types, and species of microorganisms in a water supply are limited only by the attention paid to equipment containing it. Water especially supports the growth of certain gram-negative bacilli, including *Serratia, Pseudomonas, Alcaligenes, Flavobacterium* genus. Aerosols produced during hand scrubs become airborne and contaminate. Disinfectants reduce the contamination of cleaning water.

Points in housekeeping, especially relevant to infection control and prevention of cross infection, are listed to emphasize importance of OR environmental control.

1 Faucet heads should be a type that does not hold water. They should be removed for sterilization. Handwash antiseptic containers should be sterilized before refill.

2 No surface should remain wet, thereby supporting microbial growth.

3 Organic debris should be promptly removed from walls and OR surfaces with a germicide to prevent drying and airborne contamination.

4 Lights and overhead tracks should be cleaned at least twice daily, prior to first scheduled operation and upon completion of schedule.

5 Entrance to OR suite and floors in corridors and rooms should be cleaned with the wet-vacuum system. Dry debris is removed with dry vacuum, the floor is sprayed with detergent-disinfectant solution and wet-vacuumed.

6 Housekeeping equipment should be kept clean and dry, and never stored moist in a dark area conducive to microbial growth.

7 Disposable waste should be put in covered receptacles lined with plastic liners.

8 Service elevators rather than chutes should be used to remove soiled laundry and waste disposal from OR suite. Chutes become grossly contaminated and are both an airborne contamination and a fire hazard.

9 Waste should be contained at source of origin to prevent aerosol generation during handling. Contaminated waste must be decontaminated and/or sterilized before compaction or disposal in general environment. Incineration is most effective means of waste disposal, especially infectious wastes.

10 *Adequate time must be allowed between patients for proper terminal disinfection of the room* (see Chap. 10). A patient must not be assigned to any OR of questionable environment from which the patient might acquire a wound infection.

Isolation

Isolation of patients by diagnosis or prognosis is another means of infection control. The specific technique is related to mode of transmission of pathogenic microorganisms, i.e., contact, air, or fomites. Isolation precautions and guidelines are detailed in hospital procedure books and in the CDC *Guideline for Isolation Precautions in Hospitals.* Two different methods of isolation technique are described:

1 Category-specific isolation precautions, such as strict, contact, respiratory, acid-fast bacilli (AFB), enteric, drainage/secretion, and blood/body fluids.

2 Disease-specific isolation precautions, recommendations for each specific infectious disease.

Each hospital may incorporate into its procedures whichever method is more appropriate for its particular needs and patient population. Before a patient on isolation precautions comes to the OR, the unit should inform the OR staff. A sticker on the patient's chart indicates the type of hospital isolation. For most patients, the same precautions apply in the OR as on the unit. A common sense approach is used. In all types of isolation, the most important control measure is *thorough handwashing* before and after close patient contact, after handling contaminated objects, body fluids or excretions, and between patients. Isolation techniques must not be implemented in a way that causes the patient to feel victimized. The patient should be educated to accept the regimen.

Cross Infection in the OR *Every patient in the OR should be considered potentially infected.* Specific isolation precautions are observed, in addition to routine aseptic techniques, if patient has a known infectious or communicable disease. However, the specific organism may be unknown at time of operation.

Care, caution, and competence are essential to prevent *cross infection,* which stems mainly from breaks in aseptic technique by involved personnel. The more microorganisms are prevented from entering an environment, the less chance of cross infection. *The importance of thorough frequent handwashing cannot be overemphasized.*

Tuberculosis Tuberculosis is caused by *Mycobacterium tuberculosis,* an aerobic gram-positive bacillus. Incidence of the disease in the general population has decreased, but treatment takes place in the general hospital, increasing the risk of transmission. In the hospital, the disease must be monitored and controlled to prevent cross infection. Unsuspected active cases represent a particular hazard. Patients with acute disease often are isolated for approximately two weeks following initiation of chemotherapy. For care of surgical patients, recommendation has been made to:

1 Postpone elective operation in active cases until the patient shows response to chemotherapy.

2 Use disposable anesthesia equipment as much as is feasible. Reusable equipment must be immediately sterilized after use.

3 Use respiratory isolation precautions for suspected patients and those with positive sputum.

4 Skin test OR personnel semiannually.

Hepatitis Drugs, chemicals, and viruses can produce inflammation of the liver, but acute hepatitis usually is caused by one of the hepatitis viruses: A (HAV), B (HBV), or non-A non-B (NANB). These pathogens differ remarkably.

Hepatitis A is not a major nosocomial problem. It does not involve a carrier state. It is spread by oral ingestion of fecal contaminants.

In contrast, hepatitis B (formerly known as serum hepatitis) is a major nosocomial problem. Carriers are a main source of cross infection, and may develop chronic hepatitis, cirrhosis, or liver carcinoma. Serologic tests are used to diagnose, detect carriers, and monitor high-risk groups. But it is possible for asymptomatic persons infected with hepatitis B to escape detection. Patients who have undiagnosed hepatitis, or who fail to reveal that they have chronic hepatitis or are asymptomatic carriers, potentially can transmit the virus to hospital staff. Hepatitis B is transmitted percutaneously or permucosally by blood and blood derivatives, semen, and saliva. Incubation period is six weeks to six months, producing mild to fulminant disease. The latter is rare but often fatal. Severity of disease increases with age. Individuals at high risk are health care workers who have frequent contact with blood, as in OR, ED, or hemodialysis unit. In the hospital, primary transmission from patient-to-staff is through direct contact with body fluids or via fomites.

Non-A non-B agents are responsible for about 90 percent of posttransfusion hepatitis. NANB probably includes more than one virus, and possibly three. Since NANB agents are unidentified, serologic markers do not diagnose this hepatitis. Diagnosis is made by excluding hepatitis A and B. NABA is worldwide, blood-borne, and resembles hepatitis B in transmission. As with hepatitis B, disease can be spread by IV drug abuse and sexual contact. It is frequently found in homosexual males. Incubation period varies from less than two weeks to more than six months.

Hospital-associated B and NANB hepatitis may be due to blood and serum contacts from a needle stick or scalpel injury, breaks in the skin from cut, burn or abrasion, or splash into mucosa of eye, nose, or mouth. However, special care should be taken when handling any body fluid or secretion. *Follow hospital policy for precautionary protocol. Precautions usually include:*

1 Impeccable handwashing before and after direct contact with patient or items in contact with patient's blood or feces.

2 Avoidance of parenteral exposure such as accidental self puncture with contaminated needle. Any accidental exposure should be followed up as soon as possible in the Employee Health Clinic, even if the patient is not known to have hepatitis.

3 Covering abrasions or cuts on hand.

4 Wearing gloves when handling blood, excreta, drainage, secretions.

5 Wearing gown for direct contact with blood or feces, or performing procedures in which excess blood spills or splatter may occur.

6 Meticulous decontamination of used equipment and materials followed by sterilization (see Chap. 10).

Transmission of hepatitis is preventable. Use of hepatitis B vaccine may be considered for high-risk groups prophylactically. However, the vaccine should not give a false sense of security or be a substitute for conscientious adherence to aseptic practices.

Acquired Immune Deficiency Syndrome (AIDS) AIDS is a deadly disease characterized by breakdown of the immune system in patients with no previously known immune deficiency. Without apparant explanation, victims become markedly susceptible to a wide variety of infections and certain forms of cancer. Etiology appears to be retrovirus HTLV III, human T-cell leukemia virus type III. An enzyme-linked immunosorbent assay (ELISA) may detect antibodies to HTLV III to determine whether a person has been exposed to this virus. AIDS may be infectious during the incubation period, believed to vary from six months to two years.

At present there is no known cure. The crippled cellular immune system apparently never recovers. AIDS victims may survive one infection only to succumb to another more devastating one. AIDS patients develop opportunistic infections such as *Pneumocystis carinii* pneumonia, and malignancies such as Kaposi's sarcoma or lymphomas. Other common infections are cytomegalovirus, severe mucocutaneous herpes simplex, candidiasis, cryptococcosis, and myobacterial infections. Symptoms may be specific to the opportunistic disease, but marked fatigue, severe diarrhea, weight loss, lymphadenopathy, fever, and night sweats are striking features.

Transmission is attributed to direct contact of skin or mucous membranes with the victim's blood, blood products, or semen, and possibly to contact with excretions, secretions, and tissues. Transmission appears to require intimate direct contact of mucosal surfaces or through parenteral spread. Airborne or casual contact spread seems unlikely.

Established risk groups include homo- and bisexual males, IV drug abusers, Haitians, hemophiliacs and other recipients of blood products, female sexual partners of men in these groups, and some children born to these women. Meeting the psychological and physical needs of these patients presents a special challenge. AIDS patients may come to the OR for:

1 Diagnostic procedures, e.g., biopsies of skin or lymph nodes, or bronchoscopy.

2 Palliative procedures, e.g., removal of malignant skin lesions or other cancerous growth, or tracheotomy.

CDC has recommended that precautions similar to those used for patients with hepatitis B virus be used in caring for AIDS patients. Briefly, these are:

1 Use extraordinary care to avoid accidental wounds from contaminated instruments. Avoid exposure of existing breaks in skin to potentially infected material.

2 Always wear gloves when handling specimens, blood, body fluids, secretions, or excretions of the patient, in addition to items and surfaces soiled by these contaminants.

3 Wear gown when contamination of clothing by body fluids, blood, secretions, or excretions may occur.

4 Wash hands immediately and thoroughly before and after close contact with the patient or blood, or after removing gown and gloves.

5 Double bag and label all blood and specimens with "Blood Precautions" or "AIDS Precautions." Remove blood from outside of a specimen container with disinfectant, such as 1:10 dilution of 5.25% sodium hypochlorite with water, prepared daily.

6 Clean blood spills and leakage of any body fluid with disinfectant solution.

7 Place blood-soiled articles in an impervious bag clearly labeled "AIDS Precautions" or "Blood Precautions" before sending for reprocessing or disposal. Or, place these items in special color-coded bags designated solely for disposal of infectious wastes. Dispose of infectious wastes according to hospital policy. Many hospitals incinerate these wastes. Use the hospital's hepatitis B guidelines for reprocessing contaminated reusable items.

8 Place needles and other sharp objects in a puncture-resistant container, for incineration. Do *not* recap needles before discard as this is a common cause of needle injury.

9 Use only disposable supplies when possible, especially needles and syringes. For safety, use only needle-locking syringes or one-piece needle-syringe units to aspirate body fluids. Decontaminate reusable syringes before reprocessing.

10 Private hospital room is indicated for patient too ill to use good hygiene, e.g., those with profuse diarrhea, fecal incontinence, or behavioral changes due to central nervous system infections.

In addition to the above, utilize specific precautions for the particular infections that concurrently occur in AIDS patients. Other suggested recommendations are:

1 Lensed instruments (endoscopes) *must* be sterilized after use on an AIDS patient.

2 Procedures and manipulations of potentially infectious material should be performed carefully to minimize creation of droplets and aerosols.

3 During procedures where aerosols of blood or other secretions are likely to form, e.g., endoscopy, staff should wear protective eyewear or goggles.

4 Remove unnecessary items from OR to minimize surface exposure, as feasible.

Creutzfeldt-Jakob Disease (CJD) CJD is a rapidly progressive fatal disease of the central nervous system characterized by spongiform encephalopathy, dementia, and myoclonus. The etiology is unknown, but CJD possibly is caused by a prion, virus, or spiroplasma. The causative organism is unusually resistant to disinfectants and heat. The natural means of transmission is unknown. Although very rare, nosocomial infection has been documented following ocular (corneal transplant) and intracerebral (stereotactic electrodes) contamination. It appears that the potential for noninvasive bodily contact transmission is very low.

Premortem confirmation of diagnosis often is not made, as classical clinical symptoms may be absent or appear late, although diagnosis may be suspected. Diagnostic confirmation usually is dependent on neuropathologic tissue examination at autopsy and animal transmission studies, a lengthy process.

Unanswered questions about the causative agent, mode of transmission and incubation period, and the extreme virulence of the agent raise concern among health care personnel regarding necessary precautions. But it has been suggested that extraordinary precautions be used until the etiologic agent is identified and effective disinfection/sterilization processes are established. Recommended guidelines are similar to those for patients with hepatitis B. Sterilization and disinfection cycles must be longer than for bacterial spores with respect to time and concentration. Sterilize potentially contaminated materials before discarding, cleaning, or resterilizing them. Prudent management includes the following:

1 Special care must be used in handling blood, cerebral spinal fluid (CSF), and tissue, particularly brain. Patient contact not resulting in percutaneous exposure to these materials should be followed by thorough washing of hands or other exposed parts with soap or detergent.

2 Percutaneous exposure to blood, CSF, or tissue should immediately be followed by irrigation of the wound with 0.5% sodium hypochlorite.

3 Specimens sent to the laboratory should be labeled as "biohazards" for appropriate handling.

4 Organs and tissues of these patients should not be used for transplantation.

Consult your hospital's infection control committee for specific guidelines and sterilization timing.

Toxic Shock Syndrome (TSS) TSS is a potentially fatal condition characterized by high fever over 102°F (38.9°C), hypotension, nausea, vomiting, and erythematous rash. Abnormal kidney, liver, gastrointestinal, and cardiovascular function develop. A toxin secreted by strains of *Staphylococcus aureus* appears to be the etiologic factor. The pathogen can invade any part of the body. Menstruating women seem to be the most frequently affected, but TSS can afflict any age group of either sex. Prompt diagnosis and treatment, supportive and antibiotic, are crucial. About 15 percent of cases reported to CDC involve conditions unrelated to menstruation and tampon use. These include surgical wounds infected or colonized with the implicated strain, infected burns, septic abortion, or postpartum infection.

Herpetic Whitlow This is herpes simplex virus (HSV) infection of the fingers. Transmission is by direct contact with oropharyngeal secretions from patients with active herpes labialis (lip) or genital lesions, or from asymptomatic carriers of HSV. Transmission depends on entry of the virus into the host via a cut or break in the skin or in the nail folds. It is an occupational hazard particularly to nurses, physicians, dentists, and anesthesiologists.

Operative Technique Mentioned repeatedly, operative technique is one of the most important factors influencing wound healing (see Chap. 17). The acronym GEM should apply to the surgeon: gentle, expeditious, and meticulous.

If infection is obvious at the time of operation, implantation of organisms into susceptible tissue must be avoided. Tissue traumatized during operation, such as chest or abdominal wall, can be protected by the use of fresh sterile instruments for wound closure. It is advisable to isolate wound closure materials and equipment on the instrument table so that every wound may be closed with previously unused instruments, to reduce inoculum delivered to wound.

Antibiotic Therapy

Antibiotics, also referred to as *antimicrobial drugs or agents,* are a prominent part of the surgeon's armamentarium. They act by killing or inhibiting the growth of bacteria. *Antibiotics are adjuvants to, not substitutes for, strict adherence to aseptic principles and careful operative technique.*

The penicillins, cephalosporins, and aminoglycosides are the common categories of antibiotics. The penicillins include natural penicillin G and synthetic or semisynthetic derivatives. Some are rendered inactive by penicillinase, an enzyme secreted by certain bacteria which antagonizes the action of penicillin, e.g., *Staphylococcus aureus.* Several synthetic penicillins are resistant to penicillinase. Cephalosporins also are resistant to penicillinase, but cross-sensitivity may develop between them and the penicillins. They have a broad spectrum of effectiveness and low toxicity. Aminoglycosides are effective against gram-negative organisms, e.g., *Pseudomonas, Serratia,* and *E. coli,* but are ototoxic and nephrotoxic in a dose-related manner. Aminoglycosides (acids) precipitate when mixed with heparin and are incompatible with some cephalosporins and penicillins (bases). They should be given at separate times or through separate lines. Adverse effects, such as respiratory arrest, may occur with concurrent use of aminoglycosides and neuromuscular blockers or anesthetic agents.

The incidence of allergic reactions to penicillin is relatively high. Patients should be questioned about allergies before any drug is administered, and closely watched for signs of toxicity as evidenced by skin rash, gastrointestinal disturbance, renal disorder, fever, or blood dyscrasia.

A major problem developed when indiscriminate use of antibiotics led to development of resistant strains of organisms that concentrate in patients and the environment. The efficacy of these drugs is greatly reduced when multiple organisms are involved in an infection. Sufficient risk warrants their use. Antibiotics are given:

1 *Therapeutically* to eliminate sensitive viable organisms during a period with clinical evidence of infection, including wounds with gross contamination and traumatic wounds. Choice of antibiotic and duration of therapy should be determined by clinical factors, i.e., pathogen, severity and site of infection, and clinical response. A broad spectrum drug may be given while awaiting results of cultures and sensitivity tests.

2 *Prophylactically* to prevent development of infection. Prophylaxis implies that the microorganism is attacked by the antimicrobial agent at time of lodgment and certainly before colonization takes place. A prophylactic antibiotic is given prior to surgical intervention, bacterial invasion, or clinically evident infection. These agents are effective as supplements to host defense mechanisms in selected patients. Prophylaxis is recommended for procedures:
   a Associated with brief exposure to possible infection; evidence that antibiotic can reduce infection. Example: cystoscopy following cystitis.
   b Not frequently associated with infection, but incidence would have disastrous or life-threatening consequences. Examples: clean wounds, insertion of prosthetic implant such as heart valve, vascular graft, or total joint replacement.
   c Associated with high risk of infection. Organisms are predictable and susceptible to antibiotics. Examples: clean-contaminated wounds such as biliary tract with obstruction, transection of colon.

The probability of infection is determined in the first few hours after bacterial invasion, when capillary permeability and host response are at a peak immediately after bacterial contamination. Therefore, timing and duration of drug administration is crucial. To be effective, the prophylactic antibiotic *must* be present in adequate concentration in tissues at time of wound creation or contamination. Selection of appropriate drug and early use are pertinent factors. Antibiotic regimen is governed by site of operation, potential pathogens to be found, and patient's history of drug sensitivities. Drugs may be given preoperatively and/or intraoperatively, and possibly for a short period postoperatively. The CDC recommends that:

1 Except for cesarean section, parenteral antibiotic prophylaxis should be started within two hours before operation to produce therapeutic level during operation, and not continued for more than 48 hours. A 12 hour limit is desirable for most types of wounds and operations. Parenteral use over 24 hours increases risk of antibiotic toxicity, selection of resistant strains of bacteria or superinfection, and does not further reduce risk of infection.

2 For cesarian section, prophylaxis usually is given intraoperatively after the umbilical cord is clamped.

3 Oral, absorbable prophylactic antibiotics should not be used to supplement or extend parenteral prophylaxis. They should be limited to 24 hours before operation when used prophylactically with colorectal operations.

4 When topical antimicrobial products are used in the wound, they should be free of serious local or systemic side effects.

NEED FOR STERILE TECHNIQUE

A drastic change in the pattern of life-threatening infections has occurred since the advent of broad-spectrum antibiotics and penicillinase-resistant penicillins. While gram-positive bacteria (staphylococci, pneumococci, and beta-hemolytic streptococci) continue their pathogenic activity, the resistant gram-negative bacilli, aerobic and anaerobic, deeply concern clinicians. Gram-negative infections have increased fourteenfold in 15 years. Another grave concern is the increasing incidence of gram-negative infections by bacteria of supposedly low virulence (*Serratia*), capable of causing deep, latent infections. These organisms all rapidly colonize hospitalized patients, and are transferred to other individuals by hands or equipment. Nosocomical fungal and viral infections also have become more problematic. Viruses are not usually a risk to a healthy patient having an elective procedure, but patients have died of systemic viremia following bacteremia or fungemia.

Strict aseptic and sterile techniques are needed at all times in the operating room. Freshly incised or traumatized tissue easily can become infected. Intact skin is the body's first line of defense against infection. Infraction of the integrity of the skin creates a portal of entry for microorganisms. Therefore, anything unsterile in contact with the patient is potentially dangerous. Items entering body tissue *must* be sterile. Sterility is less critical for items contacting intact mucous membranes or skin. Operative procedures are performed under sterile conditions. Conversely, terminal decontamination and sterilization of all material and equipment used during an operation is performed with the assumption that *every patient is a potential source of infection for other persons.*

It is essential that all members of the operating team know the common sources of contamination by microorganisms in the operating room, and the means by which they reach the sterile field and operative wound. Sterile technique is the responsibility of everyone caring for the patient in the OR. *All members of the operating team must be ever vigilant in safeguarding the sterility of the operative field. Any contamination must be remedied immediately.*

PRINCIPLES OF STERILE TECHNIQUE AND ILLUSTRATIONS OF APPLICATION

The patient is the center of the sterile field, which includes the areas of the patient, operating table and furniture covered with sterile drapes, and the personnel wearing sterile attire. Strict adherence to sound principles of sterile technique and recommended practices is mandatory for safety of the patient. This adherence reflects one's surgical conscience. *Principles remain the same; it is the degree of adherence to them that varies.* The principles of sterile technique are applied:

1 In preparation for operation, by sterilization of necessary materials and supplies
2 In preparation of operating team to handle sterile supplies and intimately contact wound
3 In creation and maintenance of sterile field, including prepration and drape of patient, to prevent contamination of wound
4 In maintenance of sterility and asepsis throughout operative procedure
5 In terminal sterilization and disinfection at conclusion of operation

If the principles are understood, the need for their application becomes obvious. Sterile technique is the basis of modern surgery.

Principles

Sterile persons have scrubbed and are gowned and gloved; unsterile persons have not.

Only Sterile Items Are Used within Sterile Field Some items such as linen, sponges, or basins may be obtained from stock supply of sterile packages. Others, such as instruments, may be sterilized immediately preceding the operation and removed directly from the sterilizer to the sterile tables. Every person who dispenses a sterile article must be sure of its sterility and of its remaining sterile until used. Proper packaging, sterilizing, and handling should provide such assurance. *If you are in doubt about the sterility of anything, consider it not sterile.* Known or potentially contaminated items must not be transferred to the sterile field, for example:

1 If sterilized package is found in a nonsterile workroom.
2 If uncertain about actual timing or operation of sterilizer. Items processed in a suspect load are considered unsterile.
3 If unsterile person comes into close contact with a sterile table and vice versa.
4 If sterile table or unwrapped sterile items are not under constant observation.
5 If sterile package falls to the floor, it must be discarded (see Chap. 10, p. 168).

Gowns Are Considered Sterile Only from the Waist to Shoulder Level in Front, and the Sleeves When wearing a gown, consider only the area you can see down to the waist as the sterile area. The following practices must be observed:

1 Sterile persons keep hands in sight and at or above waist level (see Fig. 7-1).
2 Hands are kept away from face. Elbows are kept close to sides. Hands are never folded under arms because of perspiration in the axillary region.
3 Changing table levels is avoided. If a sterile person must stand on a platform to reach the op-

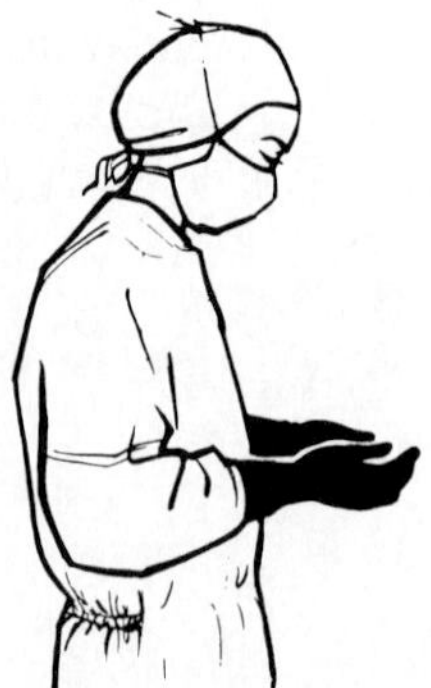

FIGURE 7-1
Sterile person keeps hands in sight and at or above waist level. Gowns are considered sterile only from waist to shoulder level in front and the sleeves.

erative field, area of the gown below waist must not brush against sterile tables or draped areas.

4 Items dropped below waist level are considered unsterile, and must be discarded.

Tables Are Sterile Only at Table Level The result is that:

1 Only top of a sterile draped table is considered sterile. Edges and sides of drape extending below table level are considered unsterile.

2 Anything falling or extending over table edge, such as a piece of suture, is unsterile. Scrub nurse does not touch part hanging below table level.

3 In unfolding a sterile drape, the part that drops below table surface is not brought back up to table level.

Persons Who Are Sterile Touch Only Sterile Items or Areas; Persons Who Are Not Sterile Touch Only Unsterile Items or Areas For example:

1 Sterile team members maintain contact with sterile field by means of sterile gowns and gloves.

2 Nonsterile circulating nurse does not directly contact the sterile field.

3 Supplies for sterile team members reach them by means of the circulating nurse who opens wrappers on sterile packages.

Unsterile Persons Avoid Reaching over a Sterile Field; Sterile Persons Avoid Leaning over an Unsterile Area For example:

1 Unsterile circulating nurse *never* reaches over a sterile field to transfer sterile items.

2 In pouring solution into sterile basin, circulating nurse holds only lip of bottle over basin to avoid reaching over a sterile area (see Fig. 7-2).

3 Scrub nurse sets basins or glasses to be filled at edge of the sterile table; circulating nurse stands near this edge of the table to fill them.

4 Circulating nurse stands at a distance from the sterile field to adjust light over it to avoid microbial fallout over field.

5 Surgeon turns away from sterile field to have perspiration removed from brow.

6 Scrub nurse drapes a nonsterile table toward self first to protect gown (see Fig. 7-3).

7 Scrub nurse stands back from nonsterile table when draping it to avoid leaning over an unsterile area (see Figs. 7-4, 7-5, 7-6).

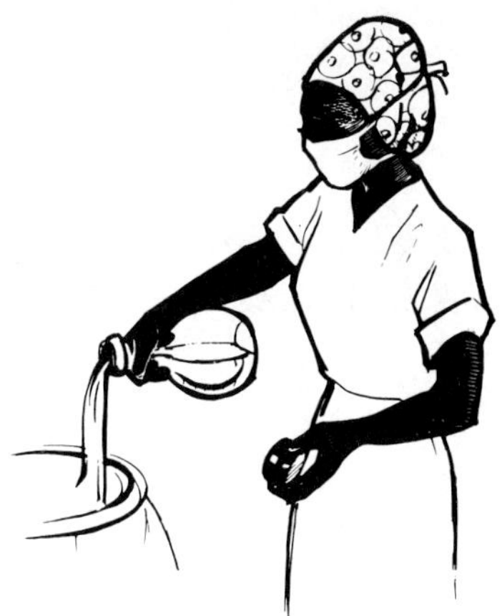

FIGURE 7-2
Circulating nurse pouring sterile solution into a sterile basin. Note that only lip of bottle is over the basin. Nonsterile person avoids reaching over a sterile field.

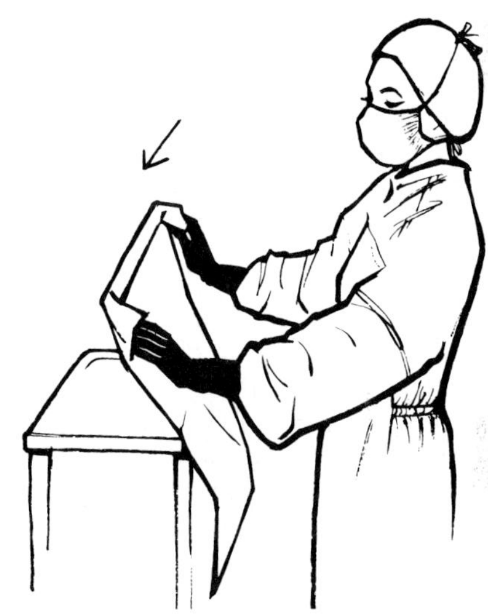

FIGURE 7-3
Sterile scrub nurse draping a small table. Sterile persons avoid reaching over a nonsterile field. The nurse, therefore, drapes nonsterile table first toward self, then away. Gown is protected by distance. Hands are protected by cuffing drape over them.

Edges of Anything That Encloses Sterile Contents Are Considered Unsterile Boundaries between sterile and unsterile are not always rigidly defined, for example, the edges of wrappers on sterile packages and caps on solution bottles. The following precautions should be taken:

1 In opening sterile packages, a margin of safety is always maintained. Ends of flaps are secured in hand so they do not dangle loosely. The last flap is pulled toward person opening package

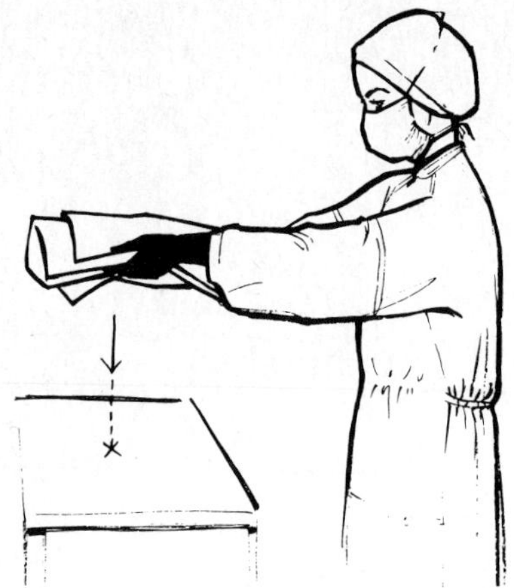

FIGURE 7-4
Draping a large nonsterile table. Scrub nurse holds the sterile fan-folded table drape high and drops it onto the center of the table, standing back from the table to protect gown.

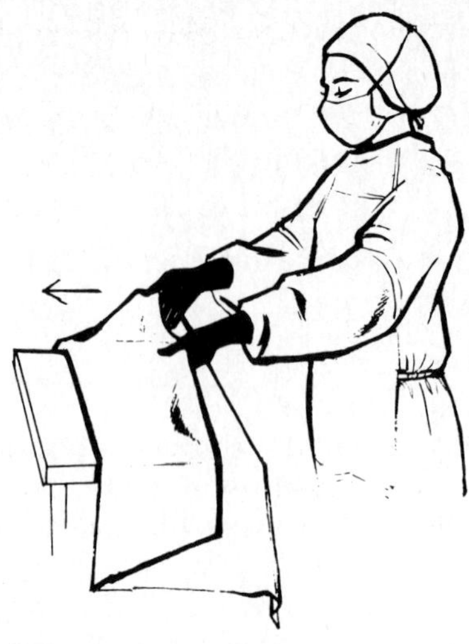

FIGURE 7-6
Nurse continuing to unfold sterile table drape. Hands are inside sterile cover for protection. Nurse may now move closer to the table, since the first part of unfolded drape now protects gown.

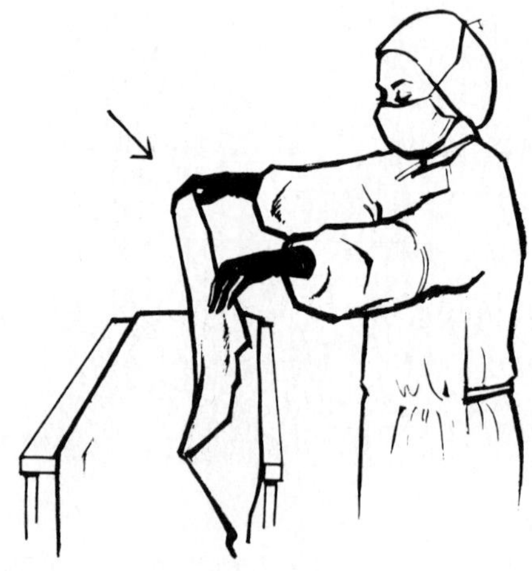

FIGURE 7-5
Scrub nurse unfolding sterile table drape. Nurse stands back from nonsterile table and unfolds drape first toward self. Note that hands are inside sterile cover to protect them.

thereby exposing package contents away from nonsterile hand.

2 Sterile persons lift contents from packages by reaching down and lifting them straight up, holding elbows high.

3 Steam reaches only the area within the gasket of a sterilizer. Instrument trays should not touch the edge of the sterilizer outside the gasket.

4 Flaps on peel-open packages should be pulled back, not torn, to expose sterile contents. Contents should be flipped or lifted upward and not permitted to slide over edges. Inner edge of the heat seal is considered the line of demarcation between sterile and unsterile.

5 If a sterile wrapper is used as a table cover, it should amply cover the entire table surface. Only the interior and surface level of the cover are considered sterile.

6 After a sterile bottle is opened, contents must be used or discarded. Cap cannot be replaced without contaminating pouring edges.

Sterile Field Is Created as Close as Possible to Time of Use Degree of contamination is proportionate to length of time sterile items are uncovered and exposed to environment. Precautions must be taken as follows:

1 Sterile tables are set up just prior to the operation (see Chap. 10, p. 160).

2 It is difficult to uncover a table of sterile contents without contamination. Covering sterile tables for later use is not recommended.

Sterile Areas Are Continuously Kept in View Inadvertent contamination of sterile areas must be readily visible. To ensure this principle:

1 Sterile persons face sterile areas.

2 When sterile packs are open in a room, or a sterile field set up, someone must remain in the room to maintain vigilance.

Sterile Persons Keep Well within the Sterile Area They allow a wide margin of safety when passing unsterile areas and follow these rules:

1 Sterile persons stand back at a safe distance from the operating table when draping the patient.

2 Sterile persons pass each other back to back (see Fig. 7-7).

3 Sterile person turns back to nonsterile person or area when passing.

4 Sterile person faces sterile area to pass it.

5 Sterile person asks nonsterile individual to step aside rather than risk contamination.

6 Sterile persons stay within the sterile field. They *do not walk around* or go outside room.

7 Movement within and around a sterile area is kept to a minimum to avoid contamination of sterile items or persons.

Sterile Persons Keep Contact with Sterile Areas to a Minimum The following rules are observed:

1 Sterile persons do not lean on sterile tables and on the draped patient.

2 Sitting or leaning against a nonsterile surface is a break in technique. If the sterile team sits to operate, they do so without proximity to nonsterile areas.

Unsterile Persons Avoid Sterile Areas A wide margin of safety must be maintained when passing sterile areas by following these rules:

1 Unsterile persons maintain at least one foot (30 cm) distance from any area of the sterile field.

2 Unsterile persons face and observe a sterile area when passing it to be sure they do not touch it.

3 Unsterile persons never walk between two sterile areas, e.g., between sterile instrument tables.

4 Circulating nurse restricts to a minimum all activity near sterile field.

Destruction of Integrity of Microbial Barriers Results in Contamination Integrity of a sterile package or sterile drape is destroyed by perforation, puncture, or strike-through. *Strike-through* is soaking of moisture through unsterile layers to sterile layers or vice versa. Ideal barrier materials are abrasion resistant, impervious to permeation by fluids or dust that transport microorganisms. The integrity of a sterile package, its expiration

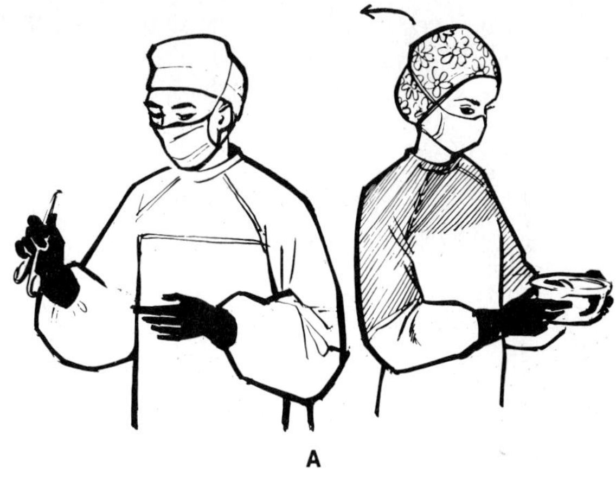

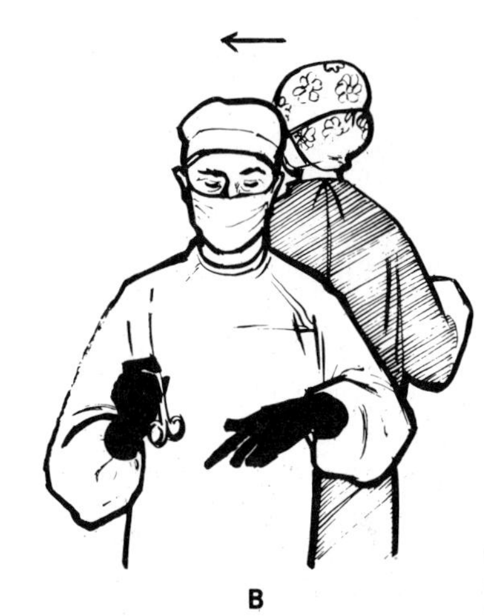

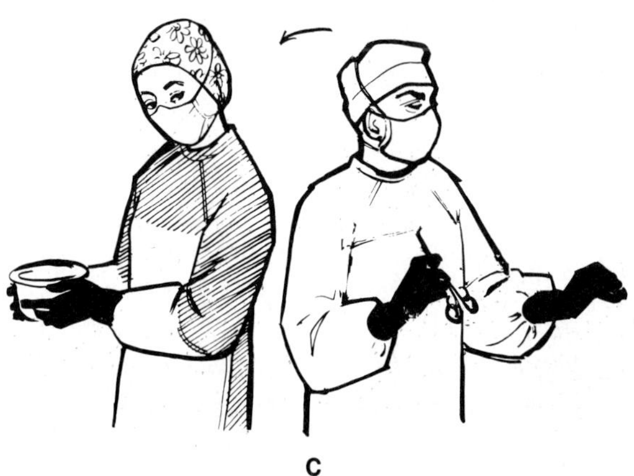

FIGURE 7-7
Sequence of one sterile person going around another. They pass each other back to back, keeping well within the sterile area and allowing a margin of safety between themselves.

date, and appearance of process monitor must be checked for sterility just prior to opening (see Chap. 10, p. 160). To ensure sterility:

1 Sterile packages are laid on dry surfaces.

2 If sterile package becomes damp or wet, it is resterilized or discarded. A package is considered nonsterile if any part of it comes in contact with moisture.

3 Drapes are placed on a dry field.

4 If solution soaks through sterile drape to nonsterile area, the wet area is covered with impervious sterile drapes or towels.

5 Packages wrapped in muslin or paper are permitted to cool, after removal from the sterilizer, before being placed on cold surface to prevent steam condensation and resultant contamination.

6 Sterile items are stored in clean dry areas.

7 Sterile packages are handled with clean dry hands.

8 Undue pressure on sterile packs is avoided to prevent forcing sterile air out and pulling unsterile air into the pack.

Microorganisms Must Be Kept to an Irreducible Minimum Perfect asepsis in an operative field is an ideal to be approached; it is not absolute. All microorganisms cannot be eliminated, but this does not obviate necessity for strict sterile technique. It is generally agreed that:

1 *Skin cannot be sterilized.* Skin is a potential source of contamination in every operation. Inherent body defenses usually can overcome the relatively few organisms remaining after patient's skin preparation. Organisms on the hands and arms of the operating team are a hazard. All possible means are used to prevent entrance of microorganisms into wound. Preventive measures include:
   - **a** Transient and resident flora are removed from skin around operative site of patient (see Chap. 16) and hands and arms of sterile team members (see Chap. 9) by mechanical washing and chemical antisepsis.
   - **b** Gowning and gloving of operating team is accomplished without contamination of sterile exterior of gowns and gloves.
   - **c** Sterile gloved hands do not directly touch skin and then deeper tissues. Instruments used in contact with skin are discarded and not reused.
   - **d** If glove is pricked or punctured by needle or instrument, glove is changed immediately. Needle or instrument is discarded from sterile field.

2 *Some areas cannot be scrubbed.* When the operative field includes the mouth, nose, throat, or anus, the number of microorganisms present is great. Various parts of the body, such as the gastrointestinal tract and vagina, usually are resistant to infection from flora that normally inhabit these parts. However, the following steps may be taken to reduce number of microorganisms present in these areas and to prevent scattering them:
   - **a** Surgeon makes an effort to use a sponge only once, then discards it.
   - **b** Gastrointestinal tract, especially colon, is contaminated. Measures are used to prevent spreading this contamination (see Chap. 21, p. 398 and p. 409).

3 *Infected areas are grossly contaminated.* The team avoids disseminating the contamination.

4 *Air is contaminated by dust and droplets.* Environmental control measures are used.

RECOMMENDED PRACTICES

Recommended practices developed by the Association of Operating Room Nurses provide guidelines for aseptic practices in the perioperative care of surgical patients. These are recommendations for optimal level of *achievable* technical and aseptic practices. They are intended to give direction and information for formulation of institutional policies. Individual hospital policies and procedures reflect variations in physical environment and/or clinical situations that determine degree to which the recommended practices can be implemented. The recommendations may not necessarily reflect current practice in individual institutions. Throughout this text referral is made to specific appropriate guidelines and/or their content is incorporated in the material presented. The AORN recommended practices are listed in the bibliography for the applicable chapters in this text.

NO COMPROMISE WITH STERILITY

Sterility is never taken for granted. It must be maintained and checked. Chapter 8 details the procedures for sterilization and handling of sterile supplies.

Basically, there is no compromise with sterility. In clinical practice, an item is considered sterile or unsterile. Always be as certain of sterility as it is possible to be. That certainty rests on the fact that the necessary conditions have been met, that all factors in the sterilization process have been observed. Obviously it is impossible to prove that every package is free from bacteria, but a single break in technique can cost the life of a patient. Operating room personnel must maintain the high standards of sterile technique they know are essential. Every individual is accountable for his or her own role in infection control.

PREVENTION OF WOUND INFECTION

Prevention of wound infection and successful outcome of surgical intervention are goals of the team administering perioperative care to surgical patients. In summary, preventive measures should focus on:

1 Control of endogenous infection

2 Use of strict sterile technique

3 Meticulous operative technique and wound closure

4 Reduction of exogenous or environmental sources of contamination such as airborne microorganisms

5 Thorough, prompt cleansing and debridement of traumatic wounds

6 Prevention of intraoperative contamination of wound

7 Appropriate use of prophylactic antibiotics in selected patients

8 Meticulous, frequent handwashing

9 Sterile technique for dressing change

10 Dissemination of wound infection statistics to surgeons and OR staff

Serious sequelae, such as wound disruption or septicemia, may follow wound infection. Therefore, it must be assiduously prevented.

CHAPTER **8**

STERILIZATION AND DISINFECTION

Pathogenic microorganisms and those that do not normally invade healthy tissue are capable of causing infection if introduced mechanically into the body. Therefore, specific standardized procedures, based upon accepted principles and practices, are necessary for the sterilization or disinfection of all supplies and equipment used in the operating room. Sterilization renders items safe for contact with tissue without transmission of infection, as long as sterility is maintained. Disinfectants are used to kill as many microorganisms in the environment as possible on items and materials that cannot be sterilized.

BIOBURDEN

Bioburden is the relative number of actual or suspected microorganisms that may be found on a specific item or in the environment at a specific time. This number may be reduced through the environmental control measures and sterile techniques described in Chapter 7.

All items that enter body tissues should be sterile. Sterilization kills microorganisms in their vegetative and spore stages. For the sterilization process to be effective, however, the bioburden on items must be relatively low. All items should be thoroughly cleaned prior to sterilization (see Chap. 10, p. 181). The cleaning process physically removes microbes and organic debris that harbors microorganisms.

Some porous materials or internal mechanisms cannot be thoroughly cleaned after use. *Single use disposable items should not be reprocessed.* Other materials deteriorate during sterilization. Manufacturers' written instructions for cleaning and sterilizing limited use items must be followed. *Limited use items* are those designed to be reprocessed only the number of times specified by the manufacturer.

MICROBIOLOGICAL SAFETY

Prior to availability of commercially packaged and sterilized products, all items were prepared in the hospital for use in a sterile field and for implantation in body tissues. Traditionally, sterility was considered by users to be the absolute absence of all microorganisms. This concept is not held today because it is known that microorganisms are killed according to a logarithmic order of death when subjected to a sterilization process. A given percentage of surviving population is killed in a unit of time, i.e., a percentage of the initial concentration will die and a percentage will survive during each subsequent unit of time of exposure. Absolute sterilization cannot be attained because it is impossible to reach zero.

The rate at which microorganisms die is expressed as the decimal reduction value (D value). The D value is time required at a constant temperature and/or dose of agent to destroy 90 percent of the microbial population, or the time required for the survivor curve to complete a logarithmic cycle. The D value is independent from the initial logarithmic reduction. The same time-agent ratio is required to reduce the microbial population tenfold: one million (10^6) to one hundred thousand (10^5) to 10^4, etc., to one to 0.1.

Sterility actually refers to the probability that an item is not contaminated. Manufacturers of sterile products employ quality control procedures to assure at least a probability that no more than one in a million products will be unsterile. Expressed scientifically as 1×10^6, this generally accepted standard refers to level of assurance that 99.9999 percent of items are sterile. A higher level of sterility assurance is sought by some manufacturers of critical implants. A manufacturer may label a product *sterile* following compliance with Federal Food and Drug Administration (FDA) and United States Pharmacopeia (USP) testing procedures. These include tests of presterilization bioburden (degree of contamination) and control tests of sterilization process variables with biological indicators or dosimeters.

A *microbiological safety/survival index (MSI)* was developed in Canada as a quality measurement for sterile products to counter the differences in user, industry, and regulatory definitions of sterility. MSI is defined as the absolute value of the logarithm (negative common logarithm) of the probability that an item is unsterile, contaminated with a viable microorganism. A MSI of 6, for example, indicates .000001 or 1×10^6 probability of nonsterility, 99.9999 percent probability of sterility. As the MSI value increases, so does assurance of sterility. An increase or decrease of one in the MSI increases or decreases the probability tenfold. Although not required, manufacturers may include the MSI on labeling of their sterile products.

Although sterility cannot be guaranteed, all items brought into the sterile field must be microbiologically safe for their intended uses. The in-hospital sterilization of supplies should be performed only by individuals who demonstrate knowledge of the principles of microbiology as they pertain to containment of contamination and sterilization processes.

PARAMETERS OF STERILIZATION

Parameters (conditions) of two types must be considered for all methods of sterilization. These are:

Product Associated

1 Bioburden, degree of contamination

2 Bioresistance, including such factors as heat and/or moisture sensitivities and product stability

3 Bioshielding, characteristics of packaging materials

4 Density, factors affecting penetration and evacuation of agent

Process Associated

1 Temperature

2 Time

3 Purity of agent and air, and residual effects or residues

4 Saturation/penetration

5 Capacity of sterilizer

METHODS OF STERILIZATION

Bacterial spores are the most resistant of all living organisms because of their capacity to withstand external destructive agents. Although the physical or chemical process by which all pathogenic and nonpathogenic microorganisms, *including spores,* are destroyed is not absolute, supplies and equipment are considered sterile when necessary conditions have been met during a sterilization process. Selection of the agent to achieve sterility depends primarily upon nature of the item to be sterilized. Time required to kill spores in the equipment available for the process then becomes critical. Each method of sterilization has its advantages and disadvantages. Sterilizing agents are:

1 Steam under pressure—moist heat (physical)

2 Ethylene oxide gas (chemical)

3 Activated glutaraldehyde (chemical)

4 Hot air—dry heat (physical)

5 Ionizing radiation (physical)

Steam under Pressure—Moist Heat

Moist heat in the form of saturated steam under pressure is a dependable physical agent for destruction of all forms of microbial life, including spores. Heat destroys microorganisms, but this process is hastened by addition of moisture. Steam in itself is inadequate for sterilization. Pressure, greater than atmospheric, is necessary to increase temperature of steam for thermal destruction of microbial life. Death by moist heat is caused by the denaturation and coagulation of protein or the enzyme-protein system within cells. These reactions are catalyzed by presence of water. Steam is water vapor. It is saturated when the steam contains a maximum amount of water vapor.

Direct saturated steam contact is the basis of the steam sterilization process. Steam, for specified time at required temperature, must penetrate every fiber and reach every surface of items to be sterilized. When steam enters the sterilizer chamber under pressure, it condenses upon contact with cold items. This condensation liberates heat, simultaneously heating and wetting all items in the load, thereby providing the two requisites: moisture and heat. *This sterilization process is spoken of in terms of degrees of temperature and time of exposure,* not in terms of pounds of pressure. Pressure increases boiling temperature of water, but has no significant effect on microorganisms or steam penetration.

Vegetative forms of most microorganisms are killed in a few minutes at temperatures ranging from 130 to 150°F (54 to 65°C); however, certain bacterial spores will withstand a temperature of 240°F (115°C) for more than three hours. No living thing can survive direct exposure to saturated steam at 250°F (121°C) longer than 15 minutes. As temperature is increased, time may be decreased. A minimum temperature-time relationship must be maintained throughout all portions of load to accomplish effective sterilization. Exposure time depends upon size and contents of load, and temperature within the sterilizer.

Advantages of Steam

1 Steam sterilization is the easiest, safest, and surest method of sterilization. Items that can be steam sterilized without damage should be processed with this method.

2 Steam is fastest method; total time cycle is shortest.

3 Steam is least expensive and most easily supplied. It is piped in from the hospital boiler room. An automatic, electrically powered steam generator can be mounted beneath the sterilizer for emergency standby when steam pressure is low.

4 Most sterilizers have automatic controls and recording devices to eliminate the human factor from the sterilization process as much as possible, when operated and cared for according to recommendations of manufacturer.

5 Many items, such as stainless steel instruments, withstand repeated processing without damage. Steam leaves no harmful residue.

Disadvantages of Steam

1 Precaution must be used in preparing and packaging items, loading and operating sterilizer, and drying load.

2 Items must be clean, free from grease and oil, and nonheat-sensitive.

3 Steam must have direct contact with all areas of an item.

4 Timing of cycle must be adjusted for differences in materials and size of load; these variables are subject to human error.

5 Steam may not be pure. Steam purity refers to amount of solid, liquid, or vapor contamination in steam. Impurities can cause wet or stained packs and stained instruments.

Types of Steam Sterilizers Sterilizers designed to use steam under pressure as the sterilizing agent frequently are referred to as *autoclaves* to distinguish them from sterilizers employing other agents. *References in this text to an autoclave mean steam sterilizer.* Personnel charged with the responsibility of operating an autoclave must fully understand the principles and operation of each type. They must be aware of problems that cause malfunction, such as attaining sterilization temperature and maintaining it for the required period of time, trapped air, and dirty traps.

Gravity Displacement Sterilizers The metal construction contains two shells, either round or rectangular, to form a jacket and a chamber. Steam fills the jacket that surrounds the chamber. After door is tightly closed, steam enters chamber at the back, near the top, and is deflected upward. Air is more than twice as heavy as steam. Thus, by gravity, air goes to bottom and steam floats on top. Steam, entering under pressure and remaining above the air, displaces air both in chamber and in wrapped items downward, and forces it out through discharge outlet at the bottom front. The air passes through a filtering screen to waste line. A thermometer, located at this outlet below the screen, measures temperature in the chamber. When steam has filled the chamber, it begins to flow past the thermometer. Timing of sterilizing period starts only when the thermometer reaches the desired temperature (see Fig. 8-1).

When air is trapped in chamber or wrapped items, the killing power of steam is decreased in direct proportion to amount of air present. Because the vital discharge of air from the load always occurs in a downward direction, never side-

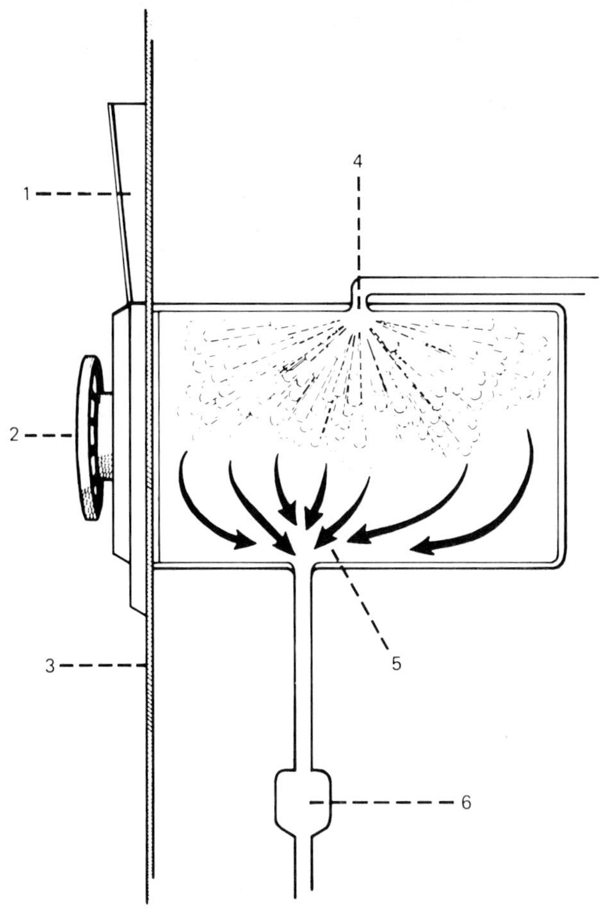

FIGURE 8-1
Schematic cross section of steam under pressure sterilizer: (1) control panel, (2) door handle of chamber, and (3) front panel of stainless steel cabinet. (4) Steam enters at top of chamber to displace air or after air is withdrawn by vacuum. (5)Air and steam are evacuated at bottom of chamber. (6) Temperature of steam is measured in air-steam drain line near vent.

wise, all supplies must be prepared and arranged to present the least possible resistance to passage of steam through load from top of chamber downward. Also, air and steam discharge lines must be kept free of dirt, sediment, or lint. The filtering screen should be cleaned daily. Discharge lines are flushed with trisodium phosphate weekly (see precautions, p. 126).

Most gravity displacement autoclaves operate on a standard cycle of 250 to 254°F (121 to 123°C) at a pressure of 15 to 17 lb per square inch (lb/in^2). Size of chamber and contents will determine exposure period; the minimum is 15 minutes.

High-Speed Pressure Sterilizer Often called a *flash sterilizer,* this autoclave operates by gravity displacement, but is designed to function rapidly at a higher temperature. It can be adjusted to operate at 27 lb pressure per square inch to increase the temperature to 270°F (132°C). *The minimum exposure time at this temperature is 3 minutes, but only for unwrapped items.* With this cycle, the entire time for starting, sterilizing, and opening the autoclave is 6 to 7 minutes. The temperature can be set for operation at 250°F (121°C) for standard cycles at 25 lb pressure.

Prevacuum Sterilizer In this high-vacuum autoclave, air is almost completely evacuated from the chamber before the sterilizing steam is admitted. This is accomplished to the desired degree of vacuum by means of a pump and a steam-injector system. A prevacuum period of 8 to 10 minutes effectively removes the air to minimize steam penetration time. The steam injector preconditions the load and helps eliminate air from packages. When the sterilizing steam is admitted to the chamber, it almost instantly penetrates to center of the packages. Provided items making up the load are easily penetrable and sterilizer is functioning properly, there is no demonstrable time differential between complete steam penetration of large or small, tight or loose packages. Air is not displaced by steam. Therefore maximum capacity can be utilized. A postvacuum cycle draws moisture from load to shorten drying time.

Temperatures are controlled at 272 to 276°F (133 to 135°C). A complete cycle takes approximately 15 minutes. Temperature, time, and degree of vacuum are recorded on a graphic chart. Although equipped with automatic controls, cycles can be operated manually or by gravity displacement of air. All items must be exposed to temperature of at least 270°F (132°C) for four minutes.

Washer-Sterilizer This sterilizer is designed to wash and terminally sterilize instruments and some other items immediately after operation is completed. Cold water fills chamber and mixes with detergent to dissolve and loosen blood and debris. Steam and air, injected through powerful jet streams located near bottom of chamber, create turbulence of the water to continue the washing process. As water is heated, it rises and carries debris to the water line. Steam then enters at top of chamber to force wash water out through the bottom drain. Steam under pressure floods chamber to sterilize items at 270°F (132°C). Although designed specifically for the combination of washing and sterilizing cycles, some units can be programmed for use as a flash sterilizer.

Precautions With all four types of steam sterilizers, the following precautions must be taken to ensure safe operation:

1 Turn valve on for steam in jacket prior to use. Steam may be kept in the jacket throughout the day. (It may be turned off at end of the operating schedule.) This maintains heat, so do not touch the inside of chamber when loading. (Check sterilizer; not all have a steam jacket.)

2 Never put heat-sensitive items in a steam sterilizer of any type; they will be destroyed.

3 Close door tightly before activating either automatic or manual controls.

4 Do not set a manually operated timer, unless it is an automatically controlled device, until desired temperature registers on thermometer and recording graphic chart. *Thermometers, not pressure gauges, are the guides for sterilization.*

5 Open door only when the exhaust valve registers zero. Stand behind door and open slowly to avoid steam escaping around the door.

6 Daily wash inside of chamber with trisodium phosphate solution, rinse with tap water, and dry with lint-free cloth.

7 Remove and clean filtering screen daily.

8 Flush discharge lines weekly with hot solution of trisodium phosphate: 1 oz (30 ml) to 1 qt (1000 ml) of hot water. Follow flush with rinse of 1 qt (1000 ml) of tap water.

Preparing Items for Steam Sterilization

Surgical Instruments Special attention must be given to cleaning surgical instruments prior to sterilization. An *ultrasonic cleaner* should be available for cleaning instruments that the washer-sterilizer has not adequately cleaned during terminal sterilization. High-frequency sound is a source of energy used for cleaning. It is not a method of sterilization. An *ultrasonic cleaner is not a sterilizer.* Therefore, instruments should be terminally sterilized before being placed in an ultrasonic cleaner.

Surgical instruments vary in configuration from plane surfaces, which respond to most types of cleaning, to complicated devices that contain box locks, serrations, blind holes, and interstices. Ultrasonic energy, high-frequency sound waves, thoroughly cleans the latter type by the process of cavitation. The tiny bubbles, generated in the cleaner solution by high-frequency sound waves, expand until they are unstable, then collapse. The *implosion* (exact opposite of explosion) of these bubbles generates minute vacuum areas that dislodge, dissolve, or disperse soil. These bubbles are small enough to get into the serrations, box locks, and crevices of instruments that are impossible to clean by other methods.

Instruments should be completely immersed in cleaning solution. The tank should be filled to a level 1 in. (2.5 cm) above top of the instrument tray. Suitable detergent, as specified by manufacturer, is added. Temperature of the water should be 80 to 110°F (26.6 to 43°C) to enhance effectiveness of detergent, but it should not coagulate protein on instruments. Instrument trays must be designed for maximum transmission of sonic energy. An important relationship exists between wire gauge, opening size, and sonic frequency. A large mesh of small wire size transmits more energy than heavy wire with narrow spacing.

Solution is degassed by turning on the ultrasonic energy. Gas, present in most tap water, impedes the transmission of sonic energy. An electric generator supplies electrical energy to a transducer. The transducer converts the electrical energy into mechanical energy in the form of vibrating sound waves that are not audible to the human ear because they are of such high frequency. If excess gas is present, it prevents the cleaning process from being fully effective because the cavitation bubbles fill with gas and the energy released during implosion is reduced. Tap water should be degassed for five minutes or longer each time it is changed.

After cleaning, instruments must be thoroughly rinsed and dried. Glassware, rubber goods, and thermoplastics also can be cleaned by this method. Instruments that are well cleaned in a detergent solution in a washer-sterilizer may not need ultrasonic cleaning after every use.

Instruments Sets Standardized basic sets of instruments or trays of instruments selected for specific operations are prepared for sterilization after thorough cleaning. Instruments must be placed in trays with *perforated* or *mesh* bottoms to allow steam penetration around instruments and to prevent trapping air in tray, or in another container designed specifically for sterilizing surgical instruments.

Instruments should be arranged in tray in a definite pattern to protect them from damage and to facilitate removal for use. Heavy instruments are placed in bottom of tray. All detachable parts must be disassembled. Hinged instruments must be open with box locks unlocked to permit steam contact on all surfaces. They can be strung on a pin or rack. Sharp and delicate instruments are placed on top. Metals should not be mixed in tray. (See Chapters 10 and 11 for further discussion of the care and handling of instruments.)

The size and density of wrapped instrument sets should not exceed a maximum weight of 16 lb (7.2 kg), or approximately 100 instruments. This is necessary to ensure adequate drying.

Basin Sets Basins and solid utensils must be separated by a porous material, if they are nested, to permit permeation of steam around all surfaces and condensation of steam from the inside during sterilization. Sponges or drapes are not packaged in basins; steam could be deflected from penetration through fabrics.

Drape Packs Freshly laundered woven textile drapes and gowns must be fanfolded or rolled loosely to provide the least possible resistance to penetration of steam through each layer of material. Packs must not exceed a maximum size of 12 by 12 by 20 in. (30 by 30 by 50 cm), and not weigh more than 12 lb (5.5 kg). Drapes are loosely crisscrossed so they do not form a dense impermeable mass. Pack density should not exceed 7.2 lb per cubic foot. The outside wrapper becomes the table drape when pack is opened (see Chap. 10, p. 160).

Rubber Goods and Thermoplastics A rubber sheet or any other impervious material should not be folded for sterilization as steam cannot penetrate it nor displace air from folds. It should be covered with a piece of fabric of the same size, both loosely rolled and then wrapped. For example, a layer of roller gauze is rolled between layers of an Esmarch's bandage.

The mechanical cleaning of tubing, including catheters and drains, is a factor in reducing microbial count inside lumen. A residual of distilled water should be left in lumen of any tubing to be steam sterilized. This becomes steam as temperature rises and helps to displace air in lumen and to increase temperature within it. Tubing should be coiled without kinks in it.

Suction tips must be removed from tubing. Detachable rubber or plastic parts should be removed from instruments and syringes for cleaning and sterilizing. Rubber surfaces should not touch each other, metal, or glassware during sterilization to avoid melting or sticking and to permit steam to reach all surfaces. Rubber bands must not be used around solid items as steam cannot penetrate through or under rubber.

Wood Products During sterilization, lignocellulose resin (lignin) is driven out of wood by heat. This resin may condense onto other items in the autoclave and cause reactions if it gets into the tissues of a patient. Therefore, wooden items must be individually wrapped and separated from other items in the autoclave.

> NOTE. Repeated autoclaving dries wood so that during sterilization it will adsorb moisture from the saturated steam. As water content of saturated steam decreases, steam becomes superheated and loses some of its sterilizing power. Because of this problem, use of wood products that require steam sterilization should be minimized and their repeated sterilization avoided.

All Items Whether washed by hand, in a washer-sterilizer, or in an ultrasonic cleaner, all items with detachable parts or parts that can be separated must be disassembled for cleaning, packaging, and sterilizing. Items must be clean and dry, except lumen of tubing, prior to sterilization. Manuals, often with photographs, or index file cards are available in the room in which supplies are packaged for ready reference during preparation and wrapping of single items, packs, or trays. Instructions must be strictly followed to assure safety in sterilizing items.

Packaging The packaging materials for *all* methods of sterilization must:

1 Permit penetration of the sterilizing agent to achieve sterilization of all items in package.

2 Allow release of sterilizing agent at end of exposure period.

3 Cover items completely and easily, and fasten securely with tape or heat seal that cannot be resealed after opening.

> NOTE. 1. At least 1 in. (2.5 cm) margin is considered standard for safety on all sealed packages.
>
> 2. Pins, staples, paper clips, or other penetrating objects must never be used to seal packages. These cannot be removed without destroying integrity of package and contaminating contents. If a staple, for example, is used to secure end of a package, it is impossible to remove it without tearing package. Scissors cannot be used to cut off the end of a package and contents drawn out over this cut end. The item would be contaminated by edge

of the packaging material. For same reason, packages are never torn open below a seal.

4 Permit identification of the contents and evidence of exposure to a sterilizing agent.

NOTE. Indicator tapes or strips on the outside of packages change color during exposure to a sterilization process. They do not indicate sterility, only that the package has been sufficiently exposed to a given parameter to turn the color. Other factors that guarantee sterility must be fulfilled (see biological testing, p. 137).

5 Provide an impermeable barrier to microorganisms, dust particles, and moisture. Items must remain sterile from time removed from the sterilizer until used.

6 Resist tears and punctures in handling. If accidental tears and holes do occur, they must be visible.

7 Maintain integrity of package at varying atmospheric and humidity levels.

NOTE. In geographic areas of high altitude or dry climates, some packaging materials are susceptible to rupture during sterilization or will dry out and crack in storage.

8 Permit easy removal of the contents with transfer to the sterile field without contamination or delamination (separation into layers).

9 Be economical.

10 Be free of toxic ingredients and nonfast dyes.

Wrapping of packages should be done in room far enough removed from sterile storage areas so mixing sterile and nonsterile packages is not possible. Nonsterile cabinets should be labeled conspicuously. A procedure for sending items to the sterilizer and receiving them from it should be set up so that sterile and nonsterile packages can never be confused en route. The procedure must be understood by everyone.

The following materials may be safely used for wrapping items for *steam sterilization.*

Muslin Although often spoken of as linen, 140-thread count unbleached muslin usually is used for wrappers. These are of double thickness sewn together on the edges only so that they are free from holes. Packages are wrapped sequentially in two layers of double-thickness muslin (four thicknesses) to serve as a sufficient dust filter and microbial barrier. This muslin wrapper is not moisture resistant. A two ply 270- or 280-thread count muslin allows a single-thickness wrapper that is moisture retardant and is an improved barrier to microbial penetration.

Small items are easily enclosed in muslin with all corners of wrapper folded in. They should be wrapped sequentially in two wrappers. After wrapping in one wrapper, turn package over and wrap in second wrapper. A small cuff turned back on first fold of each wrapper provides a margin of safety to avoid contamination when opening after sterilization. Packages can be securely fastened with pressure-sensitive indicator tape.

Advantages of muslin as a wrapper are:

1 Muslin may be the most economical material, after the initial investment, because it can be used many times.

2 A package wrapped in muslin may be opened on a table so that the wrapper becomes a sterile field drape. Muslin is memory-free so will lie flat.

NOTE. *Memory* is the ability of a material to retain a specific shape or configuration.

3 Danger of tearing or gouging holes in muslin is minimal. Small holes (not rips) can be heat-sealed with double-vulcanized patches; they should never be stitched. A sewing machine will leave needle holes in muslin. Wrappers should be discarded after four to six patchings.

4 Muslin is flexible and easy to handle.

Disadvantages of muslin wrappers are:

1 Muslin must be laundered to rehydrate, inspected on an illuminated table, patched if necessary, delinted, and folded after each use.

2 It may create free-floating lint in the OR.

3 Opacity prevents its contents from being seen.

4 Muslin has limited storage life after sterilization: 30 days maximum in closed cabinets, 21 days or less on open shelving. Sterility is not maintained for prolonged periods unless muslin-wrapped package is hermetically sealed in plastic overwrap, a dust cover.

5 Muslin wets easily and dries quickly so that water stains may not be obvious. A 270- or 280-thread count muslin may overcome this disadvantage.

NOTE. 1. Steam sterilizer cycles are based on time-temperature profile of 140-thread count muslin.

2. Heavy, tightly woven fabrics, such as canvas, duck, or twill, will retard penetration of steam so that sterility cannot be assured.

Nonwoven Fabric A combination of cellulose and rayon with strands of nylon randomly oriented through it, or a combination of other natural and synthetic fibers bonded by method other than weaving, has the flexibility and handling qualities of muslin. Nonwoven fabric is available in three weights. Lightweight is used in four thicknesses like muslin; medium is most economical for wrapping items in two thicknesses; and heavy-duty is desirable for wrapping linen packs and basin sets when the wrapper will become the table drape. Packages are wrapped in the same manner as with muslin.

Advantages of nonwoven fabric wrapper are:

1 It is disposable, eliminating the need for inspection and repair.

2 It provides an excellent barrier against microorganisms and moisture during storage after sterilization.

3 It is strong enough to be tear-resistant, yet easy to handle with very little memory.

4 It is virtually lint free.

Disadvantages of nonwoven fabric wrapper are:

1 Nonwoven wrappers may have a different time-temperature profile for steam sterilization than muslin wrappers. This must be predetermined before sterilizing cycles are established. Manufacturer should supply data for time-temperature equivalents compared to muslin profiles.

2 It is expensive because it is a one-use item. Breaks in fibers that are difficult to detect in the folds may occur after more than one sterilization cycle. Therefore, wrapper should be disposed of after use.

3 Opacity prevents contents from being seen.

4 The heavy-duty type may retain droplets of water caused by steam condensing on surface of instruments during initial phase of prevacuum sterilization. Damp or wet packages may result, but may not be noticed until the package is opened. An absorbent towel or foam placed in bottom of an instrument tray and another under the tray during the wrapping procedure will help absorb moisture for thorough drying of instruments.

Paper If paper products are used, acceptability for steam penetration must be proven. Most craft, parchment, crepe, and glassine papers are acceptable. Water-repellent paper is preferable. Available in sheets or envelopes, paper is sealed with pressure-sensitive tape.

Advantages of paper wrapper are:

1 It is disposable and inexpensive as a one-use item. Reuse is unsafe because quality may not be consistent with repeated exposure to heat.

2 It provides a good, long-term, poststerilization contamination barrier.

3 It is lint free.

Disadvantages of paper wrapper are:

1 It is difficult to spread open for removal of contents; it has memory and flips back easily and may not open flat to provide a sterile field.

2 Paper is relatively easy to puncture or tear; it is impossible to see small holes and cracks.

3 Some paper wets easily and dries quickly making contamination difficult to detect.

4 Opacity prevents contents from being seen.

Plastic Spunbonded polypropylene wrappers or polypropylene film of 1 to 3 mil thickness is the only plastic acceptable for steam sterilization. Film is usually used in the form of pouches presealed on two or three sides. The open sides must be heat-sealed after item is placed in pouch.

NOTE. Polyethylene melts in steam. Nylon (polyamide) will not permit adequate escape of condensate when package is cooling, thereby creating moisture within contents of the package. Nylon may adhere itself to contents in prevacuum sterilization so that aseptic transfer is impossible after sterilization.

Advantages of polypropylene pouch are:

1 Transparency allows contents to be seen.

2 Polypropylene provides an excellent barrier against microorganisms and moisture for prolonged poststerilization storage.

Disadvantages of polypropylene pouch are:

1 It may be difficult to seal to avoid rupture during sterilization; it requires a high heat-sealing temperature.

2 Limited flexibility makes it difficult to handle.

Combination of Paper and Plastic Pouches and tubes made of a combination of paper on one side and plastic film on the other are satisfactory for wrapping single instruments, catheters, drains, and small items. A peel-open seal, for sterile presentation, may be preformed on one end. The other end is either heat-sealed or closed with tape after the item is inserted in the pouch or tube.

NOTE. If package does not have a preformed, peel-open seal and a heat-sealing machine is not used, ends must be folded to create a sterile edge for presentation of sterile contents, and sealed with a closure tape that is easily removed without tearing package.

Advantages of paper and plastic package are:

1 Good permeability on paper side with good visibility of contents on plastic side.
2 It is generally easy to seal with peel-open access for sterile presentation.
3 It is economical and durable.
4 It provides an excellent barrier against microorganisms for poststerilization storage.

Disadvantages of paper and plastic package are:

1 Materials may delaminate during sterilizing or opening procedures.
2 Heat seals may rupture during sterilization.

NOTE. A double heat seal should be applied to ensure against accidental opening. A *double peel-open package* (an item packaged inside a peel-open package that is placed into a slightly larger outer peel-open pack) gives extra protection. The seal must not reseal itself if opened.

Loading the Autoclave All packages must be positioned in chamber to allow free circulation and penetration of steam, enhance air elimination, and prevent entrapment of air or water. When using a prevacuum autoclave, follow recommendations of manufacturer for packaging, loading, and sterilizing time. A gravity displacement autoclave must be loaded in such a way that steam can displace air downward and out through discharge line. Wire mesh or perforated metal shelves separate layers of packages. The following directions apply to this type of autoclave:

1 Flat packages are placed on shelf on edge so flat surfaces are vertical as shown in Figure 8-2.
2 Large packages are placed in one layer only on a shelf without touching each other. Small packages may be placed on shelf above.
3 If small packages are placed one on top of another, they should be crisscrossed.

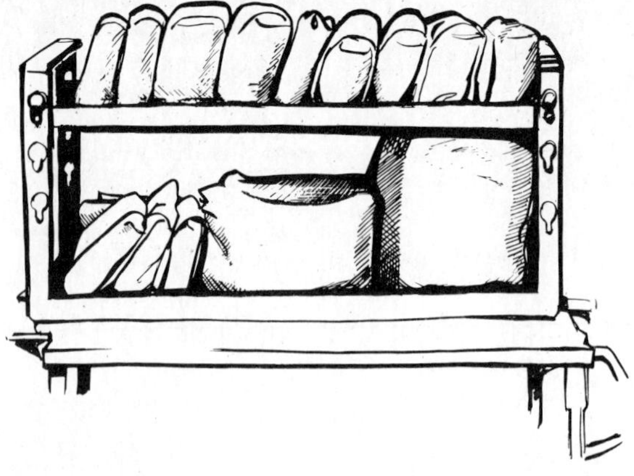

FIGURE 8-2
Proper loading of gravity displacement autoclave; place packs on edge and do not overload the rack. Steam must completely surround and penetrate every package in all autoclaves.

4 Rubber goods are placed on edge, loosely arranged, one layer to a shelf, to allow free steam circulation and penetration. No other articles should be with them.
5 Basins or any solid containers are placed on their sides to allow air to flow out of them. They should be placed so that if they contained water, it would all flow out. In a combined load with fabrics, they should be placed on lowest shelf.
6 Solutions are sterilized alone. At completion of sterilization cycle, steam should be turned off and the temperature allowed to drop to 212°F (100°C) before opening the exhaust; set the selector to "slow exhaust." Otherwise the solutions will boil over. Allow pressure gauge to reach zero before opening door so caps will not pop off.

Timing the Load Timing of a sterilization cycle begins when desired temperature is reached throughout the autoclave chamber. If autoclave does not have an automatic timing device with a buzzer that sounds at end of the cycle, an oven timer can be set after proper temperature has been reached to time the load and to alert personnel when cycle is completed.

Materials that need exposure for different lengths of time to assure sterilization in a gravity displacement autoclave should not be combined in same load if maximum time needed will be destructive to some items. Items may be sterilized wrapped or unwrapped, alone or combined with other items. Time of exposure varies depending on these factors and on temperature of the steam.

Minimum time standards, calculated after effective steam penetration of porous materials and rate of heat transfer through wrapping materials, are listed in Figure 8-3.

Most autoclaves are equipped with automatic or microcomputer time-temperature controls and a graphic recorder. Time and temperature for each load are recorded for a 24-hour period. Check the record of each load before unloading it to be certain that the desired temperature was achieved. Also, daily the temperature being recorded should be checked with the thermometer to see that the recording arm is working properly.

Drying the Load After the autoclave door is opened, a load of wrapped packages is left untouched to dry for 15 to 60 minutes. Time required depends upon type of supplies in a load; large packages require a longer time than small ones. Packages are then unloaded onto a table or cart with wire mesh shelves padded with absorbent material. Warm packages laid on a solid, cold surface become damp from steam condensation, and thus contaminated.

Time is saved in loading and unloading autoclave if the rack of wire shelves can be rolled onto a transfer carriage. The shelves are loaded and rolled into the autoclave. After sterilization, the rack can be rolled onto carriage again without handling individual packages while they cool.

Packages must be observed for water droplets on exterior or interior of package or absorbed moisture in package. Packs wrapped in moisture-permeable materials that have water droplets on outside or inside are unsafe for use as the moisture can be a pathway for microbial migration into the package. This is not a problem with moisture-impermeable wrapping materials. However, any package should be considered contaminated if wet when opened for use. Packages should be completely dry after cooling at room temperature of 68 to 75°F (20 to 24°C) for a minimum of one hour.

FIGURE 8-3
Minimum time standards for steam sterilization after effective steam penetration and heat transfer.

Materials	250°F (121°C)	270°F (132°C)
Basin sets, wrapped	20 min	10 min
Basins, glassware, and utensils, unwrapped	15 min	3 min
Instruments, with or without other items, wrapped as a set in double-thickness wrappers	30 min	15 min
Instruments, unwrapped but with other items including a towel in the bottom of tray or a cover over them	20 min	10 min
Instruments, completely unwrapped	15 min	3 min
Drape packs, 12 by 12 by 20 in. (30 by 30 by 50 cm) maximum size, 12 lb (5.5 kg) maximum weight	30 min	Not recommended except in prevacuum sterilizer. Fabrics and rubber deteriorate more rapidly with repeated sterilization at higher temperature for prolonged periods in gravity displacement autoclaves.
Linen, single items wrapped	30 min	
Rubber and thermoplastics, including small items and gloves, but excluding tubing, wrapped	20 min	
Tubing, wrapped	30 min	15 min
Tubing, unwrapped	20 min	10 min
Sponges and dressings, wrapped	30 min	15 min
Solutions, flasked	(Slow exhaust)	In the prevacuum sterilizer, the automatic selector determines correct temperature and exposure period for solutions.
75-ml flask	20 min	
250-ml flask	25 min	
500-ml flask	30 min	
1000-ml flask	35 min	
1500-ml flask	45 min	
2000-ml flask	45 min	

Ethylene Oxide Gas

Ethylene oxide gas is used to sterilize items that are heat- or moisture-sensitive. *Ethylene oxide* (EO) is a chemical agent that kills microorganisms, including spores, by interfering with the normal metabolism of protein and reproductive processes, resulting in death of the cells. Used in the gaseous state, ethylene oxide gas must have direct contact with the microorganisms in or on items to be sterilized. Because pure ethylene oxide gas is highly flammable and explosive in air, it is diluted with an inert gas such as a fluorinated hydrocarbon or carbon dioxide for use in most sterilizers. These mixtures provide a safe, nonflammable agent for EO gas sterilization.

Ethylene oxide sterilization is dependent upon EO gas concentration, temperature, humidity, and exposure time. Gas is supplied in high-pressure metal cylinder tanks or disposable cans. Mixtures contain 10 to 12 percent ethylene oxide. In the sterilization process, air is withdrawn from chamber and the gas mixture enters under pressure. In general, the EO gas concentration in the sterilizer ranges between 450 to 800 mg per liter of chamber space. Gas sterilizers normally are not equipped with gas analyzer devices. The only means for controlling EO concentration is to operate sterilizer according to manufacturer's instructions, making certain the chamber is charged to the specified pressure at the temperature designated in the operating instructions.

Gas sterilizers usually operate at 120 to 140°F (49 to 60°C). Temperature influences the destruction of microorganisms and affects the permeability of EO through cell walls as well as through packaging materials. As temperature is increased, exposure time can be decreased. However, 140°F (60°C) is the uppermost temperature limit for many heat-sensitive plastic materials. Sterilization may be achieved at room temperature, but exposure time must increase as temperature decreases to effectively kill spores.

Moisture is an essential element in achieving sterility with EO gas. Desiccated or highly dried bacterial spores are resistant to EO gas. They must be hydrated. Moisture content of the atmosphere immediately surrounding the organisms and water content of the organisms themselves are important to action of EO gas. Consequently, relative humidity of the room atmosphere where items are packaged and held for sterilization should be at least 50 percent, and not less than 30 percent, to hydrate them during preparation. Humidity of 40 to 80 percent is maintained throughout the sterilization cycle.

Time required for complete destruction of microorganisms is primarily related to gas concentration and temperature. However, cleanliness of items, type of materials, arrangement of load, and rate of penetration also influence exposure time. Drawing an initial vacuum at start of the cycle aids in penetration of gas. Generally, sterilization cycles of three to six hours are utilized. The cycle is totally automatic once the sterilizer is closed and the controls are activated.

Advantages of EO Gas

1 It is an effective substitute agent for most items that cannot be sterilized by heat.

2 It provides an effective method of sterilization for items that steam and moisture may erode; it is noncorrosive and does not damage items.

3 It completely permeates all porous materials.

> NOTE. 1. EO gas does not penetrate metal, glass, and petroleum-based lubricants. Whether or not it penetrates oils, liquids, or powder depends upon amount in containers. If material is spread thin, the gas will penetrate, but it will not go through bulk. EO gas sterilization is *not* recommended for these products.
>
> 2. Glass ampuls can be sterilized in EO as the gas does not penetrate glass. But a glass vial with a rubber stopper must not be put in the sterilizer as the gas will penetrate the rubber and may react with the drugs in solution and cause a potentially harmful chemical reaction.

4 Automatic controls preclude human error by establishing proper levels of pressure, temperature, humidity, and gas concentration. Sterilizer must be operated according to manufacturer's instructions.

5 It leaves no film on items.

6 EO gas sterilization is used extensively in preparation of packaged, presterilized items commercially available because packaging materials that prolong storage life can be used.

Disadvantages of EO Gas

1 EO gas sterilization is a complicated process so *biologic indicators should be used to verify the adequacy of every cycle.*

> NOTE. Never gas sterilize any article that can be appropriately steam sterilized.

2 EO sterilization takes longer than steam sterilization; it is a long, slow process.

3 EO gas requires special, expensive equipment. Gas is somewhat expensive per cycle.

4 Items that absorb EO gas during sterilization, such as rubber, polyethylene, or silicone, require an aeration period (see p. 135). Air admitted to the sterilizer at the end of the cycle only partially aerates the load.

5 Toxic by-products can be formed in the presence of droplets of moisture during exposure of some plastics, particularly polyvinyl chloride.

6 Repeated sterilization can increase the concentration of the total EO residues in porous items. These increased levels can be hazardous unless gas can be dissipated.

7 EO is a vesicant if it comes in contact with the skin, and may cause serious burns if not immediately removed.

8 If inhaled, EO gas can be irritating to mucous membranes. Its presence is easily detectable by odor. Overexposure to the gas causes eye and nose irritation, and long exposure may result in nausea, vomiting, and dizziness. It is not cumulative in the body. At room temperature EO is a colorless gas.

NOTE. The 1984 Occupational Safety and Health Administration (OSHA) standard governing exposure to ethylene oxide limits employee exposure to an eight hour time-weighted average of one part per million (ppm) of air. Therefore, EO gas must be vented from sterilizer to outside atmosphere to avoid personnel exposure. Following completion of cycle, the chamber door should be left open approximately six inches for about 15 minutes before unloading to allow residual gas to dissipate before personnel reach into chamber. Personnel should minimize contact with items during unloading of sterilizer. Gloves, known to be resistant to EO penetration, are recommended.

Types of Gas Sterilizers Stationary EO chambers range in size from 16 by 16 by 29 in. (40 by 40 by 73 cm) to very large units that will accommodate several mattresses. These chambers can be automatically or manually operated to achieve sterilization because the factors of gas concentration, temperature, humidity, and time are controlled. They operate at elevated temperatures and not only inject moisture to optimally control humidity, but also create a vacuum of 25 to 27 in. (625 to 675 mm) Hg to aid penetration of gas. At end of time exposure, a postvacuum helps exhaust gas from load.

Portable, small units are also available. Some of these chambers operate for a standardized time cycle at temperature and relative humidity level of the room. To compensate for room temperature, a higher concentration of gas is used. The gas flows through the chamber from an ampul broken within the chamber or from a cartridge affixed outside the chamber. Other small units are manually controlled and equipped with a heating element and a vacuum system. Another unit sterilizes and aerates items in the same chamber.

Preparing Items for Gas Sterilization

All Items All items must be thoroughly cleaned and dried, as for steam sterilization. Disassemble detachable parts. Separate syringes. Remove impermeable caps, plugs, stylets, etc.

Lumens Any tubing or other item with a lumen should be blown out with air to force dry before packaging as water combines with EO gas to form a harmful acid, ethylene glycol.

Lensed Instruments Endoscopes (see Chap. 19, p. 372) with cemented optical lenses require special cement for EO gas sterilization.

Lubricated Instruments Remove all traces of lubricant, especially a petroleum-based lubricant. EO cannot permeate the film. Air-powered instruments can be lubricated with sterile lubricant after sterilization, just prior to use.

Camera Some cameras and film can be EO gas sterilized. As a permanent record or a teaching aid, photographs are sometimes taken with a sterile camera at the operative site. An especially constructed camera is used. The film is loaded before packaging for sterilization.

Packaging for Gas Sterilization Type and thickness of wrapper used influence the time it takes for gas to penetrate. Size and shape of package and porosity of the contents also influence penetration time. Items wrapped for gas sterilization should be tagged, "for gas," to avoid their inadvertently being steam sterilized and damaged. Acceptable materials for wrapping items for EO gas sterilization include:

Muslin Double-thickness muslin is used as for steam with the same advantages and disadvantages.

Nonwoven Fabric Spunbonded olefin (polyethylene) is highly permeable to EO and moisture. It offers the same advantages as the nonwoven fabric described for steam sterilization although the two are not interchangeable; the cellulose/nylon/rayon combination should be confined to steam sterilization.

Paper Double-thickness paper is used as for steam with the same advantages and disadvantages.

Plastic Both polypropylene and low-density polyethylene of 3 mil or less thickness, film or pouches, may be used. Polyethylene is easier to handle than polypropylene, and EO gas penetrates it more rapidly. Express as much air as possible from pouches before heat sealing to avoid rupture when vacuum is drawn in the sterilizer.

> NOTE. Materials *not* to be used for EO sterilization because of inadequate permeability include nylon, polyvinyl chloride film, Saran, polyester, polyvinyl alcohol, cellophane, and aluminum foil.

Combination of Paper and Plastic Pouches and tubes can be used as described for steam, except that double wrapping may not allow adequate permeation of EO gas and moisture. Avoid combinations of materials that make a package insufficiently permeable for adequate humidification and gas penetration.

Loading the Sterilizer All packages are positioned in chamber to allow free circulation and penetration of gas. Procedures and precautions used for loading the gas sterilizer do not differ from those used for loading the autoclave. Overloading creates conditions whereby EO, moisture, and heat penetration can be retarded. Air space should be provided between chamber ceiling and topmost packages in load. Also packages should not touch walls of chamber. Do not stack packages tightly; allow air space between packages for circulation of EO gas and moisture.

Timing the Cycle Closely follow the instructions provided by manufacturer of the sterilizer.

Aerating Items Sterilized in Ethylene Oxide Gas Adequate aeration for all absorbent materials that will come in contact with the human body, either directly or indirectly, is absolutely essential. EO exerts toxic effects on living tissue. Residual products after sterilization can include:

1 *Ethylene oxide.* Porous materials, such as plastic, silicone, rubber, wood, and leather, absorb a certain amount of gas that must be removed. The thicker the walls of items, the longer the aeration time must be. Residual EO in plastic tubing or parts of a heart-lung pump oxygenator causes hemolysis of blood. Rubber gloves or shoes worn immediately after exposure can cause irritation or burns on skin. Acceptable limits for residual EO are:*
   - **a** 25 ppm for blood dialysis units, blood oxygenators, heart-lung machines, and all implants.
   - **b** 250 ppm for all topical medical devices.
2 *Ethylene glycol.* This is formed by a reaction of EO with water or moisture that leaves a clear or brownish oily film on exposed surfaces. This film on plastic or rubber endotracheal tubes or airways can cause irritation to mucous membranes. Acceptable limits of ethylene glycol are:*
   - **a** 250 ppm for blood dialysis units, blood oxygenators, heart-lung machines, and all implants.
   - **b** 1000 ppm for all topical medical devices.
3 *Ethylene chlorohydrin.* This by-product is formed when a chloride ion is present to combine with EO, such as in polyvinyl chloride plastic. Rubber, soft nylon, and polyethylene items that have been in contact with saline solution or blood can retain enough chloride ion to cause this reaction in the presence of moisture. Disposable products should be discarded after use to avoid this hazard. Acceptable limits of ethylene chlorohydrin are:*
   - **a** 25 ppm for blood dialysis units, blood oxygenators, heart-lung machines, and all implants.
   - **b** 250 ppm for all topical medical devices.

Aeration after sterilization to diffuse any residual products from porous items may be accom-

*Bureau of Medical Devices and Diagnostics: *Ethylene Oxide Sterilization: A Guide for Hospital Personnel,* Food and Drug Administration, Public Health Service, U.S. Department of Health, Education and Welfare, Oct. 1, 1975; and the Association for Advancement of Medical Instrumentation Sterilization Committee: *Good Hospital Practice: Ethylene Oxide Gas—Ventilation Recommendations and Safe Use,* AAMI, 1981.

plished with ambient (room) air or preferably in an aerator chamber designed for this purpose. Manufacturers of products suitable for EO sterilization should provide written instructions regarding sterilization exposure time and ambient or mechanical aeration time. These recommendations must be followed. Nature of the item, material in which it is packaged, intended use of item, and temperature and air flow in the area influence aeration time.

Packages may be removed from the sterilizer and placed in a clean, well-ventilated storage area. Intravenous or irrigation fluids in plastic bags must not be stored in this aeration area as residual diffusing gas could be absorbed through the plastic. At room temperature, controlled between 65 and 72°F (18 and 22°C), the following *aeration times* for various materials are recommended:*

1 Nonporous items of metal and glass may be used immediately.

2 24 hours—paper, and thin rubber products.

3 48 hours—gum rubber thicker than ¼ in. (6.35 mm) and polyethylene items.

4 96 hours (4 days)—all other plastics except polyvinyl chloride items.

5 168 hours (7 days)—polyvinyl chloride and other plastic and rubber items sealed in plastic packages; will come in direct contact with blood; will be implanted, inserted, or applied to body tissues; or will be used for assisted respiration.

Aeration at an elevated temperature enhances the dissipation rate of absorbed gases, resulting in faster removal. The entire load on the sterilizer carriage can be transferred into an *aerator.* A heater is in the upper part of the chamber. A blower system draws in air from outside and heats it. With a minimum of four air changes per minute, all materials remain in aerator for 8 hours at 140°F (60°C) to 12 hours at 122°F (50°C) or longer, depending on the temperature and instructions of manufacturer of the aerator.

Activated Glutaraldehyde

Activated glutaraldehyde solution is the method of choice for sterilizing heat-sensitive items that cannot be steam sterilized if an ethylene oxide gas sterilizer is not available or the aeration period makes EO sterilization impractical. Immersion in a 2% aqueous solution of activated, buffered alkaline glutaraldehyde is *sporicidal* (kills spores) in 10 hours (aqueous Cidex activated dialdehyde solution) or 6¾ hours (Sporicidin cold sterilizing solution). Only products that indicate on label that they are registered as a sterilant by the U.S. Environmental Protection Agency (EPA) are used for sterilization. They must be used according to manufacturers' instructions.

*Ibid

Advantages

1 Activated glutaraldehyde solution has a low surface tension; it thus penetrates into crevices and is readily rinsed from items.

2 It is noncorrosive, nonstaining, and completely safe for all instruments that can be immersed in a chemical solution.

3 It does not damage lenses or the cement on lensed instruments.

4 It is not absorbed by rubber or plastic.

5 It has low volatility so solution can be reused throughout the effective activation period.

6 Alkaline glutaraldehyde is effective at room temperature.

Disadvantages

1 Solution must be activated by adding powdered buffer to liquid.

2 Alkalinized glutaraldehyde solution changes pH and gradually loses effectiveness after date of activation. Mark expiration date on container when activated. Solution is reusable until this date, according to manufacturer's instructions.

3 Even though chemical has low toxicity and irritation, rinse items thoroughly in sterile distilled water prior to use.

4 Glutaraldehyde solution may have a mild odor.

Preparing Items for Sterilization by Immersion With this agent, as with all others, items should be clean and free of organic debris and blood. This agent will attack some organic materials. It remains highly active in the presence of protein matter in serum, mucous and soap films. The human hepatitis virus cannot be isolated, so removal of blood is critical. Items should be washed thoroughly in a nonfilming solution, rinsed, and dried prior to immersion.

Items to be sterilized should be placed in a container deep enough to completely immerse them. Be certain that items are dry before submerging so solution will not be diluted. Lumen of tubing or instruments must be completely filled with solution.

Timing the Immersion Cycle Activated glutaraldehyde solution is bactericidal, pseudomonacidal, fungicidal, and virucidal in ten minutes for disinfection, and tuberculocidal in 45 minutes. *Ten hours are required for sterilization.*

Rinsing Following Immersion Items must be thoroughly rinsed in sterile distilled water before use.

Hot Air—Dry Heat

Dry heat in the form of hot air is used primarily to sterilize anhydrous oils, petroleum products, and bulk powders that steam and ethylene oxide gas cannot penetrate. Death of microbial life by dry heat is a physical oxidation or slow burning-up process of coagulating the protein in cells. In absence of moisture, higher temperatures are required than when moisture is present because microorganisms are destroyed through a very slow process of heat absorption. Dry heat is most infrequently used method of sterilization.

Advantages

1 Hot air penetrates certain substances that cannot be steam or gas sterilized.

2 Dry heat can be used in laboratories to sterilize glassware.

3 Dry heat is a protective method of sterilizing some delicate, sharp, or cutting edge instruments. Steam may erode or corrode cutting edges.

4 Instruments that cannot be disassembled may be sterilized in hot air.

5 Carbon steel does not become corroded or discolored in dry heat as it may in steam.

Disadvantages

1 A long exposure period is required because hot air penetrates slowly and possibly unevenly.

2 Time and temperature vary for different substances.

3 Overexposure may ruin some substances.

4 It is destructive to fabrics and rubber goods.

Types of Dry Heat Sterilizers

Hot Air Oven The most efficient and reliable sterilizer is an electrically heated mechanical convection hot air oven. It has a blower within it that forces air in motion around the load to hasten heating of substances and ensure an even temperature in all areas of oven.

Autoclave The autoclave with steam only in the jacket can be used as a substitute for a hot air oven. However, this is not as reliable and demands a lengthy exposure because the maximum temperature that can be attained in the chamber is 250°F (121°C). The exposure period must be a minimum of six hours and preferably overnight.

Preparing Items for Dry Heat Sterilization

Oils The amount of mineral oil, lubricating oil for electric or air-powered instruments, etc., put in a container should not exceed 1 oz (30 ml). Preferably the layer depth of the oil is not more than ¼ in. (6.35 mm). The greater the depth, the longer the exposure period must be.

Impregnated Gauze Strips of gauze bandage covered with no more than 4 oz (120 ml) of melted petroleum jelly or other oil-base liquid should be arranged in a stainless steel container to provide a maximum layer depth of ½ in. (12.5 mm).

> NOTE. Most hospitals purchase sterile packages of impregnated gauze products to eliminate hazards inherent in preparation and sterilization of these products.

Powders An ounce (30 ml) of powder should be spread out in container so layer depth does not exceed ¼ in. (6.25 mm).

Packaging Materials for Dry Heat

Glass Petri dishes, ointment jars, flasks, or test tubes can be used. Cotton plugs or muslin are used to cover tops of flasks and tubes.

Stainless Steel Boats or Trays Covers must fit tightly. They can be held in place with indicator tape.

Muslin and Paper These materials can be used for wrapping instruments. Powders can be put in double glassine envelopes.

Loading the Sterilizer Allow space between items and along the chamber walls so hot air can circulate freely. Never load chamber to full capacity.

Timing the Load Time of exposure varies depending on characteristics of individual items, layer depth in containers, and temperature in sterilizer. If the amount in each container is kept to a minimum and sterilizer loaded according to manufacturer's recommendations, items are exposed for a minimum period of:

1 One hour at 340°F (171°C)
2 Two hours at 320°F (160°C)
3 Three hours at 285°F (140°C)
4 Six hours at 250°F (121°C)

Ionizing Radiation

Some products commercially available are sterilized by *irradiation*. Ionizing radiation produces ions by knocking electrons out of atoms. These electrons are knocked out so violently that they strike an adjacent atom and either attach themselves to it, or dislodge an electron from the second atom. The ionic energy that results becomes converted to thermal and chemical energy. This energy causes the death of microorganisms by disruption of the DNA molecule, thus preventing cellular division and propagation of biological life.

The principal sources of ionizing radiation are beta particles and gamma rays. Beta particles, free electrons, are transmitted through a high-voltage electron beam from a linear accelerator. These high-energy free electrons will penetrate into matter before being stopped by collisions with other atoms. Thus, their usefulness in sterilizing an object is limited by density and thickness of the object and by energy of the electrons. They produce their effect by ionizing the atoms they hit, producing secondary electrons that, in turn, produce lethal effects on microorganisms.

Cobalt 60 is a radioactive isotope capable of disintegrating to produce gamma rays. Gamma rays are electromagnetic waves. They have the capability of penetrating to a much greater distance than beta rays before losing their energy from collisions. Because they travel with the speed of light, they must pass through a thickness measuring several feet before making sufficient collisions to lose all of their energy. Cobalt 60 is the most commonly used source for irradiation sterilization. The product is exposed to radiation for 10 to 20 hours, depending on strength of the source.

Advantages

1 Ionizing radiation penetrates most materials to sterilize reliably. It is the most effective sterilization method.

2 Rays have very low temperature effect on materials and process is dry, so irradiation can be used to sterilize most heat- and moisture-sensitive items.

3 Products can be released for use on basis of dosimetry, measurements of radiation dose, without quarantine periods required for biological testing.

4 No residual radiation is generated.

5 Gamma rays can penetrate large bulky objects, so cartons ready for shipment can be sterilized in the cobalt 60 irradiator. This is cost effective. Irradiation sterilization presently is limited to commercial use.

CONTROL MEASURES

Biological Testing

Positive assurance that sterilization conditions were achieved by either steam under pressure, ethylene oxide gas, or dry heat can be obtained only through a biological control test. The most dependable form of biological control is a preparation of dry living spores resistant to the sterilizing agent. *Bacillus stearothermophilis* spores are used to test steam under pressure; *Bacillus subiilis var niger strain globigi* are used for ethylene oxide and dry heat.

Ampuls of spores in suspension may be used, except in prevacuum autoclave where they may explode. Biological spore strips are in especially prepared envelopes or capsule units. These are stored at room temperature and kept dry prior to use. Each of these units contains a strip to be sterilized and a control strip that is not sterilized.

An ampul or biological spore strip is placed inside, in the center, of the largest and most dense pack or packaged item that is routinely processed in a given sterilizer. For example, the test pack for steam sterilizers should contain the equivalent of three gowns, 12 towels, three gauze sponges (4 by

4 in.), five laparotomy tapes (12 by 12 in.), and one drape sheet. Test pack is placed in bottom front of steam sterilizer, or center of ethylene oxide sterilizer, and sterilized in a routine cycle. When cycle is completed, the test ampul or strip is removed from pack and sent with a control ampul or control strip to the bacteriology laboratory. If spore strips in envelopes are used, the test and control strips are aseptically transferred into a culture medium and incubated for seven days. With the closed capsule system, the incubation period is shortened to 24 hours for *B. stearothermophilis* and 48 hours for *B. subtilis. B. stearothermophilis* is incubated at 131 to 140°F (55 to 60°C); *B. subtilis* at 95 to 98.6°F (35 to 37°C).

Biological tests of all steam sterilizers and hot air ovens are conducted on a regular schedule, at least weekly. Every ethylene oxide gas sterilization cycle should be tested. Where feasible, the test results should be ascertained prior to use of EO gas sterilized items, especially implants and intravascular items. All laboratory reports are filed as a permanent record.

Process Monitors/Chemical Indicators

Process monitors are designed to indicate that packages were exposed to sterilization conditions. These chemical indicators include such devices as special tapes, chemically impregnated discs, tablets, or solutions sealed in glass tubes or plastic bags, etc., that change color. Some of these are sensitive to temperature; others to time and temperature. One type that has a bar graph to indicate "accept" or "reject" is less subject to individual interpretation than those which change color. These devices can be placed on the outside or inside of packages. Since they do not test sterility, it is advantageous to have an indicator on the outside of every package to differentiate sterilized from unsterilized items. If the indicator does not change color, it alerts personnel that the sterilization cycle may have been inadequate. Process monitors should be placed in center of every package sterilized, or at least in all packs of critical items such as implants.

To readily check for air entrapment in the prevacuum steam sterilizer, the Bowie-Dick test can be used daily. Three pieces of indicator tape, about 8 in. (20 cm) long, are crisscrossed on a record sheet placed between layers of fabric in the center of a pack of towels. This test pack must be exposed to the sterilizing cycle alone in an otherwise empty chamber. If residual air remained in the pack, which inhibited steam penetration during the cycle, the tape does not change color.

Chemical indicators monitor physical conditions within the sterilizer so personnel can check for improper packaging, loading, or performance of sterilizers.

Lot Control Number and Expiration Date

Lot (load) control number should be imprinted or labeled on every package. This number designates the sterilization equipment used, cycle, sterilization date, and expiration date. To avoid confusion, the sterilization date can be recorded as a Julian date (day 1 through 365) and the expiration date as a Georgian date (month, day, year).

An expiration date on each package sets a limit on the number of days an item will be considered sterile. The date the package was sterilized may be stamped on the package as it is removed from the sterilizer; thus an undated package is not sterile. Some hospitals write the date on the package when it is wrapped. Others use a monthly, color-coded, machine-labeling system. The expiration date on commercially sterilized products indicates the time the manufacturer can guarantee product stability and sterility based on test data approved by FDA.

SHELF LIFE

Determination of maximum *shelf life,* the time a sterile package may be kept in storage, depends on the following factors:

1 Conditions of storage
   - **a** Storage areas must be clean; free of dust, dirt, and vermin.
   - **b** Closed cabinets prolong storage of muslin- and paper-wrapped items to 30 days, as opposed to open shelving with a storage life of 21 days.
   - **c** If open shelving must be used, highest shelf should be at least 18 in. below ceiling and lowest 8 to 10 in. above floor.
   - **d** All sterile items should be stored under conditions that protect them from extremes of temperature and humidity. Prolonged storage in a warm environment at a very high humidity can cause moisture to condense inside packages and allow microorganisms to grow into and through the packaging material.

Ventilating and air-conditioning systems with filtered air should maintain temperature below 80°F (26°C) and relative humidity between 30 and 60 percent.

e Sterile storage areas should have controlled traffic patterns.

2 Material used for packaging

a Muslin- and paper-wrapped items may be stored for 21 to 30 days, then resterilization is required. However, if these items are sealed in an airtight plastic bag immediately after sterilization, following cooling or aerating, their shelf life can be prolonged from 6 to 12 months, if this dust cover does not have cracks or holes in it. The dust cover is removed before the sterile package is taken from a storage area into the OR.

b Density of nonwoven fabrics and plastic materials prolongs shelf life.

3 Seal of the package

a Tape-sealed packages wrapped in nonwoven fabrics or plastic film can be stored for three to four months.

b Heat-sealed or hermetically sealed items can be stored for six months to a year.

4 Integrity of the package

a Commercially packaged, sterilized items are usually considered sterile until the package is opened or damaged, or becomes outdated.

b The item is no longer considered sterile after accidental puncture, tear, or rupture due to crushing of a package.

c Accidental wetting of a package, except hermetically sealed plastic, contaminates the contents.

Sterile supplies must be checked daily for outdated items. Any packages that become outdated or contaminated must be resterilized. Shelf life can be minimized by inventory control and rotation of sterile supplies. By adjusting the standard number of packages kept sterile to daily needs, packages seldom become outdated. In the interest of economy and good management, stock supply of day-to-day items should be regulated to have enough for the busiest day with used items replenished daily. In this way the need for resterilization of most items is eliminated. Some items deteriorate with repeated sterilization. Many items are seldom used yet several must be kept sterile at all times. These supplies should be sterilized, or commercially sterilized items ordered, only in quantities sufficient to ensure prompt use and rapid turnover. Commercially sterilized packages can be date-stamped as they go into inventory. Some have manufacturer's expiration dates on package. Older supplies are always used first so that they do not become outdated.

NOTE. The acronym FI-FO, first in, first out, is helpful to remember as it applies to rotation of supplies, particularly sterile supplies.

DISINFECTION

Surfaces and items that cannot be sterilized must be disinfected to eliminate as many microorganisms from the environment as possible. Disinfection differs from sterilization by its lack of sporicidal power. It is utilized in the OR suite for two major purposes:

1 To kill pathogenic microorganisms on inanimate surfaces and objects that cannot be sterilized.

2 To prevent or arrest growth of microorganisms on body surfaces. (This application, referred to as *antisepsis,* for preparation of the skin of personnel and patients prior to operation is discussed in Chapters 9 and 16.)

Disinfection of inanimate surfaces can be accomplished with chemical or physical agents. These agents have two types of applications:

1 Housekeeping disinfection, which deals with floors, walls, furniture, large equipment, etc.

2 Instrument and small equipment disinfection.

NOTE. Critical items that come in contact with body tissue below the skin or mucous membranes, either directly or indirectly, *must be sterile.* Semicritical items that contact only unbroken skin or mucous membranes may be disinfected. Sterilization is *always* preferable for items that come in contact with the patient.

The best housekeeping agents are not the best instrument disinfectants and vice versa. An all-purpose disinfectant does not exist.

Chemical Disinfectants

Chemical agents, including ethylene oxide, must be registered with the Pesticide Regulation Division of the Environmental Protection Agency (EPA) to be sold in interstate commerce. An EPA registration number is granted only when all the requirements of laboratory test data, toxicity data, product formula, and label copy are approved. The product must do what the label says it does. To be labeled for hospital use, a chemical disinfectant must be proven effective against *Staphylococcus aureus* (gram-positive), *Salmonella choleraesuis* (gram-negative), and *Pseudomonas aeruginosa* (gram-negative), the most resistant gram-positive and -negative organisms. The agent can be classified as a hospital disinfectant without being pseudomonacidal, but it must be labeled whether it is or is not effective against this organism.

The EPA defines a *disinfectant* as an agent that kills growing or vegetative forms of bacteria. The terms *germicide* and *bactericide* may be used synonymously with disinfectant according to this definition. However, the tubercle bacillus has a waxy envelope that makes it comparatively resistant to aqueous germicides. Effective agents against the tubercle bacillus should be labeled *tuberculocidal.* Agents also are labeled if they kill fungi (*fungicide*), viruses (*virucide*), and/or spores (*sporicide*).

The safest products for use in the OR suite include all categories of "-cidal" action. With few exceptions, chemicals are not sporicides, however. Analysis of the label statements helps determine whether a product is appropriate for a specific purpose in the OR. Factors to be considered in the selection of an agent include:

1 Microorganisms differ markedly in their resistance to chemicals.
   - a *Low-level*: most vegetative bacteria, fungi, and lipoprotein (lipid- and protein-coated) viruses are susceptible to chemicals.
   - b *Intermediate*: tubercle bacilli and nonlipid viruses are significantly more resistant.
   - c *High-level*: bacterial spores are tremendously resistant.

2 Disinfectants differ widely in level of cidal action they produce and mechanisms involved. All are protoplasmic poisons that either coagulate or denature cell protein, oxidate or bind enzymes, or alter cell membranes. In-use culture testing must determine number of viable microorganisms after an agent is used for the intended purpose.

3 Nature of microbial contamination influences results of chemical disinfection. Bacteria, spores, fungi, and viruses are present in air and on surfaces throughout the environment. However, organic soil, such as blood, plasma, feces, and tissue, absorbs germicidal molecules and inactivates some chemicals. Therefore, good physical cleaning prior to disinfection helps reduce numbers of microorganisms present and enhances cidal action.

4 Requirements of the chemical agent vary.
   - a Housekeeping products should be *detergent-disinfectants* that meet the requirements for both cleaning and disinfection:
     - 1 Effective against a broad spectrum of microorganisms, including *Pseudomonas aeruginosa* and the tubercle bacillus, preferably in the presence of organic soil.
     - 2 Must be compatible with tap water used for use-dilution (see Note below).
     - 3 Must not leave a residual insulating film that will affect electrical conductivity.
     - 4 Should be nontoxic and nonirritating to patients and personnel.
     - 5 Should be virtually odorless.
   - b Instrument and equipment disinfectants should kill as many species of microorganisms as possible to effectively decontaminate items for handling by personnel or in preparation of semicritical items for patient use, such as stethoscopes and monitors.

5 Kill time is correlated with concentration of the agent and number of microorganisms present. Most chemicals are used in aqueous solution. Water brings chemical and microorganisms together. Without this water reaction the process stops. Increasing the concentration of the chemical may shorten exposure time, but not necessarily. Disinfectants should be premixed in required concentration and stored in properly labeled containers to ensure that personnel utilize the product in the correct concentration. *Instruments must be completely submerged for maximum time recommended by manufacturer of the product used, or used as recommended for housekeeping purposes.* All instruments should be clean and dry when put into solution. Drippy, wet items will dilute the solution and change the concentration of a chemical agent.

   NOTE. All tap water has *Pseudomonas* in it. The pH, calcium, and magnesium in tap water can inactivate disinfectants. Therefore, distilled water is recommended for use-dilution.

6 Composition of items to be disinfected varies. Nonporous items such as metal instruments are more easily disinfected than porous materials.

NOTE. Seepage of disinfectant solution into an ampul can occur if ampul has a microscopic hole or crack in it. If this material is injected or implanted, serious reactions can result. If ampuls cannot be sterilized in steam or ethylene oxide gas, a color dye must be added to a disinfectant solution. If color seeps into ampul or solution becomes cloudy, discard. Do not use any suspicious ampul.

7 Method of application influences effectiveness of chemical agent.
   a Direct application of a liquid disinfectant, either by mechanical action for housekeeping purposes or by immersion for instrument disinfection, is the most effective method of applying chemicals to the surface of inanimate objects.
   b Aerosol spray, from a pressurized container, is an effective method of spot disinfection on smooth surfaces and into crevices not otherwise accessible.
   c *Fogging* is the process of filling the air in a room with an aerosolized disinfectant solution in an attempt to control microbial contamination. Action on airborne contaminants is temporary because the agent dispersed through the air settles on surfaces or is exhausted through the ventilating system. This method is potentially toxic to personnel and patients. Unless all surfaces are completely covered by a layer of the disinfectant solution for the minimum exposure period, disinfection is incomplete. Fogging is impractical and too ineffective to be an acceptable method of disinfection in OR suites.

Chemical agents used for disinfection include:

Alcohol 70 to 95% ethyl or isopropyl alcohol kills microorganisms by coagulation of cell proteins.

Effectiveness

1 It may be used as a housekeeping disinfectant for spot cleaning, such as damp-dusting furniture and lights or wiping electrical cords, without leaving residue on treated surfaces.

2 It can disinfect semicritical instruments. To prevent corrosion of metal, 0.2% sodium nitrite must be added.

3 It is bactericidal, pseudomonacidal, and fungicidal in minimum of ten minutes exposure.

4 It is tuberculocidal and virucidal for all viruses in minimum of 15 minutes exposure.

Hazards

1 It is volatile; it will act only as long as in solution. Alcohol becomes ineffective as soon as it evaporates and loses cidal activity below 50% concentration; discard at frequent intervals.

2 It is inactive in the presence of organic soil. It does not penetrate skin oil that lodges on instruments through handling.

3 It will blanch asphalt tiles of floors.

4 It cannot be used on lensed instruments with cement mountings because it dissolves cement.

5 With long exposure, it will harden and swell plastic tubing and items, including polyethylene.

Chlorine Compounds Inorganic chlorine is valuable for disinfection of water, but it has limited use in the hospital. Chlorine compounds kill microorganisms by oxidation of enzymes. Sodium hypochlorite, 1 to 5%, has limited use.

Effectiveness

1 It is a housekeeping disinfectant for spot cleaning of floors and furniture.

2 It is bactericidal, fungicidal, tuberculocidal, and virucidal.

Hazards

1 It is unstable and dissipates rapidly in presence of organic soil.

2 Its odor may be objectionable.

3 It is corrosive to metal; cannot be used for instrument disinfection.

Formaldehyde In either solution or gas, formaldehyde kills microorganisms by coagulation of protein in cells. Solution may be 37% formaldehyde in water, or 8% formaldehyde in 70% isopropyl alcohol.

Effectiveness

1 It is an instrument disinfectant. To prevent corrosion of metal, 0.2% sodium nitrite must be present.

2 It is bactericidal, pseudomonacidal, and fungicidal in minimum of five minutes exposure.

3 It is tuberculocidal and virucidal in minimum of ten minutes in alcohol solution; in minimum of 15 minutes in aqueous solution.

4 It is sporicidal in minimum of 12 hours.

Hazards

1 Fumes are too irritating for housekeeping use.

2 It is toxic to tissues, so instruments must be thoroughly rinsed with sterile distilled water before use.

3 Rubber and porous materials may absorb formaldehyde so they should not be disinfected in this agent.

4 As a gas, it must have 70 percent relative humidity in the chamber for use as a fumigant.

Glutaraldehyde An aqueous solution of 2% activated, buffered glutaraldehyde (Cidex solution or Sporicidin) kills microorganisms by denaturation of protein. This is the agent of choice for sterilizing instruments that cannot be steam sterilized when an ethylene oxide gas sterilizer is not available, or for disinfecting semicritical instruments between patient uses. (Glutaraldehyde was discussed in detail under "Methods of Sterilization" in this chapter, see p. 135.) Glutaraldehyde is not recommended for housekeeping purposes. Both alkaline and acid glutaraldehyde solutions are available for high-level instrument disinfection in ten minutes; tuberculocidal in 45 minutes in absence of precleaning.

Iodophors A complex of iodine with detergent kills microorganisms through the process of oxidation of essential enzymes. Iodine, when properly used, is an effective disinfectant. The iodine-detergent complex enhances the cidal activity of iodine and renders the iodine nontoxic, nonirritating, and nonstaining when used as directed. A minimum of 20 minutes exposure, with a minimum concentration of 100 ppm of available iodine is needed; however, concentration varies in the products available. The manufacturer's instructions for use must be followed.

Effectiveness

1 Iodophors are used as housekeeping disinfectants for floors, furniture, walls, etc. Iodine is effective as long as it is wet. It is more effective in an aqueous rather than alcoholic solution for cleaning purposes because an aqueous solution dries more slowly.

2 An iodophor may be used as an instrument disinfectant. To prevent corrosion of metal, 0.2% sodium nitrite must be added.

3 They are bactericidal, pseudomonacidal, and fungicidal in minimum of ten minutes exposure.

4 They are tuberculocidal and virucidal in minimum of 20 minutes exposure, with a minimum concentration of 450 ppm of iodine.

Hazards

1 Some iodophors are unstable in the presence of hard water or heat, or subject to inactivation by organic soil.

2 Iodine stains fabrics and tissue, however, this is reduced or is temporary when used as an iodophor.

Mercurial Compounds Mercurial compounds bind enzymes of bacteria, but inhibit growth rather than kill the organisms. Therefore these agents are bacteriostatic, not germicidal. They have little, if any, value in hospital disinfection.

Phenolic Compounds Derivatives of pure phenol kill microorganisms mainly by coagulation of protein. Depending upon the phenol coefficient and species of organisms, phenolic compounds may cause rapid lysis of cells, leakage of cell constituents without lysis, or death by denaturing enzymes. Pure phenol, obtained from coal tar, is an extremely caustic agent and dangerous to tissue. Derivatives are used as disinfectants, usually with a minimum of a 2% phenolic compound in an aqueous solution.

Effectiveness

1 Phenolic compounds may be used as housekeeping disinfectants for cleaning floors, furniture, walls, etc. Phenolics retain a safe level of activity in the presence of heavy organic soil. They are disinfectants of choice when dealing with fecal contamination. They have good stability and remain active after mild heating and prolonged drying. Subsequent application of moisture to dry surfaces can redissolve the chemical so it again becomes bactericidal.

2 As an instrument disinfectant, 0.5% sodium bicarbonate must be added to prevent corrosion.

3 They are bactericidal, pseudomonacidal, fungicidal, and lipid virucidal in minimum of ten minutes exposure.

4 They are tuberculocidal in minimum of 20 minutes exposure.

Hazards

1 Tissue irritation precludes use for instruments that will come in contact with skin and mucous membranes, e.g., anesthesia equipment.

2 Personnel should wear gloves when cleaning with these products to avoid skin irritation.

3 Rubber may absorb phenol derivatives.

4 Product may have an unpleasant odor.

Quaternary Ammonium Compounds *Quats,* as these compounds often are called, cause gradual alteration of cell membranes to produce leakage of protoplasm of some microorganisms, primarily vegetative bacteria. These compounds possess detergent properties. Benzalkonium chloride, one of the most widely used of these compounds, should be used in a concentration of 1 to 750.

Effectiveness

1 They are rarely used as a housekeeping disinfectant for floors, furniture, walls, etc.

2 For instrument disinfection, 0.2% sodium nitrite must be added to solution to prevent corrosion.

3 They are bactericidal, pseudominacidal, fungicidal, and lipid virucidal in minimum of ten minutes exposure.

Hazards

1 Cidal effect can be reversed by adding a neutralizer, such as soap.

2 Hard water used for dilution reduces active concentration.

3 Active agent can be selectively absorbed by fabrics, thus reducing the strength perhaps to an ineffectively low level. Gauze or a towel must not be put in basin used for immersing instruments.

4 Compounds are subject to inactivation in presence of organic soil.

NOTE. Mercurial compounds and quaternary ammonium compounds are *not* recommended for hospital use because the hazards outweigh their effectiveness in the hospital environment. Other agents discussed are more efficacious.

Physical Disinfectants

Boiling Water Boiling water cannot be depended upon to kill spores. Heat-resistant bacterial spores will withstand water boiling at 212°F (100°C) for many hours of continuous exposure. Inactivation of some viruses, such as those associated with hepatitis, is uncertain.

If no other method of sterilization or disinfection is available, boiling water can be rendered more effective by adding sodium carbonate to the water to make a 2% solution, which reduces the hydrogen-ion concentration. At sea level the recommended boiling time for disinfection is 15 minutes. Rubber goods and glassware must not be boiled in sodium carbonate as it is destructive to both. If sodium carbonate is not used, the minimum boiling period is 30 minutes. At high altitudes the boiling time must be increased to compensate for lower temperature of boiling water.

Ultraviolet Irradiation Ultraviolet rays can kill microorganisms upon contact in air or water, and on surfaces of inanimate objects. Ultraviolet lights produce radiant energy in sufficient wavelengths and intensity for disinfection. The practical usefulness of ultraviolet irradiation in hospitals is very limited, however, because direct contact with the organisms must be made for this agent to be an effective disinfectant. Microorganisms are in a constant state of motion in the air currents of the ventilating system. Moving across the ray of ultraviolet light, pathogens may be exposed for only a fraction of a second or too minimal a time for effective contact with the radiant energy.

Ultraviolet rays can cause skin burns, similar to sunburn, and conjunctivitis of the eyes. Therefore, when working under exposure to ultraviolet irradiation, protective skin coverings and goggles or a visor over the eyes must be worn.

CHAPTER **9**

SURGICAL SCRUB, GOWNING, AND GLOVING

HISTORICAL INTRODUCTION

The evolution of special operating room attire as an adjunct to asepsis paralleled the realization of need for and the development of aseptic techniques in the latter half of the nineteenth century. Operating room nursing became a specialty of surgical nursing in the 1890s. As nurses assumed their place in the operating theatre, their attire changed through the years, as did the surgeon's.

One of the earliest mentions of specific OR attire appeared in that era in a nurse's training handbook that advised the nurse to bathe before operations, to take a carbolic bath before laparotomy, and to wear long sleeves and a clean apron for the operation. In the late 1800s, the surgeon often relied on his nurse to have the necessary instruments in her apron pocket. Whereas the apron has long since given way to the present scrub attire of scrub dresses, pantsuits, and jumpsuits, long sleeves are again recommended for anesthesiologists and circulating nurses to reduce the shedding of microorganisms.

The first use of caps and sterile gowns took place in Germany while the value of Lister's principle of antiseptic surgery to exclude putrefactive bacteria from wounds was still being debated on the Continent and in America. In some operating theatres, the bacteria-laden, infection-causing woolen suits and Prince Alberts were replaced by OR garb of sterilizable material to lessen the introduction of pathogenic organisms into the wound. Around 1890 the German surgeon Gustav Neuber and Hunter Robb, a gynecologist at Johns Hopkins Hospital in Baltimore, insisted on operating room cleanliness and on the wearing of caps and sterile gowns in the OR. In spite of the advances in technique and the professions, many surgeons of that time still operated in street clothes under a pus- and blood-encrusted apron. The famous Dr. William Halsted, chief of surgery of Johns Hopkins, in 1897 designed a semicircular instrument table to separate himself, in sterile gown and gloves, from observers in street clothes who watched him operate.

Also in the 1890s, while attention was being directed to the advantage of sterile gowns, Dr. William Lane developed a technique of asepsis in which only instruments, not hands, contacted tissue. Nurses trained in the Lane technique used sponge forceps for draping and even for gowning the surgeons. Special forceps were used to attach sterile towels to wound edges to occlude skin.

The use of sterile gowns antedated the routine use of caps, gloves, and masks, although in 1883 Neuber insisted on personnel wearing caps also. Emphasis on personal cleanliness expedited acceptance of special OR attire, but these standards were not rigidly practiced in all hospitals. Various styles of turbans and shower cap-style head coverings were worn from about 1908 to the 1930s, when hair was generally acknowledged to be an attraction for and shedder of bacteria. But there were no universal standards of attire at that time.

Some photographs taken in the early twentieth century show only the surgeon and instrument nurse wearing special head covering, although hair had been recognized as a contaminant years before. A 1900 photograph revealed surgeon Charles McBurney and team operating in short surgical gowns and rubber gloves but without caps or masks. Charles Mayo and team in 1913 in Minnesota were photographed operating in surgical gowns, caps, and masks. The onlookers, however, wore only a white coat over street attire. Another photo of 1918 showed the surgeon in gown, cap, gloves and a mask below his nose, the instrument nurse in gown and head cover but no mask, and the anesthetist and other nurses in gowns but regular nurses' caps.

In 1924, one of the first operating room nursing texts described the OR nurses: the circulating nurse wears OR cap, but no mask, and a gown with a pocket for pad and pencil; the scrub nurse wears both mask and gown. By the 1930s and 1940s, scrub dresses began to replace nurses' regular uniforms that had heretofore been worn under the sterile gown. Observers in the OR were gowned, capped, and masked. In the 1960s, full skirts were replaced by close-fitting scrub dresses and pantsuits that reduced the hazard of brushing against a sterile table when near or passing by it.

Rubber surgical gloves were introduced, not to protect the patient, but to protect the wearer's hands from harsh, irritating antiseptic solutions and hand soaks of the 1870s and 1880s. Their use was not popularized until the 1890s when Halsted's nurse complained of dermatitis. One of his assistants began to routinely wear gloves for clean operative procedures in 1896 although Halsted himself is known for popularizing the use of gloves to protect patients from the bacteria of ungloved hands. Mikulicz, a pioneering German surgeon, advocated wearing of cotton gloves in 1896 also, but these were soon found to lack the qualities of impermeable rubber gloves for infection control. Disposable latex gloves, introduced about 1958, were a welcome innovation that saved countless hours of daily glove reprocessing, repairing, and sterilizing. Today, the universal use of disposable gloves is well established.

Gauze masks were advocated by Mikulicz in 1896 when the droplet theory of infection (see Chap. 7) was demonstrated. Numerous types of masks were developed. Although routinely worn, gauze masks lacked high efficiency and often the nose was not properly covered. The efficiency of gauze masks decreases rapidly with use from saturation with saliva. Modern protocol demands that both mouth and nose be completely covered to exclude bacterial spray. Used masks are a potent source of contamination. The most efficient masks are disposable ones containing a high-efficiency filter.

In 1950, as restrictions became more rigid, OR personnel were required to change shoes when entering the OR suite and to wear only those shoes when within the suite. Currently disposable shoe covers are recommended and worn.

The Association of Operating Room Nurses has published recommended practices for OR wearing apparel, aseptic barrier materials for surgical gowns, and for surgical scrubs.

OPERATING ROOM ATTIRE

Purpose

The purpose of operating room attire is to provide effective barriers that prevent the dissemination of microorganisms to the patient. However, these barriers coincidentally protect personnel from infected patients. The barriers prohibit contamination of the operative wound and sterile field by direct body contact. OR attire has been shown to reduce particle count of shedding from the body from over 10,000 particles per minute to 3000 per minute, or from 50,000 microorganisms per cubic foot to 500.

Definition

Operating room attire consists of body covers, such as scrub dress, jumpsuit, pantsuit, or shirt and trouser, head cover, mask, and shoe covers. Each has an appropriate purpose to combat sources of contamination *exogenous* (external) to the patient. Sterile gown and gloves are added to this basic attire for scrubbed team members. Proper attire is one facet of environmental control.

General Considerations

1 Each OR department should have a specific complete written policy on proper wearing apparel. Protocol must be strictly monitored so that everyone conforms to established policy.

2 Only approved, clean OR attire is *worn within* the restricted area of the operating room suite. Street clothes are *never* worn within the restricted area. This policy applies to *anyone* entering the restricted area, both professional and nonprofessional personnel.
3 OR attire is *not worn outside* of the operating room suite. This protects the OR environment from microorganisms inherent in the general hospital environment and protects other persons from contamination normally associated with the OR. Blood-stained garb is unattractive as well as a source of cross infection. Before leaving the OR suite, everyone should change to other clothing. OR attire should be discarded and not hung in a locker with street clothes. Clean attire is donned on reentrance to the suite.
   a On occasion, such as preoperative visits to patients, clean laboratory coats are worn over OR attire outside the suite. This practice is not encouraged and is acceptable only when a clean, closed, knee-length lab coat is worn only once, and scrub attire is changed upon return to the suite. These coats do not protect the clothing beneath from contamination.
   b An adequate supply of clean attire should always be available so that there is no infraction of the rules. The attire is laundered daily only in the hospital's laundry facilities.
4 Dressing rooms located adjacent to the OR suite are reached through the outer corridor. Clothes and shoes must be changed before entering, or reentering, the suite. This regulation applies to *all* personnel and visitors.
5 Eyeglasses should be wiped with a tissue wet with antiseptic solution before each operation to prevent cross contamination.
6 Comfortable supportive shoes should be worn to relieve fatigue. Clogs, sandals, and tennis shoes are prohibited for reason of safety.
7 Impeccable personal hygiene must be reemphasized.
8 No person with an acute infection, such as a cold or sore throat, or skin lesion, such as a furuncle or any contagious condition, should be permitted within the OR suite. Persons with cuts, burns, or skin abrasions should not scrub or handle sterile equipment as serum, a bacterial medium, may seep from the eroded area.
9 Jewelry and fingernail polish should not be worn in the OR suite. Necklaces can grate on skin, increasing desquamation. Nail polish harbors microorganisms around nail bed. Jewelry also harbors organisms Pierced-ear studs must be contained in head cover.

Components of Attire

Each item of OR attire is a specific means of protecting the patient from the sources of contamination listed in Chapter 7, such as skin flora, nasopharyngeal flora, microorganisms on hair, fomites, and microorganisms in the air.

Body Cover A variety of scrub suits are available. All must fit the body closely. Pantsuits and trousers should have snug-fitting ankle cuffs of rib-knit or be secured with snaps or drawstrings at the ankle to contain organisms shed from the perineal region and legs. Scrub shirts and waistline drawstrings should be tucked inside pants to avoid their touching sterile areas and to reduce fallout of skin debris shed from thoracic and abdominal areas. Microorganisms multiply more rapidly beneath a covered area. One-piece jumpsuits with attached hoods and boots are convenient garb for visitors whose presence in the OR is brief, for example, pathologists.

Mask A mask is worn to contain and filter out droplets containing microorganisms expelled from the oro- and nasopharynx. One is worn at all times within the operating room. Because talking, sneezing, and coughing disperse organism-laden droplet nuclei, authorities recommend that a mask should be worn at all times by all people in the restricted area to protect the environment. This area includes inner corridors. Reusable cotton masks are obsolete. Disposable masks are far more efficient in filtering ability (up to 99 percent). Contemporary masks of soft, clothlike material, in very fine synthetic fiber mats, fulfill essential criteria. These masks are:

1 At least 95 percent efficient in filtering microbes from droplet particles.
2 Cool, comfortable, and nonobstructive to respiration.
3 Nonirritating, generally. If a person is sensitive to one type, he or she should try another brand. Masks with polypropylene, polyester or rayon fibers and fiberglas are available.

To be effective, a mask must catch all of a person's exhalations; therefore it *must be worn over both nose and mouth.* Air must pass only through the filtering system, so the mask must conform to facial contours to prevent leakage of expired air. Ejected droplets must not escape the filter action.

Masks are designed for close fit but improper application can negate their efficiency. Always tie the strings tightly, if that is the method of securing the mask, to prevent the strings coming loose during the operation. Tie upper strings at back of head; tie lower strings behind neck. Strings are never crossed over head because this distorts contours of mask along cheeks. Some types of masks have an exterior pliable strip or noseband that can be bent to contour mask over the bridge of the nose. A close-fitting mask also helps to avoid steaming of eyeglasses. To prevent cross infection, masks should:

1 Be handled only by the strings, thereby keeping the facial area of a fresh mask clean, and hands uncontaminated by a soiled mask. Do not handle the mask excessively.

2 Never be lowered to hang loosely around the neck, be placed on top of cap, or put in a pocket. Avoid disseminating microorganisms.

3 Be promptly discarded into the proper receptacle on removal. Remask with a fresh mask between patients.

4 Be changed frequently. Do not permit mask to become wet. Talking should be kept to a minimum.

Head Cover All facial and head hair must be covered in the restricted area. Various types of lightweight caps, helmets, and hoods are available for this purpose. Practically all are disposable and made of lint-free, nonporous, soft, clothlike fabric. Reusable head covers must be of a densely woven material and laundered daily. Net caps are not acceptable. If hair is long, a helmet or hood must be worn to cover the neck area. Headgear should fit well to prevent any escape of hair and to confine microorganisms. A cap or hood is put on *before* a scrub suit or dress to protect the garment from contamination by hair. Also, hair should not be combed while in scrub (basic OR) attire. Persons with scalp infection should be excluded from the OR and treated.

Hair, in addition to being a gross contaminant, is also a source of electrostatic spark.

Shoe Covers Disposable or canvas shoe covers also must be worn at all times in the restricted area. They must be safe as well as impervious to moisture. Conductive shoe covers must be worn in hazardous locations where electrical equipment is used. The black strip on conductive shoe covers must be inside of the shoe, in contact with the sole of the foot. Conductive covers provide electrical grounding for the wearer. In contact with conductive flooring, accumulated static electricity is harmlessly drained to the ground. After donning OR attire, personnel should test personal conductivity by use of a conductometer located at the entrance to any hazardous anesthetizing location.

Shoe covers should be worn on a single-use basis. They must be removed on leaving the restricted area and a fresh pair put on prior to reentrance to that area. Shoe soles are a source of gross contamination and of cross infection from one area of the hospital to another. Supportive footwear should be worn beneath the shoe covers. The bottoms of pant legs should be tucked into or connected to shoe covers to contain body shedding.

Gowns Sterile gowns are worn over scrub attire (dress or suit) to permit the wearer to create and to come within the sterile field, in order to carry out sterile technique during an operative procedure. Sterile gowns must provide an effective barrier for personnel between sterile and nonsterile areas.

Both reusable and disposable gowns, in a variety of styles, are in use. Although the entire gown is sterilized, the back is not considered sterile nor is any area below waist level, once the gown is donned. Wraparound gowns that provide sterile coverage to the back by a generous overlap are recommended. These gowns are secured at the neck and waist before the sterile flap is brought over the back and secured by ties or grips at the side or front. If the gown is closed merely by ties along the back, a sterile vest is put on over the gown to cover any exposed back area of scrub attire. The cuffs of gowns are stockinet (rib-knit) to tightly fit wrists. Sterile gloves cover the cuffs of the gown.

Gowns should be resistant to penetration of fluids and blood, and should be comfortable without excessive heat buildup. Most disposable gowns are made of spunbonded olefin or spunlaced wood pulp-polyester nonwoven, moisture-repellent materials. Reusable gowns must be of a densely woven material. Loosely woven, 140 thread count all-carded cotton muslin or similar quality permeable material is *not* a barrier to microbial migration. Pima cotton with a 270 to 280 thread count per square inch treated with a moisture-repellant finish is an acceptable woven textile. It will withstand about 100 laundering and sterilizing cycles before appreciable deterioration of the finish. Monitoring of the number of uses is necessary to remove gown from use at the sterile field when it is no longer an effective barrier. Also an additional rinse cycle may be required in the laundering process to remove residual detergent which could adversely affect the fabric. Mechanical damage from sharp instruments or snags will destroy the integrity of a gown, jeopardizing its purpose. The gown must be changed if punctured or torn during the operation. Textile gowns can be patched only with heat-applied vulcanized mending fabrics.

Gloves Sterile gloves complete the attire for scrubbed team members. They are worn to permit the wearer to handle sterile supplies or tissues of the operative wound. Surgical gloves are made of natural latex or snythetic rubber. Latex disposable gloves are used most frequently. Latex is cured with agents that may cause an allergic dermatitis. Hypoallergenic milled gloves are available that do not contain these sensitizers.

Gloves are packaged in pairs with an everted cuff on each to protect the outside of the sterile glove during donning. The inner paper wrap of the disposable glove package protects the sterility of the gloves when they are removed from the outer wrap. Glove packages are generally the peel-apart type. Prior to opening, the circulating nurse should inspect the package for damage or wetness, which indicates contamination. When the inner paper is unfolded, the wearer finds the right glove to the right, the left glove to the left, palm side up.

Both inner and outer surfaces usually are prelubricated with an absorbable dry starch powder before the sterilization process to facilitate donning, to decrease loose powder in the OR air, and to prevent adhesion of glove surfaces. Although considered absorbable and inert in tissue, this lubricant may cause serious complications, such as granulomas or peritonitis, if it is introduced into wounds. Consequently, it is important to remove the lubricant from the outside of gloves. To do this, gloves should be thoroughly wiped with a sterile damp towel or terry washcloth after donning.

If a sterile glove is punctured or torn, it must be changed immediately to prevent escape of microorganisms from the skin beneath. Some authorities estimate the incidence of glove puncture to be as high as 30 percent of unworn gloves tested. Shedders present a special threat from these imperfections.

Criteria for O.R. Attire

Attire should be:

1. Effective barrier to microorganisms. Both reusable woven and disposable nonwoven materials are used. Design and composition should minimize microbial shedding.
2. Closely woven material void of dangerous electrostatic properties. The garment must meet National Fire Protection Association Standards (NFPA-56A), including resistance to flame.
   - **a** Undergarments of synthetic material such as nylon are permissible when in close contact with the skin, such as hosiery.
   - **b** Nylon and other static spark-producing materials are forbidden as outer garments.
3. Resistant to blood, aqueous fluids, and abrasion to prevent penetration by organisms.
4. Designed for maximal skin coverage.
5. Hypoallergenic, cool, and comfortable.
6. Nongenerative of lint. Lint can increase the particle count of contaminants in the OR.
7. Pliable material to permit freedom of movement for the practice of sterile technique.
8. Able to transmit heat and water vapor, to protect the wearer.
9. Colored to reduce glare under lights. Various types of clothes in colorful prints that fulfill the necessary criteria are both attractive and functional.
10. Easy to don and remove.

Proper Attire

Clean, fresh attire is donned each time on arrival at the OR suite and as necessary at other times, if it is wet or grossly soiled.

NOTE. Showers should be available to personnel in case of gross contamination during a procedure.

Masks and head covers should be changed between patients. As extra precautions, known carriers who participate as sterile team members should:

1. Routinely bathe and scrub with an appropriate skin antiseptic agent; shampoo hair daily.

2 Change clothing frequently.
3 Wear two masks; use antimicrobial nasal ointment.
4 Use two scrub agents successively, double gown and double glove.
5 Use "no touch" technique; avoid touching any part of an instrument in direct contact with tissue.
6 Wash hands frequently and thoroughly.

Special attire is worn with laminar airflow systems in high-risk operations (see p. 109). Attire varies from hospital to hospital but may consist of a presterilized jumpsuit as basic attire, covered by sterile gown and gloves. A vacuum helmet is worn.

THE SURGICAL SCRUB

Definition

The *surgical scrub* is the process of removing as many microorganisms as possible from the hands and arms by mechanical washing and chemical antisepsis before participating in an operation.

Microorganisms

The skin is inhabited by:

1 *Transient organisms* acquired by direct contact. Usually loosely attached to the skin surface, they are almost completely removed by thorough washing with soap or detergent and water.
2 *Resident organisms* below the skin surface in hair follicles, and in sebaceous and sweat glands. They are more adherent, therefore more resistant to removal. Their growth is inhibited by the chemical phase of the surgical scrub. Resident skin flora represent the microorganisms present in the hospital environment. They are predominantly gram-negative, but some are coagulase-positive staphylococci. Prolonged exposure of skin to contaminants yields a more pathogenic resident population.

In freeing the skin of as many organisms as possible, two processes are utilized:

1 *Mechanical:* removes soil and transient organisms with friction
2 *Chemical:* reduces resident flora and inactivates microorganisms with a microbicidal or antiseptic agent

Purpose

The purpose of the surgical scrub is to remove soil, debris, natural skin oils, hand lotions, and microorganisms from the hands and forearms of sterile team members. More specifically, the purpose is:

1 To decrease the number of microorganisms on skin to an irreducible mimimum
2 To keep the population of microorganisms minimal during the operative procedure by suppression of growth
3 To reduce the hazard of microbial contamination of the operative wound by skin flora

The surgical scrub is done just prior to gowning and gloving for each operation.

Sink

Adequate scrubbing and handwashing facilities should be provided for all operating team members. The scrub room is adjacent to the operating room for safety and convenience. Individually enclosed scrub sinks with knee-operated faucets are preferred to eliminate the hazard of contaminating hands after cleansing.

The sink should be designed deep and wide enough to prevent splash. A sterile gown cannot be put on over damp scrub attire without resultant contamination of the gown by strike-through of moisture.

Scrub sinks should be used *only* for scrubbing or handwashing. They should not be used to clean or rinse contaminated instruments or equipment.

Equipment

Sterilized reusable scrub brushes or disposable sponges may be used. Single-use disposable products may be a brush-sponge combination. Some are impregnated with antiseptic-detergent agents. Disposable products are individually packaged. If reusable brushes are taken from the dispenser in which they were sterilized, each brush must be removed without contaminating the others. Brushes may be wrapped to provide sterile individual packages. The brush should not cause skin abrasion. The scrubbing solution is dispensed onto the brush or sponge by foot pedal from a container attached or adjacent to the sink. Six drops, about 2 cc or 2 to 3 ml, of solution is sufficient to generate a lather for the scrub procedure. Avoid waste of antiseptic solution.

Debris must be removed from the subungual area under nail of each finger. Metal or plastic single-use disposable products are available. Reusable nail cleaners must be sterilized between uses.

NOTE. Orangewood sticks are not used to clean under fingernails because the wood may splinter and harbor *Pseudomonas.*

Agents for Antisepsis

Various antimicrobial (antiseptic) detergents are used for the surgical scrub. The agent must be:

1 A broad-spectrum antimicrobial agent
2 Fast-acting and effective
3 Nonirritating and nonsensitizing
4 Prolonged-acting, i.e., leaves an antimicrobial residue on the skin to temporarily prevent growth of microorganisms
5 Independent of cumulative action

While the action of the agent is important in relation to its efficacy, mechanical friction and effort while scrubbing are equally influential. Most hospitals have more than one agent available in the scrub room for personnel allergic to a particular agent.

NOTE. 1. Frequent scrubbing tends to prevent rapid, complete reestablishment of resident flora.

2. Variables in skin antisepsis are mechanical factors, chemical factors, and individual differences in skin flora.

The most frequently used agents are:

1 *Chlorhexidine gluconate.* A 4% concentration of this agent exerts an antimicrobial effect against gram-positive and gram-negative microorganisms. Residues tend to accumulate on the skin with repeated use and produce a prolonged effect. This agent produces effective immediate and cumulative reductions of resident and transient flora.

2 *Povidone-iodine.* An iodine-complex detergent, frequently referred to as an *iodophor,* this agent fulfills all of the criteria for the surgical scrub. Effective cleansers, iodophors also slowly release iodine for residual effect. They are cidal with every use and effective against gram-negative as well as gram-positive microorganisms. The cidal action may be sustained for up to eight hours. Persons allergic to iodine should not scrub with an iodophor.

3 *Hexachlorophene.* This type of agent is most effective after buildup of cumulative suppressive action caused by regular use. The residual film is effective in keeping gram-positive organisms from proliferating, but is not effective against proliferation of gram-negative bacilli. Action of the agent is negated by alcohol.

4 *Triclosan.* A solution of 1% triclosan is a nontoxic, nonirritating antimicrobial agent which inhibits growth of a wide range of both gram-positive and gram-negative organisms. It develops a prolonged cumulative suppressive action when used routinely. The agent is blended with lanolin cholesterols and petrolatum into a creamy, mild detergent. It may be used by personnel sensitive to other antiseptics.

Preparation for Surgical Scrub

General Preparations

1 Skin and nails should be kept clean and in good condition, and cuticles uncut. If hand lotion is used to protect skin, a nonoil-base product is recommended.

2 Fingernails should not reach beyond the fingertip to avoid glove puncture.

3 Fingernail polish should not be worn. The lacquer may chip and peel, thereby providing a harbor for microorganisms in crevices.

Preparations Prior to Scrub

1 Inspect hands for cuts and abrasions. Skin integrity of hands and forearms should be intact, i.e., without open lesions or cracked skin.

2 Remove *all* finger jewelry. Jewelry harbors microorganisms.

3 Be sure *all* hair is covered by headgear. Pierced-ear studs *must* be contained by the head cover. They are a potential foreign body in the operative wound.

4 Adjust disposable mask snugly and comfortably over nose and mouth.

5 Adjust eyeglasses comfortably in relation to mask.

6 Adjust water to a comfortable temperature.

Length of Scrub

The length of the surgical scrub varies from one institution to another, as does the scrub procedure. Results of one study led to the estimate that microorganisms are decreased 50 percent by each six minutes of scrubbing. However, other studies have shown a vigorous five-minute scrub with a reliable agent to be as effective as a ten-minute scrub. *Variations in length may depend on frequency of scrubbing and the agent used.* The individual should scrub according to written policy of the hospital, manufacturer's recommendations for the agent used, and documentation of product efficacy in the scientific literature. A copy of the exact procedure should be posted in every scrub room. Skill and time improve with practice.

Surgical Scrub Procedure

The procedure for surgical scrub differs from one hospital to another but the recommended methods are applications of the principles of aseptic technique. These may be either the *time method* or counted *brush-stroke method.* If properly executed, they are both effective and each exposes all surfaces of the hands and forearms to mechanical cleansing and chemical antisepsis. One should think of the fingers, hands, and arms as having four sides or surfaces. Both methods follow an *anatomical pattern of scrub:* four surfaces of each finger, beginning with the thumb and moving from one finger to the next, down the outer edge of the fifth finger, over the dorsal (back) surface of the hand, the palmar (palm) surface of the hand, or vice versa, from small finger to thumb, over the wrists and up the arm, in thirds, ending 2 in. (5 cm) above the elbow. Since the hands are in most direct contact with the sterile field, all steps of the scrub procedure begin with the hands and end with the elbows.

Time Method Fingers, hands, and arms are scrubbed by allotting a prescribed amount of time to each anatomical area or each step of the procedure.

Five-Minute Scrub

1 Wet hands and forearms.

2 Apply six drops of antiseptic agent from dispenser to the hands.

3 Wash hands and arms several times thoroughly to 2 in. (5 cm) above elbows. Rinse thoroughly under running water, with hands upward, allowing water to drip from flexed elbows.

4 Take a sterile brush or sponge (from a package or dispenser), apply antimicrobial agent if it is not impregnated in the brush. Scrub nails and hands, a half minute for each hand.

5 With brush in hand, clean under fingernails under running water with a metal or disposable plastic nail cleaner. Discard after use.

6 Again scrub nails and hands with the brush a half minute for each hand, maintaining lather.

7 Rinse the hands and brush and discard the brush or sponge.

8 Reapply antimicrobial detergent and wash hands and arms with friction to the elbow for three minutes. Interlace the fingers to cleanse between them.

9 Rinse hands and arms as before.

Brush-Stroke Method A prescribed number of brush strokes, applied lengthwise of the brush or sponge, is used for each surface of the fingers, hands, and arms. A short, prescrub wash loosens surface debris and transient organisms. Scrub by brush or sponge removes resident flora.

1 Wet hands and arms.

2 Wash hands and arms thoroughly to 2 in. (5 cm) above the elbow with antiseptic agent.

3 Clean under fingernails carefully under running water with a metal or disposable plastic nail cleaner. Discard after use.

4 Rinse hands and arms thoroughly under running water, keeping the hands up and allowing water to drip from the elbows.

5 Take a sterile brush or sponge from a dispenser or package. Apply antiseptic agent to the brush or sponge if not previously impregnated.

6 Scrub the nails of one hand 30 strokes, all sides of each finger 20 strokes, the back of the hand 20 strokes, the palm of the hand 20 strokes, the arms 20 strokes for each third of the arm, to 2 in. (5 cm) above the elbow.

7 Repeat step 6 for the other hand and arm.

8 Rinse hands and arms thoroughly.

NOTE. 1. During and after scrubbing, keep the hands higher than the elbows to allow water to flow from the cleanest area, the hands, to the marginal area of the upper arms.

2. If a person scrubs frequently, some hospitals reduce the number of strokes per scrub in the brush-stroke method.

3. If policy dictates a ten-minute initial scrub, the five-minute scrub may be used for subsequent operations. Once gloves are removed, hands become contaminated from contact with inanimate items.

4. Avoid splashing water on scrub attire because moisture may contaminate sterile gown.

GOWNING AND GLOVING

The sterile gown is put on immediately after the surgical scrub. The sterile gloves are put on immediately after gowning.

Purpose

Sterile gown and gloves are worn to exclude skin as a possible contaminant and to create a barrier between sterile and unsterile areas.

General Considerations

1 The scrub nurse gowns and gloves self, then gowns and gloves the surgeon and assistants.

2 Gown packages preferably are opened on a separate table from other packages to avoid any chance of contamination from dripping water.

Drying Hands and Arms

After scrubbing, hands and arms must be thoroughly dried before the sterile gown is donned to prevent contamination of the gown by strike-through of organisms from skin and scrub attire.

The gown package for the scrub nurse contains one sterile gown, folded before sterilization, with the inside out, so that the bare scrubbed hands will not contaminate the sterile outside of the gown. A towel for drying hands is placed on top of the gown during packaging. The hands are dried as follows:

1 Reach down to the opened sterile package and pick up the towel. Be careful not to drip water onto the pack. Be sure no one is within arm's reach (see Fig. 9-1).

2 Open towel full-length, holding one end, away from nonsterile scrub attire (see Fig. 9-2). Bend slightly forward to avoid towel touching attire.

3 Dry both hands thoroughly but independently. To dry one arm, hold the towel in the opposite hand and, using an oscillating motion of the arm, draw the towel up to the elbow.

4 Carefully reverse the towel, still holding it away from the body. Dry the opposite arm on the unused (now uppermost) end of the towel.

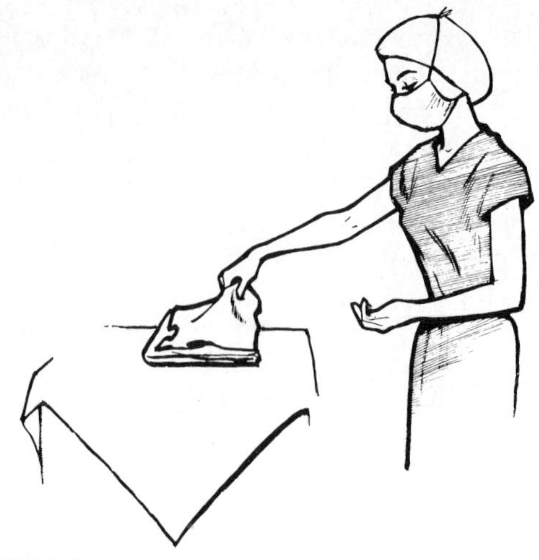

FIGURE 9-1
Scrub nurse (or technologist) preparing to gown removes the hand towel on top of the gown from the opened package. Note that mask covers both nose and mouth and skirt of scrub dress is narrow.

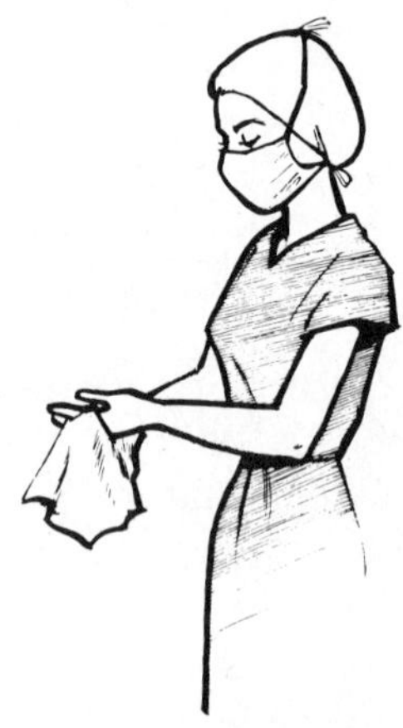

FIGURE 9-2
Scrub nurse, holding the towel out away from body, dries only well-scrubbed areas, hands first, and avoids contaminating hands on the areas proximal to elbows; then discards the towel.

NOTE. Often the towel is an absorbent, disposable one. Some hospitals package two absorbent washcloths in lieu of the towel. They are crisscrossed on top of the gown, to separate them. To use them, reach down to the sterile package and pick up one washcloth, being careful not to drip water. Holding the arms away from the washcloth, dry one hand, then the arm, as with the towel. Discard the washcloth. Use the second washcloth to dry the other hand and arm in the same manner.

Gowning and Gloving Techniques

Sterile gloves may be put on in two ways: by *closed glove technique,* or by *open glove technique.* The closed glove method is preferred except when changing a glove during an operation or when donning gloves for procedures not requiring gowns. Properly executed, the closed glove method affords assurance against contamination, when gloving oneself, since no bare skin is exposed in the process. If properly done, gloves can be put on safely either way. *The method of gloving determines how the gown is donned.*

Closed Glove Technique

Gowning for Closed Glove Technique

1 Reach down to the sterile package and lift the folded gown directly upward (see Fig. 9-3).

2 Step back away from the table, into an unobstructed area, to provide a wide margin of safety while gowning.

3 Holding the folded gown, carefully locate the neckband.

4 Holding the inside front of the gown just below the neckband with both hands, let the gown unfold, keeping the inside of the gown toward the body. Do not touch the outside of the gown with bare hands.

5 Holding hands at shoulder level, slip both arms into armholes simultaneously (see Fig. 9-4).

6 The *circulating nurse* brings gown over the

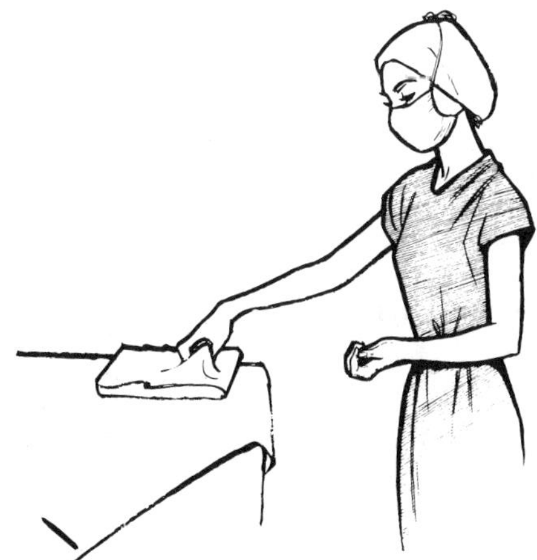

FIGURE 9-3
Scrub nurse, picking up gown below neck edge, lifts it directly upward and steps away to avoid touching an edge of the wrapper. Note that the sterile inside of the wrapper covers the table. Gown is folded inside out.

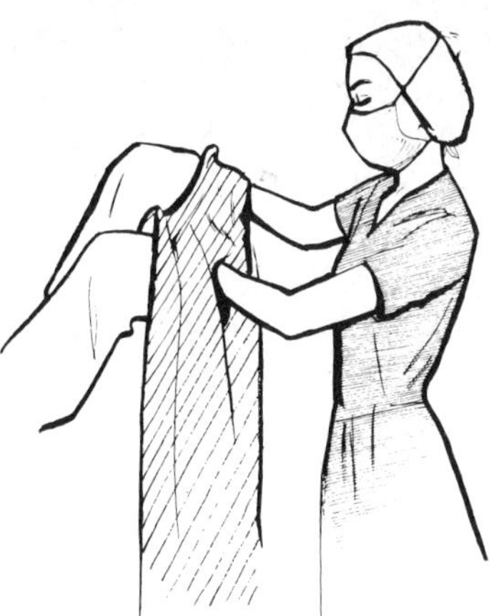

FIGURE 9-4
Scrub nurse, putting on gown, gently shakes out the folds, then slips arms into the sleeves without touching the sterile outside of the gown with bare hands.

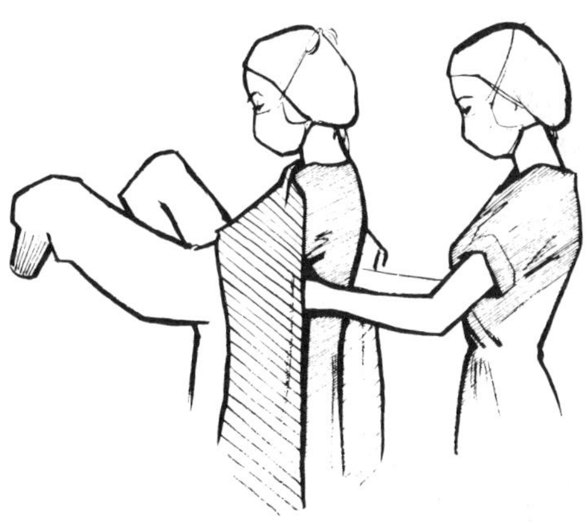

FIGURE 9-5
Circulating nurse, pulling the gown on for closed gloving technique, reaches inside the gown to the sleeve seams and pulls the gown on, leaving the cuffs of the sleeves extended over the hands.

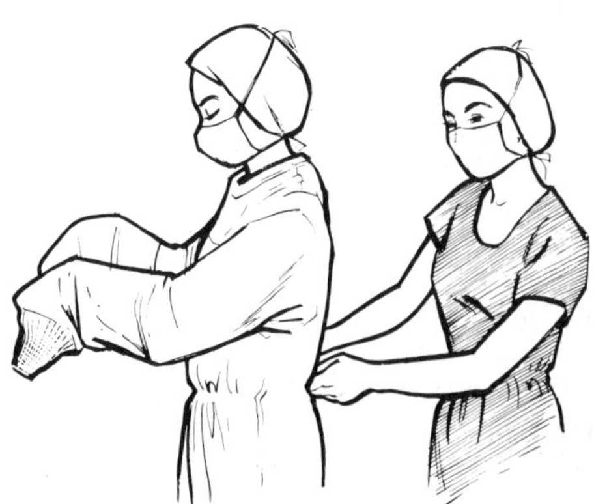

FIGURE 9-6
Circulating nurse completes pulling on the nurse's gown, ties the tapes on the inside of the back, and closes the fastener at the neck.

shoulders by reaching inside to shoulder and arm seams. *The gown is pulled on, leaving the sleeves extended over the hands.* The back of the gown is securely tied or fastened at the neck and waist, touching outside of gown at the line of ties or fasteners, in back only (see Figs. 9-5 and 9-6).

NOTE. 1. If gown is wraparound style, the sterile flap to cover the back is not touched until the person has gowned and gloved. A sterile gown may be wrapped around in various ways:

a. With gloved hands, release the fastener or untie the ties at the front or side of the gown. Hand the tie on the right to a sterile team member who remains stationary. Allowing a margin of safety, turn around to the left, thereby completely covering back with the extended flap of gown. Accept tie from the assistant and secure ties at the left side of the gown.

b. If you are the first person to gown and glove and other sterile team members are not available to assist, snap a sterile instrument such as an Allis's forceps, never a hemostat or clamp for hemostasis, to the tie on the right. Carefully hand the instrument to the circulating nurse. While he or she remains stationary, turn to the left, thereby covering the back. Take the tie in hand. The circulating nurse then releases and discards the instrument. Tie the ties at the left side.

c. Some disposable gowns have the end of one tie covered by a disposable strip. Hand strip to circulating nurse, taking care to protect hands. Turn around toward opposite side, thereby closing gown. Grasp the tie at a distance from the end. The circulating nurse pulls the strip, releasing it from the still-sterile end of the tie, and discards it. Tie the ties at front or side of the gown as indicated.

2. If the top of the gown drops downward inadvertently, discard the gown as contaminated. Never reverse a piece of sterile linen, if the wrong end is dropped toward the floor.

Gloving by Closed Glove Technique

1 Using the left hand, and keeping it within the cuff of the left sleeve, pick up the right glove, from the inner wrap of the glove package, by grasping the folded cuff.

2 Extend the right forearm with palm upward. Place the palm of the glove against the palm of the right hand, grasping in the right hand the top edge of the cuff, above the palm. In correct position, glove fingers are pointing toward you and the thumb of the glove is to the right. The thumb side of the glove is down (see Fig. 9-7).

3 Grasp the back of the cuff in the left hand and turn it over the end of the right sleeve and hand. The cuff of the glove is now over the stockinet cuff of the gown, with hand still inside the sleeve (see Figs. 9-8 and 9-9).

4 Grasp the top of right glove and underlying gown sleeve with covered left hand. Pull glove on over extended right fingers until it completely covers the stockinet cuff (see Fig. 9-10).

5 Glove the left hand in the same manner, reversing hands. Use gloved right hand to pull on left glove (see Figs. 9-11 to 9-13).

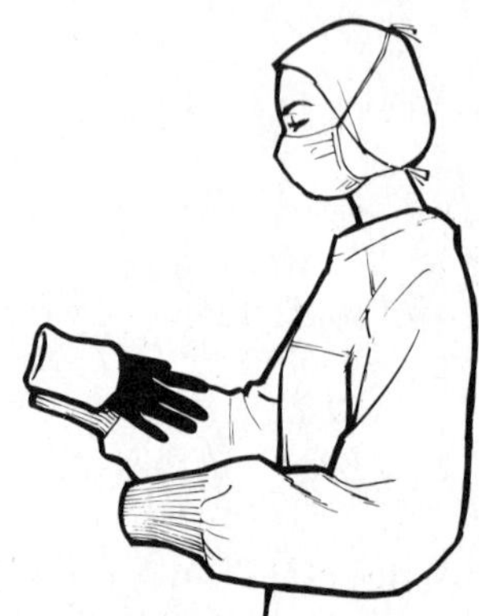

FIGURE 9-7
For closed gloving technique, using the left hand and keeping it within the cuff of the sleeve, the gowned scrub nurse picks up the right glove. The palm of the glove is placed against the palm of the right hand, grasping the top edge of the glove cuff above the palm.

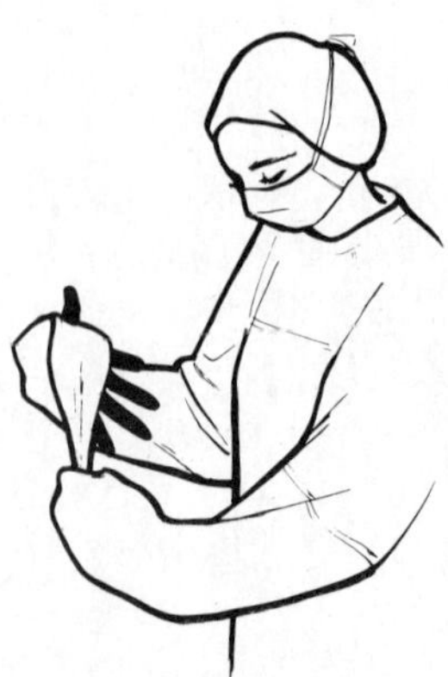

FIGURE 9-8
Back of the cuff is grasped in the left hand and turned over the right sleeve and hand.

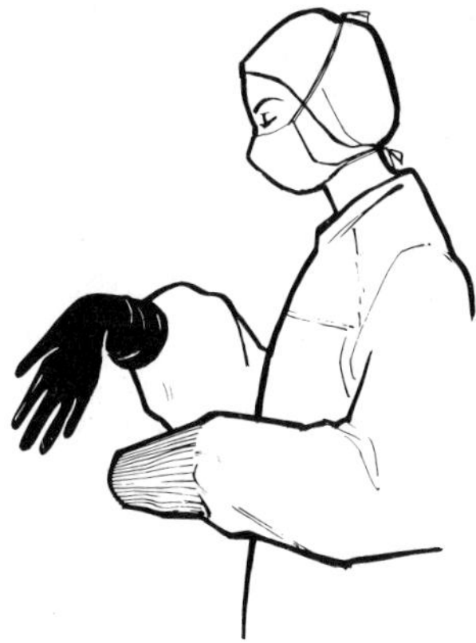

FIGURE 9-9
Cuff of the glove is now over the stockinet cuff of the sleeve, with the hand still inside the sleeve.

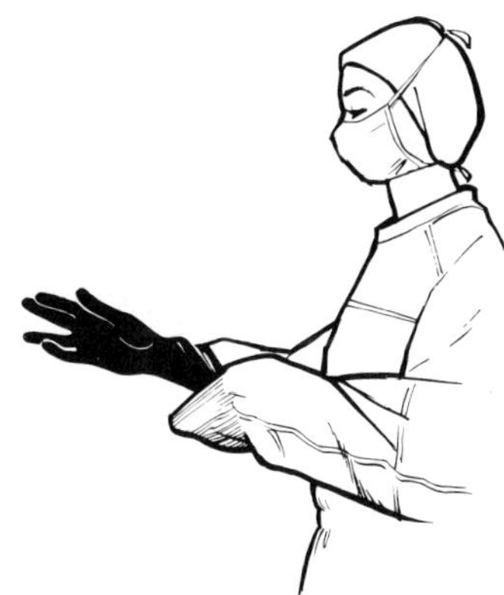

FIGURE 9-10
Top of the right glove and the underlying sleeve of the gown are grasped with left hand. By pulling the sleeve up, the glove is pulled onto hand.

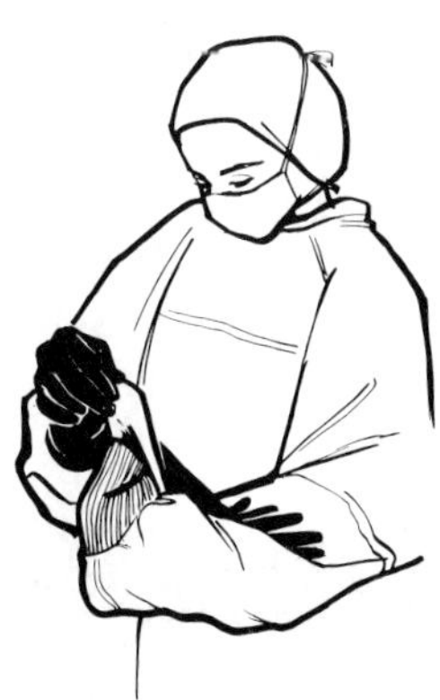

FIGURE 9-11
Using gloved right hand, the left glove is picked up and placed with the palm of the glove against the palm of the left hand. Grasp back of the cuff, above the palm, in the right hand and turn it over the left sleeve and hand.

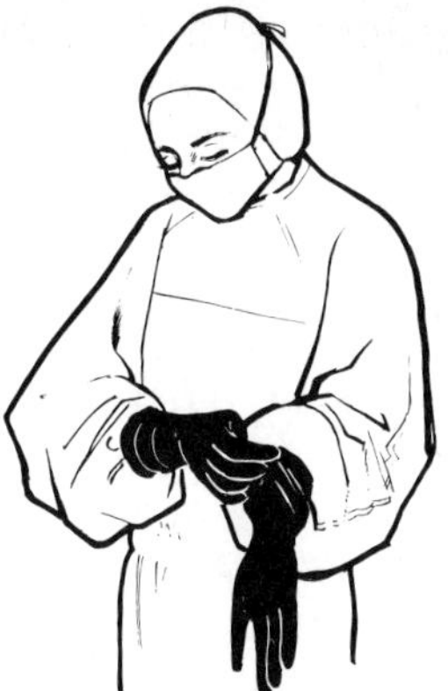

FIGURE 9-12
The cuff of the left glove is now over the stockinet cuff of the sleeve, with the hand still inside the sleeve.

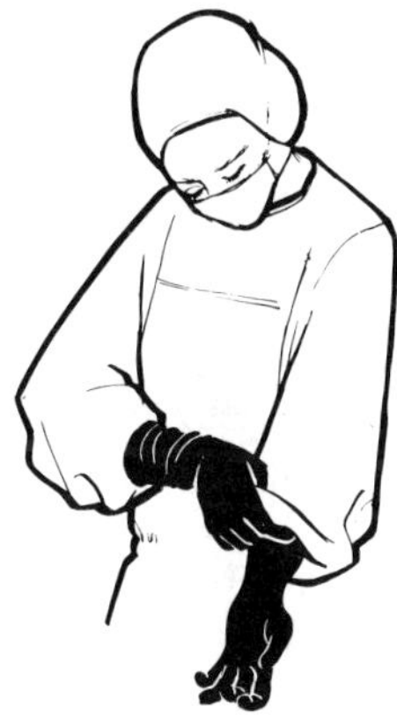

FIGURE 9-13
Grasp top of the left glove and underlying gown sleeve with right hand and pull the sleeve up, pulling the glove onto hand.

Open Glove Technique

Gowning for Open Glove Technique

1 Reach down to the sterile package and lift the folded gown directly upward.

2 Step back away from the table, into a clear area, to provide a wide margin of safety while gowning.

3 Holding the folded gown, carefully locate the neckband.

4 Holding inside front of gown just below the neckband with both hands, let the gown unfold, keeping inside of the gown toward the body.

5 Holding hands at shoulder level, slip them into the armholes simultaneously, without touching sterile exterior of the gown with bare hands.

6 The *circulating nurse* reaches inside the gown to sleeve seams, and *pulls the sleeves over the hands* to the wrists. Then back of gown is securely closed at the neck and waist with ties or fasteners, touching outside of gown at the line of ties or fasteners in the back only (see Fig. 9-14).

Gloving by Open Glove Technique This method of gloving uses a skin-to-skin, glove-to-glove technique. The hand, although scrubbed, is not sterile and must not contact the exterior of sterile gloves. The everted cuff on the gloves exposes the inner surfaces. The first glove is put on with skin-to-skin technique, bare hand to inside cuff. The sterile fingers of that gloved hand then may touch sterile exterior of the second glove, i.e., glove-to-glove technique.

1 With left hand, grasp the cuff of the right glove on the fold. Pick up the glove and step back from the table. Look behind you before moving.

2 Insert right hand into the glove and pull it on, leaving the cuff turned well down over the hand (see Fig. 9-15).

3 Slip fingers of the gloved right hand *under* the everted cuff of the left glove. Pick up the glove and step back (see Fig. 9-16).

4 Insert hand into the left glove and pull it on, leaving the cuff turned down over the hand.

5 With fingers of the right hand, pull cuff of the left glove over cuff of the left sleeve. If the stockinet is not tight, fold a pleat, holding it with right thumb while pulling the glove over the cuff. Avoid touching the bare wrist (see Fig. 9-17).

6 Repeat step 5 for the right cuff, using the left hand, and thereby completely gloving the right hand (see Fig. 9-18).

NOTE. Open glove technique is used when only sterile gloves are worn, as for intravenous cutdown or administration of spinal anesthesia. It is also used in emergency departments when donning sterile gloves for suturing lacerations, for example. It also is used for changing a glove during an operation.

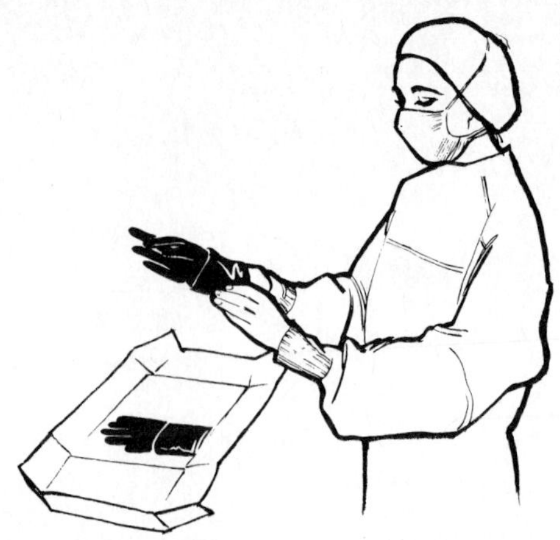

FIGURE 9-15
Scrub nurse gloving right hand with open gloving technique. With the left hand, nurse grasps the right glove on the folded-back cuff and lifts it directly up and away from the wrapper. Right hand is inserted in the glove. Note that left hand touches only the cuff or inside of the glove, skin-to-skin technique.

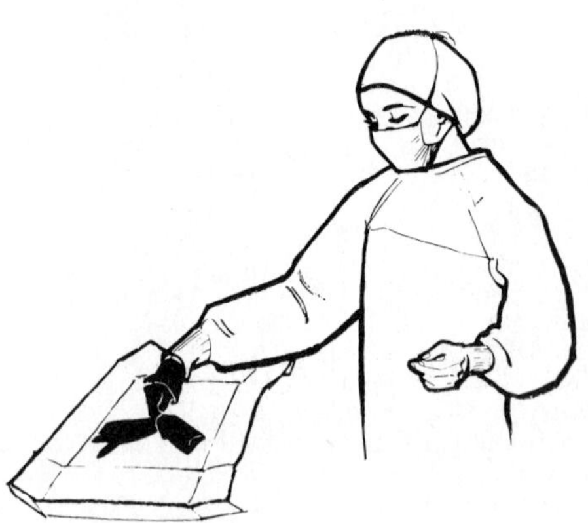

FIGURE 9-16
Picking up the left glove, scrub nurse lifts the glove from the wrapper by slipping gloved right fingers under the protective cuff, glove-to-glove technique. Bare hand does not touch the outside of the glove.

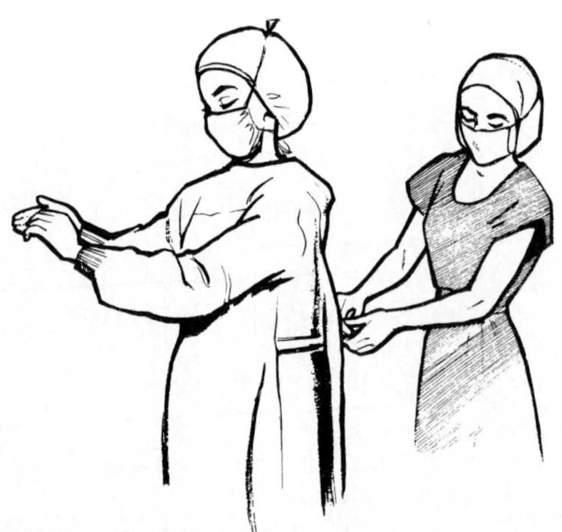

FIGURE 9-14
Circulating nurse fastens the back of the scrub nurse's gown for open gloving technique. Note that hands extend through the stockinet cuffs.

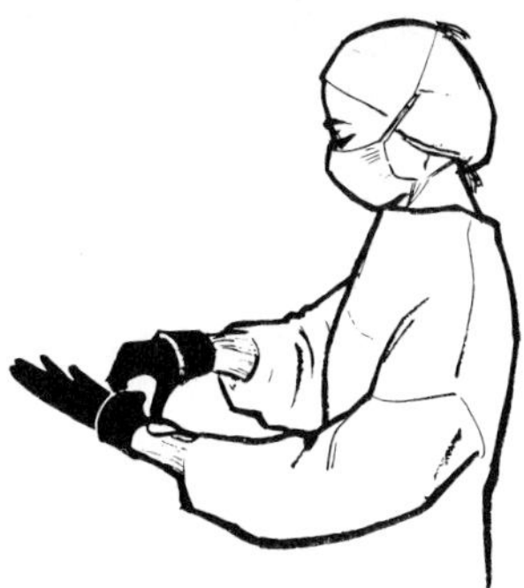

FIGURE 9-17
Pulling the cuff of the left glove up over the cuff of the sleeve, gloved fingers of the right hand touch only the outside of the left glove, near the wrist. If the stockinet is not tight, nurse folds a pleat, holding it with right thumb while pulling glove over cuff. Contact with exposed skin would contaminate the right glove.

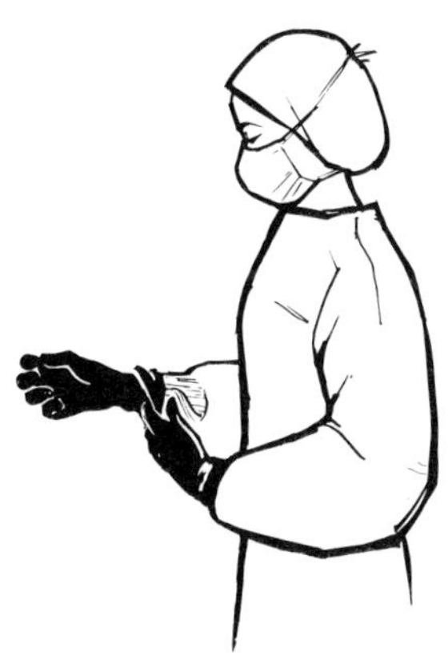

FIGURE 9-18
Using now completely gloved left hand, insert left fingers under folded-back cuff of the right glove and pull the glove cuff up over the right sleeve cuff, glove-to-glove technique.

Gowning Another Person

A team member in sterile gown and gloves may assist another team member in gowning and gloving by taking the following steps:

1 Open the hand towel and lay it on the surgeon's hand, being careful not to touch the hand.
2 Unfold the gown carefully, holding it at the neckband.
3 Keeping hands on the outside of the gown under a protective cuff of the neck and shoulder area, offer the *inside* of the gown to the surgeon. He or she slips the arms into the sleeves.
4 Release the gown. The surgeon holds arms outstretched while the circulating nurse pulls the gown onto the shoulders and adjusts the sleeves so the cuffs are properly placed. In doing so, only the inside of gown is touched at the seams.

Gloving Another Person

1 Pick up the right glove, grasp it firmly, with fingers under the everted cuff. Hold the *palm* of glove toward the surgeon.
2 Stretch the cuff sufficiently for the surgeon to introduce the hand. Avoid touching the hand by holding your thumbs out (see Fig. 9-19).
3 Exert upward pressure as the surgeon plunges the hand into the glove.
4 Unfold the everted glove cuff over the cuff of the sleeve.
5 Repeat for the left hand.
6 If a sterile vest is needed, hold it for the surgeon to slip hands into the armholes. Be careful not to contaminate gloves at neck level. If gown is a wraparound, assist the surgeon.

Changing Gown during Operation

Occasionally a contaminated gown must be changed during an operation. The circulating nurse unfastens neck and waist. By grasping it at shoulders, the gown is pulled off inside out. The gown is always removed first. The gloves are removed using glove-to-glove then skin-to-skin technique. If only the sleeve is contaminated, a sterile sleeve may be put on over the contaminated one.

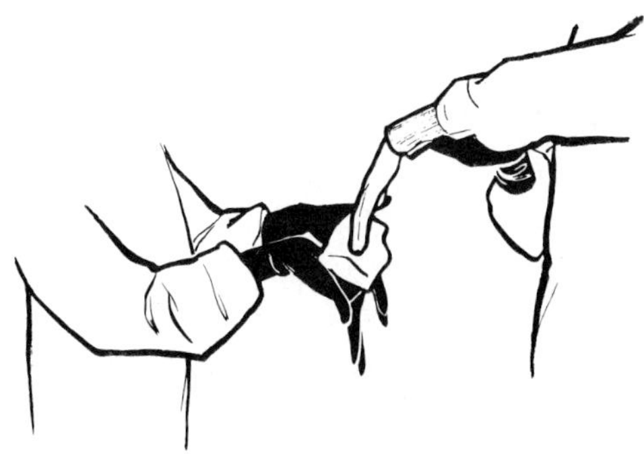

FIGURE 9-19
Nurse gloving doctor or another person holds glove with palm toward him or her. Nurse keeps thumbs extended out to avoid being touched by bare hands of person being donned.

Changing Glove during Operation

If a glove becomes contaminated for any reason during an operative procedure, it must be changed immediately. If you cannot step away at the moment, hold the contaminated hand away from the sterile area. To change the glove:

1 Turn away from the sterile field.

2 Extend the contaminated hand to the circulating nurse who grasps the outside of the glove cuff about 2 in. (5 cm) below the top of the glove and pulls the glove off inside out.

3 Preferably a sterile team member gloves another. If this is not possible, step aside and glove the hand using the open glove technique.

NOTE. The closed glove technique cannot be used for glove change during an operation without contamination of the new glove by the sleeve of the gown or without contamination of the hand by the cuff of the gown. The cuff must not be pulled down over hand. If this method is used, gloves and gown must be removed and another sterile gown donned before gloves.

Removing Gown and Gloves

The gown is always removed before the gloves. It is pulled downward from the shoulders, turning the sleeves inside out as it is pulled off the arms. Gloves are turned inside out, using glove-to-glove then skin-to-skin technique, as they are removed (see Chap. 10, pp. 184 and 185, for illustrations).

CHAPTER **10**

DIVISION OF DUTIES: SETUP, PROCEDURE, CLEANUP

PRELIMINARY PREPARATIONS

Preliminary preparations of the OR are done before each patient enters by the circulating and scrub nurses together, sometimes assisted by a nursing assistant or housekeeping personnel. It is a cooperative effort. Clean surroundings are part of the skill and care that are the patient's rights. Cleaning the room is part of total patient care. (The cleanup procedure following each operation is detailed in the last section of this chapter.)

Before First Operation of the Day

The following housekeeping duties should be done at least one hour before scheduled incision time:

1 Remove unnecessary tables and equipment from the room.

2 Damp-dust overhead operating light, furniture, flat surfaces, and all portable or mounted equipment with a disinfectant solution.

3 Damp-dust tops and rims of autoclave and/or washer-sterilizer and counter tops in substerile room adjacent to the OR.

4 Wet-vacuum floors with detergent-disinfectant (see p. 185 for technique).

Before Each Operation

After the room is clean and all surfaces are dry:

1 Put a clean sheet, arm band, and conductive strap on the operating table. Put thermal blanket or pressure mattress on table, if needed to induce hypo- or hyperthermia or to relieve pressure during a long procedure (see Chaps. 13 and 15).

2 Position operating table under overhead operating light fixture.

3 Turn on operating light to check focus and intensity, and preposition it as much as possible. The light should be positioned in relationship to location of surgeon at the operating table and to that part of the patient's anatomy that will be encountered during the operation.

4 Obtain and check electrical equipment that will be needed.

5 Connect and check suction between receptacle and wall outlet to be certain suction functions at maximum vacuum.

6 Put a waterproof linen bag or antistatic plastic bag for disposal of linen or disposable drapes in the linen hamper frame.

7 Line each kick bucket and wastebasket with an *antistatic* plastic bag with a cuff turned over the edge. These bags are not considered an explosion hazard so it is not necessary to put water in the bucket. Plastic waste disposal bags are nonconductors on which electrostatic charges may accumulate. Use care in handling them.

8 Arrange furniture with those pieces that will be draped to become part of the sterile field at least 18 in. (45 cm) away from walls or cabinets. They should be kept side by side, away from the linen hamper, anesthesia equipment, doors, and paths of traffic.

9 Put sterile drape pack on the instrument table in place so that when opened the wrapper will adequately drape the table and the drapes will be in their proper place (see Fig. 10-1).

NOTE. Although the term *linen pack* is frequently used, many hospitals use packs of disposable drapes (see Chap. 16).

10 Put a sterile basin set into the ring stand.

11 Obtain a basic set of sterile instruments or place tray of unsterile instruments in the steam sterilizer in the substerile room and sterilize them.

12 Select the correct size gloves for each member of the sterile team.

13 Collect additional instruments and supplies, according to the procedure book and surgeon's preference card, from cabinets in the room or other supply area within the OR suite.

14 Obtain special equipment, such as table appliances or pillows, needed for positioning the patient.

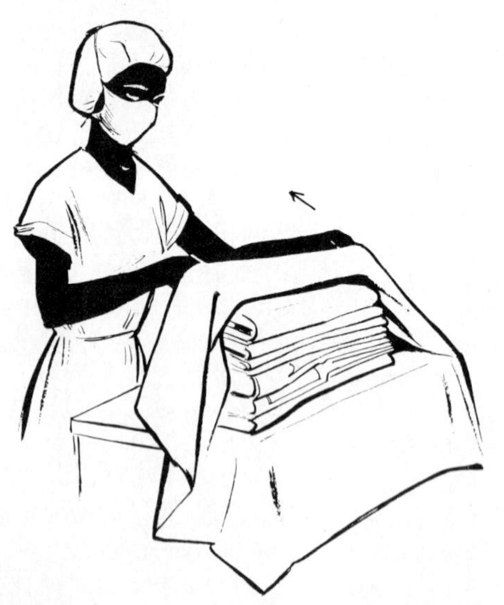

FIGURE 10-1
Circulating nurse opening sterile drape pack. Nurse lifts wrapper back while keeping hands on the outside. Hands are in a folded cuff to avoid contaminating contents of pack. The area touched falls below unsterile table level and sterile inside of wrapper (now table cover) remains sterile.

Individual Patient Setups

Each patient has a right to individual supplies prepared just for him or her. Sterile supplies should not be opened until they are ready to be used. Tables should *not* be prepared and covered for use at a later time. The scrub nurse, working with an efficient circulating nurse, has time to set up the instrument table before each operation.

The routine practice of covering sterile setups is not in the best interest of the patient. Unless under constant surveillance, sterility cannot be guaranteed. Uncovering a sterile table without contaminating it is difficult. However, should a scheduled operation be delayed, and *a sterile setup not be contaminated by the patient's presence in the room,* the setup may be covered with sterile drapes. It must remain in the room with doors kept closed, and should be used preferably within an hour from time prepared. When removing table cover, two people, one at each end, simultaneously peel back the cover. Care must be taken to avoid edges of table cover touching table contents.

If a patient is taken into the OR and for some reason the operation is canceled, the tables should be torn down and the room cleaned as if the operation had taken place.

Open Sterile Supplies

Before any sterile supplies are opened, the integrity of each package must be checked for tears and watermarks. If either are present, the package is unsafe to use. Also check expiration date and process monitor. To open packages:

1 Remove tape from packages wrapped in muslin. Check indicator tape to be certain item has been exposed to a sterilization process.

2 Open drape pack, instrument set, gown pack, and basin set so inside of each inner wrapper becomes the sterile table cover. With hands on outside of wrapper in a folded cuff, lift wrapper toward you to avoid contaminating contents of pack. The area touched falls below table level, and the inside of wrapper remains sterile. Neither reach over inside of sterile table cover or contents of pack. Always lift wrapper toward you (see Fig. 10-1).

NOTE. If packs or sets have sequential double wrappers, both layers are opened as described above by person opening supplies.

3 Open other packages, such as sponges, gloves, sutures, etc., maintaining a sterile transfer to the appropriate sterile table. Touch only the outside of the outer wrapper. Avoid reaching over sterile contents.

4 Open the gown and gloves for the scrub nurse on the Mayo stand or small table.

DIVISION OF DUTIES

The circulating and scrub nurses must plan their duties so that, through coordination of their efforts, the sterile and nonsterile parts of the operation move along *simultaneously*. From time the scrub nurse starts the surgical scrub until operation is completed and dressings applied, an invisible demarcation line separates the duties of the scrub and circulating nurses that neither nurse may cross. The duties of the two nursing positions are listed separately, but a spirit of mutual cooperation is essential to move the schedule of operations efficiently and to serve the patients' best interests.

SCRUB NURSE

When all is in readiness for arrival of the patient, the scrub nurse prepares for arrival of the surgeon.

Before Surgeon Arrives

1 Do a complete scrub according to accepted practice (refer to Chap. 9).
2 Gown and glove.
3 Drape tables as necessary according to standard procedure.
  a Sometimes a second instrument table is needed for extensive operations or special types of instrumentation.
  b The scrub nurse may drape and set a small table for the patient's skin preparation. More commonly the circulating nurse opens and prepares a disposable or prepackaged prep tray (see Chap. 16).
  c The surgeon and assistant(s) may gown and glove from a small table used only for this purpose. The scrub nurse arranges the gloves for them.

NOTE. In draping a nonsterile table, always cuff drape over gloved hands in preparation for opening it. Lift the table drape toward you to cover nonsterile front edge of table first and to minimize possibility of contaminating front of your gown. Then place drape over back of the table. After ends of the drape are unfolded over sides of the table, be careful not to lift them to table level again as you open the crosswise folds (see Figs. 7-3 through 7-6, pp. 117 and 118).

4 Move remaining contents of drape pack to a corner of instrument table if they are not preset on table drape in a convenient place. Before being wrapped for sterilization, contents of the pack can be set on table drape in the spot where they should be on the table. Then when pack is opened, contents do not need to be handled or moved. The pack contains, from top to bottom, at least:
  a One Mayo stand cover.
  b Six to eight towels.
  c One fenestrated sheet. (The types of fenestrated sheets are discussed in Chapter 16.)
5 Drape the Mayo stand. Both the frame and the tray are draped unless the tray is wrapped and sterilized separately.

The Mayo stand cover is like a long pillowcase. It is fanfolded with a wide cuff to protect gloved hands. With hands in cuff, folds of the drape are supported on the arms, in bend of the elbows, to prevent its falling below waist level. While sliding cover on, place foot on base of stand to stabilize it (see Figs. 10-2 and 10-3).

A snugly wrapped sterile tray is placed on top of the draped Mayo frame. Or a waterproof barrier, such as a nonabsorbent disposable towel or antistatic plastic film, is placed over the cover on the tray and tucked in along the edges.

6 Leave large solution basin in ring stand and take remainder of the basins to the instrument table. The wrapper on the basin set serves as the cover for the ring stand with the large basin. The surgeon and assistants may need to wash their gloves during the operation. This is no hazard in an operation devoid of frank sepsis or malignancy. The solution must be nontoxic and benign in tissues, however. Sterile normal saline or water is usually used in this

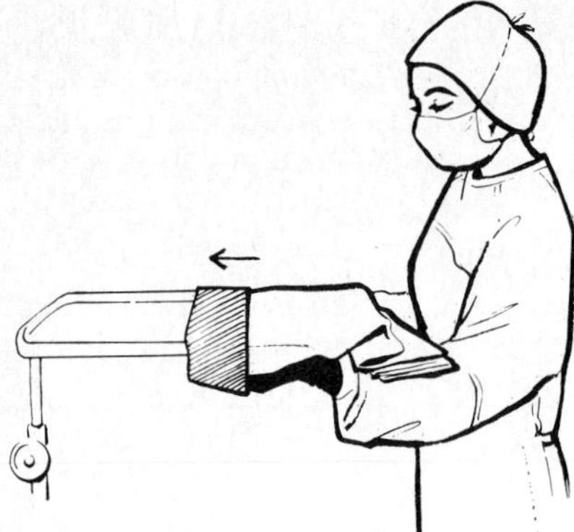

FIGURE 10-2
Starting to drape the Mayo stand. Scrub nurse's hands are protected in cuff of the drape. Folds of drape are supported on arms, in bend of elbows, to prevent their falling below waist level. Nurse may place foot on base of the stand to stabilize it.

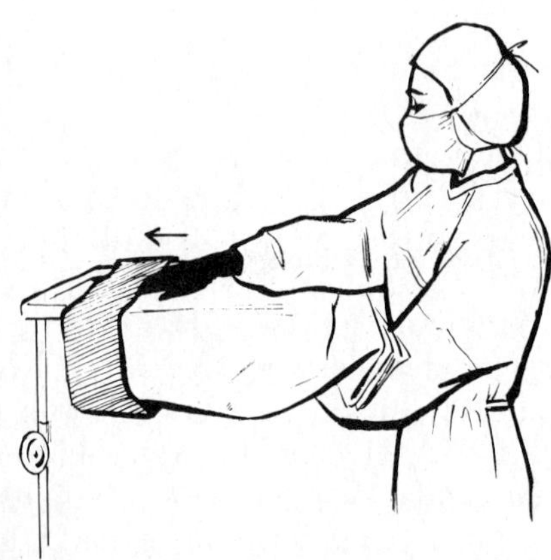

FIGURE 10-3
Completing the draping of the Mayo stand. The nurse's hands are protected in the cuff.

"splash" basin. *Splash basins are not used in many ORs.*

One basin is left on the instrument table until needed for the specimen.

A round basin will be used for moistening sponges. Place an absorbent towel on the instrument table under it.

In addition to these basins, the basin set may also contain solution cups for the skin preparation table and a basin specifically intended for trash disposal. In lieu of this extra basin, a small paper bag may be included in the basin or instrument set for trash. The bag is left standing open on the instrument table or attached with a nonperforating clip in a convenient place on the side of the table or Mayo stand.

7 Arrange instruments on instrument table and count them according to established procedure (see p. 178 later in this chapter).

Instruments for each operation are selected according to standard basic sets or an instrument book list for a given operation and the surgeon's preferences. They usually are prepared, wrapped, and sterilized several hours prior to operation so they are dry and cool for safe handling. In addition to basic sets, separate single packages of special instruments also may be sterile to be opened as indicated.

Sometimes instruments must be steam sterilized just prior to use. If so, a towel or foam is placed in bottom of tray under instruments to absorb moisture from condensation on them. (See Chapter 8, p. 131 for timing of the load.) Either the scrub or circulating nurse may lift tray from autoclave, depending on the physical location of the autoclave in relationship to the OR. *The scrub nurse should not go beyond confines of the room,* but this is the practice in some suites where the autoclave is immediately adjacent to door to the substerile room. In lifting a tray from the autoclave, the scrub nurse must be careful not to brush the sleeves or front of gown against the autoclave. The circulating nurse must not reach over the sterile instruments when lifting tray or over the sterile table when placing it.

Box locks of hinged instruments must be held open during steam sterilization. Therefore, remove them from instrument pins, racks, or holders designed for this purpose and close the instruments on the first ratchet. Handles may be hung over edge of the tray. Or take a towel from drape pack, roll it lengthwise to form a long, narrow cushion, and place hemostats and other instruments with ringed handles over it. Retractors and other heavy instruments can be left in instrument tray or laid out on table.

8 Arrange instruments on the Mayo stand for making and opening the initial incision. For each basic maneuver, a definite class of instruments of suitable size, shape, strength, and function is needed. Instruments may be classified as follows:

a Cutting or dissecting : knives and scissors
b Grasping and holding : tissue forceps

c Clamping and occluding: hemostatic forceps and clamps

d Exposing: retractors

e Suturing: needleholders

Variation in style and number of instruments will be dictated by type of operation. In addition to these basic instruments, the following accessory items may be added to Mayo stand after the supplies are prepared for use:

a Sutures and needles

b Sponges

Do not overload the Mayo stand initially (see Fig. 10-4). Additional instruments and supplies can be added as necessary as the operation progresses. Long handled forceps and clamps and deep retractors can be substituted for those used on superficial structures. The Mayo stand should be kept neat throughout the operation with instruments organized by classifications.

9 Put blades on knife handles. To avoid injury, always use an instrument, never your fingers alone. Holding the cutting edge down and away from your eyes, grasp the blade at its widest, strongest part with a needleholder and slip the blade into groove on knife handle. A click indicates the blade is in place. To prevent damage to blade, the instrument must not touch the cutting edge (see Fig. 10-5).

10 Prepare sutures in sequence in which surgeon will use them. The surgeon *ligates* (ties off) blood vessels shortly after incision is made, unless he or she prefers to use electrosurgery to seal vessels. Therefore, prepare *ligatures* (free hand ties) first, since they are used first.

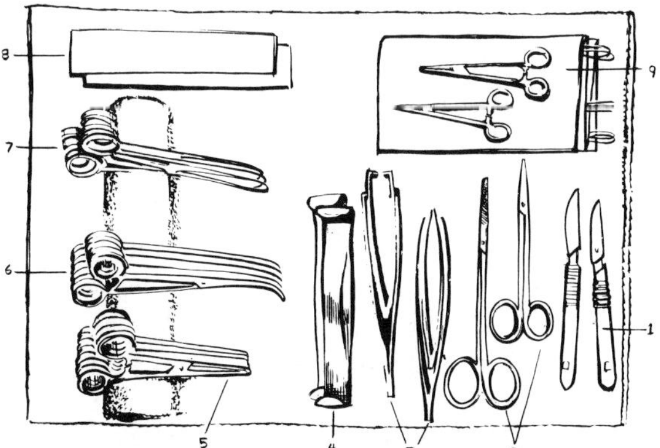

FIGURE 10-4
Contents of Mayo stand, in preparation for operation: (1) scalpels, (2) straight and curved scissors, (3) smooth and toothed tissue forceps, (4) retractors, (5) straight hemostats, (6) Kelly clamps, (7) Allis's forceps, (8) sponges, (9) suture towel and needleholders.

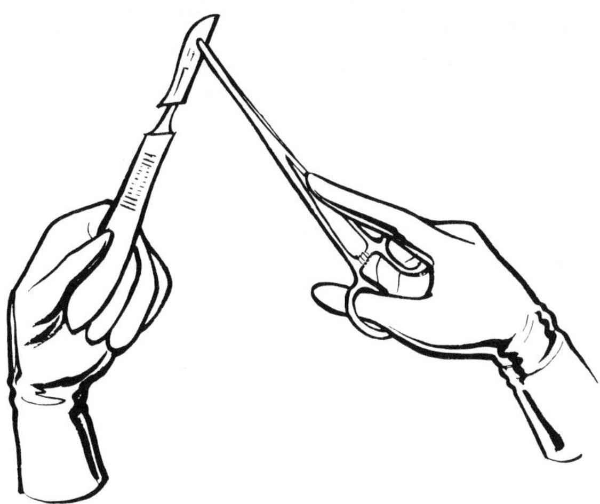

FIGURE 10-5
Putting scalpel blade on a knife handle. To avoid injury, always use an instrument, never use your hands alone. Holding it down and away from your eyes, with a strong needleholder (not a hemostat), grasp blade at its widest, strongest part, and slip the blade into groove on the handle. To prevent damage to blade, the needleholder must not touch the cutting edge.

Tear foil packets at notch in the hermetically sealed edge. Plastic packets may be torn or cut open with nurse's scissors. Remove suture material from packet, unless packet is designed for single-strand dispensing. Work over instrument table and hold onto ends to prevent strands from dropping over edge of the table, and thus becoming contaminated.

Place dispensing packets or strands of ligating material in a *suture book,* a fanfolded towel, with the ends extended far enough for rapid extraction. Place largest size in bottom layer along fold that will be farthest away when placed on Mayo stand. The next smaller size is placed in next layer so that the ends are not overriding those below; if three sizes are prepared, medium size can be placed midway between the other two. The smallest size will be along closest fold. The suture book should be placed on Mayo stand with the ends on it, *not over the edges,* and toward the sterile field. Strands are pulled out toward the operative field, *never away from it,* to prevent possible contamination.

After ligatures are prepared, a *few* packets may be opened and prepared for *suturing* (sewing or stitching). Seldom is it necessary to prepare large amounts of suture material in advance. Suture material, preparation, and handling are discussed in detail in Chapter 18.

11 Count surgical needles and other sharps with circulating nurse according to accepted practice (see p. 177).

Most hospitals use needles *swaged* (attached) to suture material. These can be left in inner folder of suture packet, after counting, until surgeon is ready to use them. The folder can be placed in a fold of the suture book.

A needle rack is prepared in advance for each operation if reusable, eyed needles are used (see Fig. 18-6, p. 350). This is sterilized with the instruments. Inspect each needle before threading for cleanliness, burrs, and integrity of the eye.

If disposable eyed needles are used, they can be threaded into top layer of suture book. *Needles should never be loose on Mayo stand* as they inadvertently could be dragged into the incision or knocked onto the floor.

Surgical needles are discussed in detail in Chapter 18.

12 Count *all* sponges with circulating nurse before doing anything else with them. Many different kinds of sponges are available. Those placed on the sterile field should have indicator radiopaque to x-ray. They are referred to as *x-ray detectable.* The following are representative of the types used:

a 3 by 3 in. (7.6 by 7.6 cm) sponges are used in small incisions.

b 4 by 4 in. (10 by 10 cm) sponges are the most common in use. They may be folded into a 2 by 2 in. (5 by 5 cm) square and used on sponge forceps.

c 4 by 8 in. (10 by 20 cm) sponges may be used for sponging or as a moist pack in a large exposed area.

d *Tapes,* also called *lap pads* or *packs,* are used for walling off the viscera and keeping them moist and warm. Either square or oblong, they have a loop of twilled tape sewed on one corner over which a metal ring, about 1½ in. (3.8 cm) in diameter, can be fastened. If rings are used, they remain outside the edges of incision while tape is inside. Tapes are usually used moist.

e Dissecting sponges:

1 *Peanut sponges* are very small gauze sponges used to dissect or absorb fluid in delicate procedures. They must be clamped into a forceps.

2 *Kitner dissecting sponges* are small rolls of heavy cotton tape. These are held in forceps.

3 *Tonsil sponges* are cotton-filled gauze with a cotton thread attached.

f Cottonoid patties, compressed rayon or cotton, are used moist on delicate structures such as nerves, brain, and spinal cord.

After the sponge count is completed (see p. 178), place on Mayo stand a few appropriate-size sponges for the initial incision. These sponges are usually opened to their full length. Fix two or three sponges on sponge forceps, but leave forceps on instrument table. Put rings on tapes, if used.

13 Fill a syringe with the correct agent if a local infiltration anesthetic is to be used. Attach an appropriate-size needle and put it on Mayo stand. This will be the first thing surgeon will use after patient is draped. State the kind and percentage of the solution when handing syringe to surgeon. The solution label must be checked by a registered nurse when it is poured and verified when it is given.

Syringes with needles are used for injection and aspiration, and syringes without needles are used for irrigation. Most hospitals use sterile disposable syringes and needles, but glass syringes and reusable needles in the same models and sizes may be used.

Syringes commonly used for injection or aspiration are:

a *Luer-Lok tip.* This has a tip that locks over needle hub. It is used whenever pressure is exerted to inject or aspirate fluid. Sizes are available from 2 to 100 cc.

b *Ring control.* This has a Luer-Lok tip. The barrel has one fingerhold and thumbhold, which give the surgeon a secure grip when injecting with only one hand. Sizes range from 3 to 10 cc.

c *Luer slip tip.* This has a plain tip that may not give a secure connection on a needle hub. It is necessary when using some catheter adaptors or a rubber connection for aspiration. Sizes vary from 1 to 100 cc.

NOTE. When using a sterile syringe be very careful not to touch plunger except at end, even with gloves on. Contamination of plunger contaminates inner wall of barrel and thus solution that is drawn into it. Glove powder can act as a contaminant.

Syringes used for irrigation are:

a *Bulb with barrel.* A plastic or rubber bulb is attached to neck of barrel. The barrel has a tapered or blunt end. This is used with one-hand control for irrigation during many types of operations. Sizes have a solution capacity of ¼ to 4 oz (7.6 to 118 cc).

b *Bulb without barrel.* This is a one-piece bulb that tapers to a blunt end. It is used to irrigate small structures.

NOTE. To fill barrel or bulb, depress bulb, submerge end in solution, and release. The bulb will reinflate, thus drawing solution into it. Warm, not hot, solution is usually used for irrigation, so check temperature before giving syringe to surgeon.

Needles for injection or aspiration:
The size of needles with a lumen is designated by length and gauge. *Gauge* is the outside diameter of needle. Although an abundance of needles are available, only a few representative sizes and their uses are mentioned.

a ½ in. (12.7 mm) by 30 gauge, for local anesthetic in plastic surgery.

b ¾ in. (19 mm) by 24 or 25 gauge, the usual needle for any subcutaneous injection.

c 1½ in. (3.8 cm) by 22 gauge, for subcutaneous or intramuscular injection.

d 2 in. (5 cm) by 16 or 18 gauge, for aspiration, or transfusion of blood products.

e 4 in. (10 cm) by 20 or 22 gauge, for deep injections of local anesthetic, or for intracardial injections.

After Surgeon and Assistant(s) Scrub

1 Gown and glove the surgeon and assistants as soon after they enter room as possible. This should take precedence over other things you may be doing. However, *do not interrupt* a sponge, sharp, or instrument count to do so. Such interruptions lead to incorrect counts. The surgeons take their gowns and gloves from a separate table set up for this purpose in some hospitals.

2 Assist in draping the patient, according to the routine procedure (see Chap. 16).

a Many surgeons use self-adhering plastic sheeting as the first drape. Stand on opposite side of operating table from surgeon to apply this drape.

b Some surgeons use towels and clips with or instead of a plastic drape. Go to same side of table as surgeon to hand towels and clips, to prevent reaching over the nonsterile operating table. Skin towels may be held in place with sutures rather than clips. Needles and needleholders are discarded from sterile field after skin towels are secured in this manner.

NOTE. Once a clip or hook has been fastened through a drape, do not remove it; points are contaminated. If it is necessary to remove one, discard it from field and cover area with another sterile drape or towel.

3 Bring Mayo stand into position over patient after draping is completed. Be sure that it does not rest on the patient. Position the instrument table at a right angle to operating table.

4 Lay a towel or magnetic pad for instruments below *fenestration* (opening) in the drape. Lay two to four sponges on this.

5 Attach suction tubing and electrosurgical cord, if either or both are to be used, to drapes with a nonperforating clamp. Allow ample length to reach both incision area and equipment. Drop ends off side of the table nearest the unit to which the circulating nurse will attach them.

During Operation

1 Hand skin knife to surgeon and a hemostat to assistant. Some surgeons do not want the knife handed to them. Lay knife on instrument towel or magnetic pad for them to pick up.

NOTE. When passing a knife always hold the handle with blade down and pointed toward your wrist, never toward surgeon. Hold hand pronated with thumb apposed against tip of index finger and flex wrist.

As soon as surgeon makes skin incision, put knife into the specimen basin. The inside of this basin is hereafter considered contaminated. Refrain from touching anything else that is put in it. Because skin cannot be sterilized, the skin knife is always considered contaminated whether surgeon has cut through an adhering plastic drape or not. The skin incision exposes deep skin flora of hair follicles and sebaceous gland ducts.

2 Hand up towels and hooks for fastening them to skin, if a plastic drape has not been applied as the first drape, as soon as subcutaneous bleeders have been ligated. These towels are placed at each side of incision and secured to cover skin completely during operation. If skin towels are used, rearrange the instrument towel to make a smooth field.

3 Watch field and try to anticipate the surgeon's needs. Keep one step ahead of him or her in passing instruments, sutures, sponges, handing up specimen basin, etc. Notify circulating nurse if you need additional supplies or if surgeon asks for something not on table. Ask quietly for supplies to avoid distracting the surgeon.

4 Pass instruments in a decisive and positive manner. When instruments are passed properly, surgeons know they have them; eyes do not have to leave operative site. When surgeon extends hand, the instrument should be slapped firmly into palm in proper position for use (see Fig. 10-6). In passing an instrument to surgeon:

   a If the surgeon is on the opposite side of the table, pass with your right hand.
   b If the surgeon is on the same side of the table and to the left, use your right hand.
   c If the surgeon is on the same side of the table and to the right, use your left hand.

   Many surgeons use hand signals to indicate the type of instrument needed. These signals eliminate need for talking, but such signs must be clearly understood. An understanding of what is taking place at the operative site makes them meaningful. When bleeding is obvious, the surgeon needs a hemostatic forceps. When a suture needs cutting, the need is for scissors.

   Keep instruments as clean as possible. Wipe blood and organic debris from them with a moist sponge. Flush suction with saline periodically to keep tip and tubing patent. Remove debris from electrosurgical tips.

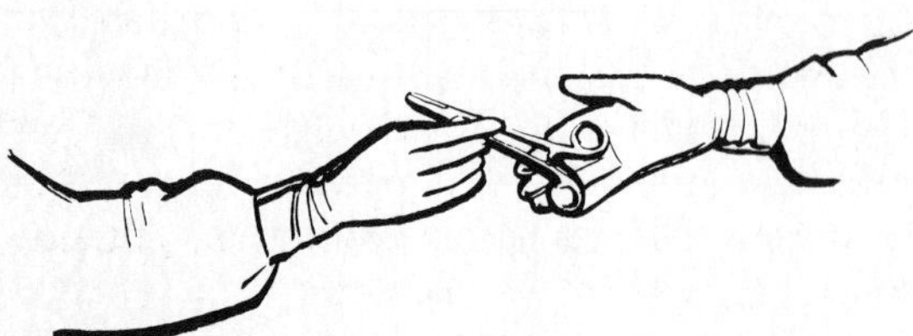

FIGURE 10-6
Passing an instrument. Tip is visible; hand is free. Handle is placed directly into waiting hand.

   Return instruments to the Mayo stand or instrument table promptly after use. Their weight could injure the patient.

5 Place a ligature in the surgeon's hand. The surgeon keeps eyes on field and does not reach for a ligature except to hold hand out to receive it. Draw a strand out of the suture book, toward the sterile field, grasp both ends, and place securely in surgeon's outstretched hand.

   Have ready, at all times during operation, a fine and a heavy suture on needles placed in needleholders. After handing a suture to the surgeon, prepare another just like it at once. The needle or suture may break. *Account for each needle as the surgeon finishes with it.* Check its integrity. Tell surgeon immediately if a needle is broken so both pieces can be retrieved.

   Repeat size of a suture or ligature when handing it to surgeon. Obviously, if surgeon is using a long series of interrupted sutures or many ligatures in rapid succession, this repetition is not necessary. Use good judgment; be logical.

   Also be logical in selecting instruments used for suturing. Give surgeon long needleholders to work deep in a cavity. Short ones may be used for surface work. Give assistant a needleholder to pull needle through tissue for the surgeon. Then, have scissors ready when knot is tied.

   Remove waste ends of suture material from the field, Mayo stand, and instrument table. Place them in trash disposal container. Put used needles on a magnet, needle rack, or into the suture book or other container for this purpose until the needle count is completed.

6 Keep two clean sponges or tapes on the field. Put up clean ones before removing soiled ones on an exchange basis. Discard soiled sponges into kick bucket. If a basin is used to accumulate soiled sponges on the field, touch only outside of it. Sponges are either potentially contaminated or grossly so. Keep basin at waist level when emptying it into kick bucket.

   If sponges or tapes are added during the operation, count them with circulating nurse before moistening or using them. Do not mix types of sponges and tapes, either on the table or in a basin of solution. Normal saline is usually used to moisten sponges and tapes because it is an isotonic solution.

7 Save all specimens of tissue according to hospital policy. Many hospitals' policies stipulate

that all tissue be sent to the laboratory, even though a piece of tissue may appear to be of no value for examination or diagnostic purposes.

Care for tissue specimen according to hospital procedure. Specimens are put in a specimen basin or attached to an instrument until put into a specimen jar. Never put a large clamp on a small specimen; this may crush cells, making tissue identification difficult. Disposable glove wrappers, marked right and left, can be used for holding bilateral specimens, e.g., right and left breast biopsies. Hand specimen from field in a basin, wrapper, or on a towel; *never place it on a sponge.* Keep specimen basin on the field until all tissue has been removed or all contaminated items are in it. Tell circulating nurse exactly what the specimen is. If you do not know, ask the surgeon to identify it.

8 Maintain sterile technique. Watch for any breaks. Observe the following points:

a Step away from sterile field if contaminated. Ask circulating nurse for another glove, gown, or sleeve—whatever is needed for yourself or another member of sterile team. If lower arm of gown becomes contaminated, a sterile gown sleeve can be drawn over it to cover the area.

b Change glove at once and discard needle or instrument if a glove is pricked by a needle or snagged by an instrument.

c Discard a piece of suture material, tubing, or a sponge that falls over edge of sterile field without touching the contaminated part of it.

d Keep hands at waist level when at rest; they should never be below waist.

e Keep contact with sterile field to a minimum. No one should lean on or against the operating table, Mayo stand, instrument table, and especially not on the patient. Remember that the patient under the drapes is unable to complain!

f Leave a wide margin of safety in moving about the room. A gown bulges, requiring more space than you are accustomed to need. In passing nonsterile objects, turn back to them.

g Do not turn back to sterile field or to members of sterile team. Face sterile areas to pass them.

h Do not reach behind a member of sterile team; go around. Pass another member of sterile team back to back (see Fig. 7-7, p. 119).

i Keep table and sterile field as dry as possible. Spread extra towels as needed. Keep strings and rings on tapes in basin, not dangling over side of it and dripping on instrument table.

j Discard soiled sponges from sterile field. A basin may be placed on the drapes near operative site to receive soiled sponges. This is handy for surgeon and avoids need to turn from the field to discard sponges. It eliminates frequent turning away from sterile field by scrub nurse also. It prevents need for rehandling soiled sponges. They can be emptied from this basin into kick bucket. Be sure to touch only outside of basin and keep it at waist level.

k Keep talking to a minimum. Avoid coughing and sneezing.

During Closure

1 Count sponges, sharps, and instruments with circulating nurse when surgeon begins closure of the wound, in accordance with established count procedures (see p. 178).

2 Clear off Mayo stand, as time permits, leaving a knife handle with blade, tissue forceps, scissors, four hemostats, and two Allis's forceps.

NOTE. Policy in many hospitals requires that Mayo stand remain sterile until patient has left the room. Cardiac arrest, tracheal collapse, hemorrhage, or other emergency can occur in the immediate postoperative-postanesthesia period. Even though sterile instrument sets are nearby, valuable time can be lost opening sterile supplies when every second counts in an emergency situation. Sterile instruments on Mayo stand, regardless of their previous use, can be used for emergency intervention. These can be lifesaving until other ones become available.

3 Have a damp sponge ready to wash blood from area surrounding the incision as soon as skin closure is completed.

4 Have dressings ready. Sterile dressings are regarded as part of operation. Their purposes are:

a To keep incision free from microorganisms. However, some surgeons prefer to leave the wound exposed in the belief that the coagulum that forms at well-approximated edges in first few minutes after wound is sutured strengthens wound and gives protection against microorganisms. Dressings are considered essential, aesthetically at least, by most surgeons.

b To protect incision from outside injury, especially in children.
c To absorb drainage.
d To give some support to incision and surrounding skin.

In considering which components to assemble for a particular dressing, keep in mind the needs of that particular wound. Some wounds require an opposite performance from a dressing than others do. A dressing's function is determined by its structure. A complete dressing must consist of at least three components:

a The *contact layer* acts either as a passageway for the secretion that emanates from a draining wound or as a barrier to protect the nondraining wound from its environment. It must conform to all body contours regardless of site and extent of wound, and must stay in intimate contact with the wound surface yet be nonadherent for painless removal.
b The *intermediate layer,* which is absorbent, serves as the storage area for the secretion passing through the contact layer from a draining wound, or as a cushion to protect a nondraining wound from further trauma. To provide adequate absorbency capacity or protection, it should be layered over the contact material to the thickness required by the particular wound.
c The *outer wrap* or *binder* holds the assembled components in proper position to serve their particular purpose.

Pressure dressings are used frequently following extensive operations, especially in plastic surgery, in operations on the knee or breast. These bulky dressings are added to the intermediate layer:

a To eliminate dead space and to prevent edema or hematoma (see Chap. 17).
b To distribute pressure evenly.
c To absorb extensive drainage.
d To immobilize a body area or to support soft tissues when muscles are moved.
e To help provide comfort to the patient postoperatively.

Materials used for pressure dressings include:

a Fluffed gauze.
b Abdominal pads. These are gauze-covered, absorbent cellulose.
c Single-piece, bulk dressings. These are available for use on trunk and extremities and save time in application.
d Cotton rolls. These are used to apply gentle pressure on each side of a knee following operation on this joint, for example.
e Foam rubber.

CIRCULATING NURSE

Circulating nurses wash hands and arms for five minutes at beginning of day before entering the OR, but do not don sterile gowns and gloves. Persons who wear sterile attire touch only sterile items; persons who are not sterile touch only unsterile items. Therefore, the circulating nurse must assist the sterile scrub nurse by providing the sterile supplies needed to prepare for arrival of surgeon.

After Scrub Nurse Scrubs

1 Fasten back of scrub nurse's gown.

2 If tray of instruments is in the autoclave in the substerile room, sterile lifting handles must be used to bring tray from autoclave to a sterile surface. Never reach over sterile instruments or sterile surface when placing tray. The tray may be set on basin in ring stand to avoid the danger of contaminating the instrument table with moisture.

3 Open packages of sterile supplies, such as syringes, suction tubing, sutures, sponges, gloves. Many of these items are prepackaged, presterilized, disposable products. Others are wrapped and sterilized by hospital personnel. Care must be taken in opening all sterile packages to avoid contamination.

> NOTE. If a sterile package drops to the floor, discard it. Compression resulting from fall can cause air and dust to enter package. It can no longer be considered sterile.

Some packages are designed so circulating nurse can flip a *rigid* item onto sterile field without reaching over it. *Many soft items do not flip.* If it does not flip easily, put item on edge of table with inside of the wrapper everted over hand. *Never reach over sterile field and shake an item from package.* An alternative method is for the scrub nurse to pick item from package as the circulating nurse opens it and holds contents exposed (see Figs. 10-7, 10-8, and 10-9).

> NOTE. *The routine use of transfer forceps is obsolete.* Should a need arise, such as for removing a single instrument from a flash sterilizer, a

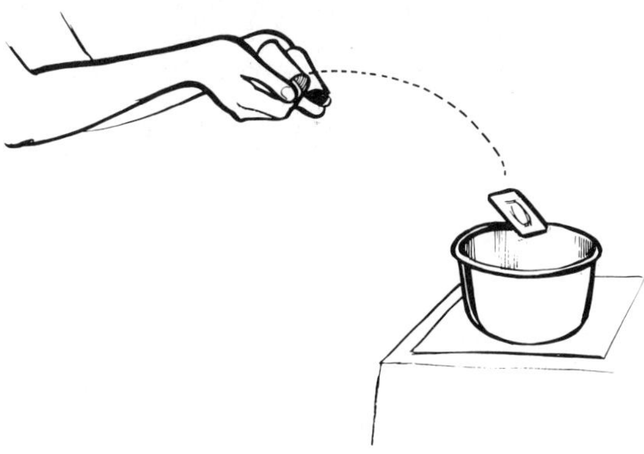

FIGURE 10-7
Circulating nurse flipping sterile suture packet from overwrap into a basin on the scrub nurse's sterile instrument table.

sterile transfer forceps may be used. At this time, a package containing a forceps is opened and used for a single transfer or placed in a sterile container, such as a dry hydrometer jar, for use as needed during remainder of *that* operation. The circulating nurse touches only the handles. Always carry a forceps high and in sight; never swing it at your side. Avoid touching tip of the instrument table when placing items.

If a forceps is placed in a container of disinfectant solution to maintain sterility during the operation, when using or holding forceps, keep tip horizontal to handle or below it. Never hold it above the horizontal level; solution will run to nonsterile handle, then contaminate tip when it is lowered again. Forceps and container are cleaned with instruments at end of operation and resterilized.

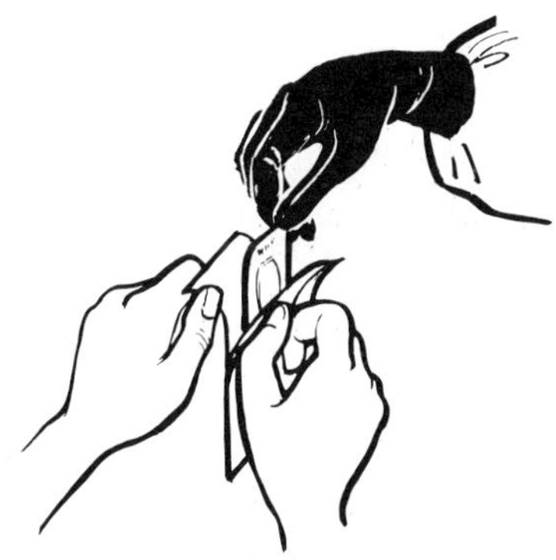

FIGURE 10-8
Scrub nurse taking contents from suture packet opened and held by circulating nurse. The scrub nurse avoids touching the unsterile outer wrapper.

4 Flip suture packets onto the instrument table, or open overwraps for scrub nurse to take packets. Check list of materials and sizes on surgeon's preference card, but verify with surgeon before opening packets. Avoid opening suture packets that will not be used. Wait until patient is in the OR before opening any packets. The operation might be canceled and then they would be wasted. Be conservative in opening packets. If you cannot anticipate the surgeon's need for sutures and do not receive instructions, you can generally keep just a packet or two ahead of actual need during the operation and thus avoid waste.

5 Pour solution (usually normal saline) into the round basin for sponges on instrument table, and into the splash basin in ring stand if this will be needed. Pour a small amount of antiseptic agent for skin preparation in solution cups to be used for this purpose.

6 Count sponges, sharps, and instruments with the scrub nurse as required by hospital policy and procedure. Record immediately (see section on counts later in this chapter, p. 177).

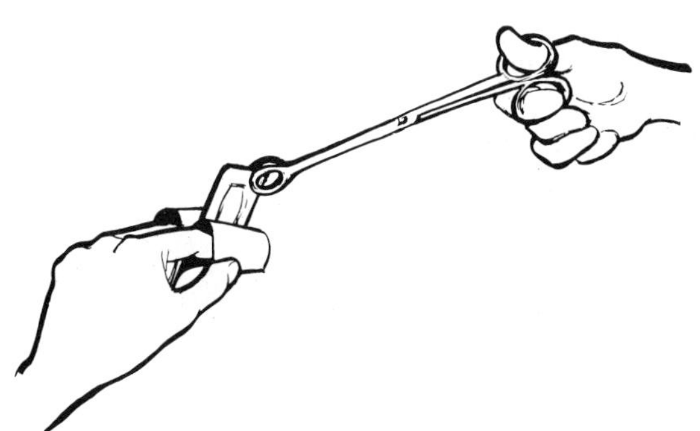

FIGURE 10-9
Circulating nurse removing sterile suture inner packet from overwrap with sterile forceps.

After Patient Arrives

While the scrub nurse continues to prepare for the arrival of the surgeon, the circulating nurse attends to the patient.

1 Greet and identify patient. Introduce yourself to the patient if you have not made the preoperative assessment. Check wristband for identification by name and hospital number.

2 Check nursing care plan and patient's chart for pertinent information, including consent.
3 Cover patient's hair with a cap to prevent dissemination of microorganisms, to protect it from being soiled, and to prevent a static spark near the anesthesia machine.
4 Take patient into the OR after surgeon sees him or her and anesthesiologist is ready for induction. The patient should see the surgeon before being anesthetized.
5 Assist patient in moving from stretcher to operating table. Both stretcher and table must be stabilized by locking the wheels when a patient is moving from one to the other. During transfer, avoid unnecessary exposure of patient. Remember that the cotton blanket and gown protect modesty as well as provide warmth. Handle blanket and gown gently to avoid dispersing lint and microorganisms into the air; they can settle on sterile tables. In moving patient, also give special caution to catheters, drainage tubes, intravenous infusions, and traction apparatus. Do not dislodge them.
6 Check to be certain a conductive strap, if used, is in contact with patient's skin, with one end of strap fastened to metal frame of the operating table. This assures an electrical connection of patient to a conductive floor.
7 Apply restraints comfortably. Place safety strap loosely over blanket 2 in. (5 cm) above knees. The patient's legs must not be crossed (see Chap. 15, p. 296). Place patient's arms at sides on the table and tuck arm band around them. If an intravenous infusion is running or will be started, place that arm on a padded armboard at a right angle to the table. Secure arm with a wrist strap. The arm must be immobilized to prevent peripheral extravasation of solution, which can cause local tissue necrosis.

NOTE. Angle of abduction of arm should *never* be greater than 90°, a right angle with the body. The brachial nerve plexus can be damaged by lengthy, too-severe abduction of arm.

8 Help anesthesiologist, as needed, to apply and connect necessary monitoring devices, headset for music, etc.
9 Assist anesthesiologist, surgeon, or assistant to start intravenous (IV) fluids. Unless this was done in holding area or is taken care of by the anesthesiologist, obtain the following equipment before patient arrives:
a Tourniquet.
b Sponges saturated with antiseptic solution for skin preparation. Thorough skin antisepsis is imperative.
c Intravenous administration set of sterile tubing with air filter and needle, cannula, or catheter. A cutdown tray may be needed.

NOTE. 1. 1½ in. (3.8 cm) by 20 or 21 gauge needles usually are used for intravenous fluids when blood transfusion is not anticipated; 1½ in. (3.8 cm) by 16 or 18 gauge needles are used when blood transfusion is anticipated.

2. When prolonged postoperative fluid therapy or hyperalimentation is anticipated, an inert, nontoxic, radiopaque plastic catheter is inserted through either a venipuncture through the skin (percutaneous insertion) or a cutdown through a skin incision to expose the vein. A venous cutdown is done in other selected situations: for central venous pressure monitoring, thrombosed superficial veins, or superficially collapsed veins due to shock or prolonged preoperative IV therapy. The cutdown site is an open wound. Catheter insertion should be considered a minor operative procedure. Sterile gloves, drapes, and tray of sterile instruments and sutures are needed. Have assorted sizes of intravenous catheters available so surgeon can choose size best suited to the vein. A soft, pliant catheter takes the contour of the anatomy and is not easily dislodged by movement of the patient.

d Parenteral infusion solution. Intravenous solutions frequently used in the OR include:
1 Normal saline.
2 Dextrose, 5 or 10%, in water.
3 Dextrose in saline.
4 *Dextran,* an artificial plasma-volume expander, acts by drawing fluid from tissues. It remains in the circulation for several hours. It interferes with cross matching of blood.
5 *Mannitol,* an osmotic diuretic agent, has an effect on renal vascular resistance. Depending on percentage of drug in solution, it can produce either an increase or decrease in renal blood flow. It may be given prophylactically to prevent renal failure. It is also used to decrease intracranial and intraocular pressure. It is rapidly excreted by the kidneys.

6 *Ringer's lactate solution,* a physiologic salt solution, is infused in patients in whom the body's supply of sodium, calcium, and potassium has been depleted or for improvement of circulation and stimulation of renal activity.

Usually, normal saline or dextrose solution is started initially.

NOTE. Gently squeeze plastic bag to detect leaks; check glass for cracks. Check solution for clarity or discoloration. A cloudy solution is contaminated. If circulating nurse hangs solution, a second registered nurse or doctor must check label on the container before it is administered. All solutions given are charted and monitored to see that they are running at the proper speed. Usually this is responsibility of anesthesiologist.

e Adhesive strips to firmly secure needle or catheter and tubing to the patient's skin to prevent motion that may cause entry of microorganisms into the skin wound or traumatize the vein.

f Stopcock to regulate or stop flow of solution through tubing into the vein.

During Induction of General Anesthesia

1 Stay in room and near patient to comfort him or her and assist anesthesiologist in the event that excitement or any other contingency occurs. The patient must be guarded during induction to prevent possible injury or fall from operating table. Further restrain or hold the patient if necessary. The circulating nurse must not leave room until anesthesiologist says the patient no longer needs to be guarded.

2 Be as quiet as possible. Excitement may occur during induction from tactile or auditory stimulation. It occurs more commonly in alcoholics. A strong startle reaction to sound can provoke life-threatening cardiac arrhythmias in any patient, however. Hearing is last sense lost. *The room must be kept completely quiet until the patient is anesthetized.* Any stimulation while patient is under light anesthesia is highly dangerous and must be avoided. A quiet, undisturbed induction makes for a much safer and easier maintenance of and recovery from anesthesia.

After Patient Is Anesthetized

1 Reposition patient only after anesthesiologist says the patient is anesthetized to extent that he or she will not be disturbed by being moved or touched. (Positioning of patient is discussed in Chapter 15).

2 Attach anesthesia screen and other table attachments as needed. These always are placed after the patient is anesthetized and positioned to prevent injury to patient.

3 Note patient's position to be certain all measures for his or her safety have been observed.

4 Place inactive electrode pad or plate in contact with patient's skin, if electrosurgical unit is to be used, to ground the patient properly. Avoid scar tissue, and hairy or bony areas. (See Chapter 19 for further discussion of electrosurgical units).

5 Expose appropriate area for skin preparation. Turn blanket downward and gown upward neatly to make a smooth area around operative site.

6 Turn on overhead spotlight over site of incision. Bright light should not be focused on the patient before he or she is asleep or eyes are covered. Preoperative medication affects pupils. Dim light is restful and not irritating.

7 Arrange sterile prep tray and pour solutions if this has not already been done. Don sterile gloves and prepare the operative site. (Patient skin preparation is discussed in Chapter 16.)

NOTE. The first assistant may be the person who preps the patient. This person first scrubs his or her own hands and arms, then puts on sterile gloves.

8 Cover or bag prep tray immediately after use. The sponges are not included in sponge count so they must not be discarded in kick bucket. A disposable tray may be bagged for disposal with trash after operation is completed.

After Surgeon and Assistant(s) Scrub

1 Assist with gowning. Reach inside gown to shoulder seam. If closed glove technique is used, pull gown sleeves only so far that hands remain covered. If open technique is used, pull each sleeve over hands so gown cuffs are at the wrists. Fasten back of gown.

NOTE. After gloving, surgeon and assistant(s) should wipe gloves with a sterile damp towel or terry washcloth to remove glove powder. Some surgeons prefer to rinse gloves in a splash basin. This basin should be removed from the sterile field immediately after use for this purpose to avoid carrying powder into operative wound if gloves are rinsed of blood and debris during the operation.

2 Observe for any breaks in technique during draping (see Chap. 16). Stand near head end of the operating table to assist anesthesiologist in fastening drape over the anesthesia screen or around IV standard next to the armboard.

3 Assist scrub nurse in moving Mayo stand and instrument table into position, being careful not to touch drapes.

4 Focus overhead operating light on site of incision, unless sterile handles will be used. The beam of light should pass the surgeon's right ear and center at tip of his or her right index finger (or left for left-handed surgeon).

5 Set platforms for team members who need them, or place stools in position for surgeon who prefers to operate seated.

6 Position kick buckets on each side of operating table and splash basin, if used, near surgeon.

7 Connect suction if necessary. Suction caps are designed so inlet for fluid is below outlet for vacuum. These connections must not be reversed. If they are, contents of the container are picked up and carried into the vacuum system, clogging it and making it nonoperational. Most hospitals use disposable suction collection units to facilitate disposal.

8 Connect electrosurgical electrode cord or any other electrical equipment to be used. Place footpedals within easy reach of surgeon's foot. Tell surgeon the settings on all machines.

During Operation

1 Be alert to anticipate needs of sterile team such as adjusting operating light, removing perspiration from brows, and keeping scrub nurse supplied with sponges, sutures, hot saline, etc. Ideally, the circulating nurse watches the operation closely enough to see when routine supplies are needed and gives them to sterile team without their having to ask for them. You must know use and care of all supplies, instruments, and equipment and be able to get them quickly. This is particularly important in emergency situations such as cardiac arrest.

2 Stay in room as much as possible. *Inform the scrub nurse if you must leave.* Be available to answer questions or offer helpful suggestions to scrub nurse. Kind help builds up a learner's confidence.

3 Keep discarded sponges carefully collected, separated by sizes, and counted. The method used depends upon provision made for care of soiled sponges in each hospital. (Refer to suggested methods of guarding sponges on p. 180 of this chapter.) It is convenient to keep them in submultiples of total number of each type of sponge in each package.

Soiled sponges should be placed in an area of room away from traffic, cabinets, and doorways, but in full view of scrub nurse and anesthesiologist. Used sponges should be kept at a level well below the sterile field on a moisture-proof surface. Do not place them on absorbent linen as it soaks through. Lint, dust, and trapped organisms will be dispersed into the air as the sponges dry and are handled for counting or disposal. Sponge forceps or gloves, *never bare hands,* are used to handle and count sponges because of danger of hepatitis transmission. Gathering them directly into plastic bags eliminates extra handling and the hazards that accompany transfer of dry, soiled sponges. Before placing them in bags, both circulating and scrub nurses should count them.

4 Weigh sponges for blood loss as requested. Some anesthesiologists and surgeons prefer to have sponges weighed for blood loss rather than visually estimating it. A scale calibrated in grams usually is used to weigh bloody sponges during operation before they dry out.

The weight of each dry sponge must be known. Usually a chart of dry weight for each type of sponge is attached to the scale. This weight is multiplied by number of sponges of each type to be weighed. The scale platform is covered with moisture-proof sheeting to protect it from contamination. Allowing for dry weights of the number of sponges to be weighed and the cover, adjust scale to register at zero. When blood-soaked sponges are weighed, the reading on scale equals the blood loss; 1 g equals 1 cc. The scale must be checked frequently for accuracy.

Record total blood loss each time sponges

are weighed, always adding new weight to preceding weight. Keep a current total. A tally board for this purpose may be mounted on wall where anesthesiologist and surgeon can read it.

Total blood volume monitoring determinations may be used for estimation of operating blood loss (see Chap. 14, p. 271).

5 Obtain blood products for transfusion as necessary. Transfusions of whole blood, plasma, packed cells, platelets, or artificial blood must be carried out according to hospital policy. Basic rules usually include the following:

a Blood products are obtained from the blood bank by a person responsible for signing them out to the proper patient. Usually a nursing assistant from the OR staff can do this.

b Blood products are started by an MD or RN after a careful comparison of label on bag or bottle with identity of patient. A second professional person confirms these data. The label stays on container while blood product is transfused.

c Another solution may be infused immediately prior to hanging a blood product. In changing from this solution to a blood product, avoid possibility of air entering the tubing. A blood-transfusion filter must be used. Filter should be changed after second or third unit of whole blood because the filter can become clogged with microaggregates.

d Anesthesiologist records on anesthesia record the following information:

1 Name of the person who started the transfusion of whole blood, plasma, packed cells, platelets, or artificial blood.

2 Time started and drops per minute.

3 Amount and information on the label: group, Rh factor, and number.

e Cold, refrigerated blood may induce hypothermia. Blood may be warmed as it is transfused by immersion of administration tubing in a controlled water bath or infused through sterile coils in a temperature-modifying device. Temperature must be controlled between 89 to 105°F (32 to 41°C).

f To have blood near patient during operation, a refrigerator with controlled temperature may be installed in the OR suite. It has a recording thermometer. An alarm bell rings if a dangerous temperature is reached. Fluctuations in temperature cause red blood cells to deteriorate. Microorganisms can multiply in unrefrigerated blood. If blood is brought into the OR and not needed, it should be returned to refrigerator in suite or blood bank immediately. Do not allow blood or its derivatives to stand unrefrigerated in the OR.

g A transfusion of wrong blood can be fatal. All established measures must be strictly observed for the patient's safety. The patient is observed closely for any type of reaction. This probability increases in direct proportion to number of units transfused. The most common type of reaction is *allergic; febrile* is almost as common; and *hemolytic* reactions are possible. Transfusion reactions under anesthesia may be accompanied by profound hypotension and temperature change. However, the common physical reactions and chills are not seen in an anesthetized patient. If any suspicious reactions occur:

1 Stop transfusion.

2 Report reaction to surgeon and blood bank.

3 Return unused blood to blood bank along with sample of patient's blood.

4 Send a urine sample to the laboratory as soon as possible.

5 Take vital signs frequently.

6 Complete an incident report covering details of the reaction to be kept on file.

Compatible bank blood is not always immediately available. Even when it is, posttransfusion hepatitis non-A non-B is a potential danger for the patient.

Autotransfusion, reinfusion of patient's own blood, may be used either during elective or emergency operations. This blood may be collected days or weeks preoperatively and stored in blood bank, or drawn just prior to or during operation. Recovery of blood as it is lost and reinfusion during operation is *intraoperative autotransfusion.* This requires sterile equipment that simultaneously suctions blood from operative site, filters, anticoagulates, defoams, and returns it to patient with minimal blood-cell damage. An autotransfusion unit for this purpose must be easily and quickly assembled as it may be lifesaving in an emergency situation. Autotransfusions can be used for a patient who will not allow blood transfusion for religious reasons but will accept his or her own blood if it is returned immediately.

Artificial blood, Fluosol, offers another altertive to transport oxygen to the brain and throughout the body when the patient's blood volume or hemoglobin level is decreased due to blood loss.

6 Know condition of patient at all times. Keep OR supervisor informed of any marked change in the patient's condition or unanticipated procedure. Also tell ORS if operation will not finish at scheduled time. This is important in a busy department as it may be necessary to rearrange the schedule.

7 Prepare and label specimens for transportation to the laboratory. Wrong patient identification on a specimen can result in wrong diagnosis for two patients. Each container is labeled with name of patient, hospital and room numbers. A requisition specifying laboratory test surgeon desires accompanies specimen. This includes date, name of surgeon, pre- and postoperative diagnoses, operative procedure, and tissue to be examined including its source.Containers for storing specimens may be plastic bags, waxed cardboard cartons, or glass jars with preservative solutions. Preservatives vary. All must be handled with care to avoid spillage. Handling of specimens should be held to a minimum and *never done with bare hands.* If instruments are used for handling, be careful not to tear or damage tissue. Routine for each type of tissue specimen may vary as follows:

a Pathological specimens should not be allowed to dry out. A solution of aqueous formaldehyde most often is used as the fixative until specimen is processed further in laboratory.

b Cultures should be refrigerated or sent to the laboratory immediately. When placed immediately into media, they can be stored in an incubator indefinitely.

Cultures are obtained under sterile conditions. Tips of swabs must not be contaminated by any other source. The circulating nurse may hold tube; however, swabs are handled only by sterile team members. OR and laboratory personnel must be protected from contamination. The circulating nurse can hold open a small paper or plastic bag for scrub nurse to drop tube into if it is handled on sterile field. This technique eliminates need for circulating nurse to handle the tube, and alerts laboratory personnel to be cautious in handling to prevent spread of microorganisms and to protect themselves.

c Smears and fluids should be taken to laboratory as soon as possible. These may be placed on glass slides or drawn into evacuation tubes.

d Stones are placed in a dry container so they will not dissolve.

e Foreign bodies should be disposed of according to hospital policy and a record kept for legal purposes. A description of the object is recorded. A foreign body may be given to the police, surgeon, or patient, depending on legal implications, hospital's policy, or surgeon's wishes.

f Amputated extremities are wrapped before sending them to a refrigerator, which is usually in the morgue.

8 Complete patient's chart, permanent operating room records, and requisitions for laboratory tests or chargeable items, as required.

a Documentation in patient's chart of direct intraoperative nursing care should include:

1 Disposition of sensory aids or prosthetic devices accompanying patient on arrival in OR.

2 Position, supports, and/or restraints used during operation.

3 Placement of monitoring and electrosurgical electrodes, tourniquets, and other special equipment, and identification of units or machines used, as applicable.

4 Skin preparation area and antiseptic agent.

5 Medications administered by RN.

b Circulating nurse documents other activities that may affect patient outcomes of surgical intervention. These may include:

1 Type, size, and manufacturer's identifying information of prosthetic implants, or type, source, and location of tissue transplants or inserted radioactive materials.

2 Disposition of tissue specimens.

3 Placement of drains, catheters, and packing.

c Requisitions are made out as a record of:

1 Charges to patients for supplies, according to hospital routine.

2 A piece of equipment sent from OR with patient to unit, e.g., an instrument such as an intestinal clamp left on patient following a colostomy, a tracheotomy set that accompanies patient following thyroidectomy, wire scissors if patient has had teeth wired together. These items are to be returned. The requisition usually is made out in duplicate; copy accompanies the item, and original is filed by lender until item is returned.

9 Be alert to any breaks in sterile technique.
  a Do not touch or reach over sterile field. When placing sterile items, transfer should be made to edge of the instrument table to avoid exposing it to contamination with microorganisms in dust or lint shed from a sleeve, arm, or wrapper.
  b Face sterile areas when passing. Just as no unsterile equipment should be placed between two sterile surfaces, no unsterile person should pass between two sterile surfaces or two sterile team members. All unsterile personnel should face and remain at least 1 ft (30 cm) from any sterile surface.
  c Do not touch unwrapped items to nonsterile rim or door when removing them from autoclave.
  d Do not touch edge of cap or lid to lip of container before or after pouring sterile solution. The outside of cap is not sterile.
  e Wash hands vigorously for at least 15 seconds after each patient contact or handling contaminated items. Hasty handwashing is better than not washing at all. Friction and water alone will remove most surface organisms from hands. However, wash hands frequently with an antiseptic agent. If you do not work up a good lather and use friction, hands will still be contaminated. Be sure to clean under fingernails; microorganisms can grow under them. Turn faucet handles off with a paper towel, if a knee or foot control is not available.
  f Keep conversation to a minimum. Do not handle mask and cap unnecessarily. Keep hair covered and mask in place.
  g Decontaminate floor and walls promptly during operation if contaminated by organic debris such as blood and sputum. A phenolic, iodophor, or other broad-spectrum detergent-disinfectant can be applied from a squeeze bottle to soilage. This prompt decontamination helps prevent microorganisms from drying and becoming airborne.

During Closure

1 Count sponges, sharps, and instruments with scrub nurse. Report counts as correct or incorrect to surgeon. Complete count records (for details of count procedures, see p. 177). Collect soiled sponges and put into plastic-lined kick bucket.

2 If another patient is scheduled to follow (TF):
  a Phone, or ask clerk-receptionist to call unit at least 45 minutes before scheduled time of operation to request that preoperative medication be given. This usually is not necessary for the first scheduled patient of day, but is the procedure for subsequent patients when the exact time of operation is uncertain. For these patients, the anesthesiologist usually orders medication "on call."
  b Send a nursing assistant for patient or notify unit to transport patient. The patient should be in the OR suite 30 minutes before time of anticipated incision. If a holding area is included in the OR suite, the patient may arrive earlier to receive preoperative medication there.
  c Check surgeon's preference card and procedure book. Collect supplies that will be needed; get them organized to extent possible. These can be assembled in substerile room or left in a cabinet. They cannot be put on furniture in room until it is cleaned after this operation is completed. Advance preparation is not necessary if a cart system is used.

3 Prepare for room cleanup so minimal time will be expended between operations, but check with scrub nurse before leaving room.
  a Remove x-rays from viewbox, place them in envelope, and take them to designated area to be returned to x-ray department.
  b Return blood not needed for transfusion to refrigerator or have it taken to blood bank by a nursing assistant.
  c Obtain washer-sterilizer tray, instrument tray, and other items necessary for the cleanup procedure (see details of procedure in last section of this chapter).

4 Send for a recovery room stretcher, ICU bed, or prepare the patient's stretcher or bed with a clean sheet, whatever is the accepted practice. Also alert nursing assistants and housekeeping personnel that operation is nearing completion, so they can be ready to assist as needed. This helps shorten time between operations.

After Operation Is Completed

1 Open neck and back closures of gowns of surgeon and assistants so they can remove them without contaminating themselves.

2 Assist with outer layer of dressing. Ideally, this outer layer should be conforming, stretchable to avoid constriction if edema develops, and capable of clinging to itself so that it will stay in position without telescoping if mobility is desired. *Adhesive tape* is used most frequently. Benzoin may be sprayed on skin around the intermediate layer, before applying adhesive tape, to increase its adhesion. Apply tape firmly but not tightly, to avoid traction on skin and wrinkling of it. Traction and wrinkling, rather than sensitivity to the tape, may cause skin irritation.

NOTE. If patient has a known sensitivity to regular adhesive tape, hypoallergenic tape should be used. It causes little or no reaction. It is lightweight yet strong, sticks well, is porous, and allows skin to breathe.

Slightly elastic bandage provides gentle, even pressure to hold bulky dressings in place. This bandage also may be used to hold other kinds of dressings or to bind a splint onto an extremity. It stretches to conform to body contours, does not constrict, yet gives firm support. The types available include:

a Four-ply crinkled-gauze bandage.

b Cotton-elastic bandage.

c Cotton-elastic bandage with adhesive on one side. This is especially useful in holding dressings on chest, as it is firm yet permits chest expansion.

Montgomery straps are used to hold bulky dressings in place that require frequent changes or wound inspections. They are made in pairs, in assorted widths, with strings. One strap is put on each side of dressing and strings are tied across dressing.

An *abdominal binder* may be needed to hold large abdominal dressings. If necessary, it usually is applied after patient is moved from operating table.

3 See that patient is clean. Wash off blood, feces, or plaster. Put on a clean gown and blanket.

4 Have nursing assistant bring in a clean recovery room stretcher or ICU bed. Check name on patient's stretcher or bed to be sure that he or she is returned to the proper one if this is the procedure. Lock wheels before moving patient.

5 Help move patient to stretcher or bed. Before moving a patient from operating table, be sure all arm and leg restraints and table appliances have been removed. A lifting frame or patient roller is a great help in moving unconscious and obese patients. The Davis patient roller consists of a series of rollers, mounted in a frame long enough to accommodate an adult patient. Edge of roller is placed under arm band and patient's side. With patient's head and feet supported, pull on arm band and roll patient onto stretcher or bed. The following precautions must be taken in lifting or rolling an unconscious patient:

a Splint arm if an intravenous is running to protect needle.

b Support arms at sides with arm band, so they do not dangle.

c The anesthesiologist guards head and neck from injury.

d Lift or roll patient gently and slowly to avoid circulatory depression. At least four people are needed; one to lift head, one to lift feet, one beside the stretcher or bed to pull, and one beside patient to lift him or her from operating table. The action of all must be synchronized.

e Remove arm band, which has been used as a lifting sheet, by rolling patient gently from side to side. Brush burns result if linen is pulled from under the patient.

f Place patient in a comfortable position most conducive to maintenance of respiration and circulation. This may vary with type of operation; usually the patient should:

1 Be semilateral following laparotomy.

2 Be semiprone following tonsillectomy, for drainage.

3 Be lateral, on affected side, following transthoracic operations, to splint the side.

4 Have an operated extremity supported on a pillow.

g Raise siderails before patient is transported out of the OR.

6 Secure IV solution bags on a standard, attached preferably near foot end of stretcher or bed, where there is less danger of injury to patient if it should fall or break.

7 Connect all drainage systems as indicated. This must be done at once to prevent extravasation of urine, bile, or other fluid with consequent irritation or infection. Attach tubing to bottom sheet, leaving a loop next to the patient. Drainage tubing should be positioned so downward flow is aided by force of gravity. Drainage bag should be kept below level of tubing to prevent retrograde flow.

8 Be sure chart and proper records, including the nursing care plan, accompany patient. Send extra units of blood as needed. Send other supplies as indicated.

Final completion of patient's chart should include documentation of:

- **a** Assessment of patient's skin condition prior to and at completion of operation, i.e., skin discoloration, rashes, pressure sores, burn.
- **b** Urinary output and estimated blood loss, if measurement during operation was appropriate.
- **c** Results of all counts. Both the scrub and circulating nurses should sign records for counts.
- **d** Type of dressing.
- **e** Time of discharge from OR and method of transport.

9 Have nursing assistant assist anesthesiologist in taking patient to recovery room, intensive care unit, or nursing unit. In some hospitals, the circulating nurse accompanies patient and anesthesiologist to give a nursing report to nurse receiving patient which includes a review of the nursing care plan.

Death in the O.R.

Although an infrequent occurrence, when a patient expires in the OR the surgeon in charge notifies the next of kin. The circulating nurse notifies the OR supervisor immediately. This may be unnecessary as the OR supervisor should be informed of any patient's deteriorating condition and all crises or emergencies.

Individual state law and hospital policy must be adhered to in caring for the body. In some states, the body of patient who expires in the OR automatically becomes property of the coroner. The circulating nurse's responsibilities in care of body include:

1 To give after-death care to body or to see that this is done according to hospital policy before transfer to hospital morgue. Some hospitals employ a mortician who assists in disposition of body and with necessary details.

- **a** Follow procedure book. Be sure identification is correct.
- **b** Body should be refrigerated within one hour of death.

2 To arrange for transportation of body to the morgue.

- **a** The nurse signs a form releasing body from the OR. The nursing assistant or person taking body also signs this form.
- **b** Extreme care should be taken in the suite to prevent other patients from seeing the body and/or the stretcher bearing it away.

SPONGE, SHARPS, AND INSTRUMENT COUNTS

The kinds and numbers of sponges, needles, other sharps, and instruments needed for different operations will vary. Each item must be considered a foreign object that can cause unnecessary harm should it be left inside the patient. Therefore, to ensure adequate patient protection, these items are counted before and after use.

A *counting procedure* is a method of accounting for items put on sterile table for use during an operation. Sponge and sharp counts are taken on every procedure performed in the OR. Sharps include surgical needles, hypodermic needles, safety pins, knife blades, electrosurgical needles and blades. Instrument counts also are recommended, although in some hospitals policy specifies that instrument counts be taken only when a major body cavity is entered, or depth and location of wound is such that an instrument could accidentally be left in patient. These would include operations within chest, abdominal and pelvic cavities, extraperitoneal spaces, vagina, hip or shoulder joint, and along the spine. Specific written policy and procedure for all counts must be followed without deviations.

Counting Procedures

Sponges, sharps, and instruments are counted at four or more different times.

First Count Person who wraps items for sterilization counts them in standardized multiple units, for example:

1 Sponges, tapes, peanuts, etc., are usually counted in multiples of 5 or 6, i.e., 10 or 12, 20 or 24 per package. If commercially prepackaged, sterile radiopaque sponges are used, this count is done by machine, usually 10 per package.

2 Needles put in racks or a suture book are counted uniformly into sets in multiples of two or three of each type and size the surgeon will need. Disposable eyed needles are precounted by the manufacturer.

3 Instruments, including sharps, are counted as they are assembled in standardized sets. Groups of six of the basic clamps facilitate handling and counting.

Second Count Circulating and scrub nurses count together when packages are opened before the operation begins and as each additional package is opened during the operation.

All Counts

1 As scrub nurse fingers each item, he or she and circulating nurse number each one aloud, quietly, until all items are counted.

2 Circulating nurse immediately records count for each type of item on count record. Preprinted forms are helpful for this purpose.

3 Count additional packages far away from the counted items already on table, in case it is necessary to repeat count or discard item.

4 Counting should not be interrupted. If uncertain about count because of interruption, fumbling, or for any other reason, repeat it.

Sponges

1 Only radiopaque sponges with an x-ray detectable element should be used on sterile field and table. Types of sponges and number of different sizes should be kept to a minimum.

2 Scrub nurse holds entire pack of sponges, of whatever type including tapes, in hand at one time.

3 Shake pack to separate sponges.

4 Holding thumb over folded edge of sponges, pick each sponge separately from pack and number it aloud while placing it in a pile on the table.

> NOTE. If a pack contains an incorrect number of sponges, scrub nurse should hand pack to circulating nurse. Danger of error is great if attempts are made to correct errors or compensate for discrepancies. Pack should be isolated and not used.

Sharps

1 All swaged and eyed, reusable or disposable, surgical needles are counted when packets are added to the table.

2 Scrub nurse retains packet with descriptive information of number and type of needles to help determine if count is correct for swaged and disposable needles.

3 Other sharps are counted as they are added to table or separated from other instruments in instrument tray.

Instruments

1 Remove top rack of instruments from instrument tray and place it on a rolled towel on instrument table or over lip of tray. Remove knife handles, towel clips, tissue forceps, and other small instruments from tray and place these on instrument table. Do not put instruments on Mayo stand until they are counted or as they are being counted.

2 Be sure all instruments left in tray are exposed for counting.

3 Detachable or disassembled parts must be counted or be accounted for during assembly.

Third Count Counts are taken in three areas when the surgeon starts the wound closure.

Sponge Count

1 *Table count.* Scrub and circulating nurses together count sponges on instrument table and Mayo stand.

2 *Floor count.* Circulating nurse counts sponges that have been discarded from sterile field. This count should be verified by scrub nurse.

3 *Field count.* Circulating nurse totals floor and table counts, subtracts this figure from total number, and tells surgeon or first assistant number needed to complete the count. One of them does operative field count. If it is desired number, the circulating nurse tells surgeon the count is correct.

> NOTE. By written policy and procedure, this sequence may be reversed. The field count may be done first, followed by table and floor counts.

Sharp and Instrument Counts Procedure is essentially the same as for sponge count. Circulating nurse adds to field count any needles, sharps, or instruments recovered from floor or passed off table. The count should be reported to surgeon as correct only after a physical count by number actually has been completed.

NOTE. If a needle or instrument has broken, both the scrub and circulating nurses must make sure all pieces are recovered.

Fourth or Final Count A fourth count is done if a discrepancy is noted in any of counts and if policy stipulates additional counts before any part of a cavity or a cavity within a cavity is closed. A final count may be taken during subcuticular or skin closure.

After final counts are completed, circulating nurse signs operative record to indicate counts are correct. A registered nurse must participate to verify that all counts are correct and to sign for all counts.

NOTE. Omitted counts due to extreme patient emergency must be documented on operative record and a patient incident report completed by circulating nurse.

When operation is completed, scrub nurse should sign operative record also. Hospital records can be subpoenaed and admitted as evidence in court. Therefore, when your name appears in a hospital record, to attest to an act you have performed, you should always write it yourself. Include your role in the act, such as "scrub nurse" signing for "sponge, sharp, instrument counts," with your signature.

NOTE. If either the scrub or circulating nurse is relieved by another person during the operation, the incoming nurse should verify all counts before nurse being relieved leaves room. Persons who take final counts are held accountable and must sign the records.

Incorrect Count

1 Entire count is repeated immediately.

2 Circulating nurse looks in trash receptacles, under furniture, on floor, in linen hamper, and throughout room.

3 Scrub nurse looks over drapes and under articles on table.

4 Surgeons recheck field and wound.

5 Circulating nurse should call supervisor, head nurse, or team leader to check count.

6 If item is not found, the surgeon may wish an x-ray taken at once, with a portable machine, to determine whether it has been left in the wound. Due to condition of patient or a reasonable assurance, based on wound exploration, that item is not in the patient, the surgeon may wish to complete the closure first. However, hospital policy should make it *mandatory* to take an x-ray *before* patient leaves the OR whenever a sponge, sharp, or instrument count is incorrect.

7 If count is wrong, circulating nurse writes up incident on appropriate form as a permanent record, even if item is located by x-ray. This record has legal significance to verify an appropriate attempt was made to find missing item. If item is not found by x-ray, the record brings to attention of personnel the need for more careful counting and control of sponges, sharps, and instruments.

Methods of Guarding Sponges

Regardless of types and numbers of sponges used, all must be accounted for expediently and conveniently. Various methods may be used to help ensure that a sponge is not left in the patient or misplaced.

By Scrub Nurse

1 Keep sponges, tapes, peanuts, etc., separated on instrument table and far away from each other and away from linen, especially towels.

2 Keep sponges far away from small items such as needles and clips that might be dragged into the wound by them.

3 Do not give surgeon or assistant a sponge to wipe powder off gloves. It may end up in linen hamper or trash.

4 Never mix sponges and tapes in solution basin at same time to avoid danger of dragging a small sponge unknowingly into wound along with a tape.

5 Do not give pathologist a specimen on a sponge to take from the room; put it on a towel instead.

6 Discard all soiled sponges into kick bucket, leaving two clean ones and one tape on field. If surgeon needs more, you must waive this rule and leave more. Keep a mental count of number of sponges or tapes on field at any given time.

7 Do not be wasteful of sponges. Besides the economy factor, the more sponges that are used, the more there are to count and the greater the chance for error.

8 Once the peritoneum is opened or the incision extends deep into a body cavity where a sponge could be lost, three alternative precautions can be taken:

a Remove all small sponges from field and use only tapes. Rings, if used, hang over wound edges.

b Use 4 by 4 in. (10 by 10 cm) sponges on sponge forceps only.

c Give sponges to surgeon one at a time on an exchange basis.

d *Do not add or remove sponges from operative field during sponge count until count is verified as completed and correct.* Prior to beginning the final count, place adequate tapes and sponges on field for use while count is taken.

By Circulating Nurse

1 To prevent possibility of a sponge being taken into the OR and causing confusion in the count, different types and sizes should be used on trays such as spinal, shave, or prep trays, and be contained before the incision is made. A tray, including the used sponges, may be bagged in plastic and stored temporarily. Sponges from these trays must never be put in kick bucket or trash receptacle until after final count is completed.

2 Unfold each discarded sponge and shake tapes to be sure no sponges are on them. To avoid transmission of hepatitis or other pathogenic organisms, soiled sponges are never touched with bare hands. Use sponge forceps or gloves to separate sponges for counting and stacking.

3 Count sponges into multiple or submultiples of total number in a package as recorded on sponge count record; count and stack into separate units for each type of sponge.

NOTE. The kick bucket is lined with an antistatic plastic bag. Therefore, either hang the sponges over rim of bucket or transfer them from kick bucket to a moisture-proof surface until count unit is completed. The number of sponges needed to complete a unit may be placed directly into a waterproof plastic or paper bag. Each bag is closed to await the final count. If this method is used, the scrub nurse should verify count as sponges are deposited in bags. Closed bags can be placed on a table or in a kick bucket under a towel placed over it to await final count. The number of sponges in each bag and number of bags are recorded so that when it is time for final count the circulating nurse has a record of the number bagged.

4 Give scrub nurse dressings after the final sponge count.

5 Trash and linen should never be taken from room until final sponge count is completed.

Method of Accounting for Sharps

By Scrub Nurse

1 Give needles to surgeon on an exchange basis; that is, one is returned before another is passed. Account for each needle as surgeon finishes with it. Never let one lie loose on field or Mayo stand. Keep them away from sponges and tapes.

2 Use needles and needleholders as a unit. Some hospitals go by the rule: no needle on the Mayo stand without a needleholder and no needleholder without a needle.

3 Secure used needles and sharps until after final count. Many methods for efficient handling are available.

a Sterile adhesive pads with or without magnets facilitate counting and safe disposal. Separate pads can be used for needles that may be used again and for those that will not be. When a large number of swaged needles will be used, the scrub and circulating nurses may determine number of needles a pad will hold and work out a unit system. When maximum number is reached and counted by them, the pad is closed. This method eliminates the hazard of handling loose needles on Mayo stand or instrument table.

b Swaged needles can be inserted through or into their original packet. An empty packet indicates an unaccounted-for needle at time of final count.

c Used needles can be returned to needle rack, or threaded into top layer of suture book.

d Accumulation of used needles in a medicine cup or other container is the least desirable method because each must be handled individually to count them. This not only potentially contaminates gloves, but may puncture them as well.

By Circulating Nurse

1 Open only number of packets of sutures with swaged needles that will be needed. Overstocking table not only is wasteful, but also complicates needle count.

2 Counted sharps should not be taken from

OR during operation. If a scalpel with a counted knife blade is given to pathologist to open specimen, it must remain in the room after gross examination, not be taken to laboratory with specimen.

Simplifying Instrument Count

Reducing the number and types of instruments and streamlining standardized sets makes counting easier. Inform the supervisor if unused, unnecessary instruments are routinely included in basic sets. Instruments peculiar to specific operations, wrapped separately, can be added to the basic set only when needed.

ROOM CLEANUP PROCEDURES AFTER OPERATION IS COMPLETED

Physical facilities influence the flow of supplies and equipment following the operation. However, basic principles of aseptic technique dictate the procedures to be carried out immediately after operation is completed to prepare OR for the next patient. Every patient merits the same degree of safety in the environment and deserves the same care as every other. In addition, personnel working in the operating room suite must be protected. Therefore, *every patient should be considered potentially a contaminant in the environment.* Some have known pathogenic microorganisms; danger of transmission of hepatitis virus or other infectious organisms may be unknown. Cleanup procedures must be rigidly followed to contain and confine organisms, known or unknown, to prevent contamination of entire suite. This is done by:

1 Destroying organisms as quickly as possible after operation is completed.

2 Protecting operating room personnel from contact with known infectious material such as frank pus, colon bacilli, gas gangrene, tetanus, or tuberculosis or any other communicable disease.

3 Preventing cross contamination of other patients.

The routine cleanup procedure can be accomplished expeditiously by circulating and scrub nurses working cooperatively. While the circulating nurse assists with outer layer of dressing and prepares patient for transport from the OR, the scrub nurse dismantles sterile field before removing gown and gloves. All instruments, supplies, and equipment must be either terminally sterilized, decontaminated, disinfected, or contained for disposal before they are handled by other personnel.

Terminal sterilization is process of sterilizing reusable items immediately after patient contact prior to handling by ungloved personnel. Items, other than disposables, that cannot be sterilized must be subjected to *high level disinfection* by a process that kills or destroys most disease producing microorganisms. Disposable items must be contained for safe handling by personnel.

By Scrub Nurse

1. Push Mayo stand and instrument table away from operating table as soon as intermediate layer of the dressing is applied. *Do not contaminate the Mayo stand* until the patient has left room (refer to Note on p. 167).
2. Assist surgeon and assistant in removing gowns and gloves. Gowns are always removed before gloves. Grasp both shoulders of gown and pull them downward over arms. Roll outside of gown inward and discard in linen or trash hamper; linen goes to laundry, disposable gown goes into trash. Using glove-to-glove technique, grasp cuff of gloves and pull them inside out over surgeon's hands. Discard in trash receptacle.
3. Check drapes for towel clips, instruments, and other items. Be sure no equipment is discarded with disposable drapes or sent to laundry with linen. Roll drapes off patient to prevent sparking and airborne contamination; do not pull them off. Disposable drapes are placed in plastic bag for disposal. Roll wettest part of linen drapes into center as far as possible to prevent soaking through linen bag, even though it is waterproof.
4. Discard soiled sponges, other waste, and disposable items in trash receptacle.
5. Discard unopened packets of suture.

   NOTE. Amount of suture put on table for the operation should be kept to a minimum so that there is very little actual waste. However, undamaged suture packets may be decontaminated and returned to manufacturer for resterilization. If a packet is grossly stained with blood or a solution, discard it. Clean packets may be soaked for a minimum of ten minutes in activated glutaraldehyde solution. They are then rinsed, dried, and placed in suture collection box to be sent to manufacturer.

6 Dispose of sharp items safely. Special care must be taken in handling all knife blades, surgical needles, and needles used for injection or aspiration. Place them in an appropriate container for either disposal or cleaning to prevent injury and potential risk of contracting hepatitis, syphilis, malaria, or aspergillosis. Primary cause of accidental cuts and punctures to personnel, both within and outside of the OR, is disposal of surgical sharps at end of operation. Those hospitals with standardized systems designed specifically for safe handling and disposal of sharps avoid virtually all accidental cuts, punctures, or lacerations. Remember, protection of yourself and other personnel is an important part of your job.

Blades and needles are never discarded loose in trash receptacles. They must be enclosed and secured so they cannot perforate the receptacle. A self-closing, adhesive pad designed for this purpose is safest device to use. Needles can cut through adhesive tape or puncture paper cups, boxes, or suture and blade packets. Sharps in these containers create a hazard. A safe disposal procedure must be implemented, and cleaning procedures adhered to.

- **a** Remove knife blades from handles. Point the blade toward table away from you, so if it breaks or slips it will not fly across the room. Remove blades with a needleholder; never use fingers. Never put knife handles in washer-sterilizer or instrument tray with blades left on them. Other instruments designed for replaceable cutting blades should have blades removed; thereafter they may be handled with other instruments.
- **b** Place reusable surgical needles, either on needle rack or loose, into a perforated stainless steel box to be run through washer-sterilizer with the instruments. Check suture book to see that it is not discarded with needles in it.
- **c** Place reusable needles used for injection or aspiration in perforated stainless steel box with surgical needles. Include those used by anesthesiologist.

NOTE. Whether or not disposable needles are run through washer-sterilizer as a safety measure before discarding depends upon individual hospital's rules and regulations. Each hospital should have a safe way of rendering them unfit for use again. Many have a needle-destruction unit available for this purpose.

7 Place instruments directly into perforated trays for processing in *washer-sterilizer.* Instruments must be terminally sterilized before they are handled for definitive cleaning in ultrasonic cleaner or by hand, and checked for proper functioning prior to reuse (see Chaps. 8 and 11).

- **a** Place heavy instruments in bottom of tray.
- **b** Turn instruments with concave surfaces, such as curettes and rongeurs, with bowl side down to facilitate drainage of the concave surface.
- **c** Open box locks and pivots of hinged instruments to expose maximum surface area.
- **d** Disassemble instruments designed to be disassembled without tools.
- **e** Sharp or pointed instruments should be carefully spaced in tray to prevent contact with other instruments that could damage their surfaces. Some hospitals prefer to wash and sterilize sharp instruments separately.

If a washer-sterilizer is not available, an alternative procedure is to carefully wash and rinse instruments and then put them into perforated trays and *autoclave* them. Any soil remaining on instruments is more difficult to remove after they have been heat-sterilized because it becomes baked on them. Soil also inhibits the sterilization process.

- **a** Obtain clean water in solution basin. Mild soap or noncorrosive, low-sudsing, free-rinsing detergent may be added to water.
- **b** Wash instruments carefully to guard against accidental spray of contaminated material around room. Brushing tends to aerosolize organisms. If brushing is necessary to remove gross soilage, keep instruments submerged beneath the level of the solution.
- **c** Load instrument tray the same way as recommended above for the washer-sterilizer tray. Autoclave with tray unwrapped. Or, after hand-washing, instruments may be placed into a solid basin, covered with a 2% solution of trisodium phosphate, and autoclaved for 45 minutes at 250°F (121°C).

8 Put glass syringes, medicine glasses, and other glassware, including those used by anesthesiologist, into a separate tray or tray with instruments. Syringes must be separated. Check for disposables and discard them in trash.

9 Place rubber goods and plastic items not to be disposed of into tray with instruments if they can be steam sterilized. Many items—gloves, catheters, tubings, etc.—are disposable. Check before putting them into washer-sterilizer.

NOTE. Disposable suction tubing is recommended over reusable tubing, which presents formidable cleaning problems. However, if tubing is reused, special care must be given to cleaning lumen prior to placing tubing with instruments for terminal sterilization. Suction detergent-disinfectant solution through lumen.

10 Wash, rinse, and dry items that cannot be immersed in water or steam sterilized. These must be wrapped for sterilization in ethylene oxide gas.

11 Invert small basins and solution cups over the instruments. Basins and trays too large for the washer-sterilizer or standard instrument sterilizer are washed, dried, and put into a double pillowcase to be autoclaved in bulk sterilizer. The circulating nurse holds pillowcase open for the scrub nurse to drop in utensils. The Mayo tray may be included.

12 Dispose of solutions and suction bottle contents in a flushing hopper. Disposable suction units simplify disposal. Wall suction units should be disconnected by the circulating nurse to avoid contamination of wall outlet. If disposable units are not used, decontaminate contents with disinfectant prior to hopper disposal. Wash container. Thoroughly wash plunger and other areas of wall-mounted suction apparatus. Containers are autoclaved along with basins and trays.

13 Put trays in washer-sterilizer and/or autoclave for terminal sterilization.

If washer-sterilizer and autoclave are in an adjacent substerile room, the circulating nurse opens doors for the scrub nurse. The scrub nurse places trays in them. The circulating nurse adds detergent to washer-sterilizer, and then starts operation of equipment.

If washer-sterilizer and/or autoclave are not in an immediately adjacent room, the scrub nurse removes gown, covers tray with a clean towel, carries it to utility room, and places it in the washer-sterilizer or autoclave there. Bring towel back to room and discard it in linen hamper, or trash receptacle if it is disposable. Care must be taken to avoid touching front of scrub clothes with either the tray or towel.

14 Discard all used disposable table drapes in plastic bag with used disposable patient drapes. Unused sponges may be put into the pillowcase with basins to be autoclaved before being placed in the stock cupboard. Some hospitals discard these.

Even if not obviously soiled, all linen from open packs should be subjected to laundering to replace moisture lost to fabric by sterilization. Therefore, put unused linen along with used linen table drapes in linen hamper to be sent to laundry.

15 Remove gown before gloves. The circulating nurse unfastens neck and back closures. Protect arms and scrub clothes from contaminated outside of gown. Grasp right shoulder of gown with left hand and, in pulling gown off arm, turn sleeve inside out. Turn outside of gown away from body with flexed elbow. Then grasp other shoulder with other hand and remove gown entirely, pulling it off inside out. Discard in linen hamper, or trash receptacle if disposable (see Fig. 10-10, p. 184).

To remove gloves, use glove-to-glove, then skin-to-skin technique to protect clean hands from contaminated outside of gloves, which bears cells of the patient. Gloves are turned inside out as they are removed and then discarded into trash (see Fig. 10-11, p. 185).

Cart System Cleanup

All reusable instruments, basins, supplies, and equipment, including suction bottles, are put on or inside cart. The cart is covered or closed and taken to the central decontamination area outside the OR suite for cleanup. A closed cart, especially if it has been used as the instrument table, is wiped off with a disinfectant solution before it is taken out of room. A cart with soiled supplies should be removed from the OR suite via the outer corridor if this is the design of the suite. If dumb-waiters are used, a separate one is provided for soiled cart. Clean and contaminated supplies are always kept separated.

The cart is designed to go through an automatic steam cart washer or a manual power wash for terminal cleaning, after it is emptied, before it is restocked with clean and sterile supplies.

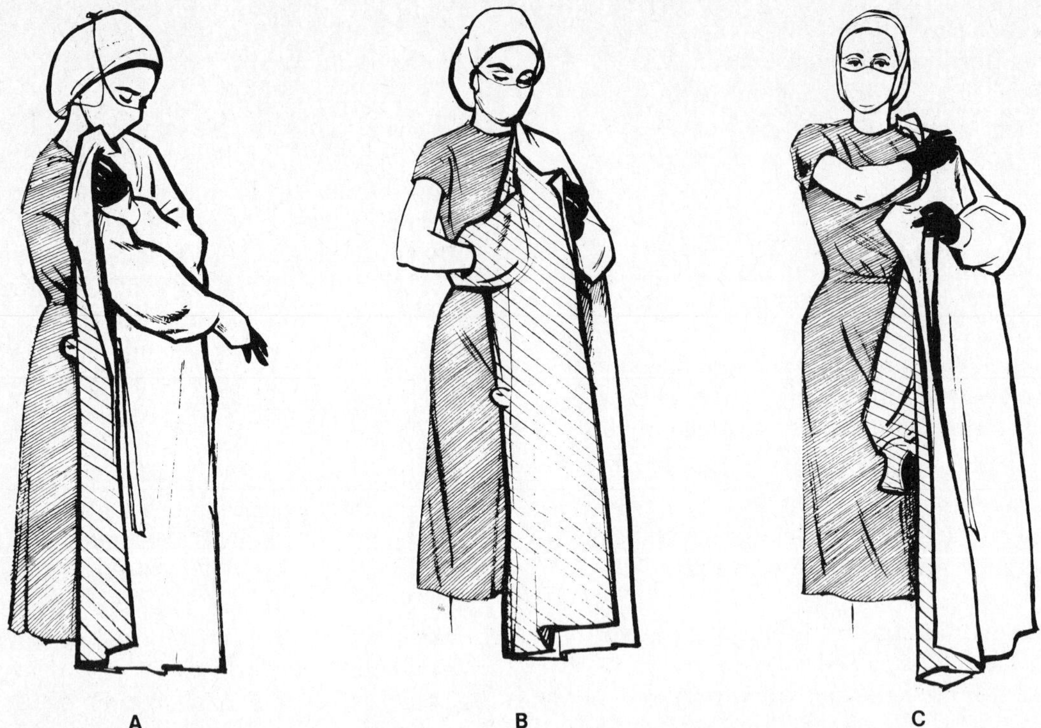

FIGURE 10-10
Sequence of scrub nurse removing soiled gown at end of operation. Clean arms and scrub dress are protected from contaminated outside of gown. (**A**) With gloves on, loosen cuffs of gown and shake them down over wrists. Then grasp right shoulder of gown (unbuttoned or untied) with left hand and, (**B**) in pulling the gown off arms, turn arm of gown away from body with flexed elbow. (**C**) Then grasp other shoulder with other hand and remove gown entirely, pulling it off inside out; thus arms are kept clean.

By Team

After the patient leaves, the circulating nurse is free to assist with cleanup of the room. Nursing assistants and/or housekeeping personnel may be available to assist also. Regardless of which member of the team performs them, specific functions must be carried out to complete room cleanup.

The personnel and areas considered contaminated during and after an operation are:

1 Members of sterile team, until they have discarded their gowns, gloves, caps, masks, and shoe covers. These remain in the contaminated area. Some hospitals require personnel to change scrub clothes after known septic operations.

2 All furniture, equipment, and floor, within and around perimeter of sterile field. If accidental spillage has occurred in other parts of room, then these areas are considered contaminated also.

3 All anesthesia equipment.

4 Stretchers used to transport patients. These should be cleaned after each patient use.

Clean, but not sterile, gloves are worn to complete the room cleanup. The scrub nurse changes gloves after the sterile field is dismantled. The following must be decontaminated:

1 *Furniture.* Wash horizontal surfaces of all tables and equipment, including anesthesia machine, with a disinfectant solution. Apply disinfectant from a pistol-grip sprayer or squeeze-bottle dispenser and wipe with a clean cloth or a disposable wipe that is changed frequently. All surfaces of mattress, pads, and screw connections of the operating table must be included. Mobile furniture can be pushed through disinfectant solution used for floor care to clean casters.

2 *Overhead operating light.* Overhead light reflectors should be wiped using a clean cloth wet with disinfectant solution. Lights and overhead tracks become contaminated quickly and present a possible hazard from fallout of microorganisms onto sterile surfaces or into wounds during each operation. Therefore, it is important to clean them.

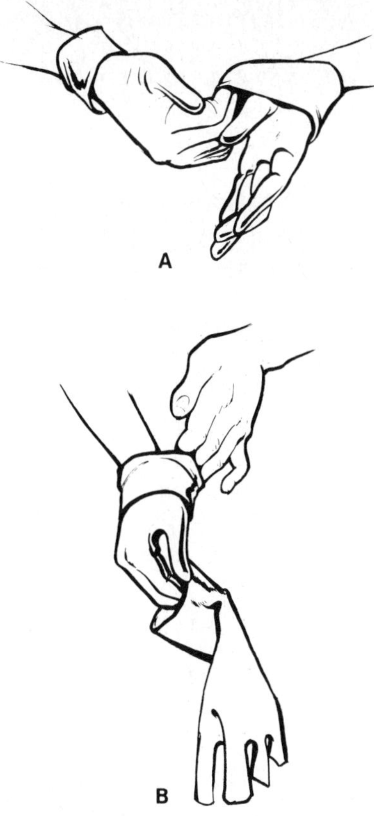

FIGURE 10-11
Sequence of scrub nurse removing soiled gloves at end of operation. Use (**A**) glove-to-glove, then (**B**) skin-to-skin technique to protect "clean" hands from the contaminated outside of gloves, which bear cells of the patient. Turn gloves inside out when removing them, keeping hands "clean."

3 *Anesthesia equipment.* All reusable anesthesia masks and tubing must be *cleaned and sterilized before reusing.* Some of this equipment can be steam sterilized; if not, it may be sterilized by ethylene oxide gas and aerated prior to reuse. If this method is not available, items should be immersed in activated glutaraldehyde solution for ten hours.

4 *Linen.* After all cleaning procedures have been completed, cloths should be discarded or put in linen bag if they are not disposable. When all linen, used and unused, has been placed inside linen bag, it is closed securely. After removal from hamper frame, someone outside room should stand at door with a clean plastic bag, holding it so that hands are covered by a large cuff in top of the bag. The sealed linen bag is placed upside down in this clean bag. Take care not to touch clean bag or other person with gloved hands. Person holding clean bag should unroll cuff and gently expel air from bag away from his or her face. A knot is tied in top of bag. This entire procedure protects housekeeping and laundry personnel since outside of bag is clean and dry for transportation from the OR suite. The hamper frame is cleaned after linen bag is removed.

5 *Trash.* All trash collected in plastic bags, including disposable drapes, kick bucket and wastebasket liner bags, is combined into one clean plastic bag, if possible, held open by a person outside of the room. It is double-bagged, as described for linen, and discarded per hospital routine.

6 *Floors.* Wet-vacuuming, with a filter-diffuser exhaust cleaner, is the method of choice for floor care in the OR. Machine cleaning is more effective than manual cleaning. If suture material and gross soilage on the floor is great, wet-vacuum equipment may be used dry for first treatment. Then floor is flooded, half of room at a time, with detergent-disinfectant solution. This may be dispensed from a pump spray or automatic spraying device attached to a central wet-vacuum equipment system. If portable equipment is used, a spray-type watering can may be used to flood floor, although this method is slower and may wet it unevenly. Hot water may hasten cidal action of the disinfectant agent, but may also soften tile adhesive. Room-temperature water requires at least a five-minute contact time for effectiveness.

Furniture is rolled across the flooded floor area to clean casters. The wet-vacuum pickup is used to pick up solution before repositioning furniture. Standing platforms are considered part of the floor and may be flooded with solution to be picked up by wet-vacuum.

The exterior of the equipment and tubing is cleaned following each use, with special attention given to cleaning the rubber blade before the next use. If the hose is equipped with a brush attachment, this is washed and autoclaved between uses.

If wet-vacuum equipment is not available, freshly laundered, clean mops can be used. The floor can be flooded with detergent-disinfectant solution. One mop is used to apply and one to take up solution. *Mops, treated or nontreated, never should be used dry in the OR.* Following *one-time use,* mop heads are removed and placed in linen hamper with other soiled linen. Mop handles may be stored in housekeeping storage area until needed again.

7 *Walls.* If walls are splashed with blood or organic debris during the operation, those areas should be washed. Otherwise walls are not considered contaminated and need not be washed between operations.

Room Ready for Next Patient

Cleaning procedures, as described, provide terminal sterilization and adequate decontamination following any operation. With appropriate care, special procedures, quarantine of a room, or discrimination of type of operative procedure scheduled to follow in the same room are rarely necessary. With a well-coordinated team, minimal turnover time between operations can be accomplished; in an average time of 15 to 20 minutes the room will be ready for the next patient.

DAILY CLEANING AFTER SCHEDULE IS COMPLETED

In O.R.

At completion of day's schedule in each OR, more stringent and rigorous cleaning is done in all areas previously discussed:

1 *Furniture* is thoroughly scrubbed, using mechanical friction in addition to chemical disinfection. Disinfectants are only adjuncts to good physical cleaning; "elbow grease" is probably the most important ingredient.

2 *Casters and wheels* should be cleaned and kept free of suture ends and debris. Equipment is available that automatically washes stretchers, tables, and platforms, then steam cleans and dries them within a matter of minutes.

3 *Equipment,* such as electrosurgical units, should be cleaned with care so as not to saturate surfaces to degree that disinfectant solution runs into mechanism, causing malfunction and repairs.

4 *Ceiling- and wall-mounted fixtures and tracks* are cleaned on all surfaces.

5 *Kick buckets, linen hamper frames, and other waste receptacles* are cleaned and disinfected; these are autoclaved when feasible.

6 *Floors* are given a thorough wet-vacuum cleaning with wet-vacuum pickup used dry and then wet.

7 *Walls* should be checked for soil spots and cleaned as necessary.

8 *Cabinets and doors* should be cleaned, especially around handles or push plates where contamination is apt to occur.

Outside O.R. Itself

1 *Counter tops and sinks* in substerile room should be cleaned.

2 *Scrub sinks and spray heads* on faucets should undergo thorough cleaning daily. A mild abrasive on sinks removes oily film residue left by scrub antiseptics. Spray heads, faucet aerators, or sprinklers should be removed and disassembled, if possible, for thorough cleaning and sterilization of parts. Contaminated faucet aerators and sprinklers can transfer organisms directly to hands or items washed under them. *Scrub sinks should not be used for routine cleaning purposes.*

3 *Walls around scrub sinks* must receive daily attention. Spray and splash from scrub antiseptics build up around sink and must be removed.

4 *Transportation and storage carts* need to be cleaned with specific attention to wheels and casters.

5 *Cleaning equipment* should be disassembled and cleaned prior to storage.

WEEKLY OR MONTHLY CLEANING

A weekly or monthly cleaning routine is set up, in addition to daily cleaning schedule, by director of environmental/housekeeping services and OR supervisor. Any routines for housekeeping must, of necessity, be based on physical construction. However, if specific schedules are not established, some areas may never be cleaned. Areas to be considered are:

1 *Walls.* Walls should be cleaned when they become visibly soiled. If they are painted or tiled with wide porous grouting, these factors must be considered in planning cleaning routines. Washing walls in the OR and throughout the suite once a week is reasonable, but less-frequent time intervals for cleaning may be acceptable if spot disinfection is assured on a daily basis. This requires adequate continuous supervision.

2 *Ceilings.* Ceilings may require regular special cleaning techniques because of mounted tracks and lighting fixtures. The types of fixtures are considered in planning cleaning routines.

3 *Floors.* Floors throughout the OR suite should be machine scrubbed periodically to remove accumulated deposits and films. Conductive flooring should never be waxed. Rounded corners and edges facilitate cleaning.

4 *Air-conditioning grilles.* The exterior of air-conditioning grilles should be vacuumed at least weekly. Additional cleaning is necessary when filters are checked and changed.

5 *Storage shelves.* Storage cabinets have been replaced in many OR suites by portable storage carts. Storage areas should be cleaned at least weekly, or more often if necessary, to control accumulation of dust, especially in sterile storage areas.

6 *Sterilizers.* Regular cleaning of all types of sterilizers must be done as recommended by the manufacturer.

7 *Dispensers.* Microbial contamination can be transferred from contaminated dispensers of surgical scrub antiseptics or hand lotions. Contents of dispensers should be drained and discarded on a weekly schedule. Dispensers should be washed, dried, and sterilized before being refilled and returned to use.

8 *Exchange and peripheral support areas.* Walls, ceilings, floors, air-conditioning grilles, lockers, cabinets, furniture, etc., should be cleaned on a regular schedule.

CHAPTER **11**

ECONOMY, WORK SIMPLIFICATION, AND SAFETY

The 1983 amendments to the Social Security Act established a prospective hospital reimbursement system for Medicare patients based on diagnosis related groups (DRGs). Historically hospitals were reimbursed for patient care on the basis of costs for room, board, and services. Under the present system, inpatients are assigned to one of the DRGs for the primary diagnosis and any secondary diagnoses. The government reimburses the hospital for care needed for the assigned DRG. If actual costs are below the determined reimbursement level, the hospital retains the difference. If costs are higher, the hospital must absorb the discrepancy. Some hospitals use DRGs for monitoring quality of care, reviewing utilization, and controlling costs.

Cost containment, one aspect of the Social Security legislation, is part of a comprehensive quality assurance program. The hospital's quality assurance program focuses on the improvement of practice. To assure quality, nursing care must be assessed in terms of outcome for the patient, actual care given, techniques and procedures used, supplies and equipment available, and efficiency within the organization.

A postoperative wound infection that prolongs hospitalization for the patient is expensive in time and money. If a consistent break in aseptic technique in the OR is identified as the cause and is corrected, this cost will be saved for other patients.

The OR staff must monitor the quality of care to determine what they are doing right, what they are doing wrong, and whether a less costly method can achieve the same or better quality nursing care. Efficiency is frequently referred to as the cost-benefit ratio. *Efficiency* is the attainment of quality reviewed in relationship of the manpower, facilities, supplies, and equipment to the appropriateness, acceptability, and cost to the patient. Quality assurance then becomes synonymous with cost containment.

EFFICIENCY OF THE O.R. STAFF

Individuals working together coordinate their efforts to accomplish the tasks necessary to achieve a common goal. In the OR suite, this common goal is to provide for the safety and welfare of every patient. Efficiency, therefore, depends primarily upon individual effort and the working relationship between team members.

Each department takes on a personality from the individuals in it. This personality gives a reputation for good or otherwise. Unethical discussions, unprofessional conduct, lapses in sterile technique, carelessness in handling expensive equipment, breakage, and forgetfulness make impressions upon patients and visitors. They may carry these impressions to others outside the hospital. Constant vigilance is necessary. Pride in one's work and in the department as a whole leads to dissatisfaction with anything less than the very best.

Musts for O.R. Nurse and Technologist

1 You must have initiative, energy, and stamina combined with honesty, dependability, and integrity.

2 You must have a responsive and pleasing personality. Make it a pleasure for others to work with you. A spirit of cooperation will make any situation tolerable and will enhance efficiency. It never hurts to say "please" and "thank you."

3 You must have a positive attitude toward everyone with whom you work. In all work situations you will find individuals from different backgrounds with a divergence of life-styles. You must possess poise and graciousness, with a genuine willingness to be compassionate and understanding of individual differences. Being considerate promotes trust and respect from others.

4 You must have a sense of humor. Situations encountered in the OR are often difficult. The ability to keep one's sense of humor aids in dealing with tension.

5 You must have an open mind and flexibility. Changes in work schedules and procedures must be made when a need for change accommodates or improves patient care. You must be adaptable and able to demonstrate efficiency in all situations.

6 You must be willing to accept and profit from constructive criticism. One who can accept criticism without becoming defensive may prevent a minor situation from developing into a real difficulty. Keep a balanced perspective. Many times it is not the incident itself, but one's reaction to it that is so devastating. Constructive criticism should be given and received tactfully and kindly. Profit by it to improve your performance.

7 You must not go off duty and discuss incidents in the day's work. Operations, patients, surgeons, and the multitude of incidents involving them are not discussed outside the OR suite. To seek advice or to unburden yourself when problems arise, discuss your work situation with your instructor, the supervisor, or the head nurse before going off duty. Any unresolved problem will affect the quality of patient care either directly or indirectly.

8 You must be properly instructed in the use and care of equipment and supplies before being given the responsibility for them. Never be afraid to say "I do not know" or to ask questions. Learning is an active process. Go out to meet it, and be eager for new experiences.

9 You must know the policies and procedures and efficiently follow them. Learn to do things right the first time and continue to do them that way. New things can be learned and much accomplished in the time wasted in correcting errors.

10 You must work rapidly. Learn to follow directions quickly and accurately to the smallest detail; carelessness or ignorance could cost the life or welfare of your patient. A change in diagnosis during operation may require an altogether different setup and a different procedure from the one anticipated. Emergencies will arise. You must be able to meet these situations quickly, calmly, and efficiently. You must know not only *what* to do in the basic situations, but also *why* you do it, to be able to exercise good judgment and to adapt to more radical situations.

11 You must be able to organize your work effectively, so that not a single minute is lost, not a motion superfluous. It is of the utmost importance to keep to a minimum the length of time a patient is under anesthesia. As the anesthesia time is prolonged, a greater burden is put on the patient's recovery. Also, the period of anxious concern is prolonged for the patient's family.

12 You must fit in and work smoothly as a member of an efficient, well-coordinated team. Each member must anticipate not only his or her own needs but also those of the others. Common interest in the goal provides teamwork in which all think and act as a unit. You must be an inconspicuous and highly efficient member of that team—inconspicuous through your alertness and anticipation and smooth, precise, and quick actions. Unrelated conversation or activities can distract team members.

13 You must enhance the atmosphere in which the surgeon prefers to work. Usually a calm, serious atmosphere with intense concentration without excessive tension is best. The surgeon must never be made to feel rushed. Show respect for the surgeon's mood and temperament that may vary with the progress of the operation.

14 You must anticipate the surgeon's needs and keep one step ahead. The surgeon is distracted from the operation when handed the wrong instrument, or when made to wait for supplies. You must be alert to intelligently read the surgeon's mind.

15 You must follow rigidly the rule that nothing is taken for granted. For example, you must know, not assume, that equipment is sterile. You must know and know that you know. While many sterile supplies are obtained commercially, some are packaged and sterilized in the OR suite or central service department. It is well to learn as much as you can about how all supplies are packaged and sterilized in order to supervise their use by others or to evaluate their level of quality and safety for the patient.

16 You must be responsible for all work assigned to you. Ask questions as necessary, and report work assignments as finished or unfinished. Your responsibility goes beyond your own assignments to those of the department as a whole. If the supervisor does not give you an additional assignment, look for ways to help others until all the work is finished. Do not waste time. Actual operations are only one part of the work in the operating room suite. Preparation and cleanup involve procedures with which you must become familiar.

TIME AND MOTION ECONOMY

Time Is Costly

Time is an important element in the OR. If time is wasted between operations, for example, the day's schedule is slowed down and later operations are delayed. The surgeons' time is wasted and they tend to come late, anticipating delays. The patients become more nervous waiting for their operations and more uncomfortable during the prolonged period without fluids.

Poor managers of time tend to become less efficient and thus drift into poor work habits. Your greatest ally is *common sense.* Take time to stop and think. Is there a quicker, easier, or more efficient way of doing the job? Most work habits can be improved.

Records of time are necessary and important to determine efficiency—when the patient arrives, when the surgeon arrives, when the anesthetic is started, when the incision is made, when the incision is closed, when the patient leaves the room, cleanup time. Undue delays are identified and may be corrected. Thus the availability of time for further operations is increased.

You must be willing to take the time to study your existing situation in a methodical manner and gather the facts needed to support the desirability of alternative methods. Recognition that a problem exists is the first step toward solving a problem. Seek to develop more efficient and economical work methods.

Associations

Association is a great aid to memory and organization of work. The mention of one article brings to mind the others used with it. For instance, the scrub nurse knows a suture calls for a tissue forceps to the surgeon, needleholder to the assistant, then scissors.

Think of the order in which instruments and supplies are going to be needed and *do first things first,* e.g., prepare sutures for closing deep tissue layers before skin sutures.

To be proficient, you must know the organization of work and the relative importance of factors in accomplishing it. For example, if, as the patient is being prepped, the surgeon requests stainless steel retention sutures for closure instead of the usual sutures, the circulating nurse should realize there is plenty of time to get them after other duties are completed. He or she must tie the gowns, supervise the draping, adjust the Mayo stand and instrument table, focus the light, etc., to start the operation before getting the closure suture. When getting steel suture, association tells nurse to also get wire scissors and bumpers or bridges.

Watch for and try to establish associations to increase efficiency. If surgeons must devote time and attention to details the nurses and technologists should know, they are distracted from their primary concerns. Time is wasted for all involved, including the patient.

Motion Economy

Wasted motion is not only time-consuming, but also adds to physical fatigue. Fatigue is the result of body movement. Ten principles of motion economy can reduce fatigue from physical activity and improve your level of efficiency.

Motions Should Be Productive Once the steps in a procedure are learned, work to increase speed and manual dexterity in carrying them out. Avoid rushed or disorganized motions. Rather make each movement count. Work quietly and quickly. Work as fast as possible without sacrificing accuracy and technique for speed.

The corollary to this principle is *a place for everything and everything in its place.* Keep an orderly work area to avoid fumbling and rehandling items. Arrange them properly and leave them there. This corollary is justification for standardization of procedures, such as a standardized instrument table setup and stocking of supplies in cabinets or on carts. If everything has a place and is in its place, you know instinctively where to put your hands on supplies when needed. A neat and orderly work area is one of the first requirements for productive motions. You should also consider the work flow so that minimal motions can be made to accomplish productive work.

Motions Should Be Simple Body movements should be confined to the lowest classification with which it is possible to perform work properly. Movements of the upper extremity are classified:

1 Class 1 involves the fingers. The knuckle provides the pivot for motion for such tasks as fingering through a card file, turning a set screw on an instrument, using a pair of scissors.

2 Class 2 involves both the hand and fingers. The wrist is the pivot for motion as in passing instruments, counting sponges, picking up or writing on an operative record.

3 Class 3 includes the forearm. Using the elbow as a pivot, more effort and time are expended in the third and succeeding classifications because the movements of any one class involve movements of all classes preceding it. It takes longer and more effort to turn the pages of a procedure book or patient's chart than to thumb through a file of surgeon's preference cards. The elbow pivots to open a peel-down package, unfold drapes, and unwrap small supplies.

4 Class 4 includes the upper arm. The shoulder pivot is used when opening a door, setting up the Mayo stand, and prepping a patient.

5 Class 5 adds the torso. The trunk bends or stretches to lift a patient, take supplies from a low shelf or drawer, reach to hang an IV bag, or bend to count the sponges in a kick bucket.

Upper extremity work should be arranged to reduce work to the lowest possible classification. Finger motion is the least fatiguing; shoulder motion is the most. The scrub nurse should be positioned at the operating table so that elbow, wrist, and finger motions can be used. He or she should be positioned opposite the surgeon so that both can work with their elbows at their sides. This avoids prolonged shoulder motion for both of them.

It is quicker for the circulating nurse to stretch to hang an IV bag than to take time to use finger action to loosen the set screw on an IV standard, lower it with shoulder movement, hang the bag with elbow action, and repeat the sequence in reverse. However, stretching is more fatiguing. The more fatigued you get, the slower your motions become as the day progresses. Maybe you saved 30 seconds with the first patient of the day, but what happens to the last patient of the day? Time is lost because energy wanes.

Motions Should Be Curved Motions should go along curved rather than straight paths whenever possible. A circular motion to clean the flat surfaces of furniture is less fatiguing than straight push-and-pull strokes.

Motions Should Be Symmetrical Motions should be rhythmic and smooth flowing, and, when possible, both hands should be used symmetrically. Damp cloths in both hands, going in opposing circles, will get flat surfaces cleaned faster and easier.

Work Should Be within Grasp Range All work materials should be arranged so they are within grasp range to avoid changes in body position. Grasp range is within the radius from the pivot point of the elbow or shoulder, either horizontally or vertically. The minimum grasp range is within the radius of the arcs formed with only forearms extended, using the elbows as pivot points on the horizontal plane (see Fig. 11-1).

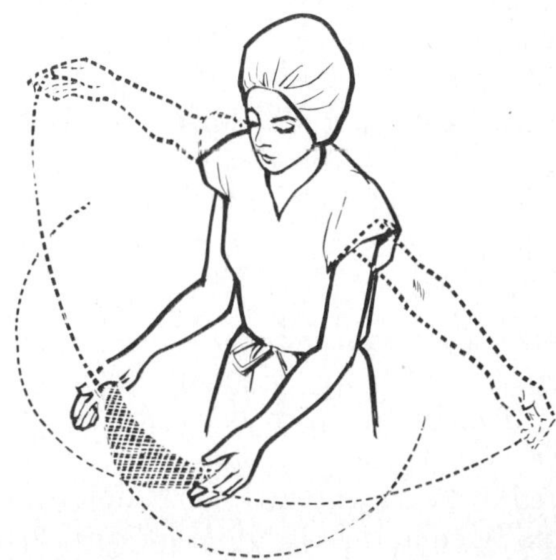

FIGURE 11-1
Grasp ranges. The minimum range is within the radius of the arcs formed with only the forearms extended, using elbows as pivotal points. The optimum range is within the area where arcs of hands overlap. The maximum range is within the arcs formed from the shoulder pivots.

The optimum grasp range is within the area where the left-hand and the right-hand arcs overlap. This is the area in which two-handed work, such as putting a needle in a needleholder, can be done most conveniently.

The maximum grasp range is within the arcs formed from the shoulder pivots. The overlapping of these arcs is the maximum extent at which two-handed work can be done within reach without changing body position.

The Mayo stand should be placed over the operating table at a height and in a position within the minimum and optimum grasp range of the scrub nurse. It must not rest on the patient, but it can be lowered to an inch or two above. The instrument table should be positioned as close to the horizontal plane within maximum grasp range as possible. Instruments or supplies requiring two-handed work should be placed on the Mayo stand and instrument table as close to the optimum grasp range as possible.

Hands Should Be Relieved of Work Hands should be relieved of any work that can be done more advantageously by other parts of the body. Many electrical instruments have foot pedals to facilitate operation.

Doors into the OR suite may be opened by stepping on a trigger mechanism or by passing an electric eye. Some people object to automatic doors due to the difficulty of holding them open if necessary. They are designed to adhere to this principle, however.

Injuries are sustained to the back, arms, or shoulders from lifting patients or equipment improperly. Lift with your legs. Bend your knees to get body weight under the load, and straighten legs to lift. A lifting frame or Davis roller helps relieve potential strain of moving unconscious or obese patients.

The Worker Should Be at Ease Tiring body motions, or awkward or strained body posture should be avoided. During standing work, when the heels are together, constant muscular effort is required by the thigh muscles to maintain an erect posture. In contrast, when the heels are apart, the ligaments of the hips and knees support the body without effort. A wide stance while standing at the operating table for prolonged periods will be less fatiguing for the scrub nurse. The circulating nurse can stand in a location to observe both operation and instrument table with upper and lower extremities in a rest position. In this standing position the arms are clasped behind the back and the feet are in a wide stance. Weight bearing on only one foot causes additional strain.

This principle includes provision of a correct and comfortable work-place height. The operating table is adjusted to the best height for the surgeon. This may not be the most comfortable position for the other members of the sterile team. Team members should be able to stand erect with their arms comfortably relaxed from the shoulders, without stooping, and should not have to raise their hands above the level of their elbows for the majority of their work motions. Platforms, standing stools, may be needed to elevate the scrub nurse and/or the assistant surgeon to a feasible working height. Platforms should be long enough to allow a wide stance.

Correct posture in the sitting position is equally important. Your back is strongest when it is straight. When you sit, sit well back in the chair or on a stool with body straight from hips to neck. Lean forward from the hips, not the shoulders or waist. This position puts the least strain on muscles, ligaments, and internal organs. Before and after the operation, the circulating and scrub nurses should rest in a sitting position between periods of standing. If work is done in a sitting position, the stool or chair should be adjusted to the correct height for the working surface.

Additional factors contribute to providing a comfortable working environment: ventilation, lighting, color, and noise. Lighting should be adequate; however, excessive glare produces fatigue. Illumination is the product of the light times the reflectance of the target. A bright, highly polished, mirror finish on an instrument tends to reflect light and can restrict the vision of the surgeon. Satin or dull-finished instruments eliminate glare and lessen the surgeon's eye strain. These instruments are made with varying degrees of dullness depending on the manufacturer. Tinted or Polaroid glasses may save the sterile team members from visual fatigue, but must not distort color of tissues.

Soft pastel colors, especially blues and green, are less reflective for linens and walls than white. Drapes with dark tones help reduce contrast between most tissues and the surrounding field. Some hospitals have a mural on a wall in the OR to enhance visual effect of the environment, particularly if the OR suite is windowless.

Although attention is given to ventilation, lighting, and color, less attention is given to the design of the OR in terms of auditory effects. Some hospitals have piped-in music. Music can be relaxing for the patient awaiting operation or undergoing an operation under local anesthesia, and stimulating for personnel. Music with a moderate rhythm and bright tone can motivate muscular activity and increase levels of efficiency. This would not be conducive to relaxation for the patient, however. Selection of music must be appropriate for the intended listener. It can be a distraction and annoyance, especially for the anesthesiologist who depends upon hearing to aid in monitoring the patient. Music should always be played at low volume in the OR. It should be turned off at request of patient, surgeon, or anesthesiologist. Constant playing of music can be more harmful than beneficial for personnel, so it should be turned off periodically to help prevent mental fatigue.

Noise can be irritating and potentially dangerous to patients and personnel. It can become intense enough to provoke peripheral vasoconstriction, dilation of the pupils, and other subtle physiologic effects, as well as interfere with necessary communication and thereby provoke irritation.

The OR should be as quiet as possible except for the essential sounds of communication between team members directly concerned with the patient's care. When it is necessary to talk, do so in low voice. Conversation unrelated to the operation is out of place. Even during deep stages, an anesthetized patient does perceive noises and conversations that occur during the operation and may remember them. If a spinal or local anesthesia is used, remember that the patient can hear the conversation. Patients interpret anything they hear in terms of themselves, so all words must be guarded. Counts or requests for supplies must be done quietly, so the patient cannot hear.

Major sources of noise in the OR involve paper, gloves, objects wheeled across floor, instruments striking one another, monitors, and high-pitched powered instruments including suction. The scrub nurse must keep these sources and their effects in mind. Avoid clattering instruments. Clamp off or kink a loop into suction tubing except while in actual use. The circulating nurse should keep doors closed to shut out noise in corridors, of water running in the scrub room, or of sterilizer operating in the substerile room. Do not crush paper wrappings. Hold a bottle of solution inches, not feet, away from basin when pouring. Monitors with audible signals should be placed as far away from patient's ears as possible, with amplifier turned away from the patient.

Remember, working in a pleasantly quiet environment is less fatiguing with fewer psychologic and physiologic adverse effects, and greater efficiency on behalf of the patient.

Work Materials Should Be Prepositioned Supplies can be arranged for convenient use and minimal handling. Drapes are packaged in order of use so they do not need to be handled by the scrub nurse, except to move the stack to a corner of the instrument table, until ready to use. Instruments can be arranged in trays so all of them do not need to be removed until needed.

Economize time and effort by placing items on the instrument table and Mayo stand in the order in which they will be used, and put them in their proper places without rearranging them. Arrange instruments on the Mayo stand in position to hand to the surgeon or assistant. In passing an instrument, place it in the surgeon's hand in the position in which it will be used, so readjustments will not be necessary (see Fig. 10-6, p. 166). Grasp it with the thumb and the first two fingers, far enough away from the handle so that the surgeon can grasp it. Hand a needle in the needleholder the same way, supporting suture so it does not drag, and with needle pointing in direction in which the surgeon will start to use it. Hand thumb forceps so the surgeon can grasp the handle; do the same with retractors.

Gravity Should Be Used Scrub sponges or brush dispensers operate on the principle that gravity should be used whenever possible. Cabinets for smaller packages in the sterile supply room can be vertical and divided into appropriate-size slots. These can be filled from the top and dispensed from the bottom of each slot. This is convenient, saves space, and assures that older items are used first. Shelves for large, heavy packs can be made of rollers and slanted slightly to facilitate handling. Gravity-feed and drop-delivery installations eliminate or reduce motions. The quickest way to dispose of an object is to drop it. This may be the quickest way to break or contaminate it too, so the application of this principle requires good judgment.

Supplies Should Be Combined Items should serve two or more purposes whenever possible. Sterilizer indicator tape, for example, will serve a dual purpose: to hold the package closed and to tell you if it has been exposed to a sterilization process. And only inches, not a yard, of tape accomplishes the job.

Disposable kits and trays are purchased, or sets are made up of reusable items, so that all the supplies and materials needed for a procedure are combined into a single unit. This eliminates opening many separate packages.

A knife blade packet can be sterilized in the instrument tray with the knife handle. This eliminates a sterile transfer to the instrument table.

Put instruments that are sterilized in sets of various sizes, such as expensive prostheses, on a small sterile table or at one side of the instrument table. When the surgeon decides which size is needed, remove it from the set without contaminating the others, and thus saving their cleanup.

ECONOMICAL USE OF SUPPLIES AND EQUIPMENT

As the cost of supplies increases, OR personnel should be conscious of ways to eliminate wasteful practices. For example, throw away disposable items only. Avoid throwing away reusable ones. Continuous emphasis on cost containment can reduce waste and result in economies of benefit to the hospital and ultimately to the patients.

The operating room suite is one of the most expensive departments of a hospital. Adequate linen, instruments, and other supplies are necessary for patient care. Dollars and cents cannot be the primary consideration. Beyond the point of safety, economy becomes a hazard. But supplies do not need to be used lavishly just because they are available. Remember the following principles.

"Just Enough Is Enough"

1 Keep the varieties and numbers of instruments and supplies needed for each operation to a minimum. If the procedure book and surgeon preference cards are kept up-to-date, articles no longer used are eliminated.

2 Do not pour an ounce of solution if a milliliter is needed. Pour just enough solution for a skin preparation according to the manufacturer's recommendation; it takes only a small amount. Do not unnecessarily open a bottle for a small amount if you know the remainder will not be used.

3 Follow procedures for draping to provide an adequate sterile field without wasting disposable draping material or opening launderable linen.

4 Do not open another packet of sutures for that last stitch. Usually a few leftover pieces are long enough to complete the closure.

5 Suction tubing, syringes, hypodermic needles, drains, catheters, extra linen, etc., are kept sterile. Supplies should be opened only as needed, not routinely "just in case" they may be needed.

6 Do not soak too much plaster when helping with cast applications. Keep just ahead of surgeon. Watch to see when it appears the cast is almost finished. Ask if more is needed before soaking an extra one or two rolls of plaster.

7 Turn off lights when they are not needed.

Use Supplies and Equipment for Intended Use

1 Use operating table appliances according to manufacturer's instructions for positioning and stabilizing patients.

2 Nonsterile gloves are available for nonsterile procedures in which the use of gloves is for hand protection. Open sterile gloves for sterile procedures only.

3 Use linen only as needed and for its intended purpose. If water runs over onto the floor, do not soak it up with good linen—use the wet-vacuum pickup or mop. But do not let it run over!

4 Do not use hemostats to clamp drapes or tubing; that ruins both the hemostat and the tubing. Use a stopcock or special tubing clamp. Use a towel clip to anchor drapes.

5 Give the assistant surgeon a needleholder for pulling needles through the tissue for the surgeon. A hemostat can be ruined by using it for this purpose. A needle can be damaged.

6 Use wire scissors for wire, tissue scissors for tissue, nurses' scissors for drains and dressings, and suture scissors to cut sutures.

Handle All Supplies and Equipment Carefully to Avoid Damage and Breakage

1 Slip the patient's gown sleeve off before the intravenous transfusion is started preoperatively to avoid having to cut off a wet, soiled gown after the operation is completed.

2 Keep older supplies moving first so that items will not deteriorate or sterility become outdated.

3 Take special care to preserve the edges of sharp instruments.

4 Follow established procedures for the proper sterilization and care of instruments, electrical equipment, etc. If you are uncertain how to sterilize or care for any equipment, find out; do not ruin items by guessing. Items for ethylene oxide gas sterilization should be plainly tagged "for gas" to help avoid possibility of inadvertently putting them into the steam sterilizer.

5 Remove all tape from packages wrapped in linen. Tape must be removed and not merely torn open and left on the wrapper, as it will clog the washers in the laundry.

6 Do not handle adhesive with rubber gloves; it sticks to the gloves and tears them.

7 Check drapes to be certain instruments are not discarded in disposable drapes or sent to the laundry in linen drapes. At end of operation, the scrub nurse should look for instruments, needles, and equipment before discarding drapes and table covers. No instrument should be consigned to the laundry or trash!

8 Carry out safe and economical practices. Careless and accident-prone personnel should be eliminated from the department.

Carelessness Can Cause Infection

1 Avoid banging furniture against walls and doors. Stainless steel guards are used on corners and sides of door frames, wherever stretchers or tables are apt to bump them. These become a hazard if loosened. Chipped walls or doors can harbor microorganisms and interfere with effectiveness of housekeeping.

2 Avoid contamination of sterile supplies in transfer to the sterile field. Watch what you are doing when opening sterile packages. If in doubt about sterility, discard the item.

3 Thoroughly clean and properly sterilize instruments. Dirty instruments corrode, do not function smoothly, and are difficult to sterilize.

4 Thoroughly clean all reusable items before sterilizing. The danger of cross infection in the reuse of cleanable, sterilizable items does not lie in the supplies themselves but in personnel practices in processing and handling them. If carelessness exists, many avenues for potential infection become a threat to the welfare of the patient.

5 Dispose of needles and knife blades safely so that housekeeping personnel or other staff members do not accidentally stick themselves or get cut. Hepatitis and AIDS can be contracted from a contaminated needle or knife blade.

PROS AND CONS OF DISPOSABLES

A disposable product is *used once* with assurance of safety and effectiveness. It is not salvaged after use; *it is discarded.* The cost of adequately and safely processing supplies is high in most hospitals. This has led to purchase of many disposable supplies for patient use. Some of these are "patient-charge" items, meaning that the cost of these items is added to the patient's bill. This requires specific and accurate records. It also requires evaluation of the advantages and disadvantages of disposable products to justify the cost to the patient.

Advantages of using disposables are:

1 When a sterile item is required, proper packaging and sterility must be assured. Sterility is guaranteed by reliable manufacturers as long as the integrity of their packages is maintained. Industry conforms to far more rigid standards of quality control than hospital conditions permit. All sterilized products are tested for sterility before they are distributed to hospitals.

2 Single-use items, such as catheters, are aesthetically more acceptable to patients. More importantly, disposable products eliminate a potential source of cross contamination.

3 Items such as needles and safety razors assure more comfort for the patient because they are always new and sharp.

4 Standardized service at reduced cost per unit may be provided. Sponges are precounted and sterilized, for example. Packs and trays become standardized, and can be customized.

5 Loss and breakage in reprocessing reusable items are eliminated.

6 Labor costs of processing supplies are reduced, particularly in the tedious, meticulous cleaning and packaging of small items, such as needles and syringes.

7 The need for expensive, mechanical cleaning equipment is reduced or eliminated.

Disadvantages of using disposables are:

1 Costly waste occurs if sterile items are contaminated or unnecessarily opened. Extreme care is needed in opening packages to maintain sterility. Handling must not cause wrappings to crack. Even though sterility of products from reliable manufacturers can be assured, their handling and storing in the hospital may pose a threat to the maintenance of this sterility.

2 Hospitals cannot be as flexible in complying with requests of individual doctors for special setups. No allowance is made for deviation from commercially supplied packs or trays, unless customized kits are purchased. Procedures may need to be revised to conform to available items and sets.

3 If a defect is found in one package, it may extend throughout the total lot requiring replacement of the total supply on hand.

4 The circulating nurse may have to open an increased number of individually packaged items. Some disposable plastic products melt so they cannot be put into instrument sets before steam sterilization.

5 In event of disaster or a sudden increase in use, adequate inventory may not be readily available.

6 An expiration date may be required for a potentially unstable product after prolonged storage, such as some disposable trays with medications or sutures in them. Unless items are rotated in storage so that oldest products are used first, unnecessary costs are incurred if a product must be discarded because its time of reliability has expired. All dated products must be routinely checked for expiration.

Many problems concerning economy, better use of personnel, storage, delivery, and disposal need to be evaluated by hospitals on an individual basis. Economy may or may not be shown with the use of disposables. Some considerations that can be argued pro or con include:

1 *Direct labor costs.* Some hospitals have saved money by reducing the labor force through conversion to as many total-disposable systems as possible, such as intravenous therapy, drapes, and special procedure trays. In some geographic areas, efficient labor may be readily available at minimum wage so that disposables become more costly than labor. If professional personnel had been used for reprocessing supplies, disposables release nurses to give more care to patients and less time to "things."

2 *Storage.* Proper and safe storage facilities must be provided. Disposables may require more storage space or more frequent deliveries to maintain adequate inventories.

3 *Disposal.* Disposal may be an ecological problem. Someone must transport used items to an incinerator, compactor, or other safe waste-disposal area. Waste must not accumulate in the OR suite or in other hospital areas.

In this era of cost containment, hospitals may attempt to salvage unused or undamaged disposable items. The risks of doing this must be seriously evaluated. Resterilization of opened, but unused sterile, single-use items is a form of reprocessing or remanufacture. Some manufacturers provide a service whereby the hospital can return clean unused and undamaged products for rewrapping and resterilizing. The manufacturer will guarantee product stability and sterility. Other manufacturers will provide written instructions for resterilizing unused but contaminated items by hospital personnel. With or without written instructions from the manfacturer, the hospital assumes legal responsibility for sterility of a resterilized item. This liability also is assumed for an item supplied sterile that is opened and placed in a tray with other items for sterilization.

Reuse of a used disposable single-use item requires cleaning and sterilizing, if it will be reused as a sterile item. Reprocessing may be potentially hazardous. Points to consider include:

1 Is the item clean? Many porous materials cannot be thoroughly cleaned after use. Cleaning must remove all traces of body fluids and organic debris.

2 Is the item toxic or pyrogenic after reprocessing? Residues from some cleaning compounds and ethylene oxide gas are toxic. Environmental contamination or conditions can support microbial growth producing endotoxins or pyrogens.

3 Is the item sterile? The sterilization method must be appropriate for the material. Sterility should be verified for each type of product that is resterilized.

4 Is the integrity of the product maintained? Physical characteristics may be altered by resterilization. Some materials deteriorate or become brittle. This can affect function.

Manufacturers use extensive controls and testing procedures to assure cleanliness, nontoxicity, nonpyrogenicity, biocompatibility, sterility, and function. The hospital must assume this same responsibility for items it chooses to reprocess and resterilize. All items must be safe and effective for their intended patient uses.

CARE AND HANDLING OF INSTRUMENTS

Surgical instruments are expensive and represent a major investment for every hospital. As operations have become more complicated and intricate, instruments have become more complex, more precise in design, and more delicate in structure. When abused, misused, or subjected to inadequate cleaning or rough handling, the life expectancy of even the most durable instrument is reduced. Cost of repair or replacement becomes unnecessarily high. With proper care, an instrument should have a life of ten years or more. Instruments do deteriorate from normal usage. However, most damage and reduced life is caused by improper cleaning, processing, and handling.

Cleaning

1 Remove blood and organic debris as soon after use as possible to prevent drying on the surfaces or in the crevices. At the operating table, the scrub nurse wipes off the surfaces of instruments that will be used again with a moist sponge. Used instruments not needed again can be immersed in a sterile basin of sterile distilled water. Sterile saline is *not* used for soaking instruments. The sodium chloride in saline is corrosive.

2 Separate delicate small instruments and those with sharp or semisharp edges for special handling.

3 Disassemble all instruments with removable parts to expose all surfaces to detergent agent.

4 Open all hinged instruments to expose box locks and serrations.

5 Separate instruments of dissimilar metals. Most surgical instruments are of high quality stainless steel, an alloy of iron, carbon, and chromium. However, some instruments are chrome plated; others are made of titanium or Vitallium, a cobalt alloy. Instruments of each type of metal should be cleaned separately to prevent electrolytic deposition of other metals.

6 Flush cold distilled water through hollow instruments or channels, such as suction tubes and endoscopes, immediately after use to prevent drying of organic debris. Clean thoroughly with warm detergent solution, rinse, and dry all endoscopes that cannot be steam or ethylene oxide gas sterilized prior to storage or disinfection.

7 Terminally sterilize all instruments that can be immersed in water and steam sterilized before they are handled for definitive cleaning and processing. They are put through a cycle in a washer-sterilizer (see Chap. 8, p. 125). Microsurgical, ophthalmic, and some lensed and powered instruments must be manually cleaned.

> NOTE. If instruments cannot be put in a washer-sterilizer immediately after operation is completed, or must be manually washed, soak them for a short time in a warm blood solvent detergent solution. Transfer those that will be put into a washer-sterilizer in an instrument tray from the OR to the cleanup area. Place the tray in a plastic bag. This delays drying and contains contamination.

8 Clean all instruments thoroughly in a noncorrosive, low-sudsing, free-rinsing detergent solution. The detergent must be compatible with the local water supply. Mineral content varies from one area to another. Some hospitals routinely use water softeners to minimize mineral deposits. Regardless of the water contents, the detergent should be anionic or nonionic and have a pH as close to neutral as possible. Alkaline detergent (pH over 8.5) will stain instruments; acid (pH below 6) corrodes or pits them. Liquid detergents are preferable as they disperse more completely than solids.

> NOTE. Do not pour liquid or put solid detergents directly on instruments. Always dilute concentration of the detergent prior to contact with instruments to avoid corrosion and staining.

9 Use a soft brush to clean serrations and box locks if manual washing is employed. A soft-bristled toothbrush may be used to clean delicate ophthalmic and microsurgery instruments. Keep instruments submerged while brushing to minimize aerosolizing microorganisms.

> NOTE. *Never* scrub surfaces with abrasive agents such as steel wool and scouring pow-

ders or pads. These will scratch and may remove the protective finish on the metal, increasing possibility of corrosion. The finish on stainless steel instruments protects the base metal from oxidation.

10 Place stainless steel instruments in an ultrasonic cleaner *after* they have been terminally sterilized in a washer-sterilizer to ensure thorough cleaning of box locks, serrations, and interstices. Always use hot water and a suitable detergent in the ultrasonic cleaner (see Chap. 8, p. 126).

NOTE. Do not put chrome-plated instruments in an ultrasonic cleaner. The plating may be cracked. Also do not put fine, delicate instruments in the ultrasonic cleaner.

11 Rinse instruments thoroughly in hot demineralized or distilled water after manual or ultrasonic cleaning to remove residual deposits and films.

12 Dry instruments completely before reassembling or storing. Instruments will corrode if they are stored with trapped moisture.

13 Immerse instruments routinely, after cleaning or before sterilizing prior to use, in an antimicrobial, water-soluble lubricant solution that is steam penetrable. The antimicrobial properties will help prevent microbial growth in the lubricant bath. A water-soluble lubricant will deposit a thin film deep in box locks, hinges, and crevices, but will not interfere with sterilization. Some lubricants also contain a rust inhibitor to prevent electrolytic mineral deposits. Use a lubricant according to manufacturer's instructions.

Processing

1 Inspect each instrument critically before and after each use for imperfections, cleanliness, and working condition. Each must be completely clean to ensure effective sterilization and proper function. Check hinged instruments for stiffness. Box locks and joints should work smoothly.

NOTE. Stiff box locks and joints are usually caused by inadequate cleaning. Lubrication eases stiffness temporarily. Only a water-soluble lubricant can be used. Mineral oil, silicones, and machine oils are *never* used because they leave a residue that interferes with steam sterilization. Oiling any surgical instrument is a break in aseptic technique. If box locks are frozen, leave the instruments in the lubricant bath overnight. Then gently work the jaws back and forth. Reinspect for cleanliness.

2 Test forceps for alignment. A forceps out of alignment can break during use. Close the jaws of the forceps slightly. If they overlap they are out of alignment. The teeth of forceps with serrated jaws should mesh perfectly. Hold the shanks in each hand, with the forceps open, and try to wiggle it. If the box lock has considerable play or is very loose, the forceps will not hold tissue securely. If a surgeon continues to use it, jaw misalignment will occur and the forceps' effectiveness is impaired.

3 Check ratchet teeth. Ratchets should close easily and hold firmly. Clamp the forceps on the first tooth only. Hold the instrument at the box lock. Tap the ratchet teeth lightly against a solid object. If the forceps springs open, it is faulty and should be repaired. Ratchet teeth are subject to friction and metal-to-metal wear by the constant strain of closing and opening. A forceps that will spring open when clamped on a blood vessel or duct is hazardous to the patient and an annoyance to the surgeon. The ratchets must hold.

4 Check the tension between the shanks. When the jaws touch, a clearance of $\frac{1}{16}$ to $\frac{1}{8}$ in. (1.5 to 3 mm) should be visible between the ratchet teeth of each shank. This clearance provides adequate tension at the jaws when closed.

5 Test needleholders for needle security. Clamp an appropriate-size needle in the jaws of the needleholder and lock on second ratchet tooth. If the needle can be turned easily by hand, the needleholder needs repair.

6 Test scissors for correctly ground and properly set blades. The blades should cut on the tips and glide over each other smoothly. Cut dissecting scissors through four layers of gauze at the tip of the blades; two layers if scissors are less than 4 in. (10 cm) in length. They should cut with a fine, smooth feel and a minimum of pressure.

7 Inspect edges of sharp and semisharp instruments, such as chisels, osteotomes, rongeurs, adenotomes, for sharpness, chips or dents, and alignment.

8 Test penetration of cataract knives, keratomes, and other fine cutting instruments on a small kidskin drum. Slide the blade by gravity through the kidskin with the handle resting on the palm of your hand. The blade should penetrate the drum as though it were passing through butter. It should not stick or tear.

9 Check chrome-plated instruments for chips, sharp edges, and worn spots. Chipped plating may harbor debris. Sharp edges will damage tissue or tear gloves. Worn spots will corrode.

10 Flatten or straighten malleable instruments such as retractors, probes.

11 Return unclean instruments to the cleaning area for ultrasonic cleaning.

12 Remove instruments in poor working condition from the sterile field or processing area. Instruments in poor working condition are a handicap to the surgeon and a hazard for the patient. Instruments should be repaired at the first sign of damage or malfunction. A place is usually designated in the OR suite for collection of instruments for repair. Do not allow a defective instrument to remain in circulation.

13 Demagnetize instruments by passing back through magnetic field. Instruments can become magnetized, although this is rare.

Handling

1 Know name and use of each instrument.

2 Watch sterile field for loose instruments. Remove them promptly after use to the Mayo stand or instrument table. Weight of instruments can injure patient or cause postoperative discomfort. Keeping instruments off the field also decreases possibility of their falling to floor.

3 Place used instruments, except sharps and delicate ones, into a tray or basin during or at the end of the operation. Careless dropping or throwing of instruments is absolutely prohibited.

General, Basic Operating Instruments

1 Hemostats, forceps, needleholders, retractors, etc., can be cleaned, assembled in trays, and sterilized together.

2 Heavier instruments always should be placed in the bottom of a tray with smaller, lightweight instruments on top.

3 Hand the surgeon the correct instrument to use for each particular task during the operation. Remember the principle, use for intended use only!

4 Instruments that must be marked for identification of ownership should be imprinted with an electro-etch device. A vibrating or impact-type marking tool breaks the finish on the instrument and can cause hairline cracks. Electro-etching should be put on the shank rather than the box lock to avoid box-lock fracture.

Sharp or Semisharp Instruments

1 Protect edges of sharp instruments, such as scissors, osteotomes, chisels, curettes, rongeurs, during cleaning, sterilizing, and storing.

2 Sharp instruments must be kept separate from dull ones and demand respectful handling.

Microsurgical and Ophthalmic Instruments

1 Each delicate instrument must be separated from adjacent ones to prevent interlocking or crushing. Never pile them on top of each other. They are easily deformed.

2 Exact alignment of the teeth is an absolute necessity in fine-toothed forceps. The microscopic teeth are very easily bent.

3 Place instruments on a firm, flat surface for sorting and cleaning.

4 Sharp blades and tips should touch absolutely nothing, not even a towel. They must never touch another instrument or any part of a receptacle in which they are placed for storage or sterilization. Most instrument manufacturers supply special sterilization-storage racks so that the blades and tips remain suspended.

5 If instrument has a protective guard, leave it on throughout sterilization. Ethylene oxide is the sterilization method of choice. Steam sterilization is also used. Tip-protecting covers or instrument-protecting plastic sleeves are made of material that does not melt or deform with heat. These guards should be left on the instruments until actual use.

6 On the Mayo stand or instrument table, support the handles on a rolled towel or gauze sponge to keep the blades and tips suspended in midair, if not in a rack.

7 Microinstruments are more susceptible to damage than standard instruments. Edges very easily are dulled and fine tips bent or broken. When instruments are in use, extreme caution is necessary not to catch the tips on any object that could bend them.

8 A nonfibrous sponge should be used to wipe off blood and debris after each use during the operation. The sponge prevents snagging and breaking of delicate tips.

9 The very small size physical appearance (like fine wires) may cause the scrub nurse to think some instruments are disposables. Avoid loss or discard at end of operation.

10 Clean and dry microsurgical and ophthalmic instruments by hand. Do *not* put in washer-sterilizer. They may be cleaned in an ultrasonic unit, separated in racks so they are not in contact with each other. They should never remain wet for long periods of time, which is conducive to corrosion and discoloration. Rather, they should be dried by hot-air blower, never a towel.

11 Inspect instruments under a magnifying glass or microscope for burrs on tips, nicks on cutting edges, and proper alignment.

12 Instrument sets are secured in holders in boxes for protection when not in use.

Lensed Instruments

1 Never handle lensed instruments with forceps. A scratch on the instrument could cause injury to tissue or the mucous membrane lining of an orifice. Also, danger of dropping the instrument is greatly increased. The forceps could crush a telescope and ruin the optical system if held too tightly. Always handle sterile instruments wearing sterile gloves.

2 Never pile these delicate instruments one on top of another or mix them with other instruments.

3 Avoid rough handling, jarring, or bending of parts. Lay them on a towel to absorb the impact and to prevent wear on the sheath.

4 Check the light source for working order before use and after cleaning.

Air- or Battery-Powered Instruments

1 Follow instructions for use, care, and sterilization recommended by the manufacturer. Each instrument has different cleaning, lubricating, packaging, and sterilizing requirements because of its various component parts.

2 Assemble appropriate instrument, attachments, power hose, regulator, power source, and footswitches. Test instrument for working condition before surgeon is ready to use it.

3 Be certain air exhaust is directed away from the sterile field. Compressed air may bring dirt into the instrument.

Electrical Instruments

1 Electrically powered instruments, such as saws, drills, dermatomes, nerve stimulators, are potential explosion hazards in the OR. Most of the motors are designed to be explosionproof. All must have sparkproof connections. However, power switches should be off when plugging electrical cords into outlets.

2 Alert the anesthesiologist if electrical equipment will be used. He or she may change the anesthetic to eliminate explosive gases if a necessary electrical item must be used and it is potentially hazardous. These instruments should be used only with nonflammable anesthetic agents. Even so, connect the power-supply cord to the wall outlet before anesthetic gases are administered and do not remove during administration.

3 Do *not* immerse motor in liquid.

4 Follow the manufacturer's recommended methods of cleaning, lubricating, sterilizing, and using each piece of electrically powered equipment.

5 Check power cords and plugs for cracks or breaks and test for working condition before surgeon is ready to use instrument and the device is applied to the patient.

ELECTRICAL HAZARDS AND SAFEGUARDS

The OR is a location fraught with hazards for both patient and personnel, namely potential electric shock, burns, fire, explosion, and mechanical injury. It is mandatory that the staff have knowledge of the equipment most often implicated in these incidents, the hazards involved in its use, and how accidents may occur. Each individual has a personal responsibility for ensuring a safe environment by correct handling of equipment and alertness to potentially hazardous situations.

Active interest in fire and explosions caused by anesthetic agents arose in 1925 with the use of ethylene gas. This was intensified in the following decade when cyclopropane anesthesia became popular. Since 1941 the United States government has issued information, recommendations, and regulations for the use of anesthetic agents. Although the potential hazard of static electricity causing combustion of flammable anesthetics has been minimized by elimination of these agents, electric shock, electrocution, and burns are potential patient injuries in the operating room and all patient care areas.

Medical electronics safety is a prime concern of hospital and industry personnel seeking safer patient care. Underlying this concern is the rapidly expanding use of electronic equipment in hospital procedures. The marketing and safety standards of medical electronic devices used in the operating room are also federally regulated. The Association for the Advancement of Medical Instrumentation (AAMI) standards and recommended practices are helpful to both manufacturers and users. Standards of the Joint Commission on Accreditation of Hospitals (JCAH) must be met for hospital accreditation as well. Inadequately trained personnel, inappropriate designs for suites, or malfunctions in equipment that cause short-circuiting of devices such as heart monitors, defibrillators, and x-ray machines are responsible for the fatalities and near-fatalities that occur. Electrical safety in hospitals is neither a major problem nor a complicated one if personnel understand appropriate terminology and a few simple principles of electricity.

Definitions Pertaining to Safety Standards

Anesthetizing Location Any area of a hospital or ambulatory care facility in which it is intended to administer any flammable or nonflammable inhalation anesthetic agents in the course of examination or treatment.

Combustible A flammable substance capable of reacting with oxygen to burn if ignited.

Conductive Materials Not only those materials that are commonly considered as electrically conductive, such as metals, but also the class of materials that, when tested in accordance with NFPA standard 56A, have a resistance to passage of electricity not exceeding 1,000,000 ohms. Such materials are required where electrostatic interconnection is necessary.[1]

Flammable Any gas or liquid that will burn or is capable, when ignited, of maintaining combustion, including oxygen.

Flammable Anesthetizing Location Any location used or intended for the use of flammable anesthetic agents where static electricity is a potential hazard.

Grounding An equipotential system of conductors that establishes a conducting connection, whether intentional or accidental, between an electrical circuit in equipment and earth or to some connecting body that serves in place of the earth to divert stray currents.

Hazardous Location The space extending 5 ft (1.5 m) above the floor during administration of a flammable anesthetic agent.

Isolated Power System An assembly of electrical devices that provides local isolated power, a single grounding point, and distinctive receptacles.

Leakage Current Any current not intended to be applied to a patient but that may be conveyed from exposed metal or other accessible parts of an appliance to ground.[1]

Line Isolation Monitor An instrument which continually checks the hazard current from an isolated circuit to ground.[2]

Macroshock Effect of large electric currents (milliamperes or larger) on the body.[2]

Microshock The effect of small electric currents (as low as 10 microamperes) on the body.[1]

Mixed Facility A hospital wherein flammable anesthetizing locations and nonflammable anesthetizing locations coexist within the same building, allowing interchange of personnel or equipment between flammable and nonflammable anesthetizing locations.[2]

Nonflammable Anesthetic Agent Inhalation agents that, because of their vapor pressure at 98.6°F (37°C) and at atmospheric pressure (760 mm Hg) cannot attain flammable concentrations when mixed with air, oxygen, or mixtures of oxygen and nitrous oxide.

Nonflammable Anesthetizing Location Any location used for, or intended for the *exclusive* use of, administration of nonflammable anesthetic agents.[3]

Patient Ground A terminal bus which serves as the single focus for grounding all electric devices serving an individual patient which are not connected by the power cord to the reference grounding point, and for grounding conductive furniture or equipment within reach of a patient or a person who may touch him.[2]

Concepts of Electrical Hazards

Electricity consists of three basic parameters:

1 *Voltage,* the driving force, forces electrons to move through material in one direction and causes current to flow.

2 *Current,* the rate of flow of electrons through a conductor.

3 *Resistance,* the measurement of the opposition to electron flow through a material. Electricity flows easily through conductors, i.e., metals and carbon. Flow is very difficult through insulators, i.e., rubber, plastic, glass. Insulators prevent equalization of potential differences. The resistance of the human body is more similar to a conductor than an insulator.

[1]From NFPA 56A, *Standard for the Use of Inhalation Anesthetics (Flammable and Nonflammable),* copyright 1980, National Fire Protection Association, Boston, Mass. Excerpted with permission.

[2]Ibid. Quoted with permission.

[3]Ibid. Adapted with permission.

Electric Shock; Electrocution Electrocution occurs when an individual becomes the component that closes a circuit in which a lethal current may flow. Lethal levels may be attained by currents through the intact body via skin or by currents applied directly to the heart. Electric shock occurs when a current is large enough to stimulate the nervous system or large muscle masses, e.g., when the body becomes the connecting link between two points of an electrical system that are at different potentials. The physiological effect of shock may range from a mere tingling sensation to tissue necrosis, ventricular fibrillation, or death. The effect is due to the electrical response of sensory cells, nerves, or muscles to electrical stimuli originating either intrinsically (within the body) or extrinsically (applied externally). Severity of the shock depends on the magnitude of current flow and path taken through the body. Two types of shock are commonly referred to:

Macroshock Shock in which the current flows through a relatively large surface of skin. It usually results from inadvertent contact of an individual with moderately high voltage sources and is expressed in milliamperes (1/1000 ampere). A current intensity of one to five amperes through the chest can cause severe burn at the point of contact. However, if the cardiac conduction system is involved, a current intensity of 50 to 100 milliamperes through the chest can cause ventricular fibrillation since the heart beat is electrically controlled. Macroshock occurs through the trunk of the body, with the current following many paths, each path carrying a fraction of the current. It may or may not be harmful depending on how much current flows through a susceptible heart along its path. Common sources of macroshock are electrical wiring failures allowing skin contact with a live wire or surface at full voltage. Never touch the victim, instrument, or surface with bare hands in case of shock. Disconnect the power supply or use an insulating material to push the victim away from the source of electricity.

Microshock Shock occurring when current is applied to a very small contact area of skin. The development of medical techniques permitting application of electrical impulses directly to the heart muscle drew awareness of the extreme danger to the electrically sensitive patient. Cardiac microshock is a potential hazard from indwelling catheters filled with conductive fluid, probes inserted into the great vessels, and electrodes implanted about the heart. These multiply the potential for electrocution because they can be conductors of electricity. The external portion of a cardiac catheter generally consists of two parts: an inner conductor(s) of wires or conductive fluid and an outer insulating sheath. When there is a highly conductive pathway from outside the body to the great vessels and heart, small electric currents may cause ventricular fibrillation and cardiac arrest. When a shock has an internal route to the heart, it takes only one-thousandth as much electricity to be fatal as when the shock is transmitted through the surface of the skin. Microshock occurs only if the current from an exterior source flows through the cardiac catheter or conductor. Conductive intravascular catheters that disperse current at the skin level diminish the risk of microshock. The most important precaution to observe is to protect the exposed end of the cardiac conductor from contact with conductive surfaces, including your body. Always wear rubber or plastic gloves when handling the external end of a cardiac catheter or conductor.

While the value of electronic devices in saving lives is unquestionable, the use of such equipment must not be allowed to cause needless death. Fibrillation and arrest may occur if the patient encounters an excess amount of accumulated small currents while connected to ground through implanted electronic devices or by contact with other grounded objects, such as electrocardiograph leads.

Electrical and Thermal Burns Electricity supplied by a defective system may cause burns. Monitors and all high-powered equipment are hazardous. Current density is highly significant. Current concentrated or of high density at the point of contact can result in a burn. An electrical burn may be severe enough to require debridement.

Electrosurgical units can be dangerous (see Chap. 19). A high-frequency current is locally applied by the small active electrode to cut or coagulate tissue. The patient is protected by a patient ground plate or pad, the inactive electrode. This must be placed under or on the patient in contact with skin at a fleshy, nonhairy area, not a bony prominence such as the sacrum. The inactive electrode provides a low current density pathway for the high-frequency current present at the active electrode back to the unit. Proper connections from the ground plate or pad to the patient and to the unit are essential to prevent burns.

Conductive surfaces must be capable of providing a return path for current other than through the operating table or its attachments. If the return circuit of high-frequency equipment is faulty, the ground circuit may be completed through inadvertent contact with the metal parts or attachments of the operating table. If the ground area is small, the current passing through the exposed area of skin contact will be relatively intense, causing a burn to the patient. For example, one such contact point may be the thigh touching the leg stirrup in lithotomy position.

Surface burns can occur when battery-operated equipment, such as peripheral nerve stimulator, is used with external electrodes. Tetanic stimuli should be limited to one or two seconds.

Other potential sources for burn include malfunctioning controls on heat-generating devices in contact with the patient, such as radio-frequency diathermy or hypo-hyperthermia machines. Factors such as the patient's nutritional state, the amount of body fat that acts as insulation, or the circulation in the body part in contact with the device influence individual reaction to a hazard.

Grounding

Grounding of all electrical equipment is essential for safety and prevention of stray leakage current. Grounding systems are designed to avoid the inadvertent passage of electric current through the patient by discharging any harmful potentials directly to the ground without including the patient in the circuit, thereby avoiding shock or burn. Electric power is brought into a hospital through two wires: *hot* and *neutral.* These wires transmit current to the three-wire outlets in the building. The third wire is the ground wire. When the cord from an electrical device is plugged into an outlet, the hot and neutral wires deliver the current. The ground wire is attached to a copper pipe driven into the ground at the point where power enters the building. An electrical connection to the ground provides a means for current to flow through the ground wire or any other conductive surface connected to the ground rather than going to the neutral wire. The copper ground wire is used to prevent the metal housings of electrical equipment from becoming electrically "hot." The ground wire within the three-wire power plug and cord connects the equipment (instrument) housing to the ground contact in the receptacle (wall outlet). This provides a constantly available return path for the current to the electrical source. If the insulation on wires is defective, such as broken or frayed cords or plugs, some current will leak or flow to other nearby conductors such as the equipment housing. When an instrument is grounded, leakage current returns through the ground wire to the earth, causing no damage. If the ground path is absent or broken, leakage current will seek another path to the ground.

Small, extraneous leakage currents can be prevented by proper grounding. Lack of grounding or use of defective electrical systems can cause microshock. This may occasion cardiac disturbances that lead to death or cause severe sparks that may be a source of ignition.

Equipotential Grounding System Current flows between points only when a voltage difference exists between them. Therefore, electric shock can be minimized by eliminating voltage differences. One system designed to do this is the equipotential grounding system, which maintains an equal potential or voltage between all conductive surfaces near the patient. To achieve equipotential grounding, all exposed conductive surfaces within 6 ft (2 m) of the patient are electrically connected to a single point that is itself connected by a copper conductor to the ground tie point at the electrical distribution center serving the area. Consequently, all exposed metal surfaces are electrically tied together and to the ground.

Isolation Power System Isolated power systems are used in hazardous locations such as operating rooms. A device, the isolation transformer, isolates the OR electrical circuits from the grounded circuits in the power mains; thus the isolated circuit does not include the ground in its pathway. The current seeks to flow only from one isolated line to the other. As a result, accidental grounding of persons in contact with the hot wire does not cause current to flow through the individual. A line isolation monitor checks the degree of isolation maintained by an isolated power system by continually measuring resistance and capacitance between the two isolated lines and ground. The meter reading is called the hazard index. The monitor, a wall-mounted meter, has an alarm that is activated at the 2-milliampere level. This warning system indicates when inadvertent grounding of the isolated circuits has occurred and alerts personnel to a dangerous situation. Since grounding can only take place when faulty equipment is plugged into ungrounded circuits, maximum safety is afforded by use of the isolation transformer. OR and obstetrical suite electrical circuits are required to be ungrounded circuits fed through isolation transformers. Permanently installed overhead operating lights and receptacles in anesthetizing locations are required to be supplied by ungrounded electrical circuits.

Static Electricity

Static electricity consists of high voltage and low ampere. An electrostatic spark develops from friction and accumulates on physical objects. When two static-bearing objects come in contact, the one bearing the higher potential discharges to the one with the lower potential. Air is a nonconductor. However, a high enough potential can overcome air resistance, jump the gap between it and a lower-potential object causing an arc across air gaps seen as a spark(s) from the heat thus generated. Sparks can ignite flammable materials or gases. Objects accumulate static in inverse proportion to their conductivity. The aim is to provide adequate channels for dissipation of static. Since the earth has a zero potential, a charge brought directly, or indirectly, through a conductor, into contact with it is discharged to the earth. A spark between two objects can occur only when there is no electrical path of good conductivity between them. If there is moderate conductivity, there is a tendency for gradual spread of charge over both objects so they come to the same potential. Generation of static electricity cannot be prevented absolutely because its intrinsic origins are present at every interface. For static electricity to be a source of ignition, there must be:

1 An effective means of static generation

2 A means of accumulating the separate charges and maintaining a suitable difference of electrical potential

3 A discharge of energy adequate to make a spark in an ignitable mixture

Explosion and Fire Hazards

Hospitals have discontinued use of flammable anesthetic agents, such as cyclopropane and ether. These are highly flammable and/or explosive when mixed with air, oxygen, or nitrous oxide. Although oxygen and nitrous oxide are nonflammable gases, they support and accelerate combustion. An explosion is the result of a combination of three factors:

1 A flammable gas, vapor, or liquid

2 A source of ignition

3 Oxygen (pure or in air) or some other substance providing oxygen such as nitrous oxide

Safeguards against Hazards

Regional, national, and federal guidelines, regulations, and laws must be adhered to in order to prevent disastrous consequences from the hazards encountered in the OR.

Elimination of Explosive Agents

1 Use nonflammable agents.

2 Air-conditioning or ventilating systems aid in the prevention of pockets of gas in the room, although concentration of the agent around the anesthesia machine is not remarkedly reduced. Heavy gas can accumulate and channel along the floor for as far as 50 ft (15 m) in explosive concentration. Air streams can carry explosive concentrations of anesthetic to an ignition source.

3 Confining potentially explosive agents by use of the closed carbon dioxide absorption technique tends to restrict the region likely to be hazardous.

Elimination of Sources of Ignition

1 Electrostatic (incendiary) spark can be an ignition source. Therefore, flammable anesthetic agents are used *only* in areas where a conductive pathway can be maintained between the patient and a conductive floor. Precautions include:

   a Use conductive flooring in flammable anesthetizing locations, in adjacent corridors and rooms, and in storage locations for flammable anesthetic agents located in operating room suite. A conductive floor must meet resistance provisions through its inherent conductive properties. The average resistance of the conductive floor shall be less than 1,000,000 ohms as measured between two electrodes placed 3 ft (1 m) apart at any points on the floor, and more than 25,000 ohms as measured between a ground connection and the electrodes placed on the floor. The resistance of conductive floors shall be initially tested prior to use and thereafter measurements taken at intervals of not more than one month. A permanent record of readings is kept.[1]

b Assure electrical connection of the patient to the conductive floor by provision of a 10-W impedance conductive strap in contact with the patient's skin, with one end of the strap fastened to the metal frame of the operating table. Mattresses and pillows are covered with conductive material.

c Discontinue administration of a flammable agent, when feasible, as soon as the ground monitor system indicates a warning. Following completion of operation, the room in which the signal functioned is not used until the electrical defect is corrected.

d Avoid contacting metals with force sufficient to produce percussion sparks.

e Use antistatic liners in kick buckets, and use caution in handling them.

f Cover all hair of patients, personnel, and visitors.

g Wear outer garments in the OR suite known to be antistatic in accordance with requirements of NFPA 56A.[1] Hose and undergarments in which the entire garment is in close contact with the skin may be of synthetic material.

h Cover patient in the OR suite or other anesthetizing location with a cotton blanket. Woolen or synthetic blankets are not permitted as they are more prone to static electricity.

i Wear conductive footwear in areas that have conductive flooring.

j Test conductivity. In hazardous areas, an instrument, known as a *calibrated ohmmeter,* is located at the entrance to the anesthetizing location and is used to measure the resistance of personnel and equipment.

k Maintain high relative humidity (weight of water vapor present); 60 percent is preferable, not less than 50 percent is mandatory in flammable anesthetizing locations. Moisture provides a relatively conductive medium, allowing static electricity to leak to earth as fast as it is generated. Sparks form more readily in low humidity.

l Do not move a patient from one area to another while a flammable anesthetic is being administered.

m Avoid unnecessary motion in the area around anesthesia equipment and patient's head.

n Dissipate static charge. Anyone who must make contact with patient or anesthesiologist does so by first touching anesthesiologist's back or stool, operating table, or patient at least 2 ft (60 cm) from the face mask. This provides for the discharge of any charge in that person before he or she is close to the mask or machine. A stool with smooth rounded feet and bare metal top or conductive cushioning is recommended for grounding anesthesiologist.

o Avoid friction on the reservoir bag of the anesthesia machine. Watch that drapes do not touch the bag or cover the machine.

p Use flammable agents only in flammable anesthetizing locations.

q Use explosion-proof receptacles and attachment plugs that cannot be pulled apart accidentally. Grounding adaptor plugs and multiple-outlet plugs are prohibited. Cords should be rubber-coated and switches explosion-proof.

2 Faulty electrical equipment may cause short circuit or electrocution.

a Particular care must be used with high-voltage equipment such as x-ray, electrosurgical unit, electronic monitoring devices.

b Hypo-hyperthermia machine must be at least 3 ft (1 m) away from anesthesia machine and both be adequately grounded.

c Electrosurgical unit should be located on the operator's side of the table as far as possible from the anesthesia machine and monitoring equipment. The power cable is not stretched across traffic lanes. If a flammable agent was employed for induction, even if followed by a nonflammable agent for maintenance, the electrosurgical unit should not be used on the neck, nasopharynx, and adjacent areas.[2]

d All electrical equipment, including a sur-

[1]Excerpted with permission from NFPA 56A, *Standard for the Use of Inhalation Anesthetics (Flammable and Nonflammable),* copyright 1980, National Fire Protection Association, Boston, Mass.; for complete details see that standard, which is published by NFPA either as a separate pamphlet or in vol. 4 of the *National Fire Codes.*

[2]National Fire Protection Association. *National Fire Codes,* vol. 15, p. 76C-45, 46, Boston, Mass., 1978.

geon's personal property, must be inspected by the engineering and maintenance department or the biomedical engineering technician prior to initial use. Every piece must meet Underwriters Laboratories (UL) or other electrical safety requirements. All equipment must be inspected, preferably monthly, and verified safe for use. Testing intervals must not exceed six months.

3 Open flames and heated objects may cause fire or explosion. Minimum ignition temperatures of anesthetic agents in pure oxygen are all lower than in air.
  a Flammable antiseptics or flammable fat solvents are not applied for preoperative preparation of the patient.
  b Only approved photographic lighting equipment shall be used with suitable enclosures to prevent sparks and hot particles from falling into a hazardous area, such as from a burst flash bulb.
  c Smoking is limited to dressing rooms and lounges with doors leading to corridors closed. Open flames and heated objects are prohibited in hazardous locations and corridors outside anesthetizing locations.
  d Lights and sources of heat must be kept at least 4 ft (more than 1 m) away from the anesthesia machine or flammable agents.

4 Spontaneous combustion can be caused by a mixture of gases under high pressure or by oil or grease in contact with cylinders containing a flammable agent.
  a Oil or grease is not used on oxygen valves or parts of anesthesia machines.
  b Anesthesia machines, cylinders of compressed gas, and flammable liquid containers must be kept away from any source of heat and not touch each other.

5 Fire should be a matter of prime concern. Fires in oxygen-enriched atmospheres (OEA) are fundamentally different in character than those occurring in normal atmosphere. The fire severity potential should be regarded as one of a high order, with extensive damage potential. The presence of flammable and combustible liquid vapors, gases, and particulate solids (dust) in OEA can result in ultrarapid combustion with explosive violence.

All hospitals have fire warning and safety systems. Staff members must be familiar with location and operation of fire alarms and fire extinguishers. They must also be familiar with evacuation routes and procedures in the event of a fire or explosion (see Chap. 6, p. 90). Fire drills are held at least quarterly.

Safeguards in Nonflammable Anesthetizing Locations

Requirements are less stringent for locations where *only* nonflammable inhalation anesthetic agents are used than for flammable anesthetizing locations. Nonconductive flooring is acceptable, for example. Antistatic clothing and conductive footwear are not required. Safeguards must still be taken, however, to prevent shock, electrocution, burns, and fire. The standards of the National Fire Protection Association (NFPA), AAMI, and JCAH must be adhered to for patient safety.

Nonflammable anesthetizing locations, whether located in a mixed facility or not, should be identified by prominently posted signs at all entrances to the operating room and within the location signifying the type of anesthetic permitted.

RADIATION HAZARDS AND SAFEGUARDS

Operating room nursing personnel may assist with invasive preoperative x-ray studies (see Chap. 20). All OR nurses and technologists are exposed to scatter radiation during intraoperative x-ray procedures (see Chap. 20), and radioactive-implant procedures (see Chap. 35). The effect of radiation exposure is directly related to the amount and length of time of exposure. Radiation has the ability to modify molecules within body cells. Therefore, constant vigilance for personal safety and strict adherence to all hospital policies and procedures are essential to avoid excessive exposure to radiation.

Radiation is measured in roentgens (R) and rads (the units of absorbed dose). The National Council on Radiation Protection and Measurements has formulated government standards for certification of x-ray equipment and for human exposure. Permissible doses of radiation are based on *units of equivalent dose,* the quantity that expresses all radiations on a common scale for the purpose of calculating their biological effects. The unit of equivalent dose is a REM (roentgen equivalent man). The maximum permissible dose for occupationally exposed persons over 18 years of age is 5 REMs per year. OR personnel rarely receive more than 2 or 3 REMs per year. However, the following precautions are taken to protect personnel:

1 Monitoring devices should be worn by all personnel who remain in the room during radiation exposure from whatever source.

a Badge dosimeters should be distributed to the entire OR team before a procedure involving radiation. These badges are worn on the torso of each person exposed. The reading is recorded for each individual at weekly intervals to monitor accumulated exposure to radiation.

b Personal radiation monitors are pocket dosimeters with an additional device that produces audible sounds when exposed to ionizing radiation. The surgeon may wish to wear this during fluoroscopy or radiation therapy procedures.

c Film badges are worn by personnel in the radiology and nuclear medicine departments, and may be used by individual OR personnel. The film badge is worn for a prescribed period. It is then developed with a second film exposed to a predetermined maximum tolerance dose for the same prescribed period and the two compared. Exposure on film badge is measured and recorded for each individual on a monthly basis.

2 To avoid overexposure of any person, especially one of childbearing age, personnel should rotate assignments on procedures that involve radiation. Sterility is a potential hazard. Exposure should not exceed 100 milliroentgen (mR) per week. A staff member may request relief from exposure during pregnancy. The maximum permissible dose to the fetus is 0.4 REM (roentgen equivalent man). All personnel who handle radioactive elements should have a complete blood count every 30 days. Anemia can result from excessive exposure.

Protection from Radiation

Radiation is not seen or felt. However, excessive exposure can cause anemia, sterility, and burns. In addition to time of exposure, shielding and distance from radiation source are key factors in protection. Safety precautions are taken to protect personnel from potential hazards.

1 Walls of rooms with fixed x-ray equipment are lined with lead to absorb emitted radiation.

2 Personnel should stand 6 ft (2 m) or more from the patient and out of the direct beam during exposure. Nonsterile team members should leave the room, and sterile team members should stand behind a lead screen if possible while x-rays are taken. Radiation from an x-ray tube is present only as long as the tube is energized. Automatic or manual collimators that confine the x-ray beam to precisely the size of the x-ray film or fluoroscopic screen are required for all equipment manufactured after August 1, 1974.

3 Lead-lined aprons and, if feasible, lead gloves should be worn during use of the image intensifier even though a lead shield is part of the installation. They also should be worn by necessary attendant personnel while injecting a substance for an invasive study, holding a cassette in position, or handling radioactive implants.

NOTE. Lead aprons should be hung or laid flat when not in use. They should *never* be folded. Folding can crack the lead, making the shield ineffective.

Safety rules for handling radioactive materials used for radiation therapy are discussed in Chapter 35, p. 625.

CHAPTER **12**

LIABILITY AND ACCOUNTABILITY

Most mistakes or accidents are preventable. Some are so slight that patients are never aware of them. Others, however, can cause injury resulting in pain, disfigurement, prolonged hospitalization and/or rehabilitation, and can even prove fatal. If negligence or malpractice is established, a nurse or technologist can be held liable for his or her own acts of omission or commission.

Along with the development of *consumerism,* a movement that focuses on consumer rights, a well-informed American public has developed an increasingly litigious attitude, demanding compensation for bodily injuries or damages to personal property. The quality of health care in this country is assessed through the outcome of services rendered. However, there is an increasing tendency for patients to take grievances to court. The severity of an injury usually determines whether a claim will arise, but other contributing factors include a breakdown of rapport between the patient and the health care team members and unrealistic expectations about the outcome of care.

The welfare and safety of the patient constitute the principles around which nursing care is built. Safe care of the patient results in safety to the nurse, the technologist, the surgeon, and the hospital. It also upholds the reputation of the professions by maintaining the confidence of the consumer public. Safeguards against the hazards peculiar to care of patients in the operating room are stressed throughout this text. Most incidents that could endanger the patient and lead to legal action can be prevented by following the accepted procedures as presented.

HISTORICAL EVOLUTION

Over 4000 years ago, King Hammurabi of Babylonia codified the laws of human behavior. These codes included penalties for physician/surgeons who did not cure. "If a physician has treated a man with a metal knife for a severe wound and has caused the man to die, or has opened a man's tumor with a metal knife and destroyed the man's eye, his hands shall be cut off."* Although this ancient punishment seems severe by contemporary judgment, it should remind the OR team that their primary consideration is still to do patients no harm, *primum non nocere.*

The first recorded medical malpractice suit was tried in England in the thirteenth century. The first one in the United States occurred in 1790. Throughout the nineteenth century and the early part of the twentieth, litigation against physicians was quite uncommon and rarely affected nurses. Malpractice suits began to increase markedly after World War II. They flourished in the 1960s and 1970s as an increasing number of people sought health care services. This automatically increased

*Code of Hammurabi, from the translation by Charles Edwards.

incidents that could lead to lawsuits. Cause for litigation lies in the thinking of patients and their families that physicians have not provided appropriate diagnosis, treatment, or results. Although the physician is professionally responsible for patient care, other professionals and paraprofessionals act as part of the health care team. Ancillary personnel and suppliers of equipment and drugs also are indirectly involved in treatment, and may be held liable.

Medical care and professional liability have become institutional problems. The primary cause of professional liability claims is *iatrogenic medical injury,* an injury or other adverse result sustained by a patient during the course of hospital and medical treatment. Many of the serious incidents that are brought to suit occur in the operating room.

In the past, the surgeon was considered the "captain of the ship" in the OR. If the surgeon had supervisory control and the right to give orders during the operation, then the operating room was like a ship and the surgeon like its captain. The captain or master was liable for the negligent acts of servants. Courts held that this doctrine, based on the master-servant relationship, was applicable by the mere presence of the surgeon. Once having entered the OR, the surgeon was considered to have complete control over other team members. Courts now recognize that the surgeon does not have complete control over the acts of the nurses and technologists on the OR team. The surgeon usually is not held responsible when a nurse or technologist fails to carry out a routine procedure as expected, since courts have decided that these procedures do not need to be supervised by the surgeon. By the *borrowed servant rule,* the surgeon is liable for acts of team members only when he or she has the right to control and supervise the way in which a nurse or technologist performs the work.

The hospital as the employer may be held responsible for its employees under the *master-servant rule.* However, the current trend is to hold an individual responsible for his or her own acts under the principle of an *independent contractor.* An alleged liability must determine whether the nurse or technologist was acting in the course of duties as a hospital employee, rendering independently contracted services such as a private scrub nurse or technologist or surgeon's assistant, or responding to instructions as a borrowed servant of the surgeon. Control over and supervision of conduct may determine who will be held liable for any resulting injury to a patient. The tendency is for plaintiffs to name all team members and the hospital as defendants in a lawsuit.

LIABILITY

To be *liable* is to be legally bound, as to make good any loss or damage that occurs in a transaction; to be answerable; to be responsible. A *tort* is a legal wrong committed by one person involving injury to another person, loss of or damage to personal property. When a tort has been committed, a patient or family member may institute a civil action against the person or persons who caused the injury, loss, or damage.

Statutory laws (laws by legislation) and *common laws* (laws based on court decisions) differ from state to state. Courts differ at times in their interpretation of laws. A nurse or technologist who is in some manner responsible for injury to a patient may be sued. The supervisor or instructor responsible for assigning duties to this individual may be included in the suit. Nurses and technologists may be considered employees of the hospital and, if the court so rules, the hospital is considered liable. However, the court may rule a learner or an experienced practitioner liable for his or her own acts. A learner may be held responsible in proportion to the amount and type of instruction received and judged by the standard of other learners in training. An individual can be held responsible for carrying out a wrong procedure if he or she has received sufficient instruction so that the correct procedure should be known.

An unqualified, unconditional general rule of law is that every person is liable for the torts he or she commits. *There is no exception to this rule.* However, liability may be imposed under one of several legal doctrines or common law precedents.

Doctrine of the Reasonable Man

A patient has the right to expect all professional and technical nursing personnel to utilize knowledge, skill, and judgment in performing duties that meet the standards exercised by other *reasonably prudent persons* involved in a similar circumstance. Every professional nurse and technologist must always carry out duties in accordance with standards and practices established by federal statutes, state practice acts, the professional organizations and regulatory agencies, and maintained in common practice throughout the country. Deviation from these standards and practices that cause injury to a patient can result in liabilities for negligence or malpractice.

Negligence is the lack of care or skills that any nurse or technologist in the same situation would be expected to use. It has been legally defined as "the omission to do something which a reasonable person, guided by those ordinary considerations which ordinarily regulate human affairs, would do, or as doing something which a reasonable and prudent person would not do."* These acts of omission or commission may give rise to tort action, which is a civil liability, as a result of injury to a patient that can be traced directly to the breach of duty.

Malpractice is "any professional misconduct, unreasonable lack of skill or fidelity in professional or judiciary duties, evil practice, or illegal or immoral conduct."* Malpractice claims usually are settled in a civil court but, depending on the severity of the injury and the extent of the misconduct, they may be taken to criminal court. Legally from the point of view of damages or fault, professional negligence usually is synonymous with malpractice in a tort action. Factors contributing to actionable negligence have been called the *four D's of malpractice:*

1 Duty to demonstrate and deliver a high standard of care directly proportional to the degree of specialty training received
2 Dereliction of that duty by omission or commission
3 Damage to a patient or personal property
4 Direct cause of a personal injury or damage because of dereliction of duty

Doctrine of *Res Ipsa Loquitor*

Translated from Latin, *res ipsa loquitor* means "the thing speaks for itself." Before this doctrine can be applied, three conditions must exist:

1 The type of injury does not ordinarily occur without a negligent act.
2 The injury was caused by the conduct or instrumentality within the exclusive control of the person or persons being sued.
3 The injured person could not have contributed to the negligence nor voluntarily assumed the risk.

This doctrine applies to injuries sustained by patients while in the operating room when foreign objects are left in the body, i.e., a sponge, needle, or instrument, or patient sustains a burn.

Doctrine of *Respondeat Superior*

An employer may be liable for an employee's negligent conduct under the *respondeat superior* master-servant employment relationship. This implies that the master will answer for the acts of a servant. If a patient is injured as a result of an employee's negligent act within the scope of that employment, the employer is responsible to the injured patient. The patient may sue both the hospital and the employee. Liability of the hospital as an employer varies, however, with its classification. A hospital is classified as:

1 Public/government
2 Private voluntary nonprofit charitable
3 Private profit-making proprietary

Although some states still uphold the immunity rule absolving charitable institutions from liability, the trend is toward holding all hospitals liable for negligent acts of employees under their control and supervision.

A hospital protects the patient, its personnel, and itself by maintaining good working conditions for a well-oriented staff. The professional and technical nursing staff members are chosen after careful screening of educational preparation and licensure or certification credentials. The staff should be adequate in size, and properly trained and assigned. A continuous program of staff orientation and education should be provided. Hospital procedures and routines are established in a manner consistent with the standards of competent nursing performance and patient safety.

Doctrine of Corporate Negligence

Under the corporate negligence doctrine, the hospital may be liable, not for the negligence of employees, but for its own negligence in failing to assure that an acceptable level of care is provided. A hospital has a duty to provide services and is responsible for:

1 Screening and verifying qualifications of staff members, including medical staff, according to

*H Creighton, *Law Every Nurse Should Know,* 4th ed, Philadelphia: Saunders, 1981.

standards established by the Joint Commission on Accreditation of Hospitals (JCAH)

2 Monitoring and reviewing performance of staff members through established personnel appraisal and peer review procedures

3 Maintaining a competent staff of physicians, nurses, and employees

Hospitals have been held liable for permitting a physician or nurse to exercise practice privileges when the hospital knew, or should have known, that the individual was incompetent or impaired.

Assault and Battery

In legal terms, *assault* is an unlawful threat to harm another physically. *Battery* is the carrying out of threatened physical harm. The lack of consent is an important aspect of an assault and battery charge. Consent may be given by words or implied by conduct, but it must be given voluntarily with full understanding of the implications. Witnessed written consents for operation and anesthesia are obtained before patient is premedicated and transported to the OR suite. The purpose of a consent is to protect surgeon, anesthesiologist, OR team members, and hospital against claims of unauthorized operations and to protect patient against unsanctioned procedures.

The surgeon and anesthesiologist must explain procedures to the patient or a family member or both, in understandable lay language, without details that might unnecessarily frighten the patient. When a patient signs an agreement, consent is given for the specific procedure that the patient understands will be done. The patient must sign the consent unless he or she is a minor, unconscious, mentally incompetent, or in a life-threatening emergency situation. The nearest of kin or other authorized person must sign for these patients. A witness is necessary to testify, if needed, that the patient signed without coercion after the surgeon explained the details of the procedure. The patient has the right to waive an explanation of nature and consequences of the procedure, and also the right to refuse treatment. (Refer to Chapter 3, pp. 41–44, for discussion of patient-physician relationship and written operative consents.)

If the surgeon goes beyond the limits to which the patient consented, liability for assault and battery may be charged. However, determination must be made whether the patient consented to a specific procedure or generally to surgical treatment of a health problem. By medical necessity and sound judgment, the surgeon may perform a different or additional operation when unexpected conditions are encountered during the course of an authorized operation. The surgeon may extend the operation to correct or remove any abnormal or pathological condition under the *extension doctrine.* This doctrine implies that the patient's explicit consent for operation serves as an implicit consent for any or all procedures deemed necessary to cope with unpredictable situations that jeopardize the patient's health.

Human experimentation with new drugs and devices requires patient consent. Department of Health and Human Services (HHS) regulations require a very specific informed consent for research carried out under HHS auspices, with strong emphasis on the need for a clear explanation of the experiment, its possible dangers, and the patient's complete freedom to refuse or withdraw from the regime at any time.

The surgeon may be approved by the Federal Food and Drug Administration (FDA) and the hospital as a clinical investigator in the controlled experimental use of new drugs and chemical agents or medical devices. Prior written, voluntary consent based on an informed decision to participate in the research must be obtained from the patient. The surgeon completes an investigator's report that is returned to the supplier of the drug or device and eventually filed with the FDA.

Invasion of Privacy

The patient's right to privacy exists by statutory or common law. Patient's chart, medical record, x-rays, and photographs are considered confidential information for use by physicians and other hospital personnel directly concerned with that patient's care. Lawsuits can be, and have been, brought to the courts by patients for violation of this right. Unauthorized persons are not permitted to observe or photograph operations or procedures of interest only to professional persons without the patient's written consent.

The patient has the right to expect that all communications and records pertaining to individualized care will be treated as confidential and will not be misused. This includes the right to privacy during interview, examination, and treatment. Every health care worker has a moral obligation to hold in confidence any personal or family affairs learned from patients.

NOTE. If a patient has been criminally assaulted or is being held in criminal custody, team members are required by law to divulge voluntarily any information concerning the patient to legal authorities. Withholding known information is punishable by law.

ACCOUNTABILITY

Accountability is the expectation that an individual may be called to account for actions taken, consistent with responsibilities contracted by virtue of employment or learner experience. Stated more succinctly, to be accountable means to answer to someone else for something one has done. OR nurses and technologists, both practitioners and learners, are accountable to:

1 Patients receiving services.

2 Hospital employing practitioners and educational institutions providing learning experiences.

3 Profession or vocation to uphold established standards of practice.

4 Public to whom nurses are licensed and technologists are certified to serve.

5 Self and other team members. The adages "to thine own self be true" and "do unto others" apply in all interpersonal relationships. Trust, honesty, and confidence are the essence of valid team member relations.

Accountability is concerned with both *efficiency and effectiveness.* Patients and the public demand quality care assurance. Documentation of nursing care given can attest to efficiency or protect against liability when an unusual incident occurs. Audit and peer review are methods for evaluating effectiveness by comparing actual care with established standards for nursing care. Perioperative nursing should include a systematic series of actions directed toward preoperative assessment of patient needs; development and implementation of a written, individualized, intraoperative nursing care plan; and postoperative evaluation of the effectiveness of the nursing care plan for continuity of each surgical patient's care.

Documentation in Patient Records

Verbal communications between patients and health care providers do not provide legal evidence in a court of law. Only the patient's medical records can be subpoenaed as legal evidence of care received or omitted. Documentation of care that has been given, including teaching provided, and patient's response to care must be complete and accurate. State facts, not conclusions, in objective terms. Some hospitals allow patients access to their records so they can review them for reliability of subjective data and clarity of plans for treatment and teaching.

During a preoperative visit, the perioperative nurse should be alert to signs that a patient does not clearly understand what is going to happen as a result of surgical intervention. This must be brought to attention of the surgeon. Significant observations or information must be recorded on the chart and reported to the unit nurse in charge. For example, if a patient verbally withdraws consent for operation or expresses a fear of death in the OR, the perioperative nurse is responsible for communicating this information to the surgeon and anesthesiologist.

The professional perioperative nursing role includes preoperative patient assessment and teaching, and postoperative evaluation of intraoperative care and reinforcement of preoperative teaching. All visits with patients are documented on the patient's chart, either in the nurses' notes or progress notes. The format for recording varies from hospital to hospital. Regardless of the format of the patient's record, all entries must be:

1 Written legibly in ink without erasures.

2 Stated factually as to what happened. Documentation of services rendered or unusual incidents should be very specific.

3 Stated in complete words. Abbreviations should be used only for very commonly accepted medical terms, e.g., T&A, D&C, TUR, O.D.

4 Dated, including the time note is written.

5 Signed with full legal signature and status of the writer.

Some hospitals use problem-oriented records; others use integrated patients' progress records, and/or written nursing care plans.

Written Nursing Care Plan Statements of identified patient needs and planned approaches for nursing care to meet these needs are formalized into a nursing care plan. This may become a permanent part of the patient's chart or may be used as an accessory guideline for implementation of nursing care. If this tool is used to document care given, it should be incorporated into the patient's medical record. (Refer to Chapter 4, pp. 73–75, for discussion of nursing care planning.)

Problem-Oriented Medical Record With the problem-oriented, goal-directed approach to care, the patient's chart is organized on the basis of problems rather than on the source of the data about them such as radiology, laboratory reports, etc. Each problem is numbered in a problem list with the initial plan for meeting each. Progress notes are charted corresponding to the problem number to facilitate assessment of the patient's response to planned intervention. Briefly, the record utilizes:

1 A defined data base of information from history, physical examination, laboratory reports, etc., to formulate a complete problem list
2 Plans for diagnostic, therapeutic, teaching, and follow-up care for each problem
3 Progress notes and flow sheets for multiple parameters that contain both subjective (symptoms) and objective (signs) information

Advantages of problem-oriented medical records are that they:

1 Check efficiency, reliability, thoroughness, and analytic sense of the professional. The nurse acquires selected assessment and communicative skills, and bases nursing judgments on scientific knowledge rather than on intuitive observations.
2 Provide better communication among health care professionals.
3 Provide systematic management of patient care by assessing, recording, and evaluating. This establishes the concept of team patient care as opposed to nursing versus medical care.
4 Enhance continuity of care and recorded data; document practice and care rendered.
5 Permit qualified participants in patient care to cooperate in compiling patient records.
6 Bring to immediate attention all essential information. Specific problems are identified, thereby furnishing immediate relevancy to data. This avoids inadvertent omission and obviates unnecessary repetition of data.
7 Facilitate audit for efficiency, performance, and effectiveness.

Problem-oriented records document information needed to accurately diagnose illness and treat patients. Some hospitals use a combined, some a separate, problem list for nurses and physicians. Critics of the system cite its emphasis on symptoms rather than prevention or improvement, and its neglect of individual strengths.

Integrated Patient's Progress Record Documentation is a vitally important aspect of continuity in patient care. A record of the patient's progress from admission to discharge guides all health care providers in planning and coordinating care. Entry of a progress note may be made by a physician or nurse on the same record. This promotes the team concept of total patient care by sharing knowledge and observations made by each team member who cares for the patient. A note is made after a treatment or procedure is initiated to document the condition and tolerance of the patient. Any change in condition, any unusual incident, complication, or deviation from the usual pattern or course of the patient must be recorded as a progress note. The nurse must document any nursing intervention and management, as well as the time the physician was notified, if this is indicated.

Intraoperative Nurses' Notes

Specific care given in the OR should be documented on the patient's chart, not only for legal reasons, but also for the benefit of recovery room and unit nurses who provide postoperative care. Information documented by the circulating nurse in the nurses' notes or progress record should include:

1 Times patient arrived in and departed from the OR and condition on transfer
2 Level of consciousness or anxiety manifested by observable physical responses
3 Site, time started, solutions administered intravenously, including blood products, and type of needle or cannula
4 Position and types of restraints and supports used for maintaining position of patient on operating table
5 Skin condition and antiseptics used for skin preparation
6 Location of electrosurgical grounding devices and monitoring electrodes
7 Operation performed and prosthetic devices implanted, if applicable
8 Specimens and cultures sent to the laboratory
9 Medications given, including local anesthetic agents, and irrigating solutions used
10 Site and types of drains and catheters

11 Type of dressing applied
12 Any unusual incident or complication

Incident Report

An injury may occur to a patient due to lack of proper care. When an accident or unusual incident occurs, whether or not it involves an injury, the person who knows the factual details should notify the supervisor at once and write an incident report. Details must be complete and accurate. They should be written as statements of facts without interpretation or opinion. For example, state that the area of the patient's skin under the inactive electrode of the electrosurgical unit was mottled and red when the electrode was removed, rather than writing that the patient's skin appeared burned by the inactive electrode. Include details of equipment used, if appropriate. Describe the action taken, care or treatment given as a result of accidental injury on both the incident report and the patient's record. Incident reports are completed per hospital policy and filed by administration. They should be reviewed as part of the overall hospital and departmental quality assurance programs.

Keep the Supervisor Informed

Policies pertaining to patients and personnel apply to nursing personnel in the operating room suite as well as to those on other units. It is very disconcerting to the OR supervisor to learn from someone outside the OR suite about events within the department that should have been communicated by the OR staff. For the safety and welfare of patients and the efficient management of the OR suite, the supervisor should learn what goes on in the department through the proper channels. Keep the supervisor informed of:

1 Any unexpected complication or change in the condition of the patient.

2 Any injury to a patient.

3 Any unusual incident, including infraction of policies or procedures by a surgeon, anesthesiologist, nurse, or technologist. Every member of the OR team has both a moral and legal obligation to report a flagrant violation of accepted standards of patient care through appropriate administrative channels.

4 Complaints about any instruments, equipment, or other supplies.

5 Broken instruments and equipment.

6 Requests for equipment not available for change of procedure.

7 Criticism that can lead to friction between team members or departments. The supervisor will discuss problems concerning another nursing unit or hospital department with the respective supervisor.

8 Any other problems that might impair efficiency within the department or leave the supervisor open to criticism if not informed about them. Seek advice and discuss minor problems before they develop into major incidents.

PATIENT SAFETY PROGRAMS

Patient safety refers to a systematic, hospital-wide program designed to minimize preventable iatrogenic physical injuries and undue psychological stress during hospitalization. Focus is on human behavior; what people are supposed to do and what they actually do. For example, whether or not a nurse or technologist is responsible for an injury to a patient due to defective equipment might depend upon whether or not the defect was noticeable and remained unrepaired when the equipment was used. Could the injury have been prevented by foresight, alertness, and good judgment? Potential hazards can be identified and eliminated, thereby reducing risks to patients.

Standards of Care

Standards provide a basic model to measure the quality of patient care. They are broad in scope, relevant, attainable, and definitive. Standards enunciate for both the practitioner and the consumer/public what the quality of health care should be. They are the criteria used to evaluate the quality of patient care rendered. Those established by national associations and regulatory agencies are recognized norms in most courts of law. Although compliance may be voluntary, because standards delineate either the optimal or minimal level of performance required, they should be achieved. Those mandated by law must be met. For operating room nursing practice, these include:

1 *Standards of Perioperative Nursing Practice.*[1] These are process standards based on problem-

[1]American Nurses' Association Division on Medical-Surgical Nursing Practice and Association of Operating Room Nurses: *Standards of Perioperative Nursing Practice,* Kansas City: American Nurses' Association, 1981.

solving techniques utilizing principles and theories of biophysical and behavioral sciences. They describe how the nursing process is used. (Refer to Chapter 4 for integration of these standards into perioperative nursing.)

2 *Standards of Administrative Nursing Practice: Operating Room.*[2] These are structural standards that provide a framework for establishing administrative practices. They include guidelines for developing philosophy, purpose and objectives, administrative accountability, policies and procedures, staffing patterns, environmental control, and quality assurance programs.

3 Joint Commission on Accreditation of Hospitals (JCAH) standards.[3] These are functional standards that relate to the optimal quality of care or services provided and the operation of hospitals and other health-related facilities, such as satellite hospital-sponsored ambulatory care services. These are the fundamental criteria used as the basis for hospital accreditation.

4 The 1965 Federal Medicare Act and the 1972 and all subsequent amendments to this Social Security Act.[4] This legislation incorporates provision that hospitals participating in Medicare must maintain the level of patient care recognized as the norm. Specific requirements are included.

5 National Fire Protection Association (NFPA) standards.[5] These standards apply to environmental safety to reduce to the extent possible hazards to patients and personnel.

6 Association for the Advancement of Medical Instrumentation (AAMI) device standards.[6] These standards provide industry with reference documents on accepted levels of device safety and performance and test methods to determine conformance. AAMI also establishes standards for sterilization, electrical safety, and patient monitoring for health care providers related to evaluation, maintenance, and use of medical devices and instrumentation.

7 Federal Medical Device Amendment of 1976. Standards and controls established by the FDA regulate the manufacture, sale, and use of many implantable medical devices.

> NOTE. The label, manufacturer's lot number, and product description of implanted devices should be attached to or included in the patient's chart, whenever feasible. If technique of implantation is inadequate, according to the manufacturer's instructions for use as approved by FDA, the surgeon is liable. If the device fails, the manufacturer is liable.

Recommended Practices

Recommended practices are optimum goals for the behavior of health care providers. They may not always be achievable, as standards are, because of limitations in a particular practice setting. Recommended practices state what ideally can be done.

The Association of Operating Room Nurses, Inc. (AORN) recommended practices for perioperative nursing concern aseptic techniques and technical aspects of nursing practice directed toward providing a safe environment for patients in the OR suite. They are based on principles of microbiology, scientific literature, validated research, and experts' opinions. Although compliance is voluntary, individual commitment, professional conscience, and the practice setting should guide OR nursing personnel in using these recommended practices.

Guidelines and recommended practices of other agencies, such as AAMI and the Centers for Disease Control (CDC),[7] also are utilized for environmental and patient safety.

Policies and Procedures

Hospital policies and procedures are established as a protection for employees and learners as well as for patients. You can protect yourself by conscientious effort and meticulous attention to learning, knowing, and following hospital policies and procedures. These vary from one hospital to another, but all are established for patient safety in that specific physical facility. Particular attention is given to policies and procedures pertaining to potentially litigious duties. Some of these are

[2]Standards of Administrative Nursing Practice: OR, *AORN J 35*(7): 1338, 1342–1343, 1346–1347, 1350–1351, June 1982.

[3]*Accreditation Manual for Hospitals* (AMH/85), Chicago: Joint Commission on Accreditation of Hospitals, 1984.

[4]*Conditions of Participation for Hospitals,* Washington, DC: Social Security Administration.

[5]Copies of NFPA standards are available from the National Fire Protection Association, 470 Atlantic Avenue, Boston, Massachusetts 02210.

[6]Copies of AAMI standards and recommended practices are available from the Association for the Advancement of Medical Instrumentation, 1901 North Fort Myer Drive, Suite 602, Arlington, Virginia 22209.

[7]Centers for Disease Control: *Guidelines for the Prevention and Control of Nosocomial Infections,* Washington, DC: U.S. Department of Health and Human Services, Public Health Service, 1981.

repeated here for emphasis because of the potential legal implications.

Identification of the Patient When a patient enters the hospital, an identification wristband is put on in the admitting office before the patient goes to the unit. The unit nurse and OR nursing assistant check the label on the identification wristband before the patient leaves the unit. The circulating nurse and anesthesiologist always check the label with the patient and surgeon, the patient's chart, and the operating schedule. The surgeon sees the patient before anesthetic agents are administered.

Protection of Personal Property Generally, it is the responsibility of unit personnel to remove valuables and prostheses before patient leaves the unit to go to the OR suite. It is the circulating nurse's responsibility to double-check the patient for contact lenses or eyeglasses, dentures, artificial extremity or eye, wig, wristwatch, rings, or religious medals. Besides the danger of losing these items, some of them constitute a hazard for the anesthetized patient.

The most frequently overlooked item on the unit seems to be dentures. These or any other item should be placed in a rigid container and labeled with the patient's name, hospital number, and room number. They should never be wrapped in a paper or linen towel, which could inadvertently be discarded in the trash or laundry hamper. The circulating nurse should immediately ask a nursing assistant to return the container to the unit. This person should obtain a receipt for the patient's personal property from the person receiving it. The receipt is given to the circulating nurse to put in the patient's chart along with a notation of the transaction in the nurses' notes.

Patients place a value on any of their property. Personnel and hospitals are liable for the care of it. A nurse can be held liable for loss or damage to a patient's personal property.

Observation of the Patient Unattended patients may fall from a stretcher or the operating table. Falls are one of the most frequent causes of avoidable injuries. Siderails and restraint straps must be used to protect patients, especially children, disoriented or sedated adults. Observe special care when moving all patients to and from the operating table.

A child or disoriented patient left alone or unguarded may sustain injury by an electric shock from a nearby outlet, or by other hazard within reach. *Abandonment* may be a cause for a lawsuit.

Since many patients receive general anesthesia and are therefore unconscious, constant vigilance is essential to safeguard patients unable to protect themselves. If a patient receives an injury while unconscious, such as a brachial nerve palsy from hyperextension of an arm on the armboard, negligence on the part of one or all team members may have to be disproved in court. Liability on someone's part would be difficult to dispute. Everyone in the operating room has a duty to monitor and protect the patient.

Dedication to Meticulous Technique Infection is a serious postoperative complication that may become life-threatening for the patient. OR team members must know and apply the principles of aseptic and sterile techniques at all times. An emergency situation in which asepsis becomes a secondary concern is a rare occurrence.

Postoperative wound infection can originate in the OR from a break in technique by a team member, from airborne contaminants of improperly cleaned floors, furniture, and ventilating systems, or from inadequately sterilized instruments and supplies. Reuse of disposable items is indefensible, as is use of an unsterile endoscope introduced into a body cavity or organ through an incision in tissues. Always carry out strict asepsis yourself and be alert to technique of other team members. Remember the principle: when in doubt about sterility, consider unsterile.

Execution of Accurate Counts Sponges left in wounds after closure are the most frequent cause for lawsuits following operations. A piece of a broken needle or a whole needle is more frequently left in the patient than an instrument; however, instruments have been left in also. The responsibility for accounting for all sponges, needles, and instruments, *before operation and at the time of closure,* rests with the circulating and scrub nurses. The surgeon and assistant take the field count before closure. If they have done their part in the count procedure, and a sponge is left in the wound because of a miscount by the circulating nurse, this nurse may be held solely responsible. In such a case the surgeon, hospital, and scrub nurse may be exonerated. Likewise, the scrub nurse may be deemed responsible for an incorrect needle or instrument count. Because exemplary hospitals recognize sponge, needle, and instrument counts to be essential to safe practice, an OR team that omits counts, and a hospital that has not established counting procedures would be in a difficult legal position. The circulating nurse should document in writing the outcome of the final counts and any unusual incidents concerning them.

Instruction for Use of Equipment All equipment and appliances must be used according to the recommendations and instructions of the manufacturer. Electrical equipment also must pass inspection of the biomedical engineering department. Exercise due caution in carrying out procedures for the use of equipment in areas of explosive or combustible agents. Electrical equipment must be properly grounded to prevent electric shock and burns. Do not use known or suspected faulty equipment. Nursing personnel who set up and operate hospital-owned equipment are negligent if a patient is injured.

Prevention of Burns Burns are one of the most frequent causes of lawsuits. A burn may occur from the use of a hot instrument such as a mouth gag or a large retractor. The scrub nurse should immerse a hot instrument in a basin of cool sterile water before handing it to the surgeon.

A patient may be burned during use of the electrosurgical unit. Inadequate skin contact or improper placement of the grounding pad or plate can cause an electrical burn. Alcohol and other flammable solutions can be ignited if pooled under the patient or allowed to saturate drapes. A thermal burn also can occur from other types of electrical equipment if improperly used or maintained.

Administration of Drugs Any drug that the surgeon uses in the operative site, such as an antibiotic or local anesthetic, is recorded by the circulating nurse and by the surgeon in the operative note. The drug is checked by two nurses, or the circulating nurse with the anesthesiologist or surgeon if a technologist is scrubbed, before it is transferred to the sterile field. The scrub nurse (or technologist) repeats the name of the drug to the surgeon when passing it. The surgeon is not held responsible if handed the wrong drug. The scrub nurse frequently has more than one drug on the instrument table. Each must be correctly identified and administered.

Preparation of Specimens All tissue removed from a patient is sent to pathology, with very few exceptions. The loss of a tissue biopsy could mean the possibility of a second operative procedure to obtain another. Specimens labeled incorrectly could mean a mistaken diagnosis, with possible critical implications for two patients. Also, the loss of a specimen could prevent determination of a diagnosis and subsequent initiation of definitive therapy. The pathological report becomes part of the patient's chart as an added record of the tissue removed and of the diagnosis.

Care for foreign bodies according to hospital policy. They may have legal significance and frequently are claimed by police, especially if the foreign body is a bullet. A receipt from the person taking them protects personnel and the hospital.

Patient Teaching

The patient and family members expect to be informed about the illness or condition and how to deal with it to restore or maintain optimum health. The patient has the right to make decisions about his or her own care. The perioperative nurse can assist, however, through preoperative teaching of deep-breathing exercises, for example, which will help the patient's postoperative recovery. Information should be provided so the patient knows how to respond appropriately. Patient teaching should be documented in the chart.

Quality Assurance Programs

Quality assurance has been defined as the establishment of criteria for measuring the degree of excellence in practice that constitutes quality, and the determination that the patient receives this level of care. Quality assurance activities attempt to identify existing or potential problems in delivery of patient care, and to resolve these problems. The 1972 amendment to the Federal Social Security Act creating the Professional Standards Review Organization (PSRO) for medical audits and utilization review in hospitals receiving federal reimbursement mandated the initiation of quality assurance programs in all hospitals. The JCAH standard for quality assurance requires "evidence of a well-defined, organized program designed to enhance patient care through the ongoing objective assessment of important aspects of patient care and the correction of identified problems."*

**Accreditation Manual for Hospitals* (AMH/84), Chicago: Joint Commission on Accreditation of Hospitals, 1983, p. 147.

The hospital quality assurance committee and/or quality assurance coordinator or risk manager (see Chap. 2, p. 33) oversee the established quality assurance programs. such as audits, and may coordinate activities of departmental quality circles.

Audits An audit is designed to measure the care received by patients as judged by established standards and criteria. The purpose is to identify both strengths and weaknesses of policies and procedures, and ultimately to correct deficiencies or deviations from accepted standards. The focus is on patient care *process criteria* or *outcome* of care.

A *process audit* focuses on a systematic series of actions that brings about an outcome. The major components of the nursing process are assessing, planning, implementing, and evaluating patient care. Through observation, a process audit determines whether or not actions taken are consistent with established standards for care in a given setting, such as the operating room. This usually includes evaluation of the environment as well as of the care rendered. Intraoperative nursing care can be evaluated through process audit.

An *outcome audit* focuses on the end result of nursing care or a measurable change in the actual state of the patient's health as a result of care received. This audit usually is done retrospectively through review of patient records. Unless every detail of nursing care is documented, an outcome audit may not reflect the actual care given in the OR, except when complications attributable to intraoperative care occur, for example, postoperative infection, nerve palsy from poor positioning, infiltration of an IV, and other complications. These may be difficult to identify unless unusual occurrences are recorded in the patient's record. Accurate and complete documentation is essential for meaningful outcome audits.

Any method that systematically examines the quality of nursing care can be termed a nursing audit. The audit must enable nurses to evaluate in an objective way the patient care they provide and to take corrective action for improvement of practice patterns on the basis of documented findings. The audit focuses on specific diagnoses and nursing tasks associated with their specific nursing problems rather than on broad, general nursing measures that apply to any patient. Preprinted audit forms used in the OR evaluate:

1 The written nursing care plan and note recorded on the patient's chart after the preoperative visit

2 Actions taken to protect the welfare and safety of the patient and to meet the identified physiological and psychological needs

3 The environment of the room used in the OR suite, including equipment and supplies

4 Records pertaining to the procedure

5 Personnel involved in care rendered

Audits encourage nurses and surgeons to coordinate their plans for patient care, improve their communications with other departments, identify needs for revision of policies and procedures, and reassess equipment, personnel, and other aspects of patient care.

Quality Control Circles A *quality control circle* is a small group of usually eight to ten staff members who work in the same department under the same supervisor. They meet voluntarily on a regular basis to identify, analyze, and develop solutions to problems in their specific work area. Each member must be committed to improving work methods, patient satisfaction, employee satisfaction, and cost containment, and be willing to work toward these objectives. This may require data collection and presentations to peers and/or management. Some problems can be solved directly by the circle; others must be presented to management with recommended solutions. The circle evaluates the success of its solutions and is committed to making them work. Documentation of quality control circle activities becomes part of the overall hospital quality assurance program.

EMPLOYEE SAFETY PROGRAMS

Orders, Judgment, and Appropriate Action

Physicians' orders must be understood and evaluated in relation to the patient's condition at the time of execution. If you do not understand an order, find out what is required of you before carrying it out. Always observe the patient closely. If a change in condition is seen, report it at once to the surgeon, anesthesiologist, or supervisor. Do not carry out an order without checking or questioning it if in your judgment it is not in the best interests of the patient. If a patient shows an adverse reaction to a medication, report this at once. You can be held liable for not reporting a patient's symptoms. They may indicate a need for special medication or treatment.

Do not assume responsibility for tasks or duties

you have not been instructed or prepared to perform. For example, the circulating nurse can refuse an anesthesiologist's request to pump the reservoir bag in the ventilating system of the anesthesia machine, or to recover a patient postoperatively. Report requests outside of your written job description to your supervisor. Your professional and legal responsibilities as well as the patient's rights dictate this course of action. The patient entrusts his or her life to others when undergoing surgical intervention. Nursing personnel must act as patient advocates when patients' rights are compromised.

Peer Review

The development of review mechanisms used for peer assessment of performance are designed to evaluate the quality and quantity of care patients receive. Peer review differs from patient care audit in that it looks at the strengths and weaknesses of an individual practitioner's performance rather than appraising the quality of care rendered by a group of professionals to a group of patients.

Peer review for OR nurses has been defined as the ongoing process whereby registered nurses with the same role expectations and job descriptions examine the nursing care provided by other individual nurse practitioners in the OR setting. The review should offer constructive criticism of the performance observed. Broad categories of tasks examined in the review should include those concerned with:

1 Patient's physiological and psychosocial needs. Are nursing actions directed toward meeting these needs?

2 Accountability and responsibility for own actions in relation to self, patient, hospital, team members, and profession.

3 Skills utilizing knowledge in application of technical, interpersonal, teaching, leadership, and communication principles.

4 Personal attributes the nurse possesses that affect professional relations with patients.

Safe Working Conditions

The Occupational Safety and Health Act (OSHA) became public law in 1970. The major purpose of OSHA is to assure safe and healthful working conditions. Although explicitly designed to protect employees rather than patients, patients do receive secondary benefits from the regulations. Reducing the frequency of work-related injuries and illnesses and making hospitals as safe as possible benefit both patients and personnel. Some of the OSHA regulations require:

1 Minimizing exposure to ionizing radiation

2 Safeguarding exposure from instruments that emit sound or radio waves, visible light, infrared, ultraviolet, and nonionizing electromagnetic radiation

3 Meeting standards of electrical codes

4 Installing ventilating systems that maintain no more than maximum allowable concentrations of atmospheric contamination from toxic and flammable chemical vapors

5 Initiating procedures for safe use, handling, storage, and dispensing of flammable and combustible liquids

6 Monitoring procedures for infection control

Puncture wounds are the leading cause of occupational injuries in hospitals. Hepatitis, AIDS, and infection can be transmitted by contaminated needles, blades, or other sharp instruments. Procedures must be established and followed for the safe handling and disposal of all sharps used in the OR. If an employee is wounded or cut, he or she must be given first aid and submit an accident report.

The OR suite is one of the most critical areas of the hospital, if not the most critical, with respect to safety control. Obvious hazards to the physical well-being of any employee should be brought to the attention of the supervisor. If the employer fails to correct a condition an employee believes to be a violation of a safety or health standard, a threat of physical harm, or an imminent danger, the employee may request an inspection by an OSHA compliance officer.

Inservice Education

Orientation of all new employees and regularly scheduled, ongoing, inservice educational programs are necessary to keep the nursing staff informed of policies, procedures, new techniques, and nursing care practices. If the quality assurance programs identify deficiencies in nursing care because of lack of knowledge, corrective action must be taken to improve performance. Audits and peer review provide specific direction for educational programs. Deficiencies in hospital policies and procedures also should be reviewed by the staff and recommendations made to revise them as necessary.

Formally organized programs of environmental safety should be included in general orientation and inservice education. Personnel must be aware of specific job hazards, and familiar with occupational safety and health programs.

Continuing Education

Professional nurses and surgical technologists have a personal responsibility for continued learning through reading and attending workshops, seminars, conferences, and other educational offerings. Education never ends with basic training. Continued learning helps the practitioner keep abreast of current trends and practices. Evidence of continuing education is mandatory in some states for renewal of RN licensure. Certified OR nurses and technologists must have evidence of continuing education for certification maintenance. Although continuing education is not a measurement for proven competence in practice, it is the most widely accepted method of self-development. Moreover, it helps maintain and update the individual's body of theoretical knowledge as a basis for sound practice and judgment.

Insurance

Liability of hospitals and individuals varies according to state laws and statutes. It is advisable to find out your own liability and that of your employer, and to protect yourself as necessary in your place of employment. Nurses and surgical technologists generally are covered by the employer's insurance. However, the hospital's insurance carrier may not be liable for malpractice exclusionary provisions in the insurance contract.

Since any patient can sue any nurse or technologist, the cost of defense may be more than you can afford even if you are not found guilty. As protection against possible financial loss from malpractice claims, nurses and technologists should have their own insurance policies. An employee may be sued individually or, if employer has to pay damages, the hospital's insurance company may seek restitution. When insured by the employer, an employee should have a certificate of insurance from the hospital. The hospital's policy protects the employee on the job only. Nurses and technologtists also should have a policy that protects them off the job.

Nurses involved in new procedures and techniques, as in teaching hospitals, are especially vulnerable to lawsuits. The hospital's insurance carrier may provide basic coverage, but hold individual employees named in a lawsuit liable for amounts that exceed this coverage.

CHAPTER **13**

ANESTHESIA: CONCEPTS, TECHNIQUES, AND AGENTS

HISTORICAL INTRODUCTION

The attempts of human beings to relieve suffering from pain are as old as the human race itself. Primitive people considered pain the torture of demons, which they attempted to frighten away by wearing charms and tattooing their bodies. The medicine men continued the use of magic.

A Babylonian clay tablet, circa 2250 B.C., gave a remedy for toothache. During the time of Nero, Greek and Roman surgeons gave their patients a mixture of wine and vinegar. It was also called a "potion of the condemned" and was used to relieve anguish such as that suffered during crucifixion. These surgeons also experimented with a form of local anesthesia by placing a carbonate stone directly over the operative area and pouring vinegar over it; they noted a numbing sensation, due to the formation of carbon dioxide. Sleep-producing inhalations were first used by the Egyptians and Arabians who concocted many potions from plants such as the poppy and the hemlock. Sponges saturated in these solutions were held to the patient's nostrils. However, death often resulted from them and from the root juices used as reviving agents because dosage was unregulated and drug action unknown. The Egyptians and Assyrians produced unconsciousness by pressing on the carotid vessels in the neck, causing cerebral anoxia.

Army surgeons have always contributed to medical advancement. Paré dulled the pain of his soldiers by compressing blood vessels and nerves near the operative area. At this time also, half-frozen soldiers were found to have a higher pain threshold. Refrigeration anesthesia was revived in 1941 for use in amputation. However, amputation often without anesthesia was the surgical trademark of the Civil War. In some instances it was performed on a kitchen table, with crude heavy knives and instruments and even table forks as retractors. If the surgeon himself was not the source of morbidity and mortality, infection and/or shock were.

Progress in anesthesia soon followed the development of chemistry and physics during the Renaissance. The modern concept of anesthesia was based on Joseph Priestley's experiments with oxygen and nitrous oxide. This combination and also ether were first used at parties for entertainment. Traveling chemists administered these agents to induce incoherence and giddy laughter, whence the term *laughing gas.* The anesthetic properties were realized when injuries sustained during inhalation of these agents were unfelt.

Dr. Crawford Long of Georgia administered the first ether anesthesia in 1842 for the painless removal of a tumor of the neck, but did not publish the results of this and subsequent cases until 1849. In 1846, however, two Boston dentists, Morton and Wells, employed nitrous oxide for tooth extraction. In October of that year, Dr. Morton first demonstrated ether for surgical anesthesia before an astounded group of clinicians; a new era in surgery was born. Dr. Oliver Wendell Holmes devised the term *anesthesia* from the Greek words meaning "negative sensation."

Sir James Simpson, a Scottish surgeon, instituted the use of chloroform anesthesia in 1847. It was administered to Queen Victoria during childbirth by England's first anesthetist. In the late nineteenth and twentieth centuries, with administration of ether and chloroform for anesthesia, operations within the abdomen, thorax, and cranium evolved. Development of the surgical specialties was concurrent with the refinement of anesthesia methods and instrumentation as science and surgery evolved.

Purification of drugs such as morphine, invention of the hollow needle, and development of gas machines hastened the finding of new anesthetic techniques and agents. Endotracheal anesthesia, first employed by open tracheotomy, was developed by Dr. Friedrich Trendelenburg. Dr. Chevalier Jackson's development of the laryngoscope greatly aided intubation. The importance of watching the patient's condition under anesthesia was realized ultimately and supportive measures were developed.

Experiments with intravenous therapy, using lamb's blood, began in the seventeenth century. The four blood types and anticoagulants were not discovered until the twentieth century. Plasma was first used during World War I to combat shock, although saline had been used earlier.

The human race is greatly indebted to the many pioneers in anesthesia. Men such as Dr. J. A. Heidbrink and Dr. Walter M. Boothby perfected gas machines and face masks. Eminent surgeons such as Dr. George Crile and Dr. Harvey Cushing emphasized the importance of keeping accurate records of the patient's condition during operation. In 1896, Dr. Cushing brought to the United States from Italy one of the first sphygmomanometers invented.

Special techniques such as hypothermia and extracorporeal circulation opened new vistas to surgeons, making possible advanced, complex surgical procedures which demand qualified anesthesiologists. Procedures lasting six to 24 hours are not uncommon.

Continuing assessment of vital functions under anesthesia, rapid pleasant induction and recovery, replacement of blood loss, and ever-developing new drugs and techniques are salient features of modern anesthesia that infinitely enhance patient recovery and the operating team's efficacy of performance. Increased specialization and utilization of computers are other facets of contemporary practice.

DEFINITIONS

Anesthesiology has been defined as "the practice of medicine dealing with the management of procedures for rendering a patient insensible to pain during surgical operations; the support of life functions under the stress of anesthetic and surgical manipulations. . ."* Understanding of common terms associated with these responsibilities is essential to comprehension of this complex specialty.

Amnesia Loss of memory.

Analgesia Lessening of, or insensibility to, pain.

Anesthesia Loss of feeling or sensation especially loss of the sensation of pain.

Anesthesiologist A doctor of medicine who specializes in the field of anesthesia.

Anesthetic A drug that produces local or general loss of sensibility.

Anesthetist A person who has been trained to administer an anesthetic.

Anoxemia Low blood oxygen; subnormal blood-oxygen content.

Anoxia Absence of oxygen.

Apnea Suspension or cessation of breathing.

Arrhythmia Lack of rhythm designating alteration or abnormality of normal cardiac rhythm.

Assisted or Controlled Respiration Maintenance of adequate alveolar ventilation by manual or mechanical means.

Biotransformation Metabolism of anesthetic drugs. They are broken down in hepatic cells where they may accelerate their own rate of metabolism or be influenced by other drugs. Metabolic products may be inert or highly reactive chemically, possibly causing destruction of liver cells. Biotransformation is a complex process. It occurs by one or more than one of four mechanisms: oxidation, conjugation, hydrolysis, reduction. Drugs are subjected to biotransformation for inactivation and elimination.

Bradycardia Slowness of heartbeat; less than 60 beats per minute.

Depolarization Neutralization of polarity; reduction of differentials of ion distribution across polarized semipermeable membranes, as in nerve or muscle cells in the conduction of impulses; to make electrically negative.

Drug Interactions Ways in which one drug affects another.

*American Board of Anesthesiology

Fasciculation Incoordinate skeletal muscle contraction in which groups of muscle fibers innervated by the same neuron contract together.

Hemodynamics Study of how the physical properties of blood and its circulation through vessels affect blood flow and pressure, i.e., the interrelationship of blood pressure, blood flow, vascular volumes, physical properties of blood, heart rate, and ventricular function.

Hyper- or Hypo- Above or below normal content, e.g., *hyperkalemia,* excess potassium level in the blood; *hypotension,* diminished or abnormally low blood pressure.

Hypercapnia Excessive amount of carbon dioxide in the blood.

Hypnosis A state of altered consciousness, sleep, or trance induced artificially in the subject by means of verbal suggestion of the hypnotist or by the subject's own concentration.

Hypnotic A drug, or verbal suggestion, that induces sleep.

Hypothermia A state in which body temperature is lower than the physiological normal.

Hypovolemia Low or decreased blood volume.

Hypoxia, Hypoxemia Oxygen want or deficiency; state in which an inadequate amount of oxygen is available to or utilized by tissue—inadequate tissue oxygenation.

Induction Period from beginning of administration of anesthetic until patient loses consciousness and is stabilized in the desired plane of anesthesia.

Lung Compliance Ability to expand.

Margin of Safety The difference between therapeutic and lethal dosage.

Narcosis State of arrested consciousness, sensation, motor activity, and reflex action produced by drugs.

Neutralization Process that counterbalances or cancels the action of an agent, rendering it inert.

P Expression for partial pressure (torr); the pressure exerted by one of the gases present in a mixture of gases. In such a mixture, the partial pressures of the gases are exerted independently of each other.

$PaCO_2$ Arterial carbon dioxide tension (partial pressure of carbon dioxide in arterial blood). Normal: 35 to 45 torr.

Pain Threshold An individual's tolerance for pain. It may be influenced by certain factors such as apprehension.

PaO_2 Arterial oxygen tension (partial pressure of oxygen in the arterial blood)—degree of oxygen transported in the circulating blood. Normal: 80 to 100 torr.

Parameter Any constant, with variable values, used as a referent for determining other variables; a constant to which a value is fixed or assigned and by which other values or functions in a given case or system may be defined.

Perfusion Introduction of fluids into tissues by their injection into blood vessels; passage of a fluid through spaces.

pH Expression for hydrogen ion concentration or acidity of blood. (Alkalemia: values above 7.45; acidemia: values below 7.35; normal: 7.4.)

Regional Anesthesia Insensitivity of a part of the body to pain caused by the interruption of the conductivity of the sensory nerves supplying that area.

Respiratory Acidosis The reduction of carbon dioxide excretion through the lungs caused by respiratory depression or obstruction, or pulmonary disease.

Tachycardia Excessive rapidity of heart action, heart beat. Pulse rate is over 100 beats per minute.

Tachypnea Abnormally rapid rate of breathing.

Tension The partial pressure exerted by a component of a mixture of gases; used interchangeably with **P**.

Ventilation The constant supplying of oxygen through the lungs.

PAIN

Pain is a perceptual phenomenon, a disturbed sensation causing suffering or distress. It is often what induces the patient to seek medical assistance. Realization of pain commences with stimulation of the nerve endings of pain fibers, which in turn produces a nerve impulse that travels to the brain. The impulse is processed and registered by the individual as an unpleasant feeling state. The quality, intensity, location, duration, and memories of pain influence one's perception and emotional response to it. No pain is undoubtedly purely organic or strictly functional; most pain also carries a psychogenic factor. Therefore, patience and discrimination on the part of health care personnel are basic to alleviation of pain.

One must also understand the anatomy and physiology of pain to assess, measure, and attempt to alleviate it. Research continues on the process and management of pain as well as in efforts to produce synthetic endogenous opiates. The discovery of opiate receptors in the brain has opened new horizons in understanding of pain control.

Any patient with trauma/tissue damage from operative procedure, ischemia (localized tissue anemia), or infarct (localized area of ischemic tissue necrosis) is a candidate for pain. Methods of surgical intervention used to relieve intractable pain are discussed in Chapter 29. Pain is beyond the domain of a single specialty.

PREOPERATIVE PREMEDICATION

Preoperative (preanesthesia) medication may be given to allay preoperative anxiety, produce some amnesia, and dull awareness of the OR environment. These drugs may decrease secretions in the respiratory tract, diminish vagal nerve effects on the heart, counteract undesirable side effects of the anesthetic, and raise the pain threshold. The preoperative medication constitutes to a greater or lesser extent a part of the overall anesthetic technique. Certain drugs may prolong the effect of anesthetic and increase a respiratory-depressant effect.

The administration of anesthetic actually begins with the giving of preanesthetic drugs. Discerning choice can lead to a smooth, effective anesthetic management and an uncomplicated postanesthetic course as opposed to a stormy, unsatisfactory experience for all concerned.

Choice of Drugs

Selection of drugs is made by the anesthesiologist based on an assessment of the patient's physical and emotional status, age, weight, medical and medication history, laboratory tests, x-ray and electrocardiograph findings, demands of the operation, and patient's concerns. If the patient is scheduled for local anesthesia (see p. 241), the surgeon may order the preoperative drugs. In choosing premedication, the anesthesiologist aims to disturb respiration and circulation as little as possible. Since more than one pharmacological response is desired, a combination of drugs is used. Most anesthesiologists prefer to have the patient arrive in the OR awake but drowsy, free of apprehension, and fully cooperative. Drowsiness and lack of fear are not synonymous; for many patients relief from anxiety is attained only by dulling the consciousness.

Time Given

The time is calculated so that maximum effect is reached before induction. It is usually given 45 to 60 minutes prior to induction. Adequate action is desired for induction and maintenance, but residual postoperative depression is to be avoided.

Drugs Used

Drugs may be classified as sedatives and tranquilizers, narcotics and antagonists, and anticholinergics. The efficacy depends greatly on the rate and extent of absorption, distribution in tissues, degree of protein binding, site and rapidity of detoxification and excretion.

Drugs taken simultaneously or in close sequence may act independently; they may interact to reduce or increase the intended effect of either; or they may produce an undesired reaction. The anesthesiologist inquires about a patient's allergies, previous drug intolerance or incidence of adverse reactions, and carefully notes any medication the patient is currently taking.

Sedatives and Tranquilizers

1 *Barbiturates*—secobarbital (Seconal), pentobarbital (Nembutal), phenobarbital—for hypnotic and sedative effect. In normal doses they cause minimal respiratory and circulatory depression, but high doses can cause respiratory depression. They do not counteract pain. Unless a narcotic is also given, painful stimuli may cause restlessness and excitation. They may be given for sleep the night before operation and to allay apprehension. Each barbiturate is metabolized or excreted characteristically. For example, phenobarbital is excreted mainly by kidneys so may be used for patients with reduced liver function. Barbiturates may react with other drugs such as Dilantin, causing variation in the latter's effectiveness. Nausea and vomiting occur less frequently postoperatively with barbiturates than with narcotics. Barbiturates may cause agitation or disorientation in the elderly.

2 *Nonbarbiturate sedatives and major tranquilizers.* Increasingly popular for sedation, amnesia, antiemetic effects, and potentiating of narcotics are the nonbarbiturate drugs such as promethazine (Phenergan), hydroxyzine (Vistaril), droperidol (Inapsine), and the benzodiazepines—diazepam (Valium) and lorazepam (Activin). Diazepam and chloral hydrate may be given orally, avoiding painful injections. Flurazepam (Dalmane) may be given for sleep.

Narcotics (Opiates) The natural alkaloids of opium (morphine, codeine), mixtures of the alkaloids (omnopon—Pantopon), semisynthetic modifications of these compounds (dihydromorphone—Dilaudid), and the synthetic narcotics (meperidine—Demerol) are analgesics. All decrease alveolar ventilation and are respiratory depressants. Lesser doses are indicated for the elderly and patients in poor physical condition or with circulatory instability because of an increased incidence of side effects related to respiration and circulation. Hepatic failure and pulmonary complications may induce unfavorable reaction.

1 *Natural alkaloids of opium,* such as morphine sulfate which is the most commonly used, produce narcosis, analgesia, and decrease of reflex irritability. They are thought to produce a moderate decrease in the amount of anesthetic needed. They pave the way for a faster, smoother induction with less anxiety, pain, and excitement. The drugs may decrease respiratory minute volume and ability of the circulation to react to stress as a result of vasodilating action on peripheral vascular smooth muscle. There is an increased incidence of hypotension. Their duration of effect may be longer than is generally expected. Narcotics are especially valuable when the patient is in pain preoperatively, but are best avoided in the asthmatic patient. Their narcotic effect may extend to the postoperative period, if the operation is of short duration, and help alleviate pain and restlessness. They constrict and stimulate smooth muscles, sometimes causing pre- and postoperative nausea, vomiting, and constipation. The latter may result because after initial stimulation, peristalsis and intestinal tone are reduced.

2 *Synthetic narcotics*—meperidine (Demerol), methadone, phenazocine (Prinadol), and fentanyl (Sublimaze). These potent drugs give good analgesia and produce fewer undesirable side effects than morphine. Meperidine is the most commonly used of these drugs. It is an effective anesthetic adjuvant and analgesic. The availability of a liquid preparation of meperidine makes it useful in postoperative pain management in pediatric patients where an oral medication is preferred to injection.

The large selection of narcotic drugs are more alike than different; one has not been found that is strikingly superior in equivalent doses. Anesthesiologists favor one or another, depending on the situation.

Narcotic Antagonist Analgesics (Agonist-Antagonist Analgesics) Naloxone (Narcan) is a specific narcotic antagonist. It has no respiratory or circulatory depressant action, whether used in the absence or presence of a narcotic. Pentazocine (Talwin) is a weak analgesic and narcotic antagonist. Adverse effects are similar to those of narcotics. Hallucinatory phenomena may occur.

Newer drugs in this group include butorphanol (Stadol), nalbuphine (Nubain), and buprenorphine (Temgesic). These drugs have antianxiety and sedative effect as well.

Anticholinergic Drugs Atropine or scopolamine are given for parasympathetic depressant action, mainly for inhibition of mucous secretion. (The routine use of less irritating anesthetic agents has diminished this problem.) The patient usually complains of dry mouth after administration. These drugs are also useful in prevention or treatment of reflex slowing of the heart, which may occur intraoperatively with stimulation of carotid sinus, intrathoracic manipulation, traction on extraocular muscles or intraabdominal viscera. While these drugs are bronchodilators, some anesthesiologists do not use them in bronchitis patients because resulting thickness of secretions and inability to cough up secretions may contribute to pulmonary problems. Dosage is reduced or drug eliminated in febrile dehydrated children, or in the presence of tachycardia.

Glycopyrrolate (Robinul) is a potent synthetic anticholinergic agent preferred by some anesthesiologists. This drug is believed not to cross the blood-brain barrier, but it reduces volume and acidity of gastric secretions.

Special Considerations in Premedication

In general, minimal, if any, premedication is given to ambulatory surgery patients. Often premedication is given just prior to operation. Agents associated with prolonged effects such as depression, vomiting, or a return to amnesia or a sedated state after awakening are best avoided. Refer to Chapter 5, p. 83.

The patient's metabolic rate varies with age, body build, and general condition. Heavy smokers, alcoholics, hyperthyroid, toxic, emotional, or high-fever patients all have a higher rate requiring more medication, oxygen, and anesthetic for effect. A lower metabolic rate, as accompanies debilitating diseases, asthenia, and hypothyroidism, requires smaller dosage.

Persons with drug addiction (abuse of barbiturates, narcotics, cocaine, or amphetamines) present the anesthesiologist with special problems concerning premedication, anesthesia, and venipuncture. These patients may have contracted AIDS, hepatitis, and in rare cases, malaria. Usually opium addicts are given their accustomed drug for premedication but they must be closely observed for premonitory withdrawal symptoms, especially during and after prolonged operative procedures. Cessation of drug intake and withdrawal may be life-threatening.

Hypnosis is valuable as a premedicant, especially in children, and for anesthesia in selected cases (see p. 251). Refer to Chapter 33 for other premedication agents more commonly used for pediatric patients.

CHOICE OF ANESTHESIA

Anesthesia selection is made by the anesthesiologist in consultation with the surgeon. The primary consideration with any anesthetic is that it should be associated with low morbidity and mortality. Choice of the safest agent and technique must be a personal decision predicated on thorough knowledge, sound judgment, and evaluation of each individual situation. The anesthesiologist aims to use the lowest concentration of anesthetic agents compatible with patient analgesia and relaxation.

Anesthetic drugs are not specific but depress activity of all cells. There is no perfect agent that would suppress only selected cells. Therefore, the ideal anesthetic agent or technique for all patients does not exist, but the one selected should include some or all of the following:

1 Provide maximum safety for the patient
2 Provide optimum operating conditions for the surgeon
3 Provide patient comfort
4 Have a low index of toxicity
5 Provide potent, predictable analgesia extending into postoperative period
6 Produce adequate muscle relaxation
7 Provide amnesia
8 Have rapid onset and easy reversibility
9 Produce minimum side effects

Ability to tolerate the stress and adverse effects of anesthesia and operation depend on respiration, circulation and function of liver, kidneys, endocrine and central nervous systems. The following factors are important:

1 Age of patient
2 Physical, mental, and emotional status of patient
3 Presence of complicating systemic disease or concurrent drug therapy
4 Previous anesthesia experience
5 Anticipated procedure
6 Position required for operation
7 Type and expected length of procedure
8 Local or systemic toxicity of the agent
9 Expertise of the anesthesiologist
10 Presence of infection at site of operation
11 Preference of the patient

THE ANESTHETIC STATE

Over the years attempts have been made to account for the action of anesthetic agents. Important theories have evolved, none of them wholly satisfactory. It is not within the scope of this text to detail these theories, only to touch briefly on them. The learner should review neuroanatomy and physiology to facilitate understanding.

Both the central nervous system and the autonomic nervous system play essential roles in clinical anesthesia.

The central nervous system possesses a powerful control system throughout the body. The effect of anesthetic drugs is one of progressive depression of the central nervous system beginning with the higher centers (cerebral cortex) and ending with the vital centers in the medulla. The cerebral cortex is not inactive during deep anesthesia. Afferent impulses continue to flow into the cortex along primary pathways and to excite cells in appropriate sensory areas. Also, the cerebral cortex is integrated with the reticular system. The brain represents approximately two percent of body weight but receives about 15 percent of cardiac output. Various factors cause alterations in cerebral blood flow and are of considerable importance in anesthesia. These factors are oxygen, carbon dioxide, temperature, arterial blood pressure, drugs, age of patient, anesthetic techniques, and neurogenic factors.

The autonomic nervous system is equally important because of its role in the physiology of the cardiovascular system, the anesthesiologist's ability to block certain autonomic pathways with local analgesic agents, specific blocking effects of certain drugs, and the sympathomimetic and parasympathomimetic effects of many anesthetic agents.

The anesthetic state involves motor, sensory, mental, and reflex functions. The anesthesiologist constantly assesses the patient's response to stimuli in order to evaluate specific anesthetic requirements. Specific drugs are used to achieve the desired results, e.g., analgesia, muscle relaxation.

KNOWLEDGE OF ANESTHETICS

Anesthesia involves the administration of potentially lethal drugs and gases. Interactions of these drugs with human physiology can be profound. Using discerning observation, astute deduction, and meticulous attention to the minutiae, the anesthesiologist provides skilled induction, careful maintenance of anesthesia, and prophylaxis to avoid postoperative complications. Responsible for vital functions of the patient, the anesthesiologist must know the physical and chemical properties of all gases and liquids used in anesthesia. These properties determine how agents are supplied, their stability, systems used for their administration, and their uptake and distribution in the body. Important factors are their diffusion, solubility in body fluids, and the relationships of pressure, volume, and temperature. The most recently synthesized general anesthetic agents are nonflammable in contrast to the older agents.

Also, operating room and recovery room nurses need to be cognizant of the pharmacologic characteristics of the most commonly used anesthetics. Anesthesia and operative trauma produce multiple systemic effects.

TYPES OF ANESTHESIA

Anesthesia may be produced in a number of ways.

1 *General anesthesia.* Pain is controlled by general insensibility. Basic elements of general anesthesia include loss of consciousness, analgesia, interference with undesirable reflexes, and muscle relaxation (see below).

2 *Balanced anesthesia.* Balanced anesthesia is a technique whereby the properties of anesthesia, i.e., hypnosis, analgesia, and muscle relaxation are produced, in varying degree, by a combination of agents. Each agent has a specific purpose (see p. 239).

3 *Local or regional anesthesia.* Pain is controlled without loss of consciousness. One area or region of the body is anesthetized. This is sometimes called *conduction anesthesia* (see p. 241).

GENERAL ANESTHESIA

Anesthesia is produced as the central nervous system is affected. Association pathways are broken in the cerebral cortex to produce more or less complete lack of sensory perception and motor discharge. Unconsciousness is produced when blood circulating to the brain contains an adequate amount of the anesthetic agent. General anesthesia permits procedures involving large operative fields usually without time limitations. It provides an immobile, quiet patient who does not recall the operative procedure.

Most anesthetic agents are potentially lethal substances. The anesthesiologist must constantly observe the body's reflex responses to stimuli and other guides to determine degree of central nervous system, respiratory, and circulatory depression during induction and operation. No one clinical sign can be used as a reliable indication of anesthesia depth. Continuous watching and appraisal of all clinical signs, in addition to other available objective measurements, are necessary. In this way, the anesthesiologist judges level of anesthesia, referred to as *light, moderate,* or *deep,* and provides the patient with optimum care (see monitoring, Chap. 14).

The three methods of administering general anesthesia are *inhalation, intravenous injection,* or *rectal installation.* The latter method is obsolete because absorption in the colon is unpredictable. Control of each method varies.

Induction of General Anesthesia

Induction is accomplished by administration of a short-acting barbiturate or other drug, or by inhalation of agent in mixture with oxygen. Induction of and emergence from general anesthesia are two crucial periods requiring maximum attention from the operating team. The following key points are critical to the patient's welfare:

1 The circulating nurse should remain at the patient's side to provide physical protection and emotional support, and to assist the anesthesiologist and closely observe the monitors. The nurse may be asked to apply gentle backward pressure to the cricoid cartilage during intubation to assist visualization of the vocal cords and occlude the esophagus, to prevent regurgitation of stomach contents (Sellick's maneuver).

2 While this period may be quiet and uneventful for most patients, untoward occurrences are possible. Excitement, cough, breath-holding, retching, vomiting, irregular respiratory patterns, or laryngospasm can lead to hypoxia. Secretions in air passages, from irritation by the anesthetic, can cause obstruction and arrhythmias. Induction must be gentle and not so rapid as to cause physiologic insult. To prevent these events, absolute avoidance of stimulation of the patient is mandatory. (Avoid venting steam from sterilizer in adjacent substerile room or clattering instruments. Do not touch patient until anesthesiologist says it is safe to do so.)

3 Precautions to be taken during induction are: continuous electrocardiography, use of chest stethoscope, readily available resuscitative equipment, including defibrillator (refer to Chap. 14).

4 Induction is individualized. For example, an obese patient may be inducted with head raised slightly to avoid pressure of the abdominal viscera against the diaphragm. The patient is placed horizontally, however, if blood pressure begins to drop. (See p. 225 concerning drug addiction.)

5 Small children need much reassurance and gentle handling. The circulating nurse can be of considerable help to the anesthesiologist in making the induction period less frightening. Sometimes a drop of artificial flavoring (orange, peppermint) put inside the face mask facilitates the child's acceptance of it.

6 Speed of induction depends on the relationship among potency of agent, administration technique, partial pressure administered, and rate at which anesthetic is taken up by blood and tissues.

Inhalation for Administering General Anesthesia

Inhalation is the most controllable method, as uptake and elimination of anesthetic agents are accomplished mainly by pulmonary ventilation. The lungs act as avenues of entrance and escape for the anesthetic although the agents are metabolized in the body in varying degrees. *The anesthetic vapor of a volatile liquid or an anesthetic gas is inhaled and carried into the bloodstream by passing across the alveolar membrane into the general circulation and on to the tissues.* Obviously, ventilation and pulmonary circulation are two critical factors involved in the process. Each can be affected by components of the anesthetic experience such as change in body position, preanesthetic medication, alteration in body temperature, or respiratory gas tensions.

In inhalation anesthesia, the aim is to establish balance between content of anesthetic vapor or gas inhaled and that of body tissues. The blood and lungs function as the transport system. Anesthesia is produced by development of an anesthetizing concentration of anesthetic in the brain. Depth of anesthesia is related to concentration.

While the respiratory system is being employed as a distributing agent for the anesthetic, it is also carrying on its normal function of ventilation, i.e., meeting tissue demands for adequate oxygenation and elimination of carbon dioxide, and helping to maintain normal acid-base balance. The amount of anesthetic vapor inspired is influenced by the volume and rate of respirations. Gas or vapor concentration and rate of delivery are also significant. Pulmonary circulation is the vehicle for oxygen and anesthetic transport to general circulation. The large absorptive surface of the lungs and their extensive microcirculation provide a large gas-exchanging surface. In optimum gas exchange, all alveoli share inspired gas and cardiac output equally (ventilation-perfusion match). Because respiratory and anesthetic gases interact with pulmonary circulation, alveolar anesthetic concentrations are rapidly reflected in circulating blood.

Alveolar concentration results from a balance between two forces: ventilation that delivers anesthetic to the alveoli and uptake that removes anesthetic from alveoli. Certain factors influence uptake of the anesthetic and therefore induction and recovery. *Uptake* has the following two phases:

1 *Transfer of anesthetic from alveoli to blood.* Rate of transfer is determined by solubility of agent in blood, rate of pulmonary blood flow (related to cardiac output), and partial pressure of anesthetic in arterial and mixed venous blood.

2 *Transfer of anesthetic from blood to tissues.* Factors influencing uptake by individual tissues are similar to those for uptake by blood. They are solubility of gas in tissues, tissue volume relative to blood flow (flow rate), and partial pressure of anesthetic in arterial blood and tissues. Tissues differ; therefore their uptake of anesthetic differs. Highly perfused tissues (heart) equilibrate more rapidly with arterial tension than poorly perfused tissue (fat), which has a slow rise to equilibrium and retains anesthetic longer. *Elimination* of anesthetic is affected by the same factors that affected uptake. As an anesthetic is eliminated, its partial pressure in arterial blood drops first, followed by that in the tissues.

Clinical Aspects of Inhalation Anesthesia

1 Pulmonary blood-gas exchange is important because defective gas exchange is the commonest cause of hypoxemia and respiratory failure. It also interferes with delivery of anesthetic.

2 Potent inhalation agents, as myocardial depressants, affect oxygenation. Most of them induce a dose-related hypoventilation, e.g., the deeper the anesthesia the more decreased the ventilation. Operative stimulation partly corrects depression and ventilation, but controlled respiration (carbon dioxide kept constant) is advised with these agents to prevent hypoventilation and reduce cardiac depression.

Controlled Respiration Respirations may be assisted or controlled. Assistance, to improve ventilation, may easily be given by manual pressure on the reservoir (breathing) bag of the anesthesia machine and implies that the patient's own respiratory effort initiates the cycle. *Controlled respiration* may be defined as the completely controlled rate and volume of respirations. The latter is best accomplished by means of a mechanical device that automatically and rhythmically inflates the lungs with intermittent positive pressure, requiring no effort by the patient. Gas moves in and out of the lungs. The combination of a volume preset ventilator with an assist mechanism maintains integrity of the respiratory center. Controlled respiration is initiated after the anesthesiologist has produced apnea by hyperventilation, or administration of respiratory depressant drugs or a neuromuscular blocker.

Controlled ventilation is used in all types of operations, especially in lengthy ones. The anesthesiologist's artificial control of respiration or the patient's respiratory efforts influences the minute-to-minute level of anesthesia. Advantages of controlled respiration are that it:

1 Provides for optimum ventilation
2 Puts the diaphragm at rest for thoracic procedures
3 Gives access to deep regions of the thorax and upper abdomen
4 Permits deliberate production of apnea to facilitate surgical manipulation below diaphragm, ligation of deep vessel, or taking x-ray

The patient is taken off a respirator gradually near the end of operation and spontaneous respiration is resumed. Or, assisted ventilation may be continued postoperatively, as in the case of an obese patient or after lengthy or open-heart procedures.

An *anesthesia machine* is used to deliver anesthetic-oxygen mixtures to the patient through a breathing system. Various types and accessories are available. Basically, the machine includes sources of oxygen and gases with flowmeters for measuring and controlling their delivery, devices to volatize and deliver liquid anesthetics, gas-driven mechanical ventilator, devices for monitoring the electrocardiogram, blood pressure, inspired or expired oxygen tension, and alarm systems to signal apnea or disconnection of the breathing circuit. Breathing tubes of corrugated rubber or plastic carry gases from the machine to the face mask and breathing system. The reservoir bag compensates for variations in respiratory demand and permits assisted or controlled ventilation by manual compression of the bag. Sterile disposable sets containing tubing, mask, Y-connector, and reservoir bag are commercially available in conductive and nonconductive materials. The elimination of waste gas, vented through an exhaust valve into a waste gas scavenger system, controls pollution of the OR atmosphere (see p. 240).

Fail-safe systems and machine design aim to eliminate delivery of a hypoxic gas mixture and to reduce possibility of human error or mechanical failure. Reference to a checklist by the anesthesiologist prior to induction enhances vigilance.

Inhalation anesthesia methods available through use of the machine may be classified as open, semiopen, semiclosed, or closed. In the *open method,* valves direct the expired gases into the atmosphere and the patient inhales only the anesthetic mixture delivered by the anesthesia machine. With this method, composition of inspired mixture can be accurately determined. However, anesthetic gases are not confined to the breathing system. High flows of gases are necessary. Water vapor and heat are lost. For children or long operations the inspired gases should be humidified for the respiratory mucosa to function properly. Also, the resistance to breathing varies. With the *semiopen system,* there is some rebreathing of the mixture; exhaled gas can pass into surrounding air with some return to the inspiratory part of the apparatus. The degree of rebreathing is determined by the volume of flow of fresh gas. Expired carbon dioxide is not chemically absorbed by the machine. The *semiclosed system,* the most widely used, is characterized by the passing of exhaled gases into the atmosphere, or else they mix with fresh gases and are rebreathed. A chemical absorber for carbon dioxide is placed in the breathing circuit. This reduces carbon dioxide accumulation in the blood. Induction is slower, but with less loss of heat and water vapor. A *closed system* allows complete rebreathing of expired gases. The expired carbon dioxide is absorbed by a chemical absorber (soda lime or barium hydroxide lime) on the machine. The body's metabolic demand for oxygen is met by adding oxygen to the inspired mixture. This system provides maximal conservation of heat and moisture. It reduces amount and, therefore, cost of gases, and reduces environmental contamination.

Techniques of inhalation anesthesia used are:

Mask Inhalation The vapor of a volatile liquid or anesthetic gas itself is inhaled from the anesthesia machine via a face mask.

Endotracheal Administration Anesthetic vapor or gas is inhaled directly into the trachea through a nasal or oral tube inserted between the vocal cords by direct or blind laryngoscopy. Endotracheal tubes are open at both ends. They have a built-in cuff that is inflated with a measured amount of air after insertion. The tube must be securely fixed in place. *Intubation* (insertion of tube directly into trachea) and *extubation* (removal of tube) are precarious times for the patient who may cough, jerk, or experience spasm of the larynx from massive tracheal stimulation. In light anesthesia cardiac arrhythmias may occur. Hypoxia is a common complication.

The patient is given oxygen before and after suctioning of a tracheal tube. Suctioning can cause adverse effects, i.e., hypoxemia, cardiac arrhythmia, tissue trauma.

Advantages: Assurance of a patent airway and control of respiration. Protection from aspiration of blood, vomitus of gastric contents, or foreign material. Minimal interference with the operative field in head and neck procedures. Airway can be preserved with many operative positions. Positive pressure can be given immediately by pressing the reservoir bag on the machine without danger of dilating the stomach. Less vapor is spilled into the room. Easy removal of secretions from trachea.

Complications: Possible trauma to teeth, pharynx, vocal cords, or trachea. Accidental esophageal or endobronchial intubation, the latter resulting in ventilation of only one side. Sore throat, hoarseness, tracheitis, laryngitis, laryngeal edema (more common in children). Ulceration and granuloma of vocal cords (late effect), ulceration of tracheal mucosa. Laryngospasm can follow extubation, especially in children. Aspiration of gastrointestinal contents can occur in patients with intestinal obstruction who are extubated before protective reflexes return. Tracheal collapse following extubation.

Inhalation Anesthetic Agents

Advantages and disadvantages of inhalation agents are entirely relative. The most important factor influencing the safe administration of any anesthetic is the knowledge and skill of the anesthesiologist. The perfect anesthetic has not yet been found, and no agent is entirely safe. With the synthesis of potent nonflammable agents, hospitals discontinued use of flammable anesthetics.

Anesthetic Gas

Nitrous Oxide (N_2O) A very commonly used inorganic gas of slight potency, it has a pleasant sweet fruitlike odor. It supports combustion. When combined with oxygen, the range over which explosion may occur is increased.

Advantages: Comfortable, rapid induction and recovery; nonirritating; few aftereffects except headache, vertigo, and drowsiness; excellent analgesic for minor operations not producing severe pain; when combined with a minimum of 20% oxygen, causes minimal physiological change.

Disadvantages: Poor relaxation; possible excitement or laryngospasm; hypoxia a hazard. Lacks sufficient potency for general surgery.

Use: As an adjunct to thiopental sodium, narcotics, and other agents. The combination of nitrous oxide with a potent agent reduces concentration of the latter needed for surgical anesthesia, thereby lessening circulatory and respiratory depressions of the more potent agents.

Volatile Liquids Volatile liquids are vaporized for inhalation by oxygen, acting as a carrier, flowing over or bubbling through the liquid in the vaporizer system on the anesthesia machine. The oxygen picks up a 0.25 to 5% concentration of the halogenated agent. This gas then mixes with nitrous oxide. Halogenation produces nonflammability. The main benefit of vaporized halogenated agents is that they allow moment-to-moment titration of anesthetic level. Known sensitivity to halogenated agents is a *contraindication* to use of these agents.

Halothane (Fluothane) A widely used synthesized halogenated compound, it has a pleasant odor. It reduces myocardial oxygen consumption more than it depresses cardiac function.

Advantages: Nonflammable, potent, versatile, chemically stable; rapid, smooth induction. High potency makes possible the use of high concentrations of oxygen for adequate ventilation. Nonirritating to respiratory tract. Depth of anesthesia can be rapidly altered. Little excitement; permits early intubation because of minimal laryngeal irritation. Spontaneous ventricular arrhythmias are rare if anoxia and respiratory acidosis are avoided. Useful for patient with bronchial asthma as it induces bronchodilatation.

Disadvantages: Potentially toxic to liver. Progressively depressant to respiration. Especially depressant to the cardiovascular system, causing hypotension, bradycardia, and, in rare cases, cardiac arrest. Sensitizes myocardial conduction system to catecholamines. Avoid concomitant use of epinephrine. May cause arrhythmias in the presence of aminophylline. Raises intracranial pressure. Limited relaxation of abdominal muscles (necessitating muscle relaxants). Has profound effect on body temperature control. May cause hypothermia. Exerts undesirable effects on rubber, some metals, and plastics. Is highly soluble in rubber and is retained in it during prolonged administration. Complete elimination of halothane takes some time.

Use: Wide spectrum—all types of operative procedures except routine obstetrics where uterine relaxation is not desired. It is a profound uterine relaxant. It is valuable as a pediatric induction agent. Because of its possible effect as a hepatotoxin, due to its metabolites, some anesthesiologists avoid repeated administration within an arbitrary time, for example, a three-month period in adults. Recent jaundice, known or suspected liver disease (past or present) are usually contraindications to its use.

Enflurane (Ethrane) A widely used, nonflammable, stable, halogenated ether, similar in potency and versatility to halothane.

Advantages: Rapid induction and recovery with minimal aftereffects. Pharyngeal and laryngeal reflexes are obtunded easily, salivation is not stimulated, and bronchomotor tone is not affected. Cardiac rate and rhythm remain relatively stable, although caution is advisable when used with epinephrine. Muscle relaxation is produced but small, supplementary doses of muscle relaxants may be required; nondepolarizing relaxants (see p. 238) are potentiated by enflurane.

Disadvantages: Respiration and blood pressure are progressively depressed with deepening anesthesia. Although biotransformation (metabolism) of enflurane is less than occurs with other halogenated agents, small amounts of fluoride ion are released. Severe renal disease is a contraindication to use. At deeper levels, an electroencephalographic pattern resembling seizures may occur. The agent is absorbed by rubber.

Use: Wide spectrum of procedures.

Isoflurane (Forane) Is the latest of the potent inhalation agents and comes closer to ideal than other inhaled agents. Isoflurane is a nonflammable fluorinated halogenated methyl ether similar to halothane and enflurane yet uniquely different. It is a more potent muscle relaxant but, unlike the others, it protects the heart against catecholamine-induced arrhythmia. Heart rhythm is remarkably stable. Blood pressure drops with induction but returns to normal with operative stimulation. A dose-related lowering of blood pressure occurs, but cardiac output is unaltered, mainly due to increased heart rate. Isoflurane potentiates all commonly used muscle relaxants, the most profound effect with the nondepolarizing type.

Advantages: Less cardiac depression; increased cardiac output, wide margin of cardiovascular safety; does not sensitize myocardium to effects of epinephrine. No central nervous system excitory effects. Rapid induction and especially recovery with minimal aftereffects (less postoperative nausea and confusion). Innocuous to organs; low organ toxicity due to low blood solubility and minimal susceptibility to biodegradation and metabolism. Provides superb muscular relaxation. Pharyngeal and laryngeal reflexes are easily obtunded. Depresses bronchoconstriction; may be used in asthmatic and COPD patients.

Disadvantages: Expensive. Is a profound respiratory depressant and reduces respiratory minute volume. Respirations must be closely monitored and supported. Assisted or controlled ventilation is used to prevent respiratory acidosis. In the absence of operative stimulation, blood pressure may drop due to peripheral dilatation. Cerebral vascular resistance decreases, cerebral blood flow increases and intracranial pressure rises, but is reversible with hyperventilation. Secretions are weakly stimulated.

Use: Induction and maintenance for a wide spectrum of procedures except routine obstetrics. Isoflurane produces uterine relaxation. Safety to mother and fetus has not been established. The drug is metabolized in the liver so may be used with minimal renal disease.

Intravenous Administration

For general anesthesia, the anesthetic agent is injected directly into circulation, usually via a peripheral vein in the arm. The drug is diluted by blood in the heart and lungs, passing in high concentrations to the organs of highest blood flow (brain, heart, liver, kidneys). Concentration in the brain is rapid. With recirculation, redistribution in the body occurs and cerebral concentration decreases. Dissipation of effects depends on redistribution and biotransformation. Since prompt removal of the agent from circulation is not possible with this method, the safety of the agents is related to their metabolism. The technique is simple and well received (often requested) by patients. Extravascular or intraarterial injection are to be avoided and it is advisable to give a small test dose at induction. Intravenous anesthesia, a widely used technique, became popular with the introduction in the 1930s of the rapidly acting barbiturates.

Nonvolatile Liquids The thiobarbituric acid derivatives are commonly used for anesthesia and offer a rapid, pleasant induction, but do not provide relief from pain, merely marked sedation and amnesia. Because solutions of them are highly alkaline and extravasation can cause thrombophlebitis, nerve injury, or tissue necrosis, they are administered via the tubing of a common intravenous solution infusion. The range of central nervous system depression produced by barbiturates is from mild sedation to coma, or cardiac arrest. Intravenous barbiturates are not appropriate for all patients, for example, those with poor superficial veins. Caution is necessary in patients with bronchial asthma, acute or chronic respiratory infections, or porphyria. Intravenous barbiturates are respiratory depressants and can also produce hypotension. Transition from consciousness to operative anesthesia is very rapid. An anesthesia machine, oxygen, and assorted airways and resuscitation equipment must always be at hand prior to administration, i.e., injection. Also, because excessive secretions in the respiratory passage predispose the patient to cough or laryngospasm, he or she should be requested to clear the respiratory passage as necessary prior to induction. Since intravenous barbiturates do not effectively block motor impulses, relaxant drugs are frequently used in conjunction with them.

Thiopental Sodium (Pentothal Sodium) The most frequently used barbiturate. It is short-acting in small dosage used for induction, but repeated administration may lead to acute tolerance and/or more prolonged effect. It is potent, has a cumulative effect, and very rapid uptake from the blood. There are wide variances in individual tolerance.

Advantages: Pleasant rapid induction (30 to 60 seconds) and recovery; nonflammable; nausea and vomiting are rare; does not irritate mucous membranes of trachea or bronchi or stimulate salivation; easy administration.

Disadvantages: Administration of large doses can cause rapid, pronounced respiratory and circulatory depression but small, divided doses are well tolerated. However, patients bear close watching as some may seem to awaken rapidly but return to an anesthetized state when undisturbed. Respiratory depression may be marked immediately following injection.

> NOTE. 1. Inadvertent intraarterial injection is evidenced by sudden excruciating pain that requires immediate treatment to prevent a chemical endarteritis with tissue destruction. Arterial spasm and ischemia must be counteracted to prevent gangrene of the fingers. Treatment: intraarterial injection of lidocaine (10 ml of 0.5% solution), which dilutes the barbiturate solution; local heparinization via the arterial needle to prevent arterial thrombosis, stellate ganglion block or general anesthesia with halothane to promote vasodilatation.
>
> 2. For extravasation, 5 to 10 ml of 0.5% lidocaine injected into the involved area dilutes the thiopental to prevent vasoconstriction.

Minor laryngeal or pharyngeal stimulation from movement of head or neck, early stimulation of the pharynx and trachea by airway insertion, blood or secretion in the pharynx, or painful peripheral stimulus can precipitate the most common complications—coughing, laryngospasm. (If spasm persists to cyanosis, a muscle relaxant and oxygen are given.) Drug cannot be removed or effect stopped once it is injected. Must be supplemented with another agent to produce analgesia and relaxation for operation. Possible excitement during recovery. Ease of administration can make it susceptible to abuse. It has been said that thiopental sodium is fatally easy to give!

Use: Excellent induction agent, its most common use, prior to administration of more potent anesthetics such as the inhalants. Short procedures not requiring relaxation, e.g., cervical dilatation, incision and drainage of abscess, closed reduction of fracture. As basal anesthetic. For control of convulsions. In patients with increased intracranial pressure. As adjunct to spinal or nitrous oxide and/or curarizing drugs. For hypnosis during regional anesthesia. Adapts to many different surgical procedures.

NOTE. Morphine sulfate and nitrous oxide have a synergistic action with thiopental sodium, i.e., when they are given together each potentiates the action of the other. They are given together with caution. Because of their combined respiratory-depressant effect, postoperative narcotics should be reduced in dosage until the patient has fully reacted. A lowered metabolic rate from the anesthetic and narcotic may also greatly prolong the usual four-hour destruction rate of morphine in the body.

Other Intravenous Barbiturates Methohexital sodium (Brevital), sodium thiamylal (Surital). Rapidity of action, duration, and potency vary. Uses are similar to thiopental sodium. These are circulatory and respiratory depressants. Methohexital sodium is used most frequently.

Dissociative Agents General anesthesia may be produced also by drugs called *dissociative agents,* the resulting state referred to as *dissociative anesthesia.* The drugs act by selectively interrupting associative pathways of the brain before producing sensory blockade. They permit operation on patients who appear to be awake (eyes remain open and movement may occur) but are anesthetized. The patient is unaware and amnesic.

Ketamine Hydrochloride A phencyclidine derivative administered intravenously (IV) or intramuscularly (IM) to yield profound analgesia. It produces rapid induction (IV—30 seconds, IM—two to four minutes); it is swiftly metabolized. Respirations are not depressed unless it is administered too rapidly or in too large a dose. It is potentiated by narcotics and barbiturates. Individual response varies depending on dose, route of administration, and age of the patient. Because of a dose-response relationship, careful selection of patient and dose are important. Its mild stimulant action on cardiovascular system may elevate blood pressure.

Use: Mainly for children two to ten years and young adults under 30, for short procedures not requiring skeletal muscle relaxation; in plastic and eye procedures when combined with local agents; for diagnostic procedures (neuroradiology); as induction agent prior to use of other general agents and to supplement low-potency agents (nitrous oxide) when adequate respiratory exchange is maintained. For longer procedures repeated doses are given that may prolong recovery time. If relaxation is needed, muscle relaxants and controlled ventilation are indicated.

Low-dose ketamine (one mg/kg) has been recommended as an induction agent for obstetrics because of rapid onset, intense analgesia and amnesia, and minimal fetal effects. With its cardiovascular stimulating properties, it is useful in hypovolemic and hypotensive patients, allowing the use of high oxygen concentration, both in obstetrics and trauma.

Contraindications: Procedures involving tracheobronchial stimulation since pharyngeal and laryngeal reflexes are usually active. If the drug is used alone, mechanical stimulation of the pharynx should be avoided. Other contraindications include hypertension, increased intracranial pressure, intraocular procedures, prior cerebrovascular accident, because this agent increases cerebrospinal fluid and intraocular pressure.

Disadvantages: Emergence reactions with psychologic manifestations may occur in the recovery period. Incidence of disturbances such as emergence delirium, vivid imagery, hallucinatory-like actions, and unpleasant dreams can be reduced by preanesthetic diazepam and by allowing the patient to lie quietly, not stimulated or disturbed except for such essential procedures as monitoring vital signs. The reactions are more common in adults. Intravenous thiopental or diazepam may be given to treat emergence delirium.

High-Dose Narcotics (Opiates) Historically the natural and synthetic narcotics have been considered analgesics given pre- and postoperatively in doses to produce analgesia and sedation. In addition they are now widely used intraoperatively as supplemental agents and/or, in combination with oxygen, for complete anesthesia in patients with little cardiovascular reserve. These include cardiac and poor-risk patients in whom cardiovascular depression must be avoided or halogenated agents are contraindicated (liver, renal disease).

The advantages of narcotic anesthesia for coronary revascularization operations are minimal myocardial depression, "stress-free" anesthesia (no increase in catecholamines and hormones), and excellent control of heart rate. Side effects include possible awareness, stiff chest, and postoperative respiratory depression. Although they are analgesics, *to reliably achieve anesthesia markedly larger doses of narcotics are needed,* for example, 10 to 30 times as much morphine (three to eight or more mg/kg body weight). High doses of fentanyl range from 50–100 micrograms (μg)/kg body weight. The drugs may be given in bolus doses or continuously via intravenous infusion. Surprisingly, side effects seem to occur less frequently as the potency of narcotics increases. In addition to reducing the adverse physiologic responses to the stress of operation such as increased work of the heart, potential arrhythmia, sodium and water retention, and increased blood glucose, the high-dose narcotic technique for complete anesthesia reduces volatile gas pollution in the OR and RR where patients exhale residue gases.

Narcotics produce a dose-related respiratory depression that can be reversed by opiate antagonists, e.g., naloxone, but this depression may recur. The respiratory effects of narcotics are:

1 Reduction of responsiveness of the central nervous system respiratory centers to carbon dioxide (less stimulation)

2 Impairment of respiratory reflexes and alteration of rhythmicity (prolonged inspiration, delayed expiration)

3 Reduction in respiratory rate before reduction in tidal volume

4 Production of bronchoconstriction (morphine, meperidine) or rigidity of chest wall (fentanyl)

5 Impairment of ciliary motion

Factors that influence narcotic respiratory actions include age, pain, sleep, urine output, other drugs, intestinal reabsorption, and disease.

The neurophysical state obtained by use of large doses of narcotics is not the same as "the general anesthesia state" resulting from use of volatile inhalation agents such as halothane. Narcotics are more selective in action. Narcotic analgesics do *not* produce muscle relaxation. Conversely, they cause an increase in muscle tone. Neuromuscular blocking agents can block or treat this action or rigidity.

The three most popular narcotics are fentanyl, morphine sulfate, and meperidine.

Fentanyl Compared to morphine, fentanyl has minimal cardiac effects—no venodilation, no histamine release, much shorter action. These effects permit deeper anesthesia without concomitant cardiovascular depression. However, the main problem with fentanyl is postoperative respiratory depression which can persist for many hours. The patient has to be ventilated for 12–18 hours postinduction. Fentanyl remains in the body long after injection, due to redistribution. Although of short duration of action, it rapidly leaves the blood stream and is highly concentrated in well-perfused tissue, such as the brain. It returns to the circulation within successive hours before it is metabolized. Thus its brevity of action is due to rapid redistribution rather than rapid metabolism. Drugs must be metabolized or excreted to get rid of their effects.

Fentanyl also can cause a drop in arterial blood pressure. It is used as a basis for controlled hypotensive anesthesia in long operations (see p. 251). However, some investigators have reported hypertension during and after sternotomy in cardiac operations using high-dose fentanyl anesthesia. Hypertension is defined as over 200 torr or an increase of 60 torr above preoperative pressure.

Fentanyl is 70 times more potent than morphine and is 1,000 times more potent than meperidine. High-dose fentanyl with oxygen can produce complete anesthesia for up to eight hours. Two synthetic fentanyl derivatives, sufentanil and alfentanil, are under clinical investigation.

Morphine Sulfate *Advantages:* Good cardiovascular stability in very ill patient, profound analgesia, only rare nausea and vomiting during induction, effective in presence of acute pulmonary edema. Morphine decreases pulmonary blood volume and increases pulmonary artery blood pressure.

Disadvantages: Incomplete amnesia, sporadic episodes of awareness, inadequate anesthesia; occasional histamine-related reactions from histamine release; significant direct dose-related vasodilatory effect on veins and arteries which increases operative blood loss and blood requirements intra- and postoperatively; severe hypotension, less common when drug is given slowly with concurrent intravenous infusion and patient in slight Trendelenburg's position; increased loss of body heat due to cutaneous vasodilatation; and antidiuretic effect, linearly related to volume of urine output; bronchoconstrictor effect that may inhibit cough and frequency of sighs, predisposing to postoperative atelectasis; tightening of some sphincters, delay in passage of gastrointestinal contents; prolonged postoperative recovery and respiratory depression.

Meperidine (Demerol) This drug causes myocardial depression and tachycardia due to peripheral vasodilatation. Following high-dose narcotic anesthesia, especially with fentanyl, the patient is awake, pain free, with adequate though not good ventilation. *These patients need very careful monitoring by a well-trained recovery room staff as renarcotization after large doses of narcotics can occur rapidly in an apparently awake and recovered patient.* The patient can hypoventilate, become hypoxic, and stop breathing when operative stimuli cease. Clinical signs to be constantly monitored include blood pressure, heart rate, respiratory rate, cardiac output, peripheral resistance, pupillary size, and skin color. The *clinical signs of narcotic toxicity* are pinpoint pupils, depressed respiration, and reduced consciousness. Naloxone is given to reverse narcotic-induced hypoventilation. The potential for delayed toxicity following intramuscular injection of narcotics, as opposed to intravenous administration, exists because absorption from muscle mass may be irregular.

Supplementary Agents Supplementary agents or drugs are used in combination with narcotics to reduce the incidence of awareness, control hypertension, and, by limiting the necessary total dose of narcotic, attenuate the extent of postoperative respiratory depression. Agents/drugs used to supplement narcotics are nitrous oxide, potent inhalation agents (halothane), diazepam, droperidal, scopolamine, small doses of thiopental. When combined with supplements, however, the relatively benign effect of narcotics on cardiovascular dynamics is no longer present. There is some loss of cardiovascular stability. Cardiovascular depression is exhibited by lowered arterial blood pressure, reduced cardiac output, and increased systemic vascular resistance. Problems occur more frequently following rapid administration or in hypovolemic, hypotensive patients.

Diazepam (Valium) A tranquilizer, anticonvulsant, muscle relaxant, amnesic drug that may be given intravenously. It is used sometimes for induction, causing less hypotension and bradycardia than thiopental. Its sedative effect facilitates awake intubation.

Etomidate (Amidate) An ultra-short-acting IV hypnotic agent for induction of general anesthesia or, in smaller amounts, for maintenance with nitrous oxide or other subpotent anesthetics for short procedures. Like thiopental, etomidate has no analgesic activity. Its main advantage is the relative absence of cardiopulmonary effects. This drug has little or no effect on cardiac output, peripheral or pulmonary circulation, or myocardial metabolism. Pain on injection and myoclonic muscle movements have been reported. But when etomidate is administered in combination with an opiate, e.g., fentanyl, skeletal muscle contractions are reduced. As with other IV hypnotics, laryngospasm, cough, and hiccup can occur during induction.

Etomidate is useful for patients sensitive to other induction agents as it does not seem to cause histamine release. Its use is contraindicated in children under ten years of age and in obstetrics, including cesarean section.

Maintenance of General Anesthesia

The anesthesiologist attempts to maintain the lightest level of anesthesia compatible with safety and good operating conditions. The anesthesiologist, as well as every other team member, must constantly watch the operative field to note color of the blood, one indication of the adequacy of oxygenation, and amount and kind of bleeding. Slow bleeding may denote poor circulation, oozing—a clotting defect, profuse bleeding—the need for transfusion. Muscle relaxation must be constantly assessed in order to provide the varying amounts of anesthesia needed at specific times. Observation of tissue manipulation is important. For example, bradycardia and cardiac arrhythmia may be caused by compression of the eye or traction on the extraocular muscles, whereas traction on abdominal viscera, placing of packs, or rapid decompression of the abdomen as from suctioning a large amount of peritoneal fluid can cause hypotension. Factors such as these affect the quality of anesthesia and patient outcome.

Emergence from General Anesthesia

The anesthesiologist aims to have the patient as nearly awake as possible at the end of the operation so that pharyngeal and laryngeal reflexes are recovered to prevent aspiration and respiratory obstruction. Retching, vomiting, and restlessness may accompany emergence, which is often similar in pattern to the patient's induction. During recovery, shivering or rigidity, slight cyanosis, or stertorous respiration are not uncommon. This is thought to be due to a temporary disturbance of body temperature control. Many agents may affect temperature-regulating mechanisms, thus altering circulation to the skin and muscle. Combined with air-conditioning, the patient is sensitive to a cool environment. These aftereffects are treated by the application of warm blankets and oxygen inhalation. Tracheal tubes are carefully removed by the anesthesiologist when the maneuver is deemed safe. Undesirable sequelae may be associated with extubation, such as cough and especially laryngospasm. The tube is not removed in the presence of cyanosis or inadequate respiratory exchange or in the absence of a means of respiratory control as when the operation endangers the airway (maxillofacial procedure). Extubation is delayed until spontaneous respiration is assured.

When it is safe to move the patient, the anesthesiologist assists in transferring the patient to a stretcher or bed, safeguarding the head and neck. Transfer must be made carefully and gently to avoid strain of ligaments or muscles. The relaxed, unconscious patient must be adequately supported. The anesthesiologist gives the recovery room nurse a verbal report, including specific problems in regard to *that* patient, and the records before transfer of responsibility.

General Considerations

1 Anesthetic agents vary in potency and therefore in the amount of analgesia they produce.

2 A deficit in pulmonary and/or cardiac function is detrimental because abnormalities of pulmonary ventilation and diffusion influence the course of anesthesia and diminish one's tolerance to stress or to insults from the anesthetic and the procedure. Subnormal cardiac reserve or oxygen-transporting ability, combined with anemia or hypoxia in an arteriosclerotic patient, for example, can be lethal. Some degree of impairment of pulmonary function accompanies general anesthesia in varying degrees.

3 Circulation is affected at many points during anesthesia, with circulatory alterations occurring both centrally and peripherally. Individual agents are associated with characteristic hemodynamic patterns. Generally, the agents are circulatory depressants that reduce arterial pressure, myocardial contractility, and cardiac output.

4 During anesthesia, respiratory patterns vary from breathholding and apnea to deep breathing or tachypnea. Drug action affecting respiratory stimulation or depression is related to changes in oxygen tension—PaO_2—or arterial carbon dioxide—$PaCO_2$. Hypoxia, anemia, and decreased cardiac output may produce inadequate tissue oxygenation.

5 The liver and kidneys are affected by general agents, for example, the rate of visceral blood flow. Alteration in liver-function tests may follow anesthesia. Halogenated hydrocarbons have been associated with hepatotoxicity. Kidney function is affected by disturbances in the systemic circulation since kidneys normally receive 20 to 25 percent of the cardiac output. Reduced renal plasma flow and glomerular filtration rate are depressions in renal function. They are related to hemodynamics and to water and electrolyte excretion. Oliguria, with reduced sodium and potassium excretion, accompanies induction. Postoperative fluid retention may result from reduction in urine volume from anesthesia and operative trauma, and use of narcotics. In the absence of renal disease, changes in renal function are usually transitory and reversible. Endocrine effects on renal function during anesthesia are important.

6 Biotransformation of agents varies with metabolites excreted by the kidneys. Urinary secretion of intravenous agents may be slow and unpredictable. Studies indicate that nitrous oxide may be exhaled as long as 56 hours after anesthesia and metabolites of halothane have been recovered from patients' urine as long as 20 days after anesthesia.

7 Agents differ in the amount of muscle relaxation produced.

8 General anesthesia is usually more complicated than local or regional anesthesia. The agents may cause nausea, emesis, or systemic complications. General anesthesia is also more expensive.

9 General anesthesia may be contraindicated for elective type procedures in a variety of medical diseases (cardiorespiratory, severe debilitation) and in emergency operations on patients who recently ingested food or fluids. Gastric suction and awake intubation are indicated. General anesthesia is avoided by some anesthesiologists for elective procedures during the first five months of pregnancy because of unknown teratogenic effects of inhalation anesthetics.

10 Endotracheal intubation is common except for the shortest of procedures.

11 Induction is usually by intravenous technique.

12 After recovery from anesthesia, the patient should be attended when he or she gets out of bed until it is safe for the patient to do so alone.

CARE OF THE ANESTHETIZED PATIENT

While safety factors are stressed throughout the text, important factors are reiterated for emphasis:

1 Team members, especially the circulating nurse and anesthesiologist, must be constantly aware of potential trauma to the patient since he or she is unable to produce a normal response to painful or injurious stimuli. Proper positioning and padding are important to avoid pressure points, stretching of nerves, or interference with circulation to an extremity (see Chap. 15). Leaning on patient during operation can be devastating.

2 The patient's position must be changed *slowly* and *gently* to allow circulation to readjust.

3 Patients' ability to detoxify anesthetic agents and tolerate stress differ greatly, but any anesthetized patient has a diminished ability to compensate for physiologic changes caused by motion or operative positions.

4 Anesthetic agents are basically depressants that affect the vasomotor and respiratory centers, predisposing the patient to postoperative respiratory complications. It is imperative that the lungs be adequately ventilated intra- and postoperatively either by voluntary or mechanical means. The patient's chest must be free for adequate respiratory excursions during operation. The airway must be patent and pressure must not be exerted on the chest. Remember that the patient under the drapes is unable to complain!

NEUROMUSCULAR BLOCKERS (MUSCLE RELAXANT DRUGS)

Use of neuromuscular blockers, skeletal muscle relaxant agents, in conjunction with anesthetics is common and has had a marked effect on clinical anesthesia. These powerful drugs give surgical relaxation in light anesthesia and are administered as adjuncts to many anesthetic agents. Deep anesthesia with its untoward effects has therefore practically been eliminated.

The drugs are administered intravenously in small amounts at intervals and may cause circulatory disturbance. They produce major alterations in respiration. The chief danger in their use is that they decrease pulmonary ventilation, thereby causing respiratory depression. Special attention to anesthesia depth, ventilation, and electrolyte balance is required.

Neuromuscular blockers may be used:

1 To increase muscular relaxation during operation; to create smoother working conditions; to shorten duration of operation

2 To widen scope of less potent anesthetics such as nitrous oxide; to lessen overall amount of anesthetic needed

3 To facilitate controlled breathing and tracheal intubation by relaxing jaw or larynx

4 To prevent contraction of the diaphragm and to give a quiet field, for example, in open-heart procedures

5 To control or prevent shivering, which accompanies systemic hypothermia

6 To facilitate diagnostic endoscopy under light general anesthesia

Types

Relaxants are classified as *nondepolarizing agents* or as *depolarizing agents.*

1 Nondepolarizing agents.
  - **a** These agents do not cause muscular fasciculation on intravenous injection.
  - **b** Their effects are decreased by anticholinesterase drugs, lowering of body temperature, acetylcholine, depolarizing relaxants, and epinephrine.
  - **c** Tetanic electrical impulses produce a gradual fade in response.

2 Depolarizing agents. These agents have the opposite effect. For example, they cause muscular fasciculation on intravenous injection.

Although theoretically antagonistic, combinations of nondepolarizing and depolarizing blockers are used during anesthesia.

Action

The neuromuscular blockers interfere with the passage of impulses from the motor nerves to the skeletal muscles. They act primarily at autonomic receptor sites, the neuromuscular junction, and at pre- and postjunctional acetylcholine binding sites causing a paralysis of variable duration. They also can affect transmission of impulses at pre- and postganglionic endings in the autonomic nervous system.

Depolarizing and nondepolarizing drugs behave differently. Depolarizing blockers generally stimulate, whereas nondepolarizing agents inhibit the autonomic receptors. Duration of action should be balanced against the duration of the clinically significant effect they produce on the muscles of ventilation. A peripheral nerve stimulator is a useful tool for assessing neuromuscular transmission as a guide to dosage, degree and nature of blockade, and evidence of muscle-response recovery during and after use of nondepolarizing agents.

Interaction with Drugs

Interaction between nondepolarizing relaxants and other drugs can result in delayed recovery. For example, antibiotics may act synergistically with nondepolarizing agents to produce prolonged paralysis. Such drug interactions are more apt to occur if the peritoneal cavity is irrigated with an antibiotic solution or the antibiotic is injected intravenously. Patients with renal failure are especially susceptible since antibiotics are excreted through the kidneys. Synergism also occurs between local anesthetic agents, inhalation anesthetics, and the nondepolarizing agents. The use of relaxants is avoided in patients with myasthenia gravis to avoid delayed recovery due to the disease state.

Neuromuscular Blocking Agents

Nondepolarizing Agents (Competitive Antagonists)

Tubocurarine Chloride (Curare) Derived from a poison obtained from certain South American plants first used centuries ago by Indians. Their poison arrows caused death by suffocation from respiratory paralysis. The action is predominantly a paralysis of voluntary muscles, resulting from blocking of transmission of nerve impulses to muscle fibers. Muscle relaxation is potentiated by halothane, enflurane, and by some antibiotics. It may be prolonged by extreme debility and widespread cancer. Autonomic blockade can cause hypotension. The drug releases histamine.

Dimethyltubocurarine (Metocurine) Has less tendency to produce hypotension than curare. *Atracurium* is a distant derivative of tubocurarine.

Pancuronium Bromide (Pavulon) A long-acting, synthetic muscle relaxant similar in action to curare but about five times more potent. It increases arterial pressure and heart rate.

Vecuronium Is related to pancuronium.

Gallamine Triethiodide (Flaxedil) Similar to curare in mechanism and duration of action. Its advantage over curare is an absence of hypotension and bronchospasm. It may cause tachycardia and increase in arterial pressure.

Depolarizing Agents

Succinylcholine Chloride (Quelicin, Anectine) An ultra-short-acting, synthetic muscle relaxant of rapid onset used mostly in intubation; it may also be used as a dilute solution to provide continuing muscle relaxation. Caution is necessary in intraocular operations, penetrating eye wounds, or in the presence of glaucoma because it increases intraocular pressure. Its use is contraindicated in recent burns, massive muscle trauma, degenerative neuromuscular disease, or electrolyte imbalance, as hyperkalemia may accompany its use. Presence of low or abnormal plasma cholinesterase (enzyme responsible for metabolism of acetylcholine) may prolong its action. Repeated intravenous administration may effect changes in heart rate and rhythm (bradycardia, ventricular arrhythmia) but this action is blocked by atropine. Return of normal function after injection is dependent on metabolism by enzymes.

Muscle contractions, caused by depolarization of the nerve-muscle end plate, are seen following injection. After this, the end plate is blocked by the drug. Muscle pain may occur after its use unless fasciculation is prevented by a small preliminary dose of a nondepolarizing agent.

Individuals susceptible to malignant hyperthermia may develop rigidity on injection (see Chap. 14, p. 276).

Decamethonium (Syncurine) A very potent, synthetic substance of rapid onset and short duration of action. It is not cumulative and has little effect on vital systems. It is used for deep relaxation of short duration such as that needed for endoscopy, treatment of laryngeal spasm, abdominal closure, endotracheal intubation. It is excreted through the kidneys and prolonged blockade may result if given to a patient in renal failure.

Blockade during Operation

The anesthesiologist must constantly verify the degree of paralysis present by noting the amount of relaxation of the abdominal wall or the limpness of extremities, or by using a nerve stimulator connected to the patient through needle electrodes. The use of neuromuscular blockers should demonstrate surgeon-anesthesiologist teamwork and communication at its best. Use of these drugs always presents the hazard of overdosage, a danger alleviated by the anesthesiologist's familiarity with the surgeon's technique and the requirements of the particular operation; thus, the anesthesiologist can regulate dosage of anesthetic and relaxant necessary to produce the conditions required at the appropriate time. For example, a major use of the blockers is in intraabdominal procedures. At different times during the operation, blockade may be more or less essential. Although tightness of tissues and inadequate exposure may be due to factors other than relaxation, such as too many packs improperly placed, it is helpful to the anesthesiologist to be told before pertinent action, such as closure of the peritoneum, is taken. Inadequate muscle relaxation makes closure difficult. Controlled respiration during upper abdominal manipulation can prevent descent of the diaphragm into the operative field.

At the conclusion of the operation the degree of residual blockade must be determined and treated if necessary for respiratory adequacy before the patient is released from the anesthesiologist's care. Sufficient ventilatory reserve must be demonstrated to overcome soft tissue obstruction and for the patient to be able to cough and breathe deeply. There must be clinical confirmation that all respiratory muscles are active.

Treatment of Residual Blockade

Although blockers are relatively safe as long as ventilation is supported, serious problems such as hypoxia, hypotension, or respiratory abnormalities may result after discontinuance. Time is required for their elimination from the body. Constant, minute-to-minute postoperative observation of patients cannot be overemphasized.

The primary treatment of residual neuromuscular blockade after anesthesia and operation is maintenance of patent airway and adequate manual or mechanical ventilation until full recovery. The action of nondepolarizing muscle relaxants may be reversed with antagonists such as neostigmine, pyridostigmine bromide, and edrophonium (Tensilon). These drugs must be accompanied or preceded by atropine sulfate to minimize side effects such as excessive secretions and bradycardia.

BALANCED ANESTHESIA

Balanced anesthesia is one of the most widely used techniques in modern anesthesia. A combination of agents are used to provide hypnosis, analgesia, muscle relaxation, and obtunding of reflexes with a minimum disturbance of physiological functions. Many variations are possible, depending upon the condition of the patient and the requirements of the operative procedure.

Induction can be accomplished with a thiobarbiturate (Pentothal, Brevital), diazepam (Valium), or a dissociative agent (ketamine). Analgesia is provided by nitrous oxide or a halogenated inhalation agent, and intravenous use of narcotics (morphine, meperidine, fentanyl). Oxygen is administered in physiologic quantities. Muscle relaxants (neuromuscular blockers) permit control of ventilation while providing muscle relaxation and optimum conditions for the surgeon. Residual effects of narcotics or relaxants may require reversal by antagonists at the conclusion of the operation.

The terms *neurolepsis* and *neuroleptoanalgesia* describe the state resulting from the combination of a narcotic (potent analgesic) and a tranquilizer (neuroleptic, psychotropic drug). The analgesia, amnesia, and sedation produced are not true anesthesia. Supplementation is necessary for extensive surgical procedures. When the narcotic-tranquilizer combination is reinforced by use of an anesthetic such as nitrous oxide (inhalation agent), the resulting state is referred to as *neuroleptoanesthesia.*

Different combinations of narcotics and tranquilizers are possible. Neuroleptoanalgesics are administered intravenously, whether used alone or in combination with inhalation of nitrous oxide. Neuroleptic drugs reduce motor activity and anxiety, produce detached apathetic state, and potentiate the hypnotic, analgesic effects of the narcotic as well as nitrous oxide. They are also anticonvulsants. The narcotic produces marked analgesia. Dosage can be regulated so that the patient can still cooperate and respond to command (neuroleptoanalgesia), e.g., as for some diagnostic procedures.

Innovar, a neuroleptoanalgesic, is a combination of droperidol, a potent long-acting (seven to 12 hours) tranquilizer, and fentanyl, a potent, short-acting synthetic narcotic. Fentanyl may cause profound respiratory depression, hypotension, bradycardia. Therefore, some anesthesiologists prefer to measure these drugs separately, individualizing doses to patient requirements and allowing more controlled injection of narcotic. An advantage of the combination is the apparent absence of toxic effects on kidneys, liver, heart (only slight cardiac depressant effect; alpha-blocking property). Droperidol also exerts an antiemetic effect. Consciousness returns within minutes but the psychotropic drug effects will persist for four to six hours after administration, causing drowsiness and indifference to discomfort. Respirations must be closely watched and patients encouraged to breathe deeply. Diazepam may be substituted for droperidol and meperidine or morphine for fentanyl. The technique is useful in aged or poor-risk patients. Neuroleptoanesthesia is one form of balanced anesthesia.

OCCUPATIONAL HAZARD AMONG OPERATING ROOM PERSONNEL

It has long been a recognized fact that substantial amounts of anesthetic gases escape into the operating room air during operative procedures and into the recovery room from patients' exhalations, thereby polluting the air. Complacency about this fact is no longer acceptable since anesthesia is thought to involve risk to all persons in the operating room as well as to the patient. Data obtained from early studies demonstrate that personnel receiving chronic exposure to waste anesthetic gas face a serious occupational health hazard, although unknown related factors, as well as stress and long working hours, may be involved. *Waste anesthetic gas* refers to anesthetic gases and vapors that escape from the anesthesia machine and equipment and those released through the patient's expirations. Possible health hazards include significantly increased risk of spontaneous abortion in females working in the OR, congenital abnormalities in their children as well as in the offspring of unexposed wives of exposed male personnel, cancer in persons administering anesthesia, hepatic and renal disease. Volunteers exposed to trace amounts of anesthetic gases corresponding to amounts present in the OR environment during a four-hour period showed significant behavioral changes including decreased perception, cognition, and motor reaction. A dose-response relationship also was seen between the least and the most exposed persons. Studies of retention of anesthetic agents in anesthesiologists following administration of clinical anesthesia have demonstrated traces of gas in expired air for varying lengths of time, from seven hours following nitrous oxide to 64 hours following halothane administration. It has been shown that high doses of nitrous oxide block vitamin B_{12} metabolism. Chronic exposure to trace levels of this gas possibly may lead to neurological problems or neuropathy.

Since an estimated multi-million inhalation anesthetics are administered annually, a substantial number of OR staff are occupationally exposed to these gases.

The United States government is concerned with the problem of the environmental effects of waste gas. In 1970, Congress passed the Occupational Safety and Health Act (OSHA). This act created the National Institute for Occupational Safety and Health (NIOSH), which has public health authority and responsibility in the research area. The responsibilities include:

1 Determination of effects of exposure to materials, processes, and stresses with potential for illness, disease, or loss of functional capacity.

2 Development of criteria for recommended standards which describe exposure levels safe for various periods of employment.

OSHA enforces the NIOSH recommendations that room air should not be contaminated by more than 0.5 parts per million (ppm) of halogenated agents when used in combination with nitrous oxide, or more than 2 ppm when used alone, over an eight-hour time-weighted exposure. Nitrous oxide should be controlled to less than 25 ppm for this same time exposure.

To reduce occupational morbidity, proper and consistently conscientious use of scavenging equipment and procedures is strongly recommended. Scavenging involves removal of waste anesthetic gases, mainly by trapping them at the site of overflow on the breathing circuit followed by disposal to the outside atmosphere and good dilution. The rate of removal of gases by the disposal system depends on the rate at which fresh air enters the OR and the patterns taken by air currents as they circulate through the room. Exposure to trace concentrations of gas can thus be reduced by 90 to 95 percent.

Personnel exposure should be reduced to the lowest practicable limits by reducing waste gas to the most technically feasible level. A waste-gas control program to ensure the continuing purity of environmental air includes the following measures:

1 Good work practices of anesthesiologists. The major source of waste gas in the OR is the intentional outflow of gases from the anesthesia breathing system. The quantity of gases discharged varies depending on the type of breathing system, gas-flow rate, and gas concentration.
2 Use of a well-designed, well-maintained scavenging system. Inexpensive, practical, effective exhaust systems are available. The gas evacuation system should be attached to every anesthesia machine and ventilator to scavenge excess gases directly into a vacuum line with a minimum flow rate of 440 ppm.
3 Use of proper anesthesia technique.
   a Different techniques of administration result in different exposure levels.
   b Components of the breathing system should fit well. Masks should fit facial contours to assure a good seal. An airway may reduce escape of gas from around mask.
   c Liquid halogenated agents should not be spilled. Gas flow should not be turned on until mask is in place or patient is intubated and connected to breathing circuit.
   d Masks, tubing, reservoir bags, endotracheal tubes should be inspected after each cleaning for leaks, holes, and abnormalities. Disposable equipment is preferable to recycled equipment.
4 Proper maintenance of anesthesia equipment through:
   a Daily routine checking of anesthesia machines for leaks. NIOSH recommends that total leak rate of each machine should not exceed 100 ml/min at 30 cm of water pressure. Leaks can be detected by use of a gas analyzer or a bubble test.
   b Periodic preventive maintenance of all machines and fittings by manufacturer's representative every six months with in-house monitoring at least quarterly.
5 Maintenance of a high flow rate of fresh air into the air-conditioning system through engineering control procedures. A good ventilating system (preferably not a recirculating one) is also important in the RR. Ventilation system should comply with HHS minimum requirements for air changes per hour.
6 Use of an OR atmospheric monitoring program to record trace anesthetic levels and to determine effectiveness of the above measures. Commercial monitors are available for each individual to wear.

Preemployment medical examination of personnel, periodic examinations for surveillance and early detection of disease, rotation of duty, and regular inservice programs to keep employees informed about hazards and current data are advocated until further research is completed. New members of the OR staff of some hospitals receive a letter explaining the risks as known at that time. When personnel leave employment in the OR area, the records should be retained in the permanent file after their termination of service.

LOCAL OR REGIONAL ANESTHESIA

Action

Local anesthesia depresses superficial nerves and blocks conduction of pain impulses from a specific area or region. Sensory nerves are affected first. The patient remains conscious. Regional anesthesia (for example: spinal) may be employed when general anesthesia is contraindicated or undesired.

Sometimes local anesthesia is used as an adjunct to general anesthesia for decreasing operative stimuli, thereby diminishing the general stress response to trauma. The local anesthetic is used during manipulation of highly sensitive tissues to reduce sensory reflexes to painful stimuli in the operative field. Injected at the site of operation, it temporarily disconnects the operative site from the central nervous system.

Preparation of the Patient

Patients who are to receive a local anesthetic need preparation that may differ somewhat from that of patients about to receive a general anesthetic. These preparations depend on extent of the procedure to be performed and on anticipated technique of administration. Although it is anticipated that the patient will remain conscious, it is sometimes desirable or necessary to supplement local anesthesia with narcosis or light general anesthesia, in which case preparation for a general anesthetic is followed. Careful preoperative assessment, history taking, preanesthetic medication, and a clear explanation of what to expect, such as paresthesias, are as essential as for general anesthesia. Preoperative orders regarding the time when the patient should cease taking anything by mouth vary with the circumstances; at least four hours prior to operation is a frequent cutoff time since the patient may vomit from apprehension or untoward reaction. Often a preoperative barbiturate or diazepam is ordered before the use of a local anesthetic agent. Medication is given as ordered. Patients are transported via stretcher.

Care of the Patient during Operation

The patient must be cooperative and willing to be awake, although drowsy from premedication. Psychological support must be given during the operation. However, supplementary agents should be available for analgesia or anesthesia as necessary. Gentle manipulation of the patient, including concern for the hearing sense, cannot be overemphasized for the patient in a conscious or semiconscious state.

These patients need careful observation throughout the operation, and for a period of time afterward, for symptoms of delayed reaction or complications. The patient may not be attended by an anesthesiologist. The surgeon may inject or topically apply the anesthetic drug. This depends, however, on the type or length of the procedure. When an anesthesiologist's presence is desired, the operation is scheduled as *attended local.*

The circulating nurse is responsible for *every* patient's safety and nursing care. *In the absence of an anesthesiologist, the circulating nurse is totally responsible for monitoring* the patient's vital signs and intravenous infusion, *and for recording* these data as well as the total amount of anesthetic and supplementary drugs administered to the patient (see Chap. 14, p. 258).

In addition, resuscitative equipment must be at hand prior to the administration of any anesthetic. If any reaction is observed, the patient is informed of it for his or her protection in future anesthesias.

Advantages of Local Anesthesia

1 Infiltration anesthetic agents are nonflammable.

2 Local anesthesia needs minimal simple equipment, provides economy.

3 Loss of consciousness does not occur, unless supplemented. Local anesthesia avoids the undesirable effects of general anesthesia.

4 It is suitable for patients who recently ingested food or fluids (as in obstetrics and emergency operation); for ambulatory patients; for minor procedures; for procedures where it is desirable to have the patient awake and cooperative.

5 The surgeon can administer the anesthetic in instances of unavailability of an anesthesiologist.

Disadvantages of Local Anesthesia

1 It is not practical for all types of procedures. For example, too much drug would be needed for some major operations; duration of anesthesia is insufficient for others.

2 There are individual variations in response to local anesthetic drugs.

3 Too rapid absorption of the drug into the blood, as in overdosage, can cause severe, potentially fatal reactions.

4 Apprehension may be increased by the patient's ability to see and hear. Some patients prefer to be unconscious and unaware.

Contraindications to Local Anesthesia

These factors are variable and exceptions may be found. Local anesthesia is generally contraindicated in patients with:

1 Allergic sensitivity to the local drug.

2 Local infection or malignancy, which may be carried to and spread in adjacent tissues by injection. A bacteriologically safe injection site should be selected.

3 Septicemia. In a proximal nerve block, a needle may open new lymph channels that drain through a region, thereby causing new foci and local abscess formation from the perforation of small vessels and exit of bacteria.

4 Highly nervous, apprehensive, excitable patients or those unable to cooperate because of mental state or age.

Techniques of Administration

Topical Application The anesthetic is applied directly to a mucous membrane, to a serous surface, or into an open wound. It is most often employed for anesthesia of respiratory passages to eliminate laryngeal reflexes and cough, for insertion of airways before induction or during light general anesthesia, or for therapeutic and diagnostic procedures such as laryngoscopy or bronchoscopy. It is also used in cystoscopy. Mucous membranes readily absorb topical agents because of their vascularity. Onset of anesthesia occurs within a minute. Volume of the topical agent in the blood may equal the same level obtained by intravenous injection. Duration of anesthesia is 20 to 30 minutes. Ointments or solutions may be used. If a spray or atomizer is used it should contain a visible reservoir so that the quantity of drug administered is clearly observed because droplets vary in size.

Preanesthetic sedation and atropine are important prior to topical application within the respiratory tract. The atropine is necessary as saliva can dilute the anesthetic and prevent adequate duration of contact with the mucous membrane. Also, a dry throat is necessary to prevent aspiration until the anesthetic effect has disappeared and throat reflexes have returned. Adverse reaction to topical anesthetic agents is not uncommon unless dosage is carefully controlled. Sudden cardiovascular collapse occurs most frequently following topical anesthesia of the respiratory tract, according to statistics.

Simple Local Infiltration The agent is injected intracutaneously and subcutaneously into the tissues at the incisional site to block peripheral nerve stimuli at their origin. It is used in suturing superficial lacerations or in the excision of minor lesions.

Regional Application The agent is injected into or around a specific nerve or group of nerves to depress the entire sensory nervous system of a limited, localized area of the body. The injection is at a distance from the operative site. A wider, deeper area is anesthetized than with simple infiltration. There are several types of regional anesthesia:

Nerve Block Anesthetizing of a selected nerve at a given point. Nerve blocks are performed to interrupt sensory, motor, or sympathetic transmission. Blocks may be used operatively, to prevent pain of the procedure; diagnostically, to ascertain cause of pain; or therapeutically, to relieve chronic pain and to prognosticate. These blocks are useful in various circulatory and neurosurgical syndromes. Each type of block carries unique complication potential. For example, *complications* of intercostal block are pneumothorax, atelectasis, total spinal anesthesia, air embolism, transverse myelitis; of brachial plexus block: pneumothorax, hemothorax, recurrent laryngeal paralysis, phrenic paralysis, subarachnoid injection, Horner's syndrome (axillary approach preferred to interscalene approach); stellate ganglion block: pneumothorax; celiac block: large vessel perforation, total spinal anesthesia. Some examples of blocks employed are:

1 Operative blocks: paravertebral (cervical plexus) block, for the area between the jaw and clavicle; intercostal block, for relatively superficial intraabdominal procedures; arm (brachial plexus, axillary) block; block at the elbow or wrist (median, radial, or ulnar nerve); hand and digital block, for fingers. In the latter, epinephrine is not added to the local agent as gangrene can result from inadequate circulation.

2 Diagnostic or therapeutic blocks: utilized to block sympathetic nerve ganglia. Desired vasodilatation is produced by paralysis of the sympathetic nerve supply to the constricting smooth muscle in the artery wall. Stellate ganglion block is used to increase circulation in peripheral vascular disease in the head, neck, arm, or hand. Paravertebral lumbar block increases circulation in the lower extremities. Celiac block may be used for relief of abdominal pain of pancreatitis or pancreatic malignancy.

NOTE. 1. With the proliferation of pain clinics concerned with the management of acute and chronic pain problems, the anesthesiologist plays an essential role as part of the multidisciplinary staff and activities. Because of familiarity with anesthetic drugs, nerve pathways, and nerve block techniques, the anesthesiologist is of great service to both colleagues and patients in assessing and treating pain, especially if amenable to nerve block.

2. Chronic intraspinal narcotic analgesia may provide sustained pain relief in patients with terminal malignancy (e.g., colorectal). This involves percutaneous epidural catheters, implanted epidural catheter with infusion port

or reservoir and pump, or implantable infusion devices.

Intravenous Regional (Bier) Block with Tourniquet Intravenous injection of a local anesthetic in an extremity. It involves draining of blood from the extremity by use of a tourniquet after placement of an intravenous catheter and subsequent injection close to site of operation of a fixed quantity of local drug that is confined to the area by tourniquet (see Chap. 17, p. 335). The tourniquet is applied to the leg for foot operation, to the forearm for hand or wrist operation, and to the arm for operation above the wrist. It is used more for upper extremity (minor arm) procedures and for those that last only one hour or less.

At the conclusion of the operation and release of the tourniquet, entry of a bolus of remaining local anesthetic into the systemic circulation may cause cardiovascular or central nervous system symptoms of toxicity.

Field Block Blocking off of operative site with wall of anesthetic solution by series of injections into proximal and surrounding tissues, as, for example, abdominal wall block for herniorrhaphy.

SPINAL ANESTHESIA

Intrathecal Block

Intrathecal block, commonly referred to as *spinal anesthesia,* is a technique of regional anesthesia. The agent is injected into the subarachnoid space, using a lumbar interspace, causing desensitization of spinal ganglia and motor roots. Absorption into the nerve fibers is rapid. The level of anesthesia attained depends on various factors: position during and immediately after injection; cerebrospinal fluid pressure; site and rate of injection; volume, dosage, and specific gravity (baricity) of the solution; inclusion of a vasoconstrictor (epinephrine); spinal curvature; interspace chosen; coughing or straining, which can inadvertently raise the level. Spread of the anesthetic is controlled mainly by solution baricity and patient position. The period immediately following injection is decisive, when the anesthetic is becoming "fixed," absorbed by the tissues and unable to travel. Further control of the anesthetic level is attained by tilting the operating table at that time. The direction of tilting depends on whether the agent is *hyperbaric* (specific gravity greater than that of spinal fluid) or *hypobaric* (lighter than spinal fluid). *Isobaric* anesthetics (same weight as spinal fluid) are made hyperbaric by the addition of 5 or 10% dextrose to the anesthetic before injection.

Immediately after injection, the anesthesiologist carefully tests the level of anesthesia by pinprick, tilting table as necessary to achieve desired level for the operation. After anesthetic fixation, with the anesthesiologist's permission, the patient is placed in operative position. The patient is asked to relax and let the team turn him or her. Straining or breathholding can precipitate hypotension or inadvertent rise in level of anesthesia. Incision is never made until it is certain that anesthesia is adequate. Supplementation of spinal anesthesia is necessary if anesthesia or muscular relaxation is insufficient or the patient is unduly apprehensive. Sometimes patient is kept in a light sleep with an intravenous agent.

Choice of Agent This depends on various factors such as duration, intensity, and level of anesthesia desired, anticipated operative position of the patient, and the operative procedure.

Duration of Agent The variable duration of anesthesia depends on physiologic, physical, and metabolic factors. It is prolonged by addition of a vasoconstrictor. Anesthesia diminishes as the agent is absorbed into systemic circulation.

Procedure

For injection, the patient is placed in the position desired by the anesthesiologist, depending on solution baricity and anesthesia to be produced.

1 *Lateral Position.* The most common, the patient's back is at edge of operating table, parallel to it, knees flexed onto abdomen, and the head flexed to the knees. Hips and shoulders are vertical to table to prevent rotation of spine.

2 *Sitting Position.* The patient sits on the side of table with feet resting on a stool. The spine is flexed, with chin lowered to sternum, arms crossed and supported on a pillow on an adjustable table or Mayo stand.

3 *Prone Position.* The patient lies face downward on table.

The circulating nurse or a nursing assistant supports the patient in position, observes and reassures him or her, and assists the anesthesiologist in any way possible. Attention to asepsis is extremely important. The anesthesiologist dons sterile gloves before handling sterile items. Sterile disposable spinal trays eliminate the need for meticulous cleaning and sterilizing of nondisposable equipment. They also avoid the hazards of sterilizing ampuls. The *tray* contains:

1 Drape
2 Ampul file
3 Ampuls of local anesthetic, spinal anesthetic, vasoconstrictor drug, 10% dextrose
4 Ultrapore filter to draw up solution
5 Sponges
6 Needles: 25-gauge hypodermic for infiltration of local anesthetic into skin; 22-gauge, 2 in. (5 cm) long, for intramuscular injection; blunt 18-gauge for mixing drugs; 22- or 26-gauge, 3½ in. (9 cm) long, spinal needles with stylets for intrathecal injection
7 Syringes: 5 cc for spinal anesthetic, 10 cc for hypobaric solutions, 2 cc for superficial anesthesia

Forceps and sponges are of a different type than those counted and used during operation. The lumbar puncture site is cleansed with an antiseptic solution and draped with a fenestrated drape. The blood pressure is checked before, during, and after spinal anesthesia as hypotension is common.

Use of Spinal Anesthesia

For abdominal (mainly lower) or pelvic procedures requiring relaxation; inguinal or lower extremity procedures; operative obstetrics (cesarean section—lacks effect on fetus); urological procedures. It is advised for alcoholics, barbiturate addicts, very muscular patients who would need large doses of general anesthetic and muscle relaxant, and for emergency operations in patients who have eaten recently. It is also used in the presence of hepatic, renal, or metabolic disease because of minimal upset of body chemistry.

Advantages Patient is conscious if desired, throat reflexes are maintained; nonirritating to the respiratory system; no difficulty with airway problems; quiet breathing; contracted bowel; excellent muscle relaxation and anesthesia if properly executed.

Disadvantages Spinal anesthesia produces a circulatory depressant effect and stasis of blood as a result of interference with venous return from motor paralysis and arteriolar dilatation in the lower extremities. Change in body position may be followed by sudden drop in blood pressure. *After fixation of anesthetic,* slight head-down position may increase venous return to the heart. Agent cannot be removed after injection. Nausea and emesis may accompany cerebral ischemia, traction on viscera, or premedication. Possible sensitivity to the agent; danger of trauma or infection. Patient can hear. Rarely, distended bowel is perforated.

Postanesthetic Complications Transient or permanent neurological sequelae from trauma, irritation by the agent, lack of asepsis, loss of spinal fluid with decreased intracranial pressure syndrome. Examples: postural dependent spinal headache; auditory and ocular disturbances such as tinnitus, diplopia; arachnoiditis, meningitis; transverse myelitis; cauda equina syndrome (failure to regain use of legs or control of urinary and bowel function); temporary paresthesias such as numbness and tingling; cranial nerve palsies; urinary retention. Late complications include nerve root lesions, spinal cord lesions, ruptured nucleus pulposus.

NOTE. 1. True spinal headache due to persistent cerebrospinal fluid leak through the needle hole in the dura usually responds to supine bed rest, copious oral or IV fluids, and systemic analgesia. Refractory postspinal headache may be treated by an epidural blood patch; five to eight milliliters of the patient's own blood is administered at the puncture site. This usually affords prompt relief.

2. If high levels of anesthesia are used, extreme caution is essential to prevent respiratory paralysis ("total spinal"), an emergency situation requiring artificial ventilation until the level of anesthesia has receded. Respiratory arrest, although rare, is thought to be due to medullary hypoperfusion. Apnea also can be produced by respiratory center ischemia due to precipitous hypotension.

3. Anesthesia machine, oxygen, and intravenous infusion must be in readiness before injection. Constant vigilance of respiration and circulation is mandatory. Blood pressure must be maintained.

4. Serial injection, "continuous" technique—intermittent injections of anesthetic given via plastic catheter—may be used for long procedures or where better control of anesthesia is desired, but is rare.

EPIDURAL (PERIDURAL) ANESTHESIA

Injection is made into space surrounding dura mater within the spinal canal. Spread of the anesthetic and duration of action are influenced by concentration and volume of solution injected (total drug mass), and rate of injection. The anesthetic diffuses toward the head and caudad. In contrast to spinal anesthesia, position, baricity and gravity have little influence on anesthetic distribution. The high incidence of systemic reactions is attributed to absorption of agent from the highly vascular peridural area and the relatively large mass of anesthetic injected. Epinephrine 1:200,000 is usually added to retard absorption. Two approaches may be used: the lumbar, the more common, and caudal.

Lumbar Approach

The lumbar approach is a peridural block. Equipment is similar to spinal, with addition of 19-gauge, 3½ in. (9 cm) long, thin-walled needle with stylet with a rigid shaft and short bevel tip to minimize danger of inadvertent dural puncture. Insertion of a catheter allows repeated injections for *continuous epidural,* requiring additional needles, stopcocks, and plastic catheter in the setup.

Caudal Approach

The caudal approach is an epidural sacral block. Injection epidurally is through the caudal canal, desensitizing nerves emerging from the dural sac. Position for injection: prone, with hips flexed, sacrum horizontal, and heels turned outward to expose injection site. Sacral area is prepared and draped, with care taken to protect genitalia from irritating solution. Lateral position is used in pregnant patients. Care must be taken in pregnant patients to avoid perforating the rectum or fetal head during labor. Spread of agents in epidural anesthesia is enhanced in pregnancy as well as in atherosclerosis and advanced age.

Spinal tray includes addition of 20-gauge, 1½ in. (4 cm) long spinal needle with stylet. Commercial sets are available. Skin and ligaments are infiltrated with a local anesthetic agent before inserting spinal needle.

Use of Epidural Anesthesia

Uses include: anorectal, vaginal, perineal procedures; intractable or prolonged pain; obstetrics. Continuous technique is sometimes employed for labor and delivery. Patient must be constantly attended by trained personnel once the block is initiated as for obstetric analgesia. Continuous electronic monitoring of fetal heart is recommended because of the patient's insensibility to uterine contractions.

Management and sequelae of epidural anesthesia are similar to spinal anesthesia.

Advantages Compared to spinal anesthesia, there is a lesser degree of hypotension, headache, and potential for neurologic complications, although a higher failure rate is reported.

Disadvantages Less controllable height of anesthesia; more difficult technique; area of potential infection from anaerobic organisms with the caudal approach; unpredictable; time-consuming—longer time for complete anesthesia; larger amount of agent injected; continuous technique may slow the first stage of labor.

Complications Intravascular injection, accidental dural puncture and total spinal anesthesia, blood vessel puncture and hematoma, profound hypotension, backache, transient or permanent paralysis (paraplegia).

LOCAL AND REGIONAL ANESTHETIC AGENTS

Local anesthetics in solution exist as hydrochloride salts of weak bases. Chemically the commonly employed agents are esters or amide compounds. They differ in structure and therefore in action. These drugs are applied to body surfaces or injected around nerves essentially to prevent the pain of surgical procedures but also to diagnose and treat pain associated with disease or trauma. They vary in potency, penetration, duration, rapidity of hydrolysis or destruction, and toxicity, detoxification occurring in the liver. All are direct myocardial depressants but central nervous system effects precede this depression.

Action

These drugs interfere with initiation and transmission of nerve impulses by mechanisms based on physical and biochemical changes, interacting with the membrane that ensheaths nerve fibers. The drugs retard and stop propagation of nerve impulses, eventually blocking conduction. This is accomplished by blocking a peripheral stimulus at its origin (topical application or local infiltration), transmission of stimuli along afferent nerves from operative site (regional anesthesia), and conducting pathways in and around spinal cord (spinal and epidural). Their duration of action depends not only on their pharmacological properties but also on volume and concentration of solution and whether it is combined with a vasoconstrictor to slow circulatory uptake and absorption, prolong anesthesia, and decrease bleeding. Epinephrine 1:200,000 or 1:400,000 may be used for these purposes, added to the local agent or commercially supplied in the solutions. If adding it to a solution, it is best to do so with a calibrated syringe rather than with a dropper, an inaccurate method. Pharmacological effects of epinephrine sometimes displayed are those of acute adrenergic response: palpitation, tachycardia, tremor, pallor, diaphoresis.

Local blood flow and vascularity can markedly influence local anesthetic action and systemic absorption. Fibrous tissue and fat contained in some injection sites act as diffusion barriers and nonspecific binding sites.

Conduction Velocity Nerve fibers vary in their susceptibility to local anesthetic agents. The larger the fiber, the greater the concentration of anesthetic required. In practice, the least amount of the lowest concentration of the anesthetic agent to achieve the desired effect should be administered.

Blocking Quality Depends on potency, latency (time between administration and maximum effect), duration of action, regression time (time between beginning and end of pain perception).

Characteristics of an Acceptable Agent

These include high potency, minimal systemic activity, prompt metabolism, lack of local irritation, reversibility of action, regional as well as topical efficacy, stability during sterilization and storage. Not every agent will possess all attributes; the perfect agent does not yet exist.

Hyaluronidase is a drug that is sometimes added to local anesthetic agents to facilitate spread of a local agent through tissues and create more certainty of reaching all desired nerves. This property also causes more rapid absorption of local anesthetic and may reduce intensity and duration of its effect. More rapid absorption may also increase the possibility of a systemic reaction (see Chap. 14, p. 255).

Types

A number of different local or regional anesthetic drugs are in use. They may be categorized by potency or duration of action, or chemical structure. The *esters* include:

Cocaine Hydrochloride The first local anesthetic introduced, cocaine is a crystalline powder with a bitter taste in solution. It is the most toxic of local drugs and, in contrast to all but lidocaine hydrochloride, is a vasoconstrictor. Cocaine reduces bleeding and shrinks congested mucous membranes. It causes temporary paralysis of sensory nerve fibers, produces exhilaration, lessens hunger and fatigue, and stimulates pulse and respiratory rates. *Administration is by topical application only* because of its high toxicity; the solution penetrates mucous membrane. Epinephrine should *not* be added. When applied to the throat, cocaine abolishes throat reflexes. The patient is awake and can cooperate, but disadvantages are its limited use and possible addiction. It is used topically in 4 to 10% concentration for anesthesia of the respiratory tract (nose, pharynx, tracheobronchial tree). Untoward reactions may occur rapidly in response to even a very small amount of the drug. Maximum dose: 200 mg or 4 mg/kg body weight.

Procaine Hydrochloride (Novocain) Similar to cocaine but less toxic. Concentrations used: 0.5% for infiltration; 1 to 2% for peripheral nerves. It is injected subcutaneously, intramuscularly, or intrathecally. It has low potency; it is of short duration; it is ineffectual topically. Its advantages include minimal toxicity, easily sterilized solution, low cost, and lack of local irritation. Newer agents are used more frequently. Maximum dose: 1,000 mg (one gram) or 14 mg/kg body weight.

Chloroprocaine Hydrochloride (Nesacaine) Possibly the safest local anesthetic from the standpoint of systemic toxicity because of its fast metabolism. It has moderate potency of short duration. It is rapidly hydrolyzed in the plasma. Its action is fast but it is not active topically. When used in obstetrics it does not detectably alter neurobehavioral responses of newborn infants. For infiltration: 0.5%; for peripheral nerves: 2%. Maximum dose: 1,000 mg (one gram).

Tetracaine Hydrochloride (Pontocaine) A very potent agent. Onset of analgesia is slow but duration of effect is longer than that of many other drugs. It has high potency of long duration. It is also more systemically toxic because of the slow rate of its destruction in the body but low total dosage tends to reduce chance of reaction. However, high incidence of reported reaction may be attributed to rapid absorption rate from respiratory tract mucosa. Use: 1 to 2% as *topical* anesthetic in the pharynx, tracheobronchial tree. Maximum dose: 80 mg; 0.5% for corneal anesthesia in ophthalmology. Infrequently for infiltration and nerve injection: 0.1 to 0.25%. Maximum dose: 100 mg.

The *amides* include:

Lidocaine Hydrochloride (Xylocaine, lignocaine) Probably the most widely used agent, this is a potent anesthetic of twice the duration of procaine. It is also more toxic, being slowly hydrolyzed in circulating plasma. It undergoes hepatic degradation. Dosage should be reduced if hepatic function or blood flow is impaired. Its major advantages are rapid onset of anesthesia and lack of local irritant effect. Allergic reactions are rare. Used extensively for operative procedures and dentistry, it has moderate potency and duration of action. For infiltration: 0.5%; for peripheral nerves: 1 to 2%. Maximum dose: 500 mg (0.5 g) or 7 mg/kg body weight. It is a good topical anesthetic although not as effective as cocaine. For topical use in respiratory tract: 2 to 4%. Maximum dose: 200 mg. It is commonly used topically prior to intubation. Lidocaine also is used in the management of ventricular arrhythmias during and after cardiac procedures, in resuscitation after cardiac arrest, and in treatment and prevention of irritability in patients who have experienced myocardial infarction. Clinical indications of lidocaine toxicity usually are related to the central nervous system (see Chap. 14, p. 256). Excessive doses can produce myocardial and circulatory depression.

Mepivacaine Hydrochloride (Carbocaine) Similar to lidocaine hydrochloride, it takes effect rapidly but produces 20 percent longer duration of anesthesia. It has moderate potency and duration of action. It is commonly employed for infiltration and nerve block. It produces minimal tissue irritation and few adverse reactions. Epinephrine may *not* be added to it because of its duration. For infiltration: 0.5 to 1%; for peripheral nerves: 1 to 2%. Maximum dose: 500 mg.

Bupivacaine Hydrochloride (Marcaine) Four times more potent than lidocaine, its high potency is of long duration. Onset of anesthesia is slow but duration is two to three times longer than that of lidocaine or mepivacaine, with toxicity approximate to that of tetracaine. Cumulation occurs with repeated injection. The drug affords prolonged pain relief following caudal block for rectal procedures. It is safely used in lower concentrations for epidural anesthesia in obstetrics because of less placental transfer than with other amide type agents. Also, bupivacaine has been shown to spare motor function while providing adequate analgesia, thus allowing more parturient participation in delivery. It produces profound relaxation for intraabdominal procedures. Used for infiltration and peripheral nerves: 0.25 to 0.75%. Maximum dose: 500 mg or 3 mg/kg body weight.

Dibucaine Hydrochloride (Nupercaine, Percaine, Cinchocaine) A very potent anesthetic producing a high rate of systemic toxicity. Lower concentrations are needed to decrease the incidence of adverse reactions. It has long duration of action. It is infrequently used topically in 0.2% concentration. Maximum dose: 30 mg.

Etidocaine Hydrochloride (Duranest) An agent similar to lidocaine but of greater potency and longer duration of action. For infiltration and peripheral nerves: 0.25 to 0.75%. Maximum dose: 500 mg.

DRUG INTERACTIONS

Anesthesiologists and/or surgeons frequently administer many drugs to patients already under the influence of several different pharmacological agents when they come to the OR. A substantial number of all hospitalized patients in the United States experience some form of an adverse drug reaction. Some seriously ill patients may receive as many as 20 drugs concurrently. Modern balanced anesthesia may involve use of eight or more different drugs, including those used for premedication. Spinal anesthesia, a relatively simple technique, usually involves at least five drugs. All drugs in use must be considered potential "interactors" with some other drug. A simple shift in pH can cause a significant alteration in action, effectiveness, distribution, and excretion of such common drugs as barbiturates and local anesthetics. Many drugs used in anesthesia are weak acids (barbiturates) and weak bases (local agents and vasopressors). Advertently or inadvertently the anesthesiologist can modify these physicochemical characteristics and thus alter effects of drugs.

In addition, many variables modify the action of anesthetic agents, such as dose, circulatory adaptation, ventilation management, effect of time, disease states, or concomitant operation. In selected patients, regional anesthesia may provide better operating conditions, safety and comfort than general anesthesia.

CRYOANESTHESIA

Cryoanesthesia involves the blocking of local nerve conduction of painful impulses by means of marked surface cooling of a localized area. It is used in topical procedures such as the removal of warts or noninvasive papular surface lesions. Cryotherapy units are commercially available.

INDUCED HYPOTHERMIA

Hypothermia is the artificial, deliberate lowering of body temperature below the normal limits. It reduces the rate of all body processes. Expert skill, knowledge, and vigilance are required, and the patient is carefully monitored.

Systemic hypothermia may be light (37 to 32°C or 98.6 to 89.6°F), moderate (32 to 26°C or 89.6 to 78.8°F), deep (26 to 20°C or 78.8 to 68°F), or profound (20°C or below, 68°F or below). Sensorium fades at 33 to 34°C (91 to 93°F).

This procedure either alone or in conjunction with extracorporeal circulation (see Chap. 31, p. 574) is used to lower body temperature in order to reduce the metabolic rate and oxygen needs of the tissues in conditions causing hypoxia or during a decrease or interruption of circulation. Bleeding is also decreased and less anesthetic is needed. The patient can therefore better tolerate the operative procedure. Hypothermia may be used:

1 For direct-vision intracardiac repair of complex congenital defects in infants and in other cardiac procedures. This is the most common usage.
2 After cardiac resuscitation, to decrease oxygen requirement of vital tissues and limit further damage to the brain following anoxia.
3 In treatment of hyperpyrexia and some other nonsurgical conditions (hypertensive crisis).
4 To increase tolerance in septic shock.
5 In neurosurgery, to decrease cerebral blood flow, brain volume, and venous and intracranial pressures.
6 To aid in transplantation of organs.

Attaining Hypothermia

To achieve hypothermia, heat must be lost more rapidly than it is produced. The following methods may be used.

1 *Surface-induced hypothermia:* attained by means of thermal blankets or mattresses circulating ice water through their coils, immersion in ice-water baths, ice packing of the body, alcohol sponging. External cooling is used for infants and small children under 20 lb (10 kg) because of their smaller surface area.

2 *Internal cooling:* achieved through decrease or interruption of blood flow by placing ice packs around a specific internal organ or cold fluids within a body cavity (ice-water enema, intragastric, intraperitoneal lavage—but carries risk of infection); drugs may be used to lower metabolism and to increase resistance to shivering.

3 *Systemic hypothermia:* bloodstream is cooled by diverting the blood through heat-exchanging devices of extracorporeal circulation and returning it to the body (continuous flowing circuit), e.g., core cooling by cardiopulmonary bypass; intravenous administration of cold fluids. Systemic hypothermia is used in adults and larger children to 26°C (78.8°F). Oxygen consumption and metabolism of different organs vary so uniform hypothermia is impossible.

> NOTE. A hypo-hyperthermia machine, an electronic system, is available. The temperature is not deliberately taken below about 29°C (84.5°F) unless arrest of the heart is desired by means of deep hypothermia (below 26°C). This is accompanied by perfusion of the rest of the body with the extracorporeal-circulation method, permitting an open, motionless dry field while the blood flow is interrupted. A noncontracting heart requires very little oxygen.

The patient is progressively rewarmed at the close of the operation until temperature is 35°C (95°F) or until consciousness returns. Sometimes a degree of hypothermia is maintained for a day or two postoperatively to allow the patient to adapt more readily. Oxygen therapy and intubation, if advised, are part of postoperative care.

Complications in Use

Hypothermia carries many inherent risks. Primarily it affects the myocardium, decreasing its resistance to ventricular fibrillation and predisposing the patient to cardiac arrest. This is more likely to happen with deep hypothermia or during manipulation of the heart itself. Other dangers are heart block, effects on the vascular system, atrial fibrillation, embolism, microcirculation stasis, undesired downward drift of temperature ("overshooting"), tissue damage and metabolic acidosis, numerous effects on other organs and systems.

Time is required for cooling and rewarming. Shivering and vasoconstriction, normal defenses of the body against cooling, can be problems during use of hypothermia. This muscle activity increases the oxygen needs greatly. Shivering can be overcome by the administration of a muscle-relaxant drug or intravenous injection of chlorpromazine or an analgesic such as meperidine. Rewarming carries certain problems such as the possibility of reactive bleeding or circulatory collapse. Rewarming can be accomplished by circulating warmed blood by means of extracorporeal circulation, or by using a mattress with circulating fluid, and warm blankets. If external heat is applied, take care not to burn the patient. "Rewarming shock" may be prevented by slow warming, adequate oxygenation, prevention of vasoconstriction and shivering.

INDUCED/DELIBERATE HYPOTENSION

Induced deliberate hypotension is the controlled lowering of arterial blood pressure during anesthesia as an adjunct to operation. Hypotensive anesthesia is used to shorten operating time, reduce blood loss and need for transfusion, facilitate dissection and visibility, especially of tumor margins in radical procedures. Visible vessels are ligated even in the absence of active bleeding.

Naturally, controlled hypotension is not indicated as a routine procedure. It is used only when the expected gain, for a particular patient requiring a specific operation, outweighs the risks involved.

Adequate oxygenation of the blood and tissue perfusion in vital organs (heart, liver, kidneys, lungs) as well as the cerebrum must be maintained to prevent damage. The degree and duration of hypotension must be carefully controlled so that the state can be rapidly terminated at any time.

Precautions in Use

1 Careful selection of patient

2 Preoperative cardiac, renal, and hepatic evaluation of patient to avoid circulatory insufficiency in vital organs

3 Choice of appropriate but not arbitrary level of blood pressure

4 Administration and evaluation by expert anesthesiologists

5 Utilization for only a short time and lowering of blood pressure only enough to obtain desired result

6 Maintenance of blood volume at optimal level by continuous infusion

7 Controlled ventilation with adequate oxygenation via endotracheal tube, as hypotension increases susceptibility to hypoxia

8 Extensive monitoring: ECG; core temperature; esophageal stethoscopy; Foley, central venous pressure and arterial catheters; electrophysiologic brain monitoring

Uses of Induced Hypotension

1 Total hip replacement.

2 Operation where excessive blood loss is anticipated, to decrease gross hemorrhage or vascular oozing.

3 Operation on head, face, neck, upper thorax, especially radical dissection, where position of patient allows blood to pool in dependent areas and reduces venous return to heart and cardiac output.

4 In neurosurgery, where control of intracranial vessel hemorrhage may be difficult. It reduces leakage, makes an aneurysm less turgid and prone to rupture, decreases blood loss in case of rupture, and facilitates placement of ligating clips.

5 Operation where blood transfusions should be avoided, as when compatible blood is unavailable or transfusion is against religious belief.

Attaining Hypotension

Several techniques are available to produce hypotension. Blood pressure may be lowered chemically by direct arterial or venous dilators or by ganglionic blocking drugs. Perfusion pressure drops in proportion to decrease in vascular flow resistance but adequate tissue blood flow exists. Fine adjustment of desired level of hypotension can be achieved by mechanical maneuvers, namely alterations in body position or changes in airway pressure, control of heart rate or blood volume, or addition of other vasoactive drugs in conjunction with hypotensive drugs. Properly used, these maneuvers can reduce the total dose of potentially toxic drugs needed for maintenance of hypotension.

Methods to produce hypotension include:

1 Deep general anesthesia with halothane or isoflurane, followed by a vasodilator for the desired minute-to-minute effect. With increased concentration, halogenated agents produce hypotension as a result of myocardial and peripheral vascular depression.

2 Vasodilators. *Sodium nitroprusside* is a potent fast-acting dilator of virtually all vascular smooth muscle (resistance vessels). It also reduces preload and afterload of the heart, and reduces pulmonary vascular resistance. To achieve safe arterial pressure control, administration is via calibrated drug pump. Acid-base status and blood cyanide level are determined frequently to guard against metabolic acidosis and SNP-induced cyanide and thiocyanate toxicity.

Nitroglycerin, primarily a venodilator, directly dilates capacitance vessels. It reduces preload and improves myocardial perfusion during diastole, a protection against potential ischemia. Nitroglycerin for infusion (Nitrostat IV), after dilution in IV 5% dextrose or physiologic saline, dilates both venous and arterial beds. Arterial pressures are reduced. Nitroglycerin migrates into plastic. To avoid its absorption into plastic parenteral solution containers, dilution and storage is made in glass parenteral solution bottles. A special nonabsorbing infusion set prevents loss of nitroglycerin.

3 *Trimethaphan camsylate (Arfonad).* Acts by blocking sympathetic ganglia which results in relaxation of resistance and capacitance vessels, and reduced arterial pressure.

4 *Fentanyl.* May be used as a basal anesthetic for hypotension. Blood pressure can be maintained at desired level by addition of small amount of a volatile agent. Fentanyl lowers arterial pressure; volatile agents reduce cardiac output.

5 *Other drugs.* Verapamil, nifedipine, phentolamine, tetrodotoxin, or adenosine triphosphate may be used.

Safe lower limits of arterial pressure may vary. Average is 50 mm Hg *mean,* 65 to 70 mm Hg systolic, with lower value for short periods only.

Potential complications of hypotensive anesthesia include cerebral or coronary ischemia or thrombosis, reactionary hemorrhage, anuria, delayed awakening, or dermal ischemic lesions. *Primary contraindications* are vascular compromise to any vital organ system or the brain.

HYPNOANESTHESIA

Hypnoanesthesia refers to hypnosis when used as a method of anesthesia. Hypnosis produces a state of altered consciousness characterized by heightened suggestibility, selective wakefulness, reduced awareness, and restricted attentiveness. Although hypnosis has a long history of misuse, modern application by highly trained medical specialists is humane. Hypnoanesthesia, although rarely used, has been successfully employed in adult and pediatric patients. Motivation is an important factor. The method may be combined with the use of a small dose of chemical anesthetic or muscle relaxant drug. *It must not be used indiscriminately in place of standard treatment.*

Hypnosis may be used as a therapeutic aid in *very selected* patients:

1 When chemical agents are contraindicated. The patient may be kept pain-free, asleep or awake, without toxic side effects.

2 When of value as an adjunct to chemical anesthesia to decrease amount of anesthesia needed.

3 When it is desirable to free the patient from certain neurophysical effects of an anesthetic.

4 When apprehension and fear of anesthetic are so great as to contribute to serious anesthetic risk.

5 When posthypnotic suggestion may be valuable in postoperative period.

6 When it is desirable to raise pain threshold.

7 When it is desirable to have the patient respond to questions or commands.

Prehypnotic Preparation

1 Careful psychiatric evaluation of patient to determine feasibility of hypnosis

2 Establishment of rapport so patient will listen to and obey commands; explanation of procedure

3 Trial trances to see if sleep is deep enough

Limitations

1 It requires skill and special training.

2 It is time-consuming and unreliable compared to chemical anesthesia.

3 Muscular relaxation is limited. Supplementation may be necessary.

4 It may release an underlying psychiatric disorder.

5 Contraindications are patient's refusal to be hypnotized or patient's being under psychiatric care.

ACUPUNCTURE

Acupuncture has a long history of use in Asia and Europe but it has not been employed extensively in the United States. This ancient medical practice is a complex phenomenon, not well understood, and numerous theories have emerged about it. Research continues in the hope of establishing credibility on a scientific or physiologic basis for its effectiveness for analgesia and anesthesia in a certain percentage of cases.

Acupuncture is a technique of providing intense stimulation at specific locations in the body known as acupuncture or meridian points. Stimulation is effected by rotation of or by electric current applied to very fine gauge needles of varying lengths inserted into these points, which generally correspond to area where the somatic nerve supply is located. Appropriate points can be selected to produce analgesia or anesthesia in the desired body region.

Acupuncture has had limited use in operative and dental procedures as well as for postoperative or intractable pain. The patient remains conscious. Procedures should be limited to use by physicians or under their direct supervision in keeping with acceptable standards of medical practice.

ANESTHESIA IN AGE-EXTREME PATIENTS

Age-extreme patients, geriatric and pediatric age groups, present a special challenge to the anesthesiologist. Physiologic function gradually deteriorates with age. The aging process is not a disease but a fundamental biologic alteration. Disease in the elderly is superimposed on senescent changes. The aged are more prone to multiple organ system failure. Central nervous system changes produce effects on other system's performance.

Characteristics of the aged include memory loss and confusion exaggerated in an institutional environment, malnutrition, anemia, osteoporosis, low blood volume, poor liver or renal function, arteriosclerosis, diminished autonomic tone and reflexes, instability of circulation, or diabetes. Reactivity to stimuli decreases with advancing years. These patients therefore experience an altered response to stress exemplified in a high pain threshold. They are more susceptible to the action of all drugs. Abnormal sleeping and breathing patterns, with production of apnea by hyperventilation, are accentuated by opioids. These phenomena translate to lower doses of opioids for analgesia and less anesthetic needed because the minimum anesthetic concentration declines progressively with advanced age.

In the elderly, mask fit may be difficult because of loss of teeth and/or jaw substance. Induction may be prolonged and ventilation difficult due to chronic obstructive pulmonary disease or emphysema. With rapid fall in blood pressure, patients are susceptible to hypoxia, stroke, and development of myocardial infarction. Anesthetization problems are augmented because operations tend to be major, take longer, and many elective ones pertain to malignancy, with reoperation necessary.

The mortality rate associated with operative procedures is higher among the aged than the general population, especially if the operation is an emergency one not allowing sufficient time for thorough preoperative evaluation and preparation. Complications related to the cardiovascular system and cerebral circulation most frequently are followed by respiratory problems, gastric aspiration, and indolent infection. Operative morbidity can be reduced, however, by skillful management of anesthesia. This is also true for the other age extreme—the pediatric patient.

Pediatric surgery involves many complex procedures that present an equal challenge for anesthesia management. Small deviations in administration of anesthetic agents can rapidly change an optimal situation into a life-threatening emergency. The uniqueness of infants, children, and pediatric anesthesia is discussed in Chapter 33.

CARE OF ANESTHESIA EQUIPMENT

Like everyone else in contact with the patient, the anesthesiologist is a potential vector in spread of infection. He or she has a personal responsibility for practicing highest standards of both personal cleanliness and asepsis in the OR. As the scope of duties takes the anesthesiologist to areas outside the OR suite, he or she must change contaminated attire on return from those areas. The anesthesiologist must also change masks between patients, and meticulously and repeatedly wash hands with antiseptic soap. It is the duty of the anesthesiologist to see that equipment used is properly cleaned and sterilized to protect the patient.

Hazards of Equipment

Anesthesia techniques encompass use of drugs for parenteral administration, as well as of gases and volatile liquids for inhalation administration by means of anesthesia machines. These machines and their component parts (reservoir bags, canisters, connecting pieces, ventilators) accumulate large numbers of microorganisms during use. Consequently, the parts that come in contact with the patient's skin or respiratory tract are sources of cross contamination. Inhalation, exhalation, and the forcible expulsion of secretions create moist conditions favorable to survival and growth of a multitude of organisms (streptococci, staphylococci, coliforms, fungi, yeasts). Therefore, the anesthesia circuit can become a veritable reservoir for microorganisms and a pathway for transmission of disease. When the apparatus is used on a patient with known respiratory disease, such as tuberculosis, the risk increases.

All used accessories must be terminally cleaned and either high-level disinfected or sterilized before reuse, as clinical respiratory cross infection has been traced to contaminated apparatus. It has been shown that valves of the anesthesia circuit become contaminated from essentially healthy patients at an average rate of 35 organisms per minute. *Pseudomonas aeruginosa* has been cultured from anesthesia absorbers. Many microorganisms accumulate in the valves and air passages, including the soda lime. While the alkalinity of soda lime inhibits many organisms, it is not a dependable germicide or effective mechanical filter, nor meant to be one. Respiratory therapy equipment, mechanical ventilators, resuscitators, suction machines and bottles present the same problems. Resistant strains of organisms, as well as opportunists, have caused nosocomial infections to become a national health problem. Patient-to-patient infection must be eliminated. One must recognize that:

1 The patient's respiratory tract is a portal of entry for pathogenic organisms as well as a source of delivering pathogens into the environment.

2 The respiratory tract loses some of its inherent defense mechanisms during anesthesia.

3 Aseptic precautions are necessary to prevent needless exposure of air passages to foreign, potentially pathogenic organisms from equipment and hands of anesthesia personnel.

4 Anesthesia machines and equipment, unless properly treated, increase danger of airborne contamination and contact transmission of pathogenic microorganisms capable of causing postoperative wound infections.

NOTE. In the presence of tuberculosis or virulent respiratory infection, the anesthesiologist may wear gown and gloves. The patient should wear a mask during transportation and until induction of anesthesia.

Disposable Equipment

Disposable equipment warrants use for reasons of safety, efficiency, and convenience. Presterilized, disposable airways, endotracheal tubes, tracheotomy tubes, breathing circuits, masks and canisters (with soda lime sealed in the plastic) reduce the hazard of infection. They are especially indicated for the compromised host and the bacteriologically contaminated patient. Single-use components of the anesthesia system are discarded after use.

Care of Reusable Equipment

All parts of the patient-exposed, reusable equipment must be thoroughly cleaned after *every* use to prevent pulmonary complications. Thorough cleaning to remove debris and drying must precede any high-level disinfection or sterilization process. Every patient is entitled to have sterile all items that can be sterilized. Manufacturers strive to make the machines that cannot be sterilized more amenable to adequate cleaning and freedom from microorganisms.

1 The anesthesia machine should be disinfected immediately whenever soiled by blood and secretions.
2 Surfaces of anesthesia machines, carts, or cabinets should be disinfected after *each* patient use, including the specific work area used for airways, endotracheal tubes, etc. The top of a cart or tray should be draped with a disposable impervious material that is *changed between patients. All* equipment for maintenance of airway should be set up on and returned to this drape. Disposable items should be discarded in suitable containers after use. Nondisposable

equipment must be set aside after use for terminal cleaning and testing, thereby diminishing the risk of contaminating clean equipment needed for subsequent patients.

3 All equipment that comes in contact with the patient and the inside of the breathing circuit must be terminally cleaned and sterilized, preferably, or high-level disinfected.
   a Endotracheal tubes, stylets, airways, laryngoscope blades, face masks, suction equipment should be sterile for each patient. Suction catheters and tubing should be sterile, single-use disposable items.
   b Interior of breathing circuits remain sterile if they stand unused in their normal position on the machine, but contamination rapidly occurs when used on patients. The parts of the circuit nearest the patient are the most heavily contaminated parts. Therefore, corrugated hoses, breathing tubes, reservoir bags are sterilized or high-level disinfected between each patient use.
   c Items located farther away, such as circle systems and ventilators, are cleaned and sterilized according to a regular schedule, at least once or twice a month.

4 For cleaning, an automated process is available for decontamination. Machines wash equipment in mild detergent and hot water, rinse and dry it. Some machines incorporate a chemical disinfection cycle. If automatic equipment is not used, anesthesia and respiratory therapy equipment must be disconnected and manually cleaned prior to sterilization. Prompt immersion in detergent-disinfectant solution prevents crusting of secretions. Tubing takes a long time to dry. Commercial dryers are available.

5 Sterilization methods (see Chap. 8).
   a Autoclaving is the preferred method for all heat-stable materials.
   b Ethylene oxide is used for materials deteriorated by heat, such as rubber, plastics, mechanical ventilators, electronic equipment. *Thorough aeration, according to the manufacturer's recommendations, is necessary before use to remove all residual gas from the material sterilized.* Otherwise, facial burns, laryngotracheal inflammation, and obstruction or bilateral vocal cord paralysis may be caused by use of the equipment.
   c Buffered glutaraldehyde solution does not impair conductivity of antistatic rubber. While the least convenient method, it is preferred if ethylene oxide is not available for heat-sensitive items. Immersion for 45 minutes in Cidex solution is recommended to ensure 100 percent kill of *Mycobacterium tuberculosis.* When glutaraldehyde is used, the items must be thoroughly rinsed with *sterile* water since tap water contains microorganisms and pyrogens.

6 Sterile packaged equipment should be stored in a closed clean dry area. Anesthesia and respiratory therapy equipment should be kept sterile until used.

7 Policies and procedures regarding processing of equipment should be written, available, and reviewed annually.

Checking Anesthesia Equipment

Inhalation systems are tested biologically at regular intervals.

CHAPTER **14**

PATIENT MONITORING, POTENTIAL COMPLICATIONS UNDER ANESTHESIA, AND CARDIOPULMONARY RESUSCITATION

The development of successful, controllable anesthesia has made modern surgery possible. The methods used are constantly being improved by research. Since anesthesia is a necessary adjunct to most operative procedures, all persons caring for surgical patients should know the pertinent facts in order to give intelligent patient care. Anesthetization is no small part of the patient's total experience. The nurse's familiarity with various anesthetic agents, their interaction with certain drugs, and their potential hazards is a necessity. The alert, informed nurse can quietly note onset of complications and help to avert an emergency or fatality.

Working with anesthesiologists in the OR gives the learner an unparalleled opportunity to master immediate resuscitative measures and their effectiveness as well as an understanding of the care of unconscious and critically ill patients. For example, the learner daily observes tracheal intubation, ventilatory control, insertion of arterial and venous cannulae, fluid replacement, sophisticated hemodynamic monitoring, and spinal tap.

It is mandatory that all persons who work in areas where electrical equipment or flammable agents are stored and used know potential explosion hazards and their control (see Chap. 11).

Finally, the fact that *no* operative procedure is minor must *never* be forgotten. Operation and anesthesia impose upon the patient certain inescapable risks, even under supposedly ideal circumstances.

ADVERSE REACTIONS TO ANESTHETICS

Adverse drug reactions occurring during anesthesia and operation are of increasing concern to both physicians and patients. These reactions are relatively frequent, often severe, potentially fatal. Reactions increase in ratio to the number of drugs used (see Chap. 13, p. 248).

Systemic reactions manifested by symptoms referable to the central nervous system and the respiratory and cardiovascular systems are caused by absorption into the circulation of toxic amounts of local or general anesthetic drugs. The main factors then in producing these reactions are vascular uptake and circulating blood level of the anesthetic. Toxic amounts of drugs can depress peripheral vessels as well as myocardium and medullary centers. Hypoxia leads to cerebral ischemia. Hypotension, apnea, coma, respiratory and circulatory collapse, and cardiac standstill may then result.

In topical anesthesia, extremely rapid systemic absorption from mucous membranes explains the relatively high frequency of toxic reactions. In local or regional anesthesia, inadvertent intravenous injection and use of fairly large quantities in highly vascular areas will contribute to local anesthetic toxicity. Allergies are thought to be more common with the ester rather than the amide group of compounds. Allergy to the preservative in the solution is also possible.

Drugs Implicated in Reaction

Many drugs release histamine, which in turn is the basis of allergic response.

1 Barbiturates, used as hypnotics or operative anesthetics, frequently cause skin rashes.

2 Nonbarbiturates, such as ketamine, may cause cutaneous eruptions.

3 Local anesthetics are associated with numerous reactions such as anaphylaxis, urticaria, dermatitis. Dermatitis is not uncommon among dentists and physicians who develop hypersensitivity because of frequent contact with an agent.

4 Adjuncts to anesthesia, such as tranquilizers and neuroleptics.

5 Neuromuscular blockers. Curare is the strongest histamine releaser.

6 Other agents: nonanesthetic drugs administered during operation such as epinephrine, antibiotics, diuretics; acrylic bone cement.

7 Blood volume expanders, such as dextran.

Predisposing Factors to Reaction

1 Overdosage—excessive amount of drug enters the bloodstream.
- **a** Inattention to maximal safe quantity.
- **b** Disregard for latent period of onset of anesthesia.
- **c** Too rapid injection.
- **d** Too rapid absorption. Intravenous is the most dangerous route of injection. Injection site is also pertinent. Hazardous sites involve vascular areas: tracheobronchial mucosa, tissues of the head, neck, paravertebral region. The least hazardous areas are subcutaneous tissue of the extremities and trunk (abdominal wall, buttocks).
- **e** Inadvertent intravascular injection. Although no antigen-antibody reaction, histamine is released to the systemic circulation.

2 True hypersensitivity (immunological sensitization) produces severe allergic responses and anaphylaxis. This can occur following very small or minimal dose. However, it is much less frequently encountered than nonimmunologic (anaphylactoid) reactions from overdosage. True allergy, mediated by antigen-antibody reaction, is accompanied by dermal reactions such as itching, skin wheals, laryngeal edema, and possibly cardiovascular collapse.
- **a** Briefly, allergic reactions are classified into four types, the response usually dependent upon prior exposure to the drug:
  - **1** Classic anaphylactic or immediate reaction (usually mediated by immunoglobulin E antibody) with release of histamine within seconds.
  - **2** Cytotoxic reaction resulting in cell destruction.
  - **3** Immune complex hypersensitivity, e.g., serum sickness.
  - **4** Delayed or cellular type hypersensitivity. (At times there is a delay of 24 hours or more before onset of reaction.)
- **b** Magnitude of allergic response is influenced by a number of factors, such as amount of antigen or antibody present and affinity of antibody for antigen. The antigen is exogenous, the other factors endogenous, which is the reason for extensive variation in individual susceptibility.
- **c** Histamine contracts smooth muscle of bronchioles and large blood vessels, dilates venules, and increases capillary permeability. Establishing the cause and mechanism for reaction, although difficult, is important in future management of the patient.

Symptoms of Systemic Reactions

Symptoms manifested may be those of central nervous system (CNS) stimulation or depression, or stimulation followed by depression and collapse. The cardiovascular system seems more resistant than the CNS to toxic effects of local anesthetics. Seizure threshold may differ enormously in individual patients as may relationship of dose to symptoms of CNS action. For example, lidocaine usually produces drowsiness prior to convulsions, whereas bupivacaine may cause sudden seizure, disorientation, decreased hearing ability, paresthesias, muscle twitching or agitation in a wide-awake patient without premonitory signs. Hypercarbia or hypoxemia from hypoventilation lowers seizure threshold. Toxicity of local anesthetics is manifested primarily by CNS effects resulting from high blood levels.

1 *Stimulation:* talkativeness, restlessness, incoherence, excitation, tachycardia, bounding pulse, flushed face, hyperpyrexia, tremors, hyperactive reflexes, muscular twitching, convulsions (focal and grand mal)

2 *Depression:* drowsiness, disorientation, decreased hearing ability, stupor, syncope, rapid thready pulse or bradycardia, apprehension, hypotension, pale or cyanotic moist skin, coma

3 *Other signs:* nausea, vomiting, dizziness, blurred vision, sudden severe headache, precordial pain, extreme pulse rate or blood pressure change, angioneurotic edema (wheeze, laryngeal edema, bronchospasm), rashes, urticaria, severe local tissue reaction

Treatment of Anesthetic Reactions

Treatment is aimed at preventing simultaneous respiratory and cardiac arrest. Treatment must be prompt. *Time is of the essence.* Administration of the agent thought to produce the reaction is stopped immediately (when possible) at the first indication of reaction. Therapy is generally supportive, the specifics dictated by clinical manifestations. *Treatment* consists of:

1 Maintaining oxygenation of the vital organs and tissues with ventilation by manual or mechanical assistance—100% oxygen with positive pressure. Tracheal intubation as indicated.
2 Reversing myocardial depression and peripheral vasodilatation before cardiac arrest occurs. Supine position with legs elevated. Intravenous fluid therapy is begun and a vasoconstrictor drug may be given intravenously or intramuscularly for hypotension or a weak pulse, signs of progressive circulatory depression. Choice of vasopressor is suggested by symptoms and used with caution. Drugs that may be used include:
   a Epinephrine (IV)—counteracts hypotension, bronchoconstriction, laryngeal edema. It also stimulates beta- and alpha-adrenergic receptors, inhibits further release of mediators. Increases arteriolar constriction and force of heart beat. When applicable, application of a tourniquet or subcutaneous injection of epinephrine in the area of drug injection may delay absorption of toxic drug.
   b Ephedrine and other vasoconstrictors such as phenylephrine (Neo-Synephrine) or mephentermine (Wyamine)—cause peripheral vasoconstriction, increased myocardial contraction, and bronchodilatation.
   c Antihistamines—block histamine release, but not generally advocated.
   d Steroids—effect is not immediate and use is directed toward late manifestations of allergic response. Enhance effect of epinephrine; inhibit further release of histamine.
   e Isoproterenol (Isuprel)—uses are predominantly in asthma and heart attack; a bronchodilator.
3 Giving antagonist drug in situations where causative agent is identified.
4 Stopping muscle tremors or convulsions if they are present as they constitute hazard of further hypoxia, possibility of aspiration, body injury. Diazepam in 5 mg doses or a short-acting barbiturate is given intravenously to inhibit cortical irritation.

NOTE. In patients in whom the adverse response is due to hypersensitivity, the previous measures are applicable. However, aminophylline may be administered to help alleviate bronchospasm, hydrocortisone (IV) to combat shock, and sodium or potassium iodide (IV) to reduce mucosal edema. See p. 284 for treatment of cardiac arrest.

The nurse must know resuscitation measures and be able to assist in or initiate them when necessary, as per hospital policy.

Precautions for preventing reactions include:

1 Questioning patient preoperatively for history of any allergies or hypersensitivities and reactions to previous anesthetics or other drugs. Extraordinary precautions must be taken for this group of patients.
   a Atopic individuals with multiple allergies are thought to be more prone to adverse reaction.
   b Any drug with known or suspected history of reaction, or any chemically related drug, is not given, e.g., penicillin.
   c If testing for sensitivity to specific drugs is done, it must be executed *very* cautiously

under *well-controlled* conditions. Prediction of allergic reactions is unreliable.

2 Knowledge of patient's general condition.
   a Many surgeons insist on seeing a patient in their office no longer than one week prior to general or local anesthesia.
   b Identification of all drugs the patient has recently received or is currently taking.

3 Administration of appropriate drugs, concentrations and dosages.

4 Constant monitoring and observing patient, including facial expressions, and noting responses to conversation and state of alertness.

5 Limiting the total amount of drug injected or applied to prescribed safe limits and recording this information. Adjust precise amount also to size of patient. Employ minimal effective concentration and smallest volume needed.

6 Immediate cessation of administration at any sign of sensitivity.

7 Slow injection to retard absorption and avoid overdosage. Use incremental titration of drug.

8 Frequent aspiration or pulling back on syringe plunger while injecting to be sure the solution is not entering a blood vessel inadvertently.

9 Cautious use of drugs that reduce ventilation (narcotics) when upper dose limit of anesthetic drug is used.

Patients receiving any significant amount of local drug should be monitored by electrocardiogram in addition to blood pressure and vital signs in case of sudden arrhythmia. Also, an intravenous lifeline should be inserted in case of reaction or inadvertent intravenous or intraarterial injection of a bolus of anesthetic. Resuscitation equipment, oxygen, Ambu bag and defibrillator must be readily available.

The anesthesiologist's or surgeon's perception of possible occurrence and readiness to treat a reaction is of great help in preventing a fatal one. The circulating nurse also shares this responsibility and that of closely observing the patient.

Care with Drug Ampuls

When you are responsible for placing drug ampuls on the table for use:

1 Be careful to read the label correctly.

2 Discard the ampul if the label is not completely legible or has been disturbed.

3 Observe the solution for clarity and discard any suspicious ampul.

4 Provide a rustproof ampul file for opening.

5 Sterile single-dose ampuls are recommended.

MONITORING OF LOCAL ANESTHESIA PATIENT

Extent of monitoring, determined in consultation with the department of surgery and anesthesiology where applicable, depends on seriousness of the procedure, sedation required and/or patient's condition. The Association of Operating Room Nurses recommended practices provide guidelines for the perioperative nurse for monitoring the patient receiving local anesthesia. They may be summarized briefly as follows:

1 Patient is monitored for reaction to drugs and for behavioral and physiological changes. The RN should recognize and report to the physician significant changes in the patient's status.

2 The perioperative nurse should have basic knowledge of the function and use of monitoring equipment and ability to interpret the information.

3 Accurate reflection of perioperative care should be documented on patient's record.

4 Institutional policies and procedures in regard to patient care, including monitoring, should be written, reviewed annually, and readily available. This information should be included in orientation and inservice. It should include policies regarding permissible drug administration by the nurse.

In addition to preoperative assessment and postoperative evaluation for continuum of care, the nursing care plan and intraoperative nursing activities should include but not be limited to the following: taking vital signs before injection of a local anesthetic drug or analgesic as well as every 15 minutes after injection, monitoring the patient's physiological status, instituting emergency measures if an adverse reaction occurs, performing additional functions on request *as per institutional policy.* For example, the latter might include attaching leads (see p. 263), identifying and reporting abnormal electrocardiograph readings, starting oxygen therapy when clinically indicated and/or administering IV therapy.

COMPLICATIONS OF LOCAL/REGIONAL ANESTHESIA

Complications of regional anesthesia are common but usually minor or transient. Serious complications, though rare, are usually permanent in nature. They may be due to a damaging mechanical effect of needles or to pharmacological effect of the anesthetic drug administered. As with general anesthesia, prevention of complication requires patient assessment and preparation, knowledge of anatomy, and attention to detail to avoid untoward reactions. Proper choice of drug, equipment, and constant monitoring are as necessary in regional as in general anesthesia. Complications of local and regional anesthesia may be summarized briefly as local effects, systemic effects, and effects unrelated to the anesthetic agent.

Local Effects

Tissue trauma, hematoma, ischemia, drug sensitivity, and infection can be minimized by the use of proper drugs and equipment, aseptic technique, avoidance of addition of vasoconstrictor drugs to local anesthetics in injection sites of impaired circulation (digits, penis), and avoidance of repetitive needling that promotes trauma, tissue necrosis, and infection.

Systemic Effects

Systemic effects are primarily cardiovascular, neurological, or respiratory, e.g., hypotension, convulsion, or respiratory depression. Drug interactions also are systemic. Following high blood levels, toxicity may occur which affects more than one system. Blood levels depend on the mass of drug used, its physical characteristics, presence or absence of vasoconstrictors, and the injection site. For example, because of the vascularity of surrounding tissue, intercostal block produces higher anesthetic blood levels in a shorter time than axillary or epidural blocks. Absorption and blood level of drugs are related to their uptake and rate of removal from circulation. A linear relationship exists between amount of drug administered via a given route and resultant peak anesthetic blood level.

When a nerve deficit occurs in the postoperative period, one must ascertain that this does not relate to a preexisting condition such as multiple sclerosis or other cause such as faulty positioning, trauma from retractors, tourniquets left inflated for inordinately long periods resulting in ischemia or pressure on peripheral nerves, or improperly applied casts.

Unrelated to Local Anesthetic

Less common, effects unrelated to an agent include bleeding, broken needle or catheter, overflow onto other nerves, pain, neuritis, epinephrine reaction.

MONITORING OF VITAL FUNCTIONS

Concurrently, operative and anesthesia techniques have become increasingly complex, allowing many critically ill patients, especially at age extremes, to experience operative procedures. The anesthesiologist keeps the surgeon instantly informed of important changes in the patient's condition, detected by precision monitoring. Monitoring implies keeping track of and/or regulating vital functions. During extensive surgery under anesthesia, the body is subjected to much stress. Bleeding, tissue trauma, potent drugs, large extravascular fluid shifts, multiple transfusions, and operative position that may inhibit breathing and circulation all contribute to disturbed physiology. These factors can induce significant cardiac dysfunction. To continuously measure the patient's responses to these stresses, clinical evaluation by listening, observing, and feeling is augmented by the use of electronic or mechanical devices. These devices reveal physiologic trends and subtle changes, give warning of an impending dangerous state, and indicate response to therapy. Most of this equipment in expensive, constitutes electrical hazard, and takes up space in the OR. Some OR suites have permanently installed apparatus with concealed wiring and conduits in a glass-enclosed room or area adjoining the operating room. Compact, precise devices with miniaturized circuitry, better visibility and easier maintenance are constantly being developed.

Personnel using electronic monitoring equipment must understand its function, be experienced in its use, and easily able to determine equipment malfunction. *Instrumentation should augment, not replace, judgment or careful observation.*

Computers in the operating room improve and expedite analysis of data. They are sophisticated data collection and management tools to assist in physical status assessment, diagnosis, and therapy. Clinical computers vary from single function devices to complex multifunction systems that acquire, store and display data, organize information, and perform calculations.

With monitoring, many aspects of respiratory,

cardiovascular, and nervous system functions can be observed constantly. Quantitative assessment is provided by periodic specific measurements. This is desirable as anesthetic agents and/or operative manipulation may initiate unwanted circulatory and respiratory reflex responses. Most anesthetics are cardiovascular and respiratory depressants. Uncorrected depression can progress to circulatory or respiratory arrest.

The spectrum of monitoring devices is broad. It ranges from noninvasive to invasive. *Noninvasive monitors* do not penetrate a body orifice. Conversely, *invasive monitors* penetrate skin or mucosa, or enter a body cavity. Some parameters can be measured by both noninvasive and invasive methods, e.g., blood pressure. Nursing responsibilities may include assisting with sophisticated hemodynamic monitoring to evaluate the interrelationship of blood pressure, blood flow, vascular volumes, physical properties of blood, heart rate, and ventricular function. Detection of early changes in hemodynamics allows prompt action to maintain cardiac function and adequate cardiac output. Monitoring facilitates rapid, accurate determination of decreased perfusion. It reflects immediate response to therapeutic measures and stress.

Abbreviations commonly used in reference to monitoring vital functions include:

ABG Arterial blood gas.
BP Arterial blood pressure.
BV Blood volume.
CI Cardiac index.
CO Cardiac output.
CSF Cerebrospinal fluid.
CVP Central venous pressure.
ECG or **EKG** Electrocardiogram.
EEG Electroencephalogram.
EF Ejection fraction.
HR Heart rate.
ICP Intracranial pressure.
LA Left atrium.
LAP Left atrial pressure.
LV Left ventricle.
LVEDP Left ventricular end-diastolic pressure.
MAP Mean arterial pressure.
P Partial pressure.
$PaCO_2$ Partial pressure of carbon dioxide in arterial blood.
PaO_2 Partial pressure of oxygen in arterial blood.
PA Pulmonary artery.
PAC Pulmonary artery catheter.
PAP Pulmonary artery pressure.
PCWP Pulmonary capillary wedge pressure.
V_t Respiratory tidal volume.
RA Right atrium.
RAP Right arterial pressure.
RV Right ventricle.
SEP Sensory evoked potentials.
SSEP Somatosensory evoked potentials.
SV Stroke volume.
SVR Systemic vascular resistance.

Invasive Monitoring

Invasive hemodynamic monitoring utilizes basic physiologic principles to detect and treat a wide variety of abnormalities. Its purpose is to avoid problems in high-risk patients, and accurately diagnose and treat patients with established life-threatening disorders. It involves direct intravascular measurements and assessments by means of indwelling catheters connected to transducers and monitors. Pressures and forces within arteries and veins are converted to electrical signals by the transducer, a device that transfers energy from one system to another. These electrical signals are then processed and amplified by the monitor into a continuous waveform displayed on an oscilloscope or monitoring screen that reproduces images received via transducer. Or, the monitor may digitally display the values. These measurements yield specific information that is otherwise not usually attainable or as accurate. Although these measurements may be pertinent in guiding patient care, they present additional risks because to obtain them requires invasion of the great vessels and/or heart. The benefits of invasive monitoring must be balanced against the risks.

Insertion of catheters into vital areas usually is performed by a physician or, in some hospitals, by certified registered nurse anesthetists (CRNA). The operator and persons caring for these patients must have precise knowledge of anatomy and physiology, must be experienced, and must understand the entire monitoring circuit. *Hospital procedure and policy manuals, and strict adherence to the manufacturers' recommendations and information in equipment manuals are essential* to minimize complications and misinterpretation of data leading to potentially erroneous therapy. In using invasive monitors, frequent checks of circuitry and calibrations are mandatory to validate the recorded data and to protect the patient.

Indwelling arterial and intracardiac catheters permit rapid accurate assessment of physiologic alterations in high-risk patients. But their use must not be abused. Cardiac arrhythmias, thrombosis, embolism, and infection are serious, sometimes fatal complications. Some hospitals require the patient to sign an informed consent form before insertion of an invasive catheter.

Various types of equipment, monitors, and catheter materials are in use. Procedures must be explained to the patient, allergies noted, and the patient reassured. Skin preparation and draping precedes the insertion of catheters. *Strict adherence to sterile techniques is absolutely essential.* Hazards involved must constantly be kept in mind. *Conscientious attention to every detail is mandatory.*

Arterial Cannulation Intraarterial access is justified in many patients because of high yield of information with minimal discomfort to the patient. An intraarterial catheter is inserted for direct measurement of arterial pressure with pulse waveform display and analysis. An arterial line facilitates taking intermittent blood samples. Blood gas monitoring (PaO_2, $PaCO_2$) is especially important in patients requiring mechanical ventilation. Samples may be taken also for other analyses, e.g., electrolytes, glucose, coagulation.

Potential arteries for cannulation include the radial, brachial, ulnar, axillary, femoral, or dorsalis pedis (continuation of anterior tibial artery). As a precaution, adequacy of perfusion to the extremity below the catheter should be established before insertion, in the event that thrombosis or occlusion should occur. A Doppler device is convenient in determining a dominant artery and in locating a weakly palpable one.

The radial artery is commonly used for cannulation if ulnar circulation to the hand is adequate. When radial artery arterial dominance exists, the ulnar artery may be used. Or, a brachial or other alternate artery is used. A radial artery distal to a prior brachial artery cutdown for cardiac catheterization is avoided because of the possibility of distorted pressures or occlusion. Some physicians cannulate a major vessel such as the femoral, if the catheter is to remain in the patient longer than one day. This is because of lower incidence of thrombosis when a large vessel is used, as compared to the radial artery.

The most common *complications of arterial cannulation* are thrombosis or occlusion of the artery, embolic phenomena, blood loss from dislodged or disconnected line, bruise or hematoma formation, arteriovenous fistula or aneurysm formation, systemic infection, ischemic fingers from arterial spasm. To minimize these complications, the important factors concerning an arterial line are:

1 Use a small-gauge nontapered catheter. The larger the indwelling catheter in relation to the artery lumen, the greater the incidence of thrombosis. Wrist circumference may be a predictor of arterial lumen size, i.e., the greater the circumference, the larger the lumen.

2 Use a continuous heparinized flush to prevent clotting in the line. For flushing, a solution containing 1 to 2 units of heparin/ml in 0.9% physiological saline or 5% dextrose in water infused at a rate of about 3.0 ml/hour is used. This slow rate reduces risk of fluid overload. Avoid forceful flushing with a large volume of solution to prevent cerebral embolism. *Routine flushing is mandatory.* The continuous flush devices are popular. The release by fast flush valve of only a small amount of fluid under limited pressure diminishes possibility of ejecting a large clot. The line usually is fast flushed both hourly and after withdrawing blood samples. Avoid rapid repeated flushing, a cause of turbulence and air bubbles. After flushing, check the drip rate of the IV bag's drip chamber.

3 Limit duration of cannulation to minimal clinical requirement. Risk of thrombosis increases significantly after three days. Thrombosis may result from irritation of the vessel wall, hypercoagulation or inadequate flushing of catheter and line. Prevent excessive manipulation.

4 Inspect the insertion site frequently for bleeding or inflammation. Bleeding may result from trauma to the vessel or improper fixation at insertion site. Should bleeding appear, apply local pressure, secure fixation site, notify doctor immediately.

Percutaneous Cannulation of Radial Artery Explain procedure and reassure patient. If patient is awake, medication for sedation may be ordered. Collect and set up the necessary equipment for cannulation and monitoring, according to the hospital policy and manufacturer's directions. Document patient's vital signs and pulse distal to selected insertion site. If pulse weakens after catherization, circulation may be inadequate and the catheter may have to be removed.

1 Affix forearm and tape thumb to armboard with hand supinated and wrist dorsiflexed 50 to 60° over a towel. Avoid extreme dorsiflexion which can obliterate pulse. Taping the thumb stabilizes the artery at the wrist.

2 Prep skin per hospital policy.

3 Assist physician as necessary during *catheter insertion.* If the patient is awake, skin and subcutaneous tissue are infiltrated with local anesthetic. Skin is incised to facilitate entrance of catheter and protect tip. Catheter is inserted in artery. Entry is indicated by spurt of bright red blood. After catheter is advanced and properly placed, cannula is connected to tubing with continuous flush device, pressure transducer and oscilloscope. Tubing is labeled as an arterial line. Connections are checked for security. Catheter is secured with tape or sutured in place. Dorsiflexion of wrist is reduced. Puncture site is dressed. Tape must not be directly over insertion site.

4 Using sphygmomanometer with blood pressure cuff on the opposite arm, check blood pressure to compare with monitor's pressure reading to verify monitor's accuracy. Monitor will probably read higher systolic and lower diastolic pressures than blood pressure cuff readings.

5 Carefully document procedure. Include insertion site; type and gauge of catheter; type of IV solution and amount of heparin added; flow rate and pressure; pulse before and after insertion; tolerance of procedure; color, sensation, and warmth of area distal to insertion site; date; time; names of insertion team.

Drawing Blood Samples When arterial or venous catheters are in place, the circulating nurse may be asked to collect blood samples for analysis or to take measurements, although this is not universal practice. These procedures require special training, skill, and knowledge of equipment and hazards involved.

Samples for arterial gas measurements (ABG) are sometimes drawn from an indwelling arterial (radial or femoral) catheter line kept open by a continuously running, intraarterial infusion, the tubing of which incorporates a plastic three-way stopcock, usually close to the catheter insertion site. One lumen of the stopcock goes to the infusion solution, one to the cannulated artery, and one to the outside air. The latter is normally closed, covered with a sterile cap, or a sterile syringe is kept inserted in the lumen to prevent bacteria and air from entering. With a three-way stopcock, two of the three lumens are always open.

In drawing blood samples from an indwelling arterial line, always *use strict sterile technique* in drawing the blood through the stopcock.

1 Use sterile gloves and tray of sterile equipment.

2 Attach sterile 5 cc syringe to stopcock lumen going to outside air. Turn off (close) infusion lumen. This automatically opens line between patient and syringe. Aspirate to clear line of fluid and close lumen to patient. Discard this diluted sample.

3 Quickly attach a second sterile syringe (coated with heparin to obtain unclotted blood) to the lumen to outside air, and open the lumen to the patient. This closes the lumen to the infusion, permitting aspiration of undiluted blood for analysis. Arterial pressure forces blood into syringe. Draw 3 to 5 cc of blood. Hold barrel as well as plunger of syringe to avoid syringe coming apart. Cap syringe for placement in properly labeled specimen bag.

4 Close lumen to patient and flush line and stopcock by letting infusion solution run through them to prevent clot formation inside catheter wall or stopcock, which could result in arterial embolization.

5 Close and recap lumen to outside air (being careful not to contaminate cap), thereby restarting infusion to patient. Regulate infusion rate with clamp on the infusion tubing.

6 If air bubbles are in the syringe, remove them. Send samples *immediately* to laboratory. If more than ten minutes elapse between blood drawing and analysis, analysis cannot be considered accurate. In event of delay, syringe with blood should be immediately immersed in ice and refrigerated at near-freezing temperature. Iced specimen bags may be used.

> NOTE. To heparinize a syringe to prevent blood samples from clotting, draw 1 ml aqueous heparin 1:1000 into a 10-cc syringe using a 20-gauge needle. While rotating the barrel, pull the plunger back beyond the 7-cc calibration. With the syringe in upright position, slowly eject the heparin while rotating the barrel. Heparinize needle also.

Parameters Monitored

Using noninvasive and/or invasive techniques, parameters are monitored to show minute-to-minute changes in physiologic variables.

Electrocardiogram (ECG, EKG) Every heart beat depends on the electrical process of polarization. Muscles in the heart wall are alternately stimulated and relaxed. Electrocardiogram is a recording of electrical forces produced by the heart and translated as waveforms. It shows changes in rhythm, rate, or conduction of the heart such as arrhythmias, appearance of premature beats, block of impulses. ECG does not provide an index of cardiac output. Cardiac monitoring has become standard procedure in the OR and RR.

Cardiac monitoring systems generally consist of a monitor screen (cathode ray oscilloscope) on which the electrocardiogram is continuously visualized and a write-out system, which transcribes the rhythm strip on paper, to permit comparison of tracings and provide a permanent record. The write-out may be controlled or automatic. A heart-rate meter may be set to write out a rhythm strip if the rate goes below a preset figure. Lights and beepers may provide appropriate visual and audible signals of heart rate. Monitor leads or electrodes, electrically conductive discs or needles, are attached to the chest and/or extremities. These electrodes detect electrical impulses the heart generates. Connecting lead wires and cables transmit them to the cardiac monitor. A complete cardiogram includes 12 different leads but usually only two or three electrodes are used. Careful placement of leads is important to show the waves and complexes of the ECG rhythm strip. Leads to the anterior, lateral, or inferior cardiac surfaces where ischemia most often occurs provide myocardial ischemia monitoring. Use of multiple leads is becoming more common, as it allows better definition of arrhythmia and ischemia, the main reason for cardiac monitoring in the OR. The choice of leads is made by the anesthesiologist, or by the surgeon in unattended local anesthesia.

In *placing disc electrodes,* be sure the skin beneath is clean and dry for *adequate adherence.* Shave sites if necessary as hair can interfere with adherence. Abrade the skin slightly with a gauze pad or rough material to facilitate conduction. Peel off the paper backing on the disc. Avoid touching the adhesive as much as possible. Check the conductive gel within the gauze pad at the center of the disc. If it is not moist, use another disc. Place the electrode on the desired site, adhesive side down, and tightly secure by applying pressure. Begin at the center and move outward to avoid expressing gel from beneath the electrode.

One ECG tracing is taken before induction as a control. An electrocardiogram is especially valuable during induction and intubation when arrhythmias are prone to occur. Rapid identification of abnormal heart rhythms makes treatment more specific. It permits early recognition of occult irregularities of the heart's action. In event of cardiac arrest, it shows when heart action ceased. It also defines type of arrest, which is of value in treatment. Changes shown may be due to the anesthetic itself, to a change in oxygenation or coronary blood flow, to hypercarbia, or to alteration in electrolyte balance or body temperature. ECG monitors should be insensitive to electrical interference but recording may be affected by use of an electrosurgical unit at high frequency. This problem is negligible in newer monitors. If a tracing problem occurs, check for lead contact, fractured lead, or choice of monitoring axis.

Stethoscopy Stethoscopy provides continuous auscultation of the chest to detect both cardiac rate and rhythm and pulmonary sounds for monitoring cardiopulmonary status. A stethoscope is taped to the precordium and attached to an indwelling plastic earpiece. Or a pressure-sensitive detecting unit may be placed within the patient's esophagus. With the trachea protected from aspiration by a cuffed endotracheal tube, the stethoscope is inserted into the esophagus to the level of the heart. Esophageal stethoscopy is especially valuable during thoracic or abdominal procedures when the team's movement can interfere with auscultatory monitoring.

Arterial Blood Pressure An *indirect method,* by means of the sphygmomanometer, is used to assess hemodynamic and respiratory status during every operation with very few exceptions. Blood pressure (BP) signifies the pressure forcing blood through the circulation, i.e., the force exerted against the vessel wall. Machines are available for automatic BP monitoring at one-minute intervals, using ultrasound (Doppler principle). Automated noninvasive BP devices function well in a noisy environment, can be programmed to sound an alarm if systolic pressure reaches a preset high or low level. At preset intervals, the ultrasonic BP monitor automatically inflates the cuff, takes a reading, and deflates the cuff. While more accurate than sphygmomanometer pressure cuff monitoring, due to amplification of blood flow sounds by ultrasonic transducer, this monitor is less accurate than direct pressure reading via an arterial line. Nor does it provide continuous BP measurement or detect extremely low systemic pressure.

Direct arterial pressure monitoring, a beat-to-beat display of arterial BP, is an invasive modality. It is extremely valuable in patients with major multiple trauma or burns, inaccessibility of an extremity, unstable vital signs, or inaudible BP. Other indications are complex extensive procedures, such as cardiopulmonary bypass, open chest, major vascular surgery with large potential fluid shifts or blood loss, total hip replacement, major neurosurgery in sitting position. Also included are patients in shock or with preexisting cardiac or pulmonary disease who must undergo major surgery. Direct pressure monitoring is mandatory in deliberate hypotensive anesthesia as well as when treating hypotensive or hypertensive crisis with continuous infusion of vasopressor or hypertensive drugs.

Direct pressures are obtained through an artery such as the radial, via an indwelling catheter inserted percutaneously (see percutaneous arterial cannulation). A very slow drip of slightly heparinized saline keeps the catheter open. The fluid-filled tubing from the catheter is connected to a mechanical electric transducer from a pressure monitor. The transducer is attached to an amplifier that displays waveform, numerical measurement and sounds an alarm. The amplified signal represents the force imposed on the transducer.

Mean arterial pressure (MAP), calculated by most monitors and shown on digital display, portrays perfusion pressure of the body. It is significant in evaluating myocardial perfusion. Normal MAP is between 70 and 90 mm Hg.

Evaluation of BP during anesthesia requires consideration of the blood volume, cardiac output, state of sympathetic tone and blood volume, since tissue perfusion is dependent on these factors. The arm used for measurements should be protected from contact with team members standing beside the operating table.

Arterial Blood Gases and pH Serial monitoring of tissue perfusion measurements is indispensable in evaluating pulmonary gas exchange and acid-base balance. In planning interventions, measurements are considered in relation to other parameters such as venous pressure, left atrial pressure, and vital signs.

Respiratory gases in the blood, oxygen and carbon dioxide, exert their own partial pressures (P). The measurements are expressed in millimeters of mercury. Identification of the gas being measured is indicated as Pa (arterial) or Pv (venous). For example, the partial pressure of oxygen in arterial blood is expressed as PaO_2—95 mm Hg. Significant decrease in PvO_2 suggests inadequate systemic perfusion and oxygen delivery. The pH, measure of blood acidity, usually is determined also when respiratory gases are measured. Monitoring techniques permit rapid analysis of pO_2, pCO_2, O_2 saturation, pH, base excess, and actual bicarbonate. Tidal volume, respiratory rate, and concentration of oxygen inhaled can be adjusted to establish adequate oxygenation and carbon dioxide elimination. Differentiation of respiratory or metabolic acidosis or alkalosis is a guide to appropriate treatment.

Hypoventilation, uneven ventilation in relation to blood flow, impairment of diffusion, venous-to-arterial shunting lead to anoxemia unless oxygen in inspired air is increased. Hypoventilation of the whole lung or a major portion leads to retention of carbon dioxide and predisposes patient to cardiac arrhythmias. Disturbances of acid-base balance have many serious consequences in many organs. They must be corrected to achieve normal physiologic functioning.

Either or both arterial and venous bloodf-gas determinations and/or pressures may be monitored.

Central Venous Pressure (CVP) Because it accurately measures right atrial blood pressure, which in turn images right ventricular blood pressure, CVP assesses function of the heart's right side. It measures the pressure under which blood returns to the right atrium, i.e., reflects pressure in the major veins as blood returns to the heart. In other words, CVP represents the amount of venous return and filling pressure of the right ventricle. This information helps to determine the patient's circulatory status.

CVP also aids in evaluating blood volume and relationship between circulating blood volume and pumping action of the heart, i.e., adequacy of volume presented to heart for pumping. Therefore, CVP is a useful guide in blood or fluid administration, to avoid circulatory overload in patients having limited cardiopulmonary reserve. Too great or too rapid replacement can cause pulmonary edema. Generally a low CVP indicates that additional fluid can be given safely. Central venous pressure may be used during shock or hypotension to judge adequacy of blood replacement. However, CVP is not a measure of blood volume per se or of cardiac output.

Some indications for CVP monitoring are: major operation in a patient with preexisting cardiovascular disease; operative procedures in which large volume shifts are anticipated, e.g., open heart; critically ill patients, e.g., massive trauma; operations in which venous air emboli are a risk, e.g., craniotomy in sitting position; or during rapid administration of blood or fluid.

Central venous pressure may be monitored via an indwelling single-lumen radiopaque polyethylene catheter inserted into the subclavian vein, internal jugular vein, or antecubital area vein and threaded into the superior vena cava or right atrium, or via the proximal lumen of a pulmonary artery catheter. The proximal lumen port or external opening of the lumen lies in the right atrium, which is the best location for CVP measurement. Either catheter can be attached to a fluid-filled manometer that obtains measurement in centimeters of water (cm H_2O), or to a transducer and monitor with the value expressed in millimeters of mercury (mm Hg). If measurement is by pulmonary artery catheter proximal lumen, the hub of this lumen is connected to the manometer or to the transducer and monitor. The latter will display a right atrial waveform. Electronic transducer systems provide continuous monitoring of venous pressure. Serial measurement, portraying a trend, is more valuable than an isolated reading. Normal CVP reading is about 3 to 10 cm H_2O or 2 to 8 mm Hg (1 cm H_2O = 1.3 mm Hg). Consideration of normal values may vary somewhat.

Although CVP monitoring provides valuable data for assessing adequacy of vascular volume, it only indirectly reflects left heart function. There is no direct relationship between right and left ventricular filling pressures. Because of distensibility (compliancy) of the pulmonary blood vessels, the lungs can accept a marked increase in blood flow before significant congestion appears. Backup of blood caused by impaired function of left ventricle and subsequent increase in pulmonary vascular resistance (PVR) may occur before this increased pressure affects right heart, as exhibited by CVP values. Thus, CVP does not correlate with left heart performance in patients with left ventricular dysfunction or pulmonary congestion.

Continuous venous pressure monitoring supplies good measurement of the right heart, which in healthy hearts is a good monitor of both sides of the heart, but when a problem exists with the left heart, CVP does not provide all the desired information.

Central venous cannulation may provide access for replacement of transvenous cardiac pacemaker, drug route to central venous system, removal of blood for autotransfusion, placement of a hyperalimentation line, access for removal of air embolism in craniotomies.

In addition to *complications* previously mentioned, catheter shearing and embolization, extravascular migration of CVP catheter have been reported. Factors influencing migration of a catheter outside a vessel are location of catheter tip, stiffness and sharpness of catheter, and movement of the patient.

Assisting with Insertion of a Central Venous Access/Pressure Line

1 Prepare for sterile procedure.
 a Collect necessary *sterile* supplies. A disposable catheter insertion tray is convenient.
 b Set up the line: connect the IV bag to the tubing; insert the manometer into the line, attached by stopcock between IV tubing and the anesthesia extension tubing; run air out of the line and clamp; secure manometer upright to IV pole. follow procedure manual.
2 Assist the physician. External or internal jugular, subclavian, brachial, or femoral vein may be used. Catheter is usually inserted percutaneously, but may be by cutdown for antecubital vein, and advanced to the superior vena cava.
 a Insertion: Position patient. For subclavian or jugular vein insertion, place patient in 25 to 30° head-down Trendelenburg's position to reduce potential for air embolism. Elevation of scapular area with padding brings vein closer to skin surface. Head is turned away from side of insertion. If awake, patient bears down (Valsalva maneuver) as vein is punctured. This increases intrathoracic pressure and counteracts negative pressure from vein, to reduce possibility of air embolism.
 b Make sure connections in the line are secure. Connections to the three-way stopcock should be taped to prevent inadvertent disconnection. As soon as the line is in place, central venous pressure reading is taken as baseline measurement and as presumptive check for proper placement of cannula tip. Since expansion of lungs will increase intrathoracic pressure (deflation decreases it), column of fluid in manometer should fluctuate with each breath while reading is being taken.
 c Chest x-ray is taken to verify accurate placement of catheter in superior vena cava or right atrium.
3 Take a CVP reading.
 a Shut off lumen of stopcock to patient,

thereby running IV fluid into manometer. At desired level, shut off stopcock lumen to IV infusion.

b Take reading on the manometer (make certain zero scale is level with patient's right atrium), then close stopcock lumen to manometer, thereby opening infusion to patient again, to keep line open. Adjust flow rate.

c Take all readings under same conditions to recognize significant changes. Replace IV bag before it runs dry.

4 Connection of catheter line to electronic monitoring device permits continuous observation of CVP.

Pulmonary Artery (PA) Pressures Because a pulmonary artery catheter (PAC) measures both right and left heart function, it provides faster more accurate indication of impending left ventricular failure than central venous pressure alone. Left heart pressures are reflected in pulmonary artery and pulmonary capillary wedge pressures, measured by the PAC. This is more sensitive to rapid changes in the cardiovascular system than CVP, and more sensitive to the ability of the heart to accommodate fluid loads. Measurement of pulmonary pressures enables precise rapid assessment of the left ventricle's ability to eject an adequate cardiac output. Continuous evaluation of left ventricular function is extremely important in patients whose left heart dysfunction has a greater direct effect on cardiac output, circulating volume, and respiratory function than impaired right heart function.

Some of the many *indications* for patient monitoring with a PAC, commonly referred to as a Swan-Ganz catheter, are:

1 Preexisting cardiac or pulmonary disease and undergoing major vascular, intraabdominal, or neurosurgical operations such as aortic aneurysm resection, sitting craniotomy. Examples: recent congestive heart failure, confirmed coronary artery disease, recent myocardial infarction, noncompliant left ventricle, chronic obstructive pulmonary disease, pulmonary hypertension.

2 Previous stability, but at risk of developing cardiopulmonary instability during or after major stress.

3 Established disorders involving one or more major organ systems. Example: acute respiratory failure, low cardiac output states, multiple trauma.

4 Other conditions: e.g., shock (to determine etiology and maintain fluid balance), burns (large fluid shifts), renal failure (low cardiac output, fluid and electrolyte imbalance), pulmonary embolism.

Relative *contraindications* to pulmonary artery catheter monitoring, an invasive modality, are abnormal cardiac anatomy in the patient, or inadequate monitors and specially trained personnel.

Use of the pulmonary artery catheter for monitoring pressures indicative of pulmonary and left ventricular status has increased considerably in the CCU, ICU, RR, and OR. In addition to revealing hemodynamic status of cardiovascular and pulmonary function, the PAC assists in prompt, individualized, rational institution of therapy. PA pressures serve as guidelines in administration of fluids, diuretics, or cardiotonic drugs to obtain optimal cardiac output. The PA catheter is a complex multiple-lumen tool. Data procured include pulmonary artery pressure (PAP), pulmonary capillary wedge pressure (PCWP), right atrial pressure (RAP) also referred to as CVP, and cardiac output computation. Various pulmonary artery catheters are available. All are made of flexible, radiopaque polyvinyl chloride, Teflon, or polyurethane. The number of lumens may vary from two to five, depending on range of functions.

The *#7F Swan-Ganz thermodilution catheter* is versatile and widely used. It is 110 centimeters (43¼ inches) long with 10 cm increments marked on the side to permit observation of how far the catheter has advanced during insertion. Like all PACs, it is a balloon-tipped flotation catheter that is inserted into a major vein and advanced to the inferior or superior vena cava. When inflated, the thin latex balloon at the tip permits the catheter to float with the flow of blood through the right atrium, tricuspid valve, right ventricle, pulmonary semilunar valve, pulmonary artery, and to wedge in a small PA branch (arteriole) for recording pulmonary capillary wedge pressure during occlusion of the vessel. When the balloon is not inflated, the catheter lies in the pulmonary artery to record PA pressures. It is essential to achieve proper catheter placement to minimize risk of vessel damage and complications as well as to validate pressure readings.

The end of catheter inserted in the patient is referred to as the distal end; the opposite one is the proximal end. The latter is comprised of the lumen ports or external openings. The PA port is used for monitoring pulmonary artery and pulmonary capillary wedge pressures. A syringe is connected to the balloon port for desired balloon inflation. The thermistor port is used for cardiac output calculation. The right atrial port is used for measuring right atrial pressure. This port also can be used to administer fluids or be connected to a flush system for maintenance of catheter patency. For cardiac output measurement, saline or dextrose is injected into the cardiovascular system via the proximal lumen. (See cardiac output, p. 270.) Pulmonary artery and right atrial ports should be labeled.

Inside the catheter are four separate lumens or passages. The pulmonary artery lumen, the largest and most distal, terminates in the opening at the catheter's tip. With proper catheter positioning, this opening lies in the pulmonary artery. In this position with the balloon deflated, PA systolic, diastolic, and mean pressures are recorded on the monitor. These are indicative of pulmonary function. When the balloon is inflated and the catheter migrates to a pulmonary artery branch to wedge, pulmonary capillary wedge pressure is recorded. PCWP is sometimes referred to as PAWP (pulmonary artery wedge pressure) or PAOP (pulmonary artery occlusion pressure). Occlusion of a PA branch creates a no-flow system, thereby blocking blood flow from the right heart to the lungs and permitting pressure equilibration in the pulmonary vascular bed distal to the catheter. Occlusion of the arteriole, and the low resistance of the pulmonary systems, gives a pressure measurement equal to left artrial pressure, which in turn is equal to left ventricular end-diastolic pressure. *The balloon is always deflated immediately after taking a reading to prevent pulmonary infarction, ischemia, or hemorrhage from prolonged wedging.* The catheter will float back into the main pulmonary artery. The PA lumen can provide blood gas samples for blood gas measurements and mixed venous blood, also of value in judging cardiac function.

The balloon lumen opening, permitting inflation and deflation, is about one centimeter from the catheter tip. When inflated, the balloon surrounds but does not cover the opening in this tip.

The thermistor lumen opening is about four centimeters from the catheter tip. This lumen contains temperature-sensitive wires that run its length and transmit the temperature of blood flowing over them from the thermistor to the computer used to determine cardiac output by the thermodilution technique (see p. 270).

The proximal (RA) lumen opening is about 30 cm from the catheter's tip. This opening lies in the right atrium to monitor right atrial pressure when the catheter is in place.

Some of the newer PA catheter models may:

1 Be heparin-coated, to reduce formation of thrombi on them. Used in patients with intracardiac shunts or requiring long-term monitoring.

2 Be multipurpose, with ventricular and atrial pacing wires. Used in several types of heart block, severe bradycardia, A-V pacing, and intracardiac ECG.

3 Be able to measure continuous mixed venous oxygen saturation (S_vO_2)—PA oximetry—to determine adequacy of cardiac output.

4 Be able to measure cardiac output without discontinuation of therapy with titrated medication, e.g., nitroprusside, because of an additional right atrial lumen (five-lumen catheter).

Interpretation of Pressures The range of normal pressure values may vary slightly from one authority to another. Characteristic waveforms appear on the oscilloscope or screen, depending on location of the catheter tip during insertion and continuous monitoring. *These waveforms must be watched carefully to ascertain that the catheter is in the desired position.* The catheter enters the right atrium via the vena cava.

Right Atrial (RA) Pressure: Normal is 3 to 6 mm Hg. Right atrial pressure (RAP) reflects RA filling (diastolic) pressure, equivalent to central venous pressure and right ventricular end-diastolic pressure (RVEDP), pressure at the end of filling just prior to contraction. Rise in right atrial pressure may indicate right ventricular failure, left ventricular failure, volume overload (hypervolemia), air embolism. Fall in RAP may indicate vasodilatation, hypovolemia, or peripheral blood pooling.

Right Ventricular (RV) Pressure: Normal is 15 to 25 mm Hg systolic, 0 to 5 mm Hg diastolic. Rise in right ventricular pressure may indicate mitral insufficiency, congestive heart failure, hypoxemia, left ventricular failure.

Pulmonary Artery Pressure (PAP): Normal pressures are 15 to 25 mm Hg systolic, 8 to 15 diastolic, mean 9 to 19 mm Hg. These pressures estimate venous pressure in the lungs as well as mean filling pressure of left atrium and left ventricle. They reflect right ventricular function unless the patient has pulmonary stenosis, because commonly pulmonary artery systolic pressure approximates right ventricular systolic pressure. Changes in PA systolic and mean pressures indicate changes in pulmonary vascular resistance. Alterations in PVR occur in a variety of conditions, namely, hypoxemia, respiratory insufficiency, pulmonary edema, pulmonary embolism, shock, or sepsis. Thus, these pressures are indices of pulmonary function. Rise in PAP may indicate left ventricular failure, increased pulmonary arteriolar resistance (present in pulmonary hypertension, hypoxia), fluid overload.

Pulmonary Capillary Wedge Pressure (PCWP, PAWP, PAOP): Normal is 6 to 12 mm Hg. Pulmonary artery diastolic and PCW pressures are prime determinants of left heart function because they reflect pressures in the left ventricle just before it contracts (LVEDP), except in patients with mitral valve impairment.

Normally, when the mitral valve between the right atrium and right ventricle is open (ventricular diastole), flow of blood from the pulmonary artery through to pulmonary veins and left heart is unimpeded. Pressures then throughout the pulmonary circulation and left heart are comparable. Since PCWP usually approximates left atrial pressure, an indicator of left heart function, it is an important determinant of left ventricle preload. Intraoperative monitoring of PCWP usually can give early disclosure of left ventricular dysfunction. Rise in PCWP may indicate left ventricular failure, mitral insufficiency, pulmonary hypertension, fluid overload, pulmonary congestion. A rise also may occur during anesthesia induction. A fall in PCWP may indicate a reduction in LVEDP and cardiac output, or hypovolemia.

Complications of Pulmonary Artery Catheter Monitoring Invasion of the great vessels and heart carries many inherent perils. Probably the most common one during insertion is cardiac arrhythmia, especially premature contractions. Other problems include local or systemic infection (septicemia, endocarditis), thrombus formation, pulmonary embolism, pulmonary infarction, pneumothorax, hemothorax, major vessel or heart chamber perforation, kinking or knotting of catheter, balloon rupture, postoperative bleeding, erroneous diagnosis from misinterpretation of data.

Although rare, pulmonary artery perforation is very serious. Predisposing factors are pulmonary hypertension, anticoagulation, hyperthermia, overinflated balloon or catheter. Hemoptysis and sudden hypotension are symptoms of pulmonary artery rupture. Equipment for endobronchial intubation, chest tube insertion, and operative intervention must be available.

Strict attention to detail can prevent or greatly reduce the incidence of complications, which are potentially life-threatening and increase markedly after 48 to 72 hours of indwelling catheterization.

Insertion of Pulmonary Artery Catheter (PAC). PAC insertion is a strictly sterile procedure. Insertion is performed by a physician with a nurse assisting. The catheter often is inserted in the OR suite by an anesthesiologist/anesthetist prior to induction or after the patient is unconscious. Insertion is a team effort. *Every precaution must be taken to ensure patient safety.*

The *nurse's responsibilities* may vary according to policy, but should include:

1 Preparing patient physically and emotionally. Checking consent form.

2 Checking the oscilloscope and gathering the necessary equipment. *Be familiar with and follow the manufacturer's directions for the brand of catheter and equipment you are using.* This cannot be overemphasized.

3 Setting up the system, initial setup similar to that of arterial lines. The type of transducer used with a balloon flotation catheter may vary. Again, *follow directions explicitly.* Check all equipment. Test for leaks. Attach stopcocks and flush devices to transducer head(s). Stopcocks control lines to transducer. Backflush transducer dome. Transducer cable attaches to monitor for readings. If patient also has a peripheral arterial line, two transducers and a triple stopcock manifold are needed. Simultaneous monitoring of pulmonary artery and right atrial pressures is thus possible. Each transducer's balancing port must be leveled with patient's right atrium. The monitor should be balanced and calibrated according to manufacturer's directions. *Be sure no air bubbles remain in the lines or system.* The catheter, after insertion, must not be attached to system until all air has been previously expelled, to prevent air embolus. Convenient pre-assembled tubing systems and disposable transducer domes are commercially available and offer advantages. Also, be sure all electrical equipment is grounded.

4 Positioning the patient as requested for access.

5 Taking vital signs before insertion and *watching the monitor during insertion.* Specially observe for arrhythmias and softly count them aloud for the physician, if desired. Have lidocaine ready to inject.

6 Observing and recording right atrial, pulmonary artery, and pulmonary capillary wedge pressures and waveforms.

7 Assisting with or applying the sterile dressing at completion.

8 Documenting the procedure and readings.

Before *catheter insertion,* the *physician* inspects the catheter for defects and tests the balloon for leakage by inflating it, submerging it in a sterile saline basin and watching for air bubbles. Balloon must then be deflated. Moistening the catheter tip with saline or lidocaine reduces possibility of venospasm at insertion. He or she uses the introducer set and after the catheter has been inserted, advances the catheter rapidly to avert loss of stiffness which can cause it to kink or knot. Continued manipulation irritates or damages vessel walls. Watching the increment markings on the side helps determine how far catheter has advanced. It is possible to keep pushing the catheter while it is not going into the right place and have it coil up and knot in the ventricle.

When the catheter tip reaches the *right atrium,* and an RA waveform appears on the oscilloscope screen or readout strip, the balloon is inflated slowly with air, using a tuberculin syringe, to enable it to float with the flow of blood. *Never inflate the balloon without visible oscilloscope trace.* If the patient is awake, a voluntary cough confirms the position of the catheter in the thoracic cavity if the RA wave fluctuates. *The amount of air is specified by the manufacturer* (usually about 1.3 to 1.5 cc). Do not overinflate, which could rupture the balloon. Carbon dioxide (CO_2) is used for balloon inflation in patients with intracardiac shunts where possible arterial circulation may be entered because CO_2 is much more soluble than air in the blood, should the balloon rupture. A feeling of resistance should accompany inflation. If there is no resistance, a sign of ruptured balloon, inflation should be stopped immediately. Fluid is *never* used for inflation because it would prevent proper catheter flotation and complete deflation.

Passing through the tricuspid valve, the catheter enters the *right ventricle.* A typical RV waveform should appear. If arrhythmia (PVC) develops or is persistent, a bolus of lidocaine may be injected. Then after floating through the pulmonary semilunar valve into the *pulmonary artery,* a PA tracing should appear on the monitor. This waveform has a steep upstroke at the beginning (right ventricle ejection and opening of pulmonic valve) followed by a dicrotic notch on the downstroke (closing of pulmonic valve). Pulmonary artery blood flow carries the balloon into one of the PA's smaller branches. When the vessel diameter becomes too narrow for the balloon to pass, the latter wedges in the vessel and occludes it. A PCWP waveform should appear. After recording of this wedge pressure, the physician permits the balloon to deflate passively. Do not aspirate the air with a syringe. The catheter will then slip back into the main branch of the pulmonary artery. A pulmonary artery pressure waveform should reappear on the monitor. Thus, the physician depends on these sequential characteristic pressure waveforms to reveal the catheter tip's location *at all times.* The nurse records the pressure at each location. *The catheter remains in the pulmonary artery with the balloon deflated, continuously recording PA pressures, except when PCWP reading is desired.* If a PAP waveform persists and a PCWP is unobtainable, or resistance is not felt at attempt to inflate the balloon, it may be that the balloon is ruptured. An x-ray is taken to confirm catheter position. In case of rupture, the catheter may be left in place to record PAP provided that it has not slipped back to the right ventricle. The physician may also elect to remove it. *The balloon is always inflated during catheter advancement and deflated during catheter withdrawal.*

After completion of the insertion procedure, the catheter is sutured in place to prevent inadvertent advancement or removal. An antibiotic ointment or skin antiseptic and sterile, preferably transparent dressing are applied to the insertion site. Be sure the dressing is not too tight and the catheter beneath it is not bent or curled. Baseline vital signs and pressures are recorded. Check all lines for security and transducer(s) and lines for patency. An x-ray may be ordered to check catheter position and patient's chest.

Catheter withdrawal usually is performed by a physician. To prevent injury to the heart valves, the balloon is slightly inflated until the catheter is withdrawn to the right atrium. Then the balloon is completely deflated for withdrawal. Arrhythmias may occur. Pressure is applied to the insertion site to prevent bleeding. Pulse and BP are checked prior to and after withdrawal. Postwithdrawal dressing is applied. Patient is monitored for at least 24 hours.

In addition to patient problems, *monitoring problems* may arise. Each requires a specific intervention. A major problem is a damped pressure or PAP waveform. This means decreased amplitude in pressure tracings or loss of sharpness in image suggestive of a defect in the circuit. Common causes are air in the system or blood in the transducer; loose connections; kinked, overwedged or malpositioned catheter; falling systolic pressure in patient or a clot in the monitor system. If the latter is suspected, gently try to aspirate blood. If no blood can be aspirated, do *not* flush. Flushing could dislodge a clot. Notify the physician who may need to withdraw the catheter.

Another problem involves sudden change in configuration of a pressure tracing. Potential causes include: transducer not at right atrium level, transducer in need of calibration, transducer connection to catheter not secure, catheter no longer in proper position, loss of pressure in pressure bag. If a PCWP waveform persists after taking a reading, the balloon may not be completely deflated or the catheter tip may be caught in the wedge position, requiring immediate attention. Nurses must be familiar with the appropriate interventions in both patient problems and monitoring problems in addition to being knowledgeable about the causes and preventive precautions. Only in this way can patient safety be maximized in invasive monitoring.

Cardiac Output (CO) Cardiac output is measured by the *thermodilution technique* to determine liters per minute of blood pumped by the left ventricle into the aorta. Normal resting value is four to eight liters per minute. A known amount of fluid at a known temperature is injected into a lumen of an arterial catheter and a temperature gradient at a point downstream is measured via a second lumen. Ten milliliters of iced cold or room temperature physiologic saline or 5% dextrose in water solution usually is used. Blood flow supplies the thermal dilution, e.g., the saline mixes with the blood in the superior vena cava or the right atrium, depending on catheter location, reducing the temperature of blood in the heart. The cooled blood flows past a transistorized intravascular thermistor in the thermodilution catheter that detects changes in blood temperatures which are then used to compute CO. When the injectate is introduced via the proximal (RA) lumen of a pulmonary artery catheter (Swan-Ganz), a digital display of CO is seen within four to five seconds.

Cardiac output reflects mechanical activity of the heart and represents total blood flow to all body tissues and vascular shunts. It depends on the rate of heartbeat (HR), contractile strength of the heart (myocardial contractility), peripheral resistance of the vessels, and venous return. Inotropic agents, such as digitalis or epinephrine, increase contractility and CO except in patients with loss of functioning ventricular muscle, e.g., myocardial infarction (MI) or aneurysm of the left ventricle. Agents such as beta blockers decrease work of the heart by reducing contractility and CO. Calculation of *left ventricular stroke work index* reflects pumping ability. During systole the ventricle does not totally eject the blood received during diastole. The amount of blood ejected with each contraction is referred to as the *stroke volume (SV).* Normal resting SV is 60 to 130 ml/beat. Determinants of stroke volume are left atrial pressure, afterload, contractile state of the myocardium, and left ventricular end-diastolic pressure (see below). *Ejection fraction (EF),* a commonly used indicator of ventricular function, is the percentage value of blood volume ejected, i.e., stroke volume. Normal EF is 60 to 70 percent. Major stroke volume determinants of cardiac output are preload, contractility, and afterload. Only in limited circumstances such as bradyarrhythmias does adjustment of heart rate therapeutically enhance cardiac output.

Preload, the amount of blood in the ventricle at the end of diastole, may be referred to as *left ventricular end-diastolic volume (LVEDV) or filling pressure (LVEDP).* Assessment of changes in volume by measurement of changes in filling pressure helps to describe cardiac function. The Starling principle concerns the relationship between volume, stretch, and contractility. It relates myocardial fiber length to the force of contraction. The greater the preload and stretch of myocardial fibers, the greater the subsequent contraction, thereby increasing stroke volume until at some point ventricular failure commences. Fiber overstretch weakens contractions. As pumping ability decreases, the left ventricle is unable to empty completely. Residual blood, combined during diastole with incoming oxygenated blood from pulmonary veins and left atrium, increases workload and elevates left ventricular volume and pressure. As ventricular efficiency declines, cardiac output falls. Unpumped blood in the left ventricle backs up into the left atrium and pulmonary circulation, increasing these pressures. Pulmonary edema and respiratory insufficiency result as fluid is impelled into alveoli. The central venous pressure catheter measures right heart preload; the pulmonary artery catheter measures the left atrial and LVED pressures.

Cardiac function may be classified as normal, compromised, or failing. In normal hearts, maximum ventricular performance seems to be achieved at 8 to 12 mm Hg filling pressure. In compromised hearts this pressure is higher.

A reduced cardiac output results in decreased perfusion of capillary circulation. During hemorrhage, when circulating blood volume is reduced, the resulting diminished venous return and preload leads to a lowered cardiac output. Atrial fibrillation also can modify filling of the ventricles. Venous dilatation contributes to pooling of blood with subsequent decreased venous return to the heart. Low CO states result from: reduced preload, as in hypovolemia, venous dilatation or cardiac tamponade; reduced contractility, as from anesthetic drugs, ischemia, infarction, or cardiac decompensation; dysrhythmias; increased afterload, as in hypertension, pulmonary embolism, or elevated or diminished heart rate. Body position can influence circulation as well as age, body surface area, oxygen consumption, body temperature, basal metabolic rate, and activity. Thus, many factors can affect cardiac output.

Afterload indicates the resistance the heart must overcome to eject blood into the systemic circulation. This impedance to flow is called *systemic vascular resistance* (SVR). Left ventricular pressure must exceed pressure in the aorta to open the aortic valve and force blood from the heart into the circulation. Afterload, not a direct measure, is deduced by calculating the SVR. Elevated afterload can produce increased left ventricle wall tension in attempt to generate adequate intracavitary ventricular pressure to overcome resistance and permit systolic ejection. The subsequent resulting increase in myocardial oxygen demand must be met by the oxygen supply or ventricular function deteriorates. Diminution of afterload reduces wall tension, thereby improving ventricular contraction. Improving cardiac function involves considering cost in myocardial oxygen consumption. Augmenting cardiac output by increasing heart rate and contractility increases myocardial oxygen consumption. Improving cardiac output by augmenting preload or by reducing afterload results in relatively little oxygen cost to the myocardium.

A comprehensive view of cardiac function can be obtained by measurement of filling pressure, cardiac output, and compilation by formula of the derivation of peripheral resistance. Repeated interval measurements offer prompt evaluation of effectiveness of treatment.

Cardiac Index (CI) Measures the volume per minute of cardiac output per square meter of body surface area. Normal CI is about 2.4 to 3.6 liters/min/m^2.

Total Blood Volume (BV) Blood volume is useful in determining the total amount of blood replacement required. Inadequate replacement can lead to decrease in cardiac output and cardiovascular collapse. Calculation of BV depends upon venous hematocrit value. The dilution principle is utilized in determination. An accurate method of BV measurement involves measuring plasma and red-cell volumes separately, then adding results together. To measure red-cell volume, cells are tagged with detectable, nontoxic, radioactive chromium, subsequently injected intravenously, and counted after an appropriate mixing time. Or radioactive iodinated human serum albumin (RIHSA), in standard-dose packages, can be injected, mixed, and counted. Counting may be done rapidly by an electronic device. This technique may be used in place of estimation of operative blood loss.

Estimation of Operative Blood Loss Is made in all operations where a major blood loss and need for replacement is necessary since a deficit of blood volume is the most frequent cause of postoperative hypotension. The gravimetric method of weighing sponges is a simple and common method. Previously dry sponges are weighed after use as they are discarded from the operative field. Dry weight is subtracted from wet weight. Blood in the suction bottle may be measured but allowance must be made for presence of irrigating solution if used. The amount of blood on drapes is visually estimated.

Respiratory Tidal Volume (V_t) Volume of air moved with each respiration may be measured with respirometer placed on the expiratory limb of the anesthesia machine or mechanical ventilator. Alarms may be incorporated to signal disconnection, failure to cycle, or excessive pressure.

Body Temperature Measures surface (skin) or deep (core) body temperatures by thermistors and thermocouples of an electronic telethermometer with dial readout. A thermistor is inserted in the patient's esophagus, nasopharynx, bladder, or rectum and connected to a meter. Changes in central body temperature can predict important incidents. Convulsions may follow hyperpyrexia, which increases metabolism and demand for oxygen. (See p. 276 for discussion of malignant hyperthermia under anesthesia.) A falling temperature, the most common change, may precede increased irritability of the heart and ventricular fibrillation. Hypothermia also delays metabolism of drugs and alters effects of neuromuscular blockers. Changes in body temperature may be marked during anesthesia. Cutaneous temperature changes are a clue to vasoactivity at a given time, helping diagnose vasoconstriction or vasodilatation. They parallel changes in cardiac output.

Hypothermia under anesthesia may result from air-conditioning, skin prep and drape saturation, massive blood replacement or cool infusion or irrigating solutions, anesthetic effect (decreased metabolic rate and increased vasodilatation), depression of thermoregulatory function by drugs or inhalation anesthetic agents, prolonged exposure of abdomen or thorax to air, high inflow anesthesia circuits with water loss from the respiratory tract, prevention of shivering. Transfusion reactions under anesthesia may be accompanied by profound hypotension and temperature change. The common undisguised physical reaction and chill are not seen in the anesthetized patient. Retention of heat and *hyperthermia* may be caused by premedication such as atropine, the sterile drapes covering the patient, a warm OR, a closed anesthesia breathing circuit, or fever and sepsis in the patient.

Surface temperature monitoring is noninvasive. Temperature sensitive chemicals are laminated within a thin plastic sheet, a sensor strip applied to the forehead. Temperature variations produce chemical and color changes which result in portrayal of a visible numerical reading. Surface temperatures show trends and indicate need for core monitoring.

Urinary Output Is measured by indwelling Foley catheter, which also prevents bladder distention. Output is valuable in assessing effective blood volume and fluid administration, except when a diuretic is given. Volume, electrolytes, osmolarity, and pH are important.

A reduction in urinary volume may indicate reduced renal perfusion. Oliguria can result from stress of operation, antidiuresis from anesthetic agent, impending renal failure, or reduced volume of circulating blood. Output above 30 to 60 ml/hour usually shows adequate intravascular volume.

The collecting system should be able to accurately measure half-hour output between one and 200 ml and provide observation of urine. Hemoglobinuria can be a manifestation of transfusion of incompatible blood. An electronic monitoring system is available, with digital display of data that can be fed into a computer. The system records output in milliliters for both the present and the immediately past hours. It also shows number of minutes elapsed in the current hour. Early warning of possible cardiovascular or renal problems is facilitated by visual alert signals if urine flow ceases. Sterile disposable collection system prevents reflux of bacteria toward patient.

Chest X-ray Essential for checking position of: pulmonary artery catheter (Swan-Ganz), central venous pressure line, endotracheal tube, chest tube; for observing changes in lung and heart during therapy.

Electroencephalogram (EEG) Electrical activity of the nervous system reflects neurologic function. Therefore, electrophysiologic monitoring provides information about the functional integrity of the central nervous system during anesthesia and operation, especially valuable in patients undergoing high-risk neurosurgical, vascular, or orthopaedic operations. EEG patterns vary among individuals, with regard to anesthetics, drugs, and pathologic and physiologic changes. They reveal the presence of organic brain damage, abnormal physiologic alterations and action of drugs.

Regional cerebral blood flow correlates well with EEG activity. Computer analysis offers visual recognition of cerebral hypoperfusion or ischemia. EEG is used particularly in operations of expected localized brain ischemia with operative occlusion. EEG also is a means of determining cessation of circulation, an index of expected prognosis and brain vitality.

Scalp electrodes, cups or discs of silver/silver

chloride, gold, or tin, are fixed in place with paste or collodion. Or subdermal platinum electrodes can be used. Electrodes are placed over areas of cerebral cortex according to a system which uses measurements of head circumference, distance between ears, and distance from nasion (point where sagittal plane intersects frontonasal suture) to inion (external protuberance of occipital bone). The small neurophysiologic signals recorded are amplified for analysis and display. Multiple channels are necessary to detect regional versus global alterations in function. As many as eight to 32 channels may be recorded simultaneously. Paper records or strip-charting provides comparisons of EEG activity during crucial periods with activity seen prior to anesthesia induction or operative manipulation. Methods of EEG analysis that permit automated pattern recognition and alarm generation enhance monitoring in the OR or ICU. Devices are available that process EEG signals to simplify and facilitate the complex EEG analysis.

Cerebral Function Monitor Provides trend recording of amplitude and amplitude variability for a single channel of EEG, mainly useful for detecting marked global alterations in EEG activity during cardiopulmonary bypass, induced hypotension, or metabolic coma. During carotid endarterectomy, paired monitors can detect EEG asymmetries. While simplifying monitoring, they may be less sensitive to ischemia than the 16-channel strip-chart recording.

Compressed Spectral Array (CSA) May give a time-compressed "mountain and valley" representation of EEG activity. CSA programs can be run on general purpose mini- or microcomputers.

Neurometrics Monitor Is also a single-channel device for displaying processed EEG signals. Four to 32 minutes of EEG can be seen at one time, but trends are less easily seen.

Somatosensory Evoked Potentials In the past, surgeons might not have known until completion of operation if healthy nerves had been injured. Intraoperative monitoring of somatosensory evoked potentials is used to continuously assess spinal cord function and to protect cord from injury during orthopaedic or neurosurgical operations on the spine or spinal cord. Since hypotension increases the insult of direct pressure on the cord and heightens damage to cord function, the spinal cord is monitored when induced hypotension is employed for spinal surgery. Impulses generated below site of operation travel over lateral afferent neural pathways, through operative spinal area, and are recorded by electrodes at brain level. Abnormal brain responses are marked by changes in arrival time of electrical impulses or amplitude of waves on a graph. Change in latency and amplitude of the recorded signal, which normally averages 30 to 50 evoked responses, alerts team to danger of spinal cord compression or ischemia. Corrective measures taken immediately can prevent serious sequelae. Evoked responses then return to normal.

COMPLICATIONS OF OPERATION UNDER ANESTHESIA

The anesthesiologist must be constantly aware of the surgeon's actions. He or she must do everything possible to ensure safety of the patient and reduce stress of operation. Continuous appraisal of the patient's overall condition helps avoid complications. Some complications may occur as a direct result of anesthesia; others may have additional contributing factors. Some conditions that may occur during the procedure are discussed in the following paragraphs. These same complications, as well as others (see Chap. 36), may appear in the postoperative period. Tragically, catastrophic emergencies may sometimes arise when least expected. Minutes can make the difference in life or death for the patient. Anticipation and preparedness may spell that difference.

Aspiration

Pulmonary aspiration of gastric contents is highly dangerous and may occur during abolition of throat reflexes when the patient is unconscious or when conscious with the throat anesthetized, as for bronchoscopy. Aspiration results in residual effects on lung function and blood-gas exchange. A chemical pneumonitis results from aspiration of highly acidic gastric juices. Edema forms, alveoli collapse, ventilation-perfusion mismatch occurs, and hypoxemia results. Aspiration of solids or particulate matter results in edema, severe hypoxia, and respiratory obstruction. Bronchospasm and atelectasis may be followed by pneumonitis or bronchopneumonia. Most aspiration is irritative, but it can be infectious if nasopharyngeal flora are aspirated. Pneumonia or lung abscess may result. Every patient who has food in the stomach is a poor risk for anesthesia; for example, a patient with traumatic injuries on whom operation is attempted without adequate preparation. Increased intragastric pressure is an aspiration hazard and may result from conditions such as pylorospasm, diaphragmatic hernia, gastrointestinal bleeding, intestinal obstruction, or gas forced into the stomach by application of positive-pressure ventilation without use of a cuffed endotracheal tube.

Symptoms Cyanosis, dyspnea, tachycardia, followed by cardiac embarrassment, lung collapse, and consolidation.

Treatment Most effective treatment occurs during the first minutes after aspiration. The strategy is to remove as much aspirate as possible and limit the spread of what is left in the lung. Lower head of table with a right lateral tilt for postural drainage. (The right mainstem bronchus take-off is the higher.) Suction oropharynx and tracheobronchial tree. If the patient has aspirated particulate matter that causes obstruction of airways, bronchoscopy must be performed to remove it. Suctioning must be interrupted every 10 to 15 seconds to give oxygen. Oxygenation and CO_2 removal are high priority. Aspiration of acid gastric content injures the alveolar capillary interface resulting in intrapulmonary shunting and pulmonary edema. Intensive pulmonary care is aimed at improving ventilation-perfusion ratios and decreasing the abnormal gas exchange. This may require tracheal intubation for mechanical ventilation with continuous positive pressure. Most severe hypoxemia is expected to occur rapidly within first 30 to 60 minutes after aspiration. Careful cardiovascular monitoring and frequent blood-gas and acid-base determinations guide therapeutic measures to maintain intravascular volume. Prophylactic antibiotics may be given for aspiration of bowel-contaminated fluid to prevent infection, and a bronchodilator to treat spasm. Most permanent injury and death result from the initial hypoxemia.

Prevention Adequate preoperative preparation (withholding oral intake eight to ten hours before induction) and careful administration of anesthetic agents. Use of nasogastric tube pre- and intraoperatively where indicated. Anesthetic is decreased near end of operation, hastening the return of throat reflexes. All obstetrical patients receiving general anesthesia should be treated as if they have full stomachs and induced with rapid sequence intubation. Gastric evacuation is delayed by labor and medications.

Laryngospasm and Bronchospasm

These spasms or abnormal narrowings of the airways are produced by marked increase in smooth muscle tone of the airway walls. Marked elevation of airway resistance profoundly alters gas flow into and out of lungs. Accompanying changes result in a decreased ventilation-perfusion ratio, with subsequent reduction in PaO_2 and rise in $PaCO_2$. Many factors can precipitate spasm.

Etiology Mechanical airway obstruction, certain anesthetics and/or drugs, allergic conditions such as asthma; vagal reflex; stimulation of pharynx and larynx under light anesthesia; traction of peritoneum; foreign material in tracheobronchial tree; movement of head or neck or traction on carotid sinus; painful peripheral stimuli. Degree of spasm varies from mild to severe.

Symptoms Wheezing respirations or stridor, reduced compliance, cyanosis, respiratory obstruction.

Treatment Depends on precipitating factor. Methods generally used: positive-pressure oxygen; tracheal intubation, neuromuscular blockers for relaxation; bronchodilator drugs such as aminophylline, isoetharine, and metaproterenol sulfate (with caution as they act as cardiac stimulators and, in the presence of hypoxia, they may contribute to cardiac arrhythmia and cardiac arrest). Patients may be refractory to bronchodilators because of acid-base abnormalities. Correction can reduce side effects and augment beneficial effects of bronchodilators. If etiology is allergic, steroids (methylprednisolone) and antihistamines may be given. Vagal reflexes are inhibited by atropine. If reflex is the cause, anesthesia is deepened. Drying agents are given for excessive secretions. Immediate effective treatment is mandatory to counteract hypoxia and prevent cardiac arrest.

Prevention Patent airway, appropriate premedication such as atropine; avoidance of factors stimulating vagal reflex; treatment of predisposing pulmonary pathology.

Respiratory Obstruction

Etiology Blocking of the airway by a foreign body, soft tissue, excessive secretions; poor position; laryngospasm or bronchospasm resulting in hypoxia and carbon dioxide retention.

Symptoms Increased respiratory effort with inadequate respiratory exchange; respiratory motion of chest and abdomen without audible air movement at the airway. Pallor and cyanosis rapidly follow hypoxia. The latter develops more slowly if the patient has been breathing high concentration of oxygen. Respirations may or may not be noisy.

Treatment Eliminate the cause; administer oxygen by positive pressure.

Prevention Patent airway; chin held up and forward if endotracheal tube is not used; adequate oxygen intake; prevention of foreign bodies in the airway; proper positioning on operating table; avoidance of pressure on chest.

Hypoxia and Hypercarbia

The ability to oxygenate depends on hemoglobin concentration, cardiac output, and oxygen saturation, therefore, any deficits in any of these factors affects oxygenation. The body compensates for mild hypoxia with increased heart and respiratory rates, bringing more oxygen to blood and tissues. If hypoxia progresses, this compensation is inadequate. If hypoxia is prolonged, cardiac arrhythmia or irreversible brain, liver, kidney, and heart damage results.

Etiology Inadequate pulmonary ventilation from depression of the respiratory center by narcotics and/or anesthetic, reduced cardiac output, severe blood loss, obstruction to respiratory passages, ventilation-perfusion ratio abnormality.

Symptoms Pallor or cyanosis; decreased volume of respirations; stertorous or labored respirations; dark blood in the operative field.

Treatment Immediate adequate oxygen intake to stimulate the medullary centers and prevent respiratory-system failure.

Prevention Patent airway, adequate oxygenation, proper positioning, intraoperative measurement of arterial pH, pCO_2, and pO_2 to enable the anesthesiologist to evaluate oxygenation and carbon dioxide removal. Patients may be given oxygen and assisted ventilation during transportation to the recovery area to prevent hypoxia from hypoventilation.

Pneumothorax

Rarely may occur from insertion of needle into the thoracic cage during nerve block or subclavian catheter insertion. The prime symptom is shortness of breath. Confirmation is made by x-ray. If extensive, and lung fails to reexpand, chest tube with underwater seal is required.

Air Embolism

May occur intraoperatively with patient in sitting position for craniotomy or posterior cervical operations. Cerebral diploic veins are noncollapsible; venous sinuses in the skull remain open. Air entering a vein is carried rapidly to the right heart and pulmonary circulation, obstructing ventricular flow. Cardiac arrhythmias or unexplained hypotension are prime symptoms. Characteristic heart murmur may be audible by precordial stethoscope or Doppler device. Air embolism may also occur during cardiopulmonary bypass, thyroidectomy, or laparoscopy.

Preoperative placement of central venous catheter (see p. 265) allows immediate aspiration of air. If no catheter is in place, the patient is placed in steep head-down position with right side up, to relieve ventricular obstruction. If cardiac arrest occurs, cardiopulmonary resuscitation is begun (see p. 284). Closed heart massage may move embolus obstructing coronary artery.

Intercostal Muscle Spasm ("Rigid Chest")

This may occur after large doses of intravenous fentanyl or on emergence from general anesthesia. It may reverse itself, or neuromuscular blockers may be needed.

Convulsions

Convulsions occur most often in patients with hyperactive metabolic rate, especially in hyperpyretic or dehydrated children. It is important to maintain as normal a body temperature as possible in all patients. Anoxia and death can result.

Etiology Severe hypoxia and carbon dioxide retention; hyperthermia; overdose of regional anesthetic drugs; air embolism; epilepsy.

Symptoms Muscular twitching, dilated pupils, rapid snorting respirations, rapid pulse, grimacing, cyanosis.

Treatment Administer oxygen to maintain respiration; diazepam or rapid-acting intravenous barbiturate or neuromuscular blocker to stop convulsions; artificial ventilation for apnea; support circulation.

Injuries

Injuries are many and varied. Some of the more common ones are injury to nerves and bones from faulty positioning and careless handling of anesthetized patients such as hyperabduction or extension of arm, which can result in paralysis, fractures, or postoperative pain. (See Chapter 10 for instructions for lifting an unconscious patient.)

Eyes can be injured from irritating anesthetics, face masks, or from drying of the cornea if the eyelids are not closed. The latter occurs most often in patients with loss of normal lubrication by eye movement, protuding eyes, or faces covered by drapes, or those in prone positions. Use of an ocular lubricant protects the cornea from drying.

Extravasation, thrombophlebitis, or air emboli are associated with intravenous infusions. Keep intravenous needles visible and not entirely hidden beneath drapes; check infusions frequently; fill tubing with solution before connecting to needle or catheter. *Precaution is the best prevention of injuries.*

Malignant Hyperthermia/Hyperpyrexia

Malignant hyperthermia (MH) is a fulminant hypermetabolic crisis triggered by anesthetic agents in susceptible individuals. This crisis results from a hereditary inability of the sarcoplasmic reticulum (SR), a skeletal muscle cell membrane, to control intramyoplasmic levels of calcium. During MH, skeletal muscle undergoes contraction as a result of releases of calcium response to drugs or stress. Rapid increase of calcium in the muscle fiber leads to generalized catabolism. MH, an often fatal complication, is characterized by uncontrolled acceleration of muscle metabolism accompanied by tremendous oxygen consumption, and heat and carbon dioxide production. Rapid progressive elevation of body temperature has been monitored as high as 47°C (117°F). Mortality rate may be as high as 60 to 70 percent in patients untreated with dantrolene. Early dantrolene therapy can reduce the mortality rate substantially.

A favorable prognosis decreases when excessive heat is noted from the patient through the surgeon's gloves or in the reservoir bag or soda lime canister as *fever may be a late sign of MH syndrome.*

The overall incidence is about one per 15,000 children and one per 20,000 of the total population. About 1,500 MH incidents are reported annually. Reported age extremes range from two months to 78 years. Onset of symptoms have been reported from one minute to as late as four and one-half hours into a general anesthetic. A number of cases did not occur until the patient arrived in the recovery room. Occurrence may be in the first anesthetic experience or a later one; one-third of cases appear in a second or subsequent anesthesia. MH crisis has occurred after as many as seven totally uneventful anesthetics. Prevalence exists in Caucasians and Orientals, in *children, young adults, and males,* perhaps due to increased muscularity.

Etiology A familial genetic transmission exists with variable penetrance. Some feel it affects 50 percent of offspring, although some cases are nonfamilial. Both rigid and nonrigid types (see p. 277) have been found in the same family. Unexplained fever during operation under anesthesia has many causes, some obscure.

Many agents may catalyze or trigger this abnormal muscular and metabolic response in susceptible individuals. Most potent volatile anesthetic agents (halogenated agents), depolarizing skeletal muscle relaxants (succinylcholine), and also local anesthetics (*amide*-type) have been associated with this catastrophe. Although MH most often occurs during general anesthesia, with halothane and succinylcholine most frequently implicated, no anesthetic agent should be presumed to be absolutely safe.

Population at Risk Suspected patients include those with any type of myopathy or muscle disease, e.g., ptosis, strabismus, hernia or area of muscle weakness, or area of muscle hypertrophy (calves of legs). Some of these patients have a history of temperature instability with minor illness, e.g., 41°C (106°F) or greater with a minor sore throat. A majority will show an unexplained preoperative elevation of creatine phosphokinase (CPK), although other conditions can produce high levels. But, *the most prominent clue to identification of an MH susceptible patient is a family history of unexplained death under general anesthesia.* A multifactoral inheritance with a wide range of susceptibilities may be present. Also, susceptibility may be acquired. One in 200 persons is possibly at risk. *Preoperative muscle biopsy is the most definitive indicator of risk for MH.*

Clinical Signs and Symptoms Signs and symptoms may be variably presented according to type of presentation of MH and swiftness of detection. The most common presenting sign is unexplained *ventricular arrhythmia,* mainly *tachycardia* or premature ventricular contractions (PVCs). This is associated with tachypnea, cyanosis or dark blood in the operative field (central venous desaturation), skin mottling, unstable blood pressure, fever, hot skin or tissues, diaphoresis. Symptoms usually, but not always, include *rigidity. Spasm of the jaw muscles with rigidity of masseter muscles or severe fasciculations following succinylcholine administration should suggest development of malignant hyperthermia.* The operation should be canceled and full therapy and monitoring for MH begun.

A sudden, generalized hypermetabolic state is produced. The temperature rises rapidly as more heat is produced than the body can eliminate. The body tries to adjust by vasodilatation and increased cardiac output. If rapidly increasing tissue demands are not met, *hypoxia, central venous hypercarbia, severe respiratory and metabolic acidosis* occur, progressing to cardiovascular collapse.

Late clinical findings include hyperkalemia, acute renal failure, left heart failure, disseminated intravascular coagulopathy (DIC), skeletal muscle swelling or necrosis from hypoxia and acidosis, pulmonary edema, neurologic sequelae (paraplegia, decerebration) and coma from ischemia secondary to hypoxia, recurrence of MH within 24 to 48 hours, inadvertent hypothermia from too vigorous cooling.

Laboratory Findings Expected values in MH include increased serum levels of potassium, magnesium, CPK, myoglobin; hypoxemia and hypercarbia (initial pCO_2 commonly 100–200 torr); respiratory and metabolic acidosis, myoglobinuria.

Treatment *Success is contingent on complete preparedness* (preplanned action, written protocol, immediate equipment supply), early diagnosis, and vigorous therapy.

1 *Discontinue anesthesia and stop operating immediately.* Replace breathing circuit and if possible anesthesia machine because of rubber/gas solubility of inhalation agents. Anesthesiologist immediately institutes *hyperventilation with 100% oxygen* at high flow rate of eight to ten liters.
2 Immediately start drug therapy. Administer:
   a *Dantrolene sodium (Dantrium IV)* one mg/kg body weight intravenously up to four times in a 15 minute period not to exceed 10 mg/kg total. Some physicians prefer to give an initial IV bolus of 2 to 3 mg/kg and repeat every five to ten minutes until a maximum of 10 mg/kg is given or the MH episode is controlled. The drug is continued for 24 hours following control of episode. Dantrolene is the first specific treatment for MH. This drug appears to directly block accumulation of calcium within muscles by interfering with release of calcium from sarcoplasmic reticulum, uncoupling excitation-contraction, thus relaxing skeletal muscle. Given IV, dantrolene has virtually no effect on cardiovascular or respiratory function.
   b *Procainamide (Pronestyl)* 15 mg/kg diluted in 500 ml physiologic saline IV. Procainamide treats cardiac arrhythmia, inhibits calcium release from the SR, and relaxes muscle rigidity.
   c *Sodium bicarbonate* one to two milliequivalents (mEq or meq)/kg IV stat and repeat as necessary with guidance from blood gas measurements (arterial pH and pCO_2). An alkali, sodium bicarbonate raises pH and combats acidosis, lowers plasma potassium level and antagonizes hyperkalemia by driving potassium into the cells. *Monitoring of pH and blood gases is mandatory.*
   d *Mannitol* 0.25g/kg IV and/or *furosemide (Lasix)* one mg/kg IV, up to four doses each. Mannitol and furosemide dislodge myoglo-

bin from renal tubules and sustain urinary flow. Maintenance of urine output greater than two ml/kg per hour may help to prevent renal failure.

3 *Begin active cooling.* Administer refrigerated or iced normal saline intravenously. Lavage stomach, bladder, and rectum. If the peritoneal or thoracic cavity is open, sterile iced saline may be poured into the opening. Cool body surface by placing patient in a plastic sheet and applying ice bags and ice water or use a hypothermia blanket. If readily available, use partial cardiopulmonary bypass (femoral to femoral) to cool viscera. Body temperature must be carefully monitored to avoid accidental cooling to arrhythmic levels. Medication may be given to limit shivering, normally a heat-retaining mechanism that also increases oxygen consumption. Surface cooling is considered more effective in children because of high ratio of surface area to body volume.

4 Administer ten units regular insulin in ten ml 50% dextrose and water IV to offset high glucose metabolic demands and improve glucose uptake for utilization, and to shift potassium back into cells. Treat hyperkalemia. Monitor blood glucose and potassium levels.

5 Correct electrolyte imbalance on the basis of immediate blood sampling of electrolytes, pH, and blood gases. Hypocalcemia and hyperkalemia followed by hypokalemia may be expected. Repeat blood gas measurements at ten minute intervals and correct on basis of results.

6 Postoperatively, continue dantrolene one mg/kg every six hours for 72 hours to prevent recurrence, which is not uncommon in the first eight hours.

NOTE. The above protocol is similar to that used in some centers. It is not intended as a standard of approved medical care but is subject to variation according to individual institutional protocol.

Mandatory Monitoring Parameters to be monitored routinely in MH at-risk and general anesthesia patients are electrocardiogram, blood pressure, core temperature by esophageal probe, and stethoscopy by precordial stethoscope. Rise in temperature greater than one-half degree centigrade per hour should raise suspicion of malignant hyperthermia.

After presumed onset of MH, an arterial line provides monitoring of blood pressure and blood sampling for pH, pCO_2, pO_2, sodium, potassium, chlorides, calcium, magnesium, and phosphate. CVP and urinary output via Foley catheter also are needed. In addition to recorded amount, urine is sampled for hemoglobin and myoglobin estimation. Also measured are creatine phosphokinase, glutamic-oxaloacetic transaminase, alkaline phosphatase, lactate dehydrogenase—indicative of muscle destruction, blood urea nitrogen (BUN)—kidney function, bilirubin—liver function, coagulation studies, blood lactate and pyruvate, serum thyroxine, as ordered.

Monitoring started in the OR should be continued in the RR or ICU. The necessary supplies that must be immediately available for both adult and pediatric patients include:

1 Monitors: ECG, electronic temperature probes and recorder

2 IV equipment: blood administration sets and pumps; CVP line setup; IV solutions—twelve 1,000 ml bottles of physiologic saline kept in refrigerator

3 Arterial line setup

4 Intubation equipment; defibrillator

5 Ice chips and plastic bags; hypothermia blankets

6 Gastric lavage set; rectal tubes; 50 cc syringes

7 Blood sampling equipment and arterial blood gas kits

8 Drugs: 12 vials, 20 mg each, of dantrolene sodium, and 12 vials, 60 ml each, of sterile water to reconstitute dantrolene; 12 vials or disposable syringes of sodium bicarbonate; 2000 mg of procainamide; two 50 ml vials of 25% mannitol; four 2 ml (20 mg) prefilled syringes of furosemide; one 100 unit vial of regular insulin; and two 50 ml vials of 50% dextrose in water

9 Associated needles and syringes

10 Anesthesia breathing circuits and soda lime canisters

11 Extracorporeal perfusion apparatus, if possible

These supplies should be kept in a specific location and those feasible (IV equipment, solutions, drugs) marked for use in malignant hyperthermia. An MH cart is convenient.

Prophylaxis/Prevention Mortality would be lowered greatly if MH could be foreseen. *Preoperative history* should routinely include questions about the patient's previous anesthesia experiences, unexplained incidents or death of family members who underwent anesthesia, and known muscular abnormalities of the patient and relatives. Hereditary predisposition has been detected in three generations. Mandatory monitoring intraoperatively should be adhered to.

Diagnosis of susceptibility to MH is now best accomplished by *preoperative muscle biopsy* and evaluation of muscle response (contracture) on exposure to caffeine and halothane in vitro (test tube). In brief, biopsied muscle from an MH susceptible patient reveals increased sensitivity to caffeine-induced contracture when exposed to halothane. Although muscle biopsy is performed under local anesthesia, a very rare MH episode may occur. Therefore, dantrolene should be readily available.

For prophylaxis, *dantrolene* should be given preoperatively to susceptible patients facing need for operation. Suggested dose is one mg/kg increments every four to six hours orally up to four mg/kg total dose; one mg/kg IV immediately preinduction.

Susceptible patients should wear a *Medic-Alert* bracelet.

Hypovolemia

Hypovolemia is low or decreased blood volume due to a deficit of extracellular fluid volume, commonly referred to as dehydration. Decreased blood volume, if present prior to operation, increases operative risk and morbidity. It should be treated preoperatively when possible and electrolyte imbalance corrected.

Etiology Reduced fluid intake, hemorrhage, extensive burns (plasma loss), loss of gastrointestinal fluids, wound drainage, fever, diaphoresis, diuresis. Impaired renal function and metabolic acidosis are predisposing factors.

Symptoms Dry skin and mucous membranes, depressed blood pressure, elevated pulse, oliguria, decreasing central venous pressure and blood volume determinations, deep rapid respirations.

Treatment Infusion of Ringer's lactate or 5% dextrose in crystalloid solution as necessary. Increase blood volume. Oxygen may be administered.

Hypervolemia

Hypervolemia is an excess of extracellular fluid in the blood, commonly referred to as *edema.*

Predisposing Factors Intravenous infusions given too rapidly or in excessive amounts, especially isotonic saline solution, or prolonged administration of adrenocorticosteroids. Edema may progress to pulmonary edema.

Symptoms Dyspnea, moist rales, elevated pulse and respiration, diminished urine output. Increasing central venous pressure may indicate fluid overload with venous distention.

Treatment Diuretics, restricted fluids, and prevention or treatment of pulmonary edema.

Arterial Hypotension

Reduced blood pressure, with resultant inadequate circulation, may accompany depression of myocardium, depression of vasomotor center in the brain, decline in cardiac output, or dilatation of peripheral vessels. Hypotension may occur also when positive pressure is applied to airway. Progressive deepening of general anesthesia usually produces peripheral vasodilatation and diminished myocardial contractility. Adequate blood flow to brain and heart, the two most vulnerable vascular beds due to their high metabolic demand, must be maintained. If arterial hypotension is uncontrolled, it may cause cerebral vascular accident, myocardial infarction, or death.

Etiology Overdosage of general anesthetic or rapid vascular absorption of local agents may be due to an actual excess of the agent for a normal patient under ordinary circumstances, or to an excessive amount at a specific time for a particular patient, exceeding the patient's tolerance. Tendency to overdosage occurs during prolonged anesthesia (large amounts of drugs absorbed), in age-extreme patients, or with unrecognized hypothermia during lengthy abdominal or thoracic procedures. Circulatory effects of spinal or epidural anesthesia, such as diminished cardiac output or reduced peripheral resistance, also produce hypotension.

Other causes are: hemorrhage, loss of whole blood, or loss of plasma into tissues during extensive operation; circulatory abnormalities such as cardiac tamponade, heart failure, hypovolemia, cerebral or pulmonary embolism (fat embolism from fracture sites, amniotic fluid emboli during delivery, or air emboli from introduction of air into circulation during infusion or procedure), myocardial ischemia or infarction; changes in position, especially if executed rapidly or roughly; excessive preanesthetic medication (postural hypotension may follow narcotic administration); potent therapeutic drugs (tranquilizers, adrenal steroids, antihypertensives) given prior to anesthetic; hypoxia.

Surgical manipulation may induce hypotension mechanically by obstructing venous return to the heart with packs, retractors, or body rests. Or, hypotension may result from vagal-induced reflex precipitated by intraperitoneal traction, manipulation in the chest or neck areas, rapid release of increased intraabdominal pressure or overdistention of bladder, or stimulation of periosteum or joint cavities. Other causes are transfusion reaction, suggested by accompanying cyanosis and oozing at operative site; septic shock; severe hyperthermia; anaphylactic reaction.

Symptoms Early reversible shock is accompanied by unstable blood pressure, vasoconstriction, elevated blood pH, and elevated catecholamine levels. Late manifestations are pallor or cyanosis, clammy skin, dilated pupils, decreased urinary output, tachycardia, decreased bleeding in operative field or pallor of organs caused by compensatory vasoconstriction, nausea, vomiting, sighing respirations, or air hunger in conscious patients.

Diagnosis Determination of arterial blood pressure and pulse rate, and estimation of pulse volume, are indicative of volume of cardiac ejection. Arbitrary figures of measured blood pressure are not as important as individual circulatory status. A specific measurement in a healthy adult may be relatively insignificant while the same figure in an aged patient could be hazardous. In critically ill patients, direct arterial pressure, central venous pressure and urine output are monitored.

Treatment Must be prompt to avoid circulatory collapse. The aim is to increase perfusion of vital organs and to treat any specific cause while giving general supportive therapy. Supportive measures include oxygen by mask with assisted respiration, elevation of the legs to increase blood pressure by draining pooled blood, especially after sympathetic blockade; rapid intravenous fluid therapy to increase blood volume. Various solutions are applicable in an emergency since the volume of fluid is more vital than its composition, in early treatment. If whole blood is not available, crystalloid solutions (e.g., Ringer's lactate), 5% dextrose in water, physiologic saline, plasma or serum albumin, or 6% dextran (plasma expander) may be given.

Vasoactive drugs are given as necessary. Vasopressor drugs exert a vasoconstrictor action through stimulation of alpha receptors of the sympathetic nervous system or increase myocardial contractile force and heart rate by activation of beta receptors. Drug selection must often be empirical. Drugs that may be used are: ephedrine, epinephrine, mephentermine (Wyamine), phenylephrine (Neo-Synephrine), methoxamine (Vasoxyl), metaraminol (Aramine), isoproterenol (Isuprel), dopamine hydrochloride (Intropin), levarterenol (Levophed). These various drugs have various actions; they increase ventricular contractile force, alter sinoatrial nodal activity, constrict vascular smooth muscles, dilate blood vessels in splanchnic bed. They may produce ventricular arrhythmia, the incidence and severity of which is intensified by hypoxia or hypercarbia. Drug effectiveness is reduced in the presence of respiratory or metabolic acidosis. Blood gases should be monitored.

Prevention Obviously the reverse of the causes, therefore: minute-to-minute observation of *all* patients receiving *any* type of anesthetic; in suspect individuals, testing cardiovascular response to proposed operative position before induction; avoiding overdosage in premedications and anesthetic drugs; gentle tissue manipulation and position change; administration of minimal amount of anesthetic needed; adequate time to induce and deepen anesthesia so as not to raise the blood level of anesthetic too rapidly; prudent application of positive pressure to airway; prompt replacement of fluid and blood loss. If major blood loss is anticipated, a large intravenous catheter (14- to 16-gauge) is inserted so blood can be rapidly infused, under pressure if necessary.

Circulatory Shock

Shock is a complex phenomenon, a life-threatening condition in which circulation fails for one or several reasons, resulting in insufficient flow of blood for adequate tissue perfusion or oxygenation. If prolonged, inadequate organ blood flow with deficient microcirculation profoundly depresses vital processes (see Chap. 36). Since the objective of circulation is achieved in the capillaries, defective cellular metabolism derived from shock interferes further with the body's inherent defenses and metabolic acidosis occurs. Normal defense mechanisms are reflex vasoconstriction and increased pulse rate, which tend to redistribute flow of blood to the heart and brain at the expense of the other vital organs. If shock is promptly recognized, treated, and reversed, permanent damage is avoided. If it progresses to irreversibility, death ensues from cellular dysfunction and organ hypoperfusion.

Multiple kinds and causes of shock present problems in relationships among the heart, circulatory system, and blood volume. Circulatory inadequacy may originate from a marked decrease in cardiac output, venous return to the heart, or peripheral vascular resistance.

Etiology Loss of circulating volume, loss of pumping power of the heart, or loss of peripheral resistance. Because of the complexity of shock, discussion is limited to the hypovolemic type.

Hypovolemic Shock Decrease in circulating blood volume from loss of blood, plasma, or extracellular fluid. Excessive fluid loss is greater than compensatory absorption of interstitial fluid into the circulation. Causes: hemorrhage; burns; severe dehydration from vomiting, diarrhea, intestinal obstruction, excessive heat or fever, withholding fluids; metabolic acidosis; prolonged cardiopulmonary bypass. Shock resulting from hemorrhage or underestimated blood loss is the type most often seen in the operating room and is usually reversed by prompt restoration of circulating blood volume.

Treatment

1 Fluid-volume replacement. Whole blood, or other intravenous fluid or plasma expander as indicated. In case of hemorrhage, if not previously done, type and cross match blood for transfusion. Hypervolemia must be avoided in replacement.

2 Position. Elevation of legs may aid venous return and cardiac output except in severe oligemia.

3 Temperature. Keep as nearly normal as possible. Keep the patient warm but not overheated as perspiration increases fluid loss.

4 Oxygen. Given when circulation is not delivering enough to the tissues (low pO_2).

5 Drugs. Administered according to the needs of the patient to maintain blood pressure, correct acidosis, protect kidneys from failure.

Venospasm

If caused by cold IV fluid infusion, venospasm may be manifested by very slow flow. It may result from pressure infusion or extravasation. Intravenous procaine relieves spasm. Thrombophlebitis may follow venospasm.

Coronary Thrombosis

This can occur from severe hypoxia and lack of oxygen to coronary vessels. Sometimes its occurrence is the reason for a patient's never regaining consciousness following an operation.

Cardiac Arrhythmias

An alteration of normal cardiac rhythm may decrease cardiac output, exhaust the myocardium, and lead to ventricular fibrillation or cardiac arrest. *Bradycardia* is the slowing of the heart or pulse rate. *Tachycardia* is an excessive rapidity of the heart's action.

Etiology Hypoxia, hypercarbia, acidosis, electrolyte imbalance, coronary disease, myocardial infarction, vagal reflexes, anesthetic agents, toxic doses of digitalis, epinephrine or other drugs, laryngospasm and coughing initiated by presence of secretions in the airway following induction. Other causes may be hypotension, hemorrhage, hypovolemia, pneumothorax, mechanical injuries. *Ventricular arrhythmias* are of major concern. An impulse originating in the ventricles must travel to rest of the myocardium from one ventricle, proceeding then to the other ventricle. Because the impulse does not travel via the rapid, specialized conduction system, depolarization of both ventricles takes longer and is not simultaneous. The complexes have an abnormal appearance on ECG compared to normally initiated and conducted impulses. Ventricular tachycardia and ventricular fibrillation are arrythmias of most serious consequence and thus most feared.

1 *Premature ventricular contractions (PVCs)* or beats (PVBs). Ectopic focus in ventricles stimulates heart before regularly scheduled sinoatrial impulse arrives. Main precipitating factors are electrolyte and/or acid-base imbalance, myocardial infarction, digitalis toxicity, caffeine. PVCs must be distinguished from premature atrial contraction (PAC). Isolated PVCs may not require treatment but those occurring in clusters of two or more or over five or six a minute require therapy. The aim is to quiet the irritable myocardium and restore adequate cardiac output. Treatment consists of a lidocaine bolus followed by a continuous drip by infusion; correction of etiology, e.g., hypoxia; other antiarrhythmic drugs if indicated, e.g., procainamide or quinidine. Temporary pacing may be used for severe bradycardia. Paired PVCs pose an increased danger of ventricular tachycardia.

2 *Ventricular tachycardia.* Rapid heart rate (100 to 220 beats per minute) resulting from ventricular ischemia or irritability, anoxia, or digitalis intoxication. The heart rate does not give time for ventricular filling and the resultant reduced cardiac output predisposes the patient to ventricular fibrillation or cardiac failure. It is treated by prompt intravenous administration of lidocaine or procainamide or intramuscular quinidine. *Synchronized cardioversion* of 10 to 200 joules may be used if blood pressure is palpable. This is the application of high-intensity, short-duration electrical shock to chest wall over heart to produce total cardiac depolarization, i.e., countershock timed to interrupt an abnormal rhythm in the cardiac cycle, thereby permitting resumption of a normal one. Cardioversion is usually applied in instances of nonarrest but nevertheless dangerous arrhythmia. It may be an elective or emergency treatment. Asynchronous cardioversion is used if patient is pulseless (see below). Treatment also includes correction of underlying cause.

3 *Ventricular flutter.* Often called fine ventricular fibrillation, the flutter appears as a transient state between ventricular tachycardia and ventricular fibrillation. Patient will show signs of poor cardiac output.

4 *Ventricular fibrillation.* The most serious of all arrhythmias, characterized by total disorganization of ventricular activity. There are rapid and irregular, uncoordinated random contractions of the small myocardial groups without effective ventricular contraction and cardiac output. Circulation ceases. It is rapidly fatal, since respiratory and cardiac arrest quickly follow, unless successful defibrillation is effected. The patient in fibrillation is unconscious and possibly convulsing from cerebral hypoxia.

Treatment

1 In a *monitored* patient, a fast sharp single blow (*precordial thump*) to the midportion of the sternum (use nipple line as a landmark) may be delivered with the bottom fleshy part of a closed fist struck from 8 to 12 in. (20 to 30 cm) above the chest. The blow generates a small electrical stimulus in a heart that is reactive, and may be effective in restoring a beat in cases of asystole or recent onset of arrhythmia.

2 Prompt defibrillation by short-duration electrical shock to the heart (*asynchronous cardioversion*). This produces simultaneous depolarization of all muscle fiber bundles after which spontaneous beating (conversion to spontaneous normal sinus rhythm) may resume if the myocardium is oxygenated and not acidotic. Defibrillation of an anoxic myocardium is difficult. *The time fibrillation started should be noted.* The electric shock is coordinated with controlled ventilation and cardiac compression. Cardiopulmonary resuscitation (see CPR, p. 284) begins as soon as the presence of fibrillation is identified. Many variables may affect defibrillation, such as body weight, paddle position, electrical waveform, and resistance to electric current flow. Procedures below follow presently established protocol.

Defibrillation: Equipment and Technique Necessary equipment for defibrillation includes: defibrillator machine, paddle electrodes, and standard electrode paste or jelly, or saline-soaked 4 by 4 gauze pads to reduce resistance to passage of electric current offered by skin. If paste is used on paddles, it should not extend beyond electrodes or on any part of electrode handles. Rapid sponge application between paddles and patient's skin provides the advantage that external cardiac compression may be resumed after defibrillation without the hand slipping on the chest. External defibrillation of the heart is used unless the chest is already open, as for intrathoracic operations. For internal defibrillation, sterile electrodes are placed on the myocardium, one over the right atrium, the other over the left ventricle. If these electrodes are gauze-covered, they are dipped in saline before use. Minimal current is needed when paddles are placed directly on the heart. *Team members must understand the functioning of the defibrillator for the patient's safety and their own.*

Available defibrillators use direct current. Most defibrillators are associated with integrated monitors, but monitor and defibrillator switches may be separate or combined. An operational monitor does not always indicate that fibrillation power supply is on. Many monitor-defibrillator units can monitor the ECG from paddle electrodes ("quick-look" paddles) as well as from separate patient leads. Quick-look paddles and patient leads cannot operate simultaneously, however. Depending on type of defibrillator system, be sure electrical cord is plugged in or batteries are charged. All defibrillators should be checked regularly with suitable test equipment.

External paddle positions. (1) Standard position: one electrode is placed just to the right of the upper sternum below the clavicle and the other electrode just to left to the cardiac apex or left nipple along left axillary line, thus delivering current through long axis of the heart. The large diameter of the paddles increases the area of skin contact, thus reducing the possibility of skin burns by spreading of the current. Paddles must be held flat against the skin and more than two inches (5 cm) apart to prevent dangerous electrical arcing. They must always be scrupulously clean as foreign material reduces uniformity of shock. (2) Anterior-posterior position: one electrode is placed anteriorly over the precordium between left nipple and sternum, the other posteriorly behind the heart immediately below the left scapula, avoiding the spinal column. This allows for more energy passage through the heart but placement is more difficult.

With the electrodes pressed firmly against the chest wall for good contact, the electric charge is delivered by person holding electrode paddles by pressing a switch on the handle, or a foot switch. The safest method is by switches on both paddles that must be pressed simultaneously for discharge of electric energy. The operator should have dry hands and stand on dry floor. *When using a defibrillator, neither the person holding the electrodes nor anyone else should touch the metal operating table or the patient as the current is applied in order to avoid possible self-electrocution. No part of the operator's body should touch the paste or uninsulated electrodes. Loud verbal warning is given before discharge.* Countershock is repeated at intervals if fibrillation persists. Transthoracic impedance falls with repetitive closely spaced electric discharges. After each countershock, reassess ECG and pulse.

Myocardial damage resulting from defibrillatory efforts is in direct proportion to the energy used, therefore maximal settings, when not required, may increasingly impair an already damaged myocardium. The energy level delivered through a specific ohm load should be indicated on the front panel of defibrillator. Delivery output ranges vary with machines. Strength of countershock is expressed in energy as joules or watt seconds, the product of power and duration. If the patient's chest muscles do not contract, no current reached the patient. Check defibrillator's connection to electrical source and "off" button to synchronizer circuit. If machine is battery operated, the battery must be charged enough to energize the capacitor. *Be familiar with and follow operating instructions for the defibrillator that you use.*

Adjunct drug therapy is used as necessary: vasopressor-cardiotonic and myocardial stimulant drugs to maintain a useful heartbeat, antiarrhythmic drugs to prevent recurrence, sodium bicarbonate to combat acidosis (see p. 290). Continuous monitoring of the heart and laboratory analysis, such as arterial blood gases, are essential.

Prevention Appropriate preoperative sedation and skillfully administered anesthesia help to avoid hazardous cardiovascular reflexes. As premature ventricular contractions are precursors to fibrillation, in itself a precursor to cardiac arrest, any cardiopulmonary emergency in a prearrest phase requires:

1 *Monitoring of heart rhythm and rate.* Ability to recognize rhythms that precede arrest permits intervention that may prevent arrest. If cardiac status is not under constant monitoring, hypoxia and acidosis may be present and require correction prior to effective use of other therapeutic modalities.

2 *Establishment of an intravenous lifeline.* Venous cannulation provides access to peripheral and central venous circulation for administering drugs and fluids, obtaining venous blood specimens for laboratory analysis, and inserting catheters into the right heart and pulmonary arteries for physiological monitoring and electrical pacing. If cardiac arrest appears imminent, or has occurred, cannulation of a peripheral or femoral vein should be attempted first so as not to interrupt cardiopulmonary resuscitation (see below). Squeeze the IV infusion bag before use to detect a puncture that could permit contamination. No drug should be added to the solution that might be absorbed by the plastic. To keep the infusion open, the rate should be kept low. The usual complications to all intravenous techniques should be guarded against.

Cardiac Arrest (Circulatory Arrest)

In cardiac arrest, there is cessation of cardiocirculatory action; the pumping mechanism of the heart ceases. Cardiac standstill represents total absence of electrical cardiac activity, reflected as a straight line on an ECG rhythm strip. It may occur as primary cardiac failure or secondary to failure of pulmonary ventilation. The types of circulatory arrest are profound cardiovascular collapse, electromechanical dissociation, ventricular fibrillation, and ventricular asystole or standstill. This may precede or follow failure of the respiratory system since the systems are interrelated.

Etiology A single or combination of factors may precipitate arrest but the general cause is inadequate coronary arterial blood flow. Defective respiratory function produces systemic hypoxemia, causing myocardial hypoxia and depression. It also increases myocardial irritability and the heart's susceptibility to vagal reflexes. Some of the specific precipitating factors are arrhythmias, emboli, extreme hypotension or hypovolemia, respiratory obstruction, aspiration, effects of drugs, anesthetic overdosage, excessively rapid, unsmooth induction, sepsis, pharyngeal stimulation, metabolic abnormalities (acidosis, toxemia, electrolyte imbalance), poor cardiac filling due to positioning, manipulation of the heart, central nervous system trauma, anaphylaxis, electric shock as from ungrounded or faulty electrical equipment.

Symptoms Loss of heart beat and blood pressure; sudden fixed dilated pupils; sudden pallor or cyanosis; cold clammy skin; absence of reflexes; unconsciousness or convulsions in previously conscious patient; respiratory standstill; dark blood or absence of bleeding in operative field.

Diagnosis Arrest is readily detected during anesthesia by the ECG monitor, absence of blood pressure and precordial heart sounds, and lack of a palpable carotid pulse. Onset of pupillary dilatation is within 45 seconds after cerebral anoxia; full dilatation is reached about 90 to 110 seconds after cessation of cerebral circulation.

Prevention Use of intraoperative electrocardiogram and temperature monitoring; insertion of intravenous line prior to operation; maintenance of intact airway, adequate oxygenation and adequate arterial blood pressure; proper timing and judicious use of medications; proper patient positioning; slow position change; no weight on patient; gentle handling of tissues with minimal traction and manipulation, especially in the region of the heart and great vessels; no stimulation during induction; skillful anesthetic administration and testing for sensitivities; optimal preoperative preparation.

Incidence Arrest may occur during induction, intraoperatively, or postoperatively. Occurrence during cardiac operations or following massive hemorrhage is not uncommon. Patients more prone to arrest include those at age extremes, those with previously diagnosed paroxysmal arrhythmias, primary cardiovascular abnormalities, myocarditis, heartblock, digitalis toxicity. Unexpected arrest is one that happens in a patient of general good health who is undergoing a low-risk or relatively routine procedure. These arrests are associated with major morbidity and mortality.

CARDIOPULMONARY RESUSCITATION

Cardiopulmonary resuscitation (CPR) is aimed at rapidly restoring oxygen delivery to vital organs to reverse the processes that lead to death. CPR is an emergency procedure requiring special training to recognize cardiac or respiratory arrest and perform artificial ventilation and circulation. Resuscitative measures must be instituted immediately within three to five minutes after arrest to prevent irreversible brain damage. *No time must be lost!* The combination of anoxia and acidosis can make restoration of normal function impossible. Resuscitation is not a one-man job. *The team must be completely familiar with the preplanned routine before the necessity for its use arises.* Success depends on prompt diagnosis and immediate effective treatment. Outcome is directly related to the rapidity with which a functional, spontaneous heart rhythm can be restored. Patients who experience arrest in an operating room may be on monitors with an intravenous line already in place, and resuscitation equipment on hand. These arrests are referred to as *witnessed arrests. Note time of onset of arrest and start the time-elapsed clock.* Basic life support is instituted *at once* to reestablish the oxygen system and restore the heartbeat.

Basic Life Support

Basic life support (BLS) is that particular phase of emergency cardiac care (ECC) that either 1) prevents circulatory or respiratory arrest or insufficiency through prompt recognition and intervention or 2) externally supports circulation and respiration of a victim of cardiac or respiratory arrest through cardiopulmonary resuscitation (CPR). BLS can and should be initiated by any person present when cardiac arrest occurs.*

The ABCs of resuscitation are:

A *Airway:* patent, free of secretions or foreign body, for effective pulmonary ventilation

B *Breathing:* prompt restoration and maintenance of oxygenation through artificial ventilation

C *Circulation:* provision of oxygen to vital tissues by means of cardiac compression (artificial circulation)

These steps should be started immediately and performed in the order given except when the patient is intubated and being monitored. A precordial thump, advanced life support, or both procedures should be instituted without delay to restore circulation. Resuscitation must be in effect until the patient can resume normal, spontaneous respiration and circulation or until their discontinuation is warranted by cardiac or central nervous system biological death.

When the arrested patient is in the operating room, anesthesiologists and other team members are present. In a witnessed arrest, the carotid pulse is palpated. Carotid artery is located in the groove between the trachea and muscles of the side of the neck. Palpation of femoral artery is an acceptable option. If the patient has respiratory arrest, four quick, full lung inflations are given without allowing for full lung deflation between breaths. Maintenance of positive pressure in lungs more effectively fills, ventilates, and prevents collapse of alveoli. If pulse and breathing are not immediately restored, CPR is begun. *If the patient is being ECG monitored at the time of arrest,* a fast precordial thump may be given and the monitor checked for cardiac rhythm while the carotid pulse is checked. If ventricular fibrillation or tachycardia without a pulse is evident, countershock is delivered as soon as possible (DC 200 to 300 joules delivered energy in adult, two joules/kg or one joule per pound in infant or child). If unsuccessful, additional countershocks and medications are given as ordered or per hospital written protocol. In open-heart defibrillation, between five and forty joules are delivered. Begin with lower energy levels. Meanwhile CPR is started. In infants and small children, a hand is placed over the precordium to feel the apical beat or brachial pulse is checked in lieu of checking a carotid pulse. Brachial pulse is on inside of upper arm midway between the elbow and shoulder. Use index and middle fingers. *Do not give precordial thump to infant or child.* In infants and children, bradyarrhythmias and heart block lead to cardiac arrest more commonly than ventricular fibrillation.

*Standards and Guidelines for Cardiopulmonary Resuscitation (CPR) and Emergency Cardiac Care (ECC), JAMA 244(5): 460–461, Aug 1, 1980. Copyright 1980, American Medical Association. Reprinted with permission.

Artificial Ventilation (Pulmonary Resuscitation) Immediate opening of the airway is mandatory to combat respiratory failure. If respiratory obstruction is present, it must be cleared. During operation under general anesthesia, either an oro- or nasopharyngeal airway or endotracheal tube is in place to maintain a patent air passage. One hundred percent oxygen can be delivered at once under positive pressure by manual ventilation. If not, ventilation by other means, such as an esophageal obturator airway or expired-air technique, should be initiated to sustain oxygenation, followed by tracheal intubation as soon as possible. A cuffed endotracheal tube permits continual delivery of high-oxygen concentration without hazard of stomach distention or aspiration. It facilitates adequate ventilation since, with its use, interposed breaths are not necessary, thereby permitting a faster, uninterrupted cardiac compression rate of 80 per minute. When a tube or airway is lacking, the most rapid means of reestablishing oxygenation is by an *expired-air technique or mouth-to-mouth or mouth-to-nose artificial ventilation.* When combined with cardiac compression, tissues receive oxygen.

Procedure With patient supine and airway patent, extend head backward as far as possible so that chin is pointed upward. Keep the head in this position to extend neck and lift tongue away from back of throat.

For *mouth-to-mouth technique,* mandible may be thrust forward also by placing fingers of one hand behind angle of the jaw and pushing it forward. Hold mouth open with thumb of this hand by retracting the lower lip. With other hand, pinch nostrils together with thumb and index finger while exerting pressure on forehead to maintain backward tilt (see Fig. 14-1). Pressure of your cheek against the patient's nose to prevent air leakage is an alternative method. Or, one hand may maintain head tilt and nostril pinch while other hand extends neck from beneath. Deliver four quick, full lung inflations in rapid succession, tightly sealing your lips over the patient's open mouth for each breath. Do not allow for full lung deflation between breaths, to maintain positive pressure. After delivering each breath, quickly turn your head toward patient's chest to take a breath of fresh air. Take a deep breath, then seal your lips over patient's mouth, and blow forcefully into it, watching for the chest to rise (see Fig. 14-2). Remove your mouth, allowing patient to exhale passively, while watching for chest to fall. Repeat this procedure every five seconds as necessary. If chest does not rise, improve jaw support and head tilt. Also blow more forcefully. Check for carotid pulse after initial four breaths and again after every 12 breaths. If absent, begin chest compression.

For *mouth-to-nose technique,* lift patient's lower jaw with one hand, thus sealing lips, and tilt patient's head back with the other hand on forehead. Take a deep breath, seal your lips around nose, and blow into it until you feel the lungs expand. Remove your mouth, allowing passive exhalation. It may be necessary to separate the patient's lips or open mouth during exhalation for air to escape as the soft palate may cause nasopharyngeal obstruction. Watch for chest to fall. Be sure to close patient's mouth before resuming ventilation. Repeat the maneuver every five seconds. For infants under one year and children one to eight years: cover both mouth and nose with your mouth and use smaller breaths (less volume) to inflate lungs every three seconds (20x/min) for infants, every four seconds for child, after initial four rapid breaths. Also, do not tilt head as much since an infant's neck is pliable and air passages may become obstructed or spinal cord injured. Head tilt-neck lift or chin lift technique is used.

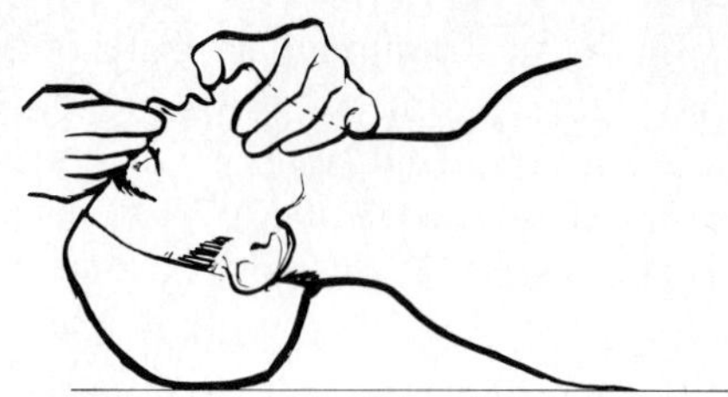

FIGURE 14-1
Positioning for mouth-to-mouth resuscitation. Patient is supine with neck hyperextended to straighten the airway. Resuscitator pinches nostrils with one hand and elevates the mandible with the other, holding the mouth open with thumb.

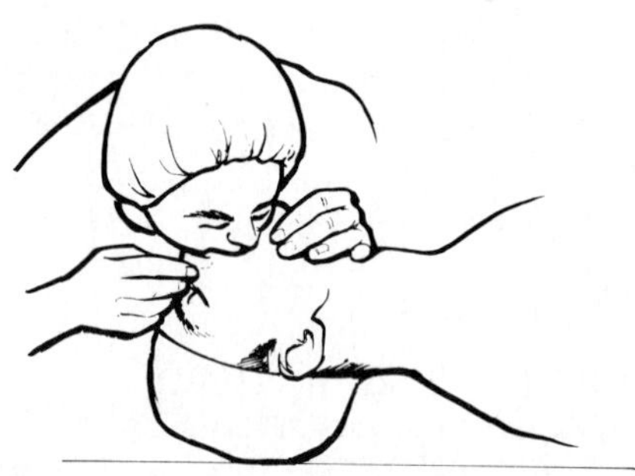

FIGURE 14-2
Mouth-to-mouth resuscitation. Resuscitator takes a deep breath and, tightly sealing lips over the patient's open mouth, blows forcefully into it, watching for the patient's chest to rise.

Apply adult techniques (nostril pinch) to child older than eight years or if child is so large that tight seal cannot be made over both nose and mouth.

Mouth-to-stoma direct ventilation is possible for patient who has a tracheostomy or laryngectomy tube. Delete head tilt or jaw thrust. Seal nose and mouth with your hand or a tightly fitting face mask to prevent air leakage when you blow into tube. This problem is prevented if the tube has an inflatable cuff. Deliver four rapid breaths etc. as above.

Mouth-to-airway technique may be used through either an endotracheal tube or oral airway.

These techniques, except when practiced through an endotracheal tube, carry a risk of inflating the patient's stomach with air, possibly followed by regurgitation and aspiration of gastric contents, as well as reduction of lung volume by elevation of diaphragm. If stomach becomes distended, recheck and reposition airway, observe rise and fall of chest, avoid excessive airway pressure. There is also danger of passing infection from patient to resuscitator. The advantages of the method are simplicity and immediate availability. In the operating room the anesthesiologist manages artificial ventilation.

NOTE. 1. If attempts to ventilate are unsuccessful despite proper opening of airway, further attempts to remove obstruction should be made. Laryngoscopy, cricothyrotomy, or tracheotomy may be indicated.

2. Tracheal suctioning should last no longer than five seconds at a time without ventilation to prevent hypoxia.

3. If spinal injury is suspected or present, extension of the neck is avoided and modified jaw thrust technique employed. Head, neck, and chest are kept aligned.

4. Ventilation is assured by seeing chest rise and fall, feeling in your own airway the resistance and compliance of the patient's lungs as they expand, hearing and feeling air escape during the patient's exhalation with your head turned and your cheek close to patient's mouth.

5. In single rescuer CPR, two quick full breaths without allowing time for full lung deflation between breaths are delivered after each cycle of fifteen chest compressions. With two-rescuer CPR, one breath is interposed during upstroke of every fifth compression.

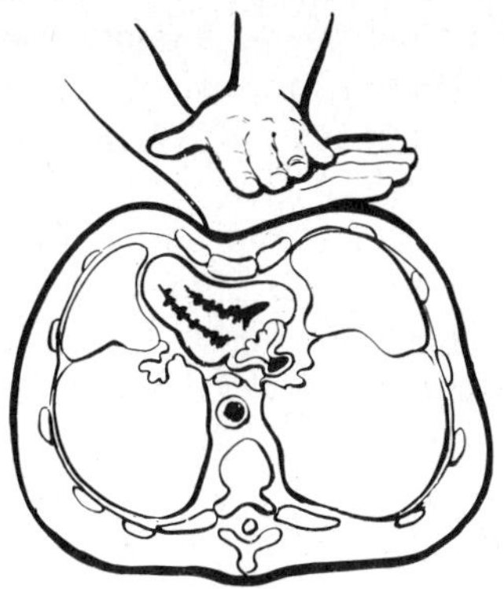

FIGURE 14-3
Manual depression of the sternum raises intrathoracic pressure and produces cardiac output. Blood is sent from heart into the pulmonary artery and aorta.

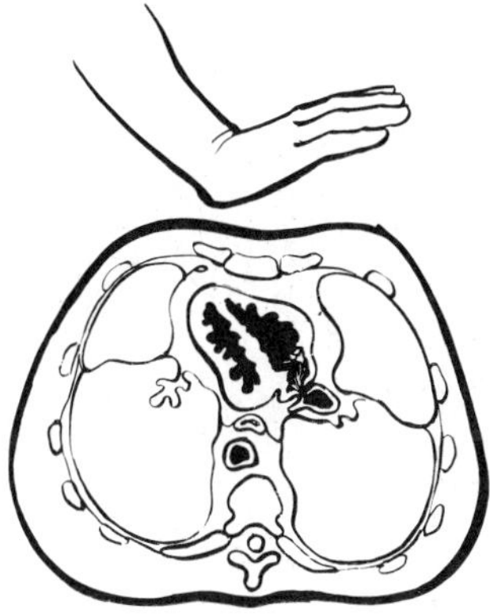

FIGURE 14-4
Releasing the pressure on the sternum allows the heart to fill with venous blood.

Artificial Circulation (Cardiovascular Resuscitation) Cardiac compression must accompany ventilation in a pulseless patient to maintain adequate blood pressure and circulation, thereby keeping tissues viable, preserving cardiac tone and reflexes, and preventing intravascular clotting. This may be accomplished by *external* (closed-chest) *cardiac compression,* the rhythmic application of pressure over lower half of the sternum, *except for the xiphoid process.* Since the heart occupies most of the space between the sternum and the thoracic spine, intermittent depression of sternum raises intrathoracic pressure and produces cardiac output (see Fig. 14-3). Blood is forced from heart into pulmonary artery and aorta. During relaxation of pressure, negative intrathoracic pressure causes venous blood to flow back into the heart from the pulmonary and systemic circulatory systems (see Fig. 14-4). Blood moves in the arterial direction through the heart valves. Carotid artery blood flow from this technique usually is only one-quarter to one-third of normal (mean BP 40 mm Hg), although systolic blood pressure is raised. It may peak to 100 mm Hg, but diastolic BP is low. Artificial ventilation is *always* required when external cardiac compression is employed as ventilation volumes from compression are inadequate for oxygenation of blood. The brain and myocardium must be perfused effectively for survival. External cardiac compression must be instituted immediately on cessation of circulation. It must be performed with knowledge and care. All physicians and appropriate nursing personnel must be trained in CPR. Many hospitals offer CPR certification courses.

Procedure The patient should lie on a hard flat surface such as the operating table. A bedboard may be needed in other locations. The resuscitator stands or kneels close beside patient. Place long axis of heel of one hand parallel to and over long axis of lower half of sternum about 1 to

1½ in. (2.5 to 4 cm) above xiphoid process. Place other hand on top of first one, parallel to it. Fingers may be interlocked for greater stability, or they should be arched upward so force will not extend to ribs (see Figs. 14-5 and 14-6). Acceptable alternative hand position is to grasp wrist of hand on the chest with other hand. Bring shoulders directly over your hands and the patient's sternum, keeping arms straight so thrust for compression is straight down. Using the weight of shoulders, exert pressure vertically downward to depress sternum at least 1½ to 2 in. (4 to 5 cm). Then release pressure, allowing heart to fill with venous blood. Compressions must be smooth, regular, and uninterrupted, not sudden or jerking. Fast jabs can cause injury and do not enhance stroke volume. Compression and relaxation should be of equal duration. Sixty intermittent compressions per minute are recommended in a two-person resuscitation team, 80 compressions per minute if one person CPR. With the other person ventilating, a 1 to 5 ratio, one breath interposed during upstroke of each fifth compression, is recommended. The heel of hand should not be removed from chest between compressions (during relaxation) but pressure should be completely released. Any interruption in compression causes cessation of blood flow and drop in blood pressure.

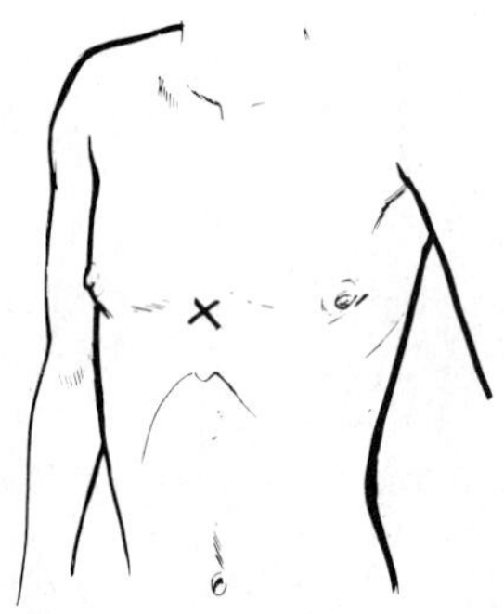

FIGURE 14-5
The cross indicates the correct spot to place the hands for performing closed-chest cardiac massage—over the lower third of the sternum but above the xiphoid process.

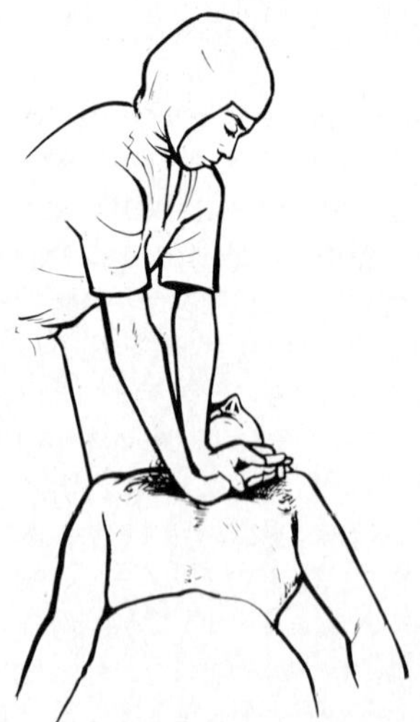

FIGURE 14-6
Closed-chest cardiac compression. Patient is supine on hard flat surface. Resuscitator places the heel of one hand over lower third of sternum, heel of the other hand on top. Fingers are arched upward so as not to exert any force on the ribs. Arms are straight with shoulders over sternum.

For infants and small children, basic principles of CPR are the same. Differences in technique are related to position of heart in the chest, small size of chest, and faster heart rate. For infants, use only the tips of two or three fingers to exert pressure over midsternum, compressing it ½ to ¾ in. (1 to 2 cm). Or, an infant's chest can be encircled with hands and midsternum compressed with both thumbs. For small children, use only heel of *one* hand to exert pressure over the *midsternum,* midway between nipples, compressing it ¾ to 1½ in. (2 to 4 cm). The rate should be 100 compressions per minute for infants, 80 per minute for children, with breath delivered as fast as possible after every five compressions (1 to 5 ratio) for both single or two-person rescue. The higher position of ventricles and liver and the greater chest pliability of these patients predisposes them to greater danger of liver laceration during compression. Since backward tilt of their heads also lifts their backs, a firm back support can be provided by putting one hand beneath a child's back while compressing chest with other hand. A folded blanket beneath the shoulders provides support. Compressions should be counted aloud by person performing compressions. Infant: one, two, three, four, five, breathe. Child: one and two and three and four and five and breathe.

Basic life support should not be interrupted for more than five seconds at a time except for endotracheal intubation or problem with transportation. If intubation is difficult, the patient must be ventilated between short attempts and CPR never suspended for more than 30 seconds. Preferably, patient should not be moved until stabilized and ready for transport or until arrangements are made for uninterrupted CPR during movement.

Elevation of the legs to a 60° angle with the trunk aids venous return and augments artificial circulation. Cardiac compression is successful only if the heart fills with blood between compressions and the resuscitator can move an adequate volume of oxygenated blood. Carotid or femoral pulse is checked every few minutes to indicate compression effectiveness or return of spontaneous effective heartbeat.

Manual cardiac pumping causes fatigue leading to variation in cardiac output; therefore it is preferable to have alternate resuscitators. Commercially available, manually operated mechanical chest compressors or automatic compressor-ventilators that provide simultaneous compression and ventilation eliminate this problem. When such devices are used, *compression must always be started with the manual method first.* Compressor-ventilators should be used only with a cuffed endotracheal tube, esophageal obturator airway or mask, and only by experienced operators. Use should be limited to adults.

Complications of external compression are minimized by careful attention to detail. Compression must be performed with extreme caution to prevent injuries such as: rib or sternal fracture; costochondral separation; fat embolism; laceration of liver; lung contusion; pneumothorax, hemothorax. *Never compress xiphoid process at tip of sternum or exert pressure on ribs to prevent fractures.*

Internal Cardiac Compression Instituted if the patient's chest is already open as during a cardiothoracic procedure. Thoracotomy may be performed and internal compression administered in some rare instances where external compression may be ineffective, e.g., internal thoracic injuries such as penetraing wounds of the heart, flail chest, pericardial tamponade due to hemorrhage, chest or spinal deformities. Internal compression may be used if the patient is salvable. The advantage of internal compression is a constantly high blood outflow. Disadvantages are delay in compression, potential trauma to lungs and myocardium, e.g., contusion of the heart, infection.

Procedure If chest is not already open, incision is made through the left fifth intercostal space. The pericardial sac is opened to permit direct manual cardiac compression. A rib spreader is placed to avoid strangulation of operator's hands. By cradling heart in hands, ventricles are compressed between thumb and fingers of one hand or fingers of both hands 60 times a minute. The heart should not be bruised to avoid impairment of myocardial function. Adequate venous filling is necessary for adequate ventricular stroke volume. The same definitive therapy applies as for external cardiac compression.

Checking Effectiveness of CPR Signs suggestive of effective compression are constricted reactive pupils; palpable peripheral pulse; audible heart beat; improvement in color of mucous membranes, skin, blood. Additional signs indicative of potential recovery are prompt return of spontaneous respiration and consciousness. Continuous compression is stopped when arterial blood pressure remains above 70 to 90 mm Hg and a strong spontaneous pulse is resumed. It may be performed intermittently as necessary to assist the restored heart.

Persistent dilatation of pupils and lack of reaction to light are ominous signs usually indicative of brain damage. Cell destruction is also manifested by convulsions, hyperpyrexia, and persistent coma. Survival in relation to these symptoms is usually accompanied by tragic consequences such as decerebration or paralysis.

If oxygenation and sternal compression (basic life support) do not promptly produce spontaneous cardiac action, additional supportive therapy is also used (advanced life support).

Advanced Cardiac Life Support

Advanced cardiac life support (ACLS) consists of *definitive therapy* intended to reinstitute spontaneous oxygenation. It includes BLS; use of adjunctive equipment and special techniques for establishing and maintaining effective ventilation and circulation; cardiac and supplemental monitoring; recognition and control of arrhythmias; defibrillation; establishing and maintaining IV infusion route; drug administration; postresuscitative care. It requires supervision and direction of a physician. It should be initiated within eight minutes of arrest to improve long-term functional survival. Subsequent insertion of an arterial line supplies access for direct pressure monitoring and arterial blood gases.

Compression is usually accompanied or followed by the judicious use of *intravenous drugs* to manipulate cardiovascular variables to improve the patient's cardiorespiratory status. The various drugs correct hypoxia, correct metabolic acidosis, increase perfusion pressure during cardiac compression, stimulate spontaneous or more forceful myocardial contraction, accelerate cardiac rate, suppress abnormal ventricular activity, treat pulmonary edema. Controversy continues concerning the use of potent vasoconstrictors to treat hypotension because of possibility of ischemic damage to organs associated with their use. Patients who do not respond to one catecholamine often respond to another. The important factor in optimal therapy is prompt recognition of causes of hypotension, shock, and cardiac arrest, and prompt correction of reversible precipitants. A number of agents are discussed below. Dosages mentioned in this text vary according to individual patient circumstances. *Follow physician's order for all drugs.*

1 *Oxygen:* 100% concentration administered immediately by inhalation. In arrest, numerous factors contribute to severe hypoxemia. Oxygen raises arterial oxygen tension, increases arterial oxygen content, and improves tissue oxygenation. Efficient ventilation combats respiratory acidosis. Supplemental oxygen is needed because mouth-to-mouth ventilation delivers only 16 to 17% oxygen and external cardiac compression provides a cardiac output only 30 percent of predicted normal.
2 *IV fluids:* given specifically as needed to increase blood volume and venous return. Circulating blood volume is expanded with whole blood, crystalloid solutions such as lactated Ringer's or physiological (0.9%) saline, or colloid solutions such as commercial plasma protein fractions, or low-molecular-weight dextran.
3 *Sodium bicarbonate:* administered in combination with ventilation to keep arterial pH near normal or to correct metabolic acidosis resulting from tissue hypoxia. Extent of acidosis depends on time interval between arrest, initiation of CPR and supplemental oxygen, and resumption of cardiac function. Acidosis impairs myocardial contractility and reduces response to countershock for ventricular fibrillation. Drug should be given according to repeated arterial blood gas analysis ($PaCO_2$, pH) and calculation of base deficit. *Dosage:* if measurement not available, one mEq/kg IV as initial dose and no more than half this dose given every 10 to 15 minutes of continued arrest. Bolus administration is preferred. Excessive dose can produce metabolic alkalosis, with reduced oxygen release from hemoglobin to tissues, sodium and water overload. Avoid mixing any drug with bicarbonate-containing preparation; e.g., catecholamines (epinephrine) may be inactivated and calcium salts precipitated.
4 *Drugs to improve cardiac output (CO) and blood pressure:* used to increase or decrease peripheral vascular tone of systemic arteries and veins, influence rate and force of cardiac contraction, and alter blood flow and BP in patients with severely reduced CO.
   a *Epinephrine hydrochloride (Adrenalin):* an endogenous catecholamine that plays an essential role in restoration of spontaneous circulation. It improves coronary perfusion pressure and CO produced during chest compression, secondary to vasoconstrictor action; improves myocardial contractility and tone; stimulates spontaneous contractions in asystole; induces "coarse" fibrillation from "fine" fibrillation to enhance defibrillation success. *Dosage:* 0.5 to 1 mg (5 to 10 ml of 1:10,000 solution) given IV. Repeat at five minute intervals as necessary because of short duration of action. Installation into tracheobronchial tree via endotracheal tube provides effective route for absorption with dosage of 1 mg (10 ml of 1:10,000 solution). Administration via these routes if accessible is preferable to intracardiac injection which requires interruption of CPR or may cause myocardial or coronary artery laceration with resultant cardiac tamponade. Inadvertent intramyocardial injection may produce intractable ventricular fibrillation. Continuous infusion may raise heart rate, BP, and CO. For infusion, 1 mg epinephrine is added to 250 ml of 5% dextrose in water. Start at rate of one microgram per minute (1 μg/min). Increase to 3 to 4 μg/min as needed. Side effects include increased myocardial oxygen demand and possible PVCs or ventricular fibrillation.
   b *Norepinephrine, levarterenol (Levophed):* a potent peripheral vasoconstrictor that elevates BP and is useful in peripheral vascular collapse such as severe hypotension or cardiogenic shock. Administration is by IV infusion catheter. Controlled by frequent, preferably direct BP measurement. *Dosage:* to prepare solution, 8 mg norepinephrine are added to 500 ml of 5% dextrose in water or saline or 16 mg of drug in 1000 ml solution, giving concentration of 16 mg/l or 16 μg/ml. Hypotension from hypovolemia is a contraindication. If norepinephrine extravasates

at site of injection, area must be promptly infiltrated with 5 to 10 mg phentolamine in 10 to 15 ml of saline solution to prevent necrosis.

c *Dopamine hydrochloride (Intropin):* dilates renal and mesenteric blood vessels in doses that may not increase heart rate or BP (1 to 2 μg/kg body weight/min). Doses from 2 to 10 μg/kg/min increase cardiac output. Peripheral vasoconstriction results from dosage greater than 10 μg/kg/min. Indications are cardiogenic shock, hemodynamically significant hypotension. Administered only by IV infusion, the initial rate varies from 2 to 5 μg/kg/min. Rate is increased until organ perfusion is evidenced by BP and urine output. The drug will maintain urine output by increasing renal blood flow and increase BP by peripheral vasoconstriction. Tachyarrhythmias are indication for reduction in dose or discontinuation of infusion. *It is inactivated in alkaline solution so must not be added to sodium bicarbonate.* Discontinuance should be gradual. *Dosage:* available in 5 ml ampuls containing 200 mg dopamine. For IV infusion, addition of 200 mg dopamine to 250 ml of 5% dextrose in water provides concentration of 800 μg/ml.

d *Dobutamine hydrochloride (Dobutrex):* synthetic catecholamine administered IV for short term only. It directly increases myocardial contractility. Usual doses produce little systemic arterial constriction. Indications for use: refractory heart failure, cardiogenic shock, hemodynamically significant hypotension. *Dosage:* 2.5 to 10 μg/kg/min. Tachycardia or other arrhythmia may result from dose larger than 20 μg/kg/min.

e *Calcium ions: calcium chloride:* augments myocardial contractility and may be valuable in treating severe hypotension associated with electromechanical dissociation. Calcium may also increase ventricular automaticity and help restore electrical rhythm during ventricular asystole. *Dosage:* IV calcium chloride 2.5 to 5.0 ml of a 10% solution (5 to 7 mg/kg) repeated as necessary at ten minute intervals. Available as a 10% solution containing 1.36 mEq Ca^{++} per 100 mg of salt (100 mg = one ml). Calcium chloride is preferred to other calcium salts given in doses: calcium gluceptate 5 to 7 ml (4.5 to 6.3 mEq); calcium gluconate 10 to 15 ml (4.8 to 7.2 mEq). *Calcium cannot be given together with sodium bicarbonate as a precipitate forms from the mixture.*

f *Metaraminol bitartrate (Aramine):* increases cardiac output and BP. Used infrequently, it produces marked vasoconstriction. *Dosage:* administered IV by continuous infusion in concentration of 0.4 mg/min of 5% dextrose in water (100 mg drug added to 250 ml solution).

g *Sodium nitroprusside (Nipride):* potent, rapidly acting direct peripheral vasodilator that affects both venous and arterial systems. It increases CO and redistributes cardiac work in patients with pump failure, but increases tissue perfusion without reflex tachycardia. It is useful in hypertensive crisis. *Dosage:* 50 mg dissolved in 2 to 3 ml of dextrose in water then added to 250 to 1000 ml of dextrose in water for infusion, preferably by infusion pump or microdrip regulating system if precise flow rate is assured. Solution deteriorates in light so must be protected by opaque material such as aluminum foil. Maximum rate should not exceed 10 μg/kg/min to avoid cyanide toxicity. Hemodynamic monitoring is mandatory.

5 *Drugs to control heart rate and rhythm:*

a *Lidocaine (Xylocaine):* commonly used for arrhythmias, especially ventricular fibrillation resistant to defibrillation effort. It increases threshold for ventricular irritability by exerting focal anesthetic effect on myocardial cell membrane. *Dosage:* bolus injection of about 1 mg/kg body weight, followed immediately by 1 to 4 mg/min by infusion pump to precisely control rate of drug delivery; or 75 mg bolus injection with simultaneous start of infusion at 2 mg/min (20 to 50 μg/kg/min) to sustain therapeutic concentration. If ectopy continues after initial bolus, an additional 50 mg bolus may be given every five minutes if needed, to total of 225 mg. Accompanying infusion started at 2 mg/min is increased by 1 mg/min after each additional bolus injection to maximum of 4 mg/min. Half of this dosage is used in presence of shock or pulmonary edema. Similar dosage can be used for prophylaxis against fibrillation, i.e., against progression of isolated ventricular ectopic beats.

b *Procainamide hydrochloride (Pronestyl):* used in suppressing ventricular premature contractions, recurrent ventricular tachycardia not controlled by lidocaine, and recurrent ventricular fibrillation resistant to attempted defibrillation. *Dosage:* 100 mg IV every five minutes at rate of about 20 mg/min until arrhythmia ceases, hypotension occurs, or total of 1 g is injected. Maintenance infusion rate is 1 to 4 mg/min. Continuous ECG and BP monitoring is essential as marked hypotension may occur if injection is too rapid.

c *Bretylium tosylate (Bretylol, Darenthin):* antiarrhythmic used for ventricular tachycardia and fibrillation unresponsive to other therapy. It may lower defibrillation threshold permitting otherwise refractory rhythms to be electrically converted. *Dosage:* 5 mg/kg given as IV bolus, followed by electrical defibrillation. If fibrillation continues, may increase dose to 10 mg/kg and repeat at 15 to 30 minute intervals until maximum dose of 30 mg/kg is given. In refractory or recurrent ventricular tachycardia, 500 mg (10 ml) is diluted to 50 ml and 5 to 10 mg/kg injected IV over eight to ten minutes. After initial dose is given drug can also be administered as continuous infusion at rate of 1 to 2 mg/min. Marked hypotension is an untoward effect.

d *Atropine sulfate:* used to reduce cardiac vagal tone, enhance atrioventricular conduction, and increase cardiac output. It accelerates cardiac rate in sinus bradycardia with severe hypotension, or bradycardia (less than 50 beats/min) without hypotension but with reduced CO. It may restore cardiac rhythm in ventricular asystole. *Dosage:* 0.5 mg IV and repeated at five minute intervals until desired rate is achieved, total dose not to exceed 2 mg which could result in full vagal blockage.

e *Propranolol hydrochloride (Inderal):* beta-adrenergic receptor blocking agent useful in treatment of supraventricular arrhythmias, for control of recurring atrial or ventricular tachyarrhythmias, or for recurrent ventricular fibrillation when control is not achieved with lidocaine or other agents. It is contraindicated in asthmatic or bronchospasm patient, and very hazardous when cardiac function is depressed. *Dosage:* IV boluses, 0.1 to 0.3 mg initial dose up to 1 mg every five minutes, usually not to exceed total dose of 5 mg. Monitor closely.

f *Verapamil hydrochloride (Isoptin):* derivative of papavarine used as antiarrhythmic agent to treat paroxysmal supraventricular tachycardia, acute atrial flutter and atrial fibrillation. *Dosage:* IV bolus of 0.075 to 0.15 mg/kg adult body weight (maximum of 10 mg) given over one minute with peak effect within three to five minutes. If response is inadequate, repeat 0.15 mg/kg (maximum of 10 mg) 30 minutes after first dose, total cumulative dose within 30 minutes not to exceed 15 mg. Monitor arterial BP closely.

g *Isoproterenol hydrochloride (Isuprel):* increases sympathetic tone, rate, and strength of heartbeat and CO. It is used for immediate control of atropine refractory bradycardia resulting from heart block. A potent cardiac stimulant, it increases CO at expense of increase in myocardial oxygen demand. It may produce tachycardia or ventricular arrhythmia. *Dosage:* IV infusion of 1 mg isoproterenol hydrochloride to 500 ml of 5% dextrose in water to produce concentration of 2 μg/ml. Recommended infusion rate is 2 to 20 μg/min titrated according to heart rate and rhythm response.

6 *Furosemide (Lasix) and ethacrynic acid (Edecrin):* potent diuretics used to treat postarrest cerebral edema or pulmonary edema. They inhibit reabsorption of sodium. Furosemide also has a direct venodilating effect. *Dosage:* for pulmonary edema: *furosemide* 0.5 to 2.0 mg/kg injected slowly IV; or *ethacrynic acid* 40 to 50 mg IV.

7 *Morphine sulfate:* analgesic used for pain from trauma or myocardial infarction and treatment of acute pulmonary edema. It increases venous capacitance, pools blood peripherally, and decreases venous return, which may help relieve pulmonary congestion and decrease myocardial oxygen requirement. It reduces systemic vascular resistance and left ventricular afterload. *Dosage:* given by titration of small IV doses at frequent intervals: 2 to 5 mg every five to 30 minutes, titrated to desired effect. Observe patient for hypotension and respiratory depression.

8 *Nitroglycerin for infusion (Nitrostat IV):* concentrated potent drug which must be diluted in IV dextrose or saline for IV infusion. A predominantly venous vasodilator, it decreases venous return to heart and reduces preload and afterload. Myocardial oxygen demand is lowered by both arterial and venous effects. Used for control of BP in hypertension associated with cardiovascular procedures or during endotracheal intubation, skin incision, sternotomy, cardiac bypass, or in immediate postoperative period. Special infusion set is used because of absorption into plastic.

In summary, oxygen, epinephrine, and sodium bicarbonate are the mainstays of pharmacologic management in CPR. Used in combination with BLS, lidocaine, and defibrillation, they correct most CPR oxygen delivery problems. Each additional drug used serves as a vital adjunct in definitive therapy and postresuscitative care.

Vasoconstrictors improve tissue perfusion by maintaining perfusion pressure, prevent or diminish blood loss, decrease tissue vascularity, and improve coronary blood flow. Among indications for use are anesthetic overdose, hypotension associated with blood loss, adrenergic insufficiency. Vasodilators improve tissue perfusion, prevent or diminish blood loss, and decrease myocardial oxygen demand. Indications for use are regional perfusion for hypo- or hyperthermia, controlled hypotension during operation, hypertensive crises such as renal failure, impaired cardiac performance such as ischemic heart disease.

Emergency Arrest/Crash Cart

An *emergency arrest cart* should be available at all times in all critical care areas, i.e., OR, ED, and intensive care units. Specific drugs and equipment vary from hospital to hospital depending on how well equipped the anesthesiologist is for emergencies. Equipment on a portable cart usually includes:

1 Oxygen and resuscitation equipment: oxygen cylinder, tubing, mask, Ambu bag

2 Laryngoscope tray, blades; endotracheal equipment and tubes; assorted airways—oral and nasal, stylet, padded tongue blades

3 Tracheotomy tray

4 Sterile gloves, sterile gauze sponges, prep swabs or spray, adhesive tape, tourniquets, sutures, armboard, drapes

5 Suction machine and catheters

6 Intravenous infusion solutions and sets, IV needles and catheters (14 and 16 gauge), tubings, stopcocks, infusion pump, additive labels

7 Cutdown tray; venous cannulas

8 Assorted sterile syringes—3, 5, 10, 20, and 50 ml

9 Assorted sterile needles—25g ⅝ in., 20g 1½ in., 18g 1½ in., 20g 3 in. (intracardiac) and spinal needles

10 Arterial blood sampling kit with needles, heparinized syringes; arterial line tray

11 Disposable scalpels, hemostats

12 Emergency thoracotomy set (scalpel with #20 blade, rib retractor, self-retaining retractor)

13 ECG monitor, leads, recording sheets

14 Cardiac arrest board

15 Defibrillator with paddles (adult, pediatric, external, internal), electrode jelly or paste, saline pads

16 Cardiac arrest record for treatment documentation/flow sheets

17 Cardiac pacemaker

18 Drugs: mainly antacids, vasoconstrictors, cardiotonics, vasopressors, cardiac depressants, anticholinergics, cerebral dehydrating agents, pulmonary dehydrating agents. (Refer to pages 290 to 293 for some specific drugs.) Many frequently used emergency drugs are available in sterile commercially prefilled syringes, to avoid delay in preparation.

19 CVP manometer

20 Nasogastric tube and bulb syringe

21 Flashlight

Personnel Responsibilities

During cardiopulmonary resuscitation, team members must *remain calm,* but react quickly and act efficiently.

1 *Director:* One person, the most knowledgeable, *usually the anesthesiologist,* commands resuscitation efforts. He/she is assisted by surgeons, nurses, and other available personnel. A cardiologist is usually summoned. Resuscitation teams are multidisciplinary. The person in charge directs lifesaving interventions which entail minute-to-minute decisions such as medications, defibrillation. To avoid confusion, the director issues orders for others to follow. Every circulating nurse should be prepared to be a team captain.

2 *Circulating nurse*

   a Start time-elapsed clock and record time of arrest.

   b Activate emergency alarm to alert OR supervisor and summon assistance.

   c Help reposition patient as necessary to supine position for CPR. Lower operating table and provide resuscitator with a standing platform to facilitate cardiac compression.

   d Obtain and prepare necessary equipment, such as medications and defibrillator, and ECG if not already in use.

e Help with and observe intravenous and monitoring lines, such as arterial line. Assist in collection of blood samples.
f Maintain accuracy of sponge, needle, and instrument counts and sterility to best of ability if wound closure progresses. But sterility is secondary to resuscitation efforts.
g Supervise termination of procedure as necessary.
h Delegate duties to assisting personnel.
i Control traffic. Exclude unauthorized personnel from room. Provide optimum environment for successful resuscitation.
j Document all medications given, time and amount, and the sequence of procedures performed. Documentation is important in guiding therapy and providing legal protection.
k Assist where needed most.
l In unsuccessful resuscitation, follow death protocol regarding notification of family, care of deceased, specimens to be saved, forms to be filled out.

3 *Scrub nurse*
a Remain sterile and keep tables sterile. If arrest occurs during operation, when chest is not open, wound is packed, covered with sterile drape, and patient repositioned as necessary for CPR. If wound can be closed rapidly during resuscitation, this may be done.
b Keep track of sponges, needles, and instruments. Counts are completed and wound closed despite outcome.
c Give attention to field and surgeon's needs. Keep syringes of medications filled and ready for use. If patient is hemorrhaging, keep suction tubing clear, tapes available.

4 *OR supervisor/charge nurse*
a Assign professional and ancillary support personnel to augment team, e.g., extra circulating nurse, medication nurse, personnel to obtain supplies or handle laboratory samples.
b Notify attending physician, if not present, and appropriate personnel, e.g., administrative services.
c Have patient placed on critical list.
d Reassign subsequent patients' scheduling.
e Keep track of resuscitation progress.
f Evaluate arrest procedure, emergency equipment, verify documentation.
g Support team as necessary. Keep surgical suite running smoothly during emergency.

Appropriate administrative personnel and services (unit, ICU, clergy) are notified of cardiac arrest as required, as well as the patient's family. In case of death, the surgeon notifies family (see Death in OR, Chap. 10, p. 177).

CPR Duration Cardiopulmonary resuscitation may be done as long as necessary to restore cardiocirculatory function if adequate ventilation and good peripheral pulse have been restored. It is not uncommon for arrest to reoccur following successful resuscitation. The time frame for survival is shortened drastically if the arrest is unwitnessed. When the patient's condition is adequately stabilized, and the wound closed, he or she is transferred to the intensive care unit.

Decision to discontinue resuscitative efforts in the OR is made by a physician. However, resuscitation team is included in this decision. It is based on assessment of cerebral and cardiovascular status. The end point of cardiovascular unresponsiveness is suggested as the most reliable basis for this decision.

Postresuscitation Care Postarrest supportive therapy depends on etiology and duration of arrest. Care centers on cardiac and cerebral preservation, maintenance of circulation and ventilation, and minimizing of sequelae, such as cerebral edema. Patient must be carefully monitored and closely observed for 48 to 72 hours postarrest. In select patients, hypothermia may be used to reduce oxygen needs. Vital signs, acid-base and electrolyte balances, and urinary output are closely watched. Seizures should be controlled to prevent further anoxia. The patient is observed for signs of embolism, pulmonary edema, fractured ribs, or hemopericardium. A chest x-ray is taken as soon as feasible after arrest. An intravenous fluid lifeline must be left in place. If there is evident cerebral damage, the prognosis is guarded.

Staff Education Practice runs of a cardiac arrest emergency and CPR with subsequent evaluation/revision are valuable to review protocol and prepare OR staff before need for implemenation.

Today's research is tomorrow's practice. The search for new anesthetic drugs tailored to suppress only selected cells continues. Research is also addressed to the development and refinement of processes for continuing automatic assessment of many vital functions. Patient and personnel safety in the operating room remains a vital concern.

CHAPTER **15**

POSITIONS

PRELIMINARY CONSIDERATIONS

Proper positioning for operation is a facet of patient care that is as important to patient outcome as adequate preoperative preparation and safe anesthesia. It requires knowledge of anatomy and *application of physiological principles* as well as familiarity with the necessary equipment.

Position for operation is determined by the procedure to be performed, with consideration of the surgeon's choice of surgical approach, and of anesthetic administration technique. Factors such as age, height, weight, cardiopulmonary status, and preexisting diseases (for example, arthritis) also influence position. See Chapter 33 for positioning and restraining of pediatric patients.

Responsibility

Choice of position for operation is made by the surgeon in consultation with the anesthesiologist and adjustments made as necessary for anesthesia. The responsibility for placing the patient in the operative position is that of the circulating nurse, with guidance, approval, and sometimes assistance of the anesthesiologist and the surgeon or assistant. In essence, it is a shared responsibility among these team members. In cases of complex positioning or obese, heavy patients, the nurse will need help in lifting and/or positioning the patient.

Time

The patient is usually supine, on his or her back face up, after transfer from the stretcher to the operating table. The patient may be anesthetized in this position and then positioned for operation, or may be positioned and then anesthetized. Factors influencing the time at which the patient is positioned are: site of operation, age and size of patient, anesthetic administration technique, pain upon moving if the patient is conscious.

Safety Measures

The safety measures included in Chapter 10 also apply while positioning patients. These include:

1 The patient must be properly identified when transferred to the operating table and the operative site affirmed.

2 The table must be securely locked in position with the brake applied, when the patient is on it and during transfer to and from the table.

3 The anesthesiologist guards the patient's head at all times and supports it during movement.

4 A physician assumes responsibility for protecting an unsplinted fracture during movement.

5 An armboard must be guarded to avoid hyperextending arm or dislodging infusion needle.

6 Anesthetized patients and the aged must be

moved slowly and gently to allow the circulatory system to adjust.

7 If a patient is on his or her back, the ankles and legs must not be crossed, which would create occlusive pressure on blood vessels and nerves.

8 If a patient is on his or her side, a pillow must be placed lengthwise between the legs to prevent pressure on blood vessels.

9 If a patient is prone, the thorax must be relieved of pressure to facilitate respiration.

10 Adequate assistance in lifting patients and constant vigilance are necessary to prevent falls.

11 The position should not obstruct tubings (catheter, intravenous, etc.) and monitors.

12 The patient is not moved without permission of the anesthesiologist.

Preparations for Positioning

Before the patient is brought into the operating room the circulating nurse should:

1 Review the proposed position by referring to procedure book and surgeon's preference card

2 Ask for assistance if unsure how to position patient

3 Consult the surgeon as soon as he or she arrives if not sure which position is to be used

4 Assemble the necessary equipment so as to expedite the procedure

CRITERIA FOR POSITIONING

The ability to tolerate the stresses of operation depends greatly on the normality of functioning of vital systems. The physical condition of the patient must be considered. Proper body alignment is important. Criteria must be met for physiological positioning.

No Interference with Respiration

Unhindered diaphragmatic movement and a patent airway are essential to maintain respiratory function, to prevent hypoxia, and to facilitate induction by inhalation. Some hypoxia is always present in a lying position. Tidal volume, the functional residual capacity of air moved by a single breath, is reduced by as much as a third when patient lies down. Therefore, there should be no constriction about the neck or chest. Patients' arms should be at their sides, on armboards, or otherwise supported, not crossed on the chest.

No Interference with Circulation

Adequate circulation is necessary to maintain blood pressure, to facilitate venous return, to prevent thrombus formation, and to prevent circulatory disturbances. Occulsion and pressure on peripheral blood vessels must be avoided. Body support and restraining straps must not be fastened too tightly.

No Pressure on Any Nerves

Prolonged pressure to or stretching of peripheral nerves can result in slight sensory and motor loss to paralysis. Extremities as well as the body must be well supported at all times. Appliances, restraints, and equipment in contact with skin must be well-padded. Most frequent sites of injury are divisions of the brachial plexus and the ulnar, radial, peroneal, and facial nerves. Axons may be stretched or disrupted. Extremes of position of the head and arm easily cause injury to the brachial plexus. The ulnar, radial, and peroneal nerves may be compressed against bone, stirrups, or operating table if the patient is improperly positioned. Femoral nerve injury may be caused by retractors during pelvic procedures. Facial nerve injury may result from too vigorous a manual effort to elevate the mandible to maintain airway, or from too tight a head strap.

Minimal Skin Pressure

Body weight is maldistributed when patient lies on the operating table. Weight concentrated over bony prominences can cause skin pressure sores. These areas must be protected from constant external pressure against hard surfaces.

Accessibility of Operative Site

The operative procedure determines the position in which the patient is placed. The surgeon must have adequate exposure to minimize trauma and operating time.

Accessibility for Anesthetic Administration

The anesthesiologist must be able to attach monitoring electrodes, administer anesthesia, observe its effects, and maintain an intravenous lifeline.

No Undue Postoperative Discomfort

Strain on muscles results in injury and/or needless postoperative discomfort. An anesthetized patient lacks protective muscle tone. If head is extended for a prolonged time, the patient may suffer more pain from a resulting stiff neck than from the operative wound.

Individual Requirements Met

If a patient is extremely obese, for example, with torso occupying the table width, his or her arms may be placed on armboards. Patients with arthritis deformans need special individualized care. An obstetric patient at term or a cardiac patient may experience dyspnea when lying flat.

EQUIPMENT FOR POSITIONING

Operating Table

Many different tables with suitable attachments are in use. Practice is necessary to master adjustments. The tables are versatile and adaptable to a number of diversified positions for all surgical specialties. However, orthopaedic, urologic, and fluoroscopic tables are utilized frequently for specialized procedures.

Most tables consist of a rectangular metal top that rests on an electric or hydraulic lift base. Some models have interchangeable tops for the various specialties. The table top is divided into three or more hinged sections. Basically, these are the head, body, and leg sections. Each can be manipulated, flexed or extended, to the desired position. This procedure is called *breaking the table.* The joints are referred to as *breaks.* Some tables have a metal crossbar or body elevator between the two upper sections that may be raised to elevate a gallbladder or kidney. The head section is removable, permitting insertion of special headrests for cranial procedures. An extension may be inserted at foot of the table to accommodate an exceptionally tall patient. An x-ray penetrable tunnel top extending the length of the table permits the insertion of an x-ray cassette holder at any area. A self-adhering, conductive rubber mattress covers table top.

Standard operating tables have posturing controls for manipulating table into desired positions. Some tables are electrically controlled, either by remote control switches or a lever-operated electro-hydraulic system; movement of others is manual. The selector controls are located at the head end of the table. By setting the selector control on *back, side, foot,* or *flex,* the desired section(s) of the table top can be articulated. By activating other selector controls, the table top may be tilted laterally from side to side and raised or lowered in its entirety. A tiltometer indicates degree of tilt between horizontal and vertical. All operating tables have a brake for stabilization in all positions.

Special Equipment and Table Attachments

Equipment used in positioning is designed to stabilize the patient in the desired position, thus permitting optimal exposure of the operative area. All attachments that come into contact with skin must be well-padded to prevent trauma or abrasion.

Safety Belt (Knee Strap) A sturdy, wide strap of conductive material, such as nylon webbing or conductive rubber, is placed over the legs, around the table top, and fastened to restrain leg movement. Some straps are attached at each side of the table and fastened together at the center. This strap or belt must be secure but not so tight as to impair circulation. It is used during all inductions and during operation except for certain positions, e.g., lithotomy. Placement depends on body position, e.g., above the knees for supine (also known as dorsal), and below the knees for prone.

Anesthesia Screen A metal bar holds the drapes from the patient's face and separates the nonsterile area from the sterile area. It is adjustable, allowing rotation or angling in any plane. It is placed after induction and positioning of patient.

Wrist or Arm Strap Narrow conductive straps placed around the wrists secure hands and arms to an armboard or to the table at the patient's side for protection. Hands must never be placed under body areas as compression results.

Arm Band (Lift Sheet) A sheet of separate layers of broad, heavy linen, stitched vertically through the middle is placed horizontally across table on top of the clean sheet before patient is transferred. The arms are enclosed in the lower flaps and the upper flaps brought down over the arms and tucked under the mattress. In this way the full length of the arm is supported at the patient's side, protected from injury, and restrained. It should be applied just before induction. The patient can be told it is to keep arms comfortable on the table when he or she is asleep and relaxed. The word "restraint" is avoided.

Armboard To support an arm not resting at the patient's side, an armboard is used when: giving intravenous infusions; arm or hand is site of operation; the arm at the side would interfere with access to the operative area; room on table for arm is inadequate; arm on the unaffected side requires support (lateral position). A self-locking type is safest to prevent displacement.

NOTE. For operation on an arm or hand, an adjustable *extremity table* may be used in lieu of an armboard. It is slipped under the mattress at one end. The other end of the table is supported by a metal leg (similar to a Mayo stand). By removing the top panel, a solution drain pan may be fit into the table top. After the skin prep or irrigation, the pan is removed and the top panel reinserted. A conductive foam rubber pad is placed and covered to receive the arm, which is then draped. The table provides a large, firm surface for operation.

Double Armboard Both arms are supported, one directly above the other, for lateral position.

Elbow Pads or Protectors Padded linen may be used to protect the elbows from pressure. A hard plastic shell with soft liner is commercially available.

Shoulder Bridge (Thyroid Elevator) A metal bar, which can be raised or lowered, is slipped onto the table under the mattress between the head and body sections by temporarily removing the head section. It is used to hyperextend the shoulder or thyroid area for operative accessibility.

Shoulder Braces or Supports Adjustable, concave metal pieces well-padded with foam rubber or conductive rubber are used to prevent the patient from slipping toward the head of the table when in Trendelenburg's position. Braces should be placed equidistant from the head of the table with a ½ in. (13 mm) space between the shoulders and the braces to eliminate pressure against the shoulders. A shoulder brace is not used when an arm is extended on an armboard to avoid nerve compression.

Shoulder Roll A solid roll of cloth placed under each side of the patient's chest raises it off the table to facilitate respiration. This type of equipment may be referred to as a *bolster.*

Elevating Pads Pads are used to elevate a specific part of the body, for example to hyperextend spine for laminectomy. Commercially available bolsters and elevating pads are commonly used. They are covered with conductive materials.

Body Rests or Braces Metal brace with a foam rubber pad covered with conductive rubber is placed in metal clamps on the side of the table and slipped in from the table edge against the body at various points to stabilize it in lateral position.

Kidney Rests Concave metal pieces with grooved notches at the base are placed under the mattress on the body elevator part of the table. They are slipped in from the table edge snugly against the body for stability in kidney position. Be careful that the upper edge of the rest does not press too tightly against the body, even though padded.

Body-Restraint Strap A belt, the center portion of which is a pad to protect the skin, is placed over the patient and secured by hooks to the sides of the table. This strap helps to hold the patient securely in position.

Hemorrhoid Strap Made of a piece of 3-in. (7.5 cm) adhesive 6 in. (15 cm) in length with a buckle and canvas strap on one end, a hemorrhoid strap is placed on each buttock, 4 in. (10 cm) lateral to the operative site, to separate the buttocks. Each strap is fastened to the table frame at the side with the patient in Kraske position.

Adjustable Arch Bar Consists of two padded rolls mounted on a frame. The rolls extend from the shoulders to the knees. The patient is placed on the abdomen on this arch. The degree of flexion desired for thoracic or lumbar vertebral operations is achieved by adjusting the height of the arch by means of a lever.

Stirrups Metal stirrup posts are placed in holders, one on each side of the table to support the legs and feet in lithotomy position. The feet are supported by canvas loops, thus suspending the legs at a right angle to the feet. During extensive surgery, special leg holders supporting the lower legs may be used. Metal knee-crutch stirrups are available. Even if well-padded, they create some pressure on the back of the knees and lower extremity, jeopardizing popliteal vessel and nerve. This is avoided with the canvas-sling stirrups.

Metal Footboard The footboard can be left flat as a horizontal extension of the table or raised perpendicular to the table to support the feet, the soles resting securely against it. It must be padded for reverse Trendelenburg's position.

Special Padded Headrests and Attachments Available for neurosurgical procedures, headrests attach to the table, supporting and exposing the occiput and cervical vertebrae. They are used with supine, prone, sitting, or lateral position.

Pillows (Soft or Hard) and Sandbags Various sizes and shapes to fit anatomic structures are used to support or immobilize parts. A donut-shaped foam rubber pad or sandbag may be used for procedures on head or face. About 10 in. (25 cm) in diameter, the occiput rests in a 3-in. (7.5 cm) hole in the center. It keeps the operative area in a horizontal plane. Foam rubber, sandbags (positioning weights), and pillows are covered with washable, conductive rubber.

Pressure Mattress To minimize pressure on bony prominences, peripheral blood vessels and nerves during prolonged operations (over two hours), an alternating pressure mattress is put over the conductive rubber mattress on the operating table before patient is transferred to table. This may be a positive pressure air mattress, circulating water mattress, or a foam rubber mattress with indentations similar to configuration of an egg crate. Thermal blankets or mattresses are used to induce hypo- or hyperthermia (see Chap. 13, p. 249, and Chap. 33, p. 592).

Surgical Positioning System A convenient, efficient, comfortable means of patient positioning is available that eliminates sandbags, bolsters, and adhesive tape. Soft pads filled with tiny plastic beads are put under or around the body part to be supported. Suction is attached to pad and, as air is withdrawn, the pad becomes firm. During air evacuation, the circulating nurse and assistant mold pad to body area with their hands. The suction is disconnected. With vacuum inside pad, the surrounding atmospheric pressure presses beads together and friction between them prevents their moving, creating a solid mass that keeps its molded shape. Various sizes and shapes of pads provide firm, yet pressure-point relieving support. To change patient's position during operation, the valve on the pad is squeezed until pad is slightly soft. The patient is repositioned, and suction is applied to remold pad.

OPERATIVE POSITIONS

Many positions for operation are used. Only the most commonly employed ones are included. If IV fluids will be infused in the arm during the operation, an arm will be on an armboard. This fact is assumed in the following discussion because IV fluids are usually given.

Supine Position (Also Known as Dorsal Position)

See Figure 15-1. This is the most natural position for the body at rest. Patient lies flat on back with arms secured at the sides, palms down. Legs are straight and parallel, in line with the head and spine. Hips are parallel with the spine. The safety belt is placed above the knees. Small pillows may be placed under head and lumbar curvature. Heels must be protected from pressure on the table by a pillow, ankle roll, or donut. Feet must not be in prolonged plantar flexion. The soles may be supported by a pillow or padded footboard to prevent foot drop. The position is used for procedures on the anterior surface of the body such as abdominal, abdominothoracic, and some lower extremity procedures.

Modifications of supine position are used:

Position 1 For procedures on *face* or *neck*. The neck may be slightly hyperextended by lowering head section of the table or by placing a narrow pad between scapulae. With patient in supine

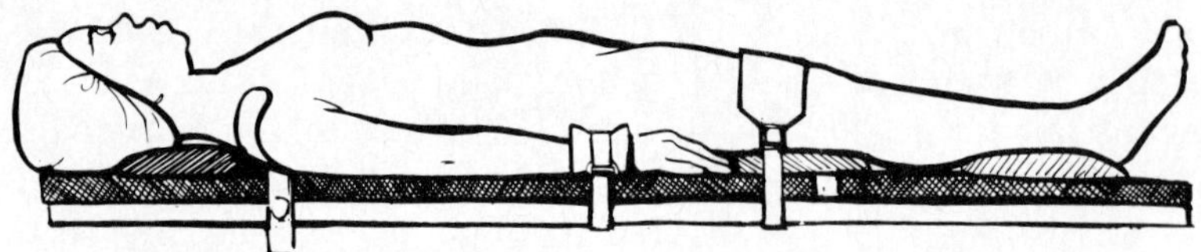

FIGURE 15-1
Supine position. Patient lies straight on back, face upward, with arms at sides, legs extended parallel and uncrossed, feet slightly separated. Strap is placed above knees. Head is in line with spine. Note small pillow supporting feet to prevent foot drop.

position, the head may be supported in a headrest or donut and/or turned toward the unaffected side. The eyes must be protected from injury or irritating solutions. They should be kept closed with eye pads taped in place during skin preparation and operation. They should be inspected at end of the operative procedure.

Position 2 For *shoulder* or *anterolateral* procedures. With patient in supine position, a small sandbag, roll, or pad is placed under affected side to elevate shoulder off the table for exposure. The length of body must be stabilized to prevent rolling or twisting of the spine. Hips and shoulders should be kept in a plane.

Position 3: Dorsal Recumbent For some *vaginal* procedures. Patient is in supine position except that the knees are flexed and thighs externally rotated. Soles of feet rest on the table. Pillows may be placed under knees if needed for support.

Position 4: Modified Recumbent (Frog-Legged) See Figure 15-2. For some operations in region of the *groin* or *lower extremity.* Patient is in supine position except that the knees are *slightly* flexed with a pillow beneath each. Thighs are externally rotated.

Position 5: Arm-Extension For *breast, axillary, upper extremity,* or *hand* operation. The patient is in supine position with arm on the affected side on an armboard that locks into position at a right angle to the body. The affected side of body must be close to table edge for access to operative area. If the axilla is involved, the arm is even with the lower edge of the armboard for accessibility. Hyperextension of arm must be avoided to prevent neural or vascular injury, such as brachial plexus injury or occlusion of the axillary artery. The armboard must be well-padded.

Trendelenburg's Position

See Figure 15-3. The patient lies on the back with knees over the lower break of the table. The knees must bend with table break to prevent pressure on peroneal nerves and veins in the legs. Shoulder braces are applied. The entire table is tilted downward about 45° at the head, depending upon the surgeon's wish. Foot of table is lowered to desired angle. This position is used for procedures in the lower abdomen or pelvis when it is desirable to tilt the abdominal viscera away from the pelvic area for better exposure. The patient remains in this position for as short a time as possible. While increasing operative accessibility, lung volume is decreased by pressure of organs against the dia-

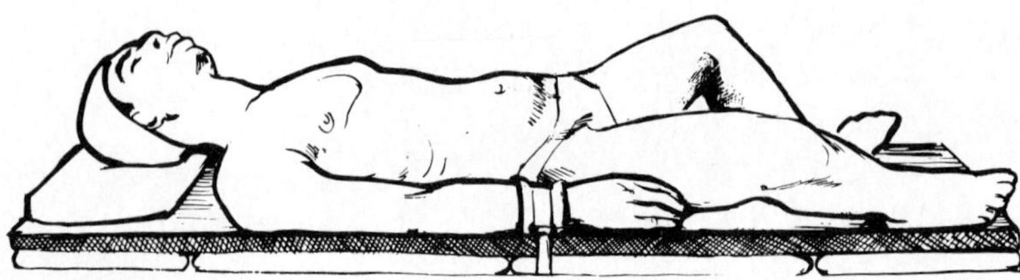

FIGURE 15-2
Modified recumbent position. Patient lies on back with arms at sides. Knees are slightly flexed, with a small pillow under each. Thighs are externally rotated.

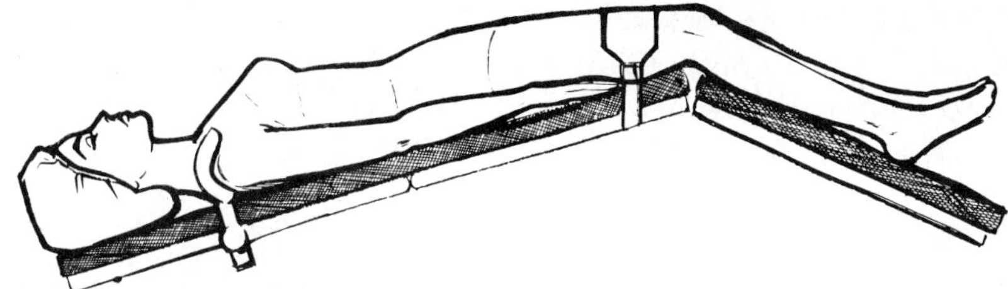

FIGURE 15-3
Trendelenburg's position. Note the knees are over the lower break in the table, knee strap is above the knees, and shoulder braces are in place.

phragm. In returning to horizontal position, *leg section should be raised first and slowly* while reversing venous status in legs. Then the entire table is leveled.

A modification of position is used for patients in hypovolemic shock. Many anesthesiologists prefer to keep trunk level and elevate legs by raising the lower part of the table at the break under hips. Others prefer to tilt the entire table downward. Either position reduces venous stasis in lower extremities.

Reverse Trendelenburg's Position

See Figure 15-4. Patient lies on back. The mattress is adjusted so operative area is over elevator bridge on the table. The entire table is tilted so head is higher than feet. A padded footboard may be used, depending on the degree of tilt. The position is used for thyroidectomy to facilitate breathing and to decrease blood supply to operative area (blood will pool caudally). It is used also for gallbladder or biliary tract procedures to allow abdominal viscera to fall away from the epigastrium, giving access to upper abdomen. Small pillows may be placed under knees and lumbar curvature. A small pillow or donut may stabilize the head. If elevator bridge is not used, the operative area may be hyperextended by a pad.

Fowler's Position

Patient lies on back with knees over lower break in the table. The footboard is raised and padded. The foot of the table is lowered slightly, flexing the knees. Body section of table is raised 45°, thereby becoming the backrest. Arms rest on a large, soft pillow on the lap. The safety belt is above the knees. The entire table is tilted slightly head downward to prevent patient slipping caudad. For cranial procedures, head is supported in a headrest.

Sitting (Upright) Position

Patient is positioned as for Fowler's except that torso is in an upright position. Shoulders and torso should be supported with body straps, but not so tight as to impede respiration and circulation. Pressure points must be well-padded. Flexed

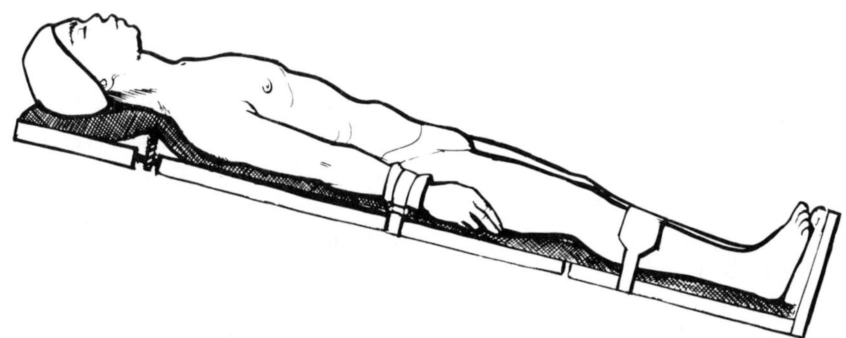

FIGURE 15-4
Reverse Trendelenburg's position. Patient lies on back. The footboard is padded and raised. The entire table is tilted so head is higher than feet. The strap is below the knees. Note operative area is over raised thyroid elevator on the table.

arms rest on a large pillow on the lap or on a pillow on an adjustable table in front of patient. Head is in a cranial headrest for neurosurgical procedures. Air embolism is a potential complication. An antigravity suit is used to counteract postural hypotension. This position is used for some otorhinology procedures.

Lithotomy Position

See Figure 15-5. Cotton boots are put on patient's legs prior to transfer to operating table for perineal, vaginal, or rectal procedures. Patient's buttocks rest along break between body and leg sections of the table. Stirrups are secured in holders on each side of the table. They must be adjusted at equal height on both sides and at appropriate height for length of the patient's legs to maintain symmetry when patient is positioned. After the patient is anesthetized, legs are raised simultaneously by two persons. Each grasps sole of a foot in one hand and supports the knee area with the other. Feet are then placed in canvas slings of the stirrups. One loop of canvas encircles sole; other loop goes around ankle. Simultaneous movement is essential as knees are flexed to avoid straining the lower back. If legs are properly placed, undue abduction and external rotation are avoided. There must be no pressure of lower leg or ankle against the stirrup. Padding is placed if necessary.

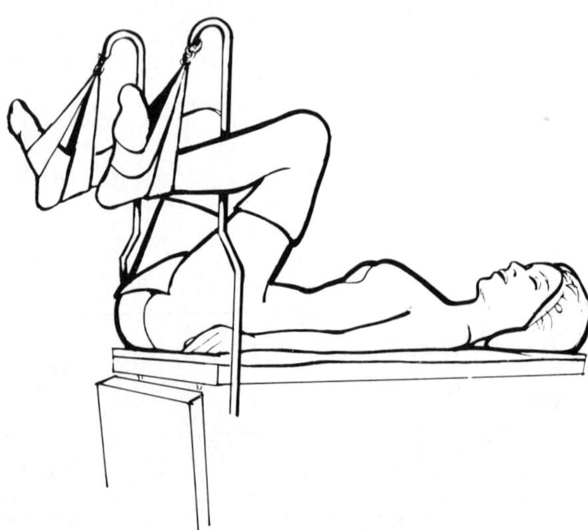

FIGURE 15-5
Lithotomy position. Patient is on back with foot section of table lowered to a right angle with body on the table. Knees are flexed and legs are on outside of metal posts with feet supported by canvas straps. Note that buttocks are even with table edge.

If legs are put in stirrups prior to induction, the patient can identify discomfort and pressure on back and/or legs.

Lower section of mattress is removed and leg section of the table lowered. The mattress is pulled down on table, as necessary, until *buttocks are even with table edge.* They must not extend beyond the edge, causing strain to lumbosacral muscles and ligaments, as body weight rests on sacrum.

Arms may be placed on armboards or loosely cradled over lower abdomen and secured by lower end of the blanket. Arms must not rest on chest and impede respiration. Lung compliance is decreased by pressure of thighs on the abdomen, which hinders descent of diaphragm. Hands should *not* extend along table where they could be injured in break during manipulation of the table or movement of the patient. Hands have been crushed in the break as leg section of table was raised at conclusion of the operation.

Legs are usually wrapped in elastic bandages prior to operation. Blood pools in lumbar region of the torso, especially during prolonged operation. Legs must be lowered *slowly* when removed simultaneously from stirrups to prevent hypotension as blood reenters legs and leaves torso. Position change places an added burden on the heart and circulation. Raise leg section of table and replace lower section of the mattress. As they are lifted from stirrups, legs are fully extended to avoid wide abduction of thighs.

Prone Position

See Figure 15-6. Patient is usually anesthetized and endotracheal tube inserted in supine position. When anesthesiologist gives permission, patient is slowly and cautiously turned onto abdomen by body rotation as a log. Shoulder rolls or bolsters under axillae and along sides of the chest raise weight of body from abdomen and thorax, facilitating respiration, although the position reduces vital capacity. Arms may be placed on armboards, lie supported along sides of the body, or raised above head. Head is turned to the side. A pillow under ankles and feet prevents pressure on toes. Safety belt is placed below knees. This position is used for procedures on the posterior chest, trunk, legs, and sometimes the rectal area.

Modified Prone Position For operation on the spine, mattress is adjusted on table so hips are

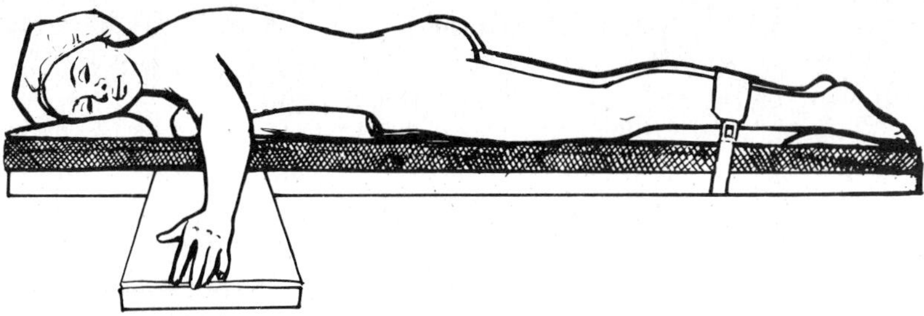

FIGURE 15-6
Prone position. Patient lies on abdomen. Note shoulder rolls under axillae and sides of chest to raise body weight from the chest to facilitate respiration, and pillow under feet to protect toes. Patient is anesthetized in supine position before turning into prone position.

over break between body and leg sections. A large, soft pillow is placed under the abdomen. Upper break of table is flexed, and table tilted so operative area is horizontal.

Prone Position on an Adjustable Arch Patient is lifted and an adjustable arch is placed under him or her with the affected part of spine at highest point of the arch. This point can be lowered or raised as desired by means of a lever. Arms are on armboards with elbows slightly flexed to prevent overextension. Head is placed in a padded headrest or supported by a roll of a cotton blanket. If electrosurgical unit ground plate is placed beneath a thigh, the scrotum may require padding for protection. A pillow protects feet and toes; bolsters protect chest and abdomen. Entire table is tilted so that operative area is horizontal. Safety belt is below knees. Some surgeons prefer a special assembly for the orthopaedic table for laminectomy rather than the adjustable arch.

Prone Position with Headrest For neurosurgical procedures, head rests in a cranial headrest exposing occiput and cervical vertebrae. Safety belt is below knees. When patient's head is in prone position or face down on a cerebellar headrest, the head should be raised from time to time to prevent pressure necrosis of cheeks and forehead. Eyes must be protected also. Prior to turning patient onto headrest, ophthalmic ointment is applied to protect the corneas and to keep lids closed. Ears also must be protected with foam support.

Kraske (Jackknife) Position

See Figure 15-7. Patient is usually supine until anesthetized, then turned onto abdomen by rotation with hips over center break of table between body and leg sections. Shoulder rolls or bolsters are placed to raise chest. Feet and toes are protected by a pillow. Head is to the side, with arms resting on armboards. Safety belt is placed below

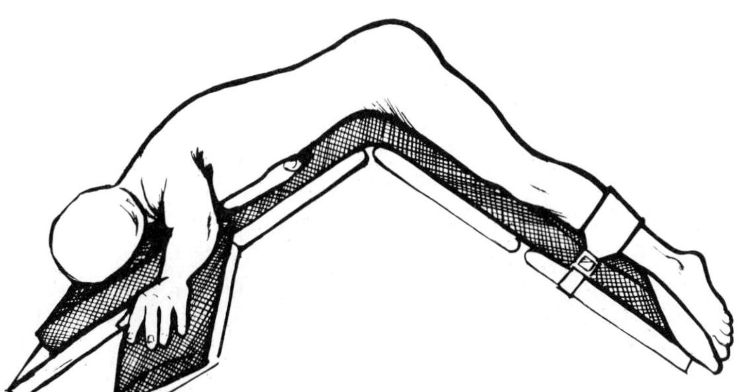

FIGURE 15-7
Kraske position. Hips are over central break in table and knee strap is below the knees. Note shoulder rolls in place and pillow under feet.

knees. Leg section of table is lowered desired amount, usually about 90°, and the entire table tilted head downward so that hips are elevated above rest of the body. Patient must be well balanced on table. For procedures in rectal area such as pilonidal sinus or hemorrhoidectomy, buttocks are retracted with hemorrhoid straps. Because of the dependent position, venous pooling occurs cephalad (toward head) and caudad (toward feet). It is very important to return patient slowly to horizontal from this unnatural position.

Knee-Chest Position

An extension is attached to foot section. Table is flexed at center break. Lower section is broken until it is at a right angle to table. Patient kneels on lower section and the entire table is tilted cephalad to elevate pelvis. Knees are thus flexed at a right angle to the body. Upper portion of table may be raised slightly to support head, which is turned to the side. Arms are placed around head with elbows flexed, with a large soft pillow beneath. Chest rests on the table. Safety belt is above knees. The table is tilted head downward so the hips are at highest point—modified jackknife. This position is used for sigmoidoscopy or culdoscopy.

Sim's Position

A modified lateral position, the patient lies on left side with upper leg flexed at hip and knee. The lower leg is straight. The under arm is extended along patient's back with weight of chest on the table. The upper arm rests in a flexed position on table. This position may be preferred for endoscopic examination performed via anus on obese or geriatric patient.

Lateral Kidney Position

See Figure 15-8. Patient is usually anesthetized in supine position, then turned to the unaffected side with back near the table edge. Kidney area is over the elevator. Arms may be placed on a padded double armboard. Knee on the unaffected side is flexed to aid in stabilization; the upper leg is straight. A large soft pillow is placed lengthwise between legs to prevent undue pressure on peroneal nerve and circulatory complications. A short kidney rest is attached to table at the patient's back. A long kidney rest is placed in front of the patient. Both must be well-padded. In an obese patient, folds of abdominal tissue may extend over end of the rest and be bruised if caution is not taken. Head should be in cervical alignment with spine. It should be supported on a small pillow between shoulder and neck to prevent stretching neck and brachial plexus. Table is flexed so kidney elevator can be raised desired amount to increase space between lower ribs and iliac crest. A kidney (body) strap is placed over the hip to stabilize patient. The safety belt is placed over legs. The entire table is tilted slightly downward toward head until operative area is horizontal. Upper shoulder, hip, and ankle should be in a straight line. Ankles and feet should be supported from pressure and foot drop. A pillow may be used to support chest and protect breasts. A chest roll may be placed to take body weight off deltoid muscle in the shoulder. Before closure, table is straightened for better approximation of tissues.

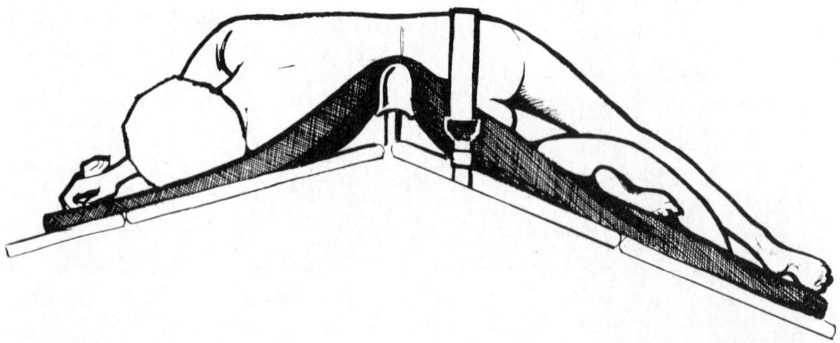

FIGURE 15-8
Right kidney position. Patient is in a lateral position with kidney region over table break. Note kidney strap across hip to stabilize body, raised kidney elevator for hyperextending operative area, and pillow between legs. Patient's side is horizontal from shoulder to hip.

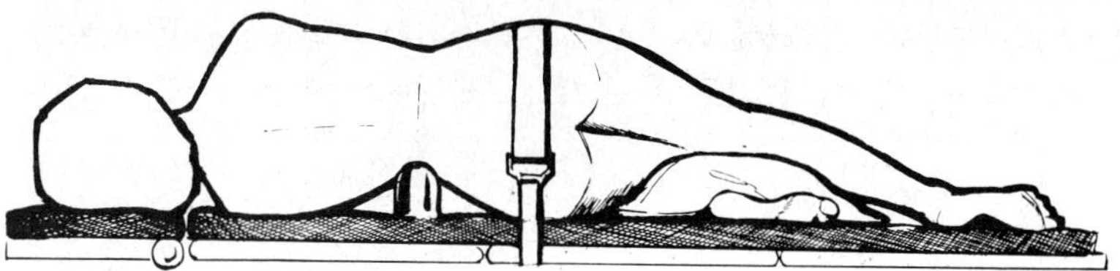

FIGURE 15-9
Right lateral position. Note strap across hip and body rest to stabilize body. Pillow between legs relieves pressure.

Used for procedures on the kidney and ureter, the position contributes to physiologic alterations and is not well tolerated. Blood tends to pool in lower arm and leg. Circulation is further compromised because of increased pressure on abdominal vessels when the kidney elevator is raised. Respiration is affected as well since gas exchange ratios in the lungs differ. Because of gravity, the lower lung receives more blood from right heart, is better perfused, has less residual air because of body weight, and is therefore more effective than the higher lung. Controlled respiration is helpful.

Lateral Chest Position

See Figure 15-9. Modifications of lateral position are used for unilateral transthoracic procedures with lateral approach. Patient is anesthetized supine, then turned onto unaffected side with back drawn to the table edge. Lower leg is flexed, upper leg straight, with a large soft pillow between them. Additional stability is provided by placing a strap over hip. A second strap may be placed over shoulder unless it interferes with skin preparation. Safety belt is placed over legs. Arms are extended on a padded, double armboard with upper arm slightly flexed, thus stabilizing shoulders; or an armboard is used for lower arm while upper arm is brought forward and down over a pad to draw the scapula from the operative area. Position depends on site and length of the chest incision. Head may be on a small pillow. A small firm pillow or pad under the operative area relieves pressure on arm of the unaffected side, permitting free flow of intravenous fluids. It also assists in spreading intercostal space for better exposure. One body rest is placed at lumbar area, another at chest at axillary level. The latter must be well-padded so as not to bruise breasts. Sandbags or towel rolls may be used instead of body rests. A pad at lumbar area facilitates respiratory movements and adds support. Shoulders and hips should be level. Lowering head of the table slightly assists postural drainage during operation. This position is restricting to cardiorespiratory systems, especially if prolonged.

Anterior Chest Position

For thoracoabdominal procedures with anterior approach, the position is more supine than the lateral chest position. After patient is anesthetized, a small firm pillow is placed under shoulder and another under buttocks on the affected side. Knee on the affected side is flexed slightly, with a large soft pillow beneath it to relieve undue strain on abdominal muscles. Safety belt is above knees. Arm on unaffected side is supported at the side. Arm on the affected side is padded well and bandaged loosely to the anesthesia screen. It must not be hyperextended to avoid injury to the brachial plexus. Head of table is lowered slightly for postural drainage.

PATIENT AS AN INDIVIDUAL

The patient's individual needs must be met in positioning as in everything else. Anomalies and physical defects are accommodated. Avoidance of unnecessary exposure, whether patient is unconscious or conscious, is an essential consideration for all patients. The nurse should objectively observe patient's position, to see if it adheres to physiological principles, before skin preparation and draping.

The circulating nurse must document in the patient's record any limitations in range of motion preoperatively, condition of skin before and after operation, and position in which the patient was positioned during operation, including special equipment used.

CHAPTER **16**

PREPARATION OF THE OPERATIVE SITE AND DRAPING

PHYSICAL PREPARATION OF PATIENT PRIOR TO OPERATION

The type of operation to be performed, age and condition of patient, and preferences of surgeon will determine specific procedures to be carried out before the incision is made. Consideration must be given to control of urinary drainage, to skin antisepsis, and to establishment of a sterile field around the operative site.

URINARY TRACT CATHETERIZATION

The patient should void to empty urinary bladder just before transfer to the OR suite, unless an indwelling retention catheter is in place. If patient's bladder is not empty or surgeon wishes to prevent bladder distention during a long procedure or following operation, catheterization may be necessary after patient is anesthetized. A retention catheter may be inserted. This maintains bladder decompression to avoid trauma during a lower abdominal or pelvic operation, to permit accurate measurement of output during or following operation, or to facilitate output and healing after operation on genitourinary tract structures. Catheterization is performed before patient is positioned, except for a patient who will remain in lithotomy position.

Urinary tract infection can occur following catheterization from contamination or traumatism of structures. Sterile technique must be maintained during catheterization. A sterile, disposable catheterization tray is used, unless the patient is being prepared for an operation in the perineal or genital area. For these latter procedures, a sterile catheter and lubricant may be added to the skin preparation setup. For other operations, the perineal area should be scrubbed (wearing clean gloves) with an antiseptic agent to reduce normal microbial flora and remove gross contaminants prior to the catheterization procedure.

Urinary catheterization is a minor operative procedure requiring aseptic technique. Sterile gloves are worn to handle sterile catheter. Catheter size should be small enough to minimize trauma of urethra and prevent necrosis of meatus; usually a 14 French is inserted in an adult female, 16 to 18 French in an adult male.

If a Foley retention catheter is to be inserted, check integrity of balloon by inflating it with correct amount of sterile water or air prior to insertion. Balloon size may be 5 or 30 cc (5 cc is used most frequently); 10 ml of sterile water are needed to properly inflate a 5-cc balloon to compensate for volume required by the inflation channel. Most Foley catheters have a rubber valve over lumen to the inflation channel that can be penetrated by a plain Luer slip tip syringe. Some require a needle on the syringe to penetrate rubber cover over the lumen. Solution or air must be evacuated prior to insertion of catheter into urethra.

Hand used to spread labia or stabilize penis is considered contaminated and should not be used to handle catheter. Sponges used to cleanse labia minora or glans penis should be handled to avoid contaminating the gloved hand used to insert catheter. To facilitate insertion and minimize trauma, lubricate tip of catheter with a sterile antimicrobial lubricant. Urine will start to flow when catheter has passed into bladder. Drain bladder. Inflate balloon of a Foley catheter.

Attach catheter to a sterile closed-drainage system. Secure tubing to patient's leg with enough slack in it to prevent tension or pull on penis or urethra. Drainage tubing should be positioned to enhance downward flow, but must not fall below level of the collection container. Attention to the catheter and tubing must be paid during positioning of patient for operation to prevent compression or kinking of the tubing. If container must be raised above level of bladder during positioning, clamp or kink tubing until container can be lowered and secured under operating table to avoid contamination by retrograde, backward flow of urine.

SKIN PREPARATION OF PATIENT

Purpose of Patient's Skin Preparation

The purpose of skin preparation (usually called *prep*) is to render the operative site as free as possible from transient and resident microorganisms, dirt, and skin oil so the incision can be made through skin with minimal danger of infection from this source.

Preliminary Preparation of Patient's Skin

Mechanical Cleansing Bathing removes many microorganisms from skin. This action can be enhanced to progressively reduce microbial population with daily use of chlorhexidine skin cleanser, or a bar or liquid soap containing hexachlorophene. The bacteriostatic action is due to the cumulative deposits that dissolve in fatty acids of skin. Many surgeons advise their patients to use such a product at home for several days prior to admission for an elective operation.

Patients whose operations will be on the face, eye, ear, or neck are advised to shampoo their hair prior to admission as this may not be permitted for a few weeks postoperatively.

All patients should shower or be bathed after hospital admission as close to time of departure from unit to the OR suite as possible. The operative site and surrounding area should be thoroughly cleansed with a rapid-acting, skin-degerming, antiseptic agent. *History of allergies must be obtained before applying any chemical agent to a patient's skin.*

The patient's general skin condition must be observed. Abnormal skin irritation, infection, or abrasion on or near operative site might be a contraindication to operation and must be reported to surgeon.

Hair Removal Hair removal can injure skin. Breaks in skin surface afford an opportunity for entry and colonization of microorganisms, and are a potential source of infection. Removal of hair from skin surrounding the operative site may be necessary, however, to prevent wound from becoming contaminated by hair. Usually the surgeon is responsible for designating in the patient's preoperative orders the limits of skin area and how it is to be prepared. Also, the procedure book specifies anatomical areas that must be mechanically cleansed and hair removed for each type of operation (see Figs. 16-1 through 16-6).

The procedure is carried out by personnel, per hospital policy, either on the unit or in the OR suite as close to time of operation as possible. Because lighting at the patient's bedside may be inadequate, shaving may be more satisfactorily accomplished in the OR under the operating lights or in an isolated well-lighted preoperative holding area in the OR suite. In the latter areas, hair must be contained to prevent a potential source of contamination. The procedure can be done in a preoperative holding area only if privacy is assured. Skin preparation may be an embarrassing procedure for patient. Drape patient to expose area to be prepared, but avoid unnecessary exposure. Hair removal after patient is anesthetized avoids this emotional trauma.

Many patients, especially women and children, do not require any form of hair removal. If necessary, hair may be removed with electric clippers, by applying a depilatory cream, or by shaving with a razor. Clippers and depilatories can be used safely before patient arrives in the OR suite.

Depilatory Cream Hair removal by depilation offers the primary advantage of intact skin free from cuts. If patient is not sensitive to depilatories, a depilatory is a safer method of hair removal than shaving. After cream has remained on skin for required number of minutes, wipe it off. Hair is removed simultaneously. Rinse skin thoroughly.

Shave Prep Time elapse between preoperative shave and operation may increase risk of postoperative infection. Shaving should be performed as near time of incision as possible.

1 Wear gloves to prevent cross contamination even though this is a surgically clean procedure.

2 Wet shaving is preferable. Wash skin from incision site to periphery to raise a generous lather. Soaking hair four minutes in the lather allows keratin to absorb three to four times its weight in water. This makes hair softer and easier to remove. Loose hair rarely strays from a lather. If dry shaving is preferred, the sticky side of adhesive tape can be used to pick up loose hair.

3 Use a sharp, clean straight or safety razor blade. Blades are either discarded after each patient use or terminally sterilized. If disposable razors are not used, razors should be terminally sterilized also between uses.

4 Hold skin taut and shave by stroking in direction of hair growth.

5 Avoid making nicks and cuts in skin. Nicks made in the OR immediately prior to operation are considered clean wounds. However, nicks made the evening before may present themselves as infected wounds at time of operation.

Skin Degreasing The skin surface is composed of cornified epithelium with a coating of secretions that include perspiration, oils, and desquamated epithelium. These surface sebaceous lubricants are insoluble in water. Therefore, a skin degreaser, or fat solvent, may be used to enhance adhesion of ECG electrodes. It also may be used prior to skin prep to improve adhesion of self-adhering drapes (p. 314) or to prevent smudging of skin markings (p. 314). Isopropyl alcohol, acetone, and halogenated hydrocarbons (Freon) are effective fat solvents. A fat solvent emollient is incorporated into some antiseptic agents.

PATIENT'S SKIN PREP ON OPERATING TABLE

Area

After patient has been anesthetized and positioned on operating table, skin of the operative site and an extensive area surounding it is mechanically cleansed again with an antiseptic agent immediately prior to draping (see Figs. 16-1 through 16-6).

Setup

A sterile skin prep tray is opened on a small table. Some disposable trays include containers of a premeasured amount of antiseptic solution. Solution of choice must be added to others. If prepackaged trays are not used, a sterile table must be prepared with the following sterile items:

1 Two towels to define the upper and lower limits of area to be prepared.

2 Small basins for solutions—usually at least two.

3 Sponges—may be 4 by 8 in. (10 by 20 cm) for large areas: 4 by 4 (10 by 10) or 3 by 3 (7.5 by 7.5) for small areas. *These must not be confused with counted sponges on the instrument table.* Textured foam sponges may be preferred.

4 Cotton applicators as necessary.

Antiseptic Solutions

The infection control committee usually determines chemical agent(s) to be used in the OR for skin antisepsis. Maximum concentration of a germicidal chemical that can be used on skin and mucous membranes is limited by its toxicity for these tissues. The agent should have the following qualities:

1 It rapidly decreases microbial count.

2 It can be quickly applied and remains effective against microorganisms.

3 It can be safely used without skin irritation or sensitization.

4 It effectively remains active in presence of alcohol, organic matter, soap, or detergent.

Chlorhexidine Gluconate Chlorhexidine gluconate significantly reduces and maintains a reduction of microbial flora for at least four hours after mechanical cleansing with this agent. A tincture of 0.5% chlorhexidine gluconate in 70% isopropyl alcohol (Hibitane Tincture) is a broad-spectrum, rapid-acting, nontoxic, antimicrobial agent. Activity is not adversely affected by traces of soap, but it is reduced in presence of organic matter. Its activity increases at elevated temperature. It is available either tinted for color demarcation of skin area being prepped, or nontinted to prevent skin staining if surgeon needs to observe skin color.

Iodine and Iodophors A solution of 1 or 2% iodine in water or in 70% alcohol is an excellent broad-spectrum, rapid-acting, cidal antiseptic. However, potential hazard of skin irritations and burns have led to a decline in its use. After application, iodine should be allowed to dry and then rinsed off with 70% alcohol to reduce potential of burns.

Iodophors, an iodine complex combined with detergents, are excellent cleansing agents to remove debris from skin surfaces while slowly releasing 1% iodine to act effectively as a cidal antiseptic. These agents are relatively nontoxic and virtually nonirritating to skin or mucous membranes. The brown film left on skin clearly defines area of application. This should *not* be wiped off after application because the cidal activity is sustained by release of free iodine as agent dries and color fades from skin. To hasten drying of skin, alcohol may be painted on area without friction before a self-adhering drape is applied (refer to p. 314).

NOTE. Iodophors must *not* be used to prep skin of patients allergic to iodine, as, for example, iodine contained in shellfish.

Alcohols Isopropyl and ethyl alcohol are useful as antiseptic agents if surgeon prefers a colorless solution that permits observation of true skin color. Since alcohol coagulates protein, it is not applied to mucous membranes or used on an open wound. Isopropyl alcohol is a more effective fat solvent than ethyl alcohol. A 70% concentration is satisfactory for skin antisepsis.

Hexachlorophene Since this agent slowly develops a cumulative suppressive action only over a period of frequent routine use, 3% hexachlorophene should only be used as the final skin prep solution on patients who have washed for several days exclusively with soap products containing this agent. Hexachlorophene is neutralized by alcohol. It is relatively ineffective against gram-negative organisms and fungi.

Triclosan A solution of 1% triclosan is a broad-spectrum antimicrobial agent. It is blended with oils and lanolin in a mild detergent. Cumulative suppressive action develops slowly only with prolonged routine use.

Basic Prep Procedure for Clean Areas

1 Expose skin area to be prepared by folding back cotton blanket and gown to 2 in. (5 cm) beyond limits of prep area. Double-check operative site.

NOTE. If operation is unilateral, be sure which is the affected side and expose the proper one. Consult chart and x-rays. Before amputation of an extremity, expose opposite one also for comparison. Check with surgeon.

2 Don sterile gloves.

3 Place sterile towels above and below area to be cleansed to mark limit of area and also to protect gloved hands from touching nonsterile blanket or gown. Also place sterile absorbent towels along each side of area to act as an absorber of runoff solution. These two towels are removed after prep is completed.

4 Wet sponge with antiseptic agent, but squeeze out excess solution.

NOTE. Solution should not run off skin area onto operating table to pool under patient. A patient lying in solution may develop skin irritation, even though the solution itself is nonirritating.

5 Scrub skin, starting at site of incision, with a circular motion in ever-widening circles to the periphery. Use enough pressure and friction to remove dirt and microorganisms from skin and pores. Effective skin antisepsis is achieved through a combination of mechanical and chemical action (see Fig. 16-1 for abdominal prep).

NOTE. Some surgeons prefer to have the antiseptic agent applied over cancerous areas by painting rather than scrubbing. During vigorous scrubbing, cancer cells may be freed, picked up by blood and lymph streams, and carried to other parts of body. To paint, secure a folded sponge in a sponge forceps, dip in solution, squeeze out excess solution, and apply to skin in circular motions from incision site to periphery.

6 Discard sponge after reaching periphery. *Never* bring a soiled sponge back toward center of area.

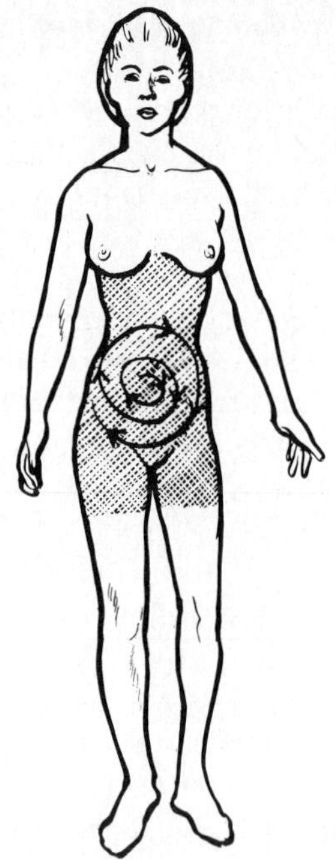

FIGURE 16-1
Abdominal preparation. The area includes breast line to upper third of thighs, from table line to table line, with patient in supine position. Shaded area shows anatomic area of hair removal. Arrows within area show direction of motion for skin preparation on operating table.

7 Repeat scrub with a separate sponge for each round. Scrub for a minimum of five minutes and apply antiseptic agent according to manufacturer's recommendations.

Contaminated Areas within Operative Field

Umbilicus The abdomen contains an area, the umbilicus, which is considered a contaminated area in relation to the surface surrounding it, because it may harbor microorganisms in the detritus that often accumulates there. Solution may be squeezed into umbilicus to soften detritus while the remainder of abdomen is scrubbed. Or, the umbilicus may be cleansed first with separate sponges and applicators to avoid run off of dirty solution over cleansed skin area. Then the abdominal prep begins with new sponges at the line of incision, moving with circular motions to the periphery and including the umbilicus again each round as it is approached within the area. The umbilicus is thoroughly cleansed with cotton applicators as final step of the abdominal prep.

Stoma The external stoma (orifice) of a colostomy, ileostomy, etc., may be sealed off from the operative site with a self-adhering towel drape. If this is not possible, follow the same rule for use of sponges as for umbilicus; come back to that area last, or use a separate sponge each round for the contaminated area only. The opening of the stoma may be packed with a sponge while surrounding area is scrubbed.

Other Contaminated Areas Draining sinuses, skin ulcers, vagina, anus, etc., are considered contaminated areas also. In all these, follow general rule of scrubbing the most contaminated area last or with separate sponges.

Foreign Substances Adhesive, grease, tar, and similar foreign materials must be removed from skin before area is mechanically cleansed with an antiseptic agent. A nonirritating solvent, such as Freon, will cleanse the skin. The solvent must be nonflammable and nontoxic. However, do not allow solution to collect underneath patient.

Traumatic Wounds When preparing an area in which the skin is not intact due to traumatic injury, wound irrigation may be part of the skin preparation procedure. The wound may be packed or covered with sterile gauze while area around it is thoroughly scrubbed and shaved if necessary.

After changing gloves, the wound itself is cleansed and irrigated. Extent and type of injury will determine the appropriate procedure. Solutions irritating to a denuded area must not be used. Small areas may be irrigated with warm sterile solution, usually normal saline, in a bulb syringe. When a bulb syringe is used, care must be taken not to force debris and microorganisms deeper into wound. The wound is irrigated gently to dislodge debris and flush it out.

Copious amounts of warm sterile solutions may be needed to flush out a large wound. A bottle of warm sterile saline or Ringer's solution attached to intravenous tubing can be hung on a standard near area to be copiously irrigated. If area is on an extremity, a sterile irrigating pan with a wire screen fitted over the top is placed under extremity. During irrigation, solution runs from wound into pan. A piece of tubing connected to an outlet on the pan carries the irrigating solution into a kick bucket on the floor near the table.

It may be necessary to place dry towels or

sheets under patient if area has not been protected during irrigation. A moistureproof pad placed under the wound before irrigation will help channel solutions into a drainage pan.

Debridement of the wound (excision of all devitalized tissue) usually follows irrigation. The surgeon may wish to have sterile tissue forceps and scissors on preparation table for removal of nonviable tissue along with the irrigation.

Areas Prepared for Grafts

1 Separate setups are necessary for skin preparation of recipient and donor sites prior to skin, bone, or vascular grafting procedures.

2 The donor site is usually scrubbed first. The recipient site for skin grafts is usually more or less contaminated, e.g., following a burn or other traumatic injury. Items used in preparation of the recipient site must not be permitted to contaminate the donor site. Also, microorganisms on skin of donor site must not be transferred to a denuded recipient site.

3 The donor site for a skin graft should be scrubbed with a colorless antiseptic agent so the surgeon can properly evaluate the vascularity of the graft postoperatively.

Special Considerations in Specific Anatomic Areas

Eye

1 Eyebrows are never shaved or removed unless the surgeon deems this essential. Eyebrows do not grow back completely.

2 Eyelashes are trimmed, if ordered by the surgeon, with fine scissors coated with sterile petrolatum to catch the lashes.

3 Eyelids and periorbital areas are cleansed with a nonirritating antiseptic agent, commonly an aqueous iodophor, then rinsed with warm sterile water. The prep starts centrally and works to periphery, i.e., from center of lid to brow and cheek. Cleansing with hexachlorophene soap or triclosan detergent and sterile water is an alternative if patient is allergic to iodophor.

4 Conjunctival sac is flushed with a nontoxic agent, such as sterile normal saline, using a bulb syringe. Patient's head is turned slightly to operative side. Solution is contained with sponges or absorbent towel. Care must be taken to prevent prep solution from entering patient's eyes or ears.

Ears, Face, or Nose

1 Usually it is not possible to define the area with towels.

2 Protect eyes with a piece of sterile plastic sheeting. If patient is awake, ask that eyes be kept closed during the prep.

3 As much of surrounding area is included as is feasible and consistent with aseptic technique. Skin surfaces should be cleansed at least to the hair line.

4 Cotton applicators are used for cleansing the nostrils and external ear canals.

Neck

1 One sterile towel is folded under the edge of the blanket and gown, which are turned down almost to the nipple line.

2 The area includes the neck laterally to the table line and up to the mandible, tops of the shoulders, and chest almost to the nipple line.

3 For combined head and neck operations, include face to the eyes, shaved areas of the head, ears, posterior neck, and area over the shoulders.

Lateral Thoracoabdominal

1 Gown is removed. Blanket is turned down well below lower limit of area to be prepared. A towel is folded under edge of blanket.

2 Arm is held up during preparation.

3 Beginning at site of incision, area may include axilla, chest, and abdomen from the neck to crest of the ilium. For operations in the region of the kidney, it extends up to axilla and down to pubis. The area also extends beyond the midlines, anteriorly and posteriorly (see Fig. 16-2).

Chest and Breast

1 Anesthesiologist turns patient's face toward unaffected side.

2 One towel is folded under blanket edge, just above pubis. Another is placed on table under shoulder and side.

3 Arm on the affected side is held up by grasping hand and raising shoulder and axilla slightly from the table.

4 Area includes shoulder, upper arm down to the elbow, axilla, and chest wall to the table line

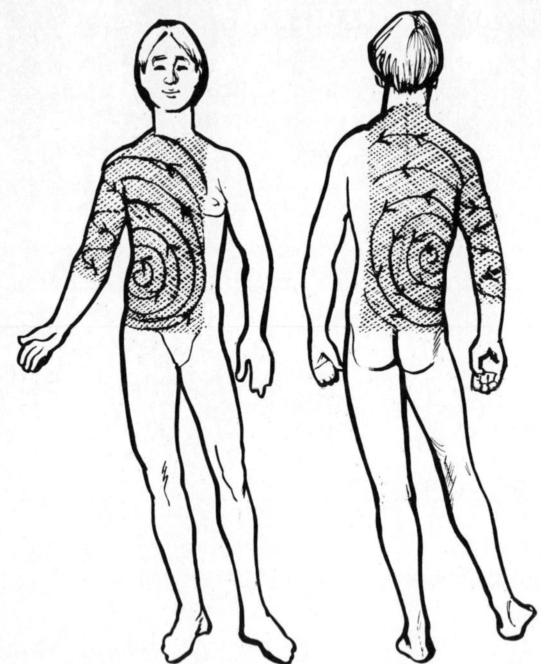

FIGURE 16-2
Lateral thoracoabdominal preparation. The area includes axilla, chest, and abdomen from neck to crest of the ilium. Area extends beyond the midline, anteriorly and posteriorly. Patient is in lateral position on operating table.

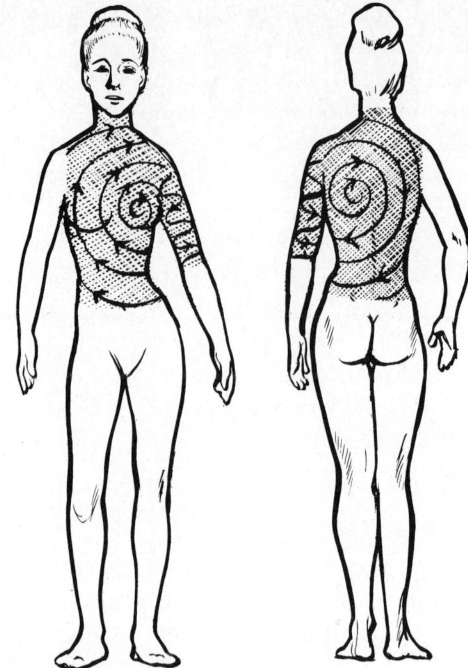

FIGURE 16-3
Chest and breast preparation. The area includes shoulder, upper arm down to elbow, axilla, and chest wall to the table line and beyond sternum to opposite shoulder. The patient may be in lateral position.

and beyond sternum to opposite shoulder (see Fig. 16-3).

Shoulder

1 Anesthesiologist turns patient's face toward opposite side.
2 Towel is placed under shoulder and axilla.
3 Arm is held up by grasping hand and elevating shoulder slightly from the table.
4 Area includes circumference of upper arm to below the elbow, from base of neck over the shoulder, scapula, and chest to midline.

Upper Arm

1 Towel is placed under shoulder and axilla.
2 Arm is held up by grasping hand and elevating shoulder slightly from the table.
3 Area includes entire circumference of arm to the wrist, axilla, and over the shoulder and scapula.

Elbow and Forearm

1 Towel is placed under shoulder and axilla.
2 Arm is held up by grasping hand.
3 Area includes entire arm from shoulder and axilla to and including the hand.

Hand

1 Towels are omitted. The anatomy of the hand furnishes sufficient landmarks to define the area, and towels are apt to slip over scrubbed area.
2 Arm must be held up by supporting it above elbow so entire circumference can be scrubbed.
3 Area includes hand and arm to 3 in. (7.5 cm) above elbow.

Rectoperineal

1 One towel is folded under edge of blanket above pubis. Another towel is placed under buttocks.

2 Area includes pubis, external genitalia, perineum and anus, and inner aspects of thighs (see Fig. 16-4).

3 Begin scrub over pubic area, scrubbing downward over genitalia and perineum. Discard sponge after going over anus.

4 Inner aspects of upper third of both thighs are scrubbed with separate sponges.

5 Rectoperineal area is prepped first, with patient in lithotomy position, followed by abdominal prep, with patient in supine position, for a combined abdominoperineal operation. Two separate prep trays are used.

Vagina

1 A sponge forceps must be included on the preparation table for a vaginal prep because a portion of prep is done internally. A disposable vaginal prep tray, with sponge sticks included, is available.

2 A moistureproof pad is placed under the buttocks and extends to kick bucket that receives solutions and discarded sponges.

3 Towel is folded under edge of blanket above pubis.

4 Area includes pubis, vulva, labia, perineum, anus, and adjacent area, including inner aspects of the upper third of thighs. *The vagina is prepped last* (see Fig. 16-4).

5 Begin over pubic area, scrubbing downward over vulva and perineum. Discard sponge after going over anus.

6 Inner aspects of the thighs are scrubbed with separate sponges from labia majora outward.

7 Vagina and cervix are cleansed with sponges on sponge forceps after external surrounding areas are scrubbed. The cleansing agent should be applied generously in the vagina because vaginal mucosa has many folds and crevices that are not easily cleansed.

8 After thoroughly cleansing vagina, wipe it out with a dry sponge to prevent possibility of fluid entering peritoneal cavity during operation on pelvic organs.

9 Catheterize, if indicated.

Hip

1 One towel is placed under thigh on the table. Another towel is placed on abdomen and folded under edge of gown, just above umbilicus.

2 Leg on affected side is held up by supporting it just below knee.

3 Area includes abdomen on the affected side, thigh to the knee, buttocks to table line, groin, and pubis (see Fig. 16-5).

Thigh

1 One towel is placed under thigh on the table. Another towel is placed on abdomen and folded under edge of gown, just below umbilicus.

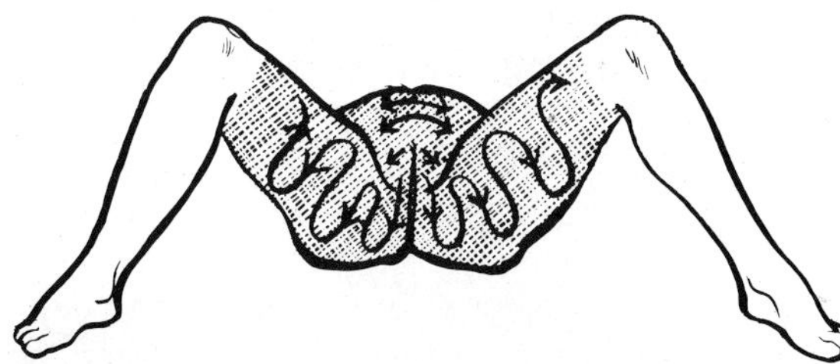

FIGURE 16-4
Rectoperineal and vaginal preparation. The area includes pubis, vulva, labia, perineum, anus, and adjacent areas, including inner aspects of upper third of thighs.

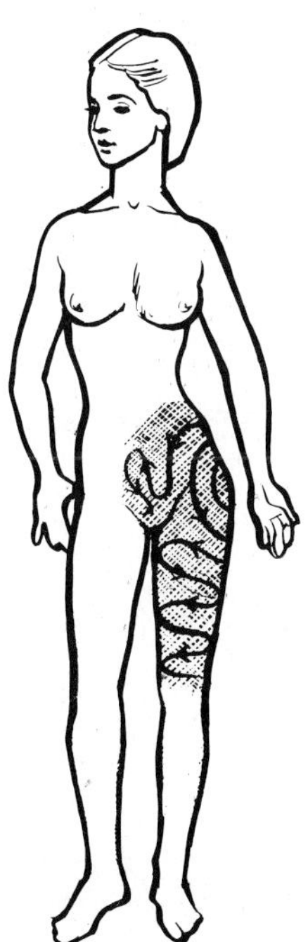

FIGURE 16-5
Hip preparation. The area includes the abdomen on the affected side, thigh to the knee, buttock to table line, groin, and pubis.

2 Leg is held up by supporting foot and ankle.

3 Area includes entire circumference of thigh and leg to the ankle, over hip and buttocks to the table line, groin, and pubis.

Knee and Lower Leg

1 Towel is placed over groin.

2 Leg is held up by supporting it at foot.

3 Area includes entire circumference of leg and extends from foot to upper part of thigh (see Fig. 16-6).

Ankle and Foot

1 Towels are omitted.

2 Foot is held up by supporting leg at knee. A leg-holder device is useful.

3 Area includes foot and entire circumference of lower leg to the knee.

NOTE. 1. A moistureproof pad should be placed on operating table under a lower extremity to retain drops of solution. This is removed after prep so table will be dry.

2. An extremity remains supported and elevated until sterile drapes are applied under and around prepped area.

3. A full extremity prep may be done in two stages to provide adequate support to joints and to assure that all areas are scrubbed. It may include the foot for hip, thigh, knee, and lower leg operations.

4. Caution must be taken to prevent solution from pooling under a tourniquet. If a tourniquet is used (refer to Chap. 17), it is positioned prior to prep. A towel tucked under the tourniquet cuff absorbs excess solution. This is removed before tourniquet is inflated.

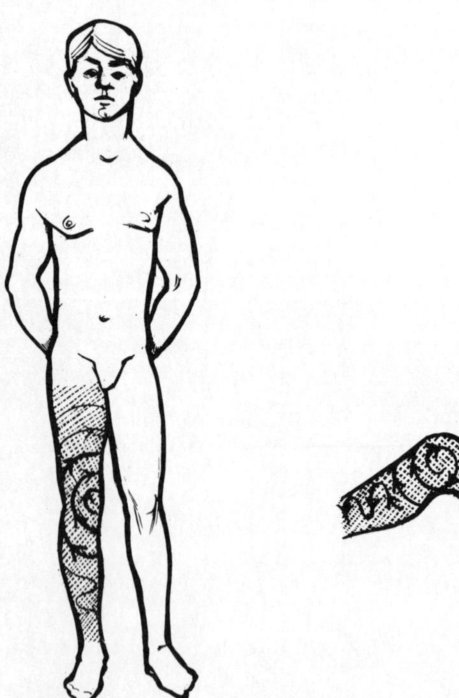

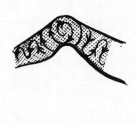

FIGURE 16-6
Knee and lower leg preparation. The area includes the entire circumference of affected leg and extends from foot to upper part of thigh.

Skin Marking

Some surgeons use a staining solution to mark the incision lines on the skin. This may be done before patient is prepped. If so, stain must withstand scrubbing without washing off. If skin is marked after prep, a sterile dye solution and applicator or sterile marking pen must be used. Methylene blue or alcoholic gentian violet are used for this purpose.

DRAPING

Draping is the procedure of covering patient and surrounding areas with a sterile barrier to create and maintain an adequate sterile field during operation. An effective barrier eliminates or minimizes passage of microorganisms between nonsterile and sterile areas. Criteria to be met in establishing an effective barrier are:

1 Blood and aqueous fluid-resistant to keep drapes dry and prevent migration of microorganisms.

2 Resistant to tear, puncture, or abrasion that causes fiber breakdown and thus permits microbial penetration.

3 Lint-free to reduce airborne contaminants or shed into the operative site. Cellulose and cotton fibers can cause granulomatous peritonitis or embolize arteries.

4 Antistatic to eliminate risk of a spark from static electricity. Material must meet standards of National Fire Protection Association.

5 Sufficiently porous to eliminate heat buildup so as to maintain isothermic environment appropriate for patient's body temperature.

6 Drapable to fit around contours of patient, furniture, and equipment.

7 Dull, nonglaring to minimize color distortion from reflected light.

8 Free of toxic ingredients, such as laundry residues, and nonfast dyes.

Draping Materials

Self-Adhering Plastic Sheeting Sterile, waterproof, antistatic, plastic sheeting may be applied to dry skin. It is available in various sizes as:

An Incise Drape The entire drape has an adhesive backing that is applied to skin. This may be applied separately or the sheeting may be incorporated into drape sheet. The skin incision is made through the plastic. An antimicrobial polymeric film is available that is coated with an iodophor-containing adhesive that slowly releases active iodine during operation to effectively inhibit proliferation of organisms from patient's skin.

A Towel Drape The plastic sheeting has a band of adhesive along one edge. Used as a draping towel, it will remain fixed on skin without towel clips. This is advantageous when clips might obscure view of a part exposed to x-rays during operation. It also is used to wall off a contaminated area, such as a stoma, from the clean skin area to prevent spilling contents and causing infection or chemical irritation.

An Aperture Drape Adhesive surrounds a fenestration (opening) in the plastic sheeting. This secures drape to skin around operative site, such as an eye or ear.

> NOTE. Caution must be used in applying this type of drape around face of patient who is awake. Be sure patient has breathing space. Some patients experience claustrophobia. Drape towels, which do not feel as confining, are used for them.

Advantages of a self-adhering plastic drape:

1 Resident microbial flora from skin pores, sebaceous glands, and hair follicles cannot migrate laterally to the incision.

2 Microorganisms do not penetrate through impermeable material.

3 Landmarks and skin tones are visible through transparent plastic.

4 Inert adhesive holds drapes securely, eliminating need for towel clips and possible puncture of patient's skin.

A nonporous material, such as plastic sheeting, should not cover more than ten percent of the body surface as it may interfere with patient's thermal regulatory mechanism of perspiration evaporation. The heat-retaining property of plastic causes the patient to perspire excessively, but its nonporous nature prevents evaporation. The material is used in the following manner:

1 Usual skin preparation is done.

2 Scrubbed area must be dried. It may dry by evaporation, or excess solution may be blotted or wiped off with a sterile sponge or towel.

> NOTE. Alcohol may be applied after an iodophor scrub to hasten drying by evaporation. Alcohol will neutralize hexachlorophene. Ether, a highly flammable agent, is not recommended for skin preparation. A combination of alcohol and Freon can produce chemical irritation on skin.

3 Transparent plastic material is firmly applied to skin with initial contact along proposed line of incision. Smooth drape away from incision area.

4 Regular fabric drapes are applied over the plastic sheeting, unless plastic is incorporated into fenestrated area of drape.

Nonwoven Fabric Drapes Often referred to as *paper* drapes, nonwoven disposable materials are compressed layers of synthetic fibers, i.e., rayon, nylon, or polyester, combined with cellulose and held together chemically or mechanically without knitting, tufting, or weaving. Material may be either nonabsorbent or absorbent. Those fabrics that comply with criteria for establishing an effective barrier have the following *advantages as disposable drapes:*

1 Moisture repellancy retards blood and aqueous fluid moisture strike-through to prevent contamination.

> NOTE. Not all nonwoven fabrics have this characteristic: only nonabsorbent materials or those laminated with plastic are impermeable to moisture.

2 Lightweight, yet strong enough to resist tears.

3 Lint-free.

4 Contaminants are disposed of along with drapes.

5 Antistatic and flame-retardant for OR use.

6 Prepackaged and sterilized by manufacturer. This eliminates washing, mending, folding, and sterilizing processes.

Some drapes have a reinforced area, roughly 2 ft

(61 cm) wide, surrounding the fenestration that contains a layer impermeable to strike-through. Other drapes are completely laminated with a plastic layer. Although lamination of nonwoven materials with a plastic layer provides a complete microbial barrier, some laminated materials can only be used for instrument table covers, but not over the entire body of the patient because of their heat-retention property.

Woven Textile Fabrics The weight and thread count of woven natural fibers determine integrity and porosity of fabric. Double-thickness, 140-thread-count muslin, as used for wrappers, is permeable to steam under pressure for sterilization. However, if used for drapes, once wet by blood or aqueous fluids even four thicknesses of muslin are ineffective as a barrier to the migration of microorganisms because of the wicking action of absorbent fibers.

Tightly woven, reusable textile fabrics are less absorbent so may inhibit migration of microorganisms. Cotton fibers swell when they become wet. This swelling action closes pores or interstices so that liquid cannot diffuse through tightly woven fibers. Tightly woven cotton cloth can be treated to repel fluids and be impermeable to moisture strike-through, for example, 270-thread count Pima cotton with a Quarpel finish. However, these fabrics have essentially the same heat-retaining qualities as plastic lamination and cannot be used for complete patient draping. The material can be used as reinforcement around fenestrations, openings, in drapes.

Points concerning textile drapes:

1 When packaged for sterilization, drapes must be properly folded and arranged in sequence of use. Drapes may be fanfolded or rolled.

2 All material must be steam-permeable.

3 Material must be free from holes and tears. It is responsibility of person who folds drape to see that it is free from holes. Those detected may be covered with heat-seal patches. Occasionally holes may not be detected until drape is laid down. A hole must be covered with another piece of linen or the entire drape discarded.

4 Drapes should be sufficiently thick to prevent moisture from soaking through them, or a plastic waterproof drape should first be placed over the operative area and the drapes placed over it.

5 Densely woven cotton treated with waterproofing will become permeable after 75 to 100 launderings. Number of uses, washings, and sterilizing cycles should be recorded, and drapes that are no longer effective as barriers should be taken out of use.

Style (Type) of Drapes

Towels May be used to outline operative site. The folded edge of each towel is placed toward line of incision. When packaging reusable linen, four towels intended for this purpose can be placed together with folded edges graduated. Nonabsorbent disposable towels are used for this technique. Towels are secured with towel clips.

Laparotomy Sheet Often called a *lap* sheet. At least 108 by 72 in. (274 by 183 cm), it has a longitudinal fenestration that is placed over the operative site on abdomen, back, or a comparable area. The opening, about 40 in. (102 cm) from the top in center of sheet, is 9 by 4 in. (23 by 10 cm), which is large enough to give adequate exposure in the usual laparotomy. A 24-in. (60-cm) reinforcement around the opening provides an extra thickness. The sheet is long enough to cover the anesthesia screen at the head and extend down over the foot of table. It is wide enough to cover one or two armboards. The sheet is unfolded toward feet first.

NOTE. Fenestrated sheets are usually marked to indicate the direction in which they should be unfolded. This may be an arrow or label designating *Top* or *Head, Bottom* or *Foot.*

Thyroid Sheet The same size as a laparotomy sheet. The fenestration is transverse and closer to top of the sheet.

Breast Sheet The same as a laparotomy sheet except the fenestration is 11 by 11 in. (28 by 28 cm), which provides for a larger exposure. Besides its use for breast procedures, it is used for operations within chest cavity.

Kidney Sheet The same size as a laparotomy sheet. The fenestration is transverse to accommodate a transverse kidney incision.

Hip Sheet The same as a laparotomy sheet except that it is somewhat longer to completely cover the orthopaedic fracture table.

Split Sheet The same size as a laparotomy sheet. Rather than fenestrated, one end is cut longitudinally up the middle at least one-third the length of sheet to form two free ends (tails). The upper end of this split may be U-shaped. Bands may be sewn on each tail approximately 8 in. (20 cm) from end of split to snug sheet around an extremity or head.

Perineal Sheet A sheet of adequate size to create sterile field with the patient in lithotomy position. It has large boots incorporated into it to cover legs in stirrups. It contains an opening 6½ to 7 in. (17 cm) in diameter with a 10-in. (25-cm) reinforcement around it.

Combined Sheet A combination laparotomy and perineal sheet, used for combined abdominoperineal resection of the rectum when the entire procedure is done with the patient in lithotomy position. The rectum is removed before the abdomen is closed.

While many hospitals use them for most operations, fenestrated sheets are not always feasible. The openings may be much too large for small incisions, such as taking specimens for biopsies, operations on hands or feet, etc. Smaller, separate sheets may be used for these purposes, leaving exposed only the small operative area, or to provide underdrapes on the operative field.

Minor Sheet This sheet is 36 by 45 in. (91 by 114 cm). It has many uses. Wrapped around an extremity, it permits extremity to remain on sterile field for manipulation during operation. It is used under an arm to cover an armboard for shoulder, axillary, arm, or hand operations.

Medium Sheet About 36 by 72 in. (91 by 183 cm). It is used to drape under legs, as an added protection above or below the operative area, or for draping areas in which a fenestrated sheet cannot be used.

Single Sheet This sheet is 108 by 72 in. (274 by 183 cm). Folded lengthwise, it is placed above the operative field to shield off anesthesiologist and anesthesia machine or other equipment near the patient's head or operating table.

Stockinet May be used to cover an extremity. This seamless tubing of stretchable material contours snugly to skin. An opening is cut through it over the line of incision. Material may be secured with a plastic incise drape before incision is made, or it may be clipped to wound edges after incision.

Techniques to Remember in Draping

Since draping is a very important step in preparation of patient for operation, it must be done correctly. The entire team should be familiar with the draping procedure. The scrub nurse must know it perfectly and be ready to assist with it. Check beforehand to see that necessary articles are arranged in proper sequence on instrument table.

Person responsible for draping patient may vary, as do materials and styles of drapes used to create a sterile field. The surgeon or assistant usually places self-adhering drape and/or towels and towel clips to outline site of incision. The scrub nurse assists with placing remainder of drapes.

During any draping procedure, the circulating nurse should stand by to direct scrub nurse as necessary and to watch carefully for breaks in technique. A contaminated drape or exposure of a nonsterile area might well be source of an infection for the patient.

1 Place drapes on a dry area. Area around or under patient may become damp from solutions used for skin preparation. The circulating nurse must remove damp items or cover area to provide a dry field on which to lay sterile drapes.

2 Allow sufficient time to permit careful application.

3 Allow sufficient space to observe sterile technique.

4 Handle the drapes as little as possible.

5 Never reach across the operating table to drape opposite side; go around table.

6 Take towels and towel clips, if used, to side of table from which surgeon is going to apply them before handing them to him or her.

7 Carry *folded drapes* to operating table. Watch front of sterile gown; it may bulge and touch the nonsterile table or blanket on patient. Stand well back from the nonsterile table.

8 Hold drapes high enough to avoid touching nonsterile areas, but avoid touching overhead operating light.

9 Hold drape high until it is directly over proper area, then lay it down where it is to remain. Once a sheet is placed, do not adjust it. Be careful not to slide sheet out of place when opening folds. If a drape is incorrectly placed, discard it. The circulating nurse peels it from table without contaminating other drapes or operative site.

10 Protect gloved hands by cuffing end of sheet over them. Do not let gloved hands touch skin of patient.

11 In unfolding a sheet from the operative site toward foot or head of the table, protect gloved hand by enclosing it in turned-back cuff of sheet provided for this purpose. Keep hands at table level.

12 If a drape becomes contaminated, do not handle it further. Discard it without contaminating gloves or other items.

13 If end of a sheet falls below waist level, do not handle it further. Drop it and use another.

14 If in doubt as to its sterility, consider a drape contaminated.

15 A towel clip that has been fastened through a drape has its points contaminated. Remove it only if absolutely necessary, then discard it from sterile setup without touching points. Cover area from which it was removed with another piece of sterile draping material.

16 If a hole is found in a drape after it is laid down, the hole must be covered with another piece of draping material or the entire drape discarded.

17 A hair found on a drape must be removed and area covered immediately. Although hair can be sterilized, the source of a hair is usually unknown when found on a sterile drape. It would cause foreign-body tissue reaction in patient if it got into wound. Remove hair with a hemostat and hand instrument off sterile field; cover area with a towel or another piece of draping material.

Procedures for Draping Patient

Draping procedures may vary from one hospital to another. However, standardized methods of application should be practiced using adequate draping materials for each operation. The most common procedures are discussed here merely to elaborate the principles. The following details procedures using only *absorbent* draping materials because it is more complex to establish a microbial barrier with them. The draping procedure is simplified when single-thickness, impermeable materials are used. Consult procedure book for specific draping procedures.

Laparotomy The term *laparotomy* refers to an incision through abdominal wall into abdominal cavity. All flat, smooth areas are draped in the same manner as the abdomen. These areas include neck, chest, flank, and back.

1 Hand up four towels and towel clips. With practice these can be held in hands at the same time and separated one by one as the surgeon takes them. Go to side of table on which surgeon is draping to avoid reaching over nonsterile table. The surgeon places these towels within scrubbed area, leaving only enough skin exposed for the incision.

2 Hand one end of fanfolded medium sheet across table to assistant, supporting the folds, keeping it high, and holding it taut until it is opened; then lay it down. Place this medium sheet below site of incision with edge of it at the skin edge, covering the draping towel. This sheet provides an extra thickness of material under area from Mayo stand to incision, where instruments and sponges are placed, and closes some of opening in the laparotomy sheet if necessary. This sheet may be eliminated if a self-adhering incise drape is used, or impermeable drapes are used.

3 Place laparotomy sheet with opening directly over skin area outlined by the towels in direction indicated for the foot or head of the table. Drop folds over sides of table. However, if an armboard is in place, hold folds at table level until the sheet is opened all the way. Open it downward over patient's feet and upward over anesthesia screen (see Figs. 16-7 and 16-8).

NOTE. Sheets with appropriate fenestrations are used to expose the operative site.

1. For neck, use a thyroid sheet.

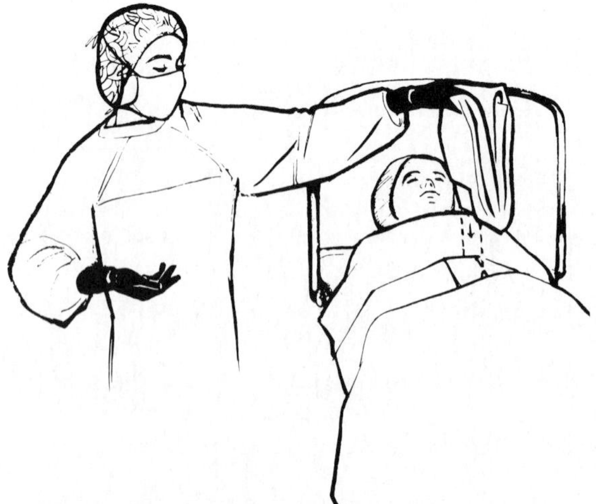

FIGURE 16-7
Draping with a sterile laparotomy sheet. Scrub nurse carries folded sheet to table. Standing far back from table, with one hand lay sheet on patient so opening in sheet is directly over prepared skin area.

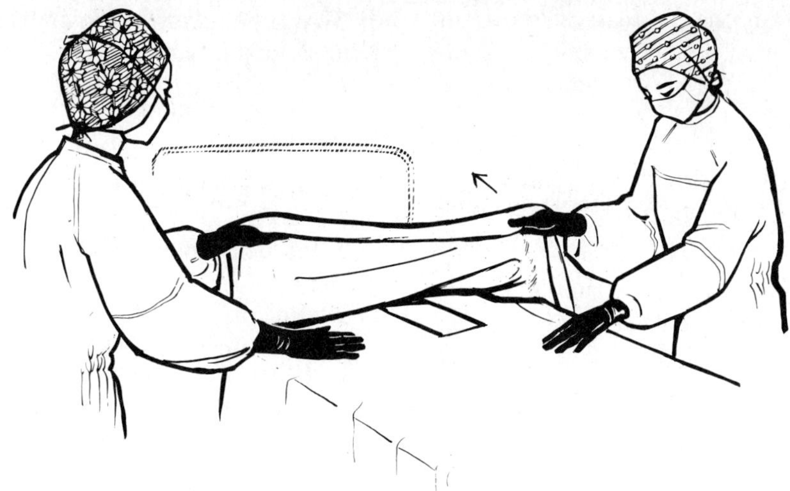

FIGURE 16-8
Unfolding upper end of laparotomy sheet over anesthesia screen. Note that hands approaching unsterile area are protected in a cuff of the drape and the sheet is stabilized with other hands.

2. For chest, with patient in either supine or lateral position, use a breast sheet.

3. For flank, with patient in kidney position for transverse incision, use a kidney sheet.

4. For back, use a laparotomy sheet the same as for the abdomen.

4 Place large, single sheet crosswise of the table above operating area. This sheet provides extra thickness above area and closes some of opening in the laparotomy sheet if necessary. It also covers the armboard if one is in use. A single sheet may be needed for this latter purpose even if an impermeable lap sheet is used.

Head An overhead instrument table may be positioned over patient. The table drape is extended down over patient's shoulders to create a continuous sterile field between instrument table and operative site.

1 Surgeon places four towels around head and secures them with towel clips or sews them in place. Towel clips are not used if x-rays will be taken during operation.

2 Hand one end of a fanfolded medium sheet to assistant. Holding it taut, unfold and secure it over the head end of operating table below operative area at skin edge of the draping towel.

3 Place a fenestrated sheet with opening over exposed skin area of the head. Unfold sheet across front edge of overhead table and secure it before allowing remainder of drape to drop over head of the operating table toward the floor.

NOTE. If a split sheet is used, the tails are placed toward head end of the operating table, draped around patient's head, and secured with towel clips.

Face Even if operation is unilateral, surgeon may want the entire face exposed for comparison of skin lines.

1 Surgeon places a drape under head while circulating nurse holds up the head. This drape consists of a towel placed on a medium sheet. Center of towel edge is 2 in. (5 cm) in from center of sheet edge. The towel is drawn up on each side of face, over forehead or at hairline, and fastened with a clip. This leaves the desired amount of the face exposed.

2 Hand up three more towels and four towel clips. These four towels surround operative site.

3 Place a medium sheet just below site. This sheet must overlap the one under the head.

4 A fenestrated drape may be placed to complete draping.

5 Cover remainder of foot of table, as necessary, with a single sheet.

NOTE. 1. If patient is receiving inhalation anesthesia, use a minor sheet instead of a towel on a medium sheet for first drape under head. A minor sheet is large enough to draw up on each side of face and to enclose tubes from the anesthesia machine for a considerable distance, thus keeping them from contaminating the sterile field.

2. If operation on face is unilateral, the anesthesiologist may sit at unaffected side, near patient's head, with an anesthesia screen placed on this side of table.

Eye After skin prep, protect unoperative eye by covering it with sterile eye pad before draping patient.

1 Surgeon places two towels and medium sheet under head while circulating nurse holds head up, as described for face drape. One towel is drawn up around head, exposing only the eyebrow and operative eye, and fastened with a clip without pressure on eyes.

2 Hand up four towels and towel clips to isolate operative site. Some surgeons prefer a self-adhering aperture drape.

3 Cover patient and remainder of table below operative site with a single sheet.

NOTE. 1. If local anesthesia will be administered, drapes must be raised off patient's nose and mouth to permit free breathing. A Mayo stand or anesthesia screen positioned over the lower face before draping will elevate drapes. Oxygen, 6 to 8 liters per minute, can be supplied under drapes by tube or nostril prongs.

2. For microsurgical operation, a sterile U-shaped steel wrist rest for surgeon and assistant is fastened to head of table after towels are put around patient's head, before rest of draping is completed.

3. If irrigation will be used, a plastic fenestrated drape is placed over the four towels to keep them dry if an aperture drape is not preferred.

Ear Basic procedure is same as draping patient for a face or eye operation, except that only ear is exposed. Head will be turned toward unaffected side. Oxygen can be supplied under drapes, as described in Note above.

Chest and Breast While arm is still being held up following skin preparation:

1 Place a minor sheet on armboard, under patient's arm, extending sheet under side of chest and shoulder. The person who has been holding arm lays it on armboard and fastens it with a wrist strap.

2 Hand up towels and towel clips; five or six are required.

3 Apply breast sheet so axilla is exposed for anticipated axillary dissection.

Shoulder While arm is still being held up following skin preparation:

1 Place a medium sheet over chest and under arm.

2 Place a minor sheet under shoulder and side of chest.

3 Surgeon outlines site of operation with towels and secures them with clips.

4 Place a minor sheet over patient's chest, covering neck. Keep this sheet even with edge of towel that limits the operative site laterally.

5 Wrap arm in a minor sheet and secure it with a sterile gauze bandage. At this point, a sterile member of team relieves person who has been holding arm.

6 Place a medium sheet above the area and secure these sheets together with towel clips.

7 A laparotomy or a breast sheet may be used. Pull arm through the opening. Or, a single sheet may be placed above area and foot of table covered with a medium sheet.

Elbow While arm is still being held up following skin preparation:

1 Place a medium sheet across chest and under arm, up to axilla.

2 Surgeon limits operative area on upper arm by placing a towel around arm and securing it with a clip.

3 Wrap hand and lower arm in a minor sheet or a double thickness of towels and secure with a sterile bandage. At this point, a sterile member of team relieves person who has been holding arm.

4 Draw stockinet over exposed operative area.

5 Place a medium sheet across chest, on top of arm, even with towel on upper arm and covering it. Secure this sheet around arm with a towel clip.

6 Lay laparotomy sheet over hand and pull arm through it, opening sheet across patient. Cover foot of table with medium sheet.

Hand While arm and hand are still being held up following skin preparation:

1 Place a minor sheet, folded in half, on armboard.

2 Surgeon places a towel around lower arm, to limit area of the site of operation, and secures it with a towel clip.

3 Pull stockinet over hand. At this stage in

draping, the nonsterile person is relieved of holding arm. The arm is laid on armboard.

4 Place a minor sheet across armboard just above operative site.

5 Place laparotomy sheet on hand with foot end toward patient. Do not drop folds *below* level of armboard. Open lap sheet across patient's body.

6 Place a medium sheet below laparotomy sheet to finish covering patient.

7 Place a single sheet over anesthesia screen.

Perineum With patient in lithotomy position:

1 Scrub nurse hangs a towel, folded in half, over a strip of 1-in. (2.5-cm) adhesive tape held by circulating nurse, if a sterile plastic towel drape is not used. Circulating nurse places this towel over the anus and fastens adhesive around patient's buttocks, if operation is vaginal or genital.

2 Hand up three towels and four towel clips.

3 Apply perineal sheet by handing one end of it to assistant, opening out folds, and drawing boots onto feet and legs. Keep hands on outside of the sheet to avoid contaminating gloves and gown.

Hip If leg will be manipulated during operation, while leg is still being held up following skin preparation:

1 Place a medium sheet on table under leg, up to the buttock.

2 Place another medium sheet on table, overlapping first one, to cover unaffected leg.

3 Surgeon wraps a towel around thigh, just below operative area, and clips it or sews it in place if x-rays will be taken.

4 Hand up additional towels to surround operative area, with towel clips to secure them.

5 Surgeon wraps foot and leg, including towel around thigh, in a minor sheet and bandages it on. The leg, held up to this point, is laid on table.

6 Place a minor sheet lengthwise of table on each side of operative site, even with the skin. Sheets under leg and above site do not overlap.

NOTE. Some surgeons prefer to omit step 6 and draw leg through opening of a hip sheet or place a split sheet under leg with the tails crossed over it toward the patient's head.

7 Place a medium sheet above operative area. Secure these last three sheets with towel clips.

8 Place a single sheet above operative area and over anesthesia screen.

If manipulation of leg is not necessary during operation, drape the same as for a laparotomy, using a hip sheet instead of a laparotomy sheet.

Knee While leg is still being held up following skin preparation:

1 Place a medium sheet lengthwise on table, under leg, up to the buttock.

2 Place another medium sheet on table overlapping first sheet to cover unaffected leg.

3 Surgeon limits sterile field above knee by placing a towel around leg and securing it with a towel clip.

4 Lay a minor sheet on sterile sheets under leg. The person who has been holding leg lays it on this minor sheet. Surgeon wraps leg in minor sheet and secures it with a sterile bandage. Stockinet may be preferred for this step.

5 Place a medium sheet above operative area, at skin edge, over draping towel, and fasten it with a towel clip.

6 Place laparotomy sheet, with opening on foot and longer part of the sheet toward table head. Open it and draw leg through the opening. A split sheet may be used.

Lower Leg and Ankle While leg is still being held up following skin preparation:

1 Place a medium sheet under leg and over unaffected leg to above knees.

2 Surgeon limits sterile field by placing a towel around leg above area of intended incision and securing it with a towel clip.

3 Put stockinet over foot and draw it up over leg to above skin edge of the towel. The person who has been holding leg is relieved and leg is held by a sterile team member.

4 Place a medium sheet above operative area and secure around leg with a towel clip.

5 Place laparotomy sheet or split sheet with leg drawn through opening.

6 Cover remainder of table over the anesthesia screen with a single sheet as necessary.

Foot The general method of draping a foot is the same as that for hand. While foot is still being held up following skin preparation:

1 Place a medium sheet on table, under foot.

2 Surgeon limits operative area on foot by

placing a towel around ankle and securing it with a towel clip.

3 Enclose foot in stockinet. A sterile team member relieves person who has been holding leg.

4 Place a medium sheet above operative area, and secure it around ankle with a towel clip.

5 Place laparotomy sheet with opening over foot and longer part of the sheet toward head of the table.

Draping of Equipment

Equipment that is brought into the sterile field but cannot be sterilized must be draped before it is handled by sterile team members.

1 Tailored disposable drapes are available to cover the operating microscope so it can be manipulated in the sterile field by surgeon.

2 If x-ray films are to be taken during operation, a cassette holder may be placed on operating table, under patient, before patient is positioned, prepped, and draped. The circulating nurse raises the drape for radiology technician to place and remove the cassette. The holder and/or cassette may be covered with a sterile Mayo stand cover or specially designed disposable cover and placed on sterile drapes when a lateral view is needed.

3 Cords, attachments, or tubings that are not sterile must be inserted into sterile coverings before they are placed on sterile field.

Nonsterile equipment that must stand near the sterile field must be excluded from sterile area by a drape shield. IV poles frequently are used to attach drapes to shield off power-generating sources of mechanical and electrical equipment, such as electrosurgical and cryosurgical units, fiberoptic lighting units, air-powered or electrical instruments. The drape over patient or a separate single sheet is extended from operating table upward in front of or over the nonsterile equipment. The circulating nurse fastens drape to IV poles on each side of equipment that stands above level of sterile field or near it.

NOTE. Heat-generating equipment must have adequate ventilation to dissipate heat. Impermeable, heat-retaining materials cannot completely encase these units.

Some nonsterile equipment, of necessity, will be moved over the sterile field. The sterile field must be protected.

1 Sterile disposable drapes are available to cover x-ray equipment, image intensifiers, etc.

2 When ready to move x-ray tube or image intensifier over sterile field, cover field with a minor sheet. Discard this sheet after use.

3 Photography and television cameras should be draped as much as feasible when used over the operative area.

PLASTIC ISOLATOR

A plastic isolator (shield around patient's bed or operating table) may be used to exclude microorganisms from the environment immediately surrounding the patient. It may isolate a patient who is highly susceptible to infection, such as a burned or immunosuppressed patient, or may isolate a patient with a gross infection as a protection for others. In the OR, plastic isolators are used to isolate operative field from both room air and OR team and thus exclude microorganisms normally in the operating room environment.

The portable, lightweight, optically transparent surgical isolator forms a bubble over patient when inflated. This surgical isolation bubble system (SIBS) has two elements: a filter/blower unit, and a prepackaged sterile, disposable bubble. Its floor provides a sterile drape that adheres to prepared skin around incision site. Built into the sides are ports (armholes) through which team works, and a port for passing sterile supplies from the circulating nurse.

A patient isolation drape may be used that is a modification of the total isolator. It isolates the sterile field from equipment, such as the C-arm image intensifier used for hip procedures. The drape is suspended from steel frame, but does not enclose the patient. The incise portion of drape may be impregnated with a time-release iodophor. Storage and irrigation pouches are incorporated into the side.

CHAPTER 17

WOUND HEALING AND METHODS OF HEMOSTASIS

HISTORY OF WOUND MANAGEMENT

From ancient times, warfare made necessary some means of controlling hemorrhage and closing wounds. It is probable that the first operation performed was surgery of trauma. Egyptian writings, dating back to 3000 B.C., tell of treatment of various injuries including all kinds of fractures. Tourniquets were used to control bleeding. Mummies have been exhumed that revealed wounds sewed together with sutures.

Early Hindu surgeons surpassed those of Egypt in their skill in treating fractures and other injuries and in performing plastic surgery. The Hindu military surgeons were responsible for the food and sanitary conditions of the army as well as for treating the wounded.

Arabian surgeons used harp strings for sutures. They were made from sheep's intestines, twisted, and sun-dried. Religious laws of the Mohammedans required caravan leaders to carry sutures and needles to take care of injuries. Sometimes camel hair was used for sutures.

Greek surgery is first mentioned by Homer in 1000 B.C. Wounds of battle were cleansed, hemorrhage was checked with crushed roots and leaves, and then covered with compresses.

Hemostasis, as practiced by early surgeons, combined styptics with pressure, bandages, and elevation of the part. Surgeons used materials at hand to cover the wound as a framework for the blood clot. Hare's fur, shredded bark of trees, egg yolk, dust, or cobwebs were bandaged on the bleeding part. The early lithotomists controlled bleeding by assigning an assistant to compress the ends of vessels between his fingers until bleeding stopped.

Hippocrates (460 to 377 B.C.) noted the analgesic action of cold as a therapeutic entity and used ice and snow to check hemorrhage. Although the effects of cold and the ligature were known to him, Hippocrates recommended hot irons to stop hemorrhage and his custom persisted for over 2000 years. He also wrote of insertion of a "hollow tin tube" with flushings of wine and tepid oil to treat empyema. This was the first wound drainage system. In his writings, he also stated that the best dressing for one side of a wound was the healthy tissue on the other side of the wound.

It was well known in early times that loss of blood meant loss of life. However, the circulation of blood was not understood. Through the writings of Aristotle (384 to 322 B.C.), veins were thought to contain all, or almost all, the blood. Arteries were thought to contain air, with only a very small amount of blood.

Celsus, a Roman of the first century A.D., described treatment of abdominal wounds. He mentioned the use of sutures as being well known and ancient. However, Celsus used clumsy, grasping forceps to stop bleeding and covered the wound with cotton lint wet with vinegar.

The doctrine of air in the arteries continued until the physiologist Galen demonstrated in the second century that arteries, like veins, contain blood. Galen wrote on the treatment of war wounds and emphasized the importance of knowing about arteries, muscles, and nerves so as not to injure them further during treatment. To stop the flow of blood from a vein, he suggested grasping it with a hook and twisting moderately. If bleeding was from an artery, a ligature of linen should be applied. He also mentioned the use of gut for sutures, although he recommended silk when it could be obtained. He used gut sutures for primary closure of wounds in Roman gladiators. Knowledge of the ligature seems to have been lost until Galen spoke of using it after trying all other known methods to stop bleeding.

Sutures fell into disuse during the Middle Ages, accompanying a general regression in surgical technique. Their use was revived by Ambroise Paré, a French army surgeon, in the sixteenth century. In his time, it was thought that gangrene was the natural result of wounds. The accepted treatment for bleeding and infection was still the use of boiling oil or hot irons. One day in treating many wounded, Paré's supply of oil was inadequate, and he was forced to use a hastily concocted poultice of egg yolk, oil of roses, and turpentine. The next day he found these men much better than the ones treated with boiling oil. The difference impressed him so much that he never used the old method again. Paré rediscovered the use of the ligature and is best known for his use of it following amputation to control bleeding. In 1552, he explained to surgeons the advantages of the ligature. He also was the first to grasp vessels with a pinching instrument. His bullet-grasping forceps is the predecessor of the hemostat in use today.

So slow was the progress of surgery that, 200 years later, surgeons were still using the inhuman, destructive irons. The use of gunpowder in warfare opened up a new field of surgery. It was thought that gunpowder poisoned the wounds, so they were cauterized and cleansed with hot oil. Mention is made of ligatures and sutures again in writings of the early eighteenth century and at various times throughout that century, as is use of pressure on bleeding points to control bleeding.

Research in wound healing did not exist before the eighteenth century, when John Hunter observed and recorded for the first time some of the various patterns of healing. He differentiated primary from secondary healing by calling the first "adhesive inflammation" and the second "suppurative inflammation." He also distinguished between epithelization and granulation. The process of coagulation was recognized also during this century, but it was believed to be the result rather than the cause of hemostasis.

Early in the nineteenth century, Dr. Philip Syng Physick found, while performing animal experiments, that the body absorbs sutures made from animal tissue. Probably the first surgeon to realize this, he wrote a paper on their use.

During this period, pus and infection were ever present in wounds. They were thought to be due to suture. The long ends of silk or flax, left hanging from wounds, sloughed out. Secondary hemorrhage from abscess formation and ulceration of ligatures through the vessels was common. Many types of devices were used to drain wounds.

William Stewart Halsted, a teaching surgeon at Johns Hopkins Hospital in Baltimore from 1893 to 1922, is acknowledged to have been one of the greatest surgeons of all times. Halsted perfected and brought into use the fine-pointed hemostat for occluding vessels, the Penrose drain, and rubber gloves. However, he is best known for his principles of tissue handling. In addition to his operative techniques, he inspired his assistants with his high ideals—as near perfection as possible in all operations. The silk suture technique he initiated in 1883, or a modification of it, is in use today. Its features are as follows:

1 Interrupted sutures are used for greater strength. Each stitch is taken and tied separately. If one knot slips, all the others hold. Halsted also believed that interrupted sutures were a barrier to infection, for he thought that if one area of a wound became infected, the microorganisms traveled along a continuous suture to infect the entire wound. A continuous suture is a running stitch tied only at the ends of the incision.

2 Sutures are as fine as is consistent with security. A suture stronger than the tissue it holds is not necessary.

3 Sutures are cut close to the knots. Long ends cause irritation.

4 A separate needle is used for each skin stitch.

5 Dead space in the wound is eliminated. *Dead space* is that space caused by separation of wound edges that have not been closely approximated by sutures. Serum or blood clots may collect in a dead space and prevent healing by keeping the cut edges of tissue separated.

6 Two fine sutures are used in situations usually requiring one large one.

7 Silk is not used in the presence of infection

(see Chap. 18 for discussion of all types of suture materials).

8 Tension is not placed on tissue. Halsted warned against bringing tissue together under tension and thus endangering blood supply.

Within reasonable limits, in the absence of hemorrhage and sepsis, wound healing is predictable. Yet abuse of the time-honored Halsted principles of operative technique can lead to such complications as hematoma, infection, wound disruption, scarring, stricture, and contracture.

Violation of tissue integrity, either by intent to explore or remove pathology or to repair traumatic injury, demands understanding the mechanism and factors that influence wound healing. Wound healing is nature's way of restoring continuity and strength to injured or incised tissue.

MECHANISM OF WOUND HEALING

When tissue is cut, the body's inherent defense mechanisms respond immediately to begin repair. Three types of wound healing are recognized: first intention, second intention, third intention. Each has practical applications in making and closing incisions or traumatic wounds.

First Intention

Healing by first intention is desired following primary union of an incised, aseptic, accurately approximated wound. It shows:

1 No postoperative swelling
2 No serous discharge or local infection
3 No separation of wound edges
4 Minimal scar formation

The rate and pattern of wound healing differ in different tissues. In general, first-intention wound healing consists of three distinct phases:

1 *Lag phase of acute inflammatory response.* Tissue fluids containing plasma, proteins, blood cells, fibrin, and antibodies exude from the tissues into the wound depositing fibrin, which weakly holds the wound edges together for the first five days. Fibrin and serum protein dry out, forming a scab that seals the wound from further fluid loss and microbial invasion. At the same time, fibroblasts, fibrous-tissue germ cells, and epithelial cells migrate from the general circulation. Subsequent adhesion of these cells, a process known as *fibroplasia,* holds the wound edges together. Leukocytes and other cells produce proteolytic enzymes to dissolve and remove damaged tissue debris.

2 *Healing phase of fibroplasia.* After the fifth postoperative day, fibroblasts multiply rapidly, bridging wound edges and restoring continuity of body structures. *Collagen,* a protein substance that is the chief constituent of connective tissue, is secreted from the fibroblasts and formed into fibers. This results in the rapid gain in tensile strength and pliability of the healing wound. *Tensile strength* is the ability of the tissues to resist rupture. Healing phase begins rapidly, diminishes progressively and terminates on about the fourteenth day.

3 *Maturation phase.* From fourteenth postoperative day until wound is fully healed, scar formation occurs by deposition of fibrous connective tissue. The collagen content remains constant, but the fiber pattern re-forms and cross-links to increase the tensile strength. Wound contraction occurs over a period of weeks up to six months. As collagen density increases, vascularity decreases, and the scar grows pale.

Second Intention

The mechanism of second-intention healing is by wound contraction rather than primary union. Granulation tissue containing fibroblasts forms in the defect and closes it by contraction with secondary growth of epithelium. In this type:

1 Infection, excessive trauma, loss of tissue, or poorly approximated tissue is present.

2 The wound may be left open and allowed to heal from the bottom toward the outer surface.

3 Healing is delayed.

4 Scar formation is excessive.

5 Healing may produce a weak union, which may be conducive to incisional herniation (rupture) later.

Third Intention

Suturing is delayed or secondary for the purpose of walling off an area of gross infection or where extensive tissue was removed, as in a debridement or by a traumatic injury. In healing by third intention:

1 Two surfaces of granulation tissue are brought together.

2 A deeper and wider scar usually results.

FACTORS INFLUENCING WOUND HEALING

Physical Condition of the Patient

Age Skin and muscle lose tone and elasticity as natural characteristics of the aging process. The rate is variable in the population, however.

Weight In obese patients, the bulk and weight of excess fat causes difficulty in confining it and securing good closure. Of all tissues, fat is the most vulnerable to trauma and infection.

Nutritional Status Wound healing is impaired by deficiencies in proteins, carbohydrates, zinc, and vitamins A, B, C, and K. Protein provides essential amino acids for new tissue construction. Carbohydrates are necessary energy sources for cells to prevent excessive metabolism of amino acids to meet caloric requirements. Vitamin B complex is necessary for carbohydrate, protein, and fat metabolism. Vitamin C permits collagen formation. Although known to be important in collagen synthesis, the mechanism of vitamin A and zinc in wound healing is not well understood. Vitamin K is involved in synthesis of prothrombin and blood clotting factors.

Fluid and Electrolyte Balance As a result of illness or injury, the patient may not be able to maintain normal fluid and electroyte balance. Changes in this balance can affect kidney function, cellular metabolism, oxygen concentration in the circulation, or hormonal function.

General Health Associated diseases such as diabetes, uremia, anemia, cirrhosis, leukemia, can delay the wound healing processes. Malignancies, debilitating injuries, and systemic or localized infections can also adversely affect wound healing.

Immune Responses The body normally responds at once to repair the inflammatory reaction of the tissues to injury or foreign substances. The cells liberate a tissue extract that starts an immune response for repair of the tissue. This is known as *tissue reaction.* Some foreign materials normally cause more tissue reaction than others. Abnormalities in function of these immune responses, such as an allergic reaction, can contribute to delayed wound healing. Patients with congenital or acquired immunologic disease are at risk. Recipients of prosthetic implants are susceptible to infection because their immune system concentrates its response around the device, thus increasing risk of systemic microbial invasion.

Drug Therapy Wound healing is basically collagen synthesis. Agents that interfere with cellular metabolism have a potentially deleterious effect on the healing process. Prolonged high dosage of steroids preoperatively, such as cortisone, inhibit fibroplasia and collagen formation.

Radiation Therapy Healing is delayed if the patient has had radiation in large doses preoperatively. The blood supply in irradiated tissue is decreased. However, little change from the normal healing pattern occurs if radiation has been given in low doses (see Chap. 35), and operation is performed within four to six weeks postradiation.

Postoperative Complications Edema, vomiting, or coughing can place stress on the healing wound before fibroplasia takes place. Complications in other parts of the body, far from operative site, such as pneumonia, thrombus, or embolus, can inhibit oxygen supply to wound site. Collagen synthesis is partly a function of oxygenation of tissues.

Physical Activity Early ambulation postoperatively is one of the most important factors in recovery of the surgical patient. Ambulation may be started immediately after recovery from anesthesia if the patient's condition does not contraindicate it. Some surgeons exempt only those whose blood pressure is not stable, those with a cardiac problem, and those whose general condition is poor. If the patient's physical condition does not safely permit ambulation, the surgeon orders otherwise.

Ambulation is started gradually by the patient first turning on his or her side. The patient then sits up with feet over side of the bed. He or she then stands on floor for a minute before returning to bed. After repeating this several times, the patient takes a few steps and finally increases the distance walked. Sitting in a chair for prolonged periods is discouraged, as this contributes to stasis of blood. A patient is fearful at first and needs a nurse at his or her side to provide confidence and safety. The nurse and patient must understand the value of early ambulation.

1 It speeds up circulation, which aids in the healing process and eliminates stasis of blood that may result in thrombus and embolus formation.

2 The patient is better able to cooperate in deep-breathing exercises to raise bronchial secretions; thus pulmonary complications are reduced.

3 Early ambulation decreases gas pains, distention, and tendency toward nausea and vomiting. Bodily functions return to normal more readily.

4 Increased exercise aids digestion. Thus the patient's oral intake progresses sooner after operation so less supplementary intravenous fluid is necessary for hydration and nutrition.

5 Early ambulation eliminates the general muscle weakness that follows bed rest.

6 Fewer pain-relieving drugs are necessary.

7 It boosts patients' morale to know they will be out of bed early after the operation, able to care for themselves, and soon ready to go home. This helps the mental outlook and through it the physical recovery.

8 It shortens hospitalization—an economic factor for the patient. From the point of view of the hospital, space is utilized more efficiently through more rapid turnover of beds.

Type of Wound

Surgical Incision The surgeon cuts through *intact* tissue. A sterile sharp scalpel (knife), scissors, or other cutting instrument may be used to separate skin and underlying tissue. Location, length, and depth of the incision is individually designed to achieve the best results for the patient following operation the surgeon has planned. A safe operative procedure requires exposure through an adequate incision.

The surgeon spreads the skin taut between thumb and index finger in preparation for making the skin incision. With one stroke of evenly applied pressure on the scalpel, a clean incision is made through skin. A number of factors influence ease with which skin incision is made:

1 Sharpness of knife blade
2 Resistance of self-adhering plastic drapes
3 Toughness of skin
4 Thickness of subcutaneous tissue

A clean stroke of a sterile surgical scalpel, followed by attention to all the principles of sterile technique and tissue handling, are the best insurances of primary healing by first intention. However, the direction of the incision may be a factor in wound healing. Wounds heal side-to-side, not end-to-end.

Traumatic Injuries Following traumatic injury, preservation of life is the first critical concern. No one specific pattern of treatment suits all patients. The patient's general condition is of prime consideration. Injuries are evaluated and the one or ones that pose greatest hazards to life or to return to normal function are cared for first. The primary objective, following life support, is wound closure with minimal deformity and functional loss. Minor injuries are cared for in the emergency department. Patients with major injuries receive treatment in the emergency department prior to going to the operating room as quickly as condition warrants.

Traumatic wounds can be classified as simple or complicated, clean or contaminated. Type of wound closure is predicated upon classification of the wound.

Simple Wounds Continuity of skin is interrupted but without loss or destruction of tissue and without implantation of a foreign body. These lacerations are usually due to a sharp-edged object cutting or penetrating at low velocity.

Complicated Wounds Tissue is lost or destroyed by crush or burn, or a foreign body is implanted by high-velocity penetration. If a penetrating wound was made by an object, such as a knife or bullet, this is not removed until the surgeon explores the wound in the operating room. Movement of a foreign object may cause further trauma. The depth of a penetrating wound is irrigated and may be excised. Skin grafting may be required following destruction of dermis (see Chap. 27).

Clean Wounds These will heal by first intention after closure of all tissue layers and wound edges. The cosmetic care of lacerated areas is important, as well as treatment to provide normal function of a part.

Contaminated Wounds Infection will result if treated by primary closure. Dirty objects have penetrated skin. Microorganisms multiply rapidly, and within six hours contamination can become infection. Debridement is done to thoroughly wash and irrigate wound. Devitalized tissue is removed because it acts as a culture medium. In excision of each area of contaminated tissue, clean instruments are used and discarded. Irrigation is continued during tissue excision.

After initial debridement to remove foreign bodies, including dirt and dead or devitalized tissue, the wound heals by second or third intention. Delayed primary closure may be performed several days later.

NOTE. Following traumatic injury that has resulted in broken skin, the patient is immunized against the tetanus bacillus. The individual is checked for sensitivity. If tetanus toxoid has been given previously, a booster dose of adsorbed tetanus toxoid may be given.

Operative Technique

Good operative technique is more important for good wound healing than any patient factor. Dr. John Deaver (1855 to 1931) of Philadelphia had a good adage: "If the surgeon cuts well and sews well, the patient gets well." Careful wound management involves the following considerations.

Aseptic Technique Healthy tissues are able to combat a certain amount of contamination. Microorganisms are normally present in skin and air. Devitalized tissues have little power of resistance. Infection may occur from any one of a variety of causes resulting in a breakdown of the wound postoperatively. The surgeon gives meticulous attention to sterile technique throughout operation to minimize contamination of operative site. The entire OR team carefully carries out the rules for aseptic and sterile techniques. In addition, many precautions are taken by all OR personnel. Strict adherence to housekeeping techniques, air engineering, sterilization procedures, and all the principles of aseptic technique is necessary. Infection may be due to a break in the chain of asepsis.

Hemostasis Complete hemostasis must be achieved to prevent loss of blood, to provide as bloodless a field as possible for accurate dissection, and to prevent hematoma (blood clot) formation. Blood loss is caused by tissue trauma. Extent of dissection and injury can affect healing if delivery of oxygen to the tissues is affected. Healing tissues consume oxygen avidly. Hence any condition that lowers circulatory flow and delivery of oxygen to the tissues impairs healing. (Hypoxia and hypovolemia were discussed in Chapter 14.)

Because they are so critical, the mechanisms and methods of hemostasis are discussed in detail later in this chapter.

Tissue Handling All tissues should be handled very gently and as little as possible throughout the operation. The surgeon plans an incision just long enough to afford sufficient operating space. Careful consideration is given to underlying blood vessels and nerves to preserve as many as possible. Retractors are placed to provide exposure, but without causing undue pressure on tissues and organs or tension on muscles. Trauma to tissue in dissecting, handling with instruments, ligating or suturing may cause edema and necrosis, death of tissue cells, with resultant slow healing. The body must rid itself of necrotic cells before the healing phase of fibroplasia takes place.

Tissue Approximation Tissue edges are brought together with precision, avoiding strangulation and eliminating dead space, to promote wound healing. Too tight a closure or closure under tension causes *ischemia,* a decrease of blood supply to tissues.

Dead space is caused by separation of wound edges that have not been closely approximated or by air trapped between layers of tissue. Serum or blood may collect in a dead space and prevent healing by keeping cut edges separated. Wound edges not in close contact cannot heal readily. A drain may be inserted to aid in removal of fluid or air from operative site postoperatively, or a pressure dressing may be applied over a closed wound to help obliterate dead space.

The choice of wound closure materials and the techniques of the surgeon are prime factors in the restoration of tensile strength to wound during the healing process. Materials used to approximate tissues are discussed in Chapter 18.

Wound Security Quality of approximated tissue and type of closure material are two factors that will determine strength of the wound. Tensile strength of the tissues themselves will vary; some are more friable than others. Drains or catheters may be placed in wound to evacuate serum or fluid from accumulating in dead space postoperatively. Drainage tubes may cause a weak spot in the incision, and underlying tissue may protrude. Also, drains may provide an inlet for microorganisms as well as an outlet for drainage. When possible, drains are placed through a stab wound in the skin rather than through the operative incision.

When sutures are used, the suture material provides all the strength of the wound immediately after closure. Closely spaced sutures give a stronger suture line. The strength of a suture should not be greater than the strength of the tissue on which it is used. To minimize tissue reaction to sutures, the least amount and the smallest size suture consistent with the holding power of the tissues is used.

Immediately after closure, tissue along the incision is at about 40 percent of its original strength. It reaches its greatest strength in 7 to 15 days. The wound is about one-third healed on the sixth postoperative day and two-thirds healed on the eighth day. The condition of the patient, type of operation, and many other factors may cause variance from the norm. As the tensile strength of the wound increases, the reliance on other support for wound security gradually lessens.

MECHANISM OF HEMOSTASIS

Hemostasis is essential to successful wound management. Literally, *hemostasis* is the arrest of a flow of blood or hemorrhage. The mechanism is *coagulation,* formation of a blood clot. The clotting of blood takes place by enzyme reaction, in several stages.

When severed by incision or traumatic injury, a blood vessel constricts and the ends contract somewhat. Platelets rapidly clump and adhere to connective tissue at cut end of a constricted vessel. Interaction with collagen fibers causes platelets to liberate adenosine diphosphate (ADP), epinephrine, and serotonin from their secretory granules. In turn, ADP causes other platelets to clump to the initial layer and to each other, forming a platelet plug. This may be sufficient in small vessles to provide primary hemostasis.

The reaction of plasma from vessels with connective tissue cells at site of injury activates clotting factors and causes a series of other reactions. *Prothrombin,* normally present in blood, reacts with *thromboplastin,* which is released when tissues are injured. Prothrombin and thromboplastin, along with calcium ions in the blood, form *thrombin.* This requires several minutes. Thrombin unites with *fibrinogen,* a blood protein, to form *fibrin,* which is the basic structural material of blood clots. This last reaction is very rapid.

The fibrin strands reinforce the platelet plug to form a resilient hemostatic plug capable of withstanding arterial pressure when the constricted vessel relaxes. Massive thrombosis within the vessels would occur, once coagulation is initiated, if it continued. However, fibrin is digested during the process. The products of this digestion, as well as the antithrombins normally present in the blood, act as anticoagulants. The coagulation mechanism rapidly and efficiently inhibits excessive blood loss so that excessive coagulation does not occur.

Hemorrhagic Disorders

Hemostasis can be effectively provided for patients with hemorrhagic disorders by giving concentrated human coagulation factors. These patients (see Chap. 3) then can undergo operation without undue risk of bleeding, and without additional risk of overloading the vascular system.

Anticoagulants In operations on the blood vessels or heart and in patients who have a history of thromboembolic disease, anticoagulants are used. The dosage is adjusted to minimize tendency of blood to clot in the vessels, yet not lead to excessive bleeding during or following operation. The following drugs are commonly used:

Heparin Acts to inhibit the reaction wherein prothrombin is converted to thrombin.

Coumarin Derivatives Depress the blood prothrombin and decrease the tendency of blood platelets to cling together, thus decreasing the normal tendency of the blood to clot.

Warfarin Sodium Interferes with the action of vitamin K to prevent synthesis of prothrombin and fibrinogen.

Low Molecular Weight Dextran Reduces platelet adhesiveness and aggregation to prevent sludge from forming in the bloodstream. It coats the blood platelets to keep them from massing together.

Aspirin Diminishes clumping of platelets by inhibiting the release reaction of platelet factors.

Vitamin K Vitamin K enables the liver to produce clotting factors in the blood. To reduce the possibility of hemorrhage during operation, it is given preoperatively to:

1 Patients who have been on anticoagulant therapy.

2 Patients having faulty metabolism or improper utilization of bile with consequent low vitamin K absorption.

3 Elderly or debilitated patients requiring eye surgery to minimize the possibility of intraocular hemorrhage.

4 Newborns who require operative procedures.

5 Mothers just before delivery to help prevent postdelivery hemorrhage. It also assures the baby of an adequate prothrombin level until a sufficient amount is produced by the liver.

METHODS OF HEMOSTASIS

Basically, two different types of bleeding may occur during operative procedures: diffuse oozing from large denuded surfaces and gross bleeding from transected or penetrated vessels. Many of the present methods of hemostasis apply principles used by ancient surgeons. However, today bleeding is controlled and wounds are closed or covered to minimize trauma to tissue and to enhance healing without complication. Numerous agents, devices, and sophisticated pieces of equipment are used to achieve hemostasis and wound closure. These various methods can be classified as chemical, mechanical, and thermal.

Chemical Methods

Absorbable Gelatin Sponge Available in either powder or compressed-pad form, gelatin sponge (Gelfoam) is an absorbable hemostatic agent made from purified gelatin solution that has been beaten to a foamy consistency, dried, and sterilized by dry heat. As a pad, it is available in an assortment of sizes that can be cut as desired without crumbling. When it is placed on an area of capillary bleeding, fibrin is deposited in the interstices and the sponge swells, forming a substantial clot. The sponge is not soluble; it absorbs 45 times its own weight in blood. It is denatured to retard absorption, which takes place in 20 to 40 days. It is frequently soaked in thrombin or epinephrine solution, although it may be used alone. Before handing a gelatin sponge to the surgeon, dip it into warm saline, if used without thrombin or epinephrine, and press it between fingers or against sides of the basin to remove air from it. Use the same procedure with thrombin or epinephrine solution, but then drop the sponge back into solution and allow it to absorb solution back to its original size.

Collagen Sponge Hemostatic sponges of collagen origin (Collastat and Superstat) are applied dry to oozing or bleeding sites. Sponges dissolve as hemostasis occurs. Residual sponge left in wound will absorb.

Microfibrillar Collagen Microfibrillar bovine collagen (Avitene) is an off-white fluffy, flour-like material used as a topical hemostatic agent. It is produced from highly purified bovine corium (dermis) via shredding, hydrochloric acid treatment, and microfragmentation into threads or fibrils less than one micron in diameter. When placed in contact with a bleeding surface, hemostasis is achieved by adhesion of platelets and prompt fibrin deposition within the interstices of the collagen. Tissue cohesion is an inherent property of the collagen itself. It functions as a hemostatic agent only when it is applied directly to the source of bleeding from raw, oozing surfaces including bone and friable tissues or from around vascular anastomoses.

Supplied sterile in glass jars, small dry quantities are picked up with dry smooth tissue forceps and applied directly to active bleeding from irregular contours, crevices, and around suture lines. Firm pressure is then quickly applied over a dry gauze sponge, held either by the fingers in accessible areas or a sponge forceps in less accessible areas. It is important that the material be firmly compressed against the bleeding surface before excessive wetting with blood can occur. Effective application is evidenced by a firm adherent coagulum with no break-through bleeding from either surface or edges. If desired, excess collagen can be removed from around the site without re-creating bleeding. The remaining coagulum absorbs during wound healing.

Oxidized Cellulose Absorbable oxidation products of cellulose are available in the form of a pad of oxidized cellulose (Oxycel) similar to absorbent cotton, or a knitted fabric strip of oxidized regenerated cellulose (Surgicel). Either of these products is laid dry on an oozing surface or held firmly against a bleeding site until hemostasis is obtained. When oxidized cellulose comes into contact with whole blood, a clot forms rapidly. As it reacts with blood, it increases in size to form a gel and stops bleeding in areas difficult to control by other means of hemostasis. Except in situations where packing is required as a lifesaving measure, only the minimal amount required to control capillary or venous bleeding or small arterial hemorrhage is used. If left on oozing surfaces, it will absorb with minimal tissue reaction. It is not recommended for use on bone unless it is removed after hemostasis as it may interfere with bone regeneration.

Oxidized cellulose is supplied in sterile vials. It cannot be steam sterilized because high temperature causes physical breakdown of the product and loss of tensile strength. It may be stored at room temperature. It is used dry; do not moisten in either hemostatic or antibiotic solutions. Oxidized regenerated cellulose has some inherent antibacterial properties.

Oxytocin Oxytocin is a hormone produced by the pituitary gland. It is prepared synthetically for therapeutic injection. This is sometimes used to induce labor and also given to cause contraction of the uterus after delivery of the placenta. It is a systemic agent used to control hemorrhage, rather than a hemostatic agent per se.

Phenol and Alcohol Some surgeons use 95% phenol to cauterize tissue when cutting across the lumen of the appendix or gastrointestinal tract. Phenol coagulates proteins and in high concentration is so extremely caustic that it can cause severe burns. Therefore it must be neutralized with 95% alcohol as soon as surgeon has used it; burning action continues until phenol is neutralized with alcohol (see Chap. 21 for use in general surgery).

Styptics A styptic is an agent that checks hemorrhage by causing *vasoconstriction,* contraction of blood vessels. Styptics, especially epinephrine, are used to some extent, but they have the disadvantage of being rapidly carried away by the bloodstream.

Epinephrine A hormone of the adrenal gland, epinephrine (Adrenalin) is prepared synthetically for use as a vasoconstrictor to prolong the action of local anesthetic agents or to decrease bleeding. Used in some local anesthetic agents to constrict the vessels locally, epinephrine keeps the anesthetic concentrated within the area injected and reduces the amount of bleeding when the incision is made. However, it is rapidly dispersed, leaving little local effect. Within the incision, gelatin sponges soaked in 1:1000 epinephrine may be applied to bleeding surfaces. These are especially useful in ear and microsurgical procedures where localized hemostasis is critical.

Silver Nitrate Crystals of silver nitrate in solution or mixed with silver chloride and molded into pencils (sticks) are applied topically. Both an astringent and antimicrobial, silver nitrate is most commonly used in treatment of burns (see Chap. 27, p. 533).

Tannic Acid A powder made from an astringent plant, tannic acid is used occasionally on mucous membranes of the nose and throat to help stop capillary bleeding.

Thrombin An enzyme extracted from beef blood is used therapeutically as a topical hemostatic agent. Thrombin accelerates coagulation of blood and controls capillary bleeding. It unites rapidly with fibrinogen to form a clot. Topically, it may be used as a dry powder to sprinkle on an oozing surface or as a solution, alone or to saturate a gelatin sponge. Topical thrombin is used on areas of capillary bleeding that do not lend themselves to other means of hemostasis, such as sealing a skin graft onto a denuded area.

Thrombin is used for local application only. *It is never injected.* When a solution of it is on the instrument table, it must be kept separated from any other solutions. Use a careful, sure means of identification. It is recommended that thrombin be mixed just before use, as it loses potency after several hours. Refer to instructions of the manufacturer for mixing solution.

Biological Dressings A biological dressing temporarily covers an open surface defect in skin and underlying tissue of complicated, contaminated wounds. It is used to arrest loss of fluid, reduce or eliminate microbial growth, and promote production of granulation tissue and epithelialization prior to healing by second or third intention. A fibrin-elastin biologic bonding system adheres dressing to exposed surfaces. Biological dressings are skin grafts (refer to Chap. 27). These may be:

Autografts Skin grafted from one part of the patient's body to another part.

Homografts Skin obtained from one genetically dissimilar person to another. A cadaver may be the source of skin for a homograft biological dressing. Controlled freezing preserves skin for use when needed.

Heterografts (Xenografts) Skin obtained from a dissimilar species placed on human tissue (refer to porcine heterografts in Chap. 18).

Controlled Hypotension In selected situations when excessive blood loss is anticipated or encountered, blood pressure may be deliberately lowered to produce an essentially bloodless field. When induced, hypotension is carefully controlled by the anesthesiologist (refer to Chap. 13).

Hyperbaric Oxygenation (OHP) *Hyperbaric oxygen therapy* is the administration of oxygen under several times greater than normal atmospheric pressure. The therapeutic aim is twofold: to raise the tissue-oxygen tension to normal levels or to raise it to above-normal levels. The physiological effects of oxygen at increased atmospheric pressure are: intense vasoconstriction, bone formation and resorption, bone marrow suppression, vascular proliferation, and a bacteriostatic or bactericidal action. These effects may be used selectively.

The therapy is administered in specially designed chambers that vary in size from one that contains a fully equipped operating room to a single-patient unit. In the larger, the patient and the OR team enter a chamber filled with compressed air. The patient is given 100% oxygen to breathe by mask. Some surgical conditions for which the chamber is used include cardiac and peripheral vascular disease, chronic pulmonary disease, crush injuries and suturing of severed extremities, and gas gangrene. These chambers are not in common use, due mainly to high cost. Hospitals that have a hyperbaric chamber accept patients from other hospitals when it is thought the treatment will benefit the patient.

Mechanical Methods

Bone Wax Composed mainly of beeswax, bone wax is used to control bleeding from bone in some orthopaedic and neurosurgical procedures, and when sternum is split for cardiothoracic procedures. The surgeon rubs a small amount of this soft material over cut bone surfaces to stop oozing. The scrub nurse places several pieces, each rolled into a ball, around the rim of a medicine cup. When needed, hold cup at the sterile field so surgeon can pick a ball of wax off the rim.

Drains Drains may be used prophylactically or therapeutically during the operation and/or postoperatively. Used prophylactically to evacuate intestinal fluids, urine, or fluids from any source, drains can stimulate a walling-off process about an operative site in which subsequent drainage may accumulate. Therapeutically, drains aid in removal of fluid or air from the operative site to obliterate dead spaces and to enhance apposition of tissues. Although technically not a method of hemostasis in the context of arresting the flow of blood, drainage of body cavities helps prevent tissue trauma and restore organs to normal function.

Drainage during Operation

1 *Gastrointestinal decompression* with a plastic or rubber nasogastric tube inserted through a nostril down into the stomach or small intestine removes flatus, fluids, or other contents. The tube has holes in several locations near the tip to permit withdrawal of contents. Several types of nasogastric tubes are used; most common are the Levin tube into the stomach and Miller-Abbott tube into the small intestine.

The surgeon may ask anesthesiologist to insert a tube to decompress gastrointestinal tract during operation when distention due to obstruction obscures operative site, to measure blood loss due to gastric hemorrhage, or to evacuate gastric seçretions during bowel anastomosis. The anesthesiologist may insert a nasogastric tube preoperatively to empty stomach before an emergency operation to prevent aspiration of stomach contents.

The nasogastric tube may remain in place postoperatively to prevent vomiting and distention caused by decreased peristalsis following anesthesia, manipulation of the viscera during operation, or obstruction from edema of tissues at the operative site. For this purpose, the tube is connected to a suction apparatus. It also may be used for nasogastric feeding during the healing process after operations on the upper alimentary canal.

2 *Urinary drainage* via urethral or ureteral catheters inserted preoperatively provides constant drainage from bladder or kidneys during operation. The purpose may be to keep the bladder decompressed or to prevent extravasation of urine into the tissues around operative site during and after genitourinary operations. Postoperatively, the inflated balloon of a Foley retention catheter maintains an even pressure on the bladder neck, which may help control bleeding following prostatectomy, for example. An indwelling urethral catheter may be connected to a bladder-irrigation or tidal-drainage system until the bladder resumes normal function postoperatively.

Postoperative Drainage

1 *Chest drainage* ensures complete expansion of lungs postoperatively. Air and fluid must be evacuated from pleural space following operations within the chest cavity. One or more chest tubes are inserted. If surgeon inserts two, the upper tube evacuates air and the lower drains fluid. After chest tube(s) is inserted during closure, end is covered with a sterile sponge until it can be connected to a sterile closed water-seal drainage system. The drainage system must prevent outside air from being drawn into the pleural space during expiration. Water in collection unit seals off outside air to maintain a negative pressure within pleural cavity.

Two tubes vent the leakproof top of the collection unit. A short air-outlet tube extends 1 in. (2.5 cm) or more above stopper to about 3 in. (7.5 cm) below it into the collection unit. The long inlet tube extends from above stopper, through it, to about 1 in. (2.5 cm) from the bottom of the collection unit. Sterile water is poured into the collection unit to a level 1 to 2 in. (2.5 to 5 cm) above end of long inlet tube. The circulating nurse marks water level on outside of collection unit. Clear sterile tubing connects the inlet tube to the tube placed into pleural space. Upon the patient's initial expiration, water rises a short distance up into the inlet tube. With each subsequent inspiration-expiration the water level in the tube fluctuates. If water level in tube remains stationary, the chest tube or connecting tubing may be clogged or kinked. *The collection unit must be kept well below chest level to prevent water entering the chest, and to keep tubing free of kinks.*

Fluid drains by gravity from the chest into the water. The collection unit should be calibrated so that drainage can be measured. Air bubbles through the water and escapes through the outlet tube.

If gravity drainage is not adequate for reexpansion of lungs, suction may be applied. This requires the addition of one or two collection units to the system, to act as a pressure regulator, and a suction machine to maintain negative pressure. Disposable chest-drainage units are available commercially, as a single unit or in a series of two or three. Some units are modifications based on the principle described for a closed water-seal system. Follow the manufacturer's direction for use. Be sure unit is properly connected before patient leaves the OR.

The chest tube may be clamped during transportation, as a safety measure with some units. Check with surgeon as to whether or not clamping is contraindicated.

2 *Closed-wound suction systems* are used when it is necessary to apply suction to a large, closed-wound site postoperatively. A constant, gentle, negative pressure vacuum evacuates tissue fluid and blood to promote healing by reducing edema and media for microbial growth. It also eliminates dead space by holding skin flaps against underlying tissue.

Sterile plastic tubing connected to a stainless steel needle is placed in the operative area, usually through a small stab wound in the skin. This tubing has several perforations along the length placed in tissues. It also has radiopaque markings to aid in checking location of tubing on x-ray if desired. The tubing is connected to a sterile, self-contained portable container. This can be attached immediately after placement of tubing and the vacuum activated. Several different units are available with containers of different capacities as well as sizes of tubings. Directions printed on each unit must be followed to activate vacuum. An anti-reflux valve guards against backflow of fluids. Calibrations on side of container measure the drainage and a line designates when it should be emptied. These units are made entirely or partially of clear plastic so surgeon can inspect drainage.

3 *Constant gravity drainage,* without negative pressure vacuum, is often used following operations on the gallbladder, bladder, kidney, or cecum. Each hospital has a supply of tubes, catheters, and various kinds of tubings and adaptors that are kept sterile. Many tubes and catheters are radiopaque. They are ready for the circulating nurse to open if needed.

A closed or semiclosed system of drainage may be used. The scrub nurse keeps end of the tube or catheter sterile until it is connected to sterile end of the constant-drainage tubing. When necessary to disconnect, protect end of each with a sterile sponge held with a rubber band. If either end becomes contaminated inadvertently, wipe tube or catheter off with an alcohol sponge. Obtain another sterile drainage tubing.

Disposable, constant-drainage bags and tubing are changed at least every eight hours. They are marked in gradations from 500 to 2000 ml.

Use tubes and catheters or any other drainage tubing for one patient only—never reuse on another. Aside from the aesthetic reasons, the wall absorbs a certain amount of irritating chemicals from the patient's tissues that causes an irritation in the next patient, even though it is thoroughly cleaned and sterilized.

4 *Penrose drain,* made of *gutta-percha,* the coagulated latex of various trees, was described by

Dr. Penrose in 1897. Sometimes referred to as a *cigarette drain,* it is still used to maintain a vent for escape of fluid or air or to wall off an area of exudate in the wound.

A Penrose drain is a thin walled cylinder of radiopaque latex. The diameter may be ¼ to 1 in. (6 mm to 2.5 cm), depending upon the surgeon's preference. It is usually supplied to the sterile field in a 6- to 12-in. (15- to 30-cm) length for the surgeon to cut as desired. Penrose drains are commercially available prepackaged and sterilized. However, if they are prepared for steam sterilization in the hospital, a gauze wick must be inserted to permit steam penetration of the lumen.

Although Penrose drains are usually used without a wick, the surgeon may prefer the wick of gauze packing left in the lumen. Without a wick, moisten drain in saline before handing it to the surgeon. After it is placed into operative area and brought out through a stab wound in the skin, the drain is secured with a skin suture, or a safety pin is attached on the outside close to the skin, to keep drain from retracting into the wound.

Penrose drains may be used to gently retract vessels and other small structures.

5 *Sump drain,* a plastic or silicone catheter, may be used for irrigation, aspiration with suction, or to introduce medication to an area. A sump drain has a double or triple lumen for these purposes. Clogging is reduced to a minimum by the large lateral openings. It is connected to a constant-drainage system, with or without suction.

Dressings Dressings give some support to incision and surrounding skin and absorb drainage (see Chap. 10 for types of dressings). Dry gauze is not used on a denuded area because it adheres and acts as a foreign body. Granulation tissue will grow into it. Bleeding can be reactivated when it is removed (refer to Chap. 27 for alternatives).

Hemostatic Clamps Clamps for occluding vessels have two opposing serrated jaws, stabilized by a box lock, and controlled by ringed handles. They are used to grasp or hold a small amount of tissue or to compress blood vessels. The *hemostat* is the most frequently used surgical instrument and the most commonly used method of hemostasis. This instrument has either straight or curved jaws that narrow to a fine point. Often the pressure of clamping the instrument is sufficient to constrict and seal a vessel with minimal trauma or adjacent tissue necrosis. A wide variety of other hemostatic clamps are used for vessel occlusion, including noncrushing vascular clamps that do not damage large vessels.

Ligating Clips When placed on a vessel and pinched shut, clips occlude the lumen and stop the vessel from bleeding. Metallic clips are small pieces of thin, serrated wire, bent in the center to an oblique angle. Absorbable polymer clips are similar in configuration. Clips are most frequently used on large vessels or those in anatomic locations difficult to ligate by other means. A specific forceps is required for the application of each type available. Single clips may be mounted in a sterile plastic cartridge that can be secured in a heavy stainless steel base to facilitate loading the applier forceps. Disposable appliers preloaded with multiple clips also are available.

Ligating clips were devised in 1911 by Dr. Harvey Cushing for use in brain surgery. Cushing clips are made of silver. Stainless steel, tantalum, and titanium clips are more common today. The serrations across the wire prevent their slipping off the vessels. Polymeric clips have a locking device to secure them on vessels. Many surgeons use clips for ligating vessels, nerves, and other small structures.

Metallic clips also may be used to mark a biopsy site or other areas to permit x-ray visualization in order to detect postoperative complications. For example, migration of a marker clip could indicate presence of a hematoma in the wound.

Ligature A ligature, commonly called a *tie,* is a strand of material that is tied around a blood vessel to occlude the lumen and prevent bleeding. Frequently the ligature is tied around a hemostat and slipped off the point onto the vessel and pulled taut to effect hemostasis. Vessels are ligated with the smallest-size strand possible and include the smallest amount of surrounding tissue possible. Ends are cut as near the knot as possible.

Large and pulsating vessels may require a *transfixion suture.* A ligature on a needle is placed through a "bite" of tissue and brought around end of vessel. This eliminates any possibility of its slipping off the vessel. All bleeding points should be ligated before next layer of tissue is incised.

Pressure Pressure is exerted on a bleeding point manually or by mechanical devices. Whether pressure promotes hemostasis or merely constricts blood vessels is questionable. However, the general belief is that it delays hemorrhage until the normal forces of blood have time to form a clot.

Digital Compression When digital pressure is applied to artery proximal to area of bleeding, such as in traumatic injury, hemorrhage is controlled. The main disadvantage of digital pressure is that it cannot be applied permanently. Firm pressure is applied on the skin on both sides as the skin incision is made to help control subcutaneous bleeding until vessels can be clamped, ligated, or cauterized. Pressure is applied while sponging the operative area to locate a bleeding vessel.

Mechanical Pressure Devices

1 *Antiembolic elastic stockings* or an elastic bandage may be applied to lower extremities to prevent thrombus or embolic phenomena. Compression on the legs helps prevent venous stasis. Stockings are available in knee- or groin-length sizes. To apply, roll stocking from top to toe. Put over patient's toes and gently unroll over leg from foot to ankle to calf, etc.

2 *Antigravity suit,* commonly known as the *G-suit,* is a method of circumferential pneumatic compression to control hemorrhage, counteract postural hypotension, and maintain venous pressure. An inflatable vinyl plastic envelope, the G-suit is wrapped and laced about patient from ankles to xyphoid process, thereby increasing pressure on walls of bleeding vessels. Section over the lower extremities is inflated first to prevent venous stasis in the legs. The entire suit can be inflated or specific sections of it as desired. It is most effective in control of intraabdominal bleeding during transport following trauma. It is also used to prevent air embolism during some head and neck operations performed with patient in a sitting position. Uniform circumferential pneumatic compression reduces volume of the vascular bed below the diaphragm, thus diverting blood to vital structures above. The increased venous filling the G-suit produces decreases possibility of air embolus.

3 *Packs* are used to sustain pressure on raw wound surfaces. The application of sponges or laparotomy tapes effectively controls capillary ooze by occluding the capillaries. The surgeon usually wants these moistened, often with cold but sometimes with hot saline solution.

Compressed rayon or cotton radiopaque patties are used for hemostasis when placed on the surface of delicate tissues such as the brain, spinal cord, or nerves. These patties have no loose fibers. They are available in an assortment of sizes. Before use, moisten with saline and press out excess, keeping them flat.

4 *Pressure dressings* are used to eliminate dead space and to prevent capillary bleeding, accumulation of serum, or formation of hematoma when closed-wound suction drainage is contraindicated. They may be used as an adjunct to wound drainage to distribute pressure evenly over the wound to minimize edema. (Refer to Chapter 10 for description of materials used.)

5 *Rubber dam,* a piece of thin latex rubber sheeting, placed over an arteriotomy site, can help hold the wound edges together until the bleeding is controlled. This rubber dam can be removed after four or five minutes of compression.

6 *Suction* is the application of pressure less than atmospheric either continuously or intermittently. It is used during operations for removal of blood and tissue fluids from operative field. An appropriate style tip is attached to sterile conductive suction tubing; many tips are disposable. The kinds of suction tips include:
   - **a** *Poole abdominal,* used for laparotomies or within any cavity in which fluid or pus may be encountered. It has an outer filter shield.
   - **b** *Ferguson-Frazier,* used when there is little or no fluid except capillary bleeding and irrigating fluid, such as in brain, spinal, plastic, or orthopaedic procedures. It keeps the field dry without the usual sponging. One model has a connection for an electrosurgical unit, and the tip can be used for fulguration.
   - **c** *Yankauer tonsil suction,* used in mouth or throat. Rather than a straight tube, like an abdominal suction tip, it is angled.
   - **d** *Plain rubber catheter,* used in the nasopharynx, especially in infants.
   - **e** *Aspirating tube,* used through an endoscope.

7 *Tourniquet* may be used on an extremity to keep the operative field free from blood and thus reduce operating time. Not generally considered a method of hemostasis, bleeding is controlled by other methods prior to wound closure. A firm dressing applied to closed wound before removing tourniquet helps prevent collection of serum in the wound. This is especially true in operations on the knee.

Regulations for and precautions with tourniquet application and usage must be observed. A tourniquet should never be used when circulation in distal part of an extremity is impaired. A tourniquet can cause tissue injury and shut off the entire blood supply to part below it, causing gangrene and loss of the extremity. Metabolic changes may be irreversible after one to 1½ hours of tourniquet ischemia. *A tourniquet is dangerous to apply, to leave on, and to remove.* A tourniquet may be applied by the surgeon, by an assistant or the circulating nurse on surgeon's orders. To apply:

a Protect the patient's skin by placing a folded towel or other padding around extremity under tourniquet. Padding must be wrinkle-free.

b Avoid vulnerable neurovascular structures. Tourniquet should be positioned at point of maximum circumference of extremity.

c Elevate arm or leg to encourage venous drainage before tightening a tourniquet.

d Record time the tourniquet is applied and removed. Inform surgeon when it has been on for one hour and every 15 minutes thereafter. The anesthesiologist may note the time with the surgeon and record it on the anesthesia sheet, thus providing a permanent record of tourniquet time. In some hospitals the circulating nurse posts tourniquet time on a tally board in view of the surgeon. It must also be recorded on the patient's chart.

Kinds of tourniquets include:

a *Blood-pressure cuff.* The surgeon determines the amount of pressure to be sustained.

b *Esmarch's bandage.* Friedrich von Esmarch, a German military surgeon, introduced an elastic bandage for the control of hemorrhage on the battlefield in 1869. As known today, this is a 3 in. (7.5 cm) latex rubber roller bandage used to compress superficial vessels to force blood out of an extremity. An Esmarch's bandage is not used, however, to empty vessels of blood preoperatively in a patient following traumatic injury or if the patient has been in a cast. Danger exists that thrombi might be in vessels because of injury or stasis of blood. These could become dislodged and result in emboli.

Starting at distal end of an extremity, an Esmarch's bandage is wrapped tightly, overlapping spirally, to level of the blood-pressure cuff or a pneumatic tourniquet. The tourniquet is then tightened and the rubber bandage removed. Or, starting at distal end of extremity, the rubber bandage can be partially removed, leaving the last three rounds, which constitute a tourniquet.

To ensure sterilization of all surfaces, a layer of roller gauze bandage is placed between layers of the rubber bandage. This must be removed and the bandage rerolled before use.

c *Pneumatic tourniquet.* Similar to a blood-pressure cuff, although heavier and more secure, the cuff consists of a rubber bladder shielded by a plastic insert inside a fabric cover. Cuff of appropriate length and width must be used; various sizes are available. Cuffs are inflated automatically with compressed gas (air, oxygen, or Freon) or ambient air by means of tubing interconnected between the cuff and a pressure cartridge, piped-in system, or battery-powered unit. The desired pressure is uniformly maintained by a pressure valve and registered on a pressure gauge. Correct pressure is minimum amount required to produce a bloodless field. The average adult arm requires 300 mm Hg (about 6 lb), the thigh 500 mm Hg (about 10 lb); thin adults and children require less. Paralysis may result from excessive pressure on nerves. Inflation time should also be kept to a minimum. If needed for more than one hour on an arm or 1½ hours on a leg, tourniquet is deflated for ten minute intervals periodically at discretion of surgeon.

Care must be taken to ensure that cuff and tubing are intact, and pressure gauge is accurate. These should be inspected prior to operation. An aneroid pressure gauge can be checked by comparing it to a mercury manometer. Pressure drifts can be detected by wrapping cuff around a rigid cylinder, inflating it to 300 mm Hg, and observing for pressure variations. During operation, gauge should be monitored to detect pressure fluctuations. A unit with a microprocessor control signals both audible and visual alarm indicators if pressure deviates from pre-set pressure.

All pneumatic tourniquets must be cleaned and inspected after each patient use.

They should be regularly tested and maintained in working order prior to storage between uses.

d *Rubber band.* This may be used as a tourniquet for a finger or toe.

e *Rubber tubing.* When starting an intravenous infusion, a small piece of rubber tubing is applied momentarily around extremity, usually an arm, while needle is being inserted. This stops venous return and makes the vein more obvious for venipuncture.

Thermal Methods

Hemostasis may be achieved or enhanced by application of either cold or heat to body tissues.

Cryosurgery Cryosurgery is performed with the aid of special instruments for local freezing of diseased tissue without harm to normal adjacent structures. Extreme cold causes intracapillary thrombosis and tissue necrosis in the frozen area. Frozen tissue may be removed without significant bleeding during or after operation. Cryosurgery is also used to alter cell function without removing tissue. It tends to be hemostatic and lymphostatic, particularly in highly vascular areas.

Extreme cold, at controlled temperatures ranging from + 20 to −60°C (+68 to −140°F) is delivered to extract heat from a small volume of tissue in a rapid manner. Liquid nitrogen is the most commonly used refrigerant, however, Freon or carbon dioxide gas may be used. The liquid or gas is in a vacuum container and comes through an insulated vacuum tube to a probe. All but the tip of the probe is insulated. Freezing of tissue at this tip is due to the liquid nitrogen becoming gaseous. In the process, heat is removed from the tissue. A ball of frozen tissue gradually forms around the uninsulated tip. Extent of tissue destruction is controllable by raising or lowering temperature of cells surrounding the lesion.

The machines vary in range of temperatures obtained according to their design and type of refrigerant used. Some are nonelectric with foot-switch operated probes. Special miniature, presterilized, disposable models for single-patient use are particularly suitable for ophthalmic applications (refer to Chap. 25, p. 488).

Because the process is rapid, involves less trauma to destroy or remove tissue, controls bleeding, and minimizes local pain, cryosurgery is used to alter the function of nerve cells and to destroy otherwise unapproachable brain tumors. Other techniques involve removal of superficial tumors in the nasopharynx and the skin, destruction of the prostate gland, removal of highly vascular tumors, removal of lesions from the cervix and anus, cataract extraction, retinal detachment, etc. The amount of tissue destroyed is influenced by the size of the tip of the probe and temperature used, duration of use, kind of tissue and its vascularity, and special skill of the surgeon.

Hypothermia Cooling of body tissues to a temperature as low as 26°C (78.8°F) in adults and large children and 20°C (68°F) in infants and small children, well below normal limits, decreases cellular metabolism and thereby decreases need for oxygen by tissues. The decreased requirement for oxygen decreases bleeding. It lowers blood pressure to slow the circulation and increases the viscosity of blood. This process results in hemoconcentration, which contributes to capillary sludging and microcirculatory stasis to provide an essentially dry field for the surgeon. Hypothermia may be localized or generalized (systemic). Refer to Chapter 13 for detailed description of methods of local and systemic hypothermia by both internal and external body cooling. Hypothermia is used as an adjunct to anesthesia particularly during operations of the heart, brain, or liver.

Diathermy Oscillating, high-frequency electric current generates enough heat to coagulate and destroy body tissues. Heat is generated by resistance of tissues to passage of alternating electric current. A short-wave diathermy machine produces a high frequency of 10 to 100 million cycles per second. The machine should not be activated until surgeon is ready to deliver this current. Diathermy is useful in stopping bleeding from small blood vessels. It is used primarily to repair detached retina (see Chap. 25) and to cauterize small warts, polyps, and other small superficial lesions.

Electrocautery A small loop heated by a steady, direct electric current to red heat will coagulate or destroy tissue on contact. Heat is transferred to tissue from the preheated wire. The hemostatic effect is a result of searing or sealing the tissues. A variety of sterile, disposable, battery-powered models are available. Hot point of cautery must be at least 24 in. (60 cm) from anesthesia machine and face mask, with a protecting screen between tip and patient's head. Cautery must *never* be used in mouth, around head, or in pleural cavity when flammable anesthetics are used. *Cautery must not be used when any flammable agent is present.* Only *moist* sponges should be permitted on the field while cautery is in use, to prevent fire.

Electrosurgery High-frequency electric current provided from an electrosurgical unit frequently is used to cut tissue and to coagulate bleeding points. The concentration and flow of current generates heat as it meets resistance in passage through tissue. Both cutting and coagulation currents are used in many open and closed operative procedures. Some surgeons prefer electrosurgery to other methods of cutting and ligating vessels. Coagulated tissue produces foreign-body reaction, however, which must be absorbed by the body during healing. If a large amount of coagulated tissue is present, sloughing may result so the wound may not heal by first intention. Refer to discussion of electrosurgery in Chapter 19.

Hemostatic Scalpel The sharp, heat-controlled steel blade of the hemostatic scalpel seals blood vessels as it cuts through tissue. Blood flow into incised area is minimal, providing surgeon with a clear, dry field. Electric current from the microcircuitry does not pass through patient, therefore, a grounding pad is not required.

Laser The laser light beam is successfully used for control of bleeding or for ablation and excision of tissues in organs that can be exposed or are accessible. The laser furnishes an intense and concentrated light beam of a single wavelength from a monochromatic source of radiation. Thermal energy of this beam may simultaneously cut, coagulate, and/or vaporize tissue. The laser wound is characterized by minimal bleeding and no visible postoperative edema. Amount of tissue destruction is predictable by adjusting width and focus of the beam. Different lasers have selective uses. Refer to Chapter 19 for detailed discussion of laser surgery.

Photocoagulation The photocoagulator utilizes an intense multiwavelength light furnished by a xenon tube to coagulate tissue. Since its use is limited to ophthalmology, refer to Chapter 25.

Plasma Scalpel The plasma scalpel vaporizes tissues and stops bleeding as it simultaneously cuts and coagulates tissue. Within the instrument, which looks like a large ballpoint pen, argon or helium gas passes through an electric arc that ionizes it into a high thermal state. These gases are inert and noncombustible. As instrument moves over tissue, the gas that flows from the tip is visible so the surgeon can see depth and extent of the incision. Tissue damage, with resultant inflammatory response during wound healing, is greater than that caused by a steel knife blade but less than that caused by other electrosurgical instruments and lasers. Because it will coagulate vessels up to 3 mm in diameter, the plasma scalpel is useful in highly vascular areas.

CHAPTER **18**

WOUND CLOSURE MATERIALS

One of the bases upon which surgery is founded as a distinct discipline of medicine is the control of bleeding and the closure of wounds. The story of sutures, in some measure, is the story of surgery itself. Many kinds of materials have been used to close wounds. Writings that are 4000 years old tell of the use of ligatures and sutures, but only since Lister's discoveries has their use been safe. Only since that time have suturing techniques and other methods of bringing tissue edges together been brought to an advanced state of development.

SUTURES

Common Terms

Suture is an all-inclusive term for any strand of material used for ligating or approximating tissue.

Ties If the material is tied around a blood vessel to occlude the lumen, it is called a *ligature* or *tie.* A *free tie* is a single strand of material handed to the surgeon or assistant to ligate a vessel. A strand attached to a needle before use is referred to as a *stick tie* or *suture/ligature.* The needle is used to anchor the strand in tissue before occluding a deep or large vessel.

Suture The verb *to suture* denotes the act of sewing by bringing tissues together and holding them until healing has taken place. A *suture,* the noun, is the strand of material used for this purpose.

Specifications for Suture Material

1 It must be sterile when placed in tissue. The principles of sterile technique must be rigidly followed in handling suture material. If the end of a strand drops over the side of any sterile surface, discard the strand.

2 It must be predictably uniform in tensile strength by size and material. *Tensile strength* is the measured pounds of tension or pull that a strand will withstand before it breaks when knotted. Minimum knot-pull strengths are specified for each basic raw material and for each size of that material by the United States Pharmacopeia (USP). Tensile strength decreases as the diameter of the strand decreases.

3 It must be as small in diameter as is safe to use on each type of tissue. The strength of the suture usually need be no greater than the strength of the tissue on which it is used. Smaller sizes are less traumatic during placement in tissue and leave less suture mass to cause tissue reaction. The surgeon ties small-diameter sutures more gently, and thus is less apt to strangulate tissue. A small-diameter suture is flexible, easy to manipulate, and leaves minimal scar on skin.

Sizes range from heavy 7 to very fine 11-0; ranges vary with materials. Taking size 1 as a starting point, sizes increase with each number above 1 and decrease with each 0 added. Thus size 7 is the largest and 11-0 is the smallest. The more 0s in the number, the smaller the size of the strand. As the number of 0s increases, the size of the strand decreases. In addition to this system of size designation, the manufacturer's labels on boxes and packets also may include metric measures for suture diameters. These metric equivalents vary slightly by types of materials.

4 It must have knot security, remain tied, and give support to tissue during the healing process. However, sutures in the skin are always removed three to ten days postoperatively, depending on the site of the incision and the cosmetic result desired. Because they are exposed to the external environment, skin sutures can be a source of microbial contamination of the wound that inhibits healing by first intention.

5 It must cause as little foreign-body tissue reaction as possible. All suture materials are foreign bodies, but some are more inert, less reactive, than others.

Choice of Suture Material

Surgical sutures as defined by the USP* are divided into two classifications: absorbable and nonabsorbable.

1 *Absorbable sutures* are sterile strands prepared from collagen derived from healthy mammals or from a synthetic polymer. They are capable of being absorbed by living mammalian tissue, but may be treated to modify resistance to absorption. They may be modified with respect to body or texture. They may be impregnated or coated with a suitable antimicrobial agent. They may be colored by a color additive approved by the Federal Food and Drug Administration (FDA).

2 *Nonabsorbable sutures* are strands of natural or synthetic material that effectively resist enzymatic digestion or absorption in living tissue. During healing process, suture mass becomes encapsulated and may remain for years in tissues without producing any ill effects. They may be colored by a color additive approved by the FDA. They may be modified with respect to body, texture, or capillarity. *Capillarity* refers to a characteristic of nonabsorbable sutures that allows passage of tissue fluids along the strand permitting infection, if present, to be drawn along the suture line. These suture materials may be untreated, or treated to reduce capillarity. *Noncapillarity* is the characteristic of some nonabsorbable sutures in which nature of the raw material or specific processing meets USP tests that establish them as resistant to "wicking" transfer of body fluids.

*United States Pharmacopeia, Twentieth Revision, Official from July 1, 1980, United States Pharmacopeial Convention, Rockville, Md., 1980.

The two classifications of suture materials are subdivided into monofilament and multifilament strands.

1 *Monofilament* suture is a strand consisting of a single threadlike structure that is noncapillary.

2 *Multifilament* suture is a strand made of more than one threadlike structure held together by braiding or twisting. This strand is capillary unless treated to resist capillarity or is absorbable.

The surgeon selects the type of suture material best suited to promote healing. Factors that influence choice include:

1 Biologic characteristics of the material in tissue, i.e., absorbable versus nonabsorbable, capillary versus noncapillary, inertness, etc.

2 Healing characteristics of tissue. Tissues that normally heal slowly such as skin, fascia, and tendons usually are closed with nonabsorbable sutures. Absorbable suture placed through the skin may cause a stitch abscess to develop as it is inclined to act as a culture medium for microorganisms in the pores of the skin. Tissues that heal rapidly such as stomach, colon, and bladder may be closed with absorbable sutures.

3 Location and length of the incision. Cosmetic results desired may be an influencing factor.

4 Presence or absence of infection, contamination, and/or drainage. If infection is present, sutures may be the origin of granuloma formation with subsequent discharge of suture and sinus formation. Foreign bodies in potentially contaminated tissues may convert contamination to infection. Foreign bodies in the presence of some body fluids may cause stone formation, as in the urinary or biliary tract.

5 Patient problems such as obesity, debility, age, diseases, that influence rate of healing and time desired for wound support.

6 Physical characteristics of the material such as ease of passage through tissue, knot tying, and other personal preferences of the surgeon.

Absorbable Sutures

Surgical Gut The early surgeons used gut strings discarded by the musicians. The strings on fiddles were called *kitstrings* because the fiddle itself was known as a *kit*. Since these strings were made of sheep intestines, they were called *kitgut*. However, a young cat is a kit, so eventually the word *catgut* replaced kitgut. The more accurate term *surgical gut* has replaced the term catgut.

Surgical gut is collagen derived from the submucosa of sheep intestine or the serosa of beef intestine. The intestines from these freshly slaughtered animals are sent to the processing plants. There they undergo many elaborate mechanical and chemical cleaning processes before ribbons are spun into strands of various sizes, ranging from the heaviest size 3 to the finest size 7-0. Although the larger sizes are made from two or more intestinal ribbons, the behavior of surgical gut is that of a monofilament suture.

Surgical gut is digested by body enzymes and absorbed by tissue; thus no permanent foreign body remains. Rate of absorption is influenced by:

1 *Type of tissue.* Surgical gut is absorbed much more rapidly in serous or mucous membrane. It is absorbed slowly in subcutaneous fat.

2 *Condition of tissue.* It can be used in presence of infection, and even the knots are absorbed. However, absorption takes place much more rapidly in the presence of infection.

3 *General health status of the patient.* Surgical gut may be absorbed more rapidly in undernourished or diseased tissue, but in old or debilitated patients it may remain for a long time.

4 *Type of surgical gut.* Plain gut is untreated, but chromic gut is treated to provide greater resistance to absorption. Surgical gut may be pliabilized to enhance its handling characteristics, but the process significantly reduces tensile strength.

Plain Surgical Gut Plain surgical gut loses tensile strength relatively quickly, usually in five to ten days, and is digested within 70 days, because collagen strands are not treated to resist absorption. Plain surgical gut is used to ligate small vessels and to suture subcutaneous fat. It is not used to suture any layers of tissue likely to be subjected to tension during healing. It is available in sizes 3 through 6-0. Usually used in its natural yellowish-tan color, it may be dyed blue or black.

Chromic Surgical Gut Chromic surgical gut is treated in a chromium salt solution to resist absorption by tissues for varying lengths of time depending on strength of the solution and duration and method of the process. The chromicizing process either bathes each ribbon of collagen before spinning into strands or applies solution to finished strand. This treatment changes color from the yellowish-tan shade of plain surgical gut to a dark shade of brown. Chromic surgical gut is used for ligation of larger vessels and for suture of tissues in which nonabsorbable materials are not usually recommended because they may act as a nidus for stone formation, as in the urinary or biliary tracts. In closure of muscle or fascia it has the disadvantage of rapidly declining tensile strength. If absorption rate is normal, chromic surgical gut will support the wound for about 14 days, with some strength up to 21 days, and will be completely absorbed within 90 days. Sizes range from 3 through 7-0. It may be dyed blue or black.

Collagen Sutures Collagen sutures are extruded from a homogeneous dispersion of pure collagen fibrils from the flexor tendons of beef. Both plain and chromic types are similar in appearance to surgical gut and may be dyed blue. Sizes range from 4-0 through 8-0. They are used primarily in ophthalmic surgery.

Handling characteristics of surgical gut and collagen:

1 Most surgical gut and collagen sutures are sealed in packets that contain fluid to keep the material pliable. This fluid is chiefly alcohol and water, *but may be irritating to ophthalmic tissues.* Hold packet over a basin and open carefully to avoid spilling fluid on the sterile field or splashing it into your own eyes. Rinsing is necessary *only* for surgical gut or collagen sutures to be implanted into the eye.

2 Surgical gut and collagen sutures should be used immediately after removal from their packets. When the material is removed and not used at once, the alcohol evaporates and the strand loses pliability. Many surgeons prefer that the scrub nurse quickly dip the strand into water or saline to soften it slightly. *Do not soak.* Excessive exposure to water will reduce the tensile strength. Before unwinding the strand, it can be dipped momentarily in water or saline at room temperature, not hot; heat will coagulate the protein.

3 Unwind the strand carefully. Handle it as little as possible. Never jerk or stretch surgical gut; that weakens it. Do not straighten suture by running fingers down its length; excessive handling with rubber gloves can cause fraying. Take the ends and tug gently to straighten.

Synthetic Absorbable Polymers Polymers, either dyed or undyed, are extruded into absorbable suture strands. These synthetic sutures are absorbed by a slow hydrolysis process in presence of tissue fluids. They are used for ligating or suturing except in tissues where extended approximation of tissues under stress is required. They are inert, nonantigenic, nonpyrogenic, and produce only a mild tissue reaction during absorption. They may be monofilament or multifilament, coated or uncoated.

Polydioxanone (PDS suture) A monofilament suture extruded from the polyester poly (p-dioxanone), PDS suture is particularly useful in tissues where both an absorbable suture and extended wound support are desirable. Absorption is minimal for about 90 days, and complete within 210 days. Approximately 50 percent of its tensile strength is retained for four weeks, and 25 percent for six weeks. Dyed violet, it is available in sizes 2 through 9-0, and clear in sizes 1 through 8-0.

Polyglactin 910 The precisely controlled combination of glycolide and lactide results in a copolymer with a molecular structure that maintains tensile strength longer than surgical gut, but not as long as polydioxanone. Approximately 30 percent of original strength is retained at three weeks. Absorption is minimal until about the 40th day, then it absorbs rapidly within 90 days. The acids of both glycolide and lactide exist naturally in the body and are readily excreted in urine. Polyglactin 910 sutures are available in two forms: uncoated monofilament and coated multifilament.

1 *Uncoated monofilament polyglactin 910 (Vicryl suture)* is available dyed violet in sizes 9-0 and 10-0 for ophthalmic procedures.

2 *Coated multifilament polyglactin 910 (Coated Vicryl suture)* is a braided strand coated with a mixture of equal parts of a copolymer of glycolide and lactide (polyglactin 370) and calcium stearate. The coating provides a nonflaking lubricant for smooth passage through tissue and precise knot placement. This absorbable coating does not affect absorption rate or tensile strength of the suture. It absorbs with the suture. Dyed violet, it is available in sizes 2 through 9-0, and undyed in sizes 1 through 8-0.

Polyglycolic Acid The homopolymer of glycolic acid loses tensile strength more rapidly and absorbs significantly more slowly than polyglactin 910. Strands are smaller in diameter than surgical gut of equivalent tensile strength. Polyglycolic acid suture loses approximately 45 percent of its tensile strength by 14 days, and absorbs significantly by 30 days. It is a braided suture material available in two forms: uncoated and coated.

1 *Uncoated polyglycolic acid (Dexon S suture)* is available dyed green in sizes 2 through 8-0, and undyed natural beige in sizes 2 through 7-0. (A 9-0 monofilament suture, dyed green, is also available.)

2 *Coated polyglycolic acid (Dexon Plus suture)* has a surfactant, poloxamer 188, on the surface that becomes slick in contact with body fluids for smooth passage through tissue. This suture requires two or three extra throws in knot tying, and ends must be cut longer than uncoated material. The coating virtually disappears from suture site in approximately seven hours. Sutures are available in the same sizes as uncoated polyglycolic acid sutures.

Handling characteristics of synthetic absorbable polymers:

1 Synthetic absorbable sutures have an expiration date on the package. Therefore, rotate stock. First in, first out is a good rule to follow.

2 Sutures are packaged and used dry. Do not soak or dip in water or saline. The material hydrolizes in water so that excessive exposure to moisture will reduce the tensile strength. It is smooth, soft, and will retain its pliability.

Nonabsorbable Sutures

Surgical Silk Surgical silk is an animal product made from the fiber spun by the silkworm larvae in making their cocoons. From the raw state, each fiber is processed to remove the natural waxes and gums. Fibers are braided or twisted together to form a multifilament suture strand. The braided type is used more frequently because surgeons prefer its high tensile strength and better handling qualities. Surgical silk is treated to render it noncapillary. It also is dyed, most commonly black, but also is available white. Sizes range from 5 through 9-0.

Silk is not a true nonabsorbable material. It loses much of its tensile strength after about one year and usually disappears after two or more years. It gives good support to wounds during early ambulation and generally promotes healing a little more rapidly than surgical gut. It causes less tissue reaction than surgical gut, but is not as inert as most of the other nonabsorbable materials. It is used frequently in serosa of the gastrointestinal tract and to close fascia in the absence of infection.

Virgin Silk Virgin silk suture consists of several natural silk filaments drawn together and twisted to form 8-0 and 9-0 strands for tissue approximation of delicate structures, primarily in ophthalmic surgery. It is white or dyed black.

Dermal Silk Dermal suture is a strand of twisted silk fibers encased in a nonabsorbing coating of tanned gelatin or other protein substance. This coating prevents the ingrowth of tissue cells and facilitates removal after use as a skin suture. It is used for suturing the skin particularly in areas of tension because of its unusual strength. It is black in sizes 0 through 5-0.

Handling characteristics of silk sutures:

1 Silk sutures are dry. They lose tensile strength if wet. Therefore, do not moisten before use.

2 If it is necessary to autoclave silk suture, do so at 250°F (121°C) for 15 minutes. Silk shrinks during sterilization and must never be sterilized on a spool, if supplied nonsterile. Some tensile strength is lost during sterilization.

Surgical Cotton Surgical cotton suture is made from individual, long-staple cotton fibers that are combed, aligned, and twisted into a smooth multifilament strand. Sizes range from 1 through 5-0. Usually white, it may be dyed blue or pink.

Cotton is one of the weakest of the nonabsorbable materials; however, it gains tensile strength when wet. Moisten before handing to the surgeon. Tensile strength is increased ten percent by moisture. Also, moisture prevents clinging to the surgeon's gloves. Like silk, cotton suture may be used in most body tissues for ligating and suturing, but it offers no advantages over silk.

Linen Surgical linen is spun from long-staple flax fibers, then twisted into tight strands and treated for smooth passage through tissue. Tensile strength is inferior to all other nonabsorbable materials. Linen suture is used almost exclusively in gastrointestinal surgery in sizes 0 and 2-0.

Surgical Stainless Steel Stainless steel sutures are drawn from 316L-SS (L for low carbon) iron alloy wire. This is the same metal formula used in the manufacture of surgical stainless steel implants and prostheses.

NOTE. *Two different kinds of metal must not be embedded in the tissues simultaneously.* Such a combination creates an unfavorable electrolytic reaction. Some implants and prostheses are made of vitallium, titanium, or tantalum. Suture material in the wound must be compatible with these metals.

Prior to the availability of surgical stainless steel from suture manufacturers, commercial steel was purchased by weight, using the Brown & Sharpe (B&S) scale for diameter variations. Many surgeons still refer to surgical stainless steel size by the B&S gauge with 18, the largest diameter, ranging to 40, the smallest. One manufacturer labels surgical stainless steel with both B&S gauge and equivalent USP diameter classifications from 7 through 6-0. Both monofilament and twisted multifilament stainless steel strands are available.

Surgical stainless steel is inert in tissue and has high tensile strength. It gives the greatest strength of any suture material to a wound before healing begins and supports a wound indefinitely. Some surgeons use stainless steel for closure following operations on the gastrointestinal tract and thus reduce the danger of wound disruption in the presence of contributing factors. It may be used in the presence of infection or in patients in which slow healing is expected. It is used for secondary repair or resuture. Following evisceration (see Chap. 36), it may be used in place of surgical gut that has been too rapidly absorbed.

Unlike most other suture materials, steel lacks elasticity. A suture tied too tightly may act as a knife and cut through tissue. Stainless steel sutures are harder to handle than any other suture material. A painstaking knot-tying technique is required. This disadvantage more than outweighs the advantages for routine use for most surgeons. However, in selected situations it fills an important need. It is widely used in the respiratory tract, in tendon repair, in orthopaedics and neurosurgery, and for general wound closure.

Handling characteristics of stainless steel:

1 Surgical stainless steel strands are malleable and kink rather easily. Kinks in the strand can make it practically useless. Therefore, care must be taken in handling to keep strand straight.

2 Use wire scissors for cutting stainless steel sutures. Barbs on the end of a strand can tear gloves, thus breaking sterile technique, or traumatize tissue.

3 If surgical stainless steel must be threaded to a needle, some surgeons prefer one or two twists of the end around the strand just below the eye of the needle to prevent unthreading during suturing.

Synthetic Nonabsorbable Polymers Although silk is the most frequently used nonabsorbable suture material, synthetic nonabsorbable materials are used because they offer unique advantages in many situations. They have higher tensile strength and elicit less tissue reaction than silk. They retain their strength in tissue. Knot tying with most of these materials is more difficult than with silk. Additional throws are required to secure the knot. The surgeon may sacrifice some handling characteristics and ease of knot tying for strength, durability, and nonreactivity of the synthetics. These advantages may outweigh the disadvantages.

Surgical Nylon Nylon is a polyamide polymer derived by chemical synthesis from coal, air, and water. It produces minimal tissue reaction. Nylon has high tensile strength, but it degrades by hydrolysis in tissue at a rate of about 15 to 20 percent per year. It may be used in all tissues where a nonabsorbable suture is acceptable, except when long-term support is critical. It is available in three forms: monofilament, uncoated multifilament, and coated multifilament.

1 *Monofilament nylon (Ethilon suture and Dermalon suture)* is a smooth single strand of noncapillary material, clear or dyed black, blue, or green. The smaller the diameter becomes, the stronger the strand becomes proportionately. Sizes range from 2 through 11-0; the latter is the smallest of all sutures manufactured for use in microsurgery. Monofilament nylon is also used frequently in ophthalmic surgery because it has a desirable degree of elasticity. Larger sizes are used for skin closure, particularly by plastic surgeons where cosmetic results are important, and for retention sutures. Wet or damp monofilament nylon is more pliable and easier to handle than dry nylon. A limited line of sutures are supplied in a moisturized state; most are supplied dry.

2 *Uncoated multifilament nylon (Nurolon suture)* is very tightly braided and treated to prevent capillary action. Usually used dyed black, but also available white, nylon looks, feels, and handles similarly to silk, but is stronger and elicits less tissue reaction than silk. Sizes range from 1 through 7-0. It may be used in all tissues where a multifilament nonabsorbable suture is acceptable.

3 *Coated multifilament nylon (Surgilon suture)* is a braided strand of nylon treated with silicone to enhance its passage through tissue. Otherwise its characteristics are similar to silk and uncoated multifilament nylon.

Polyester Fiber A polymer of terephthalic acid and polyethylene, Dacron polyester fiber is braided into a multifilament suture strand available in two forms; uncoated and coated fibers.

1 *Uncoated polyester fiber suture (Mersilene and Dacron suture)* is closely braided to provide a flexible, pliable strand that is relatively easy to handle. However, uncoated braided polyester fiber suture has a tendency to "drag" and exert a sawing or tearing effect when passed through tissue. It may be used in all tissues where a multifilament nonabsorbable suture is indicated. It is especially useful in the respiratory tract and for some cardiovascular procedures. Available white or dyed green or blue, sizes range from 2 through 10-0.

2 *Coated polyester fiber suture* has a lubricated surface for smooth passage through tissue. It is widely used in cardiovascular surgery for vessel anastomosis and placement of prosthetic materials because it retains its strength indefinitely in tissues. Sutures are available with different coating materials:

- **a** *Polybutilate* is the only coating developed specifically as a surgical lubricant. This polyester material adheres strongly to the braided polyester fiber. Polyester fiber coated with polybutilate *(Ethibond suture)* provides a strand superior to any other braided material, coated or uncoated, in decreasing drag through tissue. Colored green or white, sizes range from 5 through 7-0.
- **b** *Polytetrafluoroethylene,* a commercial product known by the DuPont trade name Teflon, is used as a coating bonded to the surface *(Polydek suture),* or impregnated into spaces in the braid of the polyester fiber strand *(Tevdek suture).* Minute particles of this coating can flake off the strand. Since they are insoluble and resistant to enzymes, foreign-body granulomas may be produced. Sutures with this material on them are white or dyed green and available in sizes 5 through 10-0.
- **c** *Silicone* is a commercial lubricant that provides a slippery coating but does not bond well to polyester fiber. It can become dislodged in the tissues as the strand is tied. Sutures with this coating *(Ti-Cron sutures)* are

available white or dyed blue in sizes 5 through 7-0.

Polyethylene (Dermalene suture) Polyethylene is a long-chain plastic polymer extruded into a blue-dyed monofilament suture strand. It is available in sizes 0 through 6-0 for use in some situations in which a monofilament material may be desired.

Polypropylene (Prolene suture and Surgilene suture) Polypropylene is a polymerized propylene extruded into a monofilament suture strand. It may be clear or pigmented with blue dye. It is the most inert of the synthetic materials and almost wholly as inert as surgical stainless steel. Polypropylene is an acceptable substitute for stainless steel in situations where strength and nonreactivity are required and the suture must be left in place for prolonged healing. It can be used in the presence of infection. It has become the material of choice for many plastic surgery and cardiovascular procedures because of its smooth passage through tissue as well as its strength and inertness. Polypropylene sutures are available from sizes 2 through 10-0.

SURGICAL NEEDLES

Except for simple ligating with free ties, surgical needles are needed to safely carry suture material through tissue with the least amount of trauma. The best surgical needles are made of high-quality tempered steel that:

1 Is strong enough so it does not break easily
2 Is rigid enough to prevent excessive bending, yet flexible enough to prevent breaking after bending
3 Is sharp enough to penetrate tissue with minimal resistance, yet need not be stronger than the tissue it penetrates
4 Is approximately the same diameter as the suture material it carries to minimize trauma in passage through tissue
5 Is appropriate in shape and size for the type, condition, and accessibility of the tissue to be sutured
6 Is free from corrosion and burrs to prevent infection and tissue trauma

Many shapes and sizes of surgical needles are available. The names vary from one manufacturer to another; general classification only, not nomenclature, is standardized. They may be straight (like a sewing needle) or curved. All surgical needles have three basic components: the point, the body or shaft, and the eye. They are classified according to these three components.

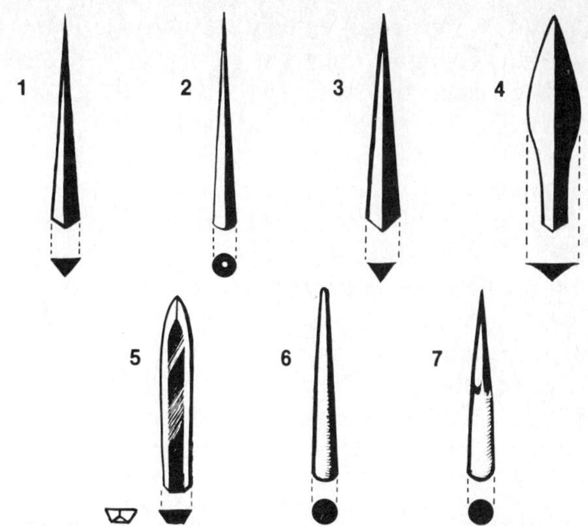

FIGURE 18-1
Configurations of needle points: (1) precision point cutting, (2) taper, (3) reverse cutting, (4) trocar, (5) side cutting, (6) blunt, (7) cutting edge at end of tapered point.

Points of Needles

Points of surgical needles are honed to configuration and sharpness desired for specific types of tissue. The basic shapes are cutting, tapered, or blunt (see Fig. 18-1).

Cutting Point A razor-sharp honed cutting point may be preferred when tissue is difficult to penetrate, such as skin, tendon, and tough tissues in the eye. These make a slight cut in tissue as they penetrate. Location and degree of sharpness of cutting edges vary.

Conventional Cutting Needles Two opposing cutting edges form a triangular configuration with a third edge on body of the needle. Cutting edges are on the inside curvature of a curved needle. Cutting edges may be honed to precision sharpness to assure smooth passage through tissue and a minute needle path that heals quickly.

Reverse Cutting Needles A triangular configuration extends along body of the needle. The edges near the point are sharpened or honed to precision points. The two opposing cutting edges are on outer curvature of a curved needle.

Side Cutting Needles Relatively flat on top and bottom, angulated cutting edges are on the sides. Used primarily in ophthalmic surgery, they will not penetrate underlying tissues. They split through layers of tissue.

Trocar Points Sharp cutting tips are at the points of tapered needles. All three edges of the tip are sharpened to provide cutting action with the smallest possible hole in tissue as it penetrates.

Taper Point These needles are used in soft tissues, such as intestine and peritoneum, which offer a small amount of resistance to the needle as it passes through. They tend to push the tissue aside as they go through rather than cut it. The body tapers to a sharp point at the tip.

Blunt Point These tapered needles are designed with a rounded blunt point at the tip. They are used for suturing friable tissue, such as liver and kidney. Because the blunt point will not cut through tissue, it is less apt to puncture a vessel in these organs than a sharp-pointed needle.

Body of Needle

The body, or shaft, varies in wire gauge, length, shape, and finish. The nature and location of tissue to be sutured influence selection of needles with these variable features.

1 Tough or fibrosed tissue requires a heavier gauge needle than the fine gauge wire needed in microsurgery.
2 Depth of "bite" (placement) through tissue determines appropriate length.
3 Body may be round, oval, flat, or triangular. The point determines the shape: round or oval bodies have trocar, taper, or blunt points; flat or triangular bodies have cutting edges. The shape also may be straight or curved (see Fig. 18-2).
   a Straight needles are used in readily accessible tissue. They have cutting points for use in skin, the most frequent use, or tapered points for use in intestinal tissue.
   b Curved needles are used to approximate most tissues because quick needle turnout is an advantage. The curvature may be ¼, ⅜, ½, ⅝ circle, half-curved with only the tip curved, or compound curved. *Curved needles always are armed in a needleholder before being handed to the surgeon.*
4 Curved needles that have longitudinal ribbed depressions or grooves along body on inside and outside curvature create a cross-locking action of the needle in the needleholder. This feature virtually eliminates twisting or turning of the needle in any position in the needleholder.
5 Body of all needles must have a smooth finish. Many needles have a surface coating of microthin plastic or silicone to enhance smooth passage through tissue.

Eye of Needle

The eye is segment of needle where suture strand is attached. Surgical needles are classified as eyed, French eye, or eyeless (see Fig. 18-3).

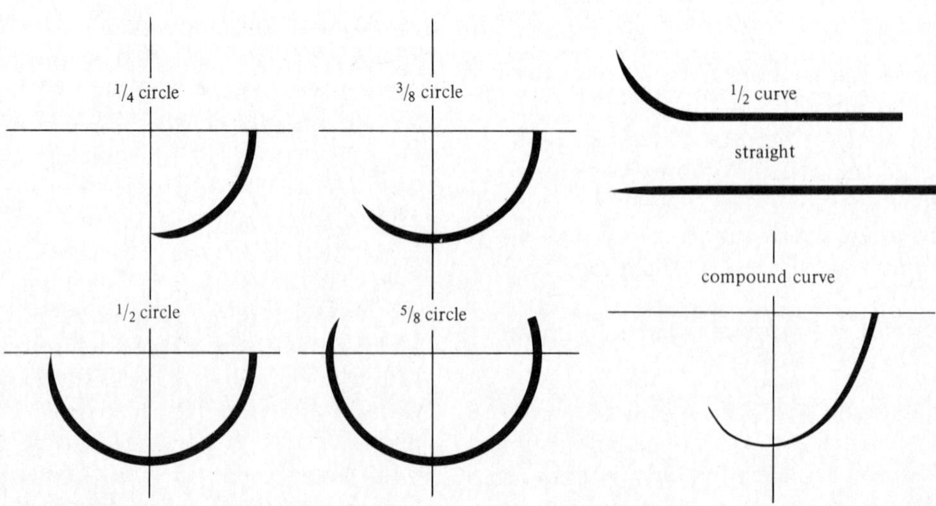

FIGURE 18-2
Shape of needle bodies.

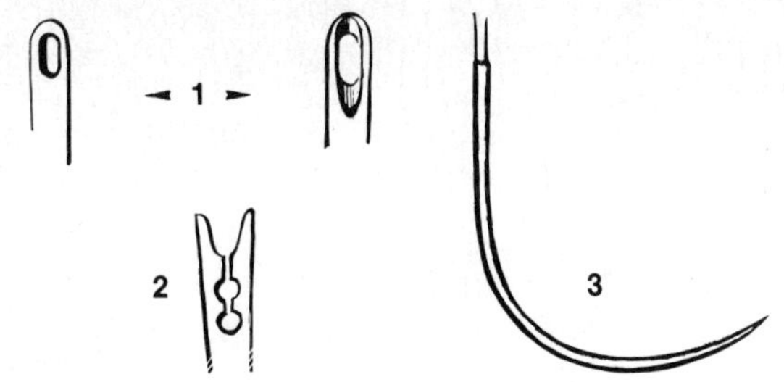

FIGURE 18-3
Eyes of needles: (1) oblong eyes, (2) French eye, (3) eyeless (swaged).

Eyed Needle The closed eye of an eyed surgical needle is like that of any household sewing needle. Shape of the enclosed eye may be round, oblong, or square. End of the suture strand is pulled 2 to 4 in. (5 to 10 cm) through the eye, so short end is about one-sixth the length of the long one.

French Eye Needle Sometimes referred to as *spring eye* or *split eye,* a French eye needle has a slit from inside of the eye to end of the needle through which the suture strand is drawn. To thread a French eye after arming needle in a needleholder, secure 2 to 3 in. (5 to 7.5 cm) of the strand between fingers holding the needleholder. Pull strand taut across center of V-shaped area above the eye and draw down through slit into the eye (see Fig. 18-4). French eye needles as a general rule are used with pliable braided materials, primarily silk and cotton, of medium or fine size. These needles are not practical for surgical gut, as strand may fray or eye may break because the diameter is usually too large for the slit.

NOTE. Eyed and French eye needles have disadvantages for the scrub nurse, surgeon, and patient.

1. Each needle must be carefully inspected by the scrub nurse for dull or burred points, corrosion, and defects in the eye before and after use.
2. Care must be taken to avoid puncturing gloves with needle point when threading.

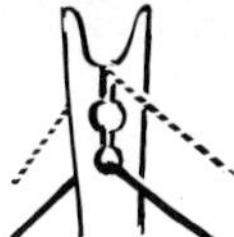

FIGURE 18-4
To thread French eye needle, pull strand taut across center of V-shaped area and draw down through the slit into the eye.

3. The scrub nurse may have to choose an appropriate needle to thread. The needle should be the same approximate diameter as the suture size requested by the surgeon.
4. Needles can unthread prematurely. This is both an annoyance to the surgeon and an uneconomical use of time for the patient. To avoid this, the surgeon may prefer the suture strand threaded double with both ends of the suture pulled the same length through the eye; the ends may be tied together in a knot, if desired. Or the scrub nurse may lock the suture strand by threading the short end through the eye twice in the same direction.
5. Two strands of suture material are pulled through tissue when threaded needles are used. The bulk of the double strand through the eye creates a larger hole than size of needle or suture material with additional trauma to tissue.

Eyeless Needle An eyeless needle is a continuous unit with the suture strand. The needle is swaged onto end of strand in the manufacturing process. This eliminates threading at the operating table and minimizes tissue trauma by drawing a single strand of material through tissue. The diameter of the needle matches the size of the strand as closely as possible. The surgeon uses a new sharp needle with every suture strand. Usually referred to as *swaged needles,* four types of eyeless needle-suture attachments are available.

Single-armed Attachment Has one needle swaged to the suture strand.

Double-armed Attachment Has a needle swaged to each end of the suture strand. The two needles are not necessarily the same size and shape. These are used when the surgeon wishes to place a suture and then continue to approximate surrounding tissue on both sides from a midpoint in the strand.

Permanently Swaged Needle Attachment Is secure so that the needle will not separate from the suture strand under normal use. The needle is separated by cutting it from the strand.

Controlled Release Needle Attachment Is secure so that the suture strand does not separate from the needle inadvertently but does release rapidly when pulled off intentionally. The surgeon grasps the suture strand just below the needle, pulling strand taut, and releases the needle with a straight tug of the needleholder on the needle. This facilitates fast separation of needle from suture when desired.

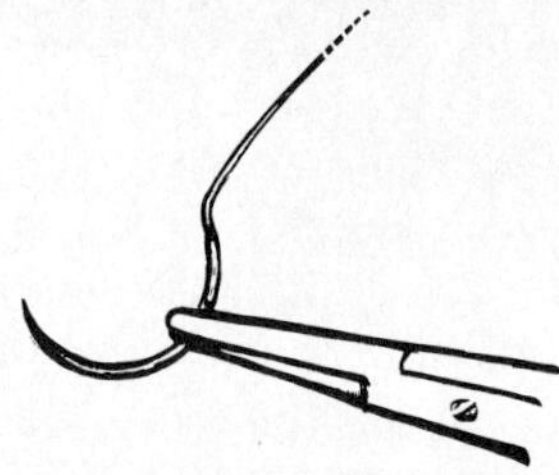

FIGURE 18-5
Correct position of a curved needle in a needleholder, about one-third down from swage or eye.

Placement of Needle in Needleholder

Needleholders have specially designed jaws to securely grasp surgical needles without damage if used correctly. The scrub nurse should observe the following principles in handling needles and needleholders:

1 Select a needleholder with appropriate size jaws for the size needle to be used. An extremely small needle requires a needleholder with very fine tipped jaws. As the wire gauge of the needle increases, the jaws of the needleholder selected should be proportionately wider and heavier.

2 Select an appropriate length needleholder for area of tissue to be sutured. When surgeon works deep inside the abdomen, chest, or pelvic cavity, a longer needleholder will be needed than in superficial areas.

3 Clamp body of the needle in an area about one-fourth or one-half of distance from the eye to the point. *Never clamp the needleholder over the swaged area.* This is weakest area of an eyeless needle because it is hollow before the suture strand is attached. Pressure on or near needle-suture juncture may break it (see Fig. 18-5).

4 Place needle securely in the tip of the needleholder jaws and close it in the first or second ratchet. If the needle is held too tightly in the jaws or the needleholder is defective, the needle may be damaged or notched in such a manner that it will have a tendency to bend or break on successive passes through tissue.

5 Hand the needleholder to the surgeon so the suture strand is free and not entangled with the needleholder. Hold the free end of the suture in one hand while passing the needleholder with the other hand. Protect the end of the suture material from dragging across the sterile field. The assistant may take hold of the free end to keep the strand straight for the surgeon and to keep it from falling over the side of the sterile field.

6 Pass needleholder with needle point up and directed toward the surgeon's thumb when grasped, so it is ready for use without readjustment.

7 Hand a needleholder to assistant to pull needle out through tissue. Do not use a hemostat or other tissue forceps for this purpose, as the instrument may be damaged or it may damage the needle. The needle should be grasped as far back as possible to avoid damage to taper points or cutting edges.

COMMON SUTURING TECHNIQUES

Primary Suture Line

The *primary suture line* refers to those sutures that hold wound edges in approximation during healing by first intention. This line may have one continuous strand of suture material or a series of suture strands. A variety of techniques are used to place sutures in tissues. The most common terms for these techniques are described.

Continuous Suture A series of stitches are taken with one strand of material tied only at ends of the suture line. This may be referred to as a *running stitch.* Closure is rapid, and less suture mass remains in the tissue. A continuous suture is used to close peritoneum because it also provides a temporary water seal. Configuration of the stitches varies with tissue and desired cosmetic result.

Interrupted Suture Each stitch is taken and tied separately. This is the technique recommended by Dr. Halsted for two reasons: if an interrupted suture breaks or loosens, the remaining sutures may still hold the wound together; in the presence of infection, microorganisms are less likely to follow the primary suture line.

Buried Suture A suture placed under the skin, buried, may be either continuous or interrupted.

Purse-String Suture A continuous suture is placed around a lumen and tightened, drawstring fashion, to close the lumen. This is used when inverting the stump of the appendix, for example.

Subcuticular Suture A continuous suture is placed beneath epithelial layer of skin in short lateral stitches. The suture comes through upper layer of skin at each end of the incision only. A perforated lead shot may be crushed tightly on each suture end. The suture is drawn tight enough to hold skin edges in approximation. It is easily removed by cutting off the shot at one end, grasping the other shot, and pulling the entire strand through the length of the incision. It was first used by Dr. Halsted. It leaves a minimal scar.

Secondary Suture Line

The *secondary suture line* refers to those sutures that reinforce and support the primary suture line, obliterate dead space, and prevent fluid accumulation in the wound during healing by first intention. They exert tension lateral to the primary suture line, which contributes to the tensile strength of the wound. Sutures used for this purpose are referred to as retention, stay, or tension sutures.

Retention Sutures Interrupted nonabsorbable sutures are placed through tissue on each side of primary suture line, a short distance from it, to relieve tension on it. Heavy strands are used in sizes ranging from 0 through 5. The tissue through which retention sutures are passed includes skin, subcutaneous tissue, fascia, and may include rectus muscle and peritoneum of an abdominal incision. Following abdominal operations, retention sutures are used frequently in patients in which slow healing is expected: due to malnutrition, obesity, carcinoma, or infection; in the elderly; for a patient on cortisone; or a patient with respiratory problems. Retention sutures may be used as a precautionary measure to prevent wound disruption when postoperative stress on the primary suture line from distention, vomiting, or coughing is anticipated. They should be removed as soon as the danger of sudden increases in intraabdominal pressure is over, usually on the fourth or fifth postoperative day. Retention sutures are also used to support wounds for healing by second intention and for secondary closure following wound disruption for healing by third intention.

Retention Bridges, Bolsters, and Bumpers To prevent the heavy suture from cutting into the skin, several different kinds of bridges, bolsters, or bumpers are used with retention sutures.

1 A *bridge* is a plastic device placed on the skin to span over the incision. The retention suture is brought through skin on both sides of the incision, through holes on each side of the bridge, and fastened over the bridge. One type allows adjustment of tension on the suture during the postoperative healing period.

2 *Bolsters* and *bumpers*—the names are used interchangeably—are segments of plastic or rubber tubing. One end of the suture is threaded through the tubing before the suture is tied. It covers all the suture strand that is on the skin surface (refer to Fig. 21-3, p. 403). Buttons and lead shot are also used as bolsters and bumpers with some other types of suturing techniques, especially in plastic and orthopaedic surgery.

Traction Suture

A *traction suture* may be used to retract a suture to the side of the operative field, out of the way, as the tongue in an operation in the mouth. Usually a nonabsorbable suture is placed through the part. Other materials may be used to retract or ligate vessels.

1 *Umbilical tape.* Aside from its original use for tying the umbilical cord on a newborn, this tape has uses in surgery. In certain cardiovascular operations, it is used as a heavy tie, or as a traction suture. It may be put around a great vessel to retract it. It is available on spools from which desired lengths are cut or as sterile strands in tubes.

2 *Aneurysm needle.* An aneurysm needle is an instrument with a blunt needle on the end. The eye is on the distal end of the needle. The needle forms a right or oblique angle to the handle, which is one continuous unit with the needle. The needles are made in symmetrical pairs—right and left. The surgeon uses them when he wishes to take a ligature around a deep, large vessel, as in a thyroidectomy or in thoracic surgery.

SURGEON'S CHOICE

The surgeon chooses from available types and sizes of sutures and needles the ones that best suit each purpose. In general, fine sizes are used for plastic, pediatric, vascular surgery; medium sizes for all kinds of surgery except the above; heavy sizes are for retention sutures and occasionally for anchoring bone. In general, cutting needles are used in tough tissue such as skin, fascia, tendon, and mucous membranes including cervix, tonsil, palate, tongue, and nose. Medium tissue calls for round taper point or cutting needles. Round taper point needles usually are used for nerve, peritoneum, muscle, and other soft tissue such as lung and intestine, subcutaneous tissue, and dura.

It is almost impossible to learn the needle-tissue-suture-surgeon combinations by memory alone because of the unlimited number of combinations. Learning the general classification of needles, sutures, and tissues is the first step; practical experience is necessary to fix in mind the combinations. Do not feel discouraged when you cannot anticipate the surgeon's wishes and do not hesitate to ask when you are uncertain of the proper combination at the proper time.

The preference card usually lists the surgeon's usual suture and needle routine by tissue layer. Some hospitals list swaged sutures by code number. Others list sutures by size and materials and needles by size and shape. Remember, suture and needle sizes are as variable as patient sizes. Therefore, the surgeon may unexpectedly request a smaller or larger size out of routine for a particular patient situation.

SUTURES AND NEEDLES: PACKAGING AND PREPARING

Most suture material is individually packaged and supplied sterile by the manufacturer. It is sterilized by cobalt 60 irradiation or ethylene oxide gas. A few materials may be steam sterilized, but most cannot. Protein in absorbable materials derived from animals will coagulate; synthetic absorbables are affected by moisture and heat. Only stainless steel can be repeatedly steam sterilized. Nylon, polyester fiber, and polyproplyene can be steam sterilized a maximum of three times without loss of tensile strength. Follow the manufacturer's recommendations for sterilization of nonsterile suture materials.

Many hospitals use only swaged-on needles. As these come in the sterile packets with the suture material, they eliminate the labor and expense of cleaning, packaging, and sterilizing needles. Disposable eyed and French eye needles are packaged and sterilized by the manufacturer.

Preparation of Reusable Needles

Standard sets of reusable eyed and French eye needles may be prepared for each operation or type of operation. This necessitates preparing many more needles in a set than any one surgeon uses if all surgeons' preferences are to be accommodated. An alternative may be to choose needles for each operation on the operating schedule according to each surgeon's preferences listed on a needle card. The basic set for the operation and the names of the surgeons who vary from this and their variations are listed. A needle card is maintained in a file for each operation and kept with the stock needle supply.

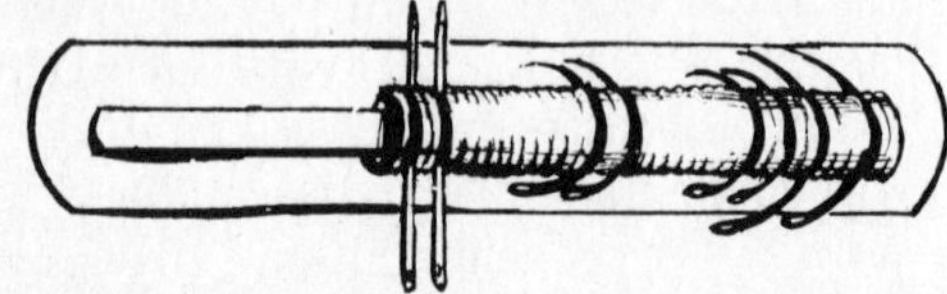

FIGURE 18-6
Metal needle rack with spring to hold eyed needles. Round and cutting needles are separated.

Eyed needles can be loaded on a metal rack with a spring to hold them (see Fig. 18-6). The rack can be steam sterilized with the instruments for that operation or it may be wrapped, labeled, and sterilized separately.

Packaging of Suture Materials

A strand of sterile suture material is supplied with as many as four coverings.

Box Each box contains one, two, or three dozen packets of sterile suture material. Label on the box may be color-coded by suture material, e.g., light blue for silk, yellow for plain surgical gut. Most boxes fit into a suture cabinet rack.

Overwrap Each packet has a hermetically sealed outer overwrap. This usually is a laminate of foil paper or coated Tyvek on one side and clear plastic film on the other. The overwrap is peeled back to expose inner primary packet for sterile transfer to the sterile table. The circulating nurse must not contaminate the sterile inner primary packet as the overwrap is peeled apart and the packet is flipped onto the sterile table.

Primary Packet Suture material, with or without swaged needles, is hermetically sealed in a primary packet that is opened by the scrub nurse. The primary packet may be made of foil, paper, plastic, or combinations of these. Labels may be color-coded by material, the same as the box. A silhouette of the needle is included on the label, if a swaged needle is enclosed, along with the size and type of suture material. A single strand of material or multiple strands may be in the primary packet. The packet may be designed for dispensing individual strands from a multiple suture packet, such as the labyrinth primary packet.

NOTE. 1. Suture packets, both overwrap and primary, should be opened only as needed. However, occasionally primary packets are removed from the overwrap, put onto the instrument table, and then not needed. If clean hermetically sealed foil primary packets are not opened or damaged, they may be returned to the manufacturer to be rewrapped and sterilized. The suture material is not resterilized, only the primary packet is; the suture remains sterile. Unopened primary packets must be decontaminated before placing in collection box or other storage container (see Chap. 10). Avoid opening overwrap unless material is needed.

2. Sterile suture packets are labeled "Do Not Resterilize." Component layers of the packaging materials do not permit exposure to heat of steam sterilization without potential physical damage to contents and packets. Ethylene oxide must be carefully controlled. The manufacturer will not guarantee product stability or sterility for packets sterilized in the hospital, or strands removed from packets and sterilized.

3. Some suture materials have an expiration date stamped on box and primary packet to indicate known shelf life of the material. Oldest sutures should be used first.

Inner Dispenser Suture material is contained within the primary packet in a manner to facilitate removing or dispensing. This may be a folder, reel, organizer, or tube that may or may not be removed with the suture strands.

Preparation of Suture Material

Length of each strand of suture material within the primary packet varies; the shortest is 5 in. (approximately 13 cm) and the longest is 60 in. (150 cm). The most commonly used lengths range from 18 to 30 in. (45 to 75 cm). Length surgeon prefers should be noted on the preference card. The scrub nurse may have to cut strands to the desired length, depending upon lengths available.

Standard Length This term refers to a 60-in. (150 cm) strand of nonabsorbable or a 54-in. (135 cm) strand of absorbable material without a swaged needle. It is never handed to the surgeon in this length. The scrub nurse may cut it into a half-length, third-length, or fourth-length for use as a free tie or thread it for a stick tie or suture as shown in Figures 18-7 and 18-8.

Ligating Reels Twelve feet (approximately 4 m) of nonabsorbable or 54 in. (135 cm) of absorbable suture are wound on disc-like plastic reels. These reels are color-coded by material and have size identification. The surgeon keeps the reel in the palm of his or her hand for a series of free ties.

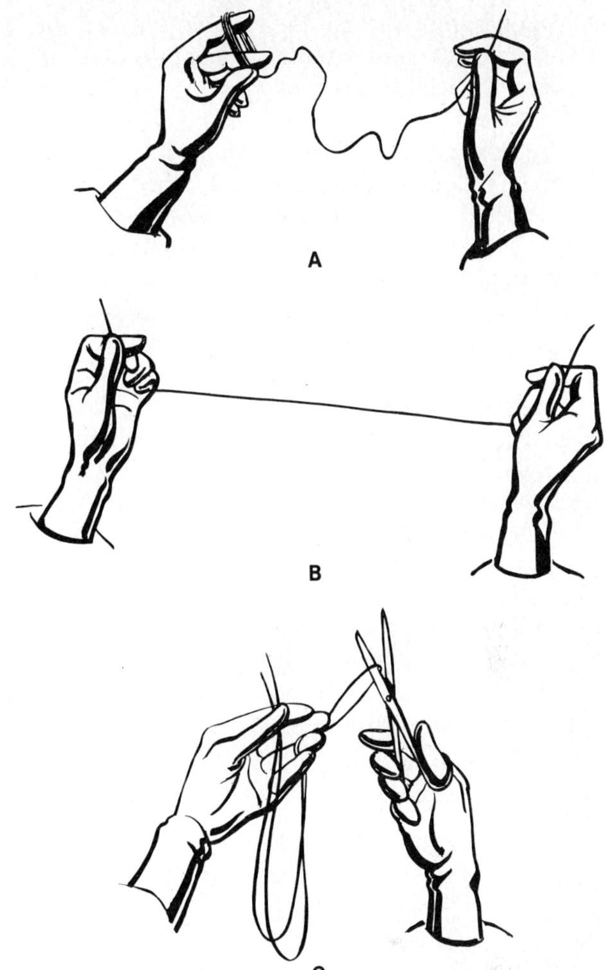

FIGURE 18-7
Sequence of scrub nurse preparing half-lengths of surgical gut suture. (**A**) The suture loops are separated by the fingers of the left hand while unwinding. (**B**) The full-length is gently unwound and straightened before cutting. The scrub nurse does not pull hard or test the strand, but keeps a firm grasp on both ends to prevent the suture from snapping away and possibly becoming contaminated. (**C**) Bend the suture in half and cut the loop.

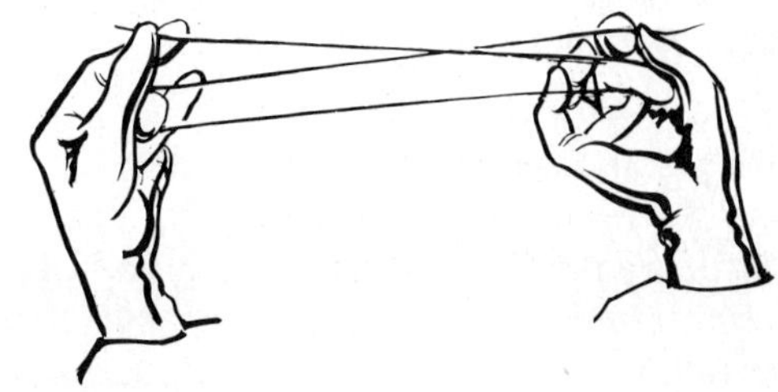

FIGURE 18-8
Scrub nurse preparing one-third length sutures. Pass one free end of the full-length strand from right to left hand, at the same time catching a loop around the third finger of right hand. Catching the other loop around the third finger of left hand while holding onto each end, adjust the suture to equal lengths (thirds), then cut each loop with scissors.

If these are not stocked, the surgeon may ask the scrub nurse to wind a standard length onto a rod or other device for this purpose.

Precut Lengths Most suture materials are supplied in lengths ready for use as free ties or for threading. These facilitate handling for the scrub nurse. They are dispensed individually from some primary packets or may be removed and placed in a fold of the suture book. Packets contain from 3 to 17 strands, depending on the material.

Swaged Needle-Suture Lengths are predetermined by the manufacturer; however, the surgeon has a wide variety of choices to meet all suturing needs. The scrub nurse must remember that a strand can be shortened but not extended. An appropriate length for the location of the tissue must be handed to the surgeon. A packet may contain one suture strand with single- or double-armed needle(s), or multiple strands with needles. The needle may be armed in needleholder and withdrawn from inner dispenser of some packets.

SURGICAL STAPLES

The first surgical stapler was introduced in Hungary in 1908 for closing the stomach. This was followed in 1924, also in Hungary, by a mechanical device for gastrointestinal anastomosis developed by Aladar von Petz. Although cumbersome and heavy, the von Petz clamp received worldwide acceptance. The Russians subsequently became the leaders in the field of stapling tissue with their refinements in instrumentation during the 1950s. Most of the reusable staplers currently in use became available in the United States in the 1960s through patents licensed from the Soviet Union. Since 1978, disposable stapling instruments have been developed. With these instruments, surgeons can join tissue together with surgical stainless steel staples.

Advantages of Using Staples

1 This is a rapid method to ligate, anastomose, and approximate tissues. The time saved over conventional suturing techniques reduces total operating time, anesthesia time for the patient, and blood loss.

2 The healing of tissues may be accelerated because of minimal trauma and nonreactive nature of the stainless steel staples.

3 They produce an airtight, leakproof closure.

4 They can safely be used in many types of tissues and have a wide range of applications.

Stapling Instruments

Each stapler is designed for stapling specific tissues, i.e., skin, fascia, bronchus, gastrointestinal tract, or vessels. The surgeon selects the correct instrument for the desired application. The consequences of an erroneous staple application are much more difficult to correct than those of manually placed sutures. The surgeon must learn when and how to use each instrument. Whether the stapler is reusable or a single-use disposable, the basic technical mechanics of stapling are the same.

Staplers fire either a single staple or simultaneously fire one or two straight or circular rows of staples. A different instrument must be used for each type of firing.

Skin Stapler To approximate skin edges, the stapler fires a single staple with each squeeze of the trigger. Edges of both cuticular and subcuticular layers must be everted, that is aligned with edges slightly raised in an outward direction, as close to their original configuration on the horizontal plane as possible. The stapler is positioned over the line of incision so that the staple will be placed evenly on each side. The staple forms a rectangular shape over the incision. As many staples are placed as needed to close the incision. Skin staplers are supplied preloaded with different quantities of staples in varying widths, i.e., crown span. The most appropriate stapler should be chosen for the selected use. For example, an average range of 28 to 35 staples is needed to close the majority of abdominal incisions. More may be needed to close the chest, fewer for an inguinal herniorrhaphy.

Skin staples must be removed, usually five to seven days postoperatively. Extractors are used for this purpose. As it heals, skin flattens out to form an even surface with excellent cosmetic results if staples have been properly placed lightly over the skin. Imbedded staples are difficult to remove and results may be less than desired.

Linear Stapler Two straight double staggered or side-by-side rows of staples are placed simultaneously in tissue with a linear stapler. This is used throughout the alimentary tract and in thoracic surgery for transection and resection of internal tissues. The tissue is positioned in straight jaws, of appropriate length, of the stapler. The gap between the jaws must be adequate for thickness of tissues. A tissue measuring device may be used for this determination in the gastrointestinal tract in conjunction with a disposable stapler, so the instrument can be adjusted to the appropriate settings for the desired staple height.

When formed, each staple is shaped like a capital letter B. This shape allows staples to hold tissues together without crushing so that tissue perfusion is maintained. The number of staples that will be fired depends on the length of stapler jaws.

Intraluminal Stapler A double row of staggered staples is placed in a circle for anastomosis of tubular hollow organs in the gastrointestinal tract with the intraluminal stapler (see Chap. 21, p. 409). Because diameter of the lumen of organs in the alimentary tract varies, the surgeon must choose stapler with an appropriate size head. The number of staples the instrument fires depends on head size. A circular knife within head of stapler trims tissue to produce a proper lumen as stapler is fired. As with the linear stapler, the staples form a letter B.

Ligating and Dividing Stapler A double row of two staples ligates tissue which is then divided simultaneously between staple lines with a cutting knife incorporated in the stapler. This stapler is used primarily to ligate and divide omental vessels, or other soft tubular structures.

Reusable Staplers

Reusable manually operated, heavy mechanical stapling instruments have many moving and detachable parts. They are expensive and not always reliable in their operation. They must be precisely aligned to fire accurately. The scrub nurse is responsible for correctly assembling Auto Suture instruments. The manufacturer's instructions for use and care must be followed to avoid technical failures.

Reusable staplers are supplied with presterilized, disposable cartridges that contain six or more staples. Quantities vary according to the stapler they fit. The number of cartridges needed varies with the procedure and/or design of the instrument. Cartridges are color-coded by size of staples.

Reusable staplers must be disassembled and cleaned after use. They should be terminally sterilized and then cleaned is an ultrasonic cleaner. They may be sterilized in steam or ethylene oxide gas, *completely disassembled,* according to manufacturer's recommendations.

Disposable Staplers

Preassembled, disposable staplers eliminate assembling, cleaning, and sterilizing processes. These self-contained, lightweight instruments, with an integral staple cartridge, are discarded after single patient use. To avoid unnecessary contamination of sterile instrument, the package should not be opened until surgeon determines correct size for intended use of the stapler.

TISSUE ADHESIVES

Synthetic, glue-like adhesive substances that polymerize in contact with body tissues effect hemostasis and hold tissues together. Methyl methacrylate is used to augment fixation of pathologic fractures and to stabilize prosthetic devices in bone. Butyl cyanoacrylate may be used on friable tissue or highly vascular tissues, such as liver and spleen, to control bleeding and approximate tissues technically difficult to manage by other means, especially following massive resections or in traumatic injuries.

Methyl methacrylate is an acrylic, cement-like substance commonly referred to as *bone cement.* It is a drug supplied in two sterile components that must be mixed together immediately prior to use. One component is a colorless, highly volatile, flammable, liquid methyl methacrylate monomer in an ampul. This is a powerful lipid solvent so it must be handled carefully. The other component is a white powder mixture of polymethyl methacrylate, methyl metacrylate-styrene copolymer, and barium sulfate in a packet. The barium sulfate provides radiopacity to the substance. When the powder and liquid are mixed, an exothermic polymeric reaction forms a soft, pliable, dough-like mass. This reaction liberates heat as high as 110°C (230°F). As the reaction progresses, the substance becomes hard in a few minutes. The mixing and kneading of the entire contents of the liquid ampul and powder packet must be thorough and at least four minutes in duration. The substance must be adequately soft and pliable for application to bone. The completion of polymerization occurs in the patient. After it hardens, it holds a prosthesis firmly in a fixed position.

A hazard to operating room personnel has been reported in regard to the use of methyl methacrylate in the operating room. Some personnel have experienced dizzy spells, difficulty in breathing, and/or nausea and vomiting following mixing of methyl methacrylate. The monomer and several of its ingredients are potent allergenic sensitizers when the vapor is inhaled. A suitable means of local exhaust should be provided that will collect vapor at the source of mixing at the sterile field, and will discharge it into the outside air or absorb the monomer on activated charcoal.

TISSUE REPAIR MATERIALS

Tissue deficiencies may require additional reinforcement or bridging material to obtain adequate wound healing. Sometimes edges of fascia, for example, cannot be brought together without excessive tension. In obese or elderly persons the fascia cannot withstand this tension because of weakness due to infiltration of fat. Biologic or synthetic mesh materials are used to fill congenital, traumatic, or acquired defects in fascia or a body wall and to reinforce fascia, as in hernia repair.

Biologic Materials

Cargile Membrane A thin membrane is obtained from submucosal layer of cecum of the ox. Cargile membrane is rarely used, although still commercially available in 4 by 6 in. (10 by 15 cm) sheet, to cover peritoneum to prevent adhesions, for isolating ligations, as a covering for packing in submucous nasal resections, and as a dural substitute.

Fascia Lata Strips of fascia lata are obtained from the fibrous connective tissue that covers the thigh muscles of beef cattle. In lieu of commercial fascia lata—*a heterogenous graft*—the surgeon may strip a piece of fascia from the thigh of the patient—*an autogenous graft.* Fascia lata also is obtained from cadavers and freeze-dried—an *allograft.* Fascia lata contains collagen. It increases the amount of tissue already present and becomes a living part of the tissue it supports. It is used to strengthen weakened fascial layers or to fill in defects in fascia. Since the advent of allografts and synthetic meshes, heterogenous strips are used infrequently.

Synthetic Mesh

Synthetic meshes offer several advantages for reinforcing or bridging fascial or other tissue deficiencies:

1 It is easily cut to desired size for the defect.

2 It is easily sutured underneath the edges of tissue to create a smooth surface.

3 Fibrous tissue easily grows through the openings to incorporate mesh into tissue to maximize tensile strength.

Polyester Fiber Mesh Polyester fiber mesh remains soft and pliable in tissue, but has limited elasticity. It is the least inert of the synthetic mesh materials. Potential complications of foreign-body tissue reaction are minimal, but it is not preferred in the presence of infection because of its multifilament construction. This mesh is machine-knitted by a process that interlocks each fiber juncture to prevent unraveling when cut. Nonsterile sheets are available in sizes 6 by 12 in. (15 by 30 cm) and 12 by 12 in. (30 by 30 cm). It may be steam sterilized *once* at 250°F (121°C) for 20 minutes, or at 270°F (132°C) unwrapped for ten minutes, immediately prior to use.

Polypropylene Mesh Polypropylene is knitted into a mesh with high tensile strength and good elasticity. It will not unravel when cut. Because it is inert it may be used in the presence of infection. It is available sterile in several sizes ranging from 2½ by 4 in. (6 by 10 cm) to 9 by 14 in. (23 by 35 cm). If sufficient skin is not available to cover it, this mesh can be used as a body wall replacement and as a support for the viscera during healing by second intention.

Stainless Steel Mesh Available nonsterile in sheets 6 by 12 in. (15 by 30 cm) and 12 by 12 in. (30 by 30 cm), steel is the most inflexible and difficult of the meshes to handle. The sharp edges may puncture gloves. Use wire scissors, not dissecting scissors, to cut it. Steel is opaque to x-ray, which may be a disadvantage for the patient in later life. Also the mesh may fragment and cause patient discomfort.

TISSUE REPLACEMENT MATERIALS

For centuries surgeons have sought materials to replace parts of anatomy. Tissue may be absent or distorted due to congenital deformity, traumatic injury, degenerative disease, or surgical resection. Replacement or substitution of tissue may be possible with biologic or synthetic prosthetic materials implanted into the body. A *prosthesis* is a permanent or temporary replacement for a missing or malfunctioning structure. Some implants replace vital structures, such as diseased heart valves and blood vessels. Devices, such as pacemakers, assist the function of vital organs. Other materials are used to repair or replace defects. Prosthetic materials implanted into the body must:

1 Be compatible with physiologic processes
2 Produce no or minimal tissue reaction
3 Be sterile so will not cause infection or become a culture medium
4 Be noncarcinogenic or other disease causative
5 Have viable and adequate tissue coverage, unless used as a biological dressing over denuded skin surfaces
6 Have adequate blood supply through or around them
7 Be stable so will not degenerate or change shape if used for permanent function
8 Contour or conform to normal tissue configuration as desired

Biologic Materials

The biologic materials are mentioned here, but detailed discussions of skin grafts and organ and tissue transplants will follow in other chapters.

Bone A bone graft affords structural support and a pattern for regrowth of bone within a skeletal defect. *Cancellous* bone is porous. Its porosity permits tissue fluid to reach deeper into it than into cortical bone, and thus most of the bone cells live. *Cortical* bone is used for bridging large defects in the skeleton, as it gives greater strength. It may be fixed in the recipient site by means of wire suture or screws.

While bone grafts become fixed to the recipient site, their main purpose is to stimulate new bone growth. *Autogenous bone,* which is obtained from the patient, usually is taken at the time of operation and may be obtained from the ilium or tibia. *Homogenous bone,* which is obtained from someone other than the patient, is stored in the bone bank until needed (refer to Chap. 24, p. 465). This bone is weaker than autogenous grafts, thus requiring a much longer time of immobilization. Homogenous bone is dead bone. The recipient bone regeneration is responsible for union with this type of bone graft. It may be desirable, however, to spare the patient the added operating time and trauma of removing an autogenous graft.

Composite bone grafts are freeze-dried homografts combined with autogenous particulate cancellous bone and marrow. A crib formed from a cadaver bone, rib for example, is packed with the patient's bone particles and marrow. When implanted to reconstruct bony defects, the composite graft induces bone regeneration in the recipient site. The freeze-dried homograft is biodegradable by slow resorption. Eventually it is replaced by mature functional bone.

Decalcified bone and demineralized bone dust or powder, prepared from homogenous bone, also are used to stimulate bone regeneration or to fill defects in bone.

Bovine Heterografts Enzymatically treated bovine carotid artery heterografts are prepared commercially. These grafts are used for blood access in patients on hemodialysis who have poor blood vessels or in whom it is difficult to create either fistulas or shunts. Femoral arteriovenous bovine shunts can be punctured innumerable times with a low incidence of thrombus formation.

Collagen Collagen is used as a biomaterial in both its natural form, such as the bovine graft and the microfibrillar hemostatic powder, and restructured into membranes or films. Collagen can be altered by a variety of techniques to change its physical properties.

An artificial skin substitute may be prepared from a layer of collagen obtained from a calf, and coated with autogenous epithelium obtained from the recipient. Another type is synthesized from a bilayered polymeric membrane. The top layer is silicone elastomer. The bottom layer is a porous cross-linked network of collagen and glycosaminoglycan. This artificial skin is biodegradable, but can be used as a temporary covering similar to porcine heterografts.

Porcine Heterografts Pig (porcine) skin is used as a temporary biological dressing to cover large body surfaces denuded of skin. Biological dressings are needed over large skin defects, such as burns, until permanent skin grafting can be accomplished (see Chap. 27). Freeze-dried preparations of split-thickness pigskin are commercially available in sterile rolls of various sizes. These are soaked in sterile water or normal saline prior to use. Vascularization of the pigskin does not occur, but it adheres tightly, while reepithelialization proceeds underneath it, for as long as two weeks before it dries up and peels off spontaneously.

Amnion Prepared from the amniotic membrane of human placenta, amnion is used as a biological dressing in treatment of burns, skin ulcers, spina bifida, and infected wounds. It is harvested by cleaning the placenta of blood and clots immediately after delivery, placing placenta in an iodophor solution, and refrigerating it at 4°C (39°F). Membrane should be stripped from placenta within 48 hours after delivery. Amnion can be used in fresh, frozen, or dried form. Some hospitals have amnion banks to prepare and store amniotic membranes.

Organ Transplants Some whole body organs can be transplanted from one human to another. This is done in an effort to sustain life by compensating for physiological deficits or inadequate function of vital organs. Refer to Chapter 34 for complete discussion of transplanation.

Tissue Transplants Skin and blood vessels are frequently transplanted from one part of the body to another. These are referred to as *autografts* since the patient is both donor and recipent. The transplanted tissue becomes a part of the living tissue in the recipient site. Refer to Chapter 27 for discussion of skin grafts and Chapter 32 for discussion of vascular grafts.

Some tissues can be transplanted from one person to another to restore function, such as the cornea, or provide support in structures, such as cartilage in nasal reconstruction. These are referred to as *allografts* or *homografts* (see Chap. 34).

Synthetic Materials

Inorganic substances are less than perfect for prostheses because they cannot unite with tissue. However, they can provide support, restore function, augment or restore body contour.

Metal Stainless steel, a cobalt alloy trade named Vitallium, and titanium are the metals used to manufacture prosthetic implants. Used primarily for stabilization or replacement of bone, metal implants must be strong enough to withstand stress of weight bearing or muscular action and must not corrode in body tissues. They are never reused due to a degree of weakening that comes with use. Refer to Chapter 24 for specific types and uses of metallic orthopaedic implants.

Special care must be taken in handling metal implants to protect the surface. A simple scratch on a metal implant can lead to corrosion in the body. It will be bathed continuously by weakly chloride body fluids. If corrosion begins, the implant may fail and have to be removed. It is very important, therefore, that all metal implants be protected from scratches. This can be accomplished by:

1 Wrapping each implant individually, or wrapping sets with each size implant in a separate compartment, for both storage and sterilization. Most prostheses come from the manufacturer in protective coverings or cases. Some of these are suitable for adequate sterilization with subsequent placement in the sterile field to minimize handling prior to implantation.

2 Preventing implants from coming in contact with other hard surfaces of metal or glass, either during storage and sterilization or on the instrument table.

3 Not handling or transferring an unprotected implant with any type of forceps.

Implants of one metal should not come in contact with those of another metal as an electrochemical reaction occurs between metals. Two different metals are not implanted in the same patient for this reason. Instruments used for insertion also should be of the same metal as the implant, e.g., a stainless steel screwdriver and screw.

Methyl Methacrylate A highly refined methyl methacrylate mixture can be molded and shaped to fit a defect in bone. When it hardens, this material looks and feels very much like bone. It is used to repair a skull defect (see Chap. 29, p. 552).

Polyester Fiber Polyester fibers woven or knitted into seamless cylinders are used to replace major arteries.

Polyethylene Struts Polyethylene tubing may be inserted into structures, such as fallopian tubes or ureters, to give support during healing or to bridge a defect in tissue continuity.

Silicone Silicone is one of the most inert of the synthetic polymers used for implantation into the body. It is used in many forms: as a gel, sponge, film, tubing, liquid, and preformed molded anatomic structures. A medical-grade silicone elastomer (Silastic) in one form or another is used in virtually every surgical specialty for tissue reconstruction or replacement.

Complete instructions for cleaning and sterilizing silicone implants before use are supplied by the manufacturer with each type of prosthesis. These instructions must be followed meticulously. After preparation, these implants are not handled with bare hands and care must be taken to ensure that they do not pick up lint and dust. Gloves worn during handling must be entirely free from powder. Skin oil, lint, dust, powder, and other surface contaminants can evoke foreign-body reactions around the implant in tissue.

Polytetrafluoroethylene (Teflon) Some prostheses or parts of prosthetic devices may be made of this synthetic polymer. Teflon may be woven into a fabric for arterial grafts, extruded into tubing for struts, or molded into a solid configuration for valves or joints. Its lubricity makes it a useful replacement for tissues when motion is desirable.

SKIN CLOSURE

In addition to sutures and staples, other materials may be used to hold skin edges in approximation.

Skin Clips

Clips made of noncorroding metal may be used to approximate skin edges. They tend to leave more scar than other methods of skin closure, but they may be applied quickly when time is a critical factor and cosmetic result in unimportant. They can be used in the presence of infection or drainage. A specially designed instrument is necessary to apply clips. Skin clips also may be used to secure stockinet or towels to the skin to isolate the incision, particularly on an extremity.

Skin Closure Strips

Strips of microporous polypropylene or nylon tape placed across the line of incision hold skin edges in approximation during healing. They may be used to close skin edges of superficial lacerations, as primary closure of skin layer in conjunction with a subcuticular suture, or in conjunction with interrupted skin sutures or staples. Often they are used following early suture or staple removal to support the wound during healing. A skin tackifier, such as tincture of benzoin, may be recommended by the manufacturer for assuring adhesion to skin.

Strips are available sterile in widths of ⅛, ¼, and ½ in. (3, 6, and 12.7 mm) and lengths from 1½ to 4 in. (3.7 to 10 cm). They are ethylene oxide gas sterilized in peel-apart packets. Skin closure strips:

1 May be used in the emergency department on superficial lacerations to eliminate need for sutures that would require local anesthesia for placement with subsequent return of the patient for suture removal.

2 Eliminate foreign-body tissue reaction of suture material in skin.

3 Have enough porosity to permit adequate ventilation of clean or contaminated wounds.

4 Permit removal of sutures within 32 to 48 hours postoperatively. Crosshatch scarring and possibility of infection are reduced when sutures are removed early. Skin closure strips provide long-term wound reinforcement and support.

5 Permit visibility of the healing wound so the surgeon can see how well the wound edges have coapted. Some strips are translucent; others have a color tone or opacity that does not afford this advantage.

6 Minimize skin irritation because they are hyporeactive.

7 Can be applied and removed rapidly.

8 Can be easily torn or cut to meet surgeon's exact length requirements.

DRUG AND MEDICAL DEVICE LEGISLATION

In 1906, the U.S. federal government enacted the Pure Food and Drug Act with the U.S. Department of Agriculture as the enforcing agency to assure introduction of safe and sanitary foods to the public. The Food, Drug, and Cosmetic Act of 1938 extended regulation to include introduction of cosmetics and drugs as well as food, and, to a minimal extent, medical devices. The Food and Drug Administration (FDA), within the Department of Agriculture, became the enforcing agency with authority to implement a preclearance mechanism requiring drug manufacturers to provide evidence of safety before a new drug could be sold. Sutures were classified as drugs.

The Kefauver-Harris Drug Amendments of 1962 added strength to the new drug clearance procedures. Drug manufacturers must prove to the FDA the effectiveness as well as the safety of drugs prior to making them commercially available. These amendments established a mechanism for clinical investigation to evaluate efficacy of drugs. Depending upon nature of a drug, clinical studies often require several years before FDA approves commercial sale of a product.

The Medical Device Amendments of 1976 gave the FDA regulatory control over all medical devices (defined as any health care product that is not a drug), in addition to the FDA's previous regulatory control of drugs. All wound closure materials are classified as either drugs or devices under these amendments. Devices are further classified into one of three categories: those complying with general established regulatory controls, those requiring development of performance standards, and those requiring premarket clearance to substantiate effectiveness. Ethical manufacturers adhere to the guidelines, standards, and regulations of the FDA prior to release of a new drug or medical device.

CHAPTER **19**

STATE OF THE ART TECHNOLOGY: SPECIALIZED SURGICAL TOOLS

Joseph Lister stated that success is attention to detail. This is the essence of the state of the art as practiced in all the surgical specialties. Advancements in technology have made possible the complex surgical techniques of the present. Continuing research will further enhance the technology of the future.

Surgical residency programs include education and training in electrosurgery, laser surgery, endoscopy, and microsurgery. Therefore, upon completion of postgraduate education, surgeons today are skilled in the use of these specialized tools. Continuing surgical educational courses, including laboratory study, are available so that practicing surgeons can learn to use the newest technology. Prior to handling, nursing personnel who function on the OR team must be equally knowledgeable about the care and use of the required equipment. Some operative procedures utilize more than one of these technologies, e.g., laser surgery through an attachment to the operating microscope directed through an endoscope. Preparing and handling these expensive pieces of equipment are major responsibilities of OR nurses and surgical technologists. In addition, all OR personnel must be aware of and safeguard against the hazards of electrical and radiation equipment (see Chap. 11). The OR environment must be safe for patients and personnel.

ELECTROSURGERY

The practice of the ancient surgeons of pouring boiling oil into a wound or searing it with hot irons to stop bleeding and infection was torture in the extreme. Patients usually were crippled if they survived. However, surgeons continued to use these techniques long after Ambrose Paré discredited their use in the sixteenth century. They recognized that application of heat accelerates the natural chemical reaction of blood to hasten clotting. This eventually lead to the development of *electrocautery,* direct contact of an electrically heated wire with tissue. Still in limited use, cautery is generated from a battery that heats the wire in a self-contained unit. *Electrosurgery,* by contrast, employs passage of high-frequency oscillating electric currents through tissue between two electrodes to coagulate or cut tissue.

In 1906, Lee DeForest, the physicist commonly known as the father of radio, discovered by accident that a high-frequency electric current could sever tissue with only slight traces of generated heat. In conjunction with his vacuum-tube generator, he patented an electrode that cut tissue with an electrical arc created at point of a dull blade. Referred to as cold cautery, pioneers like Harvey Cushing tried rather unsuccessfully to use the device.

Working with Dr. Cushing, W. T. Bovie, also a physicist, developed the first spark-gap tube generator in the 1920s. This became the universal basis of electrosurgical units, commonly still referred to as "the Bovie," prior to the 1970s when solid-state units became available. These use transistors, diodes, and rectifiers to generate current. The spark-gap generator continues to be an acceptable unit, however.

Principles of Electrosurgery

High-frequency alternating or oscillating electric currents move at more than 20,000 cycles per second (10,000 for radio frequency). Electrosurgical units operate at frequencies between 100,000 and 10,000,000 hertz (Hz). This current can be passed through tissue without causing stimulation of muscles or nerves. The heat produced is a direct result of resistance to its passage through tissue. The density of electric current flowing through a point of contact in tissue elevates temperature sufficiently to cause destruction of cells by dissolution of their molecular structure. Amount of heat produced by any amount of resistance is proportional to square of current. For example, doubling current increases heat produced four-fold. Conversely, amount of heat produced by any amount of current is directly proportional to resistance; doubling the resistance doubles heat produced. Therefore, current must be concentrated in a small area of high resistance to produce the high temperature required for electrosurgery.

Electrosurgical Unit

To complete the electric circuit to coagulate or cut tissue, current must flow from a generator (electrosurgical power unit) to an active electrode, through tissue, and back to the generator via an inactive electrode. Electrosurgery is utilized to a greater or lesser extent in all surgical specialties. Several different units are available. Some have selective uses; others are adaptable to many types of operations. Personnel must be familiar with the manufacturer's detailed manual of operating instruction for each type used.

Generator The machine that produces high-frequency or radio-frequency waves is the generator or power component of the electrosurgical unit. Solid-state generators are transistorized and use diodes and rectifiers to produce current. They usually operate at a lower output power than traditional spark-gap generators, and most have additional safety features. Both spark-gap and solid-state generators provide two separate circuits within the housing of the machine. Characteristics of current vary depending on type the generator produces. Controls on the machine allow selection of desired characteristic. The current may be identical in frequency, power (voltage), and amount (amperage), but vary in quality. Quality depends on the difference in *damping,* the pattern of waveforms by which oscillations diminish after surges of power. This difference determines tissue reaction to the current.

Coagulating Current A damped waveform has a continuous pattern of surges of current which rapidly diminishes to short time periods, gaps, in which no current is delivered. This is produced by the spark-gap circuit. *Damped* current coagulates tissue. As it approaches the active electrode, density of current increases to produce an intense heat. This sears the ends of small or moderate-sized vessels to control bleeding on contact. Attempts to coagulate large vessels can result in an extensive burn and necrosis.

Cutting Current An undamped waveform does not diminish, but retains a constant output of high-frequency current. This is produced by a vacuum tube oscillator. *Undamped* current cuts tissue. This continuous current forms an arc between tissues and an active electrode that is intense enough to divide fibrous tissue as it moves along lines of incision (reference is not to skin incision) before sufficient heat builds up to coagulate adjacent tissues.

Blended Current Undamped current can be blended with damped current to add coagulating effect to cutting current. At the same time it cuts through or across tissue, cutting current accomplishes some coagulation of cells on surface of incision and prevents capillary bleeding. Some solid-state generators have a setting for "blend" or "hemostasis" for this function. This blend can also be achieved by a slightly damped waveform from a spark-gap generator.

Controls Type and amount of current are regulated by controls on the generator. Most units provide up to 400 watts of power. It is seldom necessary to use full-power settings. A safe general rule for the circulating nurse is to start with lowest setting of current that accomplishes desired degree of coagulation or cutting, then increase current at the surgeon's request. The surgeon selects the type of current to be used with either a foot or hand control switch. The circulating nurse verbally confirms the power settings before the generator is activated. The generator should be designed to minimize unintentional activation.

In solid-state units, power output is isolated to prevent overheating and is equipped with a warning buzzer and/or light to warn of too high a setting or a break in the circuit. Flow of current to and from the generator must be balanced. A return electrode monitoring system measures and compares current flowing from active electrode with current returning from inactive electrode. The generator deactivates if continuity in the electric circuit is disrupted or inadequate in some units. The safety features should be tested before each patient use, and the generator periodically inspected by the biomedical engineering department.

The generator may be mounted on a portable stand. It must be moved carefully to avoid tipping. The machine must be cleaned before and after use. Unintentional activation or failure may occur if liquid or debris enter the generator. The hospital may be held responsible for a defect causing patient injury. The generator should have an identification number. This should be recorded in the patient's record to verify equipment used. This also provides a means of maintaining records of routine inspections and maintenance. Operational instructions should be on or attached to every unit.

Active Electrode The sterile active electrode directs flow of current to operative site. Style of the electrode tip, i.e.. blade, loop, ball, needle, will be determined by type of operation and current to be used. The electrode tip may be fixed into or detachable from a pencil-shaped handle, or it may be incorporated into a tissue forceps or suction tube. It is attached to a conductor cord, which is connected to the generator. The scrub nurse hands end of conductor cord off sterile field to the circulating nurse, who attaches it to the generator. The cord must be long and flexible enough to reach between the sterile field and generator without stress. It must be free of kinks and bends that could deviate current flow. When the unit is not in actual use, although connected, electrode tip should be kept clean, dry, and visible. It may be kept in a container to avoid possibility of a burn from one of team inadvertently stepping on foot switch or activating hand control.

The surgeon places active electrode tip on tissue, then activates foot switch or hand control on the pencil to transfer electric current from generator to tissue. Some hand switches are color-coded to identify coagulating and cutting functions. Between uses, charred or coagulated tissue should be removed from tip. This can be done by wiping with a tip cleaner or a damp sponge, or scraping with back (noncutting) edge of a knife blade.

Rather than placing tip directly on tissue, frequently multiple bleeding vessels are clamped with hemostats or smooth-tipped tissue forceps. By touching any part of metal instrument with active electrode, vessels are coagulated. The clamp tip should include as little extraneous tissue as possible to minimize damage to adjacent tissue.

The electrode and cord may be disposable. Reusable electrodes should be inspected for damage before reprocessing and before use at sterile field.

Inactive Electrode Electric current will flow to ground or a neutral potential (see Chap. 11, p. 203). Therefore, a proper channel must be provided to disperse current and heat generated in tissue. The inactive electrode disperses high-frequency current released through the active electrode and provides low current density return from tissues back to the generator. Resistance from patient to generator and from generator to wall electrical outlet must be less than one ohm. Electrosurgical units have either monopolar or bipolar, or both, mechanisms to direct flow of electric current.

Bipolar Units The inactive electrode is incorporated into forceps used by surgeon. One side of forceps is the active electrode through which current passes to tissues. The other side is inactive. Output voltage is relatively low. Current flows only between tips of forceps, returning directly to the generator. Current does not disperse itself throughout the patient as in monopolar units. This provides extremely precise control of coagulated area and is a safety factor in the use of electrosurgery. A grounding pad or plate is not needed because current does not flow through patient.

Monopolar Unipolar Units Current flows from generator to active electrode, through patient to an inactive dispersive electrode, back to generator. Because current supplied by generator is dispersed from the active electrode, it seeks completion of electrical circuit to ground or a neutral potential through the patient's body. *An inactive dispersive electrode must be used to ground patient.* This is in the form of a patient grounding pad or plate placed in direct contact with skin. Contact area must exceed 100 mm^2 or a diameter greater than 1.2 cm. The most commonly used types are disposable. Some are flexible to mold to any body surface. They must maintain uniform body contact. Some are prelubricated. If a metal plate is placed under patient, a conductive electrode lubricant (gel) must be spread evenly over entire plate to thoroughly wet skin and thus reduce its electrical resistance to a minimum. Some pads also must be lubricated. Prelubricated pads should be checked for dry spots before placement.

Current flows from active electrode through body to inactive dispersive electrode. It then returns to generator via a conductor cord. This cord must be long and flexible enough to reach without stress on attachments to electrode or generator. Attachments must be secure. The plug or adaptor at end of cord fastens into receptacle on generator. This may be labeled and/or color coded to help ensure correct attachment of inactive electrode. Unless disposable, cord should be checked before use for wire breakage or fraying. Grasp connecting plug and pull firmly on cord. If it stretches, wires inside are broken and must be repaired. Reusable cords should be inspected by the biomedical engineering department periodically for electrical integrity.

The inactive grounding pad or plate must be properly placed and connected to avoid electrical burn to the patient. The following safeguards must be taken:

1 Inactive electrode should be as close to site where active electrode will be used as possible, to minimize current through body.

2 Inactive electrode must cover as large an area of patient's skin as possible in an area free of hair or scar tissue, which tend to act as insulation. The surface area affects heat buildup and dissipation. Avoid areas where bony prominences might result in pressure points, which in turn can cause current concentration. Place pad or plate on clean, dry skin surface on or under as large a muscle mass area as possible.

3 Inactive electrode must be clean and free from bent edges. Some conductive lubricants will dry out and leave a high-resistance film that will prevent proper contact with skin.

4 A metal connection between pad or plate and conductor cord must not touch patient. Special care must be taken to ensure that cord does not become dislodged. The safest connectors are threaded or lock, and also are insulated. The connector should not create a pressure point on patient's skin.

5 Connection between inactive electrode and generator must be made properly and securely, with compatible attachments. If return circuit is faulty, ground circuit may be completed through inadvertent contact with metal operating table or its attachments. If grounded area is small, current passing through exposed area of skin contact will be relatively intense. For example, one such contact point could be thigh touching a leg stirrup while the patient is in lithotomy position.

6 Inactive dispersive electrode should be positioned and connected for generators that accommodate both bipolar and monopolar operation.

The circulating nurse should record on patient's chart the location of inactive dispersive electrode, patient's skin condition before and after electrosurgery, generator identification number, and settings used.

Safety Factors

Electrical burn through the patient's skin is the greatest hazard in the use of electrosurgery. These burns are usually deeper than flame burns, causing widespread tissue necrosis and deep thrombosis to extent that debridement may be required. Nursing personnel must be aware of hazards and safeguard against injury to patient. In addition to those noted above for preparing the electrosurgical unit and for positioning the inactive dispersive electrode used with monopolar units, other precautions should be taken:

1 Alert anesthesiologist to anticipated use of electrosurgery. Electrosurgery must never be used in mouth, around head, or in pleural cavity when high concentrations of oxygen or any flammable anesthetics are used. Follow safety regulations for use with all inhalation anesthetic agents (see Chap. 11).

2 Electrocardiogram electrodes should be placed as far away from operative site as possible. Needle electrodes should be avoided as they could transmit leakage currents into the body. Burns can occur at site of ECG electrodes and other low impedance points from invasive monitor probes if current diverts to alternate grounds.

3 Flammable agents, such as alcohol, must not be used in skin preparation. Fumes may collect in drapes and ignite when electrosurgical or cautery unit is used. Use aqueous antiseptic solutions.

4 If another piece of electrical equipment is used in direct contact with patient at same time as electrosurgical unit, connect it to a different source of current, such as a battery, if possible. Cutting current of electrosurgical unit may not work if another piece of electrical equipment is on same circuit. Or electrosurgical unit may interfere with operation of other equipment. The isolated power system of solid-state units may avoid these problems.

NOTE. Electrosurgery may disrupt operation of a patient's implanted cardiac pacemaker. The patient must be continuously monitored. A defibrillator should be on standby in OR.

5 Only moist sponges should be permitted on sterile field while electrosurgical unit is in use, to prevent fire.

6 Investigate a repeated request for more current. The inactive electrode or connecting cord may be at fault. Shock to those touching patient may result. The patient may be burned.

7 For the safety of the patient and personnel, follow instructions for use and care on the machine or in the manual provided by the manufacturer that accompanies each electrosurgical unit.

Electrosurgery causes more patient injuries than any other electrical device used in the operating room. Most incidents are due to personnel error. In addition to the foregoing precautions, refer to discussion of electrical hazards and safety in Chapter 11.

LASER SURGERY

Laser is an acronym for *light amplification by stimulated emission of radiation.* Einstein's theory purported in 1917, explaining the difference between spontaneous and stimulated emission of light, eventually led to the development of the laser. This development began in 1940 in the Soviet Union. Lasers depend on the capacity of atoms to become excited when struck by a quantum of electromagnetic energy, known as a *photon.* Photons are the basic units of radiation that constitute light. When struck by a photon, the electrons of the atom move to a high energy level. Upon spontaneous return to a lower energy level toward normal ground state, these electrons emit another photon which will strike another atom also in the transitional *pumped up* energy state. This reaction produces a second photon of the same frequency. This sets up a chain reaction of stimulated emission of photons at high energy levels. Production of this in a sustained state, known as *population inversion,* was technically difficult. The introduction of practical lasers into scientific technology finally occurred almost simultaneously in the United States and Russia around 1960.

The laser as a surgical instrument was developed in the United States. The first surgical laser, the ruby laser, was used in ophthalmology for retinal hemorrhages. As scientists discovered that other materials could be electrically stimulated to produce lasers in a variety of wavelengths, the carbon dioxide and argon gas surgical lasers were developed in the mid 1960s. The argon laser replaced the ruby laser for use in ophthalmology. However, not until after Jako adapted the carbon dioxide laser to the operating microscope in 1972 did lasers truly become viable adjuncts to surgical armamentarium.

Physical Properties of Laser

The laser focuses light upon atoms to stimulate them to a high point of excitation. The resulting radiation is then amplified and metamorphosed into the wavelengths of laser light. This light beam is *monochromatic,* one color because all the electromagnetic waves are the same length, and *collimated,* parallel to each other. The light is totally concentrated and easily focused. Unlike conventional light waves which spread and dissipate electromagnetic radiation by many different wavelengths, the *coherence* of the laser beam is sustained over space and time with wavelengths in the same frequency and energy phase.

Lasers may emit their energy in brief, repeating emissions that have a duration of only an extremely small fraction of a second. These are *pulsed laser systems.* Or they are capable of producing continuous light beams; these are *continuous wave lasers.* All lasers have a combination of duration, level, and output wavelengths of radiation emitted when activated. The power density, termed *irradiance,* is the amount of power per unit surface area during a single pulse or exposure. This is expressed as watts per centimeter squared. Regardless of beam characteristics, the components of a laser system are the same. These include:

1 *Medium* to produce lasing effect of stimulated emission. Gases, synthetic crystals, glass, liquid dyes, and semiconductors are used. Each produces a different wavelength, color, and absorption effect.

2 *Power source* to create population inversion by pumping energy into the lasing medium. This may be electrical or radio-frequency power, or an optical power source such as a xenon flash lamp or another laser.

3 *Amplification mechanism* to change random directional movement of stimulated emissions to a parallel direction. This occurs within an optical resonator or laser cavity, a tube with mirrors at each end. As photons traveling length of the resonator reflect back through the medium, they stimulate more atoms to release photons, thus amplifying the lasing effect. Power density of the beam determines the laser's capacity to cut, coagulate, or vaporize tissue.

4 *Wave guides* to aim and control direction of laser beam. The optical resonator has a small opening in one end that permits transmission of a small beam of laser light. The smaller the beam, the higher its power density will be. Fiberoptic wave guides or a series of rhodium reflecting mirrors then direct the beam to tissue.

Types of Lasers

Lasers employ argon, carbon dioxide, krypton, neodymium, or ruby as their active media. Each laser has selective uses. Laser light colors vary from visible near ultraviolet to the invisible far infrared ranges of the electromagnetic spectrum. Wavelengths also vary providing different radiation penetration depths. Lasers commonly are used in conjunction with the operating microscope and/or an endoscope. The surgeon selects appropriate type laser for the tissue to be excised or coagulated.

Argon Laser Argon ion gas emits a blue-green light beam in the visible electromagnetic spectrum at wavelengths of 488 and 514.5 nm (nanometers) or 0.5 μm (microns). This wavelength passes through water and clear fluid, such as cerebrospinal fluid, with minimal absorption. It is intensely absorbed by brown-red pigment of chromagen hemoglobin in blood or melanin in pigmented tissue and converted into heat. Thermal radiation penetrates to a depth of 1 or 2 mm in most tissue.

The argon laser operates from electrical power. A water-cooling system often is required to dissipate heat generated in the argon medium.

The argon laser beam usually is transmitted through a flexible quartz fiberoptic wave guide that is 200 to 600 microns in diameter. This can be directed to a hand piece or through an endoscope or operating microscope. Most argon laser machines deliver a nonfocused beam that vaporizes tissue poorly and scatters more radiation than other types of lasers. Irradiance may vary from less than a watt to 20 watts, depending on the model.

Argon lasers coagulate bleeding points or lesions involving many small superficial vessels, such as a port-wine stain. It is used primarily to destroy specific cutaneous lesions while sparing adjacent tissue and minimizing scarring, to treat vascular lesions, and to coagulate superficial vessels in mucosa as in the gastrointestinal tract. It is also used in ophthalmology, otolaryngology, gynecology, urology, neurosurgery, and dermatology.

Carbon Dioxide (CO_2) Laser Using a mixture of carbon dioxide, nitrogen, and helium molecular gases, the CO_2 laser emits an invisible beam from mid- to far infrared electromagnetic spectrum at wavelengths of 9,600 and 10,600 nm or 10.6 μm. This wavelength is intensely absorbed by water. It raises water temperature in cells to flash boiling point, thus vaporizing tissue. *Vaporization* is the conversion of solid tissue to smoke and gas. The vapor is removed from the operative field with suction. The intense heat of the CO_2 laser also coagulates vessels as it cuts through them. It penetrates the surface to depth of 0.1 to 0.2 mm per application to tissue with minimal thermal effect to surrounding tissue.

The CO_2 laser operates from electrical power. The machine has a self-contained cooling system.

The CO_2 laser beam must be delivered in a direct line of vision. It cannot be transmitted through a fiberoptic wave guide because its longer wavelength prevents conduction through crystal fibers. It is transmitted through an operating microscope or an articulating arm with a series of mirrors. This arm allows precise focus and direction of the beam to a pencil-like hand piece. Most machines have a helium-neon laser target beam that superimposes the invisible CO_2 beam to provide a visible red aiming light. Irradiance can vary from less than a watt up to 300 watts. A portable hand-held laser tube with a hollow needle to deliver the CO_2 beam is available for use in vascular and microsurgery.

The vaporization and hemostatic action of the CO_2 laser is of value to the surgeon in treating soft tissue and vascular lesions. Large or small masses of tissue can be removed rapidly and efficiently. This laser is used primarily in otolaryngology, gynecology, plastic surgery, dermatology, neurosurgery, orthopaedics, and general surgery.

Krypton Laser Krypton ion gas laser emits a red-yellow light beam in visible electromagnetic spectrum at wavelengths of 476.2 to 647.1 nm or 0.6 μm. It is intensely absorbed by pigment in blood and retinal epithelium. The krypton laser resembles the argon laser in construction and use. It operates from electrical power and is water cooled.

Used in ophthalmology (see Chap. 25, page 493), it is more versatile than the argon laser in selective photocoagulation of the retina. The krypton spectrum is poorly absorbed by the red of hemoglobin. Therefore it may be used effectively to treat retinal bleeding in the presence of blood in the vitreous humor. Under these circumstances the argon blue laser would be ineffective because of absorption by even a small amount of blood. Similarly, the krypton laser can be used to treat lesions much closer to the center of the macula, the zone of most distinct vision of the retina. This is due to its poor absorption of the yellow pigment of the retina.

Neodymium (Nd):YAG Laser Nd:YAG is the acronym for neodymium, yttrium, aluminum, and garnet that comprise the solid-state crystal medium which emanates the light beam of this laser. This invisible beam in the near infrared range of the electromagnetic spectrum has a wavelength of 1060 nm or 1.6 μm. It is poorly absorbed by hemoglobin and water, but is intensely absorbed by tissue protein. The wavelength penetrates to a depth of 3 to 5 mm to denature protein by thermal coagulation and shrinkage of tissue beneath the surface.

The Nd:YAG laser operates from electric current through the optical power source of xenon flash lamps. It must have a water cooling system.

The Nd:YAG laser beam can be transmitted through a flexible quartz fiber, 200 to 600 microns in diameter, which passes through an endoscope. Or it can be transmitted through a fiberoptic wave guide to a hand piece or endoscope, or focused through operating microscope. An aiming light of blue xenon or red neon-helium may be used in conjunction with the Nd:YAG beam. This laser can operate using a Q-switching mode to store energy in the resonator during pumping action followed by release of a single, short pulse of high energy. This does not burn tissue, but disrupts it with minute shock waves. Irradiance can vary from less than a watt to 120 watts.

The Nd:YAG laser has the most powerful coagulating action of all the surgical lasers. It penetrates blood clots and will coagulate large bleeding vessels. It is used to coagulate and vaporize large volumes of tissue, e.g., neoplasms. This laser has applications for vascular and mucosal lesions in the gastrointestinal tract and tracheobronchial tree. It is also used in rhinolaryngology, gynecology, urology, neurosurgery, orthopaedics, and ophthalmology.

Ruby Laser Ruby solid-state crystal laser emits a visible red light at wavelengths of 694 nm or 0.6 μm. A synthetically machined crystal rod is placed in a resonator cavity with a xenon flash lamp which, when activated, creates the optical pumping to produce the ruby laser beam. Blood vessels and transparent substances do not absorb this beam. A pulsed system, the ruby laser is capable of generating large fields of energy on impact. This shock wave effect can injure internal tissues and bone. Irradiance is one watt. Originally used in ophthalmology, the ruby laser currently is used primarily to eradicate port-wine stain lesions of the skin.

Tunable Dye Laser Liquid fluorescent dye laser can produce a visible red light with wavelengths in the 630 nm or 0.6 μm range of the electromagnetic spectrum. Tunable by a prism, from blue through tones of yellow and orange to red, the resulting visible light beam matches a ruby laser in both shade and sharpness. The patient is given an injection of hematoporphyrin derivative (HPD) in high concentrations. This is taken up by cells to photosensitize them. It remains longer in malignant cells than normal cells before it is excreted from the body. The HPD in these cells chemically reacts with the red light beam from the dye laser transmitted by an optical fiber to selectively destroy the tumor by photoradiation.

Advantages of Laser Surgery

Surgical lasers are precision tools that emit radiation. This is selectively absorbed by different tissues with resultant penetration and destruction at the focal point, but with differential thermal protection of surrounding tissues. Lasers offer the surgeon and patient many advantages over other conventional operative techniques.

1 Precise control for accurate incision and excision of tissue. The laser beam is precisely focused for localized tissue destruction. The depth of the radiation penetration is precisely regulated by duration of focus, power density, and type of tissue.

2 Access to confined areas or areas inaccessible to other surgical instruments. The beam can be directed through endoscopes or deflected off rhodium reflector mirrors.

3 Unobstructed view of operative site. The laser beam comes in contact with the tissue to be cut, coagulated, or vaporized. It can be directed through the operating microscope.

4 Minimal handling of, and trauma to tissues. Traction on target tissue is unnecessary.

5 Dry, bloodless operative field. The laser beam simultaneously cuts and coagulates blood vessels, thus providing hemostasis in vascular areas.

6 Minimal thermal effect on surrounding tissue. Essentially no permanent thermal necrosis of tissue exists beyond 100 microns from edge of area incised. This minimizes postoperative pain.

7 Reduced risk of contamination or infection. The laser beam vaporizes microorganisms, thus essentially sterilizing the contact area.

8 Prompt healing with minimal postoperative edema, sloughing of tissue, pain, and scarring.

9 Reduced operating time. Because procedures can be done more quickly, both anesthesia and operating time are shorter. Many procedures can be done without general anesthesia. Many are done in ambulatory care facilities.

Safety Factors

Despite their many advantages, surgical lasers present radiation hazards to patients and the OR team. This equipment must be used in accordance with established regulatory standards, manufacturer's recommendations, and individual hospital policy related to a laser program.

Standards The Code of Federal Regulations' *Performance Standards for Light Emitting Products*[1] provides specifications for manufacturers of medical laser systems. The federal government does not approve a laser or system. However, manufacturers must certify that their products meet all safety requirements of the federal standard. Other standards apply to the users of these products.

American National Standards Institute (ANSI) ANSI is a voluntary organization of experts who determine industry consensus standards in various fields. The standard developed for the safe use of lasers[2] is intended more for users than manufacturers, but many adhere to it in their own production facilities. The existing federal legislation and state laser safety regulations are based on the ANSI standard. Simply this standard implies that every hospital or other facility using surgical lasers must establish and maintain an adequate program for control of laser hazards. This program shall include provisions for:

1 Laser safety officer. This person should have the authority to suspend, restrict, or terminate operation of a laser system if hazard controls are inadequate. In large hospitals, a laser safety committee, often a subcommittee of the operating room committee, may appoint this surveillance officer.

2 Education of users. A safety training program must ensure that all users, including operators, nurses, surgical technologists, biomedical engineers and technicians, who work with lasers are knowledgeable of correct operation, potential hazards, and control measures.

3 Protective measures for patients, personnel, and environment. (See safety factors, p. 367.)

4 Management of accidents. This includes reporting accidents and plans of action to prevent a future occurrence.

Joint Commission on Accreditation of Hospitals (JCAH) JCAH standards[3] serve as a guide in establishing specific policies and procedures related to the use of lasers. The applicable standards include:

1 Credentialing and clinical practice privileges of medical staff. Physicians authorized to use the laser may be required to hold laser certification or to complete a postgraduate laser course in their specialties.

[1]Federal Register, *Code of Federal Regulations,* Performance standards for light emitting products, Part 1040, pp. 257–272, Washington, D.C.: United States Food and Drug Administration, 1982.

[2]*American National Standard for the Safe Use of Lasers,* ANSI Z136.1, New York: American National Standards Institute, Inc., 1980.

[3]*Accreditation Manual for Hospitals, AMH/85,* Chicago: Joint Commission on Accreditation of Hospitals, 1984.

2 Initial and ongoing educational programs for nursing personnel. They should have thorough knowledge and understanding of laser equipment, laser physics, tissue reactions, applications, and safety precautions.

3 Quality assurance. This includes appropriate care, use, and maintenance of equipment and prevention of laser-related accidents.

4 Documentation. The surgeon, procedure, type of laser used, length of use, and wattage must be recorded in the patient's medical record. This information, plus the patient's name, should also be recorded in the operating room log.

Patient Safety The surgeon must explain laser surgery and its potential complications to the patient prior to obtaining written consent. Some lasers are considered investigational devices by the Federal Food and Drug Administration. The patient must sign a specific consent form permitting data collection. With all lasers, the following precautions are taken to ensure patient safety:

1 Anesthetic agents must be noncombustible.

2 Metallic or insulated silicone endotracheal tubes are preferred for oral and laryngeal procedures. Red rubber tubes must be protected to prevent ignition (see Chap. 26, p. 512).

3 Eyes are protected with moistened eye pads taped securely in place, especially for procedures around head and neck, except ophthalmic procedures.

4 Antiseptic used for skin preparation must not have an alcohol base, i.e., isopropyl and ethyl alcohol or tincture of iodine. These are flammable.

5 Moistened woven textile or absorbent nonwoven towels should be placed over drapes in the immediate area around incision prior to use of laser.

6 Tissues surrounding the target tissue should be protected with moistened sponges or compressed patties.

7 Postoperative instructions should include care of the healing thermal wound, if on the skin.

Personnel Safety Exposure to laser radiation is hazardous for personnel. Precautions must be taken to avoid eye and skin exposure to direct or scattered radiation.

Eye Protection The eye is the most susceptible organ to laser injury. Different laser wavelengths will affect the eyes differently. Argon and Nd:YAG lasers will be absorbed by the retina, CO_2 laser by the cornea. Therefore, each type of laser requires a specific lens in safety glasses or goggles. The argon laser requires an amber-tinted lens filter; CO_2 laser requires clear glass or plastic with side guards; Nd:YAG laser requires a green-tinted lens filter. A scratch on the lens or break in frame could negate eye protection.

Skin Protection Skin sensitivities can develop from overexposure to ultraviolet radiation. The skin also can be burned from exposure to direct or reflected laser energy. These hazards are minimized if personnel are alert to warning signs in the environment and labels on the machine, and if they use appropriate instrumentation.

Environmental Safety Only properly trained persons are authorized to participate in laser surgery. Others must be aware of its hazards.

1 Warning sign, "Laser Surgery in Progress," should be affixed to the outside of the operating room door. Closed safety latches or interlocks on door prevent entry of unauthorized persons. Only those with appropriate eye protection are admitted.

2 Warning labels on the machine, affixed by manufacturer, must indicate points of danger to avoid personnel exposure to laser radiation.

3 Machine should be prepared, checked, and tested before patient is brought into the room. A preoperative checklist is helpful. Any malfunction must be reported immediately and the equipment not used until in proper working order.

4 Machine should be kept on shutter or "standby" setting with the beam terminated in a beam stop of highly absorbent, nonreflecting, fire-resistant material when not in use, to avoid accidental activation. It should be turned off and locked when left unattended for a prolonged period of time.

5 Foot switch should be operated only after throwing a master control switch. The foot pedal can be covered when not in use, so the surgeon will not inadvertently activate the laser.

6 Nonreflective instruments should be used in or near the beam. These may be of a dull blue finish titanium alloy, black chrome-plated stainless steel, or oxidized stainless steel. These defocus and disperse the laser beam.

7 Fire is a potential hazard. Precautions for patient safety are identified above. Personnel must be aware of fire safeguards (see Chap. 11, p. 206).

8 Electrical codes must be enforced to avoid electrical hazards (see Chap. 11). An isolation transformer is recommended for a high voltage laser power source to avoid dangerous overload on the existing OR power system.

9 Manufacturer's instructions for operation and care of the laser system must be followed. Proper care of lasers and accessory equipment is essential to patient, personnel, and environmental safety.

ENDOSCOPY

Endoscopy is a combined form of two Greek words, *endon* and *skopein: endon* meaning "inside," *skopein* meaning "to examine." *Endoscopy,* as term is used in medicine, is a visual examination of the interior of a body cavity, hollow organ, or structure with an *endoscope,* an instrument designed for direct visual inspection.

Although physicians sought to visualize interior of body organs, development of endoscopy was slow. It was not until the early nineteenth century that attempts were made to examine the inside of the bladder. The instruments were inadequate, however, and the light was from a candle or lamp. Finally Nitze, an Austrian, developed an instrument in 1876 that is the basis of modern endoscopy. Dr. Chevalier Jackson of Philadelphia further enhanced endoscopy with the development of the laryngoscope and bronchoscope. Only after the incandescent lamp was invented and an optical system was devised could an efficient instrument be made. Improvements started about 1878, and the precise instruments of today have evolved since that time, making possible the conservative treatment of many conditions. Endoscopic inspection of the abdominal cavity, introduced in 1902, has become a frequently employed procedure since the advent of fiberoptic illumination.

An endoscope usually is inserted into a natural body orifice, i.e., the mouth, anus, or urethra. It may be inserted through a small skin incision and/or trocar puncture, as through the abdominal or vaginal wall. An endoscopic procedure is designated by the anatomic structure to be visualized. The endoscope likewise is named for the anatomic area it is designed to visualize, e.g., a laryngo*scope* is used for laryngo*scopy.* From head to foot, nearly every area of the body can be visualized with an endoscope.

Ophthalmoscopy Direct and indirect examination of the eye
Otoscopy Auditory canal and tympanic membrane
Nasopharyngoscopy Nasopharynx
Antroscopy Maxillary sinus
Laryngoscopy Direct visualization of the larynx [Indirect laryngoscopy is an examination with a laryngeal mirror. (p. 511)]
Bronchoscopy Tracheobronchial tree (p. 517)
Mediastinoscopy Mediastinal spaces in the chest cavity (p. 565)
Pleuroscopy Pleural cavity
Thoracoscopy Pleural surfaces
Esophagoscopy Esophagus (p. 516)
Gastroscopy Stomach (p. 410)
Duodenoscopy Duodenum
Jejunoscopy Jejunum
Colonoscopy Colon from ileocecal valve to anus (p. 413)
Sigmoidoscopy Sigmoid colon and rectum (pp. 413, 415)
Proctoscopy Rectum and anal canal (p. 415)
Anoscopy Lower rectum and anal canal (p. 415)
Choledochoscopy Common bile duct (p. 405)
Nephroscopy Renal pelvis (pp. 452, 453)
Peritoneoscopy Within peritoneal cavity for visualization of abdominal and pelvic organs
Laparoscopy Through abdominal wall for visualization of abdominal organs, but usually the female pelvic organs (p. 426)
Fetoscopy Through abdominal wall and uterus for visualization of fetus in utero (p. 443)
Culdoscopy through the vaginal wall into the retrouterine space for visualization of female pelvic tissues, especially the ovaries (p. 426)
Hysteroscopy Uterus (p. 428)
Colposcopy Vagina and cervix (p. 426)
Cystoscopy Urinary bladder (pp. 454, 456)
Urethroscopy Urethra (p. 457)
Arthroscopy A joint, usually the knee (p. 474)
Vascular endoscopy Arterial or venous lumen

All the above procedures are invasive, except ophthalmoscopy, because the scope is placed into a body orifice or cavity. Endoscopy is used for many diagnostic procedures (see Chap. 20, p. 394) and in conjunction with operative procedures. Description of many of these is included in the following chapters on the page numbers noted above. Endoscopy may be described as a closed technique, as opposed to an open procedure via an incision to expose body structures.

Design of Endoscopes

Although the sizes and shapes vary according to specific uses, all endoscopes have similar working elements (see Fig. 19-1).

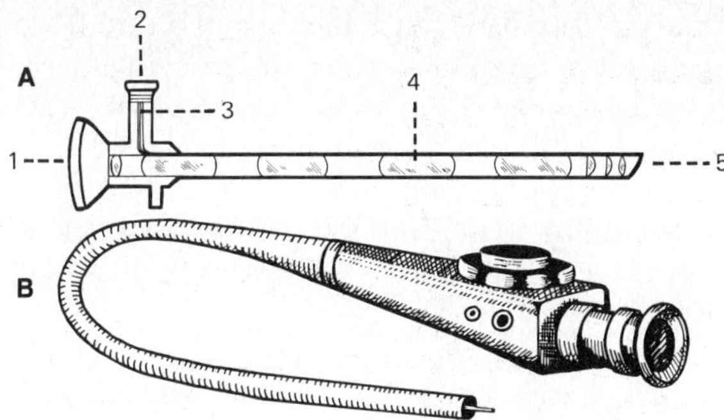

FIGURE 19-1
Schematic design of endoscopes. (**A**) Rigid scope: (1) eyepiece (ocular lens), (2) attachment for light source, (3) fiberoptic bundle, (4) telescopic lenses, (5) objective lens. (**B**) Flexible scope.

Viewing Sheath (Scope) The surgeon views anatomic structures through a round- or oval-shaped sheath. Diameter varies from the 1.7 mm needle fetoscope, to 5 mm or less of the arthroscope, to 22 mm of an anoscope. Length must be appropriate to reach the desired structure. The scope may be rigid or flexible.

Rigid Scopes These are either hollow sheaths that permit viewing through them in a forward direction only, such as laryngoscopes, or a sheath with an eyepiece and telescopic lens system that permits viewing in a variety of directions, such as cystoscopes. Most rigid scopes are metal. Disposable plastic anoscopes and otoscope sheaths are available.

Flexible Scopes These have a dial adjuster that contours the lensed tip into and around anatomic curvatures to permit visualization of all surfaces of the wall of a structure, as within the hollow organs of the gastrointestinal tract viewed through a flexible gastroscope or colonoscope. The sheath of these instruments is made of plastic material.

Light Source Illumination within the body cavity is essential for visual acuity. The light source may be through a fiberoptic bundle or from an incandescent light bulb. The light carrier may be an integral part of the viewing sheath, as in flexible scopes and rigid telescopes, or a separate light carrier accessory to a hollow rigid scope.

Fiberoptic Lighting An intense cool light illuminates body cavities including those that cannot be seen with other light sources. Light is conducted through a bundle of thousands of coated glass fibers encased in a plastic sheath. Each fiber is drawn from optical glass into a strand 10 to 70 microns in diameter that is coated to minimize loss of light by reflection. Light entering one end of the fiber is transmitted by refraction through its entire length. The light produced through the bundle of fibers is nonglaring and evenly distributed on area to be visualized. Although it is of high intensity, the light is cool, even though a minimum rise of temperature in the tissues exposed to it may occur.

Bulbs Bulbs screw into the fitting either at end of a removable light carrier or at end of a built-in lens system. Electric current is conducted through a single-filament wire to illuminate the tiny incandescent light bulb. When changing bulb, put a bit of wax on threads of bulb base to seal bulb socket from moisture to prevent short circuits. Fiberoptic lighting has replaced bulbs in most endoscopes and prevents this hazard.

Power Source Electric current must be transmitted to the light source connected to a fiberoptic bundle or a light bulb. The electric current is entirely external to the patient with fiberoptic lighting. Current flows through a power cord attached to the endoscope inserted into the patient and through the instrument to light bulb at distal end of the light carrier or sheath. The power source may or may not be connected to the electrical system in the room.

Projection Lamp A quartz-halogen or mercury-arc light bulb provides an intense light source, similar to a film projector, for transmission of light through a fiberoptic bundle to distal end of the scope. Usually a portable, compact, self-contained unit, the intensity of the light may be regulated from 400 footcandles (fc) to as much as 5200 fc, up to 5500°K daylight, in some illuminators. The bulb must be positioned securely in its socket so output focuses on center of the fiberoptic bundle. If it is not properly positioned, light output will not be of maximum value.

A fiberoptic power cable transmits light from the projection lamp to the endoscope. Both ends of the cable must have the correct fittings to attach to the lamp and to the scope or removable light carrier. Diameter of the cable varies from 2.0 to 5.5 mm to be compatible with aperture for the light source. Cable lengths also vary from 6 ft (180 cm) to 7.5 ft (234 cm) so the projection lamp can be positioned at a distance from a sterile field. Prior to use, the fiberoptic cable should be checked for damage. Hold one end of cable toward a low power light, such as the overhead operating light. With a magnifying glass, focus on the opposite end. Broken fibers in the cable will appear as dark spots. The cable must be replaced if more than 20 percent of the area appears dark.

Battery Box With one or more sets of dry-cell batteries, this may be used as the power source for light bulbs. The batteries may be recharged in some units, but eventually they must be replaced. A battery provides a good source of current, is safe, and can be used in conjunction with other electrical equipment.

Rheostat This is a resistor for regulating flow of current from the electrical system. Rapidly introduced high voltage may burn out the delicate filament in a light bulb. A rheostat reduces electrical potential and allows gradual increase of current to desired brightness of the light. However, safety precautions must be observed when using this power source to prevent shock to patient and operator. Rheostats that cannot be grounded should not be used. Also, they cannot be used when the cutting current of the electrosurgical unit is in use. Cutting current will not work if another piece of equipment is on the same circuit.

Accessories Accessories such as suction tubes, snares, biopsy forceps, grasping forceps, electrosurgical tips, sponge carriers, are used in conjunction with endoscopes. These can be passed through channels in the endoscope to remove fluid or tissue, coagulate bleeding vessels, inject fluid or gas to distend cavities, etc. Some rigid scopes have an obturator, a blunt-tipped rod placed through the lumen, to permit smooth insertion of instrument, as into the anus. The accessories that will be needed will be determined by type of endoscope and purpose of procedure.

Operating Microscope The optical system of some endoscopes can be attached to a specially designed operating microscope, such as the colpomicroscope. The illumination of the endoscope and binocular magnification of the microscope permit study of abnormal tissues and/or therapeutic procedures in areas otherwise inaccessible without open operation.

Laser Surgery A laser beam can be focused through some endoscopes. Argon and Nd:YAG lasers will pass through a fiberoptic system. The carbon dioxide laser can be directed through the interior mirror system of a multi-articulated arm of the operating microscope (see laser microadaptor, p. 379). The beam is then focused through the endoscope, usually held in a self-retaining device. A distal smoke evacuation suction device clears fumes to maintain visibility through the scope and at site of lasing. The endoscopes are specifically designed for adaptation to articulated arm of CO_2 laser, e.g., CO_2 laser laparoscope, CO_2 laser bronchoscope.

Ultrasonography A high-frequency ultrasound transducer at the end of a fiberoptic endoscope provides visualization of the heart, liver, pancreas, spleen, and kidneys. Refer to Chapter 20, p. 393, for discussion of use of ultrasonography for diagnosis of vascular diseases and for identifying location, size and consistency of abdominal organ lesions.

Cameras Lensed scopes may be equipped with a still or motion picture camera so organs or lesions can be photographed during a procedure. Video cameras with recorder/player equipment can be adapted for use with some endoscopes, such as an arthroscope. The Video Endoscope, for example, electronically transmits images to a closed-circuit television screen for viewing. The examination can be tape recorded for repeated viewing. The camera may be suspended from a mobile ceiling mount.

Hazards of Endoscopy

Endoscopy is not without its hazards. Some hospitals require the patient to sign a consent for operation prior to an endoscopic procedure in the event a complication develops. Two major complications of endoscopy are:

1 *Perforation.* This is a constant cause for concern when rigid scopes are used. Flexible fibroscopes have decreased this danger, but it remains a potential complication.

2 *Bleeding.* Bleeding can occur from a biopsy site, pedicle of a polyp, or other area where tissue has been cut.

Electrical systems used with endoscopy must conform with the standards and be subjected to routine maintenance procedures prescribed by the National Fire Protection Association code for electrical safety. Two major electrical hazards associated with endoscopy are:

1 *Improperly grounded electrical equipment.* If you expect the surgeon will use a monopolar electrosurgical unit, place the inactive electrode with adequate skin contact to allow conduction of electric current. Only solid-state generators, and preferably bipolar active electrodes, should be used to avoid variances in voltage.

2 *Unsuspected current leaks.* Corrosion or accumulation of soil can inhibit flow of current across the screw fitting between the light carrier and bulb. Current can leak through the instrument to the patient. Ideally, endoscopes should not contain electrically conductive elements or metals that can corrode. Corrosion can be caused by repeated exposure to body fluids, hard water, or chemical agents.

Microorganisms, such as *Mycobacterium tuberculosis* on a bronchoscope, can be transmitted from one patient to another. *Streptococcus pneumoniae, Pseudomonas aeruginosa,* and *Clostridium* also present potential hazards of cross contamination. All parts and accessories must be thoroughly mechanically cleaned and terminally sterilized or disinfected after use of endoscopic equipment.

Care of Endoscopes

Not all endoscopic procedures are performed as sterile procedures; some are termed *surgically clean.* When an endoscope is introduced into the gastrointestinal tract through the mouth or anus, which normally harbors resident and transient microorganisms, the procedure may not be considered sterile. However, every patient must be protected from cross infection. Endoscopes and their accessories must be thoroughly cleaned and terminally sterilized or disinfected after use, although sterility is not maintained between and during some patient uses.

If body tissue will be incised or excised, the endoscope and all accessories should be sterile, regardless of point of entry. Double standards in practice of aseptic and sterile techniques do not exist theoretically. However, practically it may not be feasible to sterilize some heat-sensitive parts, such as a lensed telescope, between patient uses when several procedures are scheduled in succession. Control of scheduling endoscopic procedures and adequate instrumentation help provide sterile endoscopes for every patient. In reality, high-level disinfection may be necessary between uses. The hospital must have written policy and procedure that states the accepted practice, i.e., sterilization vs. disinfection. *Endoscopes should be prepared in the same manner for every patient.* Legally it is not prudent to use a sterile instrument on the first patient scheduled, and a disinfected scope on succeeding patients that day. The same principles for preparation and handling apply to all patients, with exception of patients with suppressed immune systems, as from chemotherapy or steroid therapy, on whom only sterile scopes are used. If high-level disinfection is the procedure of choice, a grossly contaminated scope should be sterilized before reuse.

Cleaning Clean all parts of endoscope as soon as possible after use while organic debris is still moist. Mucus, blood, feces, and protein-type residue can become trapped in the channels of the scope. This is difficult to remove if it becomes dry and may render the scope useless.

Wash endoscopes in warm, never hot, water and a mild, nonresidue liquid-detergent solution. Use a pipestem cleaner or small brush to clean inside lumen of all channels. The stopcocks on some scopes must be thoroughly cleaned, too, as dirty ones will stick. Open them to clean; never force them but loosen them with a drop of solvent or lubricant.

Particular attention must be paid to the cleanliness of lenses or viewing will be obstructed. Debris can be carefully removed from around the lens with a fine toothpick. Special lens paper is used on the lens itself. Lensed instruments should not be cleaned with any substance containing alcohol as it may dissolve the cement around the lens.

Rinse thoroughly and dry well. If scopes are to be sterilized in ethylene oxide gas, they must be thoroughly dry. Gas combines with water on items that are damp to form ethylene glycol (refer to Chap. 8, p. 134). Use cotton on a wire stylet, or a pipestem cleaner, or force air through channels to dry inside them. Organisms will multiply in a moist environment, so all parts must be dry during interval prior to further processing.

An endoscope processor is available to clean long flexible fiberoptic scopes, such as a colonoscope. It has two modes of operation to process the viewing sheath and channels of the scope: wash and dry cycle; or wash, disinfectant soak with activated glutaraldehyde solution, rinse and dry. This equipment automatically assures safe and thorough cleaning.

All endoscopic equipment should preferably be terminally sterilized, otherwise it must be disinfected after thorough mechanical cleaning.

Sterilization After cleaning, place each endoscope with all its parts *disassembled* in a well-padded perforated tray of convenient size. Some endoscopes, such as an arthroscope, are supplied in a perforated case lined with foam cut to fit each disassembled part. Wrap the tray or fitted case for sterilization. Instruments should be packaged immediately and sent to be steam or ethylene oxide gas sterilized.

Some parts of endoscopes can be safely steam sterilized, and therefore should be. Hollow, rigid metal sheaths, such as a sigmoidoscope, can be terminally steam sterilized after use, but then may be stored to keep it clean rather than sterile for a surgically clean procedure. Some fiberoptic cables also can be steam sterilized.

Parts with lenses and some fiberoptic carriers, such as a colonoscope, cannot be steam sterilized. High temperature and moisture will soften the cement holding lenses or fiberoptic fibers in place. The flexible shafts of some accessory instruments, such as biopsy forceps, erode when steam sterilized. These parts should be sterilized in ethylene oxide gas or soaked in activated glutaraldehyde solution for *ten hours* if ethylene oxide is not available.

During ethylene oxide sterilization of a fiberoptic lighting system, the manufacturer may recommend that the pressure not exceed 5 lb. Follow manufacturer's instructions for handling, using, cleaning, and sterilizing these items.

Aeration is necessary following ethylene oxide sterilization if any part of endoscope is nonmetallic, such as the Bakelite eyepiece of a lensed instrument. EO is a vesicant if it comes in contact with skin. It also can cause eye irritation. To avoid discomfort for surgeon and patient, *parts that could retain residual gas must be aerated.*

If endoscopes and accessories are immersed for ten hours in activated glutaraldehyde solution, use a plastic tray without a towel in the bottom. Prolonged use of a stainless steel tray may create an electrolytic action between the metals and can cause metallic deposits on instruments. Scopes and all accessories must be well rinsed in sterile distilled water before they are used to prevent tissue irritation from solution.

Disinfection When necessary to immediately reuse an endoscope that cannot be steam sterilized, wash in nonresidue liquid-detergent solution, rinse, dry and immerse in activated glutaraldehyde solution for a minimum of *ten minutes. Remember this is disinfection, not sterilization.* Rinse thoroughly in sterile distilled water before use.

Storage If not immediately wrapped for sterilization and storage, endoscopes should be terminally sterilized, or at least disinfected before returning them to their respective storage cabinets. Store clean, *dry,* unwrapped instruments on a soft material such as plastic sheeting or foam. Towels hold a residue of laundry detergent that can cause tarnish on metal.

Considerations for Patient Safety

1 The patient must be observed for signs and symptoms of reaction to drugs. Endoscopy is frequently performed with the use of sedatives and a topical or local anesthetic agent or with no anesthesia at all. The patient is awake during these procedures. Psychotropic drugs such as diazepam (Valium) and narcotics such as meperidine hydrochloride (Demerol) may be administered intravenously as an adjunct to other preoperative sedation to produce relaxation and cooperation during procedure and amnesia afterward. Respiratory depression and transient hypotension can occur. Antagonistic drugs should be available to reverse narcotic depression.

2 A topical agent is frequently applied to the nasal or oral and pharyngeal mucosa prior to introduction of an endoscope into the tracheobronchial tree or gastrointestinal tract. A topical agent may be instilled into the urethra prior to introduction of a cystoscope. Refer to Chapter 14 for reactions to topical and local anesthetic agents.

3 Teeth, gums, and lips must be protected if the endoscope is introduced through the mouth. Dentures are removed. A mouthpiece is inserted.

4 Hydrogen and methane gases are normally present in the colon. These gases must be flushed out with carbon dioxide before electrosurgery through the colonoscope to avoid possibility of explosion within the colon.

5 Power sources and lights should be tested before each use, and they should be kept in working order.

6 The heat generated from the projection lamp of a fiberoptic illuminator must be dissipated. It should not be enclosed in drapes because the heat could set them afire. If the unit contains a fan for heat regulation, the direction of air flow must be away from the patient and the sterile field to minimize airborne contamination. A flammable anesthetic agent must not be used when fiberoptics is the method of lighting for any piece of equipment.

7 Endoscopes must be smooth, with no nicks on the surface. Do not handle metal endoscopes with metal lifting forceps that can scratch the sheaths. They should be handled only with the hands, usually gloved.

8 Extreme care must be taken to observe patients after endoscopies for effects of respiratory or circulatory distress due to trauma or medication. Many endoscopic procedures are performed on ambulatory outpatients. They must not leave the facility until vital signs are stable and side effects have passed.

Nursing Duties

1 Often only a circulating nurse assists the surgeon with an endoscopic procedure. The nurse sets up the supplies and equipment, as much as possible, before the patient and surgeon arrive. Consult the procedure book. Remember sterility must be maintained for a sterile procedure.

2 Explain the procedure if the patient does not understand it. It is important that the patient know the reasons for any discomfort that may be experienced so that symptoms of discomfort will be recognized as normal.

3 Explain the position and need for it before positioning the patient. The position the patient must assume during the procedure is often uncomfortable.

4 Drape the patient properly to prevent unnecessary exposure.

5 Divert the patient's attention as much as possible during the procedure. The patient may complain of pain more than is justified as a way of expressing displeasure at the invasion of the endoscope or position required during the procedure. The nurse should stay with the patient to offer reassurance and emotional support. Suggest that slow, deep breaths may help relaxation and lessen the discomfort. Soft music may help the patient relax. The surgeon may allow the patient to watch the procedure through a viewing attachment on the endoscope. The nurse evaluates the patient's level of discomfort and informs the surgeon of unusual reactions.

6 The surgeon usually wants the room in semidarkness, but not so dark that the patient's skin color and condition cannot be observed. A dimmer on the room light is helpful.

7 Be sure you can identify the different scopes and their accessories. Know how to assemble and handle them. When passing the suction tube or biopsy forceps, the nurse or assistant should place the tip directly at the lumen of the scope so that the surgeon can grasp the shaft and insert it without moving eyes from the scope.

8 Endoscopic instruments are delicate and expensive. Care must be taken not to drop them. Fiberoptic bundles are glass, so do not kink or bend them.

MICROSURGERY

Microscopy, use of a microscope, has been an essential modality in scientific investigation for centuries. Pioneers like van Leeuwenhoek, who developed in 1680 the compound microscope which magnified objects 270 times, contributed to the adoption of the germ theory. Objects as small as bacteria could be seen only through a light microscope, as viruses can be seen only through the more recently developed electron microscope. Joseph Jackson Lister, father of the English surgeon who introduced antiseptic surgery, perfected the achromatic lens to eliminate color aberrations in the compound microscope. Ernest Abbe did further work in the nineteenth century to improve refraction and illumination through the lens. A basic system for binocular eyepieces was devised in 1902.

A microscope was first used for clinical surgery in 1921 when Nylen operated on patients with chronic otitis in Sweden. He used a monocular microscope. Subsequently as binocular magnification, adequate illumination, and stable support were added, otolaryngology became the first surgical specialty to routinely use a microscope.

Ophthalmologists were the first to use the stereoscopic biomicroscope, commonly referred to as a *slit lamp,* in clinical examination to magnify objects in three dimensions. The principles employed in the biomicroscope led to the development of an operating microscope by the Carl Zeiss Company in 1953. Ophthalmologists quickly expanded applications and indications for ocular microsurgery. Most other specialties were slow to implement its use.

The simplest magnifying instrument consists of a single lens with relatively high magnification, for example, the magnifying glass or a jeweler's lens.

Surgeons requiring lesser magnification than provided by the microscope employ an operating loupe. This simple lens magnifies approximately two times. It attaches to a headband or to the surgeon's spectacles. *Loupe surgery is not microsurgery.* It terminates where microsurgery begins. However, from it and from refinements of the binocular microscope, microsurgery has evolved.

The first of the present day operating microscopes was developed in 1960 by the Zeiss Instrument Company in collaboration with Julius Jacobson, a vascular surgeon in New York. Jacobson developed microsurgical instruments, introduced microvascular techniques, and began using the term *microsurgery.* Thus began the development of clinical applications of microsurgery in every surgical specialty.

Technique of Microsurgery

Performance of operative procedures while directly viewing the operating field under magnification affords surgeons greater visual acuity of small structures. *The microscope provides a more limited, although more readily visible, operative field.* All things look considerably different under magnification. Tissues not otherwise visible can be manipulated. The use of microsurgical instrumentation and techniques does not consist of adapting formerly learned conventional methods to use under the microscope. The techniques themselves for handling instruments, sutures, and tissues are different and infinitely more complex, precise, and time-consuming because of the meticulous skill involved. Coordination must be adapted to work with minute materials in a field of altered perception and position.

Groundwork for proficiency and facility in using the operating microscope must include liberal amounts of time spent by the surgeon in special instruction and laboratory practice under relaxed conditions. This entails practice in movements and manipulation of instruments and suture materials under various magnifications. Mastery is achieved only by practice, repeated performance, and dedication to the task.

Divergence from tactile-manual to vision-oriented techniques requires of the surgeon and assistants maximum attention to detail. The most common maneuvers utilized in placing and manipulating instruments, making an incision with a scissors, and tying sutures involve a combination of several basic movements:

1 *Compression-decompression*—to close scissors and forceps

2 *Rotation*—to insert a needle, to cut, to extract, to engage or disengage

3 *Push-pull, direct or linear*—to incise with a razor knife

The surgeon also must be able to maintain a steady stationary position during remote activation of equipment such as a cryosurgical unit or laser beam. It is advisable that surgeons do no manual labor for at least a day prior to operating. Very little tremor is tolerable in microsurgery.

Advantages of Microsurgery

Microsurgery provides unique advantages in the restoration of wholeness and function of the body, such as restitution of hearing, vision, tactile sensation, circulation, and/or motion. It is utilized in many surgical specialties to improve precision of already established operations as well as to permit successful performance of procedures previously not possible. For example, blood vessels less than 3 mm in exterior diameter can be sutured. Nerves can be anastomosed. Replantation of amputated parts (see Chap. 34, pp. 617–618) and some reconstructive surgery (see Chaps. 27 and 28) are possible only under magnification. In general, microsurgery allows:

1 Dissection and repair of fine structures through better visualization.

2 Adaptation of operative procedures to individual patient requirements. Variation in anatomical landmarks is more distinct with magnification.

3 Diminution of operative trauma and complications because of safer dissection.

4 Superior focal lighting of the operative field, particularly in deep areas.

The Operating Microscope

Compound microscopes use two or more lens systems or several lenses grouped in one unit. *The operating microscope is a compound binocular instrument.* Interchangeable objective lenses combined with interchangeable eyepieces allow a wide range of magnification and working distances adjustable to the surgeon's needs. *The operating microscope employs light waves for illumination.* These waves are bent as they pass through the microscope so image seen by the viewer's eye is magnified.

One must understand the parts and their functions. Basically, all operating microscopes incorporate the same essential components: optical lens system and controls for magnification and focus, illumination system, mounting system for stability, electrical system, and accessories.

Optical Lens System The ability to enlarge an image is known as *magnifying power.* This is the ratio of size of image produced on the viewer's retina by magnification to size of retinal image when object is viewed without optical aid. To create a distinct image, adjacent images must be separated. An indistinct image remains unclear no matter how many times it is magnified. The ability to discern detail is known as *resolving power.*

Components The heart of the optical system is the *body,* which contains the *objective lens* (lens closest to the object). The *head* or *binocular oculars* (eyepieces) through which the surgeon looks are physically and optically attached to the body. The optical combination of the objective lens and the oculars determines the magnification of the microscope (see Fig. 19-2B).

Objective lenses are available in various focal lengths ranging from 100 to 400 mm, with intervening increases by 25-mm increments. The 400-mm lens provides the greatest magnification. The designation of the objective lens enumerates the *working distance,* the distance from the lens to the operating field. Distances vary from 6 to 10 in. (15 to 25 cm). For example, a 200-mm lens will be in focus at a working distance of 200 mm or approximately 8 in. (20 cm).

The oculars serve as magnifying glasses used to examine the real image formed by the objective. Most objectives are achromatic so true color of tissues can be viewed in sharp detail. The binocular arrangement provides stereoscopic viewing. Stereopsis is basically achieved through binocular viewing so each eye has a slightly different positional view of the object under examination. The observer's brain then combines the two dissimilar images taken from points of view a little distance apart, thus producing a perception of a single three-dimensional image.

Magnification The ability of the microscope to magnify depends on the design and quality of the parts in addition to the resolving power. The total magnification is computed by multiplying the enlarging power of the objective lens by that of the lenses of the oculars. The depth of the field, which is the vertical dimension within which objects are seen in clear focus, decreases with increase in magnification of power. Likewise, the width of the field of view narrows as the power of magnification increases. For example, at 20× magnification the field of view narrows to 10 mm, less than 1.25 cm (½ in.). Vertical viewing of operative field is extremely important, particularly in higher magnification ranges. It allows the surgeon more effective use of the increasingly limited depth of field.

In more complex microscopes a third set of lenses is interposed between the oculars and the objective lens to provide additional magnification in variable degrees as desired by surgeon. A continuously variable system of magnification, for increasing or decreasing images, is possible with a *zoom lens.* The faster, easier to handle zoom is preferred by most surgeons to the simpler turret magnifier that manually changes magnification by fixed increments. The zoom is usually operated by a foot control that permits the surgeon to change magnification without removing hands from the operative field. The popular range of magnification in the zoom microscope is from 3.5 to 20× magnification. At 3.5×, the depth of the field is 2.5 mm or about 1/10 in.; at 20× the depth is 1 mm or about 1/25 in. Some microscopes magnify to 40 times.

Focus Focusing is accomplished manually or by a foot-controlled motor that raises and lowers the body of the microscope to the desired distance from object to be viewed. Some microscopes divide the focus into gross and fine. Focus of ocular lens usually is set at zero; surgeon will adjust as desired.

Illumination System Illumination of the operating microscope employs light waves. The shorter the wavelength, the greater the resolving power. Intensity of illumination can be varied by controls mounted on support arm of the body. The operating microscope has two basic sources of illumination.

Paraxial Illuminators One or more light tubes, paraxial illuminators, contain incandescent bulbs and focusing lenses. The illuminators are attached to the mounting of the body of the microscope in a position to illuminate the field of view. The light is focused to coincide with the working distance of the microscope.

One of the paraxial illuminators may be

equipped with a diaphragm containing a variable-width slit aperture. This device permits a narrow beam of light to be brought to focus on the objective field. This slit image assists surgeon in defining depth perception, i.e., in ascertaining the relative distance of objects within the field (which are closer, which are farther).

Coaxial Illuminators A second source, usually fiberoptic, is transmitted through the optical system of the microscope body. This type of illumination is called *coaxial* because it illuminates the same area in the same focus as the viewing or objective field of the microscope. The fiberoptic system provides intense, though cool, light that protects the patient's tissues and the optics of microscope from excessive heat. The light intensity ranges from 600 to 2250 footcandles without creating shadows. Reflected glare may be a problem, however. Frequent wound irrigation with a cool solution is necessary to avoid tissue damage from radiant energy during long procedures.

If a fiberoptic system is not used for coaxial illumination, a heat-absorbing filter must be interposed in the illumination system. Direct heat from a high-intensity source can damage and even burn tissues.

Another type optical prism assembly provides a larger area of coaxial illumination with a brighter light than fiberoptic light bundles. Known as liquid light, it utilizes ionic, inorganic saline solution with quartz glass inserts inside a flexible aluminum spiral tube insulated with a polyvinyl chloride coating. Light is conducted throughout the cross section of the liquid, unlike a fiberoptic bundle.

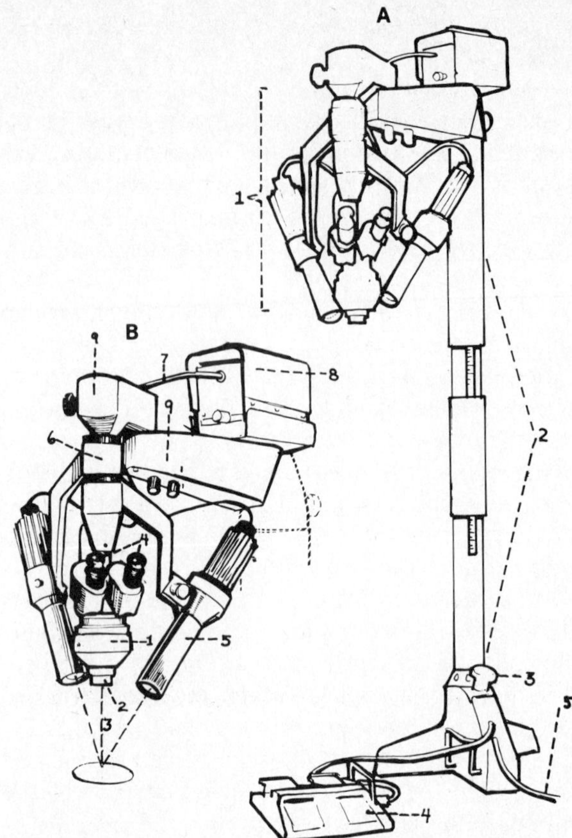

FIGURE 19-2
Floor-mounted operating microscope. (**A**) (1) optical portion, (2) vertical column, (3) brake knob, (4) foot control, (5) power cord. (**B**) Microscope detail: (1) body with zoom mechanism, (2) objective lens, (3) working distance, (4) oculars, (5) paraxial illuminator, (6) coaxial illuminator, (7) fiberoptic cable, (8) fiberoptic light source, (9) support arms.

Mounting Systems Stability of the microscope is of paramount importance. The body, optical portion, is mounted on a vertical column that may be supported by the floor, ceiling, wall, or attachment to the operating table. The body of the microscope is attached to the column by a hinged arm and a central pivot. The mounting permits positioning as desired. It may be adjusted horizontally or vertically, rotated on its axis, and tilted at different angles. The microscope can be aimed in any direction. The objective is aimed at the principal site of the operative procedure.

The floor and ceiling mounting systems are the most popular and versatile. All microscopes must have a locking mechanism to immobilize the microscope body over the operative field.

Floor Mount The base of the vertical support rests on the floor. The base has retractable casters for ease in moving the entire instrument. However, when lowered to working position, the base is locked into position (see Fig. 19-2A).

The base should be properly positioned in relation to operating table before anesthesia is administered or patient prepped. To maintain balance and control, gently push (don't pull) the microscope when moving it. Brake should be released or casters activated before moving. Arms should be folded close to the column with all attachments locked into place. Cords should be out of the way. Observation tubes should not be used as handles. Never use force in moving the microscope or in applying attachments. Check the problem instead. A floor-based microscope with column support is placed to left of a right-handed surgeon. Base should not interfere with foot controls or power cables. It must be clear of any table attachments as well.

As a safety factor, the base must not be moved when microscope is over patient because it is top-heavy. Gross adjustments, such as height in relation to operative field and focus, are made with microscope swung away from patient. Operating table height, chair, and armrest heights are adjusted at the same time gross adjustments are made. Fine focusing and adjustments are done after microscope is in position for operating. The assistant's microscope is adjusted to the same focus as that of the surgeon. During prepping and draping, microscope is rotated out of position, then brought over operative area for procedure.

Ceiling Mount This mount, subdivided into fixed and track-mounted models, provides freer floor space. The fixed unit is suspended from a telescoping column attached directly to the ceiling. The vertical support of the track-mounted unit is suspended from a ceiling rail. It can be moved out of the way when not in use (see Fig. 19-3). The microscope is positioned and focused after the patient is anesthetized. A ceiling-mounted instrument is operated by a control panel on a wall (on-off switch) and by foot controls for focusing, magnifying, raising, and lowering.

A ceiling mount is generally very stable, but it is only as stable as the supporting ceiling. Mechanical devices adjacent to the OR, such as air-conditioning units, may cause vibration. The microscope *must* be vibration-free. A ceiling mount permits the same flexibility of positioning as a floor mount.

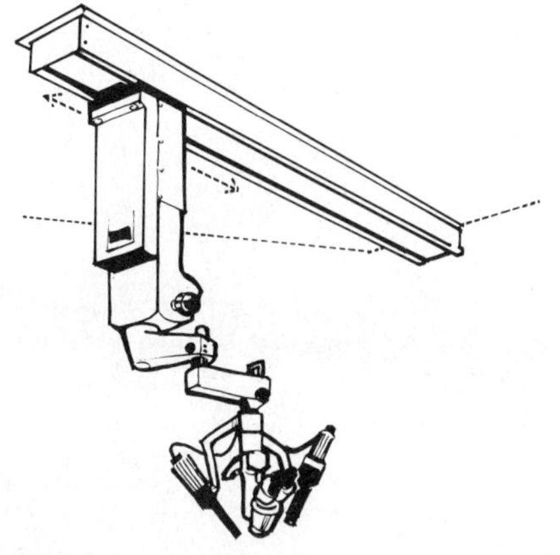

FIGURE 19-3
Ceiling-track-mounted microscope.

The vertical support has a memory stop mechanism that can be preset for a preselected operating table height. This setting should be checked and adjusted for each table-position change. The mechanism is a safety factor to prevent accidental lowering of microscope at high speed too close to the patient. High-speed lowering should be done away from patient until the memory stop is reached. As with the floor-mounted instrument, gross adjustments are never made over patient. Fine adjustment and focusing are done after microscope is over the operative field.

Wall Mount The microscope is bracketed by a flexible arm to a stable wall. The swing-arm extension permits proper positioning.

Operating Table Mount Smaller microscopes may be mounted on framework of operating table. This system has many disadvantages so is not popular.

Electrical System The same precautions are observed with the operating microscope as with any electrical equipment in the OR. Switches and wall interlocks should be explosionproof. Circuits must be protected from overload by breaker relays and fuses. All light controls should be in the off position when the power plug is inserted or removed from the wall outlet to avoid short-circuiting or sparking. A red pilot light illuminates on the control panel when the electric power is on.

Care of Microscope

Persons responsible for microscope should consult the manufacturer's manual. Any malfunction should be reported to OR supervisor or appropriate person who can arrange for repair service. A checklist to verify care and functioning of various parts prior to operation is helpful. All persons who assist with microsurgery must know how to set up and position the microscope.

1 Microscope should be damp-dusted before use.
   a External surfaces, *except the lenses,* are wiped with a clean cloth saturated with detergent-disinfectant solution.
   b Casters or wheels should be clean to reduce contamination and prevent interference with mobility.

2 Lenses should be cleaned, according to manufacturer's recommendations only, to avoid scratching or damage to antireflective lens coating.

3 Circulating nurse should prepare microscope.
  a When changing oculars, care must be taken to avoid dropping and fingerprinting the lenses.
  b Both hands should be used for attaching observation tubes. They are heavy.
  c Extra lamp bulbs and fuses should be on hand. The circulating nurse must know where they are stored and how to change them. It is advisable to check bulbs periodically to avoid necessity for replacement during a procedure. New bulbs should be inserted if a long procedure is anticipated.
  d Check electrical connections for proper fit or wire fraying. Take special care of power cables to prevent accidental breakage by heavy equipment rolling over them.
  e Check that all knobs are secured after microscope is in operating position.
  f See that foot controls are in a convenient position so surgeon does not have to search for them.

4 Properly store microscope and accessories. Store away from traffic but close to areas where used.
  a Openings into microscope body for attachment of accessory devices, such as the observer tube, should be closed with covers provided by the manufacturer when not in use to prevent accumulation of dust.
  b Lenses and viewing tubes should be protected.
  c Microscope and attachments should be enclosed in an antistatic plastic cover when not in use to keep them free from dust.
  d Power cords should be neatly coiled for storage.

Accessories

A number of accessories are available to enhance the versatility of microsurgery. The value of a good microscope is negated without proper ancillary equipment.

Assistant's Binoculars A separate optical body with nonmotorized, hand-controlled zoom can be attached to the main microscope body for use by the assistant (see Fig. 19-4). This mechanism can be focused in the same plane as the surgeon's oculars. However, its field of view does not coincide exactly with that of the surgeon. This can be rectified by using a *beam splitter,* which takes the image from one of the surgeon's oculars and transmits it through an *observer tube,* thereby providing the assistant with an identical image of the surgeon's view (see Fig. 19-5). This is particularly important in critical areas where a difference of 1 or 2 mm is crucial.

Assistant's oculars and/or observer tubes can be moved to either side. These units are heavy and so should be placed on appropriate side of microscope, right or left, before operative procedure begins.

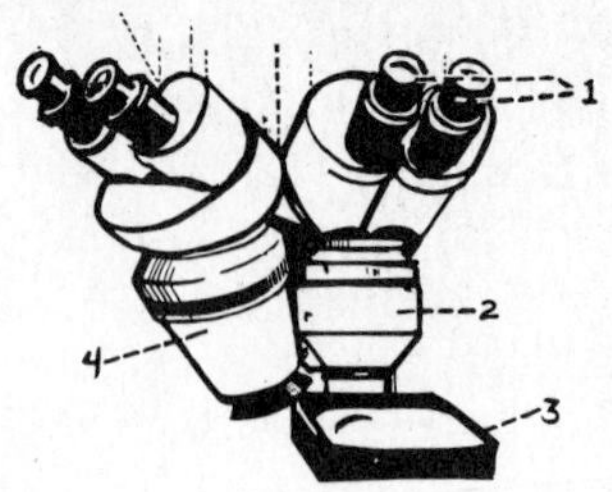

FIGURE 19-4
Surgeon's microscope on the right with assistant's attached microscope on the left: (1) oculars, (2) body with motorized zoom mechanism, (3) broadfield viewing lens, (4) body with manual zoom mechanism.

Broadfield Viewing Lens Attached to the front of the body of the surgeon's ocular, this lens is a low-power magnifying glass used for grasping needles or getting an overall view of the field adjacent to the objective (see Fig. 19-4).

X-Y Attachment An automated mechanism, this provides a precision method of controlling small movements of microscope in field of view.

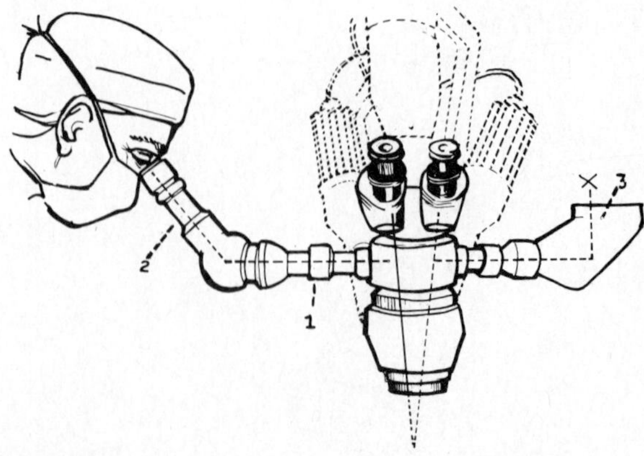

FIGURE 19-5
Microscope accessories: (1) beam splitter attachment, (2) observer tube, (3) camera attachment.

Cameras Still photographic, motion picture, videotape, and television cameras may be attached to the beam splitter, permitting filming of the operative procedure (see Fig. 19-5). Their output is useful in assisting, teaching, and research. The camera unit should be in the upright position when connected to the operating microscope. Check to be sure film is in camera by trying to rewind the film cartridge holder.

Laser Microadaptor Laser beams can be directed through the operating microscope. The microscope and laser head couplings must be perfectly aligned in the grooves and protrusions on the metal adaptors. A screw and locking pin secure the coupling. In the operating position, the laser head is at approximately a 60° angle to the microscope. It will not fire in a horizontal or upside-down position. The microadaptor must have a compatible lens, with focal length of 200, 300, or 400 mm, so surgeon can properly adjust the focal point of the laser beam.

Remote Foot Controls Simple microscopes are manually operated. However, it is more convenient for surgeon to utilize foot-controlled, motorized functions such as focus, zoom, and tilt. Foot controls may be activated by switches of the push-button type, heel-to-toe, or side-to-side motion. Number of switches corresponds to number of motor-controlled functions. There may be additional foot switches for the camera or other nonmicroscope associated equipment such as cryosurgical, bipolar electrosurgical, or laser units. Switches may be separated by a vertical bar to prevent inadvertent contact. The bar also serves as a foot rest for the surgeon. Since the surgeon and assistant frequently sit for microsurgical procedures, height of the operating table must permit them adequate knee room to operate foot controls.

Armrests and Chair It is mandatory that the surgeon's hands be adequately supported, as a shift of even 1 mm (1/25 in.) can alter the operative field, particularly at high magnifications. Support of the surgeon's arm must be continuous from shoulder to hand to give stability and to minimize tremor, especially in fine finger movements. A detachable, sterile wrist support may be affixed to the operating table, such as the Chan wrist rest.

A chair, with hydraulic foot controls for raising or lowering, provides the necessary forearm support by means of attached armrests. These are individually draped. Mayo stand covers are convenient. Armrests can be moved independently to a variety of levels and positions. They must be secured in the desired position. The surgeon must be in a comfortable position to work.

Microscope Drape The entire working mechanism and support arm of the microscope are encased in a sterile drape. Draping the entire microscope permits it to be brought into sterile field so the surgeon can position the body and adjust the optics. Disposable plastic drapes which are heat-resistant, lint-free, nonreflective, transparent, and quiet are available to fit the configuration of all microscopes and attachments. The scrub nurse slides drape over the body, with hands protected as for draping a Mayo stand. The circulating nurse helps guide drape toward the vertical column and secures it. The scrub nurse secures the drape to the oculars. Sterile lens covers or rubber bands may be supplied with the drape for this purpose.

If not heat-resistant, a plastic drape may cause heat buildup beneath it that can damage the microscope. A heat guard may be applied over the light source or heat evacuated through an opening in top of drape.

Microinstrumentation

Improved results of operative intervention utilizing microsurgical techniques are due in no small measure to the miniaturized precision instrumentation developed in association with the performance of these delicate procedures. The instruments are extremely fine, delicate, and miniature enough to handle in the very small working area. Manipulation becomes more difficult with increased size or bulk and weight. Like techniques, instruments are constantly being improved. Microsurgeons work with manufacturers to develop appropriate instruments, suture materials, and needles. Many surgeons purchase the instruments of their choice. Whether owned by the surgeon or the hospital, microinstruments require exacting care to maintain desired function (refer to Chap. 11, p. 199).

Instruments are designed to conform to the surgeon's hand movements under the microscope. They must permit secure grasp, ease of holding and manipulation, and fulfillment of their intended purpose. They are shaped to not obscure the limited field of view. While these factors are important criteria for any instrument, they are especially vital for microinstruments. Everyone assisting in or setting up for microsurgical procedures must learn and know the identification and functions of these unique instruments. Design is coincident to function.

Material and Surface Microinstruments are made of stainless steel or titanium. Titanium alloy is considerably stronger yet lighter in weight than stainless steel. Some are malleable for desired angling. Some are disposable. All are extremely vulnerable to abuse.

Finishes of at least the portions of instruments exposed to light in the operative field are deliberately dulled during manufacture to reduce glare, which is both annoying and tiring to the surgeon. Titanium microinstrments have a dull blue finish.

Shape and Tips Microinstruments are shorter than standard instruments and often angulated for convenience of approach and avoidance of obstruction of operative field.

Instrument tips have minimal separation compatible with their function. Finger pressure and movement necessary to close wide tips is undesirable because it may induce tremor.

Handles Handles are designed for secure and comfortable grasp with diameter comparable to a pen or pencil. Minimal diameter between fingers facilitates feel and accuracy of manipulation. Double-handled instruments (scissors, needleholders) have a slightly larger diameter than single-handled ones (razor knife). Shape of handle is also important to manipulation. For example, instruments rotated between fingers when in use, such as needleholders, must be turned easily. Their handles, therefore, are rounded or six-sided like a pencil. Those not rotated have finger grips or are flattened. Ring-handled instruments are not practical in microsurgery.

Many instruments, particularly scissors and some needleholders, have spring handles that return tips to open position between cutting or grasping functions. Distance from hinge to tip will vary according to function. Proper spring tension can be easily ruined by mishandling.

Handles must be long enough for comfort in the working position, but must not extend beyond the working distance to contact the unsterile objective of the microscope. Maximum length of most microinstruments is about 100 mm (4 in.). Gripping surfaces should be functionally located to prevent fingers from slipping during manipulation. These surfaces serve as a guide to accurate finger positioning. The gripping area may be six-sided, round, knurled, or flat serrated.

Primary Uses Appropriate instrumentation is used for specific types of procedures. While all surgical instruments are structured for a definitive use, function of microinstruments is even more restricted. Tissue can be severely injured by use of an improper or imperfect instrument. Instruments too can be damaged by use on inappropriate tissue. Primary usage includes cutting (knives, scissors, and saws), exposure (spatulas and retractors), gross and fine fixation (forceps and clamps), suture and needle manipulation (needleholder). Instruments must not be used for manipulations other than intended purpose.

Knives Edges of razor, diamond, and dissecting knives have different degrees of sharpness and thickness of blades appropriate to cutting function of each, i.e., to make penetrating or slicing incision. A clean cut is desired to minimize trauma and tissue destruction.

Scissors Like knives, scissors are designed to make a specific type of incision related to plane as well as to thickness. Incisions are vertical, horizontal, or of a special configuraton such as curved or two-planed. Use is governed by hinging and blade relationship. Scissors are hinged to cut vertically or obliquely. Cutting is usually done by distal part of blades for better control. Some scissors come in pairs with right and left curves. Team members must know how to tell the difference. Often a part number inscribed by the manufacturer on the handle will be an even number for a right-hand instrument and odd for a left-hand one. Scissor blades may be sharp or blunt, long or short, straight or angulated. Available straight or curved, microsurgical scissors have a spring-type handle.

Powered Instruments Microsurgical air-powered drills and saws vary in sizes and shapes. They have a fingertip control; some have an optional foot control.

Spatulas and Retractors These instruments are used to draw tissue back for better exposure or protection. Nerve hooks and elevators also are used for these purposes.

Forceps Straight and curved forceps may be toothed or smooth. They have light spring action and minimal tip separation. Teeth of some tissue forceps may be as small as $\frac{1}{10}$ mm ($\frac{1}{250}$ in.) in diameter. Therefore, many tips are barely visible to the unaided eye. Toothed forceps are used for grasping tissue, but never for grasping needles or sutures. Smooth forceps are used for tying delicate ligatures and sutures. For stability of grasp and avoidance of injury to suture strand, the forceps tips must be absolutely parallel and have perfect apposition of grasping surfaces. Suture must be grasped firmly but without trauma, often from a slippery surface. Other smooth forceps are used on friable tissues. Bipolar forceps are used for electrocoagulation.

Clamps Mosquito hemostats and various clamps are used for vascular occlusion and for approximation of edges of tissues such as nerves and vessels. Crushing of vessels must be avoided.

Needleholders Microsurgical needleholders are only for suturing, not ligating, because the very fine suture materials would break if tied with a needleholder. They should be used to hold only minute microsurgical needles so as not to ruin alignment. Handles are round to permit easy rotation between fingers. Some have spring handles. While a lock on a needleholder may cause tips to jerk when engaged or released, some have a holding catch for use in deep wounds to prevent loss of small needles. Needleholders held closed by finger pressure, rather than a catch, firmly hold a needle shaft yet permit easy adjustment of needle position.

Microsutures and Needles Microsurgical closure is unique in that the smallest sizes of sutures and needles manufactured are used. Microsuture sizes range from 8-0 (45 micron) to 11-0 (14 micron) in diameter. Because of the minute size, proportionately small needles are swaged to the suture. They range from 30 to 130 microns in diameter.

Suture materials include synthetic absorbable and nonabsorbable polymers. A strand is finer than a human hair. Packets provide ready access to the needle. When in use, needle should always be kept in view in operative field since a strand may easily be lost from view as well as difficult to pick up. The surgeon should inspect strand for damage while passing it through tissue to be sure the holding power in situ is not threatened. It is safest and easiest for the scrub nurse to keep these sutures in the packet until the surgeon is ready to use them.

Stainless steel microsurgical needles are measured in microns of wire diameter and millimeters in length. To achieve deep placement in tissue, the needle is short and sharply curved. Less curvature is required for more superficial suturing. Straight needles may be preferred for some tissues.

To arm a needle in the needleholder, some surgeons want the scrub nurse to hold the open suture packet under the accessory broadfield viewing lens so they may grasp the needle themselves. The nurse then gently removes packet from strand. Or the nurse may remove suture from the packet, letting needle rest on back or side of one hand. The surgeon grasps the needle lightly but firmly in needleholder. The nurse then releases strand, which is taken into operative field. Any readjustment of position of needle is done by surgeon under the microscope.

Closure of an incision with the least trauma to produce minimal fibrosis and scarring is enhanced by placing sutures close together to yield a firm, even apposition line and anatomically secure wound. Integrity of the sutures compensates for minimal scar tissue in supporting the wound. Use of the zoom microscope facilitates tying and cutting sutures.

Sponges Suitably small, nonfibrous sponges or lint-free patties of material such as compressed cellulose are used to accommodate the operative field. Lint readily is visible under the microscope.

General Considerations of Microsurgery

Patient The patient is prepared as for a standard operative procedure. He or she must be positioned comfortably and safely with the operating table locked in position. The operative site is immobilized if possible.

Anesthesia If general anesthesia is to be administered, the anesthesiologist should be informed in advance of the surgeon's intention to use the microscope. This is especially pertinent in procedures where patient movements under light anesthesia can result in disaster. In addition, the anesthesiologist's position in relation to the patient must be considered to allow room for the microscope. The anesthesiologist should be aware that microsurgical procedures will take somewhat longer.

With local anesthesia it is important to adequately instruct the patient to lie quietly and to tell the anesthesiologist or circulating nurse of a desire to move. Many patients sleep during procedure. A startle reflex upon awakening or unexpected movement is especially hazardous in microsurgery where the surgeon's mobility and field of view are limited. If the patient jerks or turns, he or she literally may move out of the surgeon's hands and often out of view of the operative field. Therefore, the patient must be closely monitored.

Stability A vital factor for successful microsurgery is stability of the operative field, microscope, and surgeon's hands. The complete microsurgical unit consists of the operating table with the patient, the microscope, and the surgeon's chair. They must be functionally positioned in relation to each other so that major adjustments need not be made during operation. The surgeon and circulating nurse should check that all components are properly placed before the incision is made.

Scrub Nurse Duties While a stabilized situation is crucial, a second fundamental necessity is the need for the surgeon to keep eyes on the field of view through microscope at all times. Looking away from field requires readjustment of vision to the field. Cooperation and coordination by the scrub nurse prevent the surgeon's distraction from operative site.

1 Set up Mayo stand and instrument table without touching tips of instruments. Leave protecting covers on them until ready to use. Holders are available to keep tips in the air. Place instruments on Mayo stand in anticipated order of use.

2 Place Mayo stand and instrument table conveniently to surgeon's hand so that he or she does not have to look around the microscope.

3 Pass instruments by placing in surgeon's hand in position for use and guide hand toward operative field so surgeon may keep eyes on field.

4 Keep debris, i.e., blood, mucus, or suture ends, from tips of instrments by wiping them *gently* on a nonfibrous sponge or lint-free gauze. Replace them in original position on Mayo stand not touching each other.

5 Assist efficiently but never put hands in operative field unless requested to do so.

6 Understand need for slow dissection at times. Do not let attention stray; watch television monitor if available.

The increased operating time needed for use of the operating microscope can be minimized by adequate preparation and assistance. Each team member should thoroughly understand the microscope and every facet of microsurgical techniques.

Team members can be kept up-to-date by inservice explanation of new instruments and demonstration of the microscope. It is extremely helpful, as well as contributory to understanding, if the surgeon shows nurses and technologists anatomical structures and instruments through the microscope. A comparison of microinstruments with standard instruments under the microscope is always a revelation. A television monitor is advantageous in providing scrub nurse and anesthesiologist continuous observation of the operative procedure. All members must be completely familiar with instrumentation. Not only are instruments then properly cared for, but even more importantly, operating time is reduced.

CHAPTER **20**

DIAGNOSTIC PROCEDURES

Diagnosis of pathologic disease, anomaly, or traumatic injury must be established prior to undertaking major operative procedures. Many modalities and techniques assist surgeons to assess each individual patient problem, to guide them through the operation, and to verify the results of surgical intervention. The term *diagnosis* refers to the art or the act of determining the nature of a patient's disease. Diagnostic procedures, as discussed in this chapter, include procedures that pertain to establishing or serving as evidence in diagnosis and treatment of surgical pathology. They will be classified as:

1 *Preoperative* Procedures performed prior to the patient coming to the OR suite or performed in the OR prior to incision
2 *Intraoperative* Procedures performed in the OR as a part of the operation
3 *Noninvasive* Techniques utilizing equipment placed on or near the patient's skin but outside body tissues
4 *Invasive* Techniques utilizing equipment placed into a body cavity or vessel and/or substances injected into body structures

Preoperative diagnostic procedures may be noninvasive or invasive; likewise intraoperative procedures utilize both techniques. OR nurses and surgical technologists must be familiar with modalities and equipment necessary to assist with diagnostic procedures. Seven broad categories of modalities are utilized in diagnosis:

1 *Pathology* The branch of biological science that deals with the nature of disease through study of its causes, process, and effects, e.g., biopsy
2 *Radiology* The branch of medicine that deals with x-rays, radioactive substances, and ionizing radiations for diagnosis and treatment, e.g., chest x-ray, scanning, fluoroscopy
3 *Ultrasonography* The use of sound energy for studying pulse-echo alterations of anatomic structure, e.g., vascular disease
4 *Endoscopy* A visual examination of the interior of a body cavity or viscus, e.g., bronchoscopy
5 *Plethysmography* The measurement of changes in volume of an extremity or organ caused by blood flow, e.g., oculoplethysmography
6 *Sensory evoked potentials* The measurement of somatosensory, visual and/or auditory nerve pathways, e.g., auditory brainstem evoked potential
7 *Nuclear magnetic resonance* The use of radio-frequency energy for identifying abnormalities in anatomic structures, e.g., brain scans

PATHOLOGY

Clinical pathology is the use of laboratory methods to establish clinical diagnosis of the nature of disease. *Surgical pathology* is the study of alterations in body tissues removed by surgical intervention. Tissue or body fluid may be removed for clinical diagnosis before the surgeon proceeds with a definitive operation. Procedures to obtain specimens for pathologic examinations are always invasive.

Preoperative Pathologic Studies

Biopsy Tissue or body fluid removed for diagnosis is referred to as a *biopsy*. The surgeon performs the necessary procedure to obtain a biopsy prior to scheduling further surgical intervention. The pathologist confirms the diagnosis.

Aspiration Biopsy Body fluid is aspirated through a needle placed in a lesion that contains fluid such as a cyst or abscess.

Bone Marrow Biopsy Through a small skin incision or percutaneous puncture, a trocar puncture needle or aspiration needle is placed into bone, usually the sternum or iliac crest, to aspirate bone marrow.

Excision Biopsy Tissue is cut from the body. The surgeon may remove it through an incision in the skin or mucous membrane. This may be done through an endoscopic instrument. Localization of a lesion in soft tissue, such as the breast, to be incised through a skin incision may be guided by xeroradiography or ultrasound.

Percutaneous Needle Biopsy Tissue is obtained from an internal organ by means of a hollow needle inserted through body wall. Percutaneous puncture into a lesion may be guided by fluoroscopy under image intensification, ultrasound, or computerized tomography. Special needles are used; some types are disposable.

1 *Dorsey cannula* resembles a ventricular needle except it is a bit larger and the end is open. It is used, sometimes through a burr hole, to remove a biopsy of brain tissue.

2 *Franklin-Silverman* biopsy needle is used for obtaining biopsy specimens of thyroid, liver, kidney, prostate, and other organs. It has a 14-gauge thin-wall outer cannula with a beveled obturator. An inner split needle fits into the outer cannula and protrudes beyond end of it. The distal tips of this split needle are grooved inside. They enter tissue, close on the specimen, and trap it as needle is withdrawn.

> NOTE. Slight bleeding may follow liver biopsy. Prothrombin time is checked. This method of biopsy is not used if patient has any blood abnormality.

Intraoperative Pathological Studies

Tissue or fluid specimens may be removed immediately prior to or during operation for pathologic examination to determine further therapy.

Cultures Frank pus is removed from an abscess and may be encountered in other known or suspected areas of infection. Drainage is cultured to enable surgeon to effectively prescribe antibiotics. (Refer to Chapter 10 for the procedure for handling culture specimens during operation.)

Frozen Section Special preparation and examination of tissue can determine whether it is malignant and whether regional nodes are involved. When surgeon removes a piece of tissue and wants an immediate diagnosis, the pathologist comes to the OR suite to do a frozen section. Circulating nurse should alert the pathologist that his or her services will be needed. Frozen section takes only a few minutes. If malignancy is present and the individual situation indicates, surgeon proceeds with a radical resection of affected organ or body area.

> NOTE. The specimen should be placed on a towel before circulating nurse gives it to pathologist. Never allow a counted sponge or instrument to leave the room during operation.

Surgical Specimens All tissue removed during operation is sent to the pathology laboratory for verification of diagnosis. (Refer to Chap. 10 for care of tissue specimens.)

RADIOLOGY

Wilhelm Conrad Roentgen discovered x-rays in 1895. At first they were used mainly for localization of foreign bodies or visualization of fractures. *X-ray* is a high-energy electromagnetic wave capable of penetrating various thicknesses of solid substances and affecting photographic plates. X-rays are generated on a vacuum tube when high-velocity electrons from a heated filament strike a metal target (anode), causing it to emit x-rays. The photograph obtained by the use of x-rays may be referred to as an *x-ray film, roentgenogram, radiograph,* or other "-gram" name associated either with the specific technique used to obtain the photograph or the anatomic structures identified, e.g., mammogram. X-rays are also used for diagnostic imaging with fluoroscopy, developed in the 1950s, the scanning techniques of computerized tomography introduced in the early 1970s, and digital radiography of the 1980s. As the science of radiology has advanced, the diagnosis of disease in all surgical specialties has progressed. The treatment to be followed frequently is based upon radiologic findings.

Noninvasive Preoperative Studies

The following noninvasive radiologic studies are performed in the radiology department preoperatively. The surgeon may request that the x-ray films or radiographs be sent to the OR for reference during operation.

Chest X-Ray Most surgeons consider a chest x-ray an extension of the patient's history and physical examination, even though chest disease is not associated with the patient's clinical symptoms. A chest x-ray may be part of the admission procedure for elective surgical patients to rule out unsuspected pulmonary disease that could be communicable or would contraindicate use of inhalation anesthetics. This may be routine for patients over age 40. It is always a part of the diagnostic workup in patients with suspected or symptomatic pulmonary abnormalities.

Mammography A technique for projecting an x-ray image of soft tissue of the breast, mammography is the most effective screening method for early diagnosis of small, nonpalpable breast tumors. Three views of each breast are exposed to conventional x-rays. Tumors appear on mammogram as opaque areas or occasionally as areas of punctate calcification.

Xeroradiography The patient is positioned between an x-ray source and a photosensitive aluminum plate. The plate has an electrically charged selenium surface. The pattern of the charge remaining on plate after exposure to x-ray beam corresponds to densities of tissues and amount of radiation absorbed. A negatively charged blue toner powder is dusted on plate. A pale blue on white image is transferred by photoconduction rapidly and permanently to a sheet of plastic-coated paper. Xeroradiography minimizes radiation exposure, is performed rapidly, and produces detailed images easier to interpret than on x-ray film. It is used for diagnosis of breast disease, bone disorders, laryngeal disorders, to name a few anatomic structures, and for detection of foreign bodies in soft tissue.

Tomography An x-ray beam moves across the body in one direction, usually an arc, to photograph structures in a selected plane of tissue. The roentgenograms show detail of the structures within this single plane while blurring the images above and below the selected plane.

Computerized Tomography (CT and CAT Scan) Special, complex, expensive equipment employs an x-ray beam in conjunction with a computer. Because the x-ray beam moves back and forth across the body to project cross-sectional images, the technique is referred to as *computerized tomography* (CT), *computerized axial tomography* (CAT), or simply *scanning.* It produces a highly contrasted, detailed study of normal and pathologic anatomy. The x-ray tube and photomultiplier detectors rotate slowly around the patient's head, chest, or body for 180° in a linear fashion along the vertical axis. The computer processes the data and constructs a picture on a cathode-ray tube in shades of gray (on a black and white monitor) or in colors that correspond to the density of tissue. Structures are identified by differences in density. This picture is photographed for a permanent record. The computer also prints out on a magnetic disc the numerical density values related to the radiation-absorption coefficients of substances in the area scanned. The radiologist uses this printout to determine whether a substance is fluid, blood, normal tissue, bone, air, or a pathologic lesion. Exact size and location of lesions in the brain, mediastinum, and abdominal organs are identified. Although it becomes an invasive procedure, a radiopaque contrast medium may be injected intravenously to enhance visualization of the vascular and renal systems, in order to determine size of an aortic aneurysm or a renal mass. Computed tomography presents a hazard to the patient from ionizing radiation and a potential allergic reaction to IV contrast medium (see p. 388), if used. To ensure proper utilization of this complex equipment, as well as to protect the patient from excessive or unnecessary radiation, the procedure is done under the supervision of a qualified radiologist.

Emission Computed Axial Tomography (ECAT) Head of a rectangular field gamma camera in this scanner rotates 360° around patient. This capability provides multi-planar images of an organ. A computer program then reconstructs images from these multiple angles and processes them as in CAT scan. The field of view is enlarged with the ECAT.

Total-Body Scanning Total-body scanning does not refer to computerized tomography but to a scanning procedure following intravenous injection of a radionuclide material (see p. 391). Uptake of the radionuclide within the tissues depends on blood flow. Therefore, the imaging procedure may be delayed for several hours after the dose is given, not because it takes long for the material to localize in a tumor or inflammatory lesion where the uptake is high, but rather because differentiation is achieved after washout from normal structures. Scanning may include the whole body or only areas of specific interest. Total-body scanning includes identification of structures in the skeletal and vascular systems for diagnosis of pathology such as metastatic bone tumors or thrombotic vascular disease.

X-Ray for Trauma In addition to being an aid in determining the extent of traumatic injury, x-rays and scans may be entered as legal evidence in a court of law to establish injuries sustained by the patient or to justify medical care given. Conventional x-rays will show:

1 Fractures of bones
2 Presence and location of some kinds of foreign bodies, e.g., a bullet
3 Air or blood in pleural cavity
4 Gas or fluid in abdominal cavity
5 Outline of abdominal and chest organs and any deviation from normal size or location

Invasive Preoperative Studies

Invasive studies require the ingestion or injection of a radiolucent gas, a radiopaque contrast medium, or a radionuclide element prior to exposing the patient to radiation. The procedures that require injection of these substances must be performed under aseptic conditions using sterile equipment. Many hospitals have one or more rooms within the OR suite equipped for diagnostic as well as intraoperative radiologic procedures. In other hospitals, OR nursing personnel must go to the radiology department to assist with these preoperative diagnostic procedures.

Types of Equipment

Fixed X-ray Equipment A fixed overhead x-ray tube with housing may be mounted on a ceiling track for unrestricted movement of the x-ray beam into desired position over the patient. When not in use, it can be moved against a wall and retracted toward the ceiling. Some units are fixed to specially designed tables, such as the urological table for cystoscopic examinations (refer to Chap. 23). The controls are in an adjacent room or behind a lead shield. These are activated by the radiologist or radiology technician.

Portable X-ray Machine An x-ray tube mounted on a portable electric- or battery-powered generator of a nonexplosive design approved for use in hazardous locations may be moved from one room in the OR suite to another. It offers the advantages of flexibility in scheduling procedures and of availability when and where needed. However, it also has the disadvantage of being a source for cross contamination. All portable equipment must be thoroughly disinfected before being brought into a room and again after use. It should be stored within the OR suite between uses.

Cassette The lightproof holder for x-ray film is referred to as a *cassette.* The patient is positioned between the x-ray tube and the cassette. Holders for cassettes may be built into or attached to the operating table.

Processing Equipment Conventional x-ray equipment projects a black and white image on x-ray film that must be developed by a chemical process. Some OR suites have a darkroom where x-ray film is developed after exposure so surgeon can see results of the study without excessive delay. Others have an automatic processor in which film can be developed in 90 seconds to three minutes.

Fluoroscope Similar to an x-ray generator, a fluoroscope has an additional screen composed of fluorescent crystals, which lies in contact with a photocathode. When x-ray beam passes through this screen, it fluoresces. Fluorescent light sets electrons free from adjacent photocathode to produce an electron image. Rather than photographing this image of body structures on x-ray film, it is reproduced as an optical image on a luminescent screen. The image can be projected on a television monitor or retained on film or videotape by using a television camera. Known as *fluoroscopy,* examination under a fluoroscope allows visualization of both form and movement of internal body structures. Fluoroscopy is used frequently for both preoperative and intraoperative procedures. It is an invasive technique because a fluorescent substance must be injected or a radiopaque device inserted. Fluoroscopy exposes patient and personnel to radiation at higher levels than do conventional x-rays when exposure time is prolonged to perform a procedure with visual fluoroscopic control, e.g., cardiac catheterization. Personnel must wear lead aprons during fluoroscopy even though a lead shield is part of the installation. Patients should be protected with gonadal shields.

Image Intensifier The image intensifier amplifies the fluoroscopic optical image projected onto a television screen. The surgeon activates the image intensifier with a foot pedal. Clarity of the image is an aid in diagnosis, particularly of vascular, neurologic, and bone disorders. The surgeon and radiologist can observe the progression of an injected fluorescent substance as it moves through internal structures or the placement of a device into the body. When connected to other closed-circuit television facilities, the image can be transmitted to other rooms for teaching purposes. Also, the image can be filmed for a permanent record and for teaching. The monitoring screen may be ceiling-mounted above the operating table to save space in the OR, or it may be portable.

Mobile C-arm Image Intensifier Designed primarily for orthopaedic operations, foreign body and calculi localization, and catheter placement, mobile image intensifiers offer the same advantages and disadvantages as do portable x-ray machines. The *C-arm,* so named by its shape, keeps the image intensifier and x-ray tube in alignment; the intensifier is directly under the tube. It can be moved from an anterior to a lateral position. Utility of the mobile C-arm image intensifier is enhanced when the system is capable of making electronic radiographs for permanent records. An additional formatting device is required.

Computerized Digital Subtraction Processor (Digital Radiography) Following intravenous injection of a radiopaque contrast medium (see p. 388), the computerized digital subtraction x-ray imaging system visually records perfusion within the cardiovascular system, e.g., extra- and intracranial vessels. Prior to arrival of contrast medium to body region to be visualized, fluoroscopic images are converted to digital data for storage in one of the memory units in the processor. Termed the *mask image,* these digitized data are integrated into a single or multiple video frames. The video signal is logarithmically amplified and digitized. The mask image electronically is subtracted from subsequent images with the contrast medium. This process removes unwanted background, thus providing optimal visualization of vessels with contrast density that cannot be achieved by other image intensifiers. The resultant images are displayed on a video screen and can be recorded on film or tape.

Radiographic Table The table top the patient lies on must be Bakelite, acrylic, or some other material capable of being penetrated by x-rays. Some operating tables have a tunnel top the length of the table that permits insertion of x-ray cassette at any area. For fluoroscopy with image intensification, the entire top must be radiolucent, because the image intensifier is positioned underneath the table. If the entire operating table is not radiolucent, the foot section can be lowered and a radiolucent extension attached that will accommodate the C-arm.

Nursing Duties

1 Sterile technique of operative procedures in general applies also to invasive diagnostic procedures.

2 Each hospital has its own supply list for the procedures routinely performed. It is convenient to keep a stock of routine supplies on a portable cart if procedures are done in the radiology department. In general, the following items should be readily available:
   - **a** Sterile tray for the specific procedure
   - **b** Skin prep tray and solutions
   - **c** Intravenous administration sets and solutions
   - **d** Local anesthetic agents
   - **e** Radiopaque contrast material
   - **f** Sterile gowns, gloves, linen, and dressings
   - **g** Extra sterile syringes and needles
   - **h** Plastic tubing and catheters

   Because an element of risk is associated with some of these procedures, there should also be available:
   - **i** Stimulants

j Cardiac resuscitation equipment, including defibrillator

3 An explanation of procedure must be given to patients to allay fears and ensure their understanding of the value of procedure in making a diagnosis. During procedure, explanation should be given of equipment being used and of the necessity to remain quiet while films are being taken.

4 Patients must be carefully observed during all procedures for any change in condition. Even if a procedure is done under local anesthesia, a stand-by anesthesiologist should be available to check vital signs.

Types of Invasive Studies The most common agents and some of the more commonly performed procedures are discussed. Each agent may have many more uses than are described here.

Radiolucent Gases Filtered room air, oxygen, nitrogen, carbon dioxide, or a combination of gases may be injected into body spaces or structures normally containing *fluid other than blood.* Gases are radiolucent, transparent to x-rays, so that gas-filled spaces appear less dense on x-ray film than do surrounding tissues.

The first visualization of the ventricles of the brain was accidental and was reported by W. H. Luckett in 1913. The patient had sustained a skull fracture about three weeks previously, and x-rays showed the ventricles to be filled with air. Luckett explained that the patient in sneezing had forced air through fracture lines and lacerated dura, thus filling the ventricles.

Walter E. Dandy first thought of replacing fluid in the ventricles with air and x-raying them. Since most lesions in the brain modify size and shape of ventricles, this procedure would aid in localizing a lesion. In 1919, Dandy first injected air into the spinal canal to visualize the subarachnoid space. Modifications of his technique are still employed to determine appropriate neurosurgical access to brain lesions.

Ventriculography is the study of the ventricles following injection of gas directly into the lateral ventricles of the brain. It is used in patients with signs of increased intracranial pressure as a result of blockage of cerebrospinal fluid circulation. Ventricular needles or catheters may be inserted into one or both lateral ventricles through holes made in the skull. The ventricular needle has a blunt, tapered point that prevents injury to the brain as it is inserted into the ventricle. Openings on the side near the point permit removal of spinal fluid and injection of gas. If the patient is an infant whose suture lines in the skull are not yet closed, needles are inserted through these.

The entire procedure may be done, or may begin, in the OR to drill the holes and insert the ventricular needles or an intraventricular catheter. The patient may then be transferred to the radiology department or diagnostic room within the OR suite. If a lesion is identified, the diagnostic procedure may be followed immediately by operation because of the possibility of a further increase in intracranial pressure. If the patient is returned to the unit following the procedure, sterile ventricular needles should accompany the patient. If intracranial pressure becomes too great after gas injection, needle can be inserted to remove the gas.

Arthrography is the study of a joint following the injection of gas into it. Conventional x-rays show only the bony structure of a joint. By injection of a gas, injury to cartilage and ligaments may be visualized. A radiopaque, iodinated contrast medium may also be used for a double contrast study, particularly useful in knee arthrograms.

Radiopaque Contrast Media Agents composed of nonmetallic compounds or heavy metallic salts that do not permit passage of radiant energy are *radiopaque.* When exposed to x-ray, the lumina of body structures filled with these agents appear as dense areas. Radiopaque contrast media frequently used for the procedures described below include:

1 Cardiografin, for angiography
2 Hypaque, for arteriography, cardiography, cholangiography, intravenous pyelography and venography
3 Renografin, for angiography, cystography, myelography, and pyelography
4 Angio-Conray, for arteriography
5 Dionosil, for bronchography
6 Barium sulfate, for gastrointestinal studies
7 Pantopaque, for myelography
8 Renovist, for cystography, retrograde pyelography, and ureterography

Some of these agents are fluorescent dyes. Most contain iodine. A history of sensitivity to iodine-related substances, such as shellfish, or other allergies must be obtained before these agents are injected. A test dose of 1 or 2 ml may be given before dose required for x-ray study. The patient must be observed for allergic reaction throughout procedure.

Egas Moniz, a Portuguese physician, was the first to do cerebral angiography in 1927. In 1929, in Germany, Forssman catheterized the right atrium by passing a ureteral catheter into it through a vein in the right arm. He was not successful in his attempt to inject a radiopaque substance through the catheter to visualize the pulmonary vessels. In 1931, Moniz was able to visualize right chambers of the heart and pulmonary vessels using Forssman's technique. Poor visualization of areas and reaction of patients to the substance discouraged pioneers in this procedure. However, by 1937 Robb and Steinberg had worked out the technique as it is used today, but enhanced by advantages of more sophisticated equipment.

In 1935, the vertebral artery was first exposed and injected, and in 1949 it was first injected percutaneously. Although the latter technique is generally preferred, both methods are used for angiography.

Angiography is a comprehensive term for studies of the circulatory system following injection of radiopaque substance to permit visualization of a specific blood vessel system. These procedures are useful in the differential diagnosis of arteriovenous malformations, aneurysms, tumors, or vascular accidents due either to traumatic injury or acquired structural disease.

1 *Aortography* is the study of the aorta and its branches to determine site and size of lesions within the aorta or its major branches such as the renal vascular system. A 7-in. (17.7-cm) × 15-, 16-, or 17-gauge needle may be inserted into the aorta through a translumbar approach with the patient in prone position. The more selective aortographic procedures are performed by positioning a catheter under direct fluoroscopic visualization via the femoral artery into a branch of the aorta.

2 *Arteriography* is the study of the arterial circulation of a specific vascular system. It is identified by reference to the major blood vessel to be injected: i.e., right or left carotid or vertebral arteriogram to study cerebral circulation; via right brachial artery to study coronary arteries of the myocardium; right or left femoral arteriogram to study circulation in a lower extremity. Various routes of entrance for a needle or intraarterial catheter exist for injection of these major vessels.

3 *Cardiography* is the study of the chambers in the heart. A catheter is positioned under direct fluoroscopic visualization through one of the great vessels into the heart. Cardiography is done usually in conjunction with other cardiac catheterization procedures. *Cardiac catheterization* includes the recording of pressure measurements within the heart chambers and withdrawing blood samples for analysis (refer to Chap. 31, p. 573).

4 *Venography* is the study of veins to show inflow, filling, and emptying to determine venous blood flow and valve action.

Techniques and equipment to be used will vary according to specific procedure, but all types of angiography have the following commonalities:

1 The procedures may be done under local or general anesthesia.

2 Access to vessel to be injected with a radiopaque contrast medium may be made by percutaneous puncture or by a cutdown. An intravenous drip is maintained on all patients when latter approach is used.

- **a** Cannulated needles with or without a radiopaque plastic catheter, similar to types used for intravenous infusions, may be used for percutaneous puncture. Cannulated needles used for these procedures have an obturator that remains in place until the contrast medium is injected to prevent backflow of blood. Long catheters have a guide wire to assist threading through vessel.
- **b** Seldinger needle, 18 gauge, has a sharply beveled inner and a blunt outer cannula. The blunt end of outer cannula prevents trauma to vessel. After insertion, inner cannula is replaced with a guide wire and outer cannula removed. A 20-cm vessel dilator is threaded over guide wire to create a track for a radiopaque catheter. After it is removed, the catheter is positioned and the guide wire is withdrawn. This *Seldinger method* is generally preferred for angiography, because blood vessels other than the one punctured can be injected with contrast medium.
- **c** Cournand needle has a curved flanged guard that contours to the body. It is particularly useful in carotid arteriography to hold needle in position in neck during injection.
- **d** Robb cannula is blunt with large lumen and a stopcock at the hub. It is inserted via a cutdown. It is used with a Robb syringe that has a large opening in tip for fast injection.
- **e** Sheldon needle has an occluded point with an opening at 90° to the lumen. When verte-

bral artery is entered, a right-angle injection is made into lumen of the artery.

3 Dosage of radiopaque contrast substances injected into blood vessels is computed for infants and children according to weight. In adults, dose is measured so it can be repeated safely for more exposures if necessary. Radiopaque agents dissipate very rapidly in the bloodstream.
4 Radiopaque contrast material should be warmed to body temperature to prevent precipitation and to reduce viscosity.
5 If awake, patient should be told to expect a warm feeling and possibly a burning sensation when contrast medium is injected.
6 Plastic tubing, 30 in. (76 cm) long with syringe on one end and adaptor on the other, is connected to needle or catheter in the vessel to prevent jarring during pressure of injection and to keep hands of operator out of the x-ray beam.
7 Automatic high-pressure injector may be used instead of injecting contrast medium by hand. This device correlates injection and x-ray exposure. When an automatic injector is used, special high-pressure nylon tubing is used, since this does not pull apart with pressure. When this tubing is used, a stopcock is placed on the end for closing it off at the syringe connection, because nylon tubing cannot be clamped.
8 Automatic seriogram equipment takes rapid multiple exposures while the contrast medium is in sufficient concentration to visualize the vessels. It can be set at ½- to 2-second intervals to take multiple pictures in succession. Or a roll-film changer, like a movie camera, may be used. This can be set for multiple exposures per second also. These devices are used for angiography with the image intensifier.
9 Digital subtraction angiography converts x-ray beam into a video screen image (see p. 387). A small amount of contrast medium is injected IV. Vessel catheterization is unnecessary and less contrast medium is used. This procedure may be done on an ambulatory basis.

Bronchography is a study of the tracheobronchial tree performed to aid in diagnosis of bronchiectasis, cancer, tuberculosis, and lung abscess or to detect a foreign body. Location of a lesion can be determined and operation planned accordingly. The procedure should be explained in detail to the patient, because cooperation is necessary to accomplish the desired result (refer to Chap. 26).

Gastrointestinal x-ray studies are performed to identify lesions in the mucosa of the gastrointestinal tract, such as an ulcer or tumor. Inflammatory lesions and partial or complete obstructions caused by a variety of lesions may also be identified. Barium sulfate is either swallowed by the patient or instilled by enema to outline the lumen of segments of the tract to be studied. These studies are done in the radiology department, but surgeons often refer to films during operation.

Myelography is a study to identify lesions in the spinal canal. It is helpful to localize a filling defect, a spinal cord tumor, or herniated nucleus pulposus. Most surgeons do not rely entirely on this method of diagnosis. The patient's symptoms and signs are important in final diagnosis. Arachnoiditis is a potential complication of intrathecal injection of iophendylate (Pantopaque). Therefore, a water-based contrast medium such as metrizamide may be preferred.

Urography is a comprehensive term for radiological studies of the urinary tract. Most procedures are performed in the radiology department, but some are done in conjunction with cystoscopic examinations (refer to Chap. 23).

1 *Cystography* is study of bladder following instillation of a contrast medium. It is valuable in detecting ureterovesical reflux, a malfunction of the sphincter valves.

2 *Cystourethrography* is study of bladder and urethra to determine obstruction or abnormality in contour or position. X-rays may be taken as contrast medium is injected into the bladder or when the patient voids the material.

3 *Intravenous pyelography* is the study of structures of the urinary tract and a study of kidney function. Contrast medium is introduced into circulatory system by rapid intravenous injection or slow infusion IV drip. It is excreted through the kidneys. X-rays are taken at carefully timed intervals. If medium is poorly excreted through the kidneys, the last film may be taken as many as 24 hours after injection. Tomograms also may be taken while the contrast material is still in the urinary tract. These procedures are done in the radiology department rather than in the cystoscopy room.

4 *Retrograde pyelography* is study of shape and position of kidneys and ureters. Contrast medium

is injected through catheters placed in each ureter. This procedure is used to visualize renal pelves and calyces.

5 *Ureterography* is the study of one or both ureters to identify position and patency of the lumina. Contrast medium is injected through ureteral catheters (refer to Chap. 23, p. 454).

6 *Urethrography* is a study of the contour and patency of the urethra. Contrast medium may be instilled into bladder. X-rays are taken as the patient voids. The medium must flow well but be viscous enough to distend the urethra to give good detail of it on the x-ray. If patient is anesthetized, a very viscous contrast medium is injected into the urethra and films taken. Because the urethra is quite short, the latter technique is of little value in female patients.

Radionuclides Radioactive elements utilized in medicine are referred to as *radionuclides.* A *nuclide* is a stable nucleus of a chemical element, such as iodine, plus its orbiting electrons. A nuclide bombarded with radioactive particles becomes unstable and emits radiant energy; it becomes a *radionuclide.* Except for the emission of energy, action of a radionuclide is the same in the body as is its stable counterpart. Radionuclides that emit electromagnetic energy are used for diagnostic studies to trace function and structure of most organs of the body. They may be given orally or intravenously or by infusion. These agents may be used to visualize specific areas rather than radiopaque contrast media in some of the procedures previously described. They are particularly useful in studies of bone marrow, liver, spleen, biliary tract, thyroid, brain, urinary tract, and peripheral vascular system. Because they provide better quantification of arrival times for vascular perfusion above and below lesions, radionuclides may be a more accurate index of the functional significance of a lesion than are other radiopaque contrast media.

Noninvasive Intraoperative Studies

Noninvasive x-rays are taken during operation most frequently to verify position of a body structure, a metallic implant or instrument, or to identify presence of a foreign body. The need for x-rays can be anticipated and scheduled for:

1 Closed reduction of fractured bones, with or without internal fixation devices (refer to Chap. 24)

2 Open reduction of hip fractures and fractures of some other bones when internal fixation devices are implanted (refer to Chap. 24)

3 Sterotaxic neurosurgery to identify landmarks as instruments are introduced into the brain (refer to Chap. 29)

Unanticipated need for x-rays occurs when a sponge, needle, or instrument is unaccounted for at the time the final count is taken during wound closure. An x-ray will confirm whether item is still in patient. Unless patient's condition demands immediate wound closure, an x-ray should be taken before closure is completed (refer to count procedures in Chap. 10).

Invasive Intraoperative Studies

The surgeon may wish to inject a radiopaque contrast medium into a blood vessel or other anatomic structure during operation to ascertain operative results prior to wound closure or to obtain further guidance for operative procedure. Some operations are performed with patient positioned on a fluoroscopic table equipped with an image intensifier for radiographic visualization of anatomic structures as operation progresses. Examples of procedures that utilize radiologic control include but are not limited to the following.

Angiography Intraoperative studies often are essential to assess the results of vascular reconstruction. Angiography is one method of assessment to confirm position and patency of an arterial or venous graft or the quality of a restored vessel lumen. Intraoperative angiography frequently is indicated for these assessments in the peripheral vessels of the extremities. After insertion of a bypass graft or endarterectomy, patency of the graft or vessel is checked by pulsations and also by arteriography (refer to Chap. 32 for further discussion of these operations).

Angiography is also utilized at the time of operation to identify vascularity or exact location of some types of lesions in extremities, brain, and thoracic and abdominal cavities. After injection of radiopaque contrast medium, radiological studies are made.

Cholangiography In addition to preoperative diagnostic x-ray studies, some surgeons routinely request radiological studies in conjunction with cholecystectomy or cholelithotomy (refer to Chap.

21, p. 404) to identify gallstones in the biliary tract. Other surgeons selectively include cholangiography at time of operation in patients in whom they suspect stones might be present or retained in the bile ducts. Conventional x-ray equipment or an image intensifier may be used for these intraoperative studies.

The basic difference between preoperative and intraoperative cholangiography is site of administration of the radiopaque contrast medium. For preoperative invasive cholangiography, the contrast medium injected intravenously, through percutaneous venipuncture, is excreted by the liver into the bile ducts. During open operative procedures, the medium is injected directly into bile ducts. When intraoperative cholangiography is scheduled, add to the usual sterile setup:

1 50-cc syringe
2 Radiopaque contrast medium
3 Radiopaque cholangiocath (a plastic catheter for insertion into common or cystic duct)

All other precautions for patient and personnel safety must be observed.

Considerations for Patient Safety in OR All precautions for patient and personnel safety from hazards of radiation exposure must be observed when x-rays are taken or fluroscopy is used in OR. The patient is exposed to the primary beam. Personnel are exposed to scatter radiation in the room. Refer to Chapter 11, p. 206, for detailed discussion of radiation hazards. Other factors to be considered for the welfare of the patient are:

1 X-ray film cassette holder, often called a bucky, must be properly positioned on operating table under area to be exposed to x-ray beam. If table does not have a built-in tunnel or compartment for cassette, part of mattress may be removed and the holder, a Bakelite or wooden frame, placed on table in the appropriate section. A scout film or brief fluoroscopic exposure may be taken after patient is positioned, but before operation begins, to check position of cassette or C-arm. The floor can be marked so that a portable x-ray machine, or the C-arm of image intensifier, will be repositioned correctly when films are taken during operation. The operating table must be correctly positioned under a fixed unit.

2 X-ray tube or C-arm that will extend over the operative site must be free from dust. It should be damp-dusted with a disinfectant solution before patient arrives and operation begins. It may be covered with a sterile drape or sleeve before moving it into the sterile field.

3 Draping towels may be sutured on rather than secured with towel clips, which might interfere with the view.

4 Aseptic technique must be maintained at all times. The scrub nurse covers the operative field with a sterile minor sheet to protect it from contamination while x-ray tube is over it. The circulating nurse removes the sheet after radiographs have been taken.

5 If a lateral x-ray will be taken, as during fixation of a hip fracture, a lateral cassette holder or C-arm may be positioned before patient is draped and covered with the drape. The circulating nurse raises drape for radiology technician to place and remove the cassette. Or the holder may be left on outside of sterile drapes and covered with a sterile Mayo stand cover when ready to swing it into place for the lateral view.

6 Scrub nurse must enclose cassette with a sterile cover if it must be placed within the sterile field. Disposable covers designed for this purpose are available or a Mayo stand cover may be used. Be certain gloved hands are well protected in a cuff of the cover while the circulating nurse places cassette into it.

7 Radiopaque contrast medium used for injection must be sterile. The outside of ampuls or vials must also be sterile if they are placed on sterile instrument table before withdrawing contents into a sterile syringe. Warm radiopaque contrast medium to body temperature to overcome viscosity.

8 Remove all instruments and metallic or radiopaque items from operative site.

9 The radiologist or radiology technician must be notified well in advance so that he or she is standing by when surgeon is ready. Delays waiting for radiology personnel prolong operation unnecessarily for patient.

Time, distance and shielding are the key factors in minimizing radiation exposure. Personnel must stand at least 6 ft away from x-ray beam and/or wear lead aprons or sternal and gonadal shields. Patients should be protected with gonadal shields.

ULTRASONOGRAPHY

Vibrating high-frequency sound waves, beyond the hearing capability of the human ear, can detect alterations in anatomic structures or hemodynamic properties within the body. The basic component of any diagnostic ultrasound system is its specialized transducer, which is a piezoelectric crystal. The transducer converts electric impulses to ultrasonic waves at a frequency greater than a million cycles per second. These ultrasonic frequencies are transmitted into tissues through a transducer placed on the skin. A water-soluble gel is applied to the skin to maintain airtight contact between skin and transducer because ultrasonic waves do not travel well through air. A portion of the transmitted ultrasonic waves is reflected back as real time images to a receiving crystal. The transducer is held on the skin long enough to obtain a graphic recording of the reflected high-frequency sound waves. Connected to a microprocessing computer, uniform imaging of a wide range of body tissues is possible. Ultrasound is not effective in the presence of bone or gases in the gastrointestinal tract. Whether used as a preoperative or intraoperative diagnostic technique, ultrasonography is a rapid, painless, noninvasive procedure. It distinguishes between fluid-filled and solid masses.

Preoperative Studies

Alterations in Anatomic Structures Ultrasonic frequencies are reflected when the beam reaches target anatomic structures of different density and acoustical impedance. The reflected signal is picked up by the transducer/receiver as an echo. The intensity of the returning echo is determined not only by the angle formed between the ultrasound beam and the reflecting surface of the anatomic structure but also by the acoustic properties of that surface. The resulting echo is described in terms of time and intensity. The echo can be displayed on a sonarscope, a cathode-ray oscilloscope, for immediate interpretation of movements and dimensions of structures. The image can be recorded on videotape or printed out to provide a permanent record known as an *echogram* or *sonogram*. Sonograms can be obtained on multiple planes. Ultrasonography is a useful adjunct in the diagnosis of:

1 Space occupying lesions in the neonatal brain. The echoencephalogram will show a shift of the brain due to tumor.

2 Lesions in the breast, thyroid, and parathyroid glands, and in abdominal or pelvic organs. Ultrasound can distinguish between a cystic and a solid tumor mass in the kidney, pancreas, liver, ovary, and testis. It is the best imaging method in gallbladder disease.

3 Emboli, either blood or fat. This is particularly useful in the early diagnosis of pulmonary embolism. Fat embolus syndrome can develop following long bone fractures.

4 Fetal maturation. Fetal head size is an aid in determination of fetal maturation. This can be measured by ultrasound prior to an elective cesarean section or to determine need for C-section because the head is too large for vaginal delivery. Ultrasonography is also used to determine position of fetus and placenta, and to detect fetal abnormalities.

5 Cardiac defects. Structural defects, insufficient valvular movement, and blood-flow volumes within the heart chambers and myocardium can be detected. This diagnostic technique is known as *echocardiography*.

Hemodynamic Properties of the Peripheral Vascular System Blood-flow velocity and pressure measurements are possible with ultrasound because moving blood cells produce a sufficient interface with surrounding vessels to independently reflect high-frequency sound waves. The Doppler ultrasonic velocity detector emits a beam of 5 to 10 megahertz (MHz) ultrasound that is directed through the skin into the bloodstream. A portion of the transmitted ultrasound is reflected from moving particles in the blood. Known as the *Doppler effect*, the reflected sound wave changes in frequency because the source of the sound is in motion. This shift in frequency is proportional to blood-flow velocity. Originally introduced for use in detecting obstruction in arterial blood flow, the Doppler instrument is used extensively to locate and evaluate blood-flow patterns in peripheral arterial and venous diseases or defects.

1 *Arterial disease.* Detection of altered hemodynamics in arterial flow is significant in diagnosis of obstructive or occlusive arterial lesions. For example, the Doppler instrument will indicate regions in the neck where carotid artery blood flow to the brain is obstructed by atherosclerosis. Operation can be performed to remove or bypass the obstruction to avoid the patient suffering a cerebral vascular accident (stroke). It also may help the surgeon determine the appropriate level of lower extremity amputation for ischemia caused by peripheral arterial occlusive disease. It is useful in diagnosis of aortoiliac aneurysms.

2 *Venous disease.* Occlusion of superficial or deep veins and presence of incompetent valves can be located and identified by sounds made by the flow of blood through the peripheral venous system. The Doppler instrument can qualitatively demonstrate the abnormal venous hemodynamics in patients with varicose veins and thrombotic disease. This information helps the surgeon plan surgical intervention.

Intraoperative Uses

Air Embolus The Doppler instrument can be used to monitor patients during open-heart surgery or operations on the great vessels in the chest to detect the escape of air into the circulation. Air entering an artery to the brain (cerebral air embolism) may cause brain damage or death. If an air embolism is detected at the time it occurs, therapy can be initiated immediately.

Localization of Lesions Ultrasound is used for intraoperative localization of subcortical brain lesions, spinal cord lesions, pancreatic tumors, and lesions in other soft tissues to determine whether lesion is resectable. Exact location of gallbladder and kidney stones can also be identified. Ultrasonography is less time-consuming and requires less tissue manipulation than do other intraoperative diagnostic procedures, and does not expose patient to radiation and contrast medium.

Percutaneous Puncture Direction and depth of needle punctures to locate lesions in various abdominal organs, such as pancreatic cyst, can be determined by following the ultrasound beam continuously visualized on the sonarscope. The echo from the tip of the needle is easily visible on the scope when the lesion is entered. These procedures are performed to aspirate cytologic specimens for diagnosis.

ENDOSCOPY

Direct visualization within body cavities and structures aids in determination of appropriate course of therapy for many conditions. Endoscopes were discussed in Chapter 19, including their basic design, care and handling, and patient safety considerations. Specific endoscopic procedures will be discussed in the following chapters when pertinent to diagnostic and operative procedures in the appropriate surgical specialties.

Preoperative Endoscopy

Diagnostic endoscopy is frequently performed in conjunction with radiologic studies or to obtain specimens for pathologic examination. A radiolucent or radiopaque contrast material may be injected through the endoscope or an accessory prior to radiologic studies. Fluid and secretions may be withdrawn for culture or chemical analysis. Biopsies are frequently obtained. Direct visualization alone may confirm presence or absence of a suspected lesion or abnormal condition. This may be enhanced by an ultrasonic transducer at the end of a flexible fiberoptic scope. Endoscopic diagnosis often provides the information necessary to proceed with open operation or results in cancellation of anticipated operation.

NOTE. History of allergies and previous drug reactions must be obtained. This history should include allergy to shellfish if a radiopaque contrast medium containing iodine will be injected for radiologic study in conjunction with endoscopy.

Intraoperative Endoscopy

Vascular endoscopy and visualization of other vessels, such as the biliary and hepatic ducts, following either removal or bypass of an obstruction, confirm the patency of the vessel before completion of the operation. Colonoscopy may be performed intraoperatively to locate soft nonpalpable tumor masses that must be removed transabdominally. Flexible fiberscopes are used for these procedures.

Therapeutic procedures are performed through endoscopes without subjecting the patient to open operation. Removal of a foreign body, excision of a small tumor or polyp, application of a medication, aspiration of fluid, permanent hemostasis of bleeding, and ligation of a structure are examples of therapeutic procedures. Electrosurgery, cryosurgery, and the laser beam may be used through an endoscope to destroy or remove tissue following confirmation of diagnosis.

PLETHYSMOGRAPHY

Pressure-sensitive instruments placed on an organ or around an extremity record variations in volume and pressure of blood passing through tissues. Tracings reflect pulse-wave impulses transmitted from moving currents within the arteries or veins. A quantitative, noninvasive, diagnostic technique, plethysmography does not provide anatomic information regarding exact location, extent, or characteristics of vascular disease.

Oculoplethysmography

The instrument is placed on each eyeball to record pulse waves in the eye emanating from the cerebrovascular system for diagnosis of cerebral vascular obstruction. Sometimes the carotid arteries are compressed momentarily for comparative pressure evaluations in both eyes.

Strain Gauge Plethysmography

Pneumatic cuffs are placed snugly around both thighs, calves, ankles, and/or great toes. An electronically calibrated strain gauge attached to the plethysmograph and pulse-volume recorder is secured around each foot. Each cuff is inflated in sequence to measure changes in blood flow and systolic pressures in the lower extremities. Changes in blood-flow volume are measured by changes in circumference of the calf, foot, or toe. Systolic pressure is noted when the strain gauge registers a change in volume on a pen recorder. The test is usually done before and repeated after exercise. This test provides an index of peripheral vascular resistance in the lower extremities due to venous thrombosis, varicose veins, or arteriosclerotic disease.

SENSORY EVOKED POTENTIALS

Used to measure neural pathways, the procedure involves placement of multiple recording electrodes over peripheral nerves or scalp and ears. The evoked potentials generated in response to stimulation are recorded. Components of the computerized system provide sensory stimulation; acquisition, amplification, and filtering of electrophysiologic signals; signal processing; and display, measurement, and storage of sensory evoked potential (SEP) waveforms. These noninvasive measurements may be taken preoperatively to assist in diagnosis of pathology, such as acoustic neuroma, or assessment of trauma. The techniques may also be used for intraoperative monitoring (see Chap. 14, p. 273) to assess status of central nervous system. Multimodality evoked potentials aid in assessment of patients with trauma. Three modalities are used.

1 *Somatosensory evoked potential* is objective evaluation of peripheral and central neural pathways. Pairs of surface or needle skin or scalp electrodes are placed in desired patterns over appropriate peripheral nerves and areas of spinal cord and cerebral cortex. These electrodes record somatosensory responses elicited upon application of electrical stimuli, as to the peroneal peripheral nerve at the knee or from over the spinal column or scalp. These impulses along neural pathways are charted to determine if nerve is functioning properly or if a lesion is impeding impulses to the brain. Testing time can range from 45 minutes to 4 hours, depending on number of peripheral nerves stimulated and sites necessary to assess neural pathways.

2 *Auditory brainstem evoked potential* is test of eighth cranial nerve and auditory pathway to cerebral cortex. The patient, wearing headphones or earphones, responds to auditory clicks or tones. Multiple electrodes on scalp and ears record responses. This is used to assess physiologic condition of brainstem and patient's hearing threshold.

3 *Visual evoked potential* is test of responses to visual pattern-reversal stimulation of optic nerve and its associated pathways to the cerebral cortex. The patient receives stimuli via a television monitor or special eye goggles. Multiple electrodes on scalp and ears record the evoked potentials.

NUCLEAR MAGNETIC RESONANCE

Like the CAT scan, the nuclear magnetic resonance (NMR) scanner for diagnostic imaging was developed in England. First installed there in 1975, NMR was introduced in hospitals in the United States in 1982. Unlike CAT scan, NMR does not use radiation. The patient lies flat inside a large electromagnet. In this static magnetic field, patient is exposed to bursts of alternating radiofrequency energy waves. The magnetic nuclei of hydrogen atoms in the water of body cells are stimulated from their state of equilibrium. When the radio signal is turned off, nuclei return to their original state. As they do so, they emit radio-frequency signals related to their quantity and environment. These signals are recorded and measured, and converted to a visual image by a digital computer. Three-dimensional images of clear resonance can be obtained with one measurement. The major applications of this noninvasive technique are detection of tumors, inflammatory diseases, infections and abscesses, and evaluation of body chemistry of the cardiovascular and central nervous systems and other organs. NMR images bone and soft tissue. Metal ligating clips cannot be used as markers, however. NMR has the capacity to diagnose some abnormalities not readily apparent with other diagnostic modalities.

CHAPTER **21**

GENERAL SURGERY

The discipline of general surgery provides the fundamentals for surgical practice, education, and research. The definition of general surgery agreed upon by the American Board of Surgery and the Residency Review Committee for Surgery serves as the basis of graduate education and certification as a specialist in surgery. Inherent in general surgery is:

1 A central core of knowledge of and skills common to all surgical specialties; viz., anatomy, physiology, metabolism, pathology, wound healing, shock and resuscitation, neoplasia, and nutrition.

2 Diagnosis and preoperative, operative, and postoperative care of patients with diseases of the alimentary tract; abdomen and its contents; breast; head and neck; vascular system, excluding intracranial vessels, heart, and vessels intrinsic and immediately adjacent thereto; and endocrine system. Also responsibility for all phases of care of an injured patient, including musculoskeletal, hand, and head injuries, is an essential component of general surgery.

3 Employment of endoscopic techniques, such as proctosigmoidoscopy and operative choledochoscopy, and familiarity with such endoscopic techniques as laryngoscopy, bronchoscopy, gastroscopy, colonoscopy, and peritoneoscopy for diagnosis and treatment.

4 An understanding of the principles of and clinical experience in operative care in the more common problems in thoracic, cardiac, gynecologic, neurologic, orthopaedic, plastic, neonatal, and urologic surgery, and anesthesiology.*

HISTORICAL INTRODUCTION

The earliest time in which surgical procedures were done is not known, but in 5702 B.C. an Egyptian physician put into writing his knowledge of anatomy.

The Greeks were noted for their written records concerning bowel obstruction, hernias, and amputations. Gastric ulcers were recorded as early as the fourth century B.C. Hippocrates was recognized as the medical authority for 2000 years.

Revolutionary discoveries by Semmelweis, Pasteur, and Lister marked the beginning of present-day aseptic surgery. The introduction of surgical specialties was the outgrowth of increased knowledge of etiology of disease and specialized treatment of all parts of the body. *General surgery,* the basis for all specialties, decreased in breadth as specialization increased. The parts of anatomy not specifically delegated to the specialists have remained in the realm of the general surgeon. However, other surgical disciplines depend on general surgeons for clinical collaboration in reconstruction involving the gastrointestinal and vascular systems. The scope of this chapter will focus on procedures commonly categorized as general surgery.

*Adapted from definition of American Board of Surgery adopted in 1983.

SPECIAL FEATURES OF GENERAL SURGERY

Frequently, the operation performed depends on the biopsy and frozen section report at the time of operation, while the patient is still under anesthesia. Although the patient has been informed preoperatively of an anticipated procedure, the unknown factor is cause for apprehension. The operating room nurse must convey sincere concern.

1 Malignant lesions account for a large percentage of surgical interventions, especially those of the breast, thyroid, and gastrointestinal tract. Operability of the lesion sometimes may be determined only after thorough exploration at operation.
2 Frequently the nurse must be prepared with two draping and instrument setups depending on diagnosis established after the operation begins. Anticipated equipment and supplies must be available without delay.
3 Positioning and draping of the patient for a general surgical procedure are as varied as are the operations. Extra pillows, padding, and accessory positioning aids must be available (see Chap. 15).
4 All types of anesthesia may be administered. Occasionally none is needed.
5 Instrumentation is quite varied and suited to function in a specific anatomical area. For example, gastrointestinal procedures require the addition of crushing clamps used to occlude the intestinal lumen before resection, and rubber-shod clamps to protect delicate tissues. Included in all procedures are instruments for exposing, dissecting, grasping, holding, clamping, occluding, and suturing. Various lengths of umbilical tape, hernia tape, or thin strips of disposable radiopaque material may be placed around vessels to retract them. These are nontraumatic to blood vessels, nerves, and ureters.
6 A number of general operative procedures are adaptable to ambulatory surgery; others are extremely extensive.
7 The electrosurgical unit frequently is used; a laser beam, endoscope, and/or ultrasound transducer may be used.
8 In abdominal and pelvic procedures:
   a Indwelling or ureteral catheters are often inserted preoperatively.
   b A nasogastric tube is frequently passed before or during the operation.
   c After the abdominal cavity is entered, single free 4 by 4 sponges should be removed from the field. They are used only folded and secured on a sponge stick. Wet or dry tapes (laparotomy packs) are used in the abdominal cavity. A small dissector is always clamped in a forceps before handing to the surgeon.
   d Suction must always be available and immediately ready to use before the peritoneum is incised, especially in biliary or intestinal procedures or when fluid or blood may be anticipated in the peritoneal cavity.
   e Before the gastrointestinal or biliary tract is resected, lap packs are used to isolate the area to prevent contamination of the peritoneal cavity.
   f A drain may be exteriorized through the incision or a stab wound in the adjacent abdominal wall prior to closure.
   g Contaminated items such as those used to anastomose intestinal segments are placed in a discard basin on the sterile field. Only the outside of the basin is touched.
   h The wound is often irrigated prior to closure to remove blood and debris.
   i Retention sutures may be used to give additional strength to wound closure (refer to Chap. 18).
9 Assorted sizes of drains, tubes, drainage bags, and wound-suction apparatus should be available.
10 Irrigating solutions should be at body temperature before using. All radiopaque dyes, anticoagulants, and solutions on the instrument table must be clearly labeled to avoid any error in administration.
11 Blood loss and urinary output frequently are recorded.

NECK PROCEDURES

Operations are conveniently classified by anatomical location. The head, face, and parts of the neck belong to other specialties, but general surgery claims the thyroid, parathyroid, cervical, and scalene node areas. For operations in these areas, the patient is positioned with neck extended, usually over thyroid elevator attachment to the operating table (see Chap. 15. p. 298). Arms are secured at sides of body and not on armboards, to prevent distortion of body contour in the neck region. The table may be tilted into reverse Trendelenburg's position.

Thyroid Procedures

The *thyroid gland,* located in the anterior aspect of the neck, is composed of two lobes that lie on either side of the trachea and are united by a narrow band, the isthmus. The *thyroid hormone* controls rate of body metabolism and may influence physical and mental growth.

Hyperthyroidism (Grave's disease), hypothyroidism, and an enlarged gland (goiter) are the main disorders of the thyroid. Drugs, radioactive iodine, and/or surgical resection are used to treat hyperthyroidism. This disease, rare in elderly patients or the very young, affects females more frequently than it does males. Replacement of the thyroid hormone with drug therapy is specific treatment for hypothyroidism. Oral administration of thyroid extract or iodine may reduce glandular size, but surgical excision is frequently necessary.

Thyroid Biopsy A needle biopsy or an excisional biopsy may be performed to aid in establishing a diagnosis of thyroiditis or differentiating between nodular goiter and carcinoma.

Subtotal Thyroidectomy The usual operation for hyperthyroidism is removal of approximately five-sixths of the thyroid gland. This procedure generally relieves symptoms permanently, because the remaining thyroid tissue secretes sufficient hormone for normal function.

Thyroid Lobectomy The removal of a lobe of the thyroid is adapted especially for toxic diffuse goiter, which is usually benign. In case of malignant growth, the lobe and the lymph nodes in the neck that drain into the involved area may be dissected. Care must be exercised not to damage the recurrent laryngeal nerve and parathyroid glands that lie in close proximity, because trauma can result in temporary or permanent laryngeal paralysis. Voice disturbance with hoarseness occurs with paralysis of one vocal cord.

Substernal Intrathoracic Thyroidectomy Goiters invading the substernal and intrathoracic regions occur less frequently, but their size and location often cause tracheal obstruction. The sternum may have to be split to remove a large adherent intrathoracic goiter.

Postoperative complications of thyroidectomy and associated procedures include hemorrhage, edema of the glottis, injury to the recurrent laryngeal nerve, tetany, and acute thyrotoxicosis. A tracheotomy set (refer to Chap. 26) must remain at the patient's bedside postoperatively per hospital routine or until released by the surgeon, usually for at least 24 hours, in case of respiratory obstruction.

Thyroglossal Duct Procedures

Thyroglossal Duct Cystectomy Excision of a thyroglossal cyst requires removal of the entire cystic sac and a portion of the hyoid bone.

Parathyroid Gland Procedures

Parathyroidectomy The *parathyroids,* the four or more small endocrine glands attached to or within the thyroid, regulate metabolism of calcium in the body. Diseased glands are surgically excised; however, resection of all parathyroid tissue may cause severe tetany.

Cervical and Scalene Node Procedures

Biopsy Cervical and/or scalene nodes are biopsied for diagnosis of metastatic extension of cancer or tuberculosis into these lymphatic nodes. The procedure may also be performed by thoracic surgeons.

BREAST PROCEDURES

The *mammary glands* are bilateral organs lying in the superficial fascia of the pectoral area. They are attached to the underlying muscles by loose areolar tissue. The breasts extend from border of the sternum to anterior axillary line and from approximately the first to seventh rib.

General surgery on the breast includes diagnostic procedures and those performed for known pathology. Diagnostic techniques include mammography, xeroradiography, and thermography, as well as the traditional tissue biopsy. Self-examination by the patient plays an important role in detection of potential breast problems. The desired operative procedure should be determined on an individual basis after careful diagnostic studies and histologic diagnosis. Size, location, and type of diseased tissue or stage of malignancy are important considerations. No single operation is suitable for all patients.

Incision and Drainage

Surgical opening of an inflamed and suppurative area is most frequently carried out because of infections in the lactating breast. The cavity is usually irrigated and the wound packed and allowed to heal by granulation. The causative organism is often staphylococcus. The patient may be placed on drainage/secretion isolation precautions.

Biopsy of the Breast

To determine exact nature of a mass in the breast, tissue is removed for histologic examination. Until proven benign, all breast masses are considered malignant. A *needle biopsy,* a type of incisional biopsy, is done by inserting a large bore needle attached to a syringe into the mass and withdrawing a core of suspected tissue for cytological examination. Any retrieved fluid is also sent to pathology. If an *incisional biopsy* is performed, the mass is incised and only a portion is removed.

An *excisional biopsy* consists of removal of the entire mass. Biopsy is carried out for the presence of a tumor mass detected by palpation, x-ray diagnostic studies, skin changes such as dimpling, and nipple discharge. Excisional biopsy is usually the procedure of choice because it permits examination of the whole mass and avoids entering the lesion with accompanying risk of seeding or implantation of malignant cells. A Penrose drain may be inserted.

A patient may be scheduled for breast biopsy and frozen section. The surgeon may intend to proceed directly with the indicated dissection if results of the frozen section warrant it. Preoperatively, the surgeon discusses with the patient possible findings and treatment and the patient agrees to definitive operation. When a patient has a biopsy and immediate extended operation, two separate prepping, draping, and instrument sets are necessary.

Partial Mastectomy (Lumpectomy)

Partial mastectomy (lumpectomy) is recommended only for patients with small peripherally located lesions and consists of removal of the entire tumor mass along with at least 2.5 cm (1 in.) of surrounding nondiseased tissue.

Subcutaneous Mastectomy (Adenomammectomy)

Subcutaneous mastectomy may be performed for patients with chronic cystic mastitis who have had multiple previous biopsies, patients with multiple fibroadenomas or hyperplastic duct changes, and patients with central tumors of the breast that are noninvasive in origin. Removal of all breast tissue is carried out with the overlying skin and nipple remaining intact. A prosthesis may be inserted at time of operation, depending on the surgeon's decision and the patient's wishes (see Chap. 27, p. 530).

Simple Mastectomy (Total Mastectomy)

In simple mastectomy, the entire breast is removed but without lymph node dissection. Simple mastectomy may be performed if the malignancy is confined to breast tissue with negative nodes, as a palliative measure for an advanced ulcerated malignancy, or to remove extensive benign disease. Skin grafting may be necessary if primary closure of skin flaps would create unacceptable tension. Skin flaps are then loosely approximated and grafts taken from the thigh are applied to the remaining defect. A latissimus dorsi or rectus abdominus myocutaneous flap may be preferred for reconstruction (see Chap. 27, p. 525).

Modified Radical Mastectomy

Modified radical mastectomy is usually done for localized small malignant lesions. The term *modified* encompasses various techniques but all include removal of the entire breast (total mastectomy). In addition, all axillary lymph nodes are resected. The underlying major pectoral muscle is left in place. The minor pectoralis muscle may or may not be removed. Breast reconstruction may be performed immediately, or a few days following modified radical mastectomy, in patients with small lesions and no metastases (see Chap. 27, p. 529).

Radical Mastectomy

Radical mastectomy is performed for larger infiltrating cancers to control the spread of malignant disease. Following a positive tissue biopsy, the entire involved breast is removed along with axillary lymph nodes, pectoral muscles, and all adjacent tissues. During operation, skin flaps and extensive exposed tissue are covered with moist packs for protection. The chest wall and axilla are irrigated before closure.

Extended Radical Mastectomy (Urban Procedure)

Extended radical mastectomy is indicated when malignant disease is present in the medial quadrant or subareolar tissue, because it tends to spread to the internal mammary lymph nodes. Cancer is a disease that grows deeply as well as laterally. The involved breast is removed en bloc along with underlying pectoral muscles, axillary contents, and upper internal mammary (mediastinal) lymph node chain. This procedure is more difficult than is classical radical mastectomy.

Considerations for Female Breast Procedures

Patients for breast procedures are placed in supine position with the involved side close to edge of the table with arm on the affected side extended on an armboard. General anesthesia is usually preferred for mastectomy. Local infiltrate may obscure a tumor.

Because of vascularity of breast tissue, mastectomy patients should be watched for excessive bleeding. A compression dressing usually is applied in the OR. A closed-wound suction system may be inserted depending on amount of tissue resected, to remove extravasation of blood and serum and prevent necrosis of skin flaps.

Patients who have undergone mastectomy are frequently referred to the Reach to Recovery rehabilitative program. Under this program, volunteers who have had mastectomies visit patients and share information with them, as well as give encouragement.

Reduction of the Male Breast

This procedure is carried out for *gynecomastia,* a pathologic lesion consisting of bilateral or unilateral enlargement of the male breast. It occurs primarily after the age of 40 or during puberty and is usually related to alterations in normal hormonal balance. All subareolar fibroglandular tissue is removed, followed by reconstruction of the resultant defect. Carcinoma can also occur in the male breast.

OPERATIVE ABDOMINAL INCISIONS

Surgical opening of the abdominal wall and entering of the peritoneal cavity is called *laparotomy.* Various types of incisions are used, but each follows essentially the same technique. The exact position of incision is determined before the surgeon begins. The skin and subcutaneous tissue are incised and blood vessels are ligated. Fascia covers the muscles anteriorly and posteriorly. The anterior fascia is incised and each muscle layer is separated and/or divided with bleeding vessels ligated. The layers are retracted. The peritoneum is the thin serous membrane lining interior of the abdominal cavity (*parietal peritoneum*) and surrounding the organs (*visceral peritoneum*). It lies beneath the posterior fascia. Both posterior fascia and peritoneum may be cut at the same time, thus exposing the contents of the abdominal cavity (refer to Fig. 21-1).

The surgeon chooses the most suitable incision for the procedure to be performed. All incisions incorporate with varying degrees of success certain characteristics that include:

1 Ease and speed of entry into the abdominal cavity
2 Maximum exposure
3 Minimum trauma
4 Least postoperative discomfort
5 Maximum postoperative wound strength

Types of Incisions

The two main factors governing incisions are direction and location. Incisions may be vertical, horizontal, or oblique, in various areas of the torso (see Fig. 21-2). The following incisions are applicable to abdominal or pelvic procedures.

Paramedian Incision Paramedian incision is a vertical incision about 4 cm (approximately 2 in.) lateral to the midline on either side, in the upper or lower abdomen. After skin and subcutaneous tissue are incised, the rectus sheath is split vertically and muscle retracted laterally. This incision allows quick entry into the abdominal cavity with excellent exposure, limits trauma, avoids nerve injury, is easily extended, and gives a firm closure. Examples of use: right upper quadrant, biliary tract or pancreas; left lower quadrant, resection of sigmoid colon.

Longitudinal Midline Incision A longitudinal midline incision can be upper abdominal, lower abdominal, or a combination of both going

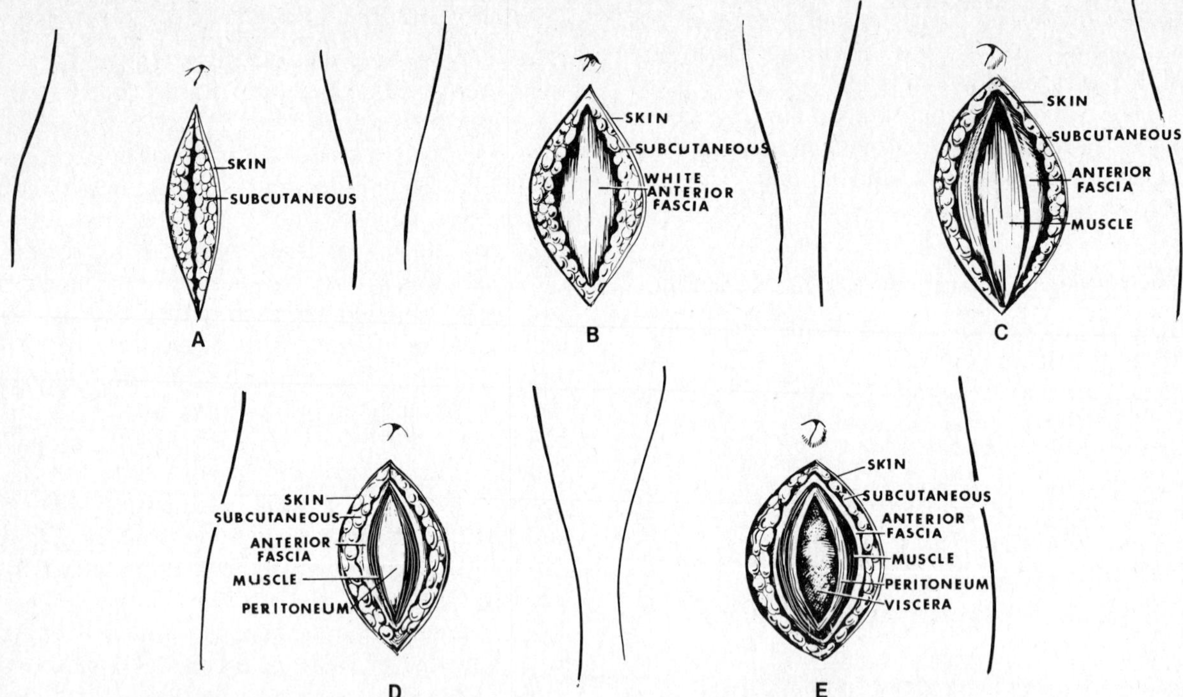

FIGURE 21-1
Dissecting tissue layers of the abdomen. **(A)** Subcutaneous fat (yellow). **(B)** Anterior fascia (white). **(C)** Muscle (red). **(D)** Skin through muscle dissected. Thin white peritoneum presenting for dissection. **(E)** Opened peritoneum with viscera beneath.

around the umbilicus. Depending on length of incision, it begins in the epigastrium at level of the xiphoid process and may extend vertically to suprapubic region. After incision of the peritoneum, the falciform ligament of the liver is divided.

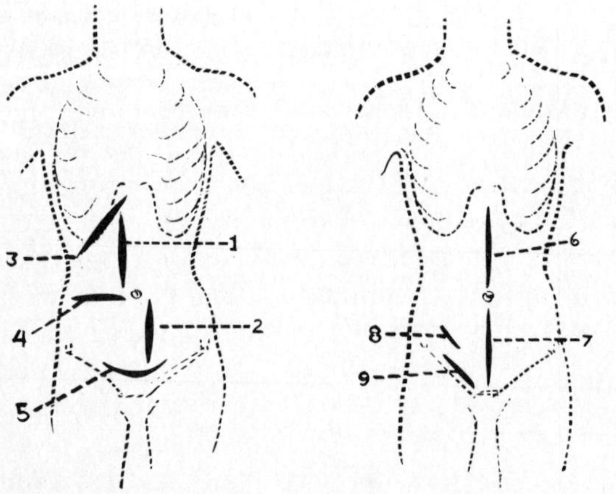

FIGURE 21-2
Abdominal incisions: (1) right upper paramedian, (2) left lower paramedian, (3) right subcostal, upper quadrant oblique, (4) right midline transverse, (5) Pfannenstiel's, (6) upper longitudinal midline, (7) lower longitudinal midline, (8) McBurney's, (9) right inguinal, lower oblique.

Upper midline incision offers excellent exposure of upper abdominal contents and rapid entry but is not a strong incision and may disrupt. The *lower midline incision* provides exposure of pelvic organs and rapid entry. It is not as strong as a paramedian incision. Examples of use: upper for gastrectomy; lower for intestinal resection.

Subcostal, Upper Quadrant Oblique Incision A right or left oblique incision begins in the epigastrium and extends laterally and obliquely just below the lower costal margin. It continues through the rectus muscle, which is either retracted or transversely divided. Although the incision affords limited exposure except for upper abdominal viscera, cosmetically it provides good results, since it follows the skin lines and produces limited nerve damage. It is a strong incision postoperatively, although a painful one. Examples of use: biliary procedures, splenectomy; or bilateral incisions joining in the midline for stomach and/or pancreas procedures.

McBurney's Incision The area just below the umbilicus and 4 cm (about 2 in.) medial from the anterior superior iliac spine marks McBurney's point in the right lower quadrant. A muscle-splitting incision extending through fibers of the external oblique muscle is made. The incision is deepened, and internal oblique and transversalis muscles split and retracted. Then the peritoneum is entered. This is a fast, easy incision, although exposure is limited. Primary use: appendectomy.

Thoracoabdominal Incision With patient in lateral position, either a right or left incision begins at a point midway between xiphoid and umbilicus and extends across abdomen to the seventh or eighth costal interspace and along the interspace into the thorax. The rectus, oblique, serratus, and intercostal muscles are divided in the line of incision down to peritoneum and pleura. This converts the pleural and peritoneal cavities into one main cavity, thus allowing excellent exposure for upper end of the stomach and lower end of the esophagus (see Fig. 30-2, p. 565). Examples of use: esophageal varices, repair of hiatus hernia.

Midabdominal Transverse Incision The midabdominal transverse incision starts on either right or left side slightly above or below the umbilicus. It may be carried laterally to the lumbar region between the ribs and crest of the ilium. Intercostal nerves are protected by cutting posterior rectus sheath and peritoneum in direction of the divided muscle fibers. Advantages are rapid incision, easy extension, provision for retroperitoneal approach, and secure postoperative wound. Examples of use: choledochojejunostomy or transverse colostomy.

Pfannenstiel's Incision Pfannenstiel's incision is a curved transverse incision across lower abdomen within hairline of the pubis. Rectus fascia is severed transversely and the muscles are separated. The peritoneum is incised vertically in the midline. This lower transverse incision provides good exposure and strong closure for pelvic procedures. Example of use: abdominal hysterectomy.

Inguinal Incision, Lower Oblique An oblique incision of right or left inguinal region extends from the pubic tubercle to the anterior crest of the ilium, slightly above and parallel to the inguinal crease. Incision of external oblique fascia gives access to the cremaster muscle, inguinal canal, and cord structures. Example of use: inguinal herniorrhapy.

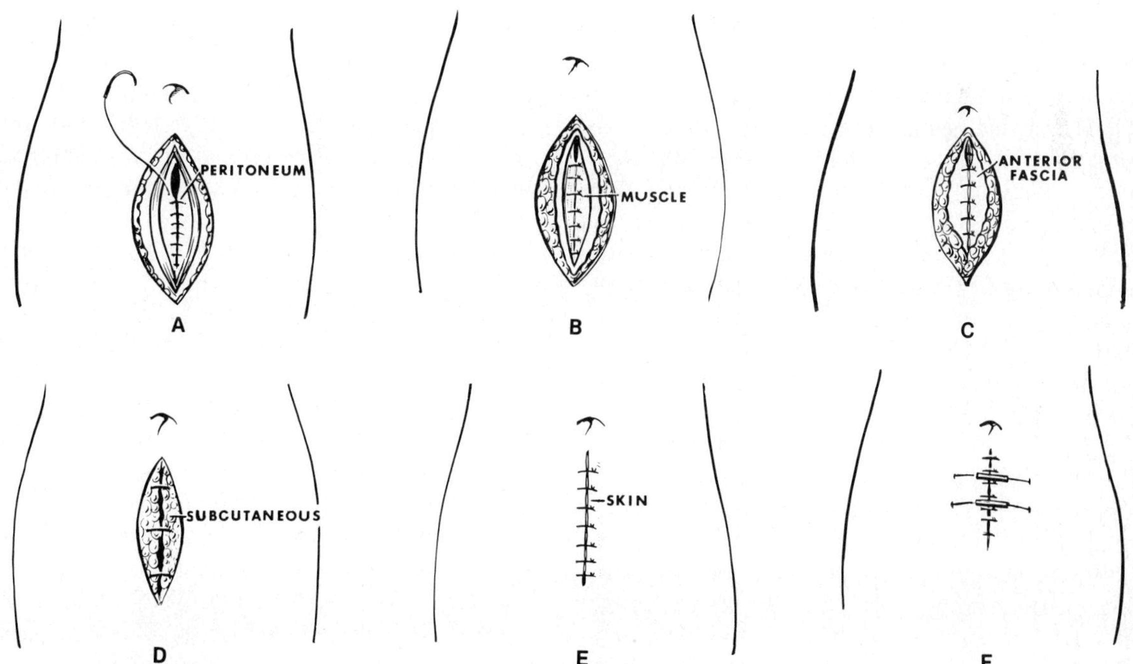

FIGURE 21-3
Suturing incised tissue layers. (**A**) Peritoneum (continuous stitch, taper point needle). (**B**) Muscle (interrupted stitch). (**C**) Anterior fascia (interrupted stitch, cutting needle). (**D**) Subcutaneous (not always sutured, taper point needle). (**E**) Skin (interrupted stitch, cutting needle). (**F**) Retention sutures. Note bumpers to protect skin.

Wound Closure

Closure is done in reverse order of incision. Each layer is closed with interrupted or continuous sutures (see Fig. 21-3). Separation of tissues produced by failure to approximate wound edges closely results in dead space, which delays healing. Absorbable material is usually used if peritoneum is sutured. Either absorbable or nonabsorbable material is used on muscle and fascia. It may be necessary to place a few absorbable sutures in subcutaneous layer. Skin edges are approximated with nonabsorbable suture, skin clips, or staples. Sometimes the suture line is supported by retention or stay sutures.

Many surgeons prefer the Smead-Jones far-and-near technique for abdominal wound closure. This is a single layer closure through both layers of fascia, abdominal muscles, and peritoneum with interrupted sutures, either monofilament stainless steel or polypropylene. These sutures resemble the figure 8 when placed. This closure is rapid and strong.

BILIARY TRACT PROCEDURES

The *gallbladder* is located in a fossa on the undersurface of the right lobe of the liver (see Fig. 21-5, p. 406). It is a thin-walled sac with a normal capacity of about 50 to 60 ml of bile. Bile, which is secreted by the hepatic cells, enters the intrahepatic bile ducts and progresses to the common bile duct. When not needed for digestion, bile is diverted through the cystic duct into the gallbladder, where it is stored. When needed, the gallbladder contracts, emptying bile into cystic duct from which it flows to common bile duct, and on into the duodenum. *Gallstones,* concretions of elements in bile, particularly cholesterol, may be found in the gallbladder or any portion of the hepatic duct system. Incidence of stones or calculi increases with age, and is more prevalent in women. Ultrasonography is used for diagnosis of gallbladder disease. Oral and intravenous cholecystography may also be used for visualization of gallbladder in initial evaluation of patients with biliary symptoms. Acute or chronic inflammation, common duct stone (*choledocholithiasis*), carcinoma, or congenital absence of bile ducts (*biliary atresia*) are the most common indications for operation. Obstructive jaundice, potentially fatal, may be a sign of ductal cholelithiasis or presence of a neoplasm. Cause of jaundice must be determined and condition relieved to spare patient irreversible progressive liver damage.

Cholecystostomy

Cholecystostomy is operative formation of an opening into the gallbladder to permit drainage and to avoid rupture. It is usually done under local anesthesia in patients whose general condition prohibits a prolonged procedure. A purse-string suture is placed in the fundus. Gallbladder is decompressed and aspirated by inserting a trocar with suction attached inside the purse string. After removal of the contaminated trocar, the opening is enlarged to permit insertion of a stone forceps or spoon and any calculi are removed. A drainage catheter is placed in the opening and the purse string closed around it. The catheter may be secured with additional suture and fundus of gallbladder sutured to the abdominal wall to reduce hazard of bile leakage. A Penrose drain is placed in the abdominal cavity and the wound closed. A specimen of the aspirated fluid is sent for culture.

Cholecystectomy

Removal of the gallbladder is the most common operation performed on the biliary tract. It is done to relieve gastrointestinal distress common in patients with acute or chronic cholecystitis with or without calculi. Also, it removes a source of recurrent sepsis. Persistent infection in the biliary tract may be the cause of recurrent calculi.

Supine position is used with the gallbladder rest elevated. The table may be tilted slightly so that abdominal contents tend to gravitate downward away from the operative area. The gallbladder usually is reached through a right subcostal or right paramedian incision.

Following exploration of the abdominal cavity, laparotomy packs are used to wall off surrounding organs from the gallbladder. Infected contents must not be spilled into the peritoneal cavity, to prevent peritonitis. No attempt is made to remove the gallbladder until biliary tract structures are identified accurately. These include the cystic duct, cystic artery, hepatic ducts, and common bile duct. *Operative cholangiograms,* injection of radiopaque solution into the cystic duct or into a tube placed in the common duct, frequently are done intraoperatively to permit identification and removal of overlooked stones. The x-ray department is notified in advance if cholangiography is anticipated. Scout films should be taken when the patient is initially positioned on the operating table, which must have a radiographic top or be equipped for x-rays or fluoroscopy (see Chap. 20, p. 391). Intraoperative ultrasonography may be preferred rather than operative cholangiography to detect stones.

Concomitant *exploration of the common duct* is often done during cholecystectomy. Curved stone forceps, small malleable scoops, dilators of various sizes, and Fogarty balloon-tipped catheters are useful in clearing ducts of stones to prevent their lodging in the duct, with subsequent obstructive jaundice. *Intraoperative biliary endoscopy* by use of the choledochoscope gives image transmission and illumination, allowing the surgeon visual guidance in exploring the biliary system. After the scope is introduced into the common duct, a flexible stone forceps or a Fogarty biliary catheter may be inserted through the instrument channel to allow manipulation of a stone under direct vision. A biopsy forceps may be inserted to obtain a tissue sample.

Blunt dissection with dry dissector sponges is used to separate adhesions caused by previous inflammation. If the gallbladder is tightly distended, it may be aspirated before removal. After palpation of the ducts for stones, and ligation and division of the cystic duct and artery, the gallbladder is removed. Penrose drains and/or T tubes (in ducts) are usually inserted and brought out through the incision or stab wound to the right of the incision. Complications of cholecystectomy include hemorrhage and injury to the common duct.

Choledochostomy; Choledochotomy

Choledochostomy is drainage of the common bile duct through the abdominal wall. A T tube is used for drainage. *Choledochotomy* is incision of the common bile duct for exploration and removal of stones. Intraoperative cholangiography may be performed before and after exploration and/or stone removal. The duct is irrigated after removal of calculi. Patency of duct and of ampulla of Vater is investigated. If a neoplasm is found during exploration, resectability is determined. However, many tumors of the liver or pancreas are inoperable. A T tube is placed in the common duct and a Penrose drain inserted before abdominal closure if a cholecystectomy is also performed.

Cholecystoduodenostomy; Cholecystojejunostomy

Cholecystoduodenostomy or cholecystojejunostomy is done to relieve an obstruction in the distal end of the common duct. These procedures establish continuity, by anastomosis, between the gallbladder and duodenum or gallbladder and jejunum. Careful evaluation precedes operation. These are bypass procedures to avoid further obstructive jaundice, but do not solve problem. Common causes of obstruction are calculi, stricture of the duct, or neoplasms of the duct, ampulla of Vater, or pancreas.

Choledochoduodenostomy; Choledochojejunostomy

Side-to-side anastomoses between the duodenum or jejunum and the common duct are carried out when the surgeon is not totally satisfied that all stones have been removed or is concerned about the possibility of subsequent reexploration.

LIVER PROCEDURES

The *liver,* the largest gland in the body, is divided into left and right segments or lobes. It is located in the upper right abdominal cavity beneath the diaphragm (see Figs. 21-4 and 21-5). Part of the stomach and duodenum, and the hepatic flexure of the colon lie directly beneath the liver. A tough fibrous sheath, *Glisson's capsule,* completely covers the organ. The tissue within the capsule is very friable and vascular. The hepatic artery, a branch of the celiac axis, maintains the arterial supply. Blood from the stomach, intestine, spleen, and pancreas is carried to the liver by the portal vein and its branches.

The many functions of the liver include forming and secreting bile, which aids digestion, transforming glucose into glycogen, which it stores, and helping to regulate blood volume. The liver is vital in metabolic function of the body. This organ

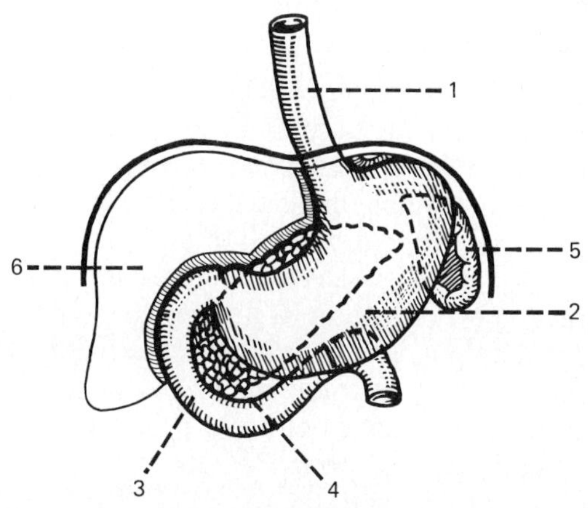

FIGURE 21-4
Organs in upper abdominal cavity: (1) esophagus, (2) stomach, (3) duodenum, (4) pancreas, (5) spleen, (6) liver.

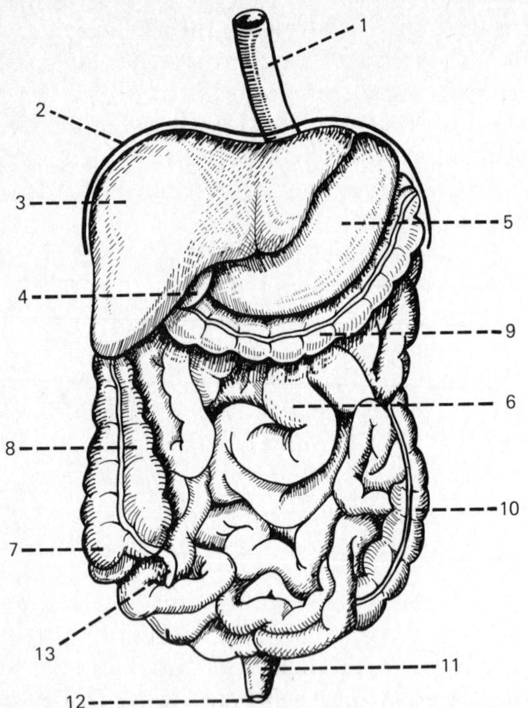

FIGURE 21-5
Abdominal organs within peritoneal cavity: (1) esophagus, (2) diaphragm, (3) liver, (4) gallbladder, (5) stomach, (6) small intestine, (7) cecum, (8) ascending colon, (9) transverse colon, (10) descending colon, (11) rectum, (12) anus, (13) appendix.

has remarkable regenerative capacity and up to 80 percent may be resected with little or no alteration in hepatic function. Liver function tests are used to assess degree of functional impairment and evaluate liver activity and reserve. Most of these tests involve taking a series of blood samples from the patient for specific studies. Ascites may result from impaired liver function.

Liver Needle Biopsy

A needle biopsy may be done to help establish diagnosis of hepatic disease. Since the procedure is done under local anesthesia, during explanation the patient must be instructed to take several deep breaths and to hold the breath and remain absolutely still while the needle is inserted. Failure of patient cooperation can cause needle penetration of the diaphragm or liver injury resulting in hemorrhage, a serious complication. Leakage of bile into the abdominal cavity may produce chemical peritonitis, an additional hazard. After prep and local anesthesia, with the patient supine, a Silverman biopsy needle is introduced into the liver via intercostal (transthoracic) or subcostal (transabdominal) route. After insertion, the needle is rotated, thus separating a fragment of tissue about 1 to 4 cm (½ to 1½ in.) in length. The needle is withdrawn and the specimen is removed and sent to pathology. As soon as the needle is removed, the patient is told to resume normal breathing and is assisted in turning onto the right side to compress the chest wall at the penetration site to prevent bile or blood seepage.

Drainage of Subphrenic and Subhepatic Abscesses

Abscesses in and about the liver may be caused by a variety of pyogenic microorganisms, secondary amebic types, or as secondary infections from abdominal organs. They generally are treated by incision and drainage. Care must be taken to avoid contamination of the pleural or peritoneal cavity. Location of the abscess determines approach, i.e., transpleural, subpleural, transperitoneal, or retroperitoneal.

Hepatic Resection

Indications for right or left hepatic lobectomy or wedge resection include cysts, benign or malignant tumors, or severe lacerations of the liver caused by trauma. Lacerations may cause intraperitoneal hemorrhage and shock.

The abdominal cavity is entered through a right subcostal incision that is extended through the seventh or eighth interspace. Or, a right upper abdominal vertical incision is used for laceration, to permit incision extension if necessary, and for exploration. It is necessary to divide the appropriate ligamentous attachments and ligate the anatomical veins and arteries before rotating the liver forward and segmentally excising the diseased or injured portion.

Liver tissue is very friable and hemostatic substances are often used to control bleeding. Prevention or arrest of hemorrhage is a prime concern. Large, blunt, noncutting needles are used to suture the organ. Drains usually are placed in the wound and brought out through the incision or adjacent drain sites. Equipment for blood replacement, portal pressure measurement, and thoracotomy drainage should be readily available.

Portosystemic Shunts

Portal hypertension, bleeding esophageal varices, or massive gastrointestinal hemorrhage may necessitate an emergency operation for decompression of the portal venous system. Often the patient is alcoholic with cirrhosis, poor nutrition, and unstable blood volume, or generally a poor operative risk. A portosystemic shunt is a vascular anastomosis between portal and systemic venous systems. The surgeon may select one of several techniques for a portacaval or mesocaval shunt. A splenorenal shunt may be performed in conjunction with a splenectomy in patients with portal hypertension and hypersplenism for portal decompression. Refer to Chapter 32, p. 588, for discussion of these shunt procedures.

SPLENIC PROCEDURES

The highly vascular *spleen* is located in the upper left abdominal cavity, protected by lower portion of rib cage, and lies beneath the dome of the diaphragm (see Fig. 21-4). The capsule of the spleen is covered with peritoneum and held in place by numerous suspensory ligaments. The splenic artery furnishes arterial blood supply. The splenic vein drains into the portal system. As the largest lymphatic organ of the body, it has an intimate role in immunologic defenses of the body and acts as a blood reservoir. The spleen has several functions, chiefly concerned with formation of blood elements. X-ray examination and radionuclide scanning provide information for diagnosis.

Splenectomy

The most common cause for removal of spleen is *hypersplenism,* overactivity that causes reduction in the circulating quantity of red cells, white cells, and platelets or a combination of them. Splenectomies frequently are scheduled at specific times, since these patients often require administration of whole blood immediately prior to operation. Often the patients are also on steroid treatment and provisions must be made to maintain therapy during operation and postoperatively. Traumatic ruptures, tumors, or accessory spleens may also be cause for operative intervention. Splenic rupture requires immediate operation to prevent fatal hemorrhage.

A left rectus paramedian or subcostal incision is used to enter the peritoneal cavity. The spleen is displaced medially by careful manual manipulation and the splenorenal, splenocolic, and gastrosplenic ligaments are ligated and divided. Great care must be exercised in ligating the splenic artery and vein because these vessels are frequently very friable. Hemorrhage is the principal hazard encountered intraoperatively. After removal of the spleen, careful inspection for bleeding from the splenic pedicle and retroperitoneal space is essential before closure. A drain, exteriorized through a stab wound, may be inserted in the left subdiaphragmatic space in patients with extensive trauma.

> NOTE. After splenectomy, patients are prone to infection, sometimes with catastrophic results. Therefore, surgeons attempt to save the organ to protect the immune competence of patient following splenic trauma. The spleen may be sutured, packed with microfibrillar collagen hemostat (Avitene), or pulled together in a network of surgical gut sutures to compress it.

PANCREATIC PROCEDURES

The *pancreas* is both an endocrine and exocrine gland. Islets of Langerhans comprise the endocrine division and secrete insulin and glucagon, hormones essential to carbohydrate metabolism and storage of calories. Acini and ducts leading from them constitute the exocrine portion that secretes pancreatic juice into the duodenum. Pancreatic juice neutralizes stomach acid. Loss of it results in severe impairment of digestion and foodstuff absorption.

The pancreas lies transversely across the posterior wall of upper abdomen behind the stomach. The head or right extremity is attached to the duodenum and the tail or left extremity is in close proximity to the spleen (see Fig. 21-4).

Disorders of the pancreas generally include acute and chronic inflammation, cysts, and tumors. The head of the pancreas is most common site of malignant tumor. Accuracy of diagnosis in pancreatic problems is difficult, but evaluation by ultrasound and scanning has led to significant improvement in planning operative treatment. Pancreatitis is most often associated with gallstones or alcoholism. Corrective biliary tract operations usually alleviate gallstone pancreatitis.

Pancreaticojejunostomy

Pancreaticojejunostomy may be performed for relief of pain associated with chronic alcoholic pancreatitis and pseudocysts of the pancreas. There are several types of procedures for drainage of obstructed ducts or pseudocysts. These involve anastomosing a loop of the jejunum (Roux en Y loop) to the pancreatic duct. Hemorrhage or leakage of bile are complications to be avoided.

Pancreaticoduodenectomy (Whipple Operation)

Pancreaticoduodenectomy, an extensive procedure, is performed for patients with carcinoma of head of the pancreas or ampulla of Vater. A gastrointestinal setup is used. The abdominal cavity is exposed through one of several possible anterior incisions, but a long right paramedian incision is usually made. The abdominal and pelvic cavities are explored for distant metastases. Since many vital structures and organs are involved in resecting diseased portion of pancreas, careful dissection of vessels is necessary to prevent hemorrhage, which complicates the procedure. Resection includes all but tail of pancreas, distal stomach, duodenum distal to pylorus, and distal end of common bile duct. Several methods of reconstructing the digestive tract are possible, but all include anastomosis of pancreatic duct, common bile duct, stomach, and jejunum. After pancreatic and biliary reconstruction, the divided end of the duodenum is anastomosed to side of jejunal limb used for the reconstruction. Watertight seal of all anastomoses is essential to prevent peritonitis or pancreatitis. Drains are inserted.

Postoperatively, the most common complications are shock, hemorrhage, renal failure, and pancreatic or biliary fistula. If a fistula should occur, wound suction is continued until the fistula closes. It will generally close spontaneously if adequate nutrition and electrolyte balance are maintained.

Improvements in pre- and postoperative care and refinement of technical details have increased the survival rate of this potentially hazardous radical operation.

Pancreatectomy

Subtotal distal pancreatectomy is usually done to resect benign tumor or for chronic pancreatitis. The distal tail is resected to the head of the pancreas. Splenectomy is usually performed with this procedure because blood supply to tail of pancreas comes from splenic vessels which must be sacrificed.

Total pancreatectomy allows a wide resection of a primary malignant tumor and its multifocal sites in the pancreas. This operation leaves the patient with some endocrine and exocrine pancreatic insufficiency, however.

ESOPHAGEAL PROCEDURES

The *esophagus* is the musculocutaneous canal between the pharynx in the throat and the stomach in the abdomen. It passes through the thoracic cavity and enters the abdominal cavity through the esophageal hiatus, opening, in the right crus of the diaphragm. It joins the right medial surface of the stomach. Within the abdominal cavity the esophagus lies between the liver anteriorly, aorta posteriorly and slightly to the left, with spleen on the left, and the right and left branches of the vagus nerve (see Figs. 21-4 and 21-5).

Esophageal Hiatus Herniorrhaphy

The abdominal esophagus and a portion of the stomach may slide through the esophageal hiatus into the thoracic cavity when intraabdominal pressure exceeds pressure in the chest. Although the condition is quite common, referred to as hiatus or diaphragmatic hernia (see p. 417), operation is indicated when resultant esophagitis causes ulceration, bleeding, stenosis, or chest and back symptoms. Reflux esophagitis and sphincter incompetence may also have other causes necessitating operation.

The abdominal approach to correct the problem is through a midline or left subcostal incision. Visualization of the hiatal area may be difficult, so incision may be extended over the lower rib cage. The patient may be placed in slight Trendelenburg's position. Organs and vital structures must be protected with moist tapes and gently retracted to expose the hiatus. Long-handled clamps are needed. Following mobilization, the hiatus is narrowed with heavy sutures and the fundus of the stomach is anchored against the diaphragm to prevent recurrent herniation and gastroesophageal reflux. Prevention of reflux is one of the prime objectives of operation, because it was the cause of the patient's previous esophagitis. Lengthening the intraabdominal esophagus and increasing pressure on lower esophageal sphincter also help control reflux. Pressure is augmented by wrapping proximal stomach around the gastroesophageal junction, the *Nissen fundoplication* procedure.

Operations for Esophageal Varices

Esophageal varices are tortuous dilated veins in the submucosa of the lower esophagus, although they may extend up in the esophagus or down into the stomach. This condition is caused by portal hypertension due to obstruction within a cirrhotic liver. Rupture of esophageal varices can cause massive hemorrhage. The patient may come to the OR with a Sengstaken-Blakemore tube in place to control bleeding by pressure from the inflated balloon in the tube. At operation, varices may be ligated or coagulated by laser beam through an esophagoscope. The lower esophagus may be transected and the distal segment anastomosed with a stapler just proximal to the stomach. A portosystemic shunt procedure may be performed for portal decompression.

GASTRIC PROCEDURES

The *stomach,* a hollow muscular organ, is situated in upper left abdomen between esophagus and duodenum (see Figs. 21-4 and 21-5). Anatomically it is divided into fundus, body, and pyloric antrum. The two borders of the stomach, the *lesser* and *greater curvatures,* are important surgically because of their relation to the major vascular and lymphatic systems supplying the stomach. A double fold of peritoneum attached to the lesser and greater curvatures loosely covers the intestines. The autonomic nervous supply from the vagus nerve controls reflex activities of movement and secretions of the alimentary canal and is significant in rhythmic relaxation of the pyloric sphincter.

Food entering the stomach must be reduced to a semiliquid to pass through the duodenum and small intestine. Interference of gastric activity or muscular contractions results in gastrointestinal complaints of abdominal pain, nausea, vomiting, hemorrhage, and dyspepsia. Some diseases, such as cancer, may not produce symptoms until the condition is far advanced. Operation is indicated when the presence of disease is established following laboratory tests such as gastric analysis, gastroscopy, and/or radiographic studies.

Advances in surgical management of patients with gastrointestinal problems have lessened mortality rate, although treatment may be palliative rather than curative.

Interference with the gastrointestinal tract affects its functioning and specific deficiencies may result from gastrointestinal surgery, depending on the site and extent. Massive resection of the small intestine can produce long-term nutritional problems, such as weight loss and malabsorption of most nutrients, thus endangering compatibility with life. Metabolic bone disease may follow gastric surgery, due to poor absorption of calcium and vitamin D. Patients who have undergone extensive gastric operation should have periodic nutritional evaluation. Biochemical tests monitor nutritional status. These include serum proteins, albumin-globulin ratio, and blood urea nitrogen. Body weight is significant also. If caloric intake is inadequate, protein is converted to carbohydrate for energy and protein synthesis then suffers.

The *dumping syndrome* may be experienced by patients shortly after eating following gastric surgery. This complication occurs because of rapid empyting of food and fluids into the jejunum. It is characterized by nausea, vomiting, sensations of weakness and dizziness, pallor, sweating, palpitations, and diarrhea. It usually subsides within six months to a year.

Considerations for Gastrointestinal Surgery

Separation of instruments used for resection and anastomosis, and abdominal closure is essential. Two distinct setups may be used, but the single setup, most commonly used, consists of identifying and using only selected instruments and supplies for resection, anastomosis, and abdominal closure, and discarding contaminated instruments and equipment from the field after use. Acid secretions from the resection site are very irritating and may cause peritonitis. Gloves are changed before closure, and in some hospitals gowns also are changed.

It is necessary to have a variety of gastrointestinal tubes available for irrigation and aspiration. Electrosurgery frequently is used. Intestinal forceps jaws should be protected with soft rubber tubing to reduce tissue trauma. Stapling devices are preferred by some surgeons to mechanically anastomose organs. Normal saline is always required in abdominal procedures for laparotomy packs. Saline or other solutions, such as oxychlorosene (Chlorpactin XCB) or antibiotics, may also be needed for irrigation.

NOTE. An intraluminal stapler can be used for end-to-end, end-to-side, or side-to-side anastomoses from the esophagus to the rectum (see

Chap. 18, p. 353). The stapler is introduced into the lumen through a gastrotomy or enterotomy site, except in low anterior colon resection when entry is through the anus (see p. 415). Because the size of the lumen varies in different organs of the gastrointestinal tract, the circulating nurse should not open a sterile disposable stapler until the surgeon determines the appropriate head size for the instrument to be used.

Gastric Procedures

Gastroscopy Passage of a fiberoptic gastroscope, via mouth, allows operator to visually inspect mucosal walls of the stomach. Sometimes tissue specimens are obtained, thus allowing differential diagnosis. Bleeding points may be coagulated with laser beam or by electrosurgery.

Gastrostomy The establishment of a temporary or permanent opening in the stomach may be indicated to provide alimentation for a prolonged period when nutrition cannot be maintained by other means. The patient may not be able to tolerate major operation or may have an inoperable lesion, such as an extensive esophageal tumor. Through a small upper left abdominal or midline incision the stomach is exposed and a catheter or tube is inserted into the anterior gastric wall. It is held in place with a purse-string suture. Foleys and various mushroom catheters are frequently used. Whenever feasible, a small-bore nasogastric polyethylene catheter for enteral hyperalimentation is preferred rather than gastrostomy.

Total Gastrectomy The entire stomach is excised through a bilateral subcostal, long transrectus, or thoracoabdominal incision. This procedure is done for malignant lesions. The operation necessitates reconstruction of esophagointestinal continuity by establishing an anastomosis between a loop of the jejunum and the esophagus. Leakage at site of anastomosis leads to peritonitis. Gastric carcinomas are frequently inoperable due to extended metastases to the liver and surrounding tissues. The appropriate operation is determined after thorough exploration of the abdominal cavity by the surgeon.

Partial Gastrectomy, Billroth's Operations, Subtotal Gastrectomy The presence of a benign or malignant lesion located in the pyloric half requires removal of the lower half to two/thirds of the stomach. In patients with peptic or duodenal ulcer, the operation relieves pain, bleeding, vomiting, and weight loss and limits gastric acidity. The peritoneal cavity is entered through a right paramedian abdominal incision. A variety of operations may be used to reestablish gastrointestinal continuity. Anastomosis of remaining portion of the stomach to the duodenum, gastroduodenostomy (Billroth I), or to a loop of the jejunum, gastrojejunostomy (Billroth II), frequently is performed.

Common modifications of the Billroth I operation are the Schoemaker and the von Haberer-Finney techniques. The Schoemaker operation involves end-to-end anastomosis of the stomach and duodenum after the lesser curvature of stomach is sutured to make the anastomosis site the same size as the duodenum. With the von Haberer-Finney method, the lateral wall of the duodenum is brought up to the stomach so entire end of stomach is open for direct anastomosis.

The popular modifications of Billroth II operation include Polya and Hofmeister techniques. These involve variations of end-to-side gastrojejunostomy.

Vagotomy Chronic peptic, gastric, and duodenal ulcers that do not respond to medical treatment cause patients severe pain and difficulty in eating and sleeping. Vagotomy may be recommended to interrupt vagal nerve impulses, thus lowering gastric hydrochloric acid production and hastening gastric empyting. *Vagotomy* is division of the vagus nerves. *Proximal gastric vagotomy,* also known as *parietal cell vagotomy,* divides vagal nerves to proximal stomach, but maintains entire stomach and vagal nerves to the antrum. These nerves inhibit the release of gastrin, a stimulant of gastric secretion.

Truncal vagotomy and *selective vagotomy* require a concomitant drainage operation because these procedures denervate the stomach. A gastroenterostomy is done with truncal vagotomy, which divides the vagal trunks at the distal esophagus. Antrectomy is performed with selective vagotomy, which transects the gastric branches. Vagotomy with drainage is a compromise operation restricted to high-risk patients or those with severe duodenal deformity.

Pyloroplasty, enlarging the pyloric opening between the stomach and duodenum, may be done in elderly patients with an obstructing pyloric ulcer, or in conjunction with vagotomy to treat bleeding duodenal ulcers.

Conservative operative therapy as compared with gastrectomy, vagotomy procedures decrease operative risk for selected patients with chronic ulcers.

Gastrojejunostomy (Roux en Y Gastroenterostomy) A procedure may be necessary to reestablish continuity between the stomach and intestinal tract, such as following partial gastrectomy or obstruction of lower end of stomach due to ulcer or nonresectable tumor. A gastrojejunostomy may be performed to treat alkaline reflux gastritis, postgastrectomy syndromes, such as postvagotomy diarrhea, and dumping syndromes. Except in elderly patients, a concomitant vagotomy is necessary when the acid-forming portion of the stomach is not resected, to prevent postoperative gastrojejunal ulcer.

A loop of jejunum may be anastomosed to the anterior or posterior wall of the stomach. Both approaches have advantages and disadvantages. In a Roux-Y gastrojejunostomy, the jejunum is divided. The distal end is anastomosed to side of stomach and the proximal end to side of jejunum at a lower level. The result is a Y-shaped double anastomosis which diverts flow of bile and pancreatic enzymes directly into the jejunum, bypassing the created gastric stoma. An adaptation of a Roux-Y anastomosis is also used to drain the biliary tract or other organs, such as the pancreas or esophagus, directly into the jejunum to bypass the stomach and prevent reflux of intestinal contents.

Bariatric Surgery

Interest in the study of morbid obesity, *bariatrics,* has led to the development of subspecialization in general surgery in the field of bariatric surgery. Persons who weigh more than 100 lb over ideal weight, have no serious disease, and have failed to lose weight despite years of medical treatment are potential candidates for bariatric surgery.

The physical size of the patient presents special needs with respect to transporting and positioning, selecting instrumentation, and providing psychological suppport. These procedures are not without risks. Neurologic and metabolic disturbances, liver disorders, and failure of staple lines have occurred postoperatively.

Gastric Bypass The size of the stomach is reduced by creating a small pouch in the proximal segment. The stomach is transected with a linear stapler. A gastrojejunostomy is constructed between the pouch and jejunum, bypassing remainder of the stomach, to establish intestinal continuity for passage of gastric contents.

Gastroplasty (Gastric Partitioning) The capacity of the stomach is reduced to 30 to 60 ml by placing two transverse linear staple lines across proximal stomach just distal to the cardia. An unstapled outlet channel is left along the greater curvature for passage of gastric contents from proximal to distal segments. The stomach is divided between the staple lines and oversewn with sutures. The undivided channel may be enclosed with synthetic mesh to prevent dilatation.

Jejunoileal Bypass The proximal jejunum is anastomosed end-to-end to the distal ileum, thus bypassing a portion of small intestine. This produces a malabsorption state that initiates weight loss. It may also cause diarrhea, fluid and electrolyte imbalance, and liver changes. Gastric operations have largely replaced jejunoileal bypass for morbid obesity.

INTESTINAL PROCEDURES

Intestines is an inclusive term referring to the continuous muscular tube of the bowel, which extends from the lower end of the stomach to the rectum (see Fig. 21-5). Food and products of digestion pass through this section of the alimentary canal during the processes of digestion, absorption, and elimination of waste products. Anatomically, the intestines are divided into the small (upper) and large (lower) intestine, with subdivisions of each.

The small intestine extends from the pylorus to the ileocecal valve. The three sections include the *duodenum* or proximal portion, the *jejunum* or middle section, and the *ileum* or distal portion that joins the large intestine. The *ileocecal valve,* a sphincter muscle, prevents return of material that has been discharged to the large intestine.

The large intestine or *colon* extends from the ileum to the rectum and is generally divided into ascending, transverse, descending, and sigmoid colon. A blind pouch, the *cecum,* is formed where the large intestine joins the small intestine.

The *mesentery,* a peritoneal fold, attaches the small and large intestines to the posterior abdominal wall, and contains the blood vessels that nourish the intestines.

Inflammation, intestinal obstruction, and disruption in absorption and motility are disorders that may lead to surgical intervention. Etiology of the disorder determines the operative procedure.

Resection of Small Intestine

Certain tumors, strangulation from adhesions, volvulus, obstruction, and regional ileitis usually are treated by resection of the involved segment. An abdominal incision is made over the suspected or known site of pathology. After exposure, clamps are placed above and below the diseased segment of bowel and mesentery to avoid spillage. The involved area is resected. An end-to-end, end-to-side, or side-to-side anastomosis is done to restore continuity. Variations of this technique are used for other related problems of the small intestine such as extensive perforation. Bowel strangulation and obstruction necessitate immediate operation to prevent necrosis, peritonitis, and death.

Hemicolectomy, Transvere Colectomy, Anterior Resection, Total Colectomy

Colitis, diverticulitis, obstruction, and neoplasms are the most frequent reasons for operative intervention to remove a diseased segment of the colon. Fundamentally all operations involve opening the abdomen, walling off the peritoneal cavity, incising and clamping at the points where resection is to be carried out, and finally reestablishing continuity by anastomosis. The separate instrument technique must be employed in intestinal procedures (see p. 409).

Bowel procedures are major ones requiring pre- and postoperative supportive care of the patient. Specifically, this care includes preoperative administration of intestinal antibiotics, bowel-cleansing methods, and diet restrictions. Postoperatively, nasogastric tubes inserted before operation remain in place until partial healing of anastomosis occurs and effective peristalsis returns. Fluid and electrolyte balance must be maintained.

Intestinal Stomas

An intestinal *-ostomy* is a surgically created opening, stoma, from a portion of the bowel to the exterior, via the abdominal wall. The procedure may be done to divert intestinal contents so as to permit healing of inflamed bowel, to decompress pressure caused by an obstructive lesion, or to bypass an obstruction such as a benign or malignant tumor. The type and level of the lesion determine whether an ileostomy, cecostomy, or colostomy is indicated. The opening may be permanent or temporary, depending on the etiology and course of the disease or obstruction. In patients with a temporary stoma, intestinal continuity is reestablished following healing by closure of opening in the bowel and anastomosis of the previously resected ends.

Patient acceptance of these procedures is as varied as are an individual's emotional reactions. Each patient requires a rehabilitation plan based on personal needs. These plans should include care of collection device, maintenance of skin integrity, proper diet, odor control, and comfortable concealing clothing. Patient participation is an integral part of preparation for self-care and enhances self-confidence.

Ileostomy Performed for a condition such as chronic ulcerative colitis, or following removal of the colon (colectomy), the proximal end of transected ileum is exteriorized through the abdominal wall. The liquid or semisolid discharge is collected in an ileostomy bag. The skin around the stoma requires special care, such as use of karaya gum, to prevent excoriation and irritation.

Operations are performed to create a *continent ileostomy.* In the endorectal-ileoanal pull-through operation, the entire cecum and colon, as well as rectal mucosa (mucosal proctectomy), are resected. The ileum is anastomosed to the anus. The rectal and anal muscles are preserved for anal continence. In modified techniques, a pouch is constructed from the terminal ileum proximal to the anal anastomosis. These procedures offer an acceptable alternative to an ileostomy stoma, especially in children and young adults.

Cecostomy An opening is created between the cecum and lower right side of the abdomen. This may be performed as an emergency decompression prior to subsequent colon resection.

Colostomy An opening in either the transverse or descending colon to the exterior creates an artificual anus. Either a double-barreled or loop colostomy may be performed. In a *double-barreled* *colostomy,* the transverse colon is divided and both ends are brought out to margins of the skin incision. The proximal stoma serves as an outlet for stool, while the distal opening leads to the non-functioning bowel. In a *loop colostomy,* a loop of transverse colon is brought out onto the abdominal wall. A glass rod or ostomy bridge is placed under loop to hold it out on the exterior abdominal wall. A short length of rubber tubing is connected to each end to stabilize the rod in position. The peritoneum is closed and the wound around the colostomy sutured. Some surgeons prefer to leave an intestinal clamp in place. This is exteriorized until the stoma is opened and then it is removed.

Following combined abdominoperineal resection for rectal carcinoma, a permanent colostomy in the sigmoid colon forms an artificial anus. A collection device for fecal material is not needed after a patient's bowel evacuation becomes regulated.

Appendectomy

Appendicitis can occur at any age but is seen most frequently in adolescents and young adults. It may imitate other conditions such as ruptured ovarian cyst or ureteral calculus. Some appendices are retrocecal, making diagnosis more obscure. Classical symptoms of early appendicitis include right lower quadrant pain, rebound tenderness, nausea, and moderate temperature and white blood count elevation.

Emergency operative removal of an acutely inflamed vermiform appendix is necessary to prevent progression to gangrene and perforation of friable tissue, with subsequent peritonitis. A right lower quadrant muscle-splitting incision is made over McBurney's point. The blood supply is ligated and severed. A crushing clamp is applied to appendiceal base, which is then ligated and severed from the cecum. Following amputation, the surgeon may elect to cauterize the stump with phenol and alcohol or wipe it with a sponge soaked with an iodophor (Betadine) to reduce contamination. Then the stump is inverted into the cecum as a purse-string suture is tightened around the stump. Since the intestinal tract is laden with bacteria, a culture is generally taken in case of future infection.

Drainage is indicated in the presence of an abscess, rupture of the appendix, or any gross contamination of the wound.

Usually appendectomy is an uncomplicated procedure with rapid convalescence unless life-threatening peritonitis results.

COLORECTAL PROCEDURES

Colorectal carcinoma is one of the most common abdominal malignancies. It affects approximately 100,000 persons annually, with females having the highest incidence. Almost two out of three who die of it might be saved by early diagnosis and prompt treatment. Resection of carcinoma is the operation of choice; however, electrocoagulation, laser, and cryosurgery have proven valuable in elderly or high-risk patients who have low-lying rectal cancers.

Various procedures aid diagnosis and are performed in patients with bowel or rectal bleeding, chronic diarrhea, or history of polyps and/or carcinoma of the colon. These procedures routinely are done before rectal or colorectal surgery. Serial guaiac stool tests are valuable in testing for occult blood. Barium enema, which frequently follows endoscopy, provides complete radiographic study of the colon. Some therapeutic procedures also may be accomplished through endoscopes.

Sigmoidoscopy

Sigmoidoscopy is direct visual inspection of sigmoid and rectal lumens by means of a flexible fiberoptic or rigid lighted sigmoidoscope. The flexible scope is more comfortable for patient, and gives surgeon better visualization of mucosal surface to evaluate left colon and rectosigmoid. It may be used intraoperatively, as well as for preoperative diagnosis.

The patient is prepared preoperatively with enemas. Knee-chest or Kraske position allows the sigmoid colon to fall forward into the abdomen. Sims or lithotomy position may be used for an extremely obese or extremely ill patient. The surgeon may inflate air to better visualize the mucosal walls. This causes a feeling of desire to defecate, which necessitates reassurance of the patient.

Colonoscopy

Colonoscopy provides visual inspection of the lining of the entire colon. The scope is flexible and consists of two channels, one for suctioning and one for operating. Its greatest use is for survey of the cancer-prone colon, especially search for and excision or ablation of polyps. Other indications are for study of inflammatory bowel or diverticular disease, passage of blood in the feces (hemochezia), change in bowel habits, preoperative screen prior to colostomy closure, confirmation of x-ray findings, and follow-up of patients who had intestinal procedures performed. Argon and Nd:YAG lasers are used through colonoscope to treat polyps, arteriovenous malformations, and bleeding disorders.

Preparation consists of clear liquids for 48 hours, castor oil at bedtime, and saline enemas until clear the morning of the procedure. Lateral position is used, and the scope introduced through the anus.

Contraindications are the precariously ill or uncooperative patient. If perforation is likely, relative contraindications may include acute, severe, or radiation inflammatory disease or complete obstruction.

Among the complications are electrical burn during polypectomy, tear or perforation of the colon by tip pressure, tear of the liver or the spleen by air pressure, tear of diverticuli by introduction of air into them.

Polypectomy

Polypectomy is often performed through a sigmoidoscope or colonoscope. However, in some patients polyps are excised or the involved segment of colon removed by abdominal approach, although the development of colonoscopy has reduced need for laparotomy.

Many surgeons and pathologists believe that every mucosal polyp in the terminal colon is a potential malignancy and should be removed. Intestinal polyps may be single or multiple. Although benign and often of familial tendency, they frequently undergo malignant changes. Polyps are easily excised at the base. If they are pedunculated, they are cauterized and retrieved. Electrocoagulation or lasing of the base provides hemostasis. These patients are followed for the remainder of their lives because adenomatous polyps, common in the colon, are prone to become malignant.

Abdominoperineal Resection

Abdominoperineal resection is an extensive procedure for carcinoma, mainly in lower third of rectum but sometimes in the anal canal. Preoperative preparation is meticulous for verification of the diagnosis, search for metastases, and optimal condition of the patient. Prior to operation, a Levin or Miller-Abbott tube is inserted, ureteral catheters are often inserted, and an indwelling bladder catheter is attached to a closed-drainage system.

Two approaches, abdominal and perineal, are required, necessitating prep and drape of both areas. After resection of the sigmoid, contaminated instruments are removed from the field, because the colon is a reservoir of bacteria. Two sets of instruments are necessary. With the patient in Trendelenburg's position, the peritoneal cavity is entered through a lower abdominal incision. Preliminary exploration is done to seek metastases. If the tumor is resectable, the sigmoid colon is mobilized, clamped, and divided. The proximal end of the sigmoid is exteriorized through a stab wound in the left lower quadrant to create a permanent colostomy. The mesentery may be sutured to the abdominal wall to prevent internal hernias. The distal end of the sigmoid is tied to prevent contamination and is placed deep in the presacral space for ultimate removal. The pelvic floor is reperitonealized and the abdomen closed. Dressings are placed on the abdominal incision and the colostomy.

The second phase of the operation is closure of the anus with a purse-string suture to prevent contamination, and removal of the anus, rectum, rectosigmoid, surrounding nodes and lymphatics through a perineal incision. Drains are placed and the perineum is closed.

When the abdominal and perineal procedures are done simultaneously, two teams are employed. The patient is initially positioned supine in modified lithotomy position. This approach reduces operating time and blood loss and provides simultaneous exposure of abdominal and perineal fields.

Patients must be carefully monitored to prevent hypovolemic shock because of the great amount of blood loss from vascular areas and length of the procedure.

Low Anterior Colon Resection

The sigmoid colon and rectum lie within the bony pelvis, making resection of tumors in the lower sigmoid colon, rectosigmoid, and rectum technically difficult. The objective is to achieve wide local excision with en bloc resection of lymphatics and perirectal mesentery. An abdominoperineal resection with a permanent colostomy may be necessary for lesions in the lower third of the rectum. The intraluminal and linear staplers offer an alternative to low anterior colon resection in some situations by facilitating colorectal anastomosis. The distal colon is transected after closure with a linear stapler. The intraluminal stapler, with the anvil removed, is introduced through the anus and the rectal stump either through or adjacent to the linear staple line. After anvil is replaced, the intraluminal end-to-end or end-to-side anastomosis with the proximal segment of bowel is completed. Total excision of the mesorectum is necessary to prevent recurrence of tumor in pelvis or at the staple line. At least a 2-cm distal tumor clearance is necessary. Colorectal continuity is restored and anal sphincter control maintained with this technique for low anterior colorectal anastomosis.

ANORECTAL PROCEDURES

Hemorrhoids, abscesses, fissures, and fistulas are frequently indications for surgical intervention. The anal region is well supplied with nerves and these procedures often cause much discomfort. Patients are also sensitive and embarrassed because of the operative site. Following rectal surgery, patients may have initial difficulty voiding and usually experience considerable pain, requiring medication and sitz baths.

Anoscopy, Proctoscopy, Sigmoidoscopy

Endoscopic diagnostic procedures as anoscopy, proctoscopy, and sigmoidoscopy are used to visually examine the mucosa of the anus, rectum, and sigmoid. Sigmoidoscopy is routinely done before rectal surgery. Fiberoptic equipment has aided in early detection of tumors, polyps, and ulcerations.

Hemorrhoidectomy

Hemorrhoidectomy is surgical excision and ligation of varicosities of the veins of the anus and rectum that do not respond to conservative treatment. Hemorrhoids are classified as *internal,* occurring above internal sphincter and covered with columnar mucosa, or *external,* appearing outside external sphincter and covered with skin. Often both types are present in the patient. External hemorrhoids cause pruritis and pain. The internal type frequently bleed and may become thrombosed and edematous. Rectal bleeding cannot be assumed to be from hemorrhoids, but requires thorough investigation to rule out gastrointestinal disease.

The usual procedure consists of dilating the sphincter, ligating the hemorrhoidal pedicle with suture ligatures, and excising each hemorrhoidal mass. The electrosurgical or cryosurgical unit may be employed. Kraske position usually is used, with the patient's buttocks retracted by hemorrhoid straps fastened to the edges of the operating table. Petrolatum gauze packing is inserted in the anal canal, or a compression dressing and perineal binder are applied at completion of operation.

As an alternative to operation, rubber-band ligation of internal hemorrhoids as an office procedure has become very popular.

Incision and Drainage of Anal Abscess

Localized infection in tissues around the anus results in abscess formation. Early incision and drainage are essential to prevent infection from spreading.

Fistulotomy, Fistulectomy

Formation of a fistula-in-ano often results following incision and drainage or spontaneous drainage of an abscess. A fistulous tract may be opened to allow drainage and healing by granulation, or the tract may be excised. Injection of a dye or use of a probe and grooved director aids in identifying the tract.

Fissurectomy

When a benign ulcerative lesion occurs in the lining of the anal canal, the anus is dilated and infected tissue excised. Fecal incontinence due to damage to the anal sphincter is a potential complication the surgeon tries to avoid by midline sphincterotomy.

Treatment of Rectal Tumors

Surgeons prefer to study a small rectal cancer under anesthesia (often caudal) and not hasten into a radical operation. Many cancers are amenable to local treatment using an operating endoscope, laser, and microsurgical technique. Electrosurgical cutting and coagulation can also be combined to remove a superficial cancer. For electrosection, the lesion should be small, mobile, polypoid, and posterior, with no palpable rectal lymph nodes. Protocol includes external radiation therapy, electrocoagulation, and reevaluation in six weeks. Sometimes interstitial radiation therapy is used for small anorectal squamous-cell carcinoma.

EXCISION OF PILONIDAL CYST AND SINUS

A painful draining cyst with fistulous tract(s) may occur in soft tissues of the sacrococcygeal region. When they become infected, drainage is necessary to relieve pain, swelling, and suppuration. The cyst and sinus tracts must be *excised* or *marsupialized* to prevent recurrence. Marsupialization is suturing of cyst walls to edges of the wound, following evacuation, to permit the packed cavity to close by granulation. Surgical judgment determines whether primary closure or healing by granulation is chosen. A compression dressing is applied.

HERNIA PROCEDURES

A *hernia* is the protrusion of an organ or part of an organ through a defect in supporting structures that normally contain it. A hernia may be congenital, acquired, or traumatic. The majority occur in the inguinal or femoral region; however, umbilical, ventral, and hiatus hernias do occur.

A hernia is usually composed of a sac (covering), hernial contents, and an aperture, but in some locations a sac is absent.

When hernial contents can be returned to the normal cavity by manipulation, the hernia is called *reducible.* If the hernial contents cannot be reduced, it is called *irreducible* or *incarcerated.* Bowel present in an incarcerated hernia not only may lack adequate blood supply but may also become obstructed. This is referred to as a *strangulated* hernia. Immediate operation is necessary to prevent necrosis of the strangulated bowel.

Inguinal Herniorrhaphy (Hernioplasty)

Repair of inguinal hernias involves two types, indirect and direct.

Indirect The peritoneal sac containing intestine protrudes through the internal inguinal ring and passes down the inguinal canal. It may descend all the way into the scrotum. Indirect inguinal hernia, more common in males, originates from a congenital defect in the fascial floor of the inguinal canal.

Direct The hernia protrudes through a weakness in the abdominal wall in region between rectus abdominis muscle, inguinal ligament, and inferior epigastric artery. This hernia is the most difficult type to repair and appears more frequently in men. An acquired weakness of the lower abdominal wall, a direct inguinal hernia often results from straining, such as heavy lifting, chronic coughing, or straining to urinate or defecate. Prompt operative repair avoids possible discomfort and threat of later complications.

NOTE. In both indirect and direct inguinal herniorrhaphy in males, the spermatic cord and blood supply to the testis must be protected from injury. If herniorrhaphies are performed bilaterally, severance of the cords will cause sterility. Infarction of a testis can occur if blood supply is compromised.

Femoral Herniorrhaphy

Femoral herniorrhaphy involves repairing the defect in the transversalis fascia as well as removing the peritoneal sac protruding through the femoral ring. The transversalis fascia is normally attached to Cooper's ligament, which prevents the peritoneum from reaching the femoral ring. To repair this defect it is necessary to reconstruct the posterior wall and close the femoral ring. These hernias appear more frequently in women.

Umbilical Herniorrhaphy

Repair of an umbilical hernia consists of closing the peritoneal opening and uniting the fascia above and below the defect to reconstruct the abdominal wall surrounding the umbilicus. This type of hernia, seen most frequently in children, represents a congenital defect of protrusion of peritoneum through the umbilical ring. It also may be acquired by women following childbirth.

Ventral (Incisional) Herniorrhaphy

Impaired healing of a previous operative incision, usually a vertical abdominal one, may cause incisional hernia. Often the result of weakening of abdominal fascia, projections of peritoneum carrying segments of bowel protrude through fascial perforations. It is necessary to reunite the tissue layers to close the defect. After excising the old scar, the peritoneal sac is opened, the hernia is reduced, and the layers are firmly closed. If existing tissue is not sufficient for repair, synthetic mesh may be used to reinforce the repair. Incisional hernias are sometimes the aftermath of postoperative hematoma, infection, or undue strain.

Hiatus (Diaphragmatic) Herniorrhaphy

A hiatus hernia results when a portion of the stomach protrudes through the hiatus of the diaphragm. The *hiatus* is the opening for the esophagus through the *diaphragm,* which is the chief muscle of respiration. A weakening in the hiatus permits violation of the muscular partition between abdomen and chest. Symptoms largely are due to inflammation and ulceration of the adjacent esophagus, caused by reflux of gastric juices from the herniated stomach. Symptoms include pain, blood loss, and difficulty in swallowing (*dysphagia*). Diagnosis is made by radiologic and endoscopic studies.

Surgical treatment is appropriate when medical therapy fails to alleviate the problem. Operative approach may be via the abdomen or chest, or thoracoabdominal. Each offers certain advantages. The abdominal approach is generally preferred (see p. 408). However, the better view of hiatal region afforded by opening the chest may favor this approach (see Chap. 30, p. 568).

AMPUTATION OF EXTREMITIES

Amputation is the total or partial removal of any extremity. Necessity for amputation is associated most frequently with massive trauma, presence of malignant tumor, extensive infection, and vascular insufficiency. (Refer to Chapter 34 for discussion of replacement of traumatically severed extremities.)

In preparing patient for a lower extremity amputation, expose both legs for comparison before skin preparation in addition to checking the chart. *Be absolutely certain correct leg is prepared.*

Many lower extremity amputations are done under spinal anesthesia. Ensure that the specimen is never, at any time, within the patient's sight. Follow hospital policy in regard to patient's permission for disposal of an extremity.

Two types of amputation generally are performed, *open* (*guillotine*) and *closed.*

The guillotine operation, rarely performed, is regarded as an emergency procedure. Tissues are cut circularly with the bone transected higher to allow soft tissues to cover the bone end. Blood vessels and nerve endings are ligated, but the wound is left open. The operation frequently is followed by prolonged drainage and healing, muscle and skin retraction, and excessive granulation tissue. A second operation is often required for final repair. Patients who are severely ill or toxic, or experience severe trauma, such as an extremity caught under an immovable object, are candidates for this operation.

The conventional flap or closed type of amputation is more desirable. Fashioning curved skin and fascial flaps prior to amputating the bone allows for deep and superficial fascia to be approximated over the bone end before loose skin closure. Drainage by catheter or suction apparatus may or may not be required. The wound usually heals in about two weeks.

Amputations of the Lower Extremity

Amputations of the lower extremity are classified as above the knee (AK), below the knee (BK), toe, transphalangeal, transmetatarsal, and Syme amputation. The level of amputation is determined by the patient's general health, vascular status, and rehabilitative potential.

AK Amputation Amputation at lower third of the thigh is selected when gangrene or arterial insufficiency extends above the level of the malleoli. Mid-thigh amputation involves circular incision over the distal femur, creating large anterior and posterior skin flaps, transecting fasciae and muscles. Vessels and nerves such as the femoral and sciatic, respectively, are ligated and severed. Sharp bone edges of the stump are smoothed by filing. The wound is well irrigated with sterile saline before closure of tissue layers. Hemostasis is important to prevent massive hemorrhage or painful hematoma. Depending on surgeon's preference, drains may be used. A noncompressive dressing is applied. A longer time is required for rehabilitation than after BK amputation since AK is a more extensive procedure. A prosthesis is generally fitted four to six weeks after amputation.

BK Amputation Amputation at middle third of the leg provides for more functional prosthesis fitting and reduction of phantom limb pain. It permits a more natural gait. An immediate postoperative prosthesis (IPOP) can be applied in the operating room. The IPOP dressing requires a stump sock, felt and lamb's wool for padding, twill Y straps that are attached to a fitted corset, and a rigid plaster dressing. This dressing not only protects the stump but aids in controlling the weight placed on it. The prosthesis is metal and provides a pull on the stump. The pylon (foot) may be attached before patient returns to the unit. However, if the patient is obese or debilitated, weight bearing may be delayed several days.

Toe, Transphalangeal, and Transmetatarsal Amputations Toe and partial foot amputations are generally performed for gangrene and osteomyelitis.

Syme Amputation Syme amputation is usually performed for trauma and involves the distal part of the foot. The amputation is above the ankle joint. The skin of the heel is used for the flap.

Hip Disarticulation and Hemipelvectomy Hip disarticulation and hemipelvectomy are radical procedures involving total removal of a posterior extremity including the hipbone. They are indicated for malignant bone or soft tissue tumors and extensive traumatic injuries. These operations are most often performed by orthopaedic surgeons. Specialized prosthetic devices are available to permit ambulation.

Amputations of the Upper Extremity

Amputations in the Hand Hand amputations usually result from trauma and include part or all of the distal phalanges of the digits. Attention is directed to keeping hand as a working unit when one or more fingers are removed. Every effort should be made to save the thumb, since the smallest stump is better than a prosthesis. (Refer to digital transfer in Chapter 27, p. 526).

Forearm and Forequarter Amputation Wrist, elbow, and humerus disarticulations are radical procedures performed for malignant tumors or extensive trauma.

Rehabilitation

Postoperative considerations of any amputation include control of bleeding and phantom limb sensations, stump care, immediate fitting and functional terminal prosthesis, exercises to prevent flexion contractures, and ambulation or use of a hand or arm.

The loss of an extremity involves major adjustment psychologically and physically. The rehabilitative process, so important, is often affected by the emotional reactions of the amputee. Patients with an early postoperative prosthesis have a more positive outlook about their loss. Being able to walk the first postoperative day or soon thereafter (which will depend on the surgeon's orders for the weight-bearing program in the case of a leg amputee) boosts morale. This in turn aids in ambulation.

The combined efforts of patient, family, and interdisciplinary professional personnel are needed for successful rehabilitation.

CHAPTER **22**

GYNECOLOGY AND OBSTETRICS

From its inception in 1930, the American Board of Obstetrics and Gynecology has emphasized the inseparability of the two phases of this specialty because of their anatomical and physiological relationships. *Gynecology,* commonly referred to as "gyn" (GYN), is the science of diseases of the female reproductive organs. Gynecological surgery also includes certain problems of the female genitourinary tract. *Obstetrics* (OB) concerns the care of women during pregnancy, labor, and puerperium (period from delivery to time uterus regains normal size, usually about six weeks). Although all surgeons certified by this Board are competent in both disciplines, some limit their practice to either obstetrics or gynecology. Specialty certification boards have also been established in gynecological oncology, endocrinology and infertility, and perinatal medicine. This text limits discussion to the most common surgical procedures performed by gynecologists and/or obstetricians in the operating room.

HISTORICAL DEVELOPMENT

Ancient interest in diseases of women is recorded in the Egyptian *Ebers papyrus* of the sixteenth century B.C. Hippocrates was familiar with the use of gynecological instruments centuries later. During the Greco-Roman period, Galen, Celsus, and Soranus dealt with gynecological conditions. The writings of Soranus, who practiced in Rome in the second century A.D., were regarded as authority for 1500 years. During that time, removal of a prolapsed uterus by cautery was advocated. Writers on gynecology in the fourth and fifth centuries merely compiled the work of predecessors. Practice remained bound by ancient authority and tradition and even regressed during the medieval period. It was not until the Renaissance that new interest developed. In 1566, Caspar Wolf of Switzerland issued a large encyclopedia of gynecology entitled *Gynecia.*

Writings by Hendrik van Roonhuze in the seventeenth century on extrauterine pregnancy, uterine rupture, and vesicovaginal fistula are regarded as the first on operative gynecology having modern connotation. In the following century, practitioners advocated treatment of ovarian cysts by tapping or excision. Retroversion of the uterus and removal of extrauterine pregnancy were also described.

Operative gynecology became an independent specialty in the early nineteenth century. In 1809, Ephraim McDowell removed an ovarian cyst by abdominal approach and the patient survived for 31 years. James Sims became famous for treating vesicovaginal fistulas. A limited variety of gynecological procedures such as oophorectomy and salpingectomy were developed by succeeding pioneers. The first successful vaginal hysterectomy was performed in 1818.

Early gynecologists fought public prejudice against exposure of female organs for examination. Clergy, midwives, and even physicians were among those attempting to deter such practice. Examination by speculum was a notable advance.

The progress of surgery in general, which followed development of antisepsis and anesthesia, eventually overcame opposition.

Obstetricians and gynecologists were influential in introducing the concept of periodic health examination on a large scale. Obstetricians aim to protect the pregnant woman and unborn fetus from unnecessary complications. The intent of gynecologists is to discover and treat pelvic disease, especially carcinoma, in early stages.

ANATOMY AND PHYSIOLOGY

The genitourinary system comprises the organs, glands, secretions, and other elements of reproduction. Components of female reproductive system are both external and internal organs.

External Genitalia

Vulva is a collective term for the female external genitalia. This sensitive, delicate area is highly vascular, with an extensive lymph supply and rich cutaneous sensory innervation. It includes the following.

Labia Majora The labia majora are two large folds, or lips, containing sebaceous and sweat glands imbedded in fatty tissue covered by skin. They join together anteriorly in a fatty pad, the *mons veneris,* which overlies the pubic bone. Sebaceous secretions of the labia lubricate the proximal area. The labia majora atrophy after menopause, making the labia minora more prominent.

Labia Minora The labia minora, small lips, lying within the labia majora, are flat folds of connective tissue containing sebaceous glands. Anteriorly these labia split into two parts. One part passes over the clitoris to form the protective prepuce or foreskin. The other passes under the clitoris to shape a *frenulum,* a fold of mucous membrane. Posteriorly they join across the midline to form the *fourchette,* a fold of skin just inside the posterior vulvar commissure.

Clitoris The clitoris, an erectile organ, is the female homologue of the penis. The mucous membrane covering the glans contains many nerve endings. The urethra opens just below the clitoris.

Vestibule The vestibule is the space, or shallow elliptical depression below the clitoris, enclosed by the labia minora. The fourchette bounds it posteriorly. Opening into the vestibule are four canals: the urethra, the vagina, and the bilateral ducts from the Bartholin's glands.

Bartholin's Glands Bartholin's glands are small bilateral glands that lie deep in the posterior third of the labia majora, within the bulbocavernosus muscle. The mucous secretion is a coital lubricant.

Hymen The hymen is a thin vascularized connective tissue membrane that surrounds and may partially or completely occlude the vaginal orifice. It varies individually in thickness and elasticity. The central aperture permits passage of menstrual flow and vaginal secretions.

Perineum The perineum is a diamond-shaped wedge of fibromuscular tissue between the vagina and the anus. It is divided by a transverse septum into an anterior urogenital triangle and a posterior anal triangle. It consists of the perineal body and perineal musculature. With fibers of six muscles converging at its central point, the perineum forms the base of the pelvic floor and helps support the posterior vaginal wall. These muscles are the bulbocavernosus (vaginal sphincter), the two superficial transverse perineal, the two levator ani, and the external anal sphincter. The levators ani are the largest muscles and, in contrast to the other superficial muscles, are deep. The most important muscles in the pelvis, the levators ani (pelvic diaphragm) form a hammock-type suspension from anterior to posterior pelvic wall, beneath the

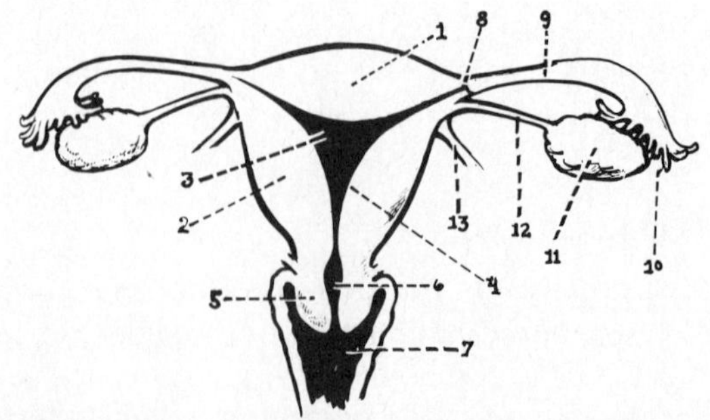

FIGURE 22-1
Female reproductive system: (1) uterine fundus, (2) corpus uteri, (3) uterine cavity, (4) endometrium, (5) cervix, (6) endocervical canal, (7) vagina, (8) cornu, (9) fallopian tube, (10) fimbria, (11) ovary, (12) ovarian ligament, (13) round ligament.

pelvic viscera. These muscles retain the organs within the pelvis by offering resistance to repeated increases in intraabdominal pressure, such as coughing, respiring, bearing down in labor, and straining at stool.

Internal Genital Organs

The internal organs (see Fig. 22-1) lie within the pelvic cavity, protected by the bony pelvis. Bones and ligaments form the pelvic outlet. The dilated cervix of the uterus and the vagina constitute the birth canal.

Vagina The vagina is a thin-walled, fibromuscular tube extending from the vestibule obliquely backward and upward to the uterus, where the cervix projects into the top of the anterior wall. Constituting a copulatory and parturient canal, the vagina is capable of great distention. The bladder lies anteriorly to it, the rectum posteriorly. It is lined with mucous membrane and contains glands that produce a cleansing acid secretion.

The anterior vaginal wall is shorter than is the posterior. The upper third of the posterior wall is covered by peritoneum reflected onto the rectum. Normally the anterior and posterior walls relax and are in contact. However, the lateral walls remain rigid because of the pull of the muscles and therefore are in close contact with pelvic tissues.

A rich venous plexus in the muscular walls makes the organ highly vascular. Uterine and vaginal arteries supplying the area are branches of the internal iliac artery. Branches of the vaginal artery extend to the external genitalia and the adjacent bladder and rectum. Lymphatic drainage is extensive. The upper two-thirds of the vagina drains into the external and internal iliac nodes, the lower third into the superficial inguinal nodes.

The *vault,* dome or upper part of the vagina, is divided into four *fornices,* or arches (see Fig. 22-2). During digital pelvic examination, the gynecologist can palpate pelvic contents through the thin walls of the vault. The anterior fornix, in front of the cervix, is adjacent to base of the bladder and distal ends of the ureters.

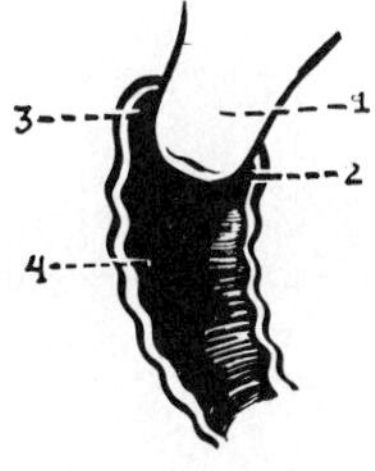

FIGURE 22-2
Cervix in vaginal vault. (1) Cervix, (2) anterior fornix, (3) posterior fornix, (4) vagina.

The *pouch of Douglas* (retrouterine cul-de-sac) directly behind the larger posterior fornix lies behind the cervix. This pouch separates the back of uterus from the rectum: anteriorly by uterine peritoneal covering, which continues down to cap the posterior vaginal fornix, and posteriorly by anterior wall of the rectum. Lateral boundaries are uterosacral ligaments, as they embrace the lower third of the rectum in their course. Floor of the pouch, about 7 cm above the anus, is formed by reflection of the peritoneum from the rectum to the upper vagina and uterus. The posterior fornix is the route of entry for a number of diagnostic or operative procedures because the pouch of Douglas, lowest part of the peritoneal cavity, is separated from the vagina only by thin vaginal wall and peritoneum of the fornix.

The lateral fornices lie on either side of the cervix, in contact with anterior and posterior sheets of the broad ligaments surrounding the uterus. Proximal structures are the uterine artery, ureters, fallopian tubes, ovaries, and sigmoid colon.

Uterus The organ of gestation, the uterus, receives and holds the fertilized ovum during development of the fetus and expels it during childbirth. Resembling an inverted pear in shape, this hollow muscular organ is situated in the bony pelvis. It lies between the bladder anteriorly and the sigmoid colon posteriorly. It is divided by a slight constriction into a wider upper part, the body or *corpus uteri,* and a narrower lower part, the *cervix uteri* or neck. The corpus meets the cervix at the *internal os.* Peritoneum covers the corpus externally; the endometrium lines it internally. This mucous membrane is uniquely adapted to receive and sustain the fertilized ovum. The *fundus,* or domelike portion of the uterus, lies above the uterine cavity.

The *uterine cavity,* flattened from front to back, is roughly triangular in shape in the nonpregnant female. The upper lateral angles extend out toward the openings of the fallopian tubes, which enter through the uterine walls at the *cornua.* The apex of the triangle is directed downward to the cervix. The cavity within the cervix, the *endocervical canal,* narrows to a slit at the end where the cervix communicates with the vagina via the *ex-*

ternal os. The *endocervix* is the glandular mucous membrane of the cervix. The corpus and cervix are considered individually in relation to disease and therapy because they differ in structure and function.

As the incubator and nurturer of the developing embryo, the uterus is capable of expansion. Much of the bulk of the corpus consists of involuntary muscle, the *myometrium,* composed of three layers. The inner layer prevents reflux of menstrual flow into the tubes and peritoneal cavity, which could result in endometriosis. It also contributes to the competency of the internal os sphincter to prevent premature expulsion of the fetus. The middle layer encloses large blood vessels. These muscle fibers act as living ligatures for hemostasis after delivery. The outer layer has expulsive action, ejecting menstrual flow and clots, aborted embryo, or the baby at term.

Usually the uterus lies bent forward at a right angle to the vagina and resting on the bladder. While the cervix is anchored laterally by ligaments, the fundus may pivot about the cardinal ligaments widely in an anterior-posterior plane. Mobility rather than position is the criterion for normality.

Fallopian Tubes (Salpinges) The fallopian tubes, small, hollow musculomembranous tubes, sometimes called *oviducts* or *uterine tubes,* run bilaterally like arms from each side of the upper part of uterus to the ovaries. Near each ovary, the open end of each tube expands into the *infundibulum,* the edges of which are divided into *fimbriae,* fingerlike projections that are thought to sweep up the *ovum* (the female reproductive cell) as it is expelled from the ovary. Fertilization of ovum by sperm takes place in one tube. Within the tube are ciliated cells that move the fertilized egg toward the uterus. The lumen of the tube becomes very narrow where it penetrates the uterine wall to reach the uterine cavity. Contractions in the muscular walls change shape and position of the tubes. At ovulation they move the fimbriated ends into close apposition with the ovarian surfaces.

Ovaries The ovaries are oval-shaped and lie in a shallow peritoneal fossa on the lateral pelvic walls from which they are suspended by the infundibulopelvic ligaments. They are attached to posterior layer of the broad ligament by the *mesovarium,* a peritoneal fold, and to uterus by the *ovarian ligament,* a fibromuscular cord.

The ovaries, counterpart of the male testes, give rise to ova. Every ovary consists of a center of cells and vessels surrounded by the *cortex,* the main portion which contains the stroma or fibrous framework in which the ovarian follicles are imbedded. Of the approximately 200,000 primordial follicles present at birth, less than 400 are likely to produce a mature ovum *(graafian follicle)* during the reproductive years. A serous covering derived from peritoneum surrounds the ovaries.

In addition to producing ova, the ovaries, which atrophy after menopause, produce female sex hormones.

The ureters course along the peritoneum and lie close to the ovarian blood supply.

Muscles and Ligaments Muscles and ligaments support the uterus and fallopian tubes in normal position in the center of the pelvic cavity.

Broad Ligaments Bilateral broad ligaments are composed of a broad double sheet of peritoneum extending from each lateral surface of the uterus outward to the pelvic wall. Between these two layers of peritoneum are a number of important structures, such as the fallopian tubes enclosed in the free upper borders (mesosalpinges) with the tubal ostia opening directly into the peritoneal cavity.

Round Ligaments The round ligaments are fibromuscular bands that extend from the anterior surface of the lateral borders of the fundus to the labia majora. They run beneath the peritoneum and anterior sheet of the broad ligament down, outward, and forward through the inguinal canal to the labia.

Cardinal Ligaments The lower portion of the broad ligaments, the cardinal ligaments are attached to the lateral vaginal fornices and supravaginal portion of the cervix. They act as a supportive pivot.

Uterosacral Ligaments The uterosacral ligaments are peritoneal folds containing connective tissue and involuntary muscle. They arise on each side from the posterior wall of the uterus at the level of the internal os, pass backward around the rectum, and insert on the sacrum at the level of the second sacral vertebra. Their course describes an archlike curve with concavity toward the midline. They pull on the cervix to keep the uterus anteverted and, through the cervix, the vagina in position as well.

Physiology

The function of the female reproductive organs is to conceive, nurture, and produce offspring. The development and function of these organs are influenced by the hormonal secretions of the ovaries, adrenals, thyroid, and pituitary. The organs also affect sex characteristics.

The physiological cycle prepares the womb for the fertilized ovum. Hormone production stimulates the endometrium and breasts, resulting in thickening and increased blood supply.

Each month during the years from puberty to menopause, one of the ovaries produces on its surface a follicle from within. When the matured graafian follicle ruptures, it discharges the enclosed ovum, which enters the fallopian tube at the fimbriated end. The process of maturation and discharge of the egg is called *ovulation,* a fertile period that lasts several days. Changes in cervical mucus and vaginal epithelium also accompany ovulation. Union of the ovum with a viable mature male germ cell *(spermatozoon),* which has ascended to the fallopian tube from the vagina, results in *fertilization.* The fertilized ovum normally proceeds to the cornu of the uterus, where it enters to implant in the endometrium. Pregnancy has occurred.

The ovarian hormone estrogen together with progesterone cause a sequence of changes in the endometrial lining of the uterus to prepare for implantation of the fertilized ovum. Estrogen also produces the development of secondary sexual characteristics. Progesterone is responsible for maintaining pregnancy until hormones from the placenta assume this role.

Menstruation is the end result of lack of fertilization. It is the periodic discharge of blood, mucus, disintegrated ovum, and uterine mucosa formed during the cycle. Duration of menstrual period varies, but the average is three to five days. The amount of blood lost varies greatly. The menstrual cycle, the time between the onset of each period, is approximately 28 days in length. Regularity of menstruation can be disturbed by disease conditions and emotions in addition to onset of pregnancy. This physiological cycle continually recurs throughout the reproductive life of the woman.

GYNECOLOGY

The emotional preparation of gynecologic patients presents a special challenge to the perioperative nurse. Some operations destroy reproductive ability and produce the menopausal state. Many alter self-image. Anticipation of physical exposure, potential loss of sexuality, infertility problems, or termination of a pregnancy can create severe anxiety. The patients must be able to express concerns, ask questions, and receive reassurance and support.

Special Features of Gynecologic Surgery

Diagnostic and operative procedures may be carried out through a vaginal or abdominal approach or the two approaches may be combined. Each requires a different position and different preparation, drapes, and setup. Operative techniques for abdominal surgery discussed in Chapter 21 apply to gynecologic surgery. However, diagnostic and operative procedures are often combined and done in one operation. In both vaginal and abdominopelvic procedures:

1 Spinal or, more commonly, general anesthesia is used.

2 Patient is catheterized in the OR unless she has an indwelling catheter. Usually a Foley catheter is inserted to prevent bladder from becoming distended during operation, and to record urinary output. The circulating nurse should check the collection bag regularly and report evidence of blood. This could indicate injury to bladder or ureters. Insertion of a cannula directly into the bladder (suprapubic cystostomy) provides an alternative indwelling drainage system in selected patients.

3 Electrosurgical unit is frequently employed, with either monopolar or bipolar electrodes.

4 Argon, carbon dioxide, and Nd:YAG lasers are used, usually in conjunction with colposcope (p. 426) or laparoscope (p. 427) and the operating microscope. A special suction device removes fumes from operative site and scope. All accessories and attachments must be properly assembled and secured. Safety precautions must be taken when laser is used (see Chap. 19, p. 367).

5 Closed-wound suction drainage, or another type of drain, is commonly used to prevent hematoma or serum accumulation in pelvis and/or wound.

6 Prophylactic anticoagulation with heparin, antiembolic stockings, and early ambulation are especially important in pelvic surgery because of the anatomic relationship of deep major vessels to the operative field. In addition, lithotomy position slows circulation. Postoperative thrombosis is a serious complication.

Vaginal Approach

1 Procedures approached through vagina generally are performed with the patient in lithotomy position.

2 Instrumentation includes implements of sufficient length for use within the vaginal canal and uterine cavity, e.g., long curved dressing forceps for insertion of vaginal packing. In addition to cutting, holding, clamping and suturing instruments, vaginal setups include *D&C (dilatation and curettage) instruments* (see Fig. 22-3).

3 Cryosurgical unit or laser beam may be used to remove hypertrophied tissue or certain benign neoplasms.

4 Suction tubing and apparatus are part of setup.

5 Sponges should be secured on a sponge forceps in deep areas. Long narrow gauze pads with tape on the end are used for packing off abdominal viscera in vaginal procedures. All counts are very important in these procedures.

6 Vaginal packing is inserted following certain procedures. Antibiotic cream may be applied to the packing during insertion. The packing should be recorded on the patient's chart and removed at the surgeon's order.

7 At completion of operation, a belt is placed on the patient to hold the perineal pad in place postoperatively.

Abdominal Approach

1 Supine or Trendelenburg's position is used for abdominopelvic procedures. Preparation and drapes are same as for abdominal laparotomy.

2 When a large abdominal mass is present or the pelvic organs are pushed from their normal relationships, ureteral catheters may be inserted prior to operation to permit easy identification of the ureters in proximity to or within the dissecting area. Inadvertent severing of ureters during operation greatly increases postoperative morbidity and mortality if the injury is not immediately detected and corrected.

3 Instrumentation includes basic laparotomy setup with the addition of long instruments for deep manipulations within the pelvis. Some surgeons prefer a double Mayo stand with instruments for superficial work on one and supplies for deeper areas on the other.

Combined Vaginal-Abdominal Approach

If vaginal as well as abdominal surgery is indicated, a combined procedure is planned. For example, the patient may be scheduled as prep vault, vaginal plastic, abdominal hysterectomy. In such instances the vaginal procedure is performed first. Then the patient is removed from lithotomy position, repositioned in supine, and the abdominal prep and operation are carried out.

1 Because of the hazard of infection, separate sterile setups are used for vaginal and abdominal procedures performed concurrently.

FIGURE 22-3 D & C instruments.

To expose	Vaginal speculum Posterior retractor Weighted posterior retractor Narrow lateral Heaney retractors
To grasp and hold	Single- and double-toothed tenaculi Jacobs tenaculum
To measure uterine cavity	Uterine sound (graduated probe)
To dilate cervix	Graduated dilators Goodell dilator
To scrape tissue	Sharp and blunt, large and small uterine curettes
To obtain specimen	Endometrial biopsy suction curette
To carry sponges	Sponge forceps
To remove polyps and biopsy tissue	Polyp and biopsy forceps
To insert packing	Uterine dressing forceps

2 Vaginal preparation precedes exploratory pelvic laparotomy in readiness for the unexpected, or for D&C scheduled to precede an abdominal operation. A separate sterile prep table is used for the external genitalia and vagina. Another sterile setup is used for the abdominal prep.

DIAGNOSTIC TECHNIQUES

The gynecologist employs both noninvasive and invasive diagnostic techniques. Some are performed as office or ambulatory procedures, especially those using the vaginal approach.

Pelvic examination includes inspection and palpation of external genitalia; bimanual abdominovaginal and abdominorectal palpation of the uterus, fallopian tubes, and ovaries; and speculum examination of the vagina and cervix. This inspection is augmented by a cytologic study of smears of cervical and endocervical tissue obtained by scrapings. The *Papanicolaou (Pap) smear* has facilitated a significant increase in diagnosis of patients with cervical cancer or premalignant lesions. Characteristic cellular changes in cervical epithelial cells may be identified. Cytologic aspiration from within the endocervical canal may reveal unsuspected carcinoma of the endometrium, tubes or ovaries as well as occult cervical cancer.

Schiller's test involves staining the vaginal vault and cervical squamous epithelium with Lugol's solution. The glycogen in normal epithelium takes up the iodine. Abnormal tissues, with little or no glycogen, do not stain brown and therefore pinpoint sites for biopsy. Abnormal cytology is an indication for further evaluation by histological tissue study.

NOTE. Uterine cancer consists of two entities: cervical cancer and endometrial cancer. These differ by age groups, types, and consequences. Cancer of the cervix appears most often in association with coitus at an early age, multiple partners, nonbarrier contraceptives, poor sexual hygiene, chronically infected cervices, or a history of sexually transmitted diseases. These include infection with herpes simplex virus, human papillary virus, and cytomegalovirus, *Chlamydia trachomatis,* and *Trichomonas vaginalis.* A higher frequency of abnormal Pap smear is associated with these infections and with herpes virus and papillary virus which produce condylomata, identified as possible causes of carcinoma. Prompt early treatment of cervical malignancy yields an excellent rate of cure. Follow-up is extremely important.

Each form of therapy for cancer has certain advantages and limitations. Factors affecting response to treatment are host factors, clinical stage of malignancy, histological grade of malignancy, and therapy employed. Pretreatment workup is extensive for all modes of therapy. Refer to Chapter 35 for discussion of oncology.

Biopsy of Cervix

Cervical cancer may not present symptoms in the early stage and may progress to invasion before discovery. Intermenstrual *(spotting)* or postmenopausal bleeding may be the first visible sign. The condition may be suspected by cytologic examination or visual inspection, but diagnosis must be made by biopsy. Methods that may be used are:

Excisional Biopsy In excisional biopsy, an attempt is made to excise the entire lesion.

Incisional Biopsy Incisional biopsy involves use of scalpel, punch biopsy, or other instrument to obtain tissue for diagnosis, but not to remove lesion. If a malignancy is diagnosed, additional evaluation of the patient and further treatment must be carried out by surgery or radiation therapy.

Cone Biopsy (Conization of the Cervix) Patients diagnosed by Pap smear as having severe cervical dysplasia or intraepithelial carcinoma of the cervix require conization to remove the lesion and rule out invasive carcinoma. The biopsy, taken with a scalpel or cervitome *(cold knife conization),* includes the squamocolumnar junctions of the ectocervix (transformation zone) and is tapered to include the endocervical canal to the level of the internal os. Most of the lesions categorized as cervical intraepithelial neoplasia (CIN), dysplasia, and carcinoma in situ are found in this area. Conization of the cervix provides the most comprehensive specimen to diagnose a premalignant or malignant lesion.

Hemostasis is secured by sutures. Multiple blocks and sections are examined by the pathologist to rule on invasive disease. General anesthesia is used. Risks include hemorrhage and infection. Cone biopsies obtained by laser minimize these risks.

Colposcopy Directed precision biopsy may obviate conization. Multiple specimens may be taken from the cervix and vagina for histological examination and diagnosis. The illumination and binocular magnification afforded by the *colpomicroscope,* focused on the cervix, permit study of abnormal epithelium on the *ectocervix* (portion of cervix that protrudes into the vagina), the lower part of the cervical canal, and the vagina. Wiping the cervix with 3% acetic acid eradicates mucus and facilitates view of the surface and vasculature. Endocervical curettage may also be performed.

Following confirmation of histologic diagnosis, remainder of lesion may be destroyed by laser. Vaginal condylomas and adenoses, preinvasive lesions of the cervix, cervical dysplasia, CIN, and other vaginal and cervical lesions can be treated by laser through the colpomicroscope. Visualization is excellent, unobstructed by instruments. The laser permits selective destruction of large areas of vaginal epithelium without vaginal and cervical stenosis. It cuts, coagulates, seals, and sterilizes simultaneously. This results in less blood loss, shorter period of vaginal discharge after treatment of the cervix, and lower incidence of infection than do other surgical treatment modalities.

Culdocentesis and Colpotomy

Culdocentesis Blood, fluid, or pus in the cul-de-sac may be aspirated by needle via the posterior vaginal fornix for suspected intraperitoneal bleeding, ectopic pregnancy, or tuboovarian abscess.

Posterior Colpotomy (Culdotomy) A transverse incision is made through the posterior vaginal fornix into the posterior cul-de-sac to facilitate diagnosis by intraperitoneal palpation, inspection of pelvic organs, or determination of free fluid, blood, or pus in the pouch of Douglas. Pus from a pelvic abscess or blood, possibly a sign of ectopic pregnancy or ruptured ovarian cyst, is evacuated. The tubes and ovaries are inspected, and if they are normal, the incision is closed. A drain may be inserted.

Some operative therapy, such as aspiration of ovarian cyst or sterilization by tubal ligation, can be performed through the incision, although exposure and visualization are limited. A tube or ovary is sometimes removed through the vagina.

Pelvic Endoscopy

Pelvic endoscopy is an established part of the gynecologist's diagnostic and therapeutic armamentarium. It permits detailed intraperitoneal inspection of pelvic organs without laparotomy. The procedure is not without danger, however, and requires an experienced operator, careful patient selection, and adequate anesthesia. Two methods are employed: culdoscopy by vaginal approach and laparoscopy by abdominal approach.

Culdoscopy For direct visualization of pelvic organs and adjacent structures, a culdoscope is introduced into the peritoneal cavity via the posterior vaginal fornix and the pouch of Douglas. It is useful in patients where laparoscopy is contraindicated or unavailable but contraindicated in patients with fixation of organs adjacent to the cul-de-sac, e.g., large pelvic tumors, pelvic inflammatory disease (PID), or endometriosis. Indications are unexplained pelvic pain, questionable pelvic masses, ovarian disorders, or infertility.

Local or caudal anesthesia is used, with the patient in knee-chest or lithotomy position. Inadvertent perforation of the bowel or rectum is a major hazard. Vaginal preparation and empty bowel and rectum are prerequisites to the procedure. With posterior lip of the cervix held by a tenaculum and retracted anteriorly, the uterus is elevated while counterpressure is applied to posterior vaginal wall by speculum. This maneuver stretches the posterior vaginal fornix while a trocar and cannula or sheath penetrate the thin wall and enter the pelvis between the uterosacral ligaments. When the trocar is removed with the cannula in place, air enters the cul-de-sac because of the negative intraabdominal pressure produced by knee-chest position. Air displaces the bowel and the scope may be inserted through the cannula.

To check for tubal patency, an aqueous solution of dye such as methylene blue or indigo carmine in saline can be instilled via a cervical cannula. The dye is observed dripping from the fimbrial end of the tube. Or, if obstruction is present, the nature of the block may be demonstrated.

At completion of the procedure, the culdoscope is removed. Before the cannula is removed, the operating table is straightened and the patient flattened while as much air as possible is evacuated by hand pressure on the abdomen. Some surgeons place a suture in the puncture site.

Laparoscopy Laparoscopy, or peritoneoscopy, is insertion of a fiberoptic laparoscope into the peritoneal cavity for diagnostic and/or therapeutic purposes. It permits direct observation and selective biopsy of pelvic and upper abdominal organs and peritoneal surfaces. This technique is used to diagnose ectopic pregnancy; inspect the ovaries for evidence of follicular activity; visualize pelvic masses; and determine etiology of pain, internal bleeding, infertility, endocrinopathies, or amenorrhea. It often obviates the need for laparotomy. Pelvic diseases such as endometriosis, adhesions, and tubal occlusions may be identified. Because it allows a view of the anterior surface of the uterus, bladder, and cul-de-sac, laparoscopy is preferred to culdoscopy in many patients.

Operative procedures such as tubal sterilization by electrocoagulation with or without division or partial resection, placement of a metal clip or silicone ring on the tube, biopsy, or lysis of adhesions can be performed. The argon laser will pass through the fiberoptic system to ablate endometriosis. The carbon dioxide laser may be used to vaporize tissue in conjunction with the operating microscope attached to the laparoscope. Laparoscopy also is used to recover ova for in vitro fertilization (see p. 441).

Equipment in addition to laparoscope and its accessory parts includes D&C instrument tray; uterine sound fixed to a cervical clamp to manipulate cervix; laparoscopic tray with trocars, cannulas, tubing, and instruments for viewing viscera; and operating instruments such as graduated probe, electrosurgical probe, and biopsy forceps. Extra instrumentation may be needed for microsurgical procedures. Unsterile equipment includes CO_2 pump, fiberoptic power source, and laser or electrosurgical unit. Only a solid-state electrosurgical generator should be used with the laparoscope. High peaks of voltages from spark-gap generators may cause excessive tissue destruction. Prior to use, fogging of the distal lens of the optic by intraperitoneal temperature and moisture can be prevented by warming the tip of the scope in warm towels or saline.

Usually general anesthesia by intubation is administered. Vaginal prep, catheterization, and D&C are often performed first. A special cannula or catheter may be inserted into the cervix for instillation of a dye solution to observe tubal patency and for manipulation of the uterus to afford greater visibility. The vaginal area is covered with a sterile drape, and with the patient in modified lithotomy position (stirrups adjusted so the legs are at a 45° angle to the axis of the operating table), the abdomen is prepped and draped as for laparotomy. A combined sheet (double fenestration) also may be used.

Insertion of the scope is preceded by pneumoperitoneum to produce abdominal distention. The subumbilical midline area is most commonly used if no scars, with possible adherent viscera beneath, are present. This area is preferred because it has no abdominal wall vessels that might be injured. The firm attachment of fascia to peritoneum facilitates entry. However, great care must be taken to avoid injury to the great vessels or intraabdominal organs.

To produce pneumoperitoneum, a Verres needle is introduced percutaneously into the peritoneal cavity. This needle has an outer sharp trocar with an inner blunt hollow retractable cannula or a stylet with a spring at its base. The needle also has a two-way stopcock at the base for control of gas flow. A plastic tube with adaptor to fit the needle hub connects to the carbon dioxide insufflation apparatus. Carbon dioxide is used as the insufflation medium because it is nontoxic, highly soluble in blood, and rapidly absorbed from the peritoneal cavity. The gas is slowly introduced into the cavity under controlled flow and pressure, monitored by the circulating nurse and surgeon. The volume injected varies according to need, but overdistention must be avoided to prevent complications.

After insufflation, the valve is closed and the patient placed in Trendelenburg's position. A small subumbilical incision is made in the anterior abdominal wall and through it the trocar and cannula (sleeve) are introduced into the peritoneal cavity via puncture. The sharp tip must be carefully guided to avoid inadvertent perforations. The trocar is removed and the scope of the same caliber is inserted through the sleeve, which remains in the cavity. The fiberoptic cable is connected to the light source and the gas tube is reconnected to the cannula.

Although operating scopes permit insertion of accessory instruments, these may be introduced through a second small incision in the lower abdomen. Another smaller trocar and cannula are inserted into the peritoneal cavity under direct vision through the laparoscope, which offers good transillumination for the puncture when the room lights are dimmed. After removal of the trocar, an operating instrument is inserted through the cannula. Accessory instruments include calibrated metal probe for assessment of organ size or distance between organs, insulated electrosurgical unit electrodes for unipolar or bipolar coagulation, aspirating tube, and biopsy forceps.

At completion of operation, the accessory instrument and cannula are removed. Hemostasis is surveyed and the scope removed from the primary puncture site. The valve of its sleeve is opened to allow escape of intraperitoneal gas while gentle pressure is applied to the abdomen. The skin incisions are sutured and a small dressing is applied.

While numerous complications have been reported, the most common are perforation of a hollow viscus such as the intestine, hemorrhage from a punctured vessel or a biopsy site, gas embolism from intravascular injection, and burns of the abdominal wall and bowel. The patient requires close monitoring by the anesthesiologist because increased intraabdominal pressure may lead to cardiovascular disturbances from vagal reflex due to stretching of the peritoneum, retention of carbon dioxide, or compression of the inferior vena cava.

Postoperative shoulder pain may follow use of pneumoperitoneum. This is referred pain caused by pressure on the diaphragm, which is somewhat displaced by carbon dioxide during the procedure. Slight elevation of head after recovery from anesthesia relieves this pain.

> NOTE. Laparoscopy is a sterile procedure. Except for the telescope with the optical system of the laparoscope and some trocars and forceps with plastic components, laparoscopic instruments can be steam sterilized. The recommendations of manufacturer should be followed prior to sterilization in steam under pressure or in ethylene oxide gas if preferred. Meticulous cleaning with a detergent, followed by high-level disinfection with activated glutaraldehyde solution may be an accepted alternative to sterilization. *Laparoscopic instruments should be prepared in the same manner for every patient, per written hospital policy and procedure.* Inconsistent sterilization procedures may be a source of liability. Refer to Chapter 19, p. 371, for further discussion of care of endoscopes.

Hysteroscopy Hysteroscopy is direct inspection of the uterus by means of a fiberoptic hysteroscope to diagnose or treat intrauterine disease. It may be used to supplement curettage of the uterine cavity, and in the management of infertility, abnormal uterine bleeding, lost intrauterine devices (IUDs), or intrauterine synechiae. It also provides an intrauterine approach for ablating endometrial hyperplasia with the Nd:YAG laser. Adequate dilatation of the cavity is a prerequisite for careful viewing of endometrial surfaces. To provide distention, 5% glucose in water, carbon dioxide, or viscid dextran solution is used.

Hysteroscopy is not widely performed because of the availability of other diagnostic methods and its own disadvantages. These disadvantages include the need for extensive training in the method, the danger of tumor cell dissemination in the presence of malignancy, and the obscuration of the visual field by bleeding.

Tubal Perfusion

To test tubal patency, methylene blue dye in a solution of normal saline is introduced into the uterine cavity via a 50-cc syringe or IV tubing attached to a cervical cannula. The surgeon views the ends of the fallopian tubes through a laparoscope. Dye sighted coming from one or both tubes indicates patency.

Uterotubal Insufflation (Rubin's Test)

In addition to hysterosalpingography and pelvic endoscopy, uterotubal insufflation may be used to study infertility. It is done to test the patency of the fallopian tubes. The test is preferably done prior to ovulation, so as not to interfere with potential fertilization.

After vaginal prep, a uterine sound is passed to discover depth of the cervical canal. A special cannula with airtight seal is inserted into the cervicouterine canal, the seal is adjusted, and the cannula is connected to an insufflation apparatus. Carbon dioxide is introduced slowly under controlled flow. Resistance to flow—back pressure—is measured on a mercury manometer. A relationship exists between stenosis and the pressure required to force gas into the tubes. The manometer is watched closely for fluctuations in pressure, which indicate tubal patency. A sudden drop in pressure after initial rise to about 100 mm of mercury suggests patency of one or both tubes as gas flows out of them into the peritoneal cavity. In a normal test, as flow slowly continues, the pressure fluctuates between 40 and 80 mm of mercury, reflecting tubal peristalsis.

Sudden, sharp, transient shoulder pain when the patient sits up, after conclusion of the procedure, is characteristic of a positive test. This is referred pain due to irritation from subdiaphragmatic carbon dioxide before total absorption from the peritoneal cavity. If pain is delayed, the tubes may be patent but ascent of gas is retarded by intraabdominal adhesions. The test may be therapeutic in relieving minor obstructions.

Contraindications include genital tract infection, possible pregnancy, or any uterine bleeding because of danger of gas embolism. To prevent embolism, a Rubin's test should precede, never follow, a D&C (see p. 432).

Hysterosalpingography

Radiologic investigation of the uterus and tubes may afford further evaluation of infertility following repeated negative Rubin's tests. Tip of a catheter is inserted into cervical canal and a water-soluble radiopaque dye is instilled. The contrast medium ascends into corpus uteri and tubes to yield information about structure and function.

VULVAR PROCEDURES

Benign growths, although rare, mainly consist of fatty and fibrous tumors. These are excised if large. Suspicious lesions should be removed for pathological examination. Cancerous lesions may be multicentric, with the majority found on the labia majora and a lesser percentage on the labia minora, vestibule, clitoris, and posterior commissure. Vaginal smears should be taken to determine presence of metastatic growth to the vaginal wall. Treatment depends on size of primary lesion, involvement of nodes, and extent of metastasis. Mutilative procedures require emotional adjustment to permanent change. Therapeutic procedures include the following.

Excision of Lesion Wide local excision of only the lesion may be done in a single, well-localized area with no premalignant changes elsewhere. Leukoplakia and preinvasive lesions of the vulva may be treated with laser.

Simple Vulvectomy without Node Dissection Simple vulvectomy without node dissection is performed for premalignant lesions and early cancer of limited penetration *(microinvasive cancer).* The labia majora and minora, part of the mons veneris, hymenal ring, including the clitoris, may be removed. Occasionally the clitoris and perianal region are spared if the lesion is small. Incision must be wide to avoid local recurrence.

Total Vulvectomy Basal cell carcinoma usually does not metastasize but is often locally extensive and prone to recur. Treatment consists of wide total vulvectomy, also without node dissection.

Radical Vulvectomy with Bilateral Inguinal-femoral (Groin) Lymphadenectomy Radical vulvectomy is performed for invasive vulvar cancers and is usually done in one stage. Resection lines may vary depending on location and size of the lesion. Since the procedure involves adbominal and perineal dissection, both areas, including thighs to knees, are prepped. Structures generally removed include all from anterior surface of the pubis to perianal region posteriorly, with wide lateral excision beyond the vulva, to fascial depth. More specifically, these include large areas of abdominal and groin skin, labia majora and minora, the mons, clitoris, Bartholin's and periurethral glands, superficial and sometimes deep inguinal-femoral lymph nodes, and portions of the saphenous veins. In early cancers with no superficial node involvement, deep pelvic node dissection may be avoided. If the urethra and anus are involved, or they are near the tumor, they are also removed. Anal involvement may require a colostomy. Involvement of the vagina may require resection of part of vagina.

Lymphadenectomy is carried out en bloc with the patient in supine position. Suction drains are inserted and inguinal incisions are closed. The patient is then placed in lithotomy position for vulvectomy. Reconstruction of the pelvic floor and vaginal walls may be necessary. Vaginal packing is inserted and suction drainage used postoperatively to avoid fluid collection beneath skin flaps. Postoperative care emphasizes open-wound management for prevention of infection.

Marsupialization of Bartholin Cyst or Abscess The cyst enlarges as secretions accumulate. Obstruction of the excretory duct of Bartholin's gland may be postinflammatory and the cyst may be prone to secondary infection or abscess formation. Marsupialization establishes drainage from within the vagina by creation of a new enlarged ductal opening. The cyst is incised linearly in the region of the normal opening and evacuated. Edges of vaginal mucosa and cyst wall are sutured together to produce epithelization. After epithelization no cyst recurrence can occur.

VAGINAL PROCEDURES

Excision of Adenosis Lesion A benign epithelial tumor should be biopsied and studied histologically to rule out adenocarcinoma. Vaginal adenosis and gross cervical abnormalities, such as collar or hood, as well as clear cell adenocarcinoma of the vagina have occurred in female offspring of women who received diethylstilbestrol (DES) or similar synthetic estrogen during the first trimester of pregnancy to avoid miscarriage. Adenosis may be treated with laser (see colposcopy, p. 426).

Vaginectomy Vaginectomy (partial or complete) is performed for carcinoma in situ or carcinoma of the vagina. Vaginoplasty is necessary for reconstruction. External radiation and radium application (refer to Chap. 35), with possible eventual pelvic exenteration (p. 434), is the treatment for advanced invasive malignancy. The proximity of bladder and rectum makes therapy difficult.

Radical vaginal or abdominal hysterectomy and vaginectomy with extraperitoneal lymphadenectomy sometimes are combined for carcinoma of the upper and middle thirds of the vagina if the bladder or rectum is not involved.

Construction of Vagina Vaginal construction is utilized in patients with congenital absence of entire vagina, or more commonly stenosis after radiation therapy, or after operative removal of the vagina. Care must be taken to avoid damage to urethra, bladder, and rectum. The vaginal space is created by blunt and sharp dissection. If a large part of the surface of the space is denuded, a skin graft is shaped around a vaginal mold and the mold is placed in such a way that the graft will take. With the use of dilators to prevent stenosis and estrogen cream to assist in epithelization of cavity, an adequate functional vagina can be created in many patients.

Procedures for Repair of Pelvic Outlet Injury to muscles and fascia of the perineum and/or genital tract, usually during childbirth, may result in extensive vaginal relaxation. Manifestation of perineal herniae may be delayed until later years, when generalized loss of elastic tissue develops. Downward pressure is exerted on other structures, such as the bladder. Moderate to severe degrees of herniation of viscera require surgical intervention to restore pelvic floor integrity and sphincter competency. Vaginal plastic procedures for genital prolapse consist of narrowing and reconstructing the damaged pelvic floor. Vaginal repairs are referred to as *vaginal plastic procedures.*

Anterior Colporrhaphy Anterior colporrhaphy is performed for prolapse of the anterior vaginal wall to repair *urethrocystocele,* a herniation of the bladder into the vaginal canal. With the patient in lithotomy position, the wall is incised and a strip of redundant vaginal mucosa is excised, the extent of which depends on severity of prolapse. The bladder is dissected free from the vaginal septum and returned to normal position by suturing the pubocervical ligaments beneath it. Approximation of the pubococcygeus muscles provides further suburethral support. The vaginal wall is closed by sutures. By improving support to the bladder neck region, restoring the posterior urethrovesical angle, and narrowing the urethral opening, stress incontinence (urinary loss with strain) is relieved. The operation also prevents voiding difficulty and recurrent cystitis that accompanies retention of urine due to a cystocele hanging below the bladder neck.

Posterior Colpoperineorrhaphy Repair of the posterior vaginal wall for *rectocele,* a herniation of the rectum into the vagina, consists of triangular excision of redundant vaginal mucosa and separation of the vagina from the rectum. Support is reestablished by suturing together rectovaginal fascia, as well as the levator ani, as high as possible. Perineal muscles are reconstructed to restore continuity of support. A lacerated perineum may also be sutured. The operation relieves fecal incontinence and/or constipation.

Repair of Enterocele An abnormally deep hernial sac may contain a segment of intestine, referred to as *enterocele,* or cul-de-sac hernia. Repair consists of opening the sac, reducing its contents, excising the sac, closing the aperture or weakness that allowed the sac to descend into the rectovaginal septum, and strengthening the normal anatomical coverings. Approximation of uterosacral ligaments and levator ani in the midline removes the cul-de-sac defect.

Repair of Prolapsed Uterus or Procidentia Various operations correct and restore support. In complete prolapse both cervix and uterine body protrude through the vaginal aperture and the vaginal canal is inverted. Bleeding ulceration of exposed tissue may occur. Often cystocele and rectocele are present and are simultaneously repaired. Correction of prolapse anteverts the uterus and shortens an elongated cervix and the cardinal ligaments. Most patients, however, are treated by vaginal hysterectomy.

Colpocleisis (Le Fort Operation) Colpocleisis, obliteration of vagina by denuding and approximating the anterior and posterior walls, is generally reserved for elderly patients or those who are a poor operative risk.

NOTE. 1. A vaginal pessary to support a retrodisplaced or prolapsing uterus may be inserted in women who are poor operative risks.

2. Vaginal hysterectomy (p. 432) is done for severe prolapse or prolapse accompanied by stress incontinence when childbearing is no longer desired.

Procedures for Repair of Genital Fistulas A fistula is an abnormal communication between a part of the genital canal and either the urinary or intestinal tract. Various dye tests, cystoscopy, and pyelography help pinpoint a urinary tract fistula. Injury during parturition, operative trama (especially radical procedures for cancer), penetrating extension of cervical carcinoma, and radiation necrosis are common etiologic factors.

Repair of Vesicovaginal Fistula The most common type, a vesicovaginal fistula is between the bladder and vagina. A small opening permits seepage of urine, although the patient may void normally. Total incontinence may result from a large fistulous aperture and cause irritation of vagina, vulva, and thighs. Through vaginal approach the anterior vaginal wall is dissected free. The fistula to the bladder is closed and the bladder to vagina attachment is reestablished. The repair should be made with at least three layers of tissue and the bladder should be decompressed by indwelling Foley catheter for at least 14 days. Antibiotics may be administered judiciously to prevent infection in healing site.

If the vesicovaginal fistula is high in the vagina, a better result will be obtained by entering the bladder via suprapubic incision for direct repair rather than using a vaginal approach. Care must be taken not to occlude ureteral orifices. This is accomplished by insertion of ureteral catheters which can be removed following operation. Attention is given to excision of any infected tissue, closure with multiple layers, and bladder decompression by catheter.

Repair of Ureterovaginal Fistula A ureterovaginal fistula is between the ureter and vagina; its repair depends on location. If the fistula is near the junction of ureter and bladder, the ureter can be divided above the defect and reimplanted in the bladder. If the fistula is not proximal to the bladder, it can be excised and the severed ureteral ends anastomosed. Occasionally a nephrectomy on the involved side is necessary.

Repair of Urethrovaginal Fistula A urethrovaginal fistula is between the urethra and vagina; repair consists of layered closure. If the neck of the bladder is involved, the area must be reconstructed. This may include transplant of the bulbocavernosus muscle.

Repair of Rectovaginal Fistula A fistula between the rectum and vagina may follow episiotomy, obstetrical perineal lacerations, vaginal surgery such as culdoscopy, or rectal surgery such as hemorrhoidectomy. Fecal incontinence and fecal material in the vagina are characteristic, although the anal sphincter is intact. Preoperative bowel preparation, including prophylactic antibiotic therapy, is important because of the contaminated operative area. A temporary colostomy may be advisable before the operation to divert the infective fecal stream from the repair site. Using a vaginal approach, a plastic repair of the perineum is done. Scar tissue and the fistulous tract are excised and the edges of the perineal muscles and fascia are approximated.

Cervix

Treatment of an abnormal cervix should be preceded by tests to rule out early malignant change. Operative treatment of the cervix involves a number of procedures.

Electrocautery The cervix may be cauterized to treat chronic inflammation and/or leukorrhea.

Trachelorrhaphy Lacerations of the cervix may result from childbirth. Repair involves reconstruction of the cervical canal as necessary. A vaginal plastic setup is used.

Conization Employed therapeutically for chronic inflammation and for premalignant lesions in women of child-bearing age, conization may be performed by scalpel, electrosurgery, or laser.

Amputation The cervix may be amputated to remove an intraepithelial cancer. However, because this procedure leaves the corpus uteri, which may become cancerous, some surgeons prefer total hysterectomy to cervical amputation.

Uterus

Examination under Anesthesia Bimanual examination of the pelvis with patient in lithotomy position and relaxed from anesthesia allows more thorough inspection, especially in women experiencing pain, nervous tension, or obesity. This examination should precede every gynecological operative procedure, since it allows the size, outline, consistency, position, and mobility of the uterus, tubes, and ovaries to be assessed accurately. The examination also helps the surgeon determine the stage of malignancy and whether or not a lesion is resectable. It is a routine prelude to vaginal and abdominal operations. In patients for laparotomy, the vaginal vault is prepped and examination performed prior to the abdominal preparation.

Dilatation and Curettage (D&C) The most frequently performed gynecologic operation, dilatation of the cervix and curettage is done for diagnostic and/or therapeutic purposes. Sometimes both are accomplished by the same operation. Fractional curettage specimens differentiate between the endocervix and the endometrium of the corpus, which helps locate a lesion. The main purpose of D&C is to establish the etiology of abnormal uterine bleeding so that the gynecologist can plan definitive treatment. The procedure is mandatory in women with postmenopausal bleeding or symptoms suggestive of endometrial cancer, even when cytological smears are negative. It may be performed in infertility studies, or to confirm preoperative diagnosis before amputation of the cervix or hysterectomy. Therapeutic applications are to relieve dysmenorrhea by cervical dilatation only, to remove polyps or benign endometrial pathology, to remove residual tissue and arrest bleeding following incomplete abortion, or for voluntary or therapeutic abortion before the thirteenth week of pregnancy. A regional paracervical block or general anesthesia is required.

Schiller's test of the cervix utilizing Lugol's solution may precede D&C performed for multiple biopsy or cervical conization. The test aids in localizing areas for biopsy. Then, with the anterior lip of the cervix held in a tenaculum and the posterior vaginal wall retracted, a small curette is introduced into the endocervical canal, which is scraped from the internal to the external os. The specimen is placed on a Telfa pad and both are put into a container. The scraping precedes cervical dilatation to avoid dislodging tissue from above. A uterine sound is then introduced into the uterus to determine length and direction of the intrauterine cavity. It is important that the surgeon know the shape and position of the uterus to avoid perforation and injury to it and to other pelvic organs, the primary complications. Successively larger dilators are then passed through the cervix and internal os to permit insertion of a curette into the uterine cavity for curettage of the endometrium. Submucous fibroids are usually discernible as the curette passes over them. The endometrial curettage specimen is kept separate from the endocervical one. Both specimens are identified and sent to pathology for histological examination. Exploration of the fundus with a polyp forceps usually extracts any polyps present in the endometrium. The cervix may be biopsied if indicated by the Schiller's test in association with D&C.

NOTE. Separate instruments should be used for fractional curettage specimens. (Refer to listing of D&C instruments, Fig. 22-3, p. 424.)

Vaginal Hysterectomy (Standard) Vaginal hysterectomy is performed for severe uterine prolapse, prolapse accompanied by stress incontinence, and occasionally for sterilization of patients with pelvic relaxation or history of myomata, irregular uterine bleeding, or treated premalignant lesion.

The uterus is removed through the vagina, with incision of the vaginal wall and the pelvic cavity. D&C may be done prior to hysterectomy. Urinary incontinence, enterocele, and/or rectocele may be simultaneously repaired by anterior and posterior colporrhaphies and with reconstruction of the pelvic floor. Advantages of the procedure include restoration of normal anatomic relationship and preservation of vaginal function. The ovaries are not usually removed. Contraindications are immobility of pelvic organs, large uterus, pathology such as ovarian mass, or pelvic malignancy.

The vaginal wall is incised anteriorly and the bladder is separated from the cervix. The incision is continued around the cervix. The peritoneal cavity is entered through the posterior cul-de-sac and the anterior uterovesical pouch. Ligaments supporting the uterus and uterine vessels are ligated and cut. The fundus is delivered, upper pedicles sutured, uterus removed, and peritoneum closed. Suturing the cardinal and uterosacral ligaments together and to the vaginal vault supports the vault and prevents prolapse of the vagina. Potential complications include injury to ureters, bowel, or bladder, and massive hemorrhage from uterine vessels. An unopened laparotomy setup should be available.

Radical Vaginal Hysterectomy (Schauta Operation) An operative approach to early carcinoma of the cervix, radical vaginal hysterectomy does not permit pelvic lymph node dissection but is useful in selective patients, e.g., obese patients. It includes vaginal removal of uterus, upper third of vagina, parametria, fallopian tubes, and ovaries. Damage to the ureters or bladder is a potential complication.

ABDOMINAL PROCEDURES

The abdominal approach is used for fixed or enlarged uterus, exploration, inflammatory disease, and most malignant lesions of the uterus, fallopian tubes, and ovaries. This approach permits inspection of pelvic and abdominal organs as well as lymph glands for biopsy or treatment. Laparotomy set is used.

Abdominal Cavity

Exploratory Pelvic Laparotomy ("Lap") Exploratory pelvic laparotomy is performed for diagnosis but may be followed immediately by a therapeutic procedure such as hysterectomy. Significant pelvic pain, uterine bleeding, or pelvic mass are frequent indications for differential diagnosis from abdominal disease.

The appendix may be removed incidentally unless the patient's condition precludes this. The patient should be informed preoperatively that this procedure may be performed at the discretion of the surgeon.

Uterus

Abdominal Hysterectomy Abdominal hysterectomy is removal of the uterus through abdominal incision and opening of the peritoneal cavity. The most frequent indication is leiomyofibroma, commonly known as benign fibroids or myomas. The most common gynecologic tumors, fibroids are composed of muscle and fibrous connective tissue. They may be single or multiple and most often are present in the wall of the uterus. Some may be attached by pedicle, protrude into and distort the uterine cavity. Fibroids, which are usually slow-growing, are treated conservatively if small and presenting no problems. The tumor ceases to grow at menopause. If symptoms such as menometrorrhagia, bladder or bowel pressure, pelvic discomfort, or rapid tumor growth develop, operative treatment is essential. Differential diagnosis includes dysfunctional bleeding due to disturbed endocrine function, tubal or ovarian masses, and pelvic malignancy. In addition to these indications, hysterectomy is performed for uterine prolapse, extensive endometriosis, and cervical or uterine malignancy. Various types of hysterectomy are performed.

Supracervical (Subtotal, Partial) Hysterectomy) Rarely performed, partial hysterectomy involves removal of the corpus uteri only and is reserved for poor-risk patients or difficult operations in which total hysterectomy would increase morbidity or mortality. Leaving the cervix subjects the patient to risk of possible future cervical cancer. The operation may also be performed in disseminated ovarian carcinoma with removal of the primary ovarian tumor. Reduction of the total mass facilitates radiation therapy.

Total Hysterectomy The entire uterus, the corpus uteri and cervix uteri, is resected. If normal, ovaries are preserved whenever possible in patients under 45 years of age for hormone production.

After vaginal and abdominal preparation, the abdominal peritoneal cavity is entered through a vertical midline or horizontal Pfannenstiel's incision. Vertical incision facilitates exploration. The patient is placed in deep Trendelenburg's position. Incision through the uterine peritoneum is carried laterally. Abdominal organs are retracted and protected with warm saline laparotomy packs. The fallopian tubes, round and broad ligaments are clamped, cut, and ligated. The ovaries, when not removed, are suspended to avoid adherence to the vaginal vault. With the uterus forward, posterior sheets of the broad ligaments are incised, ureters are identified, and uterine vessels and uterosacral ligaments are clamped, divided, and sutured. All uterine-supporting ligaments must be divided and ligated. The bladder is mobilized from the cervix and vagina, the vaginal vault incised, and cervix dissected from the vagina. After the uterus is removed, the connective tissue ligaments are anchored to the vagina. The vaginal mucosa and muscular wall are approximated by sutures, and the bladder, vault, and rectum (pelvic floor) reperitonealized or covered with peritoneum. Abdominal layers are closed as for laparotomy.

NOTE. When the surgeon is closing the vaginal vault following removal of the uterus, the needle, suture, needleholder, and all instruments used on the cervix and vagina are considered contaminated. The scrub nurse holds the specimen basin to receive them and does not touch them. Separate instruments are used for abdominal closure.

Wide Cuff Hysterectomy Wide cuff hysterectomy is removal of the total uterus and a generous cuff of the vagina. Surgeons employ this procedure for cervical carcinoma in situ or early stromal invasion (microinvasion) if invasion is less than 5 mm and no tumor cells appear within lymphatic or vascular channels. Preservation of ovaries depends mainly on the patient's age.

Radical Hysterectomy with Pelvic Node Dissection (Radical Wertheim Operation) The radical Wertheim operation may be performed for early stages of invasive cervical cancer and sometimes for endometrial cancer. It involves wide en bloc removal of paracervical, parametrial, and uterosacral tissues (uterus, tubes, ovaries, ligaments), and at least the upper third of the vaginal canal. Bilateral pelvic lymph nodes and channels surrounding the external iliac artery and vein, hypogastric artery and vein, and obturator fossae are also dissected and removed.

Some surgeons perform a *modified Wertheim operation* for microinvasive carcinoma. This is somewhat less extensive than is the radical procedure and may omit lymphadenectomy.

Total Hysterectomy and Bilateral Salpingo-oophorectomy Fallopian tubes and ovaries are removed along with the uterus. The procedure is done for endometrial, tubal, or ovarian cancer. It is also performed in postmenopausal women when total hysterectomy is indicated to avoid potential for future ovarian malignancy.

NOTE. Endometrial malignancy, which is increasing in incidence, is essentially a disease of peri- or postmenopausal years. It is characterized by intermittent spotting between periods or after menopause, or steady bleeding. Postmenopausal bleeding is considered to be due to cancer until proven otherwise. Most patients are treated by preoperative radiation.

Complications of hysterectomy include injury to the ureters with possible fistula formation or renal failure, injury to the bladder or bowel with fistula formation, or massive hemorrhage from damage to major vessels.

Medical, psychosocial, and sexual ramifications must be considered when contemplating hysterectomy. Medically the procedure may be lifesaving in patients with malignancy or severe hemorrhage. The gynecologist has an obligation to consider the individual patient's attitudes when more than one mode of therapy is available as an alternative to hysterectomy.

Signaling as it does the end of the patient's reproductive potential, hysterectomy may cause psychological stress and a sense of incompleteness, even though sexual responsiveness is not dependent on the uterus. Patients whose families are complete, however, may welcome reproductive sterilization.

Myomectomy Single or multiple fibroid tumors can be removed from the uterine wall in premenopausal women who may still desire pregnancy. The operation is especially adaptable to pedunculated tumors, which may become necrotic from interference with blood supply. Removal of large submucous fibroids may require opening the uterus.

Pelvic Exenteration An ultraradical procedure for invasive persistent carcinoma, exenteration is not performed for palliation but only when a possibility of cure exists. Extent of disease determines the amount of exenteration. In *anterior exenteration,* the reproductive organs, distal part of the ureters, bladder, and vagina are removed. This modification is performed for cancer of the cervix, vagina, or vulva with extension to the bladder. The ureters are diverted to an ileal conduit while the bowel remains intact. *Posterior exenteration* removes the reproductive organs, sigmoid colon, and rectum. It is done for cervical carcinoma involving the rectum, or advanced rectal carcinoma involving the uterus and posterior vaginal wall. The urinary system remains intact; fecal diversion is by colostomy. *Total or complete exenteration,* rarely performed, involves en bloc dissection of the bladder, reproductive organs, perineum, rectum, and pelvic lymph nodes. Two setups are needed: abdominal and perineal. These mutilative operations change structure, function, body image, and sex life and must be preceded by intensive physical and psychological preoperative preparation.

Numerous complications may occur involving any major system. Anesthesia and operating times are long. Blood replacement and extensive monitoring are essential. Multiple stoma and gross pelvic defect with much dead space predispose to infection; therefore wound drainage is used.

Fallopian Tubes

The fallopian tubes are also referred to as the *uterine tubes, oviducts,* and *salpinges.*

Tubal Ligation Sterilization should be considered permanent, because reversal cannot be guaranteed. Thorough preoperative counseling of the patient and her husband or partner should preface this procedure. A number of operative techniques are used for tubal ligation. They are essentially similar in removal of a portion of the middle part of the fallopian tube on each side for pathological confirmation, and ligation of both the distal and proximal ends to prevent the cut ends from growing together. Frequently performed by laparoscopy, tubal ligation by open abdominal approach may be done alone, in conjunction with other indicated abdominal surgery, or in cases where previous operations interfere with laparoscopic technique. Ligation may be performed through a small horizontal incision in the pubic hairline area. This is referred to as *minilaparotomy.* Or tubal ligations are often performed postpartum, following cesarean delivery and closure of the uterine wall (see p. 440). No additional instruments are required other than those used for the C-section.

The *Pomeroy technique* of ligation is the safest, provides a surgical specimen of each tube, and causes minimal tubal destruction. The tube is tied with suture material and a section is removed. The tube eventually pulls apart, destroying the passage between ovary and uterus.

Sterilization may also be performed following vaginal delivery, on the first to third postpartum day. In the cauterization technique, the bipolar electrosurgical electrode transects and seals ends of fallopian tube, or excises a section of tube and seals the ends. Application of a stretchable Silastic band or a ligating clip may also produce occlusion. In some patients, however, Pomeroy type and occlusion techniques may be reversible by subsequent reparative operation.

Tuboplasty An estimated one percent of sterilized women will seek reversals because of sterilization at an early age, remarriage, or death of a child. Improved tubal reconstructive techniques, fine suture materials, and particularly microsurgery and lasers have vastly improved results. Success depends on extent of tubal destruction, amount of tube left, location of previous cut or ligation, and normality of tissue at severed ends of tube. For example, chance for success is slight if fimbriectomy was performed. Preoperative assessment may include hysterosalpingogram, to determine length and patency of tubal segments, and/or laparoscopy. The average success rate is 60 to 70 percent if tubes do not show major damage. Some subspecialists claim a success rate of 30 percent for the latter group. By removal of the occlusion, tuboplasty may reverse infertility caused by diseased or damaged tubes. Although tubal patency may be restored, function may remain abnormal, limiting the chance of successful uterine pregnancy and increasing the risk of tubal pregnancy.

The procedures, dependent on the site of obstruction, are tubal resection for excision of abnormal tissue and anastomosis, cornual resection and replantation, and fimbrioplasty. These are microsurgical techniques. An abdominal approach is used. A cervical cannula may be inserted, with patient in lithotomy position, prior to laparotomy if demonstration of tubal patency by injection of methylene blue is desired before anastomoses of tubes. A laser beam may also be used through the microscope to open fimbriated ends and to divide adhesions in blocked fallopian tubes.

Salpingectomy, Salpingo-Oophorectomy Acute tubal infections may be diagnosed by laparoscopy. Operative treatment is indicated when a pelvic infection such as salpingitis does not respond to antibiotic therapy. Removal of large tuboovarian abscesses is essential to prevent rupture and dissemination of pus in the abdominal cavity. *Salpingectomy,* removal of a fallopian tube, is often performed in association with partial or total removal of corresponding ovary. It is then referred to as *salpingo-oophorectomy.* Procedures may be uni- or bilateral. Indications are:

1 Extensive damage to the tube and ovary such as chronic tuboovarian abscess from repeated pelvic inflammatory infections. Since this is a bilateral disease, it is often treated by total abdominal hysterectomy and bilateral salpingo-oophorectomy.

2 Tubal ectopic pregnancy. This is life-threatening, and must be diagnosed early. Treatment consists of removal of the affected tube.

3 Primary adenocarcinoma of the tube. Total hysterectomy and bilateral salpingo-oophorectomy are performed.

4 Large adnexal cysts.

Salpingostomy An incision of the fallopian tube may be performed to evacuate an early small tubal pregnancy and preserve the tube in a woman desiring children. The involved portion of the tube is resected and the ends anastomosed using a polyethylene splinting catheter. If the pregnancy is in the cornual region, and other portions of the tube are normal, cornual resection and tubal replantation are done. Salpingostomy is also performed for infectious occlusion of the fimbriated ends of the tubes.

Ovaries

Ovarian pain usually is referred to the lower abdomen just above either groin, making differential diagnosis from abdominal disease pertinent. Ovarian mass due to cyst or tumor requires exploration for evaluation. Ovarian tumors may be benign or malignant, cystic or solid. Some secrete hormones. Cysts are by far the most frequent. Cysts may simulate abdominal disorder or ruptured ectopic pregnancy. Pelvic endoscopy and ultrasonography assist diagnosis. The cyst may rupture, causing massive bleeding that necessitates laparotomy.

Genuine neoplastic cysts, such as dermoid, persist and increase in size. Dermoid cysts are encapsulated and often contain embryonal remnants. Rupture or leakage of their content is very irritating to the peritoneal cavity.

Cysts of considerable size or solid tumors, even if asymptomatic, should be removed as a precaution because they may degenerate into malignancy, increase in size, or lead to twisting of the pedicle. The type of operation depends on type of cyst, age of patient, and importance of preserving pregnancy potential.

Oophorocystectomy, Cystoophorectomy, Ovarian Cystectomy (Removal of Ovarian Cyst) Many benign ovarian cysts and tumors are treated by local excision with preservation of the ovary. A large cyst may be aspirated before removal. Immediately after removal, the surgeon incises the cyst for examination to determine its character, since gross appearance as well as frozen section is important. If there is reasonable assurance that the lesion is benign, removal of only the cyst or resection of a diseased portion, e.g., endometrioma, is justified, with preservation of normal tissue.

Oophorectomy (Removal of an Ovary) The most frequent indications for oophorectomy are benign ovarian tumors. Many gynecologists believe that cystadenomas and all solid benign ovarian tumors should be treated by unilateral salpingo-oophorectomy because of the difficulty of clean dissection and the questionable assurance of their benign nature. In postmenopausal women, both ovaries, tubes, and uterus are removed to avoid future cancer. Ovarian cancer is the fourth leading cause of cancer deaths in women in the United States.

If there is a strong probability or proof of malignancy in any ovarian cyst or mass, total hysterectomy and bilateral salpingo-oophorectomy are usually performed, regardless of age. Partial or complete omentectomy may be included because the rich blood supply of omentum contributes to rapid metastases. Extent of operation is determined by the lesion. In malignant tumors, a differentiation is made between primary and metastatic ovarian cancer, which influences treatment (see Chap. 35). The cure rate of ovarian cancer has not been significantly lowered. Metastasis is often present by the time symptoms present. Advanced ovarian carcinoma can obstruct the urinary and intestinal tracts.

Incision or Biopsy Biopsy is performed as indicated for diagnosis. Sometimes when a benign cyst is found in one ovary at laparotomy, the gynecologist carefully transects the other ovary to rule out any small neoplasm.

Muscles and Ligaments

Urinary stress incontinence may be corrected abdominally by suspending the bladder. Sometimes it is treated by a combined abdominoperineal procedure. Differential diagnosis from fistulas, bladder neuropathies, and primary lesions may be established by cystoscopy (see Chap. 23), urethrocystography, and urodynamics.

Marshall-Marchetti Vesicourethral Suspension Marshall-Marchetti vesicourethral suspension is done by extraperitoneal abdominal approach through the prevesical space. After mobilization, the urethra and bladder neck are suspended to the posterior surface of the pubis by sutures. These are placed through the anterior vaginal wall on each side of the urethra and then through the retropubic periosteum. Sutures may also be placed adjacent to the bladder neck and through the rectus muscle fascia to prevent descent of the bladder neck. Marshall-Marchetti suspension, an effective procedure for correction of stress incontinence, may be performed in conjunction with other pelvic surgery. Variations of the procedure have been devised. Refer to Chapter 23, p. 457, for discussion of Peyrera procedure for urinary incontinence.

SEX REASSIGNMENT

Sex transformation (gender transformation) is an established phenomenon in modern society. The patient shows an anxious desire to change from one physical status to another. A sex change, however, requires a stable personality, psychiatric counseling for feasibility, and careful preparation and support. While the majority of transformations are from male to female (see Chap. 23), female to male cross gender is also possible in satisfactory candidates; however, the management of this change is more complex. A treatment schedule of hormonal substitution, i.e., androgens (male hormone) in the female patient, is begun well in advance of the operation.

In a one-stage procedure, bilateral subcutaneous mastectomy, total abdominal hysterectomy, and bilateral salpingo-oophorectomy are performed. Three additional stages are necessary to complete transformation. These are:

1 Urethral reconstruction, to tip of enlarged clitoris

2 Transfer of the labia for penile lengthening and scrotal reconstruction

3 Prosthetic testical implantation

An understanding, nonjudgmental, unembarrassed attitude on the part of health care personnel can help the patient adjust mentally, as well as recover physically, after the radical change.

OBSTETRICS

Diagnostic techniques such as ultrasound, specialization in fertility problems, and techniques of fetal monitoring and management have brought significant changes in the field of reproductive biology. Consequently, OR nursing personnel become involved in care of obstetric patients both in elective and emergency procedures.

Threatened Pregnancy

Cerclage A tape is placed around an incompetent internal cervical os in an attempt to retain a pregnancy. The procedure is employed following diagnosis of incompetent cervix from a history of rapid, painless second- or early third-trimester spontaneous abortions in apparently normal pregnancies. Preferably elective in patients with typical history, cerclage is performed after the sixteenth week of pregnancy. Occasionally it may be an emergency procedure when the cervix is dilating and membranes are bulging, as long as membranes have not ruptured or premature labor has not begun. This operation may be performed in the nonpregnant patient with incompetent cervix.

Shirodkar Procedure A small incision is made in the anterior vaginal mucosa at the level of the bladder reflexion and at the posterior cervico–cul-de-sac junction. A tunnel under the cervical mucosa is then made to join the anterior and posterior incisions. Using an aneurysm needle, a synthetic polyester tape is placed around the internal os and tied, and the knot is secured by a suture. The mucosal incisions are closed. At term, the patient is usually delivered by cesarean section. The operation is not indicated in the presence of bleeding, premature rupture of the membranes, or premature labor.

Aborted Pregnancy

Suction Curettage (Dilatation and Evacuation, D&E) Suction curettage is the aspiration of intrauterine contents performed for termination of pregnancy, usually in first trimester (1 to 12 weeks), or for early incomplete spontaneous abortion. It is sometimes performed in the second trimester (13 to 24 weeks), but potential for complication is greater. The cervix must be opened wider, instruments must be larger, and the chance of perforation or hemorrhage is greater. Ultrasound may be used to determine stage of pregnancy. Cervical dilatation is adjusted to stage of pregnancy and the necessary cannula. A laminaria tent, cone-shaped plug, may be inserted preoperatively to gradually dilate the cervix, usually for 4 to 24 hours. The laminaria, removed before operation, is gentler than instrument dilatation, which can cause cervical tearing. A vacuum aspirator-cannula is connected by tubing to an electric vacuum pump. With gentle suction, the specimen is collected in the vacuum bottle and removed for examination. Following incomplete abortion, it is vital to remove all retained products of conception to prevent infection, especially anaerobic, which may proceed to septic shock (see Chap. 36). The removed tissue is sent for culture and pathologic examination.

D&C setup is used. Anesthesia is local or general. Disposable equipment for suction curettage not requiring dilatation or anesthesia is commercially available.

Ectopic Pregnancy A fertilized ovum may become implanted outside the uterus. Referred to as an *ectopic pregnancy,* rarely does the fetus develop to term. Although it may reach the ovary, abdominal cavity, or cervix uteri, the ovum usually implants in a fallopian tube. Symptoms of tubal pregnancy are abdominal pain and menstrual irregularity. The fetus grows to a size sufficient to rupture the tube. Diagnosis is made by laparoscopy or by detection of blood in the cul-de-sac by aspiration (see culdocentesis, p. 426). Hemorrhage results from extensive trauma to the tube and mesosalpinx. The patient often goes into severe shock. Immediate operation and blood replacement are mandatory. *Ruptured ectopic pregnancy is a true obstetric/gynecologic emergency.* At operation, the affected tube and fetus are removed, the pelvic cavity is aspirated, and bleeding is stopped. Removal of the associated ovary depends on extent of damage from the rupture.

Cesarean Section

Commonly referred to as C-section, a cesarean section is a method of delivery by abdominal and uterine incisions. Cesarean delivery may take place in the obstetric labor-delivery suite or in the OR suite. Pregnancy and labor produce many physiological alterations. Both mother and newborn have specific obstetric needs requiring comprehensive care. The OR nurse must be cognizant of these physiological and psychologcal needs, and the reasons for abdominal delivery, in order to promote a positive experience. C-section is a significant family event. Husbands may be permitted in the OR, and mothers are usually awake.

The frequency of cesarean section has increased markedly. It is the tenth most common surgical procedure in the United States. This is attributed mainly to diagnosis and management of uterine dystocia (ineffective labor) and to fetal monitoring. It is performed when safe vaginal delivery is questionable or immediate delivery is crucial because of threatened well-being of the mother or fetus. Indications may include hemorrhage, placenta previa, abruptio placentae, toxemia, fetal malpresentation, disproportion of fetus to birth canal, chorioamnionitis, genital herpes in the mother within six weeks of delivery, fetal distress, prolapsed cord, or previous cesarean birth. However, the traditional rule "once a section, always a section" is no longer true. Selected patients are now able to deliver vaginally following a section with a low uterine segment transverse incision, but delivery should be done only in situations where immediate surgical intervention is possible. The risk of uterine scar rupture during labor is not as great as was formerly believed. To reduce incidence of C-section, planning for twin pregnancy, breech presentation, and high-risk mothers should be individualized. Regional perinatal care centers have drastically changed the care of high-risk patients. Some educational programs offer cesarean childbirth classes.

Cesarean delivery may be scheduled or an emergency. Severe unexplained complications during late pregnancy or labor which adversely affect the mother or fetus, for example, massive third trimester bleeding or severe fetal distress, create an emergency. In these patients, preparations must be rapid. The patient easily senses a loss of control, especially if she participated in a childbirth education program for vaginal delivery. She needs special support. Most mothers fear more for the survival of the fetus than for themselves.

Admission procedures vary. Some hospitals admit an elective patient the morning of surgery. The patient is prepared by maternity personnel and taken to the OR or to an OR in the delivery suite. An emergency patient may go directly to the OR from the labor area. The trend is to perform C-sections in the obstetric suite. In any situation, the pediatrician and neonatal personnel from the nursery are notified before operation, to resuscitate and care for the infant in the OR. Sterile pediatric equipment and supplies must be available instantly. Notification is a responsibility of the circulating nurse and/or obstetrician. The circulating nurse must also communicate with the obstetrical unit where the patient will go.

Oxygen consumption increases about 20 percent during pregnancy, and as much as 100 percent above normal during labor in response to increased metabolic demand. Hypoxia and hypercapnia develop very rapidly. Fetal oxygenation varies in direct relation to that of the mother in normal and abnormal situations. In treating fetal distress, continuous 100% oxygen is administered to the mother until delivery or relief of the distress. Hypo- and hyperventilation are potentially harmful because they induce hypoxemia and hypercarbia in both the parturient and fetus. Maternal hypotension and hypovolemia diminish uterine blood flow and fetal perfusion. Hypoxia and acidosis threaten fetal well-being. Fetal acid-base status is the difference between scalp capillary and umbilical artery blood. The mother is safeguarded by appropriate anesthetic technique and selection of drugs. The fetus is protected by adequate uteroplacental perfusion and fetal monitoring.

Setup Routine laparotomy skin prep, drape, and setup are used. Instruments are essentially those for major gynecological laparotomy with addition of delivery forceps, cord clamp, and aspirant bulb for the infant. Foley catheter provides intraoperative bladder drainage. The patient should not be left alone in the holding area or OR. Fetal heart rate and uterine contractions are monitored continually. *The procedure involves care of two patients.*

Position Uterine displacement to the left during transport and until after delivery is necessary to shift the uterus away from pelvic vessels. Positional effect on cardiac output is of major importance in avoiding maternal hypotension and maintaining fetal well-being. In supine position, the enlarged uterus compresses the inferior vena cava and aorta, resulting in diminished venous return to the heart, stroke volume, and cardiac output. Operative position is supine with the right side slightly elevated by a wedge to tilt the uterus to the left. The OR table may be tilted 30° to the left. Slight Trendelenburg's position assists venous return.

Anesthesia Conduction anesthesia is most commonly employed. Anesthesia is selected on an individual basis, however. Regional is advantageous in diabetics because of reduced metabolic expenditure, low incidence of vomiting, and earlier return to oral intake. It is also advantageous for the asthmatic or sickle cell anemia patient. General anesthesia is advised when mother or fetus are in jeopardy and delivery is crucial, as in the presence of hemorrhage or severe fetal distress. Choice also depends on reason for operation, degree of urgency, and patient's condition and wish. The anesthesiologist chooses the method safest for mother and fetus. Gastric motility and emptying is inhibited by fear, pain, labor, and narcotic administration. Emergency patients may have eaten recently. *A parturient should always be regarded as having a full stomach.*

Spinal or epidural anesthesia allows the mother to see her newborn in the OR. It also reduces neonatal depression and risk of maternal aspiration. Hypotension is treated with intravenous infusion and/or ephedrine given in IV increments. Ephedrine, mephentermine (Wyamine), and metaraminol (Aramine) do not cause undesired uterine vasoconstriction. Other vasopressors can cause fetal hypoxia. Placentally transmitted drugs depressant to the fetus are avoided. A single injection of morphine may be given through the epidural catheter at conclusion of operation. With injection into the pain path, the drug significantly reduces postoperative pain for 24 to 36 hours with minimal side effects.

General anesthesia provides more rapid induction, less hypotension, greater cardiovascular stability, and better control of airway and ventilation. Preoxygenation precedes induction. Rapid-sequence induction and intubation is used. Pressure to the cricoid during intubation occludes the esophagus to prevent regurgitation. Induction to delivery (I-D) and uterine incision to delivery (UI-D) intervals must be minimized. I-D time is directly related to fetal hypoxia. UI-D intervals greater than three minutes may lead to lower pH of blood, and depression of infant from altered uteroplacental perfusion. All efforts are made to deliver the newborn as rapidly as possible consistent with safety, to minimize anesthesia and operating time, and to protect the fetus. With general anesthesia, all preparations, such as patient skin prep and gowning and gloving, are done prior to induction.

Incision and Delivery Low transverse Pfannenstiel's or low or high midline vertical incision is made. Length varies with size of the fetus. Dissection is expeditious. Suction must be ready for amniotic fluid. Uterus is incised while the bladder is retracted. Retractors are removed and fetal head is gently delivered as pressure is applied to the fundus. Immediately on emergence of the head, the nares and mouth are aspirated with a bulb syringe to clear them of amniotic fluid. Cesarean newborns have respiratory secretions. Delivery is completed and umbilical cord is clamped and cut. The newborn is transfered via a sterile sheet to the neonatal resuscitation team.

After delivery of the shoulders, IV oxytocin is administered to the mother to promote uterine contraction, minimize blood loss, and facilitate expulsion of the placenta and membranes. The placenta is delivered and placed in a specimen basin. The uterine fundus is palpated for firmness and massaged as necessary to prevent hemorrhage from relaxation. The patient is returned to horizontal supine position. The uterine incision is closed and hemostasis assured. After inspection of the pelvic organs and possible tubal ligation, the peritoneum and abdominal incision are closed.

Intraoperative assessment is the same as for any major surgical patient. However, sponges, tapes, and needles are counted before closure of the uterus and again before closure of the peritoneum and skin.

Postpartum surveillance of the patient is essential. Lochia is observed. Abnormal bleeding, such as rapid saturation of the perineal pad, is reported and recorded. Nurses' notes should include mother's contact with the infant, emotional reaction to operation, and persons in attendance, in addition to the physical information.

The Neonate Immediate postdelivery care is given in the OR by the neonatal team. The baby is taken to the nursery after careful examination by a pediatrician. The neonate traditionally has been evaluated by the Apgar score, acid-base status, and neurobehavioral examination. Apgar score is an excellent screening tool for vital functions immediately after birth, but subtle effect of drugs may be overlooked. The Neurologic and Adaptive Capacity Score does not use noxious stimuli but emphasizes neonatal tone. Use of drugs and dosages during labor and delivery which will produce significant neurobehavioral changes in the newborn must be avoided.

In the newborn, apical or umbilical pulse is the most accurate. Oxygenation is extremely important. Too little oxygen, hypoxia, can lead to intracranial hemorrhage, brain damage, or necrotizing enterocolitis. Too much oxygen, hyperoxia, can cause bronchopulmonary dysplasia or retrolental fibroplasia.

Father in OR Paternal participation in the birthing process is well-established for vaginal delivery, to provide support to the mother, a family-centered birth, and immediate bonding with the infant. However, presence of the father in the OR during cesarean delivery is not universal. Hospitals adopting this policy report favorable experiences. Valid concerns include increased risk of postpartum infection and team responsibility for handling adverse physical reaction, accident, injury, or behavior of the father. Paternal presence during operation must be approved by the obstetrician. The father is informed of the conditions permitting and excluding his presence. Those who have attended a structured childbirth education course have more understanding of pregnancy and birth. In compliance with hospital policy, donning of OR attire and supervised hand wash with antiseptic scrub agent before entrance to the OR are mandatory. A request signed by both parents may be essential. After delivery the father may choose to accompany the baby to the newborn examining area or stay with the mother. If condition of newborn permits, both baby and father can rejoin the mother in the OR or in the recovery room for this critical period of the family-centered experience.

In Vitro Fertilization

Infertility, lack of a couple's ability to have a biological child after one year of knowledgeable attempt, can be physically and emotionally devastating. Both husband and wife undergo extensive testing to determine etiology of the problem. Possible causes may be organic or functional. These include structural defect in either partner, e.g., irreparable tubal damage; past infections; genetic and/or immunologic abnormalities; endocrine imbalance or deficit; hostile cervix; female antibodies to sperm; endometriosis; exposure to diethylstilbestrol (DES) in utero; or inadequate number, quality, or mobility of sperm. Tubal occlusion is the most frequent indication for in vitro fertilization.

The perioperative nurse is an integral member of the team that aids in achieving pregnancy and live birth of a mature live infant through in vitro fertilization. The first birth from in vitro fertilization and embryo transfer occurred in England in 1980. The procedure is accepted therapy for women with severely damaged or nonfunctioning fallopian tubes, husbands with scarcity or absence of live spermatazoa in semen, or infertility of unknown cause. In vitro fertilization refers to removal of ovum from the prospective mother at the proper time, placement in a culture dish, and addition of sperm from the prospective father in hope that under controlled conditions fertilization will take place. The fertilized embryo is subsequently transferred to the mother's uterine cavity. In vitro means "in glass." The process is carried out in a culture dish or test tube, as opposed to in vivo, which means in the living organism.

Preoperative Determinations

1 Evidence of ovulation.

2 Normal uterine cavity and accessible ovary, evaluated by screening laparoscopy to evaluate pelvis and endometrial biopsy to assess tissue normalcy and estrogen levels, and a hysterosalpingogram to show uterine cavity.

3 Normal male factor. Semen analysis to check sperm.

Contraindications include uterine myoma, only one cornu, or septate uterus.

Induction of Ovulation Following screening, the first step is to time the ovulatory cycle. From the fifth to the ninth day of the menstrual cycle, the patient takes clomiphene citrate, a synthetic hormone to stimulate development of multiple ovarian follicles. Maturation of several ova improves chances of retrieving at least one. Ova harvested from the graafian follicle must be mature or they will not divide normally and fertilize properly. During drug therapy the patient is monitored to determine when an ovum is ready to be harvested. Serum estradiol is measured daily. Estradiol is the hormone produced by granulosa cells which surround ova and envelop the entire follicle. Size of developing follicles also is monitored daily by ultrasonic examination. Just before maturity, about the thirteenth day of the cycle, the patient is given human chorionic gonadotropin by injection to mimic rise in systemic luteinizing hormone, which causes final maturation and induces release of the follicle. About 36 hours later, laparoscopy is performed for retrieval of mature ovum or ova before spontaneous ovulation occurs.

Ovum Retrieval Usually an ambulatory procedure, laparoscopy is performed with the patient in supine position under general anesthesia. Equipment includes the usual laparoscopy setup plus an ovum retrieval needle kit, culture medium, test tubes, flushing medium, and grasping forceps. The instruments must be kept at normal physiologic temperature [98.6°F (37°C)]. The laparoscope is supported by a self-retaining retractor. The surgeon visualizes the ovaries. To harvest the ovum, the mature egg follicle is punctured with a special 8-in. × 14-gauge needle. Ovum and surrounding fluid are aspirated directly into a test tube through a catheter attached to the needle. As the clear fluid enters the test tube, the ovum may appear as a white speck. To avoid contamination, the egg and fluid are not exposed to the environment. After completion of aspiration, the circulating nurse labels the specimen. It is immediately taken to the laboratory for confirmation of ovum retrieval while instrumentation is still in place in the patient. The laboratory immediately reports back to the OR. If report is negative, the search for another ovum continues until the lab gives a positive response of retrieval. Multiple oocytes can be fertilized and embryos may be stored in frozen state for later implantation, if desired. During laparoscopy, contact with the uterus is avoided to prevent uterine irritation.

The procedure is completed and the patient moved to the recovery room. Postoperative care is the same as following any laparoscopy, but the patient may experience more discomfort because of abdominal manipulation. Minimal vaginal bleeding and high level of anxiety are normal reactions. The patient is discharged after meeting discharge criteria and receiving written postoperative instructions and information about follow-up.

Fertilization What normally happens to the egg in the fallopian tube is simulated in the laboratory. The aspirated ovum is placed in a culture dish containing a nutrient mixture similar to tubal secretions at midcycle, which prepares the egg for fertilization. Fresh semen, or a previously collected specimen frozen at the sperm bank, is added to the ovum. The culture dish is placed in an incubator for 36 to 40 hours for fertilization to take place. If the egg is fertilized, cell division will be detected by microscopic examination. When four-to-eight-cell embryonic development has occurred, the embryo is ready for transfer to the patient's uterus.

Embryo Transfer and Implantation The patient returns to hospital for embryo transfer. Instrumentation includes Graves speculum to expose cervix, single-toothed tenaculum to grasp cervix, and long smooth forceps to wipe mouth of uterus to cleanse it prior to implantation. Sterile technique is used, but the procedure may be performed in a nonsterile environment. The patient, supported by the nurse, is placed in knee-chest position for the media to approach the uterine fundus by gravity. A narrow catheter threaded through a metal cannula is used to transfer the fertilized egg into the upper uterine fundus. This catheter, which contains the embryo and culture medium, is prepared by the laboratory. The procedure is painless, requiring no anesthesia or cervical dilatation. The patient remains in knee-chest position with instrumentation in place while laboratory personnel check to be certain the embryo is gone from the catheter. Immediately following embryo transfer the patient is given an injection of progesterone, necessary for implantation. The patient remains in knee-chest position or on the abdomen with pillows under the abdomen from knee to breast for six to eight hours to prevent loss of the embryo. During the next 12 to 15 days she receives a daily injection of progesterone. The embryo must implant itself into the uterus to become a fetus and to grow and develop. The patient's own ovarian function sustains early gestation. Sonography reveals intrauterine gestation. The patient is referred to a high-risk pregnancy obstetrician.

About 20 percent of conceptuses become implanted in the uterus for pregnancy. Failure to implant may be due to escape of the embryo from the uterus with removal of the catheter, excess uterine contractility, inadequate luteal phase affecting the endometrium, mechanical disturbance of the endometrium, or encapsulation of embryo in blood or mucus.

In vitro fertilization is an expensive, time-consuming, and often frustrating trial-and-error last-option procedure. Many implants may precede favorable outcome. Nevertheless, the procedure has fulfilled hope for many couples worldwide.

Vaginal Ovum Retrieval In a nonsurgical method of obtaining ova for in vitro fertilization, a 10-in. needle is inserted through the vaginal wall under local anesthesia. While watching ultrasound imaging, the surgeon penetrates the ovary with the needle and gently suctions out the mature egg cells. Before undergoing the procedure the patient receives fertility drugs to induce production of more than one ovum. Used in selectively difficult patients with extensive scarring whose ovaries are inaccessible by conventional approach, vaginal approach carries a risk of accidental perforation of internal organs, such as the bladder. Fewer ova are removed per procedure as compared with the number typically removed through the surgical approach.

In Vivo Fertilization and Embryo Transfer

Research continues in in vivo fertilization by artificial insemination of semen from a male to fertilize an ovum in a fertile female. The embryo is then transferred to the uterus of the infertile female who brings the pregnancy to term and gives birth. This procedure may be used for women with damaged tubes or without ovaries.

Prenatal Testing

Potentially useful for management of some congenital developmental disorders or genetic defects, prenatal diagnostic studies are performed during pregnancy in selected patients. Disorders in the fetus may be cause for therapeutic abortion, elective cesarean delivery, or intrauterine fetal surgery.

Ultrasonography Ultrasound is the standard tool for fetal imaging in utero. This noninvasive technique permits accurate location of placenta and reliable diagnosis of structural defects, e.g., hydrocephalus or spina bifida.

Amniocentesis Amniocentesis is aspiration of amniotic fluid from the amniotic sac, under ultrasound direction at 16 to 20 weeks gestation, for chromosomal analysis. This highly accurate test is indicated for known or suspected risk of chromosome abnormality due to advanced maternal age, known parental translocation carrier, or history of previous pregnancy with chromosomal defect in the fetus or infant. Maternal serum alpha-fetoprotein measurement can predict neural-tube disorders, e.g., meningomyelocele in the fetus.

Fetoscopy Fetoscopy permits direct visualization of the fetus. A fiberoptic needle scope (fetoscope) is inserted into the amniotic cavity to view fetal parts, biopsy skin, or sample fetal blood. The fetoscope is 1.7 mm in diameter with a visual field of 70°. To ensure an adequate volume of amniotic fluids, fetoscopy is done after 16 weeks of pregnancy. Because of intent to view specific structures, position of the fetus must first be determined and the procedure performed under sonographic visualization. Placental localization is important, especially in the area of umbilical cord insertion. Hemoglobinopathies and coagulation problems, for example, hemophilia, may be rapidly diagnosed by aspiration of fetal blood from the placenta or umbilical cord insertion. Biopsies may detect congenital skin disorders and albinism. Direct viewing of the fetus may reveal characteristic abnormalities of various congenital syndromes. The procedure is not without complications, and should be employed only by trained physicians when genetic information is critical.

Intrauterine Fetal Surgery

Improvement and expansion in prenatal diagnosis has led to rapidly developing antenatal surgical intervention, *intrauterine fetal surgery.* The aim is to provide optimal prenatal development, a crucial factor in determination of ultimate health. For example, diagnostic screening by sonogram during gestation reveals abnormalities heretofore diagnosed postdelivery. Some medical disorders can be treated in utero. Other conditions fall within the province of the surgeon. Prerequisites for fetal therapy include accurate diagnosis, known pathophysiology, workable treatment, and technical capability. Radiologists, perinatologists, pediatric surgeons, anesthesiologists, and perioperative nurses comprise fetal surgery teams.

Most correctable malformations may be detected in utero but are best remedied by operation after delivery at term. The full-term infant is a better operative risk than is the fetus. Other anomalies, such as giant omphalocele or conjoined twins, can cause dystocia or require cesarean delivery. Operative treatment in utero is reserved for fetuses in which impaired organ development could be normal if treated, e.g., obstructive hydrocephalus, diaphragmatic hernia, or bilateral hydronephrosis due to urethral obstruction. As these complex procedures are attempted, OR nurses may participate in preoperative patient assessment and coordination of efforts intraoperatively.

CHAPTER **23**

UROLOGY

"Urology is that branch of medicine and surgery concerned with the study, diagnosis, and treatment of abnormalities and diseases of the urogenital tract of the male and the urinary tract of the female. The practice of urology involves, aside from routine diagnostic and surgical work, special knowledge and skills in the treatment of pediatric urologic problems, infections of the urinary tract, infertility and sterility, male sexual problems, renal dialysis and renal transplantation, renal hypertension, endocrine problems as they relate to the adrenal, testes and prostate, and cancer immunology and therapy. Because of shared responsibility in patient care with pediatricians, internists, nephrologists, endocrinologists, surgeons, and chemotherapists, close association with specialists in these disciplines is essential."*

DEVELOPMENT OF UROLOGY

Writings that date back to 3000 B.C. tell of urinary diseases. The earliest known specimen of a bladder stone was found in the grave of an Egyptian dating back to 4000 B.C. Around 2000 B.C. people in India are known to have suffered from bladder stones. Removal of a stone from the bladder through an incision is one of the earliest known operations. It was often performed by itinerant lithotomists, who flourished from the time of Hippocrates to the early eighteenth century. Hippocrates wrote that he did not remove stones but left them for those trained for such work. For centuries this operation was not considered a part of surgery.

While enlarged prostates were noted in the time of Hippocrates, the attempts to remove part of them perineally during lithotomy or to tunnel through them with a sharp instrument were extremely dangerous.

Urethral sounds and bronze catheters were found in the ruins of Pompeii, buried since 79 A.D. Metal catheters were used until the advent of rubber ones in the late nineteenth century.

The first urologists were mainly venereologists and "instrumenteurs" of the urethra. However first attempts to visualize the interior of the bladder were not made until the early nineteenth century. But the source of light and the instruments were inadequate. In 1876, Nitze, an Austrian, developed an instrument that is the basis of our modern cystoscope and urologic endoscopy.

Urologists have contributed to the evolution of medicine in general. Swick's development of intravenous pyelography is the foundation of modern angiography. Huggins opened a new vista to oncology when he identified that prostatic cancer was not fully autonomous. The use of antibacterial drugs by urologists freed all physicians from time-consuming treatment of venereal disease. Urology has been and continues to be a supporting speciality within medicine and surgery and is interdependent with other specialties.

*Definition of the American Board of Urology.

ANATOMY OF THE URINARY TRACT

The urinary system provides the vital life-sustaining functions of extracting waste products from the bloodstream and excreting them from the body. Organs of this system include bilateral kidneys and ureters, the bladder, and urethra (see Fig. 23-1).

The *kidneys* are large bean-shaped glandular organs located bilaterally in the retroperitoneal space of the thoracolumbar region behind the abdominal cavity. Each kidney is enclosed in a thin fibrous capsule. The *renal parenchyma,* the substance of the kidney within the capsule, is composed of an external cortex and internal medulla. The *medulla* consists of conical segments called *renal pyramids.* Each pyramid and its surrounding cortex forms a lobe. Within these pyramids are the essential components of renal function: the nephrons.

Each *nephron* consists of a glomerulus, glomerular capsule, and tubules. A *glomerulus* is an aggregation of capillaries formed by an afferent branch of the renal artery. These capillaries unite to form an efferent vessel. This capillary network is enclosed in a *glomerular capsule* (capsule of Bowman), which is the dilated beginning of the *renal tubule.* From the capsule, the tubule becomes tortuous and forms the proximal convoluted tubule. The distal portion forms the descending and ascending limbs of the *medullary loop* (loop of Henle). Nitrogenous wastes, salts, toxins, and water filtered from the capillary network form urine that flows through the medullary loop into the collecting tubule. The collecting tubules converge at the papilla (apex) of each renal pyramid. Urine flows continuously from each papilla into a *calyx.* Each kidney has between four and thirteen minor calices leading into two or three, rarely four, major calices that form the renal pelvis. The *renal pelvis* forms the dilated proximal end of the ureter.

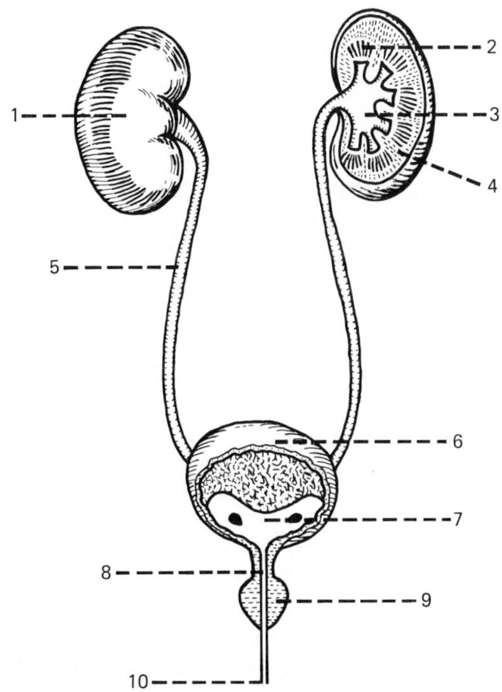

FIGURE 23-1
Male urinary tract: (1) renal capsule of kidney, (2) renal calyx, (3) renal pelvis, (4) renal cortex, (5) ureter, (6) bladder wall, (7) trigone of internal bladder between ureteral orifices and bladder neck, (8) urethra, (9) prostate, (10) urinary meatus.

The *ureters* are connecting tubes, 4 to 5 mm in diameter and about 12 in. (27 to 30 cm) long, between the kidneys and bladder. They lie bilaterally beneath the parietal peritoneum and descend along the posterior abdominal wall to the pelvic brim. From there, they pass along the lateral wall of the pelvis and curve downward, forward, and inward along the pelvic floor to the bladder. The wall of each ureter is composed of mucous membrane, longitudinal and circular muscles, and an outer layer of fibrous and elastic tissue. Slow, rhythmic, peristaltic contractions carry urine from kidneys to bladder.

The *bladder* is a hollow muscular reservoir lined with mucous membrane located in the anterior pelvic cavity behind the symphysis pubis. The ureters enter the bladder wall obliquely on each side. The triangular area between ureteral and urethral orifices is called the *trigone.* Valves formed by folds of mucous membrane in the bladder wall prevent backflow of urine into the ureters. Urine collects in the bladder until nerve stimulus causes micturition (urination) through the urethra. This stimulus opens the muscle fibers that form an internal sphincter at the *bladder neck,* the vesicourethral junction.

The *urethra* in the male is about 8 in. (20 cm) long and consists of three portions: prostatic, membranous, and cavernous. The *prostatic urethra* passes from the bladder orifice to the pelvic floor through the prostate gland. The *membranous urethra* passes through the pelvic floor to the penis. The *bulbous and anterior urethra* pass through the penis to the external urethral orifice. The membranous and anterior urethra also serve as passageway for excretions from the male reproductive system.

The female urethra is about 1½ in. (3.5 cm) long. It is firmly embedded posteriorly in the anterior vaginal wall.

An obstruction to blood flow in the renal arteries or in any part of the urinary system can cause renal damage, ultimately resulting in uremia (biochemical imbalance) or renal failure, if undiagnosed and untreated. Vascular hypertension, tumors, infection, trauma, and other systemic or neurogenic disorders are of major concern to the urologist.

UROLOGIC ENDOSCOPY

Cystoscopic diagnostic and some conservative urologic procedures approached through the urethra are performed in an especially designed and equipped area, often referred to as the *cysto room* or *suite.* This may be within the OR suite or in the urology clinic. X-ray control booths and developing units are adjacent to or within the area. Because x-ray procedures are frequently performed, walls and doors of the room must be lead-lined.

All safety regulations apply in the cysto room, just as they do elsewhere in the OR suite, to protect the welfare of the patients and personnel. All lighted instruments and electrical equipment should be checked for proper function before and after each use. Personnel who must remain in the room with the patient while x-rays are taken should wear lead aprons. Patients should be protected with gonadal shields whenever feasible.

Proper OR attire is worn by all personnel entering the room. Most urologists don a conductive water-repellent apron before scrubbing, unless sterile water-repellent gowns are provided. The urologist wears sterile gown and gloves. Procedures performed in the cysto room must maintain a sterile field. Adherence to all the principles of aseptic technique is mandatory to prevent nosocomial urinary tract infection.

Preparation of the Patient

1 The patient should be encouraged to drink fluids before coming to the cysto room, unless the procedure will be done under general or regional anesthesia. Fluids ensure a rapid collection of urine specimens from the kidneys.
2 Frequently procedures are done without anesthesia, with topical agents, or with local infiltration anesthesia. The patient should be reassured that the procedure usually can be performed with only mild discomfort. Respect the patient's modesty, and try to avoid embarrassing him or her.
3 Patient is assisted into lithotomy position with knees resting in padded knee supports. Pads avoid undue pressure in popliteal spaces. Some cystoscopic procedures are performed with patient in supine position.
4 The drainage pan is pulled out of the lower break of the urologic table after patient's legs are positioned on knee supports and foot of the table is lowered.

   NOTE. The urologic table differs from the standard operating table in that it must provide an x-ray unit with a film cassette holder, a drainage pan, and knee supports. Some tables are equipped with hydraulic or electric controls to adjust height and tilt, tray attachments for the light source and electrosurgical unit, and hooks for irrigating solution containers.

5 The pubic region, external genitalia, and perineum are mechanically cleansed with an antiseptic agent according to routine skin preparation procedure (refer to Chap. 16). Warm solution before applying it to an unanesthetized patient.
6 Topical anesthetic agents are instilled into urethra at end of prep procedure. A viscous liquid preparation of lidocaine hydrochloride, 1 or 2%, may be used. This medium remains in urethra rather than flowing into bladder.
   a *For female.* The female urethra is most sensitive at the meatus. Thus, a small sterile cotton applicator dipped into the anesthetic agent and placed with cotton tip in the meatus is sufficient. It is removed when the urologist is ready to introduce an instrument.
   b *For male.* A disposable cylinder with an acorn tip is used for intraurethral insertion. Agent is injected into urethra and the penis compressed with a penile clamp for a few minutes to retain drug.
7 A sterile stainless steel filter screen is placed over the drainage pan. The patient is draped as for other perineal procedures in lithotomy position. The urologist may want to have access to the rectum. A disposable O'Connor sheet is

used. This has a synthetic rubber rectal sheath that protects the finger during rectal palpation. The perineal sheet has two fenestrations: one exposes the genitalia; the other fits over the screen on the drainage pan. A gauze filter is incorporated into this latter fenestration in a disposable cystoscopy drape.

The urologist may prefer to wear a sterile disposable plastic apron over his or her gown. Attached to the table, this provides a sterile field from the urologic table to the urologist's shoulders. A receptor kit that attaches to the apron eliminates the need for the drainage pan. Tissue specimens are collected as irrigating fluid passes through a collecting basket.

Urologic Endoscopes

Urologic endoscopic instruments and catheters are available in sizes to suit infants, children, and adults. Size of these instruments and catheters is measured on the French scale: the diameter in millimeters multiplied by 3. Ureteral catheters are available in sizes 3 to 14 French, as described on page 454. The smallest is 1 mm in diameter times 3, or 3 French.

Specific endoscopic equipment is required to perform all the procedures under the broad term *cystoscopies.* All urologic endoscopes have the same basic components as follows.

Sheath The hollow sheath may be concave, convex, or straight in configuration at the distal end inserted into the urethra. The other end has a stopcock attachment for irrigation. Sizes range from 11 French for infants to 30 French for adults. Within the sheath, space is provided to accommodate instruments for work in the bladder or urethra. Other instruments and catheters can be inserted through the sheath into the ureters and kidneys for purposes of diagnosis or treatment.

Obturator The stainless steel obturator, inserted into the sheath, occludes the opening and facilitates introduction into the urethra without trauma to the mucosal lining.

Telescope Telescopes are complex precision optical systems. Each telescope contains multiple, finely ground optical lenses that relay the image from the distal end inside the bladder or urethra to the ocular of the urologist. Additional rod-shaped elements, known as *field lenses,* are between each pair of relay lenses. Properly spaced throughout the length of the telescope, the lenses give an undistorted clear vision at the desired angle with some magnification. Telescopes are costly delicate instruments that must be handled gently at all times. The optical systems provide several angles of vision:

1 Direct forward or 0° vision is useful for viewing urethra, and for use with optical urethrotome.

2 Right angle is most suitable for viewing the entire bladder, and for ureteral catheterization.

3 Lateral, which deviates 70° but includes right angle in line of vision, is used for wide-angle viewing within the bladder.

4 Foroblique, which is a forward vision with an oblique view somewhat in front of right angle, is used to examine the urethra, and for transurethral operative procedures.

5 Retrospective, which provides an approximate 55° angle of retrograde vision, is used to inspect the bladder neck.

All telescopes are stainless steel with a Bakelite ocular. Some have operating or working elements incorporated into them.

Light The light source may be either a fiberoptic bundle or an incandescent bulb (see Chap. 19). This may be an integral part of the sheath or the telescope. A cord connects instrument to a fiberoptic projection lamp, rheostat, or battery. Fiberoptics have largely replaced incandescent lamps.

Types of Urologic Endoscopes While many different urologic endoscopes and accessories are in use, only the most commonly used are described.

Brown-Buerger Cystoscope The stainless steel sheaths range in size from 14 to 26 French. Size 21 French is used most frequently in adults with a right-angle examination telescope for routine inspection of the bladder. Size 24 or 26 French is used to accommodate larger instruments and catheters that cannot be used through size 21. The sheath contains the light carrier.

A Brown-Buerger cystoscope set usually consists of two sheaths, one concave and one convex, each with its own obturator, and two or three right-angle telescopes. Along with the basic examination telescope, the set may have a combination operating and double catheterizing telescope, known as a *convertible telescope,* or the operating and double catheterizing functions may be in separate telescopes. The convertible operating and catheterizing telescopes have a small deflectable lever on the distal end to aid in directing ureteral catheters or flexible stone baskets into the ureters (see pp. 453 and 454). All corresponding parts of each set must be the same French size.

McCarthy Panendoscope The stainless steel sheaths range in size from 14 to 30 French. These are used most frequently with the foroblique telescope for viewing the urethra. Other telescopes are available for bladder visualization. The telescopes are interchangeable with all sizes of sheaths. A bridge assembly is required to fit the telescope properly to the sheath. The light is supplied through the telescope.

Wappler Cystourethroscope The Wappler cystourethroscope combines the functions of the Brown-Buerger cystoscope and the McCarthy panendoscope. The stainless steel sheaths range in size from 17 to 24 French. The foroblique and lateral telescopes, which also supply the light, are interchangeable with all sheaths. A visual obturator may be used to permit visualization and irrigation during introduction of sheath into urethra.

NOTE. Verify with the urologist the type and size of the available endoscopes preferred for examination and/or treatment prior to placing instrumentation on sterile instrument table.

Resectoscope The resectoscope uses electric current to excise tissue from bladder, urethra, or prostate. Components of this instrument include the sheath, obturator, telescope, working element, and cutting electrode. The sheath, usually 24 to 28 French, must be made of Bakelite or fiberglass to prevent short circuit of the electric current. If the short beak post sheath is used with a wide-angle telescope, a Timberlake obturator must be used to introduce sheath into urethra.

The working element of the resectoscope, inserted through the sheath, has a channel for the telescope and cutting electrode. The types of working elements differ by the method in which the cutting electrode moves.

1 The *Iglesias* resectoscope uses a thumb control on a leaf spring-lock mechanism. The working element can be adapted for simultaneous irrigation and suction to control hydraulic pressure in the bladder.

2 The *Nesbit* resectoscope uses a thumb control on a spring.

3 The *Baumrucker* resectoscope uses finger control on a sliding mechanism.

4 The *Stern-McCarthy* resectoscope uses a rack and pinion to move the loop forward and back. This requires two hands.

The cutting electrode is the most critical component of a resectoscope. Because it must both cut and coagulate tissue, the electrode must be stabilized in the working element so that it retracts properly into the sheath after each cut. The electrode has a cutting loop from which electric current is passed through tissue, an insulated fork, an insulated stem, and a contact that is inserted into the working element. Several loop sizes are available; the stem is usually color-coded by size. Loop size corresponds to French size of the sheath. The electrode is malleable; therefore, it must be checked before use to be certain insulation is intact and the loop is not broken. Electric current is applied only when loop is engaged in tissue and inactivated after a cut is completed. The sheath can be charred if electric current is maintained after the cutting loop has been retracted into it.

Conductive lubricants must never be used on the sheath. They may provide a pathway for electric current. Cleanliness of the sheath and all other components is essential to proper function.

Electrodes

In addition to the cutting loops used with the resectoscope primarily for transurethral resections, other types of electrodes are used in the bladder. These are inserted through the operating telescope of the Brown-Buerger cystoscope or Wappler cystourethroscope. They are used mainly for fulguration of bladder tumors, coagulation of bladder vessels to control bleeding following biopsy, and ureteral meatotomy. More electric current is needed when working in solution, as in the bladder, than in air. The power control settings on the electrosurgical unit should be as low as possible, however. All precautions and safeguards for the use and care of electrosurgical equipment apply to urologic procedures (refer to Chap. 19). A spark-gap generator should be used for transurethral resection and fulguration, which require high-voltage arcing described as spray coagulation.

Lasers

Argon and Nd:YAG lasers can be adapted for use with cystoscopes (refer to Chap. 19). These are particularly useful for ablation of hemangiomas and vascular tumors in the bladder.

Irrigating Equipment

Continuous irrigation of the bladder is necessary during cystoscopy to:

1 Distend the bladder walls so that the urologist can visualize them
2 Wash out blood, bits of resected tissue, or stone fragments to permit continuous visibility and collection of specimens

A sterile disposable closed irrigating system is used because it prevents airborne contamination of the solution. Two to four or more liters of sterile irrigating solution may be needed for a single examination. Ten to twelve liters are needed for a transurethral resection (TUR, see p. 459). Disposable tandem sets may be used to connect several containers together. Tandem sets allow for a continuous flow and for replacement of containers without interruption of flow. Sterile disposable irrigating tubing is connected to the irrigating solution container before hanging it on a hook on the urologic table, in the ceiling, or on a stand placed beside the table. The solution container should be at a level 2½ ft (0.75 m) above the table: a lower level decreases flow; a higher level increases hydraulic pressure with consequent fluid absorption by patient's tissues. Tubing should be filled with solution before it is attached to sheath of the cystoscope or resectoscope. The plastic tubing from the container to the instrument is for individual patient use only.

Sterile isosmotic irrigating solutions that are nonhemolytic and nonelectrolytic are generally preferred by most urologists. However, sterile distilled water may be used for observation procedures and during resection or fulguration of bladder tumors. If a sufficient amount enters circulation through open blood vessels, water may hemolyze red blood cells. As much as three to six liters of solution may be absorbed during a transurethral prostatectomy. Minerals in water or saline act as a conductor and disperse the current when the electrosurgical unit is used. Saline must *never* be used.

Isosmotic solutions of 1.5% glycine, an amino acid, or sorbitol, an inert sugar, premixed in distilled water are commercially available in 1.5- and 3-liter containers. A glycine solution, Urogate or Uromatic, is more commonly used for TUR.

During the procedure, the flow of solution into the endoscope is controlled by the stopcock on the sheath where the tubing attaches. Rubber tips or nipples are used to seal other openings on the instrument to prevent escape of solution during a procedure. The openings through which catheters or instruments are to be inserted are closed with tips containing a hole. The accessory can be inserted through this hole with the seal maintained.

When the urologist wishes, the irrigating solution flows away from the instrument into the drainage pan through the filter screen. The solution drains from the pan, through tubing, into a collecting bucket that is emptied after each patient use. Some cysto rooms have floor drains. These may be a source of environmental contamination unless cleaned thoroughly. If large quantities of solution are used, observe the level of drainage into the bucket to avoid overflow on the floor or around the foot pedal of the electrosurgical unit.

Evacuators

Evacuators may be used to irrigate bladder and to aspirate stone fragments, blood clots, or resected tissue. The two most commonly used types are the Ellik and Toomey.

Ellik The Ellik is a double bowl-shaped glass evacuator containing a trap for fragments so that they cannot be washed back into the sheath of the endoscope while irrigating with pressure on the rubber-bulb attachment.

Toomey The Toomey is a syringe-type evacuator with a wide opening into the barrel. It may be used with any endoscope sheath. A metal adaptor permits its use with a catheter.

Care and Preventive Maintenance

1 Adequate sterilization is mandatory; therefore, all endoscopes and reusable accessories must be free of debris and residue.
   a Disassemble all parts and open all outlets.
   b Clean all parts in a warm nonresidue liquid-detergent solution, rinse in clean water, and dry thoroughly.

c Clean the interior of sheaths and openings with a soft brush.

d Wipe lenses gently with a soft, dry cloth.

2 Place endoscopes on a towel, to act as padding, in the sink, on countertops, and in trays to protect them from hard surfaces during handling and storage.

3 In cleaning the inside of a sheath or telescope, take care not to break the glass window over the light. These windows should be inspected each time the endoscopes are used, because the urethra may be lacerated by a broken window.

4 Check function of all moving parts, clarity of vision through telescopes, and patency of channels through instruments and catheters.

5 Keep sets of sounds, bougies, and filiforms and followers together so that the urologist will have a complete range of sizes readily accessible.

6 After cleaning, wrap items for sterilization. Flexible instruments should be protected by a rigid container.

7 Clean, dry stone baskets may be sealed in a peel-open package and sterilized in ethylene oxide gas. Retractable stone baskets must be sterilized in the open position.

8 The principles and methods of sterilization discussed in Chapter 8 apply to urologic instrumentation. Steam sterilizable items should be steam sterilized. However, with the exception of nylon and rubber catheters, bougies and nonflexible stainless steel instruments that do not have lenses, urologic endoscopes and accessories must be sterilized in ethylene oxide gas or activated glutaraldehyde solution. All items should be sterilized after cleaning and then placed in sterile storage. Aeration following ethylene oxide sterilization is essential for Bakelite parts of endoscopes and for woven and synthetic materials.

SPECIAL FEATURES OF UROLOGIC SURGERY

The genitourinary tract is often referred to as the *GU tract.* Open operation is performed only after conservative treatment fails or examination of the GU tract confirms a condition that does not yield to this treatment. Fortunately, the majority of urologic conditions can be diagnosed and treated conservatively through a urologic endoscope and its accessories. The urologist performs open operations to repair, revise, reconstruct, or remove organs when a congenital or acquired condition will not respond to conservative therapy. Obstructive and neuromuscular disorders are common problems of the urinary tract.

Many patients seen by urologists are in the preadolescent and older age groups. Congenital and common pediatric problems are discussed in Chapter 33. This discussion focuses on adult problems. Most of these occur in men over 50 with prostatic disease. In middle age, renal calculus disease and tumors in the urinary tract are most commonly diagnosed. All these conditions may cause obstruction and subsequent infection in the kidneys, ureters, or bladder.

COMMON OPERATIONS IN URINARY TRACT

Kidney

Definitive renal operations are justified for management of renal neoplasms, large cystic lesions that compromise renal function and/or produce obstruction, inflammatory diseases that necessitate drainage, or renal vascular disease. The kidney is usually approached posteriorly with the patient in a lateral position elevated on the kidney rest. A flank incision is made parallel to and just below or over the eleventh and twelfth ribs. Sections of the ribs may be removed. The kidney is frequently approached trans- or thoracoabdominally, especially for tumors or trauma, when prompt control of blood supply is important.

Nephrectomy Removal of a kidney is indicated when tumor, chronic degenerative disease, or severe traumatic injury has produced irreparable damage to renal cells resulting in absence of renal function in one kidney.

Nephrectomy also is performed in the OR on a living donor (unilateral) or cadaver (bilateral) to harvest a kidney(s) for transplantation. Meticulous dissection is necessary to free the kidney, its blood vessels, and the ureter with minimal trauma. The ureter is dissected free and transected while the renal blood supply remains intact to ensure adequate urinary output. This operative procedure may last much longer than does the usual nephrectomy.

Bilateral nephrectomy may be indicated pretransplant for a patient maintained on chronic hemodialysis (see p. 451) but who has prolonged, severe hypertension. Following kidney transplantation, if rejection is uncontrollable, the patient may require transplant nephrectomy and return to chronic hemodialysis. This is less likely following transplant from a live donor than from a cadaver. Transplantation is discussed in Chapter 34.

Partial or Heminephrectomy Partial excision may be sufficient when one lobe has been destroyed by localized disease but the remainder of the kidney is functional.

Nephrostomy or Pyelostomy Incision through renal parenchyma or into renal pelvis may be necessary to establish temporary or permanent drainage when an obstruction prevents flow of urine from the kidney. A tube placed in the kidney exits through the skin. A cutaneous nephrostomy tube may be used to drain a kidney postoperatively during healing following renal reconstruction or revascularization. Silastic tubes placed internally through a cystoscope eliminate need for open operation for temporary urinary diversion. More frequently this is done percutaneously (see p. 452), under fluoroscopic or ultrasound guidance, by radiologist and/or urologist.

Pyeloplasty Revision or reconstruction of the renal pelvis is performed to relieve an anatomic obstruction in the flow of urine by creating a larger outlet from the renal pelvis into the ureter. This may be done to repair or excise damaged tissue so that kidney function will be restored without a partial or total nephrectomy.

Renal Hemodialysis *Hemodialysis* is the process of removing waste products from the blood of a patient in renal failure by diffusion through the semipermeable membrane of a *dialyzer* (artificial kidney machine). This treatment modality alleviates the acute manifestations of uremia and controls many of the chronic long-term complications of end-stage renal disease. Grossly undernourished and anemic patients with severe electrolyte imbalances must be adequately stabilized by hemodialysis prior to kidney transplantation. Some patients will remain on periodic weekly dialysis the remainder of their lives. Therefore, patients undergoing chronic dialysis must have a means of dialysis access established.

External Arteriovenous Shunt Shunts can be placed in either an arm or leg. The Quinton-Scribner shunt, the oldest and simplest device, consists of two Teflon tips attached to Silastic tubing. One tip is placed in the artery and the other in a nearby vein. Tubing from each tip is exteriorized through a subcutaneous tunnel to the skin and connected together. Blood flows from the artery to the vein between periods of dialysis. Variations and modifications of this basic external shunt are used. Each provides access to patient's circulation for hemodialysis. Clotting and infection are potential problems that must be avoided. Needles must never be inserted into the Silastic tubing. Blood samples must be obtained for blood-gas analysis under strict aseptic conditions.

Subcutaneous Arteriovenous Fistula An anastomosis, usually between the radial artery and the cephalic vein in the forearm, creates an arterialized peripheral vein that permits dialyzer connections to be made by venipuncture. Needles are placed in the venous limb of the fistula for blood outflow and return. Saphenous vein grafts may be used in either the arm or thigh to create an arteriovenous fistula.

Bovine Heterograft A segment of sterile processed bovine carotid artery is a biologically acceptable graft material that may be used to create an arteriovenous fistula in either the forearm or thigh. These grafts tolerate repeated venipuncture well. They are prepackaged sterile and are handled much like a human artery. They can be inserted under local anesthesia.

Patients with chronic renal failure can tolerate extensive operative procedures with minimal complications. Their management in the OR must include strict attention to maintenance of a patent dialysis access shunt or fistula, careful monitoring of fluid and electrolyte balance, and avoidance of postoperatve infections. Following kidney transplantation, the patient may require postoperative dialysis, so the access must remain patent during and after operation.

Renal Revascularization Stenotic lesions of the renal arteries are the predominant etiology in surgically correctable forms of hypertension. Renovascular reconstructive procedures (renal angioplasty) are designed to improve blood flow through the stenotic area to kidney, or to bypass stenotic area. Revascularization procedures may have a dual purpose: to correct hypertension and to preserve renal function. The patient is in supine position for these procedures because the renal arteries are approached through an abdominal incision.

In Situ Vascular Reconstructive Techniques Renal artery obstruction most often occurs from atherosclerotic stenosis at origin of the artery or fibromuscular dysplasia (abnormal development) confined to the main renal artery. The obstruction is most often resected and replaced by an aorto-renal-saphenous vein bypass graft. A reversed segment of proximal saphenous vein, gently distended and irrigated, is anastomosed first to aorta and then to renal artery. Prosthetic woven Dacron grafts may be used rather than an autogenous vein graft for renal artery bypass combined with distal aortic replacement (see Chap. 32 for discussion of vascular grafts). Segmental resection of diseased arterial segments with primary end-to-end anastomosis may be performed. However, thromboendarterectomy (see Chap. 32, p. 585) is more frequently performed than is the latter procedure. All these procedures may be performed bilaterally or as staged bilateral renal artery reconstructions. Percutaneous transluminal angioplasty may be preferred to these open procedures (see Chap. 32, p. 585).

Ex Vivo Extracorporeal Kidney Surgery When stenotic disease or other obstructive lesion extends into branches of the renal artery, in situ reconstruction may be difficult, hazardous, or impossible. In these patients, temporary nephrectomy with microvascular repair followed by autotransplantation of kidney may be performed. Referred to as *workbench surgery,* the kidney is completely mobilized from the retroperitoneal space. If one kidney is to be reconstructed, the ureter can remain intact and reconstruction performed on a sterile bench placed over patient's lower abdomen. For bilateral reconstruction, one kidney is detached from its ureter to permit complete removal from the abdomen. A second team works on contralateral kidney while other is reconstructed at an adjacent dissecting bench.

Extracorporeal perfusion is necessary for renal preservation during reconstruction. This may be accomplished either with perfusion of cold Ringer's lactate or other hyperosmolar solution by gravity flow, or with a continuous hypothermic perfusion through a Belzer pump machine. Or, simple cold storage in saline slush may be used for renal preservation.

A kidney may be autotransplanted into the patient's groin or pelvis for revascularization of the kidney, removal of renal tumors or calculi, or repair of ureteral injuries.

Traumatic Injury If a kidney is ruptured or injured by blunt trauma, bullet or stab wound, fatal or near-fatal hemorrhage may be associated with the accident. This requires immediate operation. The surgeon makes every effort to save kidney tissue and ureter. A Foley catheter is inserted to keep an output record as well as to check for presence of hematuria pre- and postoperatively. Gross hematuria preoperatively usually indicates injury of bladder or urethra. Kidney damage is diagnosed by the presence of blood seen microscopically.

Urolithiasis (Urinary Calculus)

A renal calculus, kidney stone, is a solid deposit or deposits (calculi) of minerals and salts that accumulate in the renal collecting system. Calculi may form as a result of a metabolic disorder. But more commonly they are concentrations of excess substances such as calcium oxalate, calcium phosphate, or uric acid in the blood that are filtered through the kidneys, or crystals of salts that form around fragments of organic matter as from chronic infection. Renal colic is perhaps the most intense pain experienced by human beings. It is due to a calculus or fragments of calculi partially or completely obstructing the calices or renal pelvis. Renal calculi frequently dislodge and move from the renal pelvis into the ureter. A nidus, such as infection or an exposed suture postoperatively, can be the focal point for formation of a calculus in the ureter. If calculi are small enough they will pass into bladder and be voided. Those that remain lodged, causing obstruction to outflow from any part of the urinary tract, must be removed. Preservation of renal function is the primary objective of operations for urolithiasis. *Lithotomy* is removal of a calculus. *Lithotripsy* is fragmentation of a stone followed by removal. *Chemolysis* is dissolution with a chemical substance.

Percutaneous Nephrostolithotomy or Nephrolithotripsy Using fluoroscopy, a guide wire is introduced inside a transluminal angioplasty needle, through flank and into renal pelvis, carefully closing the access point. This may be done in the radiology department under local anesthesia. In the OR, dilators are placed over the guide wire to enlarge a nephrostomy tract for introduction of a nephrostomy tube or nephroscope. Either a rigid or a flexible fiberoptic scope may be used to visually inspect the renal collecting system. Renal calculi may be removed with stone baskets or forceps, or fragmented with lithotriptors. Lithotripsy is necessary for large calculi such as a staghorn calculus, which branches from renal pelvis into calices and may extend down into ureter.

Ultrasonic Lithotripsy An ultrasonic lithotriptor generates ultrasonic sound waves that shatter the calculus into fragments. These are removed by suction. This procedure is usually done under spinal or general anesthesia.

Electrohydraulic Lithotripsy An electrohydraulic lithotriptor creates an electric discharge in fluid. This discharge is transformed into a hydraulic shock wave. A calculus disintegrates when the probe is directed at it. Larger fragments may be removed with Randall stone forceps; smaller ones are flushed out with irrigation. A tube is left in the nephrostomy tract for continued irrigation for several days postlithotripsy. This procedure may be performed under local anesthesia with IV sedatives and analgesics.

Nephrolithotomy or Pyelolithotomy A large staghorn renal calculus that does not dislodge from the calices or renal pelvis may have to be removed through an open incision. A nephroscope may be used during the operation for direct visual examination of the nephrons to locate and remove residual calculi. Ultrasound may also be used to identify retained fragments. Localized hypothermia provides the surgeon with a bloodless operative field and extends the period of time in which the renal artery may safely be clamped without loss of renal function during search for and extraction of calculi.

Percutaneous Chemolysis Hemiacidrin may be instilled through a small nephrostomy tube to alkalinize cysteine and uric-acid calculi and dissolve debris remaining following other lithotomy procedures.

Extracorporeal Shock Wave Lithotripsy A noninvasive procedure, focused spark-induced shock waves fragment calculi within the kidney. After receiving epidural anesthesia, the patient is placed in a tank of water. The calculi must be visualized by x-ray to focus waves. Over a period of 30 to 60 minutes, 500 to 1500 shock waves produced by an underwater high-voltage condenser spark are synchronized with R waves of patient's ECG to avoid disrupting cardiac rhythm. A loud report sounds in the OR each time a spark is fired. Both patient and personnel must wear protective earplugs.

Percutaneous Ureterolithotomy A calculus originating from or lodged in the renal pelvis or upper tract of the ureter can be extracted or fragmented through a ureteropyeloscope, as described for percutaneous nephrolithotomy and lithotripsy.

Ureteral Stone Extraction A flexible-shaft basket-type stone dislodger (stone basket) is inserted into ureter through a cystoscope in the bladder for extraction of ureteral calculus. Several types of *stone baskets* are available, including the Dormia, Johnson, Levant, Pfister-Schwartz, and Lomac. These have a fine wire or nylon basket that can be expanded through the shaft to ensnare a calculus located in lower third of the ureter.

Stone baskets must be cleaned promptly after use in a nonresidue liquid-detergent solution to remove debris. Removable parts must be disassembled. Debris should be brushed *away* from the junction of basket and shaft with a small soft brush. During cleaning, inspection of the basket wires is critical. If they are cracked or broken at end closest to the shaft, the basket may be passed into the ureter but it cannot be withdrawn without trauma.

Ureterolithotomy If a calculus fails to pass spontaneously through the ureter or cannot be removed with a stone basket, open operation may be necessary. The patient is positioned for a lateral flank incision below the twelfth rib if the calculus is high in the ureter near the kidney. An abdominal incision is used to reach one in the lower segment near the bladder. When exposed, the ureter will be dilated proximal to the calculus and collapsed distal to it. The surgeon makes a small incision directly over the calculus and extracts it from the ureter with a stone forceps.

Cystolithotomy and Litholapaxy Calculi usually can be removed from the bladder through the urethra. Crushing a urinary calculus in the bladder is referred to as *litholapaxy* or *lithotrity.* A lithotrite, introduced into the bladder through the urethra, is used to pulverize and remove calculi. This may be an instrument with hinged jaws, an ultrasound lithotriptor, or an electrohydraulic lithotrite. The electrohydraulic lithotrite generates energy shock waves at the tip of a flexible probe inserted through a cystoscope. With either instrument a telescope enables the urologist to work under vision. The stone fragments are irrigated from the bladder.

If a litholapaxy is unsuccessful or contraindicated, the removal of a calculus by incision into the bladder may be necessary. This operation is a *cystolithotomy.*

NOTE. Following removal from any location in the GU tract, urinary calculi should be placed in a dry container and sent to pathology for chemical analysis.

Ureter

The ureters are the vital anatomic structures for the flow of urine produced in the kidneys to the bladder. An obstruction to urinary flow must be corrected or diverted. The ureters may be approached either through an endoscope or through open incision.

Ureteral Endoscopy Both rigid and flexible fiberoptic *ureteropyeloscopes* allow direct visualization of upper ureteral tumors, calculi, and strictures. These scopes are introduced percutaneously or cystoscopically. Strictures can be corrected by balloon dilatation. Ureteral calculi can be extracted with stone baskets or forceps, or fragmented with lithotriptors.

Percutaneous endoscopic techniques can be used in conjunction with cystoscopy. *Complete cystoscopy* implies that the procedure extends beyond the bladder into the ureters. This procedure may be performed for:

1 Drainage of the renal pelvis for differential diagnosis or renal function
2 Insertion of ureteral catheters to provide constant drainage for one or both kidneys or to outline ureters for a difficult pelvic operation
3 Insertion of a ureteral stent for internal drainage of an obstructed ureter
4 Dilation of a stricture in the ureter
5 Manipulation and removal of calculus
6 Ureteral meatotomy to enlarge the opening of one or both ureteral orifices into the bladder

The endoscopic instruments introduced into the urinary bladder were discussed (see p. 447). Only accessories used for diagnostic or therapeutic procedures within the ureters are mentioned here.

Ureteral Catheters Made of flexible woven nylon or other plastic material, ureteral catheters range in caliber from size 3 to 14 French and are about 30 in. (76 cm) long. Sterile, prepackaged, disposable catheters are available. Most are radiopaque so that they can be visualized on x-ray.

The urologist visualizes the ureteral orifice through the cystoscope. The catheter is then inserted through the scope and introduced into the ureter. The catheter has graduated markings in centimeters so that the urologist can judge the distance the catheter has been inserted. The urologist will request size and style of catheter tip best suited for the intended purpose. The most common tips are:

1 *Whistle tips,* which are used for drainage, as ureteral markers, or for injection of radiopaque contrast medium for retrograde pyelography (refer to Chap. 20, p. 390). Largest sizes are used to dilate ureters to facilitate passage of a calculus.
2 *Olive tips,* which may be used for same purposes as whistle tips.
3 *Round tips,* which may be preferred for drainage.
4 *Flexible filiform tips,* which may be used to bypass an obstruction for drainage.
5 *Blassuchi curved tips,* which may be used to bypass a ureteral stricture more easily than straight tips.
6 *Braasch bulb, whistle tips,* which are preferred to dilate ureter or to inject contrast medium for a ureterogram (refer to Chap. 20, p. 391).
7 *Acorn or cone tips,* which may be preferred for a ureterogram.
8 *Garceau tapered tips,* which are used to dilate ureter.

If left indwelling to provide drainage, ureteral catheters must be attached to a sterile closed urinary drainage system. Since they are smaller in diameter than standard urinary drainage catheters, an adaptor must be used. This may be a small rubber tip or nipple placed on one end of a straight connector or both ends of a Y connector. The catheters are put through the hole in the tip(s). The other end of connector is attached to constant drainage system with a piece of sterile tubing.

A separate drainage system for each catheter may be desired by the urologist. Each drainage container must be labeled to identify right and left ureteral catheters.

Ureteral Stent Catheter The Gibbons silicone indwelling stent catheter is inserted for long-term drainage in a wide variety of benign and malignant diseases causing ureteral obstruction. The stent is passed through the cystoscope over a ureteral catheter used as a guide. When the catheter guide is withdrawn, the stent remains fixed in the ureter for internal urinary drainage through the obstructed area.

Cutaneous Ureterostomy Diversion of urinary flow into the bladder can be accomplished by bringing end of the ureter closest to the bladder through the abdominal wall to the skin. Ureterostomy can be performed unilaterally or bilaterally with a single cutaneous stoma for permanent diversion or a double-loop stoma for temporary diversion. The patient must be fitted postoperatively with an appliance for collection of urine directly from the ureter to exterior of the body. This procedure may be performed as a temporary emergency measure following trauma to the bladder, such as a ruptured bladder.

Ureteroenterocutaneous Loops Bilateral transplantation of the ureters for permanent urinary diversion is performed when neoplasms, congenital anomalies, chronic infecton, trauma, or other etiology impairs bladder function. The ureters are implanted into the intestinal wall, or more commonly into an isolated segment or loop of the intestine. This loop becomes a conduit for urinary flow.

Ureterosigmoidostomy or Ureteroileosigmoidostomy The ureters may be anastomosed to a nonrefluxing segment of sigmoid colon. The ureteroileosigmoidostomy operation implants the ureters into an isolated segment of the ileum anastomosed to the sigmoid colon. Urine diverted into the colon may cause physiologic complications; however, the patient retains an intact body image.

Ileal Conduit The external stoma of an ileal conduit creates the psychological stress of altered body image for the patient. Both ureters are anastomosed to an isolated (6- to 10-cm) segment of the terminal ileum, near its proximal end. The distal end is everted and sutured to a predetermined stomal site on the skin. The stoma is usually located on the right side of the abdomen, below the waist. A urinary collection appliance is secured over the stoma before the patient leaves the OR.

Ureteroneocystostomy Implantation of the ureters into the bladder wall can be performed to relocate the ureters into a different site for correction of ureterovesical reflux, to reestablish urinary flow following temporary diversion, or to establish urinary flow from renal transplant following bilateral nephrectomy and ureterectomy.

Ureteroureterostomy Anastomosis of two segments of one ureter is usually performed to reestablish ureteral continuity following traumatic injury. A ureteral catheter may be inserted as a stent and the ureter sutured over it. This procedure, or *transureteroureterostomy* anastomosis, may be indicated to bypass a ureteral stricture or to eliminate ureteral reflux that also may be the result of trauma to a ureter. Injury to a ureter can occur as a complication of pelvic or abdominal operations, as well as from external penetrating wounds. Ideally, a transureteral anastomosis can be made 2 to 4 cm above the pelvic brim, since ureters are close at this point and the recipient ureter has a straight course into the bladder.

Bladder

The bladder may be opened through a suprapubic incision when a neoplasm, calculus, obstruction of the bladder neck, or traumatic injury is not amenable to treatment through the cystoscope. Diagnosis is usually established through direct visualization prior to operation.

Cystectomy Total or partial removal of the bladder and adjacent structures is usually performed to excise a carcinoma within the bladder wall. If a urinary diversion procedure (previously described) has not been performed prior to removal of the bladder, transplantation of the ureters into the skin or into the intestinal tract for urinary drainage is required at the time of cystectomy.

Cystometrogram A cystometrogram may be done to measure voiding pressure within the bladder to determine muscular tone and to check nerve supply. A calibrated recording tidal irrigator cystometer is used. When 350 ml of solution are put into the bladder, the patient should feel a desire to void. Carbon dioxide gas is used with some electronic transducers or radio pressure gauges. Normal maximum capacity is 500 ml. Normal pressure is 40 to 50 ml of water. If the problem is neurogenic, cystometric findings are not higher than normal. If the problem is a hypertonic bladder, they are higher than normal.

Cystoscopy *Cystoscopy* is a visual examination of interior walls and contents of the bladder. The term is used broadly, because various concurrent procedures may be carried out by using especially designed instruments through the cystoscope.

Plain cystoscopy is a routine examination of the bladder. Complete cystoscopy and litholapaxy have been described. In conjunction with plain cystoscopy, the following other procedures may be performed within the bladder.

1 Biopsy of tumor with a flexible-shaft biopsy forceps to obtain specimens
2 Cystogram for diagnostic x-ray studies (refer to Chap. 20, p. 390) after injection of contrast medium into bladder
3 Fulguration of a tumor by use of an electrode (see p. 448) to destroy tissue
4 Resection of or incision into a bladder neck obstruction with electrosurgical equipment (refer to resectoscope on p. 448)
5 Coagulation of hemangiomas and vascular tumors of bladder wall with argon or Nd:YAG laser
6 Removal of foreign body with flexible-shaft foreign-body forceps
7 Insertion of interstitial radionuclide seeds (refer to Chap. 35, p. 624)

Suprapubic Cystostomy Urinary drainage from the bladder may be provided via a catheter inserted through a suprapubic incision or trocar puncture into the bladder. If the bladder or urethra is injured due to trauma associated with bony and soft tissue injuries of the pelvis, the bladder may be drained with a catheter placed above the pubic arch. This method of drainage is also preferred following some ureteral, bladder, prostatic, and urethral operations to decrease tension on sutures and to ensure a patent route for urinary drainage. Suprapubic catheters are connected to a sterile closed constant-drainage system before the patient leaves the OR. The most commonly used catheters for cystostomy drainage are:

1 Foley, 30-cc balloon, French sizes 20, 22, or 24.
2 Foley, 5-cc balloon, French size 24, three-way irrigating catheter. The third lumen can be used for continuous irrigation.
3 Bonanno suprapubic catheter.

Cutaneous Vesicostomy Urinary drainage can be established directly from the bladder into a collecting device affixed on the abdomen, rather than through a suprapubic catheter. The bladder is opened through a transverse suprapubic incision and a flap raised at the dome. A skin flap is raised in the midline of the abdomen below the umbilicus. The bladder flap is sutured to the defect created in the skin and then covered with the skin flap. A transparent adhering skin dressing and collection device form a seal around the resultant bladder stoma. Cutaneous vesicostomy may preserve renal function and/or improve upper urinary tract structure in patients with neurogenic or atonic bladder, urinary incontinence, or bladder outlet obstruction.

Cystotomy An incision into the urinary bladder through a suprapubic incision may be performed to repair a bladder laceration or rupture due to trauma. The bladder is also incised to perform a Y-V plasty to relieve a stricture or contracture of the bladder neck by broadening the outlet of the bladder into the urethra.

Urinary Incontinence

Involuntary, uncontrollable voiding is distressing for a patient. Urinary incontinence may be due to congenital or acquired physiologic conditions, such as loss of bladder control following spinal cord injury or neurogenic disease. Incontinence occurs in males following some operations, most commonly a prostatectomy (see p. 459). It can develop in females due to obstetrical injury. Surgical intervention is often necessary for *stress incontinence,* the intermittent leakage of urine as a result of sudden increase in intraabdominal pressure, as during coughing or sneezing, on weakened urethral sphincter muscles at the bladder neck. Various operative procedures are performed depending on individual patient circumstances as determined by *urodynamics,* study of vesical function. Some bladder suspension procedures are done by gynecologists (refer to Marshall-Marchetti vesicourethral suspension, Chap. 22, p. 437).

Artificial Urinary Sphincter A prosthesis may be implanted to apply pressure to the urethra to maintain continence between periods of voiding. The pressure-regulating mechanism has a balloon, cuff, and pump constructed of silicone rubber. A balloon with desired predetermined pressure is positioned intraabdominally beside the bladder. The cuff encircles either bladder neck or bulbous urethra, depending on preferred surgical approach. The pump is placed in the subcutaneous tissue of the scrotum (in male) or labium (in female). A control assembly, constructed mainly of stainless steel, lies subcutaneously adjacent to the external inguinal ring. Tubing connects the components. A radiopaque isotonic solution is used to fill the prosthesis. When patient squeezes the pump, solution is transferred from cuff into balloon, thus releasing pressure on urethra to permit urine to flow.

Teflon Injection Teflon paste (Polytef) may be injected into tissues surrounding the urethra proximal to external sphincter. The injection swells the tissue, narrowing the urethra sufficiently for sphincteric control. This is done in selected patients, such as a male following TUR or a female in whom a suspension procedure has been unsuccessful. The injection is made transurethrally with a flexible syringe through a fiberoptic cysto-urethroscope.

Modified Peyrera Needle Suspension Procedure With female patient in lithotomy position, the vaginal wall is dissected from overlying urethra through an inverted U or midline vaginal incision. Dissection is carried superiorly to above level of bladder neck and laterally into the retropubic space. A suspension suture anchors the musculofascial vaginal tissue adjacent to urethra. A Peyrera ligature carrier needle is passed through a small suprapubic incision, down through rectus fascia and muscle into retropubic space and out into vagina. The ends of the suspension suture are drawn by this needle out through the suprapubic incision. Before ends are tied to suspend urethra, a cystoscope is inserted into bladder to assess success of suspension without injury to bladder. This procedure relocates proximal urethra and bladder neck into zone of intraabdominal pressure without necessity for open pelvic surgery.

Bladder Flap-Urethroplasty When urodynamics show a resistance to urinary flow in a female with neurogenic bladder, a bladder flap-urethroplasty procedure is advisable.

Urethra

The urethra funtions as the outlet for urine to pass from the bladder. Obstruction or dysfunction of the urethra may cause urinary retention or incontinence. Enlargement of the prostate may cause obstruction. Gonorrhea, other disease processes, or traumatic injury may cause a stricture. Problems associated with congenital displacement of the urethra are discussed in Chapter 33.

Perineal Urethrostomy When indwelling or intermittent urethral catheterization is contraindicated in a male patient with an obstructed or traumatized urethra, urinary drainage may be established through a perineal incision. An indwelling catheter is inserted into the bladder through an incision into the membranous urethra.

Urethral Dilatation Periodic dilatation may be necessary for weeks to years following infection or trauma that has caused a urethral stricture. Either woven filiforms and followers, bougies, or metal sounds are used. If the latter are preferred, curved metal sounds are used to dilate a male urethra; straight sounds are used on females.

Urethrotomy An Otis urethrotome may be used to cut into a urethral stricture. After this instrument is passed into urethra, the blade is released to cut the stricture. If a specimen of the urethra is taken for biopsy, a rigid biopsy forceps is used through a cystourethroscope. This scope may also be used with a laser to open a urethral stricture.

Urethroplasty Reestablishment of continuity without stricture is the ultimate objective following traumatic urethral injury, usually associated with pelvic fracture in men. Scrotal-inlay urethroplasty or other method of urethral reconstruction is usually delayed until the extent of the injury can be fully evaluated by urethrograms. A suprapubic cystostomy catheter, inserted as an emergency measure, can maintain urinary drainage for several weeks to months. Insertion of a urethral catheter into a ruptured urethra in the immediate posttraumatic period can produce periurethral infection, stricture, and other irreparable damage.

ENDOCRINE GLANDS

Two pairs of glands in the endocrine system are of primary interest to the urologist: the adrenals in both sexes and the testes in the male.

Adrenal Glands

The adrenal glands secrete substances that help regulate fluid and electrolyte balance, influence metabolism and sexual organs, and assist the body in coping with stress. These glands are located in the retroperitoneal spaces immediately above the superior pole of each kidney. Total or partial excision of one or both adrenal(s) is usually performed by the urologist. However, in some hospitals, this operation has become the province of endocrinologic surgical specialists.

Adrenalectomy may be indicated for the removal of a benign, malignant, or metastatic tumor within the adrenal medulla, or to eliminate adrenal hormonal secretions. The adrenal glands are a rich source of estrogens. Bilateral adrenalectomy may be performed as supplemental treatment of advanced prostatic or breast cancer to reduce the hormonal environment within the body. Estrogens may stimulate recurrence or metastasis from prostatic or breast cancer.

For a unilateral adrenalectomy, the adrenal gland is usually approached posteriorly through a lateral incision into the retroperitoneal space. The surgeon may also prefer a posterior approach for a bilateral adrenalectomy with the patient placed in a modified prone position for bilateral incisions. Other surgeons prefer an anterior thoracoabdominal or transabdominal incision into the retroperitoneal space with the patient in supine position. The circulating nurse must verify with the surgeon the preferred position before the patient is positioned, prepped, and draped. The thoracoabdominal incision may be preferred to extend the incision across the costal margin into the eighth or ninth intercostal space for exposure and exploration of the extra-adrenal paraganglion system, depending on the preoperative diagnosis.

Testes

The *testes* are the pair of male reproductive glands suspended in the scrotum that after sexual maturity are the source of spermatozoa. They also secrete hormones that influence growth and development, sexual activity, and secondary sex characteristics. When both testes are excised, the castrated patient becomes sterile and deficient in male hormones.

Bilateral orchiectomy is usually performed as adjunctive therapy in patients with prostatic cancer to alter the hormonal environment. Control of the disease following this relatively simple procedure is attempted before the urologist considers adrenalectomy. Psychological preparation is important to help the patient accept sterilization and other body changes, such as breast enlargement, which may occur as a result of alteration in the hormonal system.

Bilateral oblique incisions in the inguinal canals extend into the upper anterior surface of the scrotum over the testes. Following ligation of the spermatic cords at the external or internal inguinal rings, the testes are removed from the scrotum. Silicone rubber prostheses may be implanted in the scrotal sac to improve cosmetic appearance for psychological rehabilitation of the patient.

MALE REPRODUCTIVE ORGANS

Testes

The testes are both hormonal glands and male reproductive organs. Disorders in or around one (or both) testis that inhibit sexual activity, reproductive capability, or cause discomfort in the scrotum may necessitate an operative procedure.

Unilateral Orchiectomy Removal of one testis does not sterilize the patient. This procedure may be performed (unilaterally as described for bilateral orchiectomy) to remove a testicular tumor, or may be indicated following traumatic injury or infection.

Hydrocelectomy A *hydrocele* is an accumulation of fluid in the sac of the tunica vaginalis of the testis. Through an anterior incision into the scrotum, the hydrocele sac is dissected away from the testis and removed from the scrotum.

Scrotal-Testicular Trauma A scrotal-testicular injury may require exploration to ligate bleeding vessels or to insert a Penrose drain. Infection is apt to occur following a penetrating wound, so the extraperitoneal spaces in the scrotum must be drained thoroughly.

Varicocele Ligation Dilatation of the spermatic veins of the pampiniform plexus of the spermatic cord can cause a soft, elastic, often uncomfortable swelling in the scrotum. This condition, known as *varicocele,* occurs more frequently on the left side. It can cause loss in testicular mass and a decrease of sperm density associated with male infertility. Ligation of the spermatic vein can improve the sperm count if the testis has not atrophied.

The spermatic vein is ligated above the inguinal canal lateral to inferior epigastric vessels or in retroperitoneal space lateral to iliac artery. In the latter approach, a transverse abdominal incision starts at the anterior superior iliac spine and extends toward the lateral aspect of the rectus abdominis muscle. The hemiscrotum must be manually emptied of all blood before the vein is ligated or the varicocele may persist postoperatively.

Vas Deferens

The *vas deferentia* are the small fibromuscular excretory ducts that carry sperm upward through the spermatic cords from the epididymides lying along the upper portion of each testis to the seminal vesicles, the pouchlike glands in front of the urinary bladder near the prostate gland. Interruption of or obstruction to the vas deferens inhibits normal spermatogenesis.

Vasectomy Elective bilateral vasectomy is an established method of male sterilization. This is usually performed as an ambulatory surgical procedure. A segment of each vas deferens is removed. Cut ends are either ligated with suture or clips or fulgurated by coagulating epithelium of lumen, depending on preference of the urologist. Techniques vary, but all patients should be informed that spontaneous regeneration of a severed vas deferens does occur in a small percentage of patients.

Vasovasostomy Recannulization of the vas deferens for restoration of fertility requires a nonobstructed anastomosis. The tough 2-mm outer diameter with an inner diameter of 1 mm or less at distal end, plus dilation of proximal end, makes precise anastomosis under the operating microscope preferable to nonmicrosurgical techniques in which it is difficult to see the lumen of the vas deferens on the distal side. One-layer anastomosis and splinting techniques for vasectomy reversal often result in a stricture caused by scarring within lumen of the vas deferens that inhibits passage of sperm. After a scrotal incision exposes vas deferens above and below site of previous ligation, the two ends are cut to excise scar tissue and to open lumen. Under magnification of the operating microscope, interrupted sutures are placed in mucosal lining of the lumen to create a fluid-tight nonstrictured anastomosis. Muscularis is approximated separately. Sperm counts return to normal soon after operation.

Prostate Gland

A musculoglandular organ encased in a fibrous capsule, the *prostate gland* surrounds the posterior urethra at the bladder neck. It is divided into five lobes. Normal function of this gland provides secretions to the seminal fluid for sperm mobility during ejaculation.

Though this gland normally weighs 20 g, it will enlarge to some degree in most men by the time they reach age 50. Enlargement of the prostate gland can obstruct the urethra. Difficulty in voiding most often brings men with prostatic disease to a urologist. The entire gland or one or more lobes can be resected from its capsule transurethrally. Prostatectomy can also be performed through a suprapubic or retropubic abdominal approach or a perineal incision. A radical prostatectomy, performed through a retropubic abdominal or perineal incision, includes extirpation of prostate, periprostatic tissue, seminal vesicles, and vas ampullae en bloc. The approach and procedure depend on the urologist's preference for removing the pathology. Carcinoma of the prostate is the second most common cancer in all males and the most common in men over 50 years of age. Benign prostatic hypertrophy (BPH) is also a common indication for prostatectomy in males over 50.

Transurethral Prostatectomy A *resectoscope* (see p. 448) is introduced into prostatic urethra. Transurethral resection (TUR) of the prostate refers to electroresection or cryosurgical removal of all or part of the glandular tissue within the prostatic capsule. BPH of glands under 50 g in size is the usual indication for TUR. This approach is not without potential complications of impotence and urinary incontinence. The technique is one of the most difficult for a urologist to master.

After a TUR, the urologist may insert a three-way 30-cc Foley catheter. The third lumen provides a means for continuous irrigation for a time postoperatively to prevent formation of clots in the bladder.

Suprapubic Prostatectomy The suprapubic approach is limited almost exclusively to removal of a large benign hypertrophied gland over 50 g. Through a midline vertical incision above the symphysis pubis, the superior bladder wall is opened to expose the prostatic urethra. The prostatic lobes are enucleated with a finger inserted through an incision into the mucosa of the urethra. This procedure may be termed *transvesicocapsular prostatectomy* because the prostatic capsule is approached through the bladder. Hemostatic agents are usually packed into the extremely vascular prostatic fossa to help control bleeding. Pressure from the Foley catheter balloon inserted after closure of the urethra also helps obtain hemostasis. A cystostomy tube is inserted to facilitate urinary drainage from the bladder during the healing process.

Retropubic Prostatectomy The prostate gland is exposed below the bladder neck through a vertical or transverse abdominal incision above the symphysis pubis. The gland is removed through an incision in the prostatic capsule; this is a *transcapsular prostatectomy.* The periprostatic tissue, seminal vesicles, and vas ampullae also may be excised if operation is performed for carcinoma with no evidence of spread beyond the prostatic capsule. This latter radical procedure may be carried out as a second stage following either a diagnostic transurethral or suprapubic prostatectomy.

Perineal Prostatectomy With the patient in an extreme lithotomy position, the perineum affords the most direct open operative approach to the prostate through a relatively avascular field. The urologist incises the perineum above the anal sphincter and dissects the rectum from the posterior surface of the prostate, or dissection may be carried out between the external anal sphincter and the rectum. The perineal approach may be used to enucleate the prostate gland from its capsule or for total prostatovesiculectomy. The latter radical procedure includes removal of the entire prostate gland, its capsule, the seminal vesicles, and a portion of the bladder. The classical radical perineal prostatectomy may be the urologist's operation of choice to reduce morbidity from early or advanced prostatic carcinoma.

Pelvic Lymphadenectomy Through a lower abdominal incision into the extraperitoneal space, lymph nodes are dissected bilaterally from the iliac vessels, the obturator spaces, and the hypogastric vessels. These nodes may be examined by frozen section to detect early and subtle metastases from prostatic carcinoma. If several positive nodes are present, the patient is unlikely to benefit from radical prostatectomy. If nodes are negative, the urologist may proceed with a radical retropubic prostatectomy. Pelvic lymphadenectomy also may be done as a staged procedure prior to radical perineal prostatectomy.

Penis

The *penis* is the male organ of copulation. Because it contains the urethra, a deviation or malformation in structure may affect normal urinary flow from the bladder. Operations to repair congenital anomalies of the penis and circumcision are discussed in Chapter 33 because these procedures usually are performed during infancy and childhood. In the adult, however, erectile impotency frequently brings a male to a urologist. Etiology of impotence can be classified as *organic* or *psychogenic.* Patients must be thoroughly evaluated and properly selected for surgical therapy.

Implantation of a penile prosthesis can enable some impotent men to achieve a satisfactory return of sexual activity. Penile prosthetic implants are of three types: semirigid silicone, semiflexible silicone-braided silver, and an inflatable hydraulic device.

1 The Small-Carrion semirigid prosthesis consists of two foam-filled silicone rods inserted into the corpus cavernosum on each side of the penis, usually through a vertical incision in the perineum underneath the scrotum. The suitable-size prosthesis is selected from lengths available. The prosthesis maintains a permanent semierection.

2 The Finney Flexirod is similar to the Small-Carrion prosthesis except that it is hinged at the penoscrotal junction when implanted. This allows penis to hang in a dependent position when erection is not desired.

3 The Jonas prosthesis is constructed of malleable braided silver and silicone. It is semiflexible.

4 The Scott-Bradley inflatable hydraulic device is inserted through a midline incision extending from the base of the penis to a point midway between the symphysis pubis and the umbilicus. Silicone cylinders are implanted into each corpus cavernosum. Tubing connected to these cylinders at the base of the penis is brought into left inguinal canal, into prevesical space, and into right inguinal canal, where it is connected to tubing from the pump-release mechanism placed in the scrotum. A reservoir, filled with a radiopaque solution, is sutured into the abdominal fascia of the prevesical space. Tubing from this reservoir is also connected to the pump-release mechanism. To achieve erection of the penis, the patient squeezes the pump in the scrotum.

Transsexual Surgery

Transsexual surgery is the only cure for a patient who is psychologically possessed with the desire to physically and emotionally become a member of the opposite sex. This type of surgery presents extreme challenges to the urologist and gynecologist. Operative techniques have been developed to eliminate the obvious external genitalia of a male by dissection of penile structures, shortening of the urethra, and removal of the testes. The penile and scrotal skin are preserved for construction of a pseudofemale vaginal orifice. This procedure is done as the final stage following change of secondary sexual characteristics by hormonal and/or surgical therapy to produce breast enlargement, suppression of beard and body hair, redistribution of adipose tissue, voice change, and removal of pronounced thyroid cartilage (the Adam's apple). This final stage of transsexual surgery, from male to female, creates a vagina by inverting the hollow penis into the hypogastrium between the new urethral orifice and the rectum. Because the nerve endings from the penis are intact, the newly constructed vagina is capable of experiencing orgasm postoperatively. The prostate and seminal vesicles are retained so that orgasm with emission is possible. The scrotal skin forms the labia.

CHAPTER **24**

ORTHOPAEDICS

Orthopaedics is derived from two Greek words: *ortho* (straight) and *paed* (child). Orthopaedics, as the name implies, began with the treatment of crippled children by means of rest, braces, and exercises. As a contemporary surgical specialty, it is "that branch of surgery especially concerned with the preservation and restoration of the functions of the skeletal system, its articulations and associated structures."* Diseases and disabilities affecting the neuromusculoskeletal system cause loss of function and impair the activity of many individuals. The increasing age of the population has added numbers to those suffering from these diseases and disabilities. Congenital deformities of the musculoskeletal system are frequent. Conservative, noninvasive methods are nearly always used first, but patient care must be individualized to restore both form and function.

DEVELOPMENT OF ORTHOPAEDICS

Records tell of the treatment of fractures in Egypt 4500 years ago. Mummies have been found with splints still in place. Some of these were made from the bark of trees; others were strips of linen impregnated with a gluelike substance. Egyptian mummies and murals show evidence of crippling diseases. One drawing, over 800 years old, shows a man using a crutch.

Hippocrates described scoliosis, congenital dislocation of the hip, clubfoot, and tuberculosis. His writings included the accumulated knowledge of past centuries, so no doubt many of the treatment methods he advocated date back beyond his time. Almost all the principles of treating fractures currently followed are included in his book *On Fractures*. He discussed the use of traction, countertraction, bandages, splints, and treatment of compound fractures. He used mixtures of gelatinous substances and clay to coat bandages. He recognized the necessity of immobilizing a joint above and below a fracture. He described the proper position of fixing joints for the best possible future function. He wrote that exercise strengthens but inactivity wastes a part. He advocated mobilization of fractures as much as possible, to prevent atrophy. For centuries much of the wisdom in the books of Hippocrates was ignored or forgotten, then rediscovered.

Galen described muscles and their function as a motor system directed by the brain through nerves. He named the spinal deformities still known as lordosis, scoliosis, and kyphosis.

In the sixteenth century, Paré described appliances to support or correct orthopaedic conditions. He wrote a book on dislocations. His description of fractures of the spine was the beginning of modern spinal surgery.

Modern orthopaedic surgery began to evolve in the eighteenth century. The earliest known institute for treatment of skeletal deformities was founded in Switzerland in 1790. The development

*American Board of Orthopaedic Surgery.

of orthopaedic surgery has been enhanced by expenditures of governments and societies for the care of the crippled and disabled, and by the growth of hospitals and rehabilitation centers.

Of the orthopaedic surgeons in the late nineteenth century, no one contributed more to the development of the specialty than Charles Fayette Taylor (1827–1899). His investigations in *kinesiatrics* (movement therapy) and surgical mechanics contributed to the undertaking of exercise and rest in the treatment of musculoskeletal disorders. Fundamental concepts of these and other early teachers have not changed; their methods of treatment have changed as new knowledge has been gained and materials have been improved. Knowledge of skeletal tissue led orthopaedists to attempt operations of tendons and joints. An increased knowledge of bone regeneration, the concept of aseptic technique, the discovery of x-ray, the introduction of sulfonamides and antibiotics, the development of instrumentation and appliances all have contributed to the advancement of orthopaedic surgery.

The multidisciplinary approaches of physics and biology created a surge of interest in neuromusculoskeletal science and technology for orthopaedic surgery. Attempts were made in the 1950s to replace the components of the hip joint. In 1959, John Charnley suggested in England that methyl methacrylate, used in dentistry, might be used to hold prosthetic components in place. The field of biomechanics really began to develop, however, when Charnley introduced the low-friction torque prosthesis for total hip replacement in 1962. Since then biomechanics has revolutionized orthopaedic surgery.

SPECIAL FEATURES OF ORTHOPAEDIC SURGERY

The orthopaedic surgeon, also referred to as an *orthopaedist* or *orthopod,* attempts to restore the mechanical function of the body. Operations may be performed to correct congenital deformities (refer to Chap. 33), reconstruct or eradicate degenerative disease processes, or repair traumatic injuries. The orthopaedist is basically concerned with the bones, ligaments, tendons, muscles, and capsule tissues of the extremities, including the shoulder and hip joints, and the vertebral column. A large percentage of the operations involve contaminated wounds or tissues highly susceptible to infection. An infection in bone may remain for life or may cause loss of an extremity. Therefore, meticulous attention to sterile technique is critical in all orthopaedic procedures.

Instrumentation

Each orthopaedic operation must have the correct instrumentation for *that* particular bone, joint, tendon, or other structures the orthopaedist will encounter. An instrument used on a hip procedure is not appropriate for a hand. Orthopaedic instruments are heavy, often large and bulky, but also delicate. Each instrument has a specific purpose and requires special care and handling. Orthopaedic instruments can be divided into categories by functional design.

Exposing Instruments To expose a bone or joint, special retractors and elevators are used. Retractors are contoured to fit around the bone or joint without cutting or tearing muscles. Periosteal elevators are semisharp instruments used to strip periosteum from bone without destroying its ability to regenerate new bone.

Grasping Instruments Grasping instruments are required to hold, manipulate, or retract bone. Bone-holding forceps should be selected appropriately for size of the bone in the operative field. Bone hooks are used for retraction and leverage. Heavy clamps are needed to hold smaller bones or to grasp a joint capsule, such as a meniscus clamp for fibrocartilage in knee.

Cutting Instruments Cutting instruments are used to remove soft tissue around bone; to cut into, cut apart, or cut out portions of bone; or to smooth jagged edges of bone. The orthopaedist's armamentarium includes osteotomes, gouges, chisels, curettes, rongeurs, reamers, bone-cutting forceps, meniscitomes, rasps, files, drills, and saws. These have sharp edges. Take extra care not to nick or damage cutting edges by protecting them on the instrument table and during cleaning, sterilizing, and storing. Fitted sterilizable racks, trays, foam towels or canvas cases are used to keep sets together by sizes, e.g., osteotomes, gouges, chisels, and curettes, as well as to protect cutting edges.

NOTE. Cutting instruments must be sharp. Osteotomes, chisels, gouges, and meniscitomes can be sharpened by OR personnel with hand-held hones or a honing machine designed for this purpose. Most manufacturers provide a service for sharpening and repairing instruments. Curettes, rongeurs, and reamers should be returned for sharpening. Small drill bits and saw blades usually are discarded when dulled.

Power-driven Cutting Instruments Powered instruments increase speed and decrease fatigue of manually driven drills, saws, and reamers. The power source may be electricity from direct current or a battery, or compressed air or nitrogen.

1 *Electric saws and drills* that are explosion-proof should be used. Observe rules for use of electrical equipment (refer to Chap. 11).

2 *Air-powered instruments* use compressed nitrogen that is either piped into the OR or supplied from a cylinder on a stable carrier. The pressure must be set and monitored by the operating pressure gauge of the regulator. The instruments are small, lightweight, and easy to handle for pinpoint accuracy at high speed, free of vibration.

These instruments offer precision in drilling, cutting, shaping, and beveling bone. Blood loss from bone is reduced by the tiny particles packed into the cut surface. The instrument may have rotary, reciprocating, or oscillating action. Rotary movement is used to drill holes or insert screws, wires, or pins. Reciprocating movement, a cutting action from front to back, and oscillating cutting action from side to side are used to cut or remove bone. Some instruments have a combination of movements and can be changed from one to the other. In some the change may be made by adjusting the chuck forward or backward and locking it in the desired position. Power instruments are not used without some inherent dangers.

1 Heat generated can damage bone cells. Air-powered instruments cause minimal heating by comparison with electric instruments because they operate at a faster and higher speed. When using electric saws or drills, the orthopaedist usually has the assistant drip saline solution on the area from a bulb syringe, to cool the bone and wash away particles. Care must be used so the syringe does not touch the blade, especially if it is glass. Plastic bulb syringes are less hazardous.

2 Normal tissue, including the orthopaedist's or assistant's finger, can be caught in a rapidly spinning drill or oscillating saw unless carefully controlled. The instrument may cut more than desired. When a power instrument is being used, particularly with rotating movement, all team members must be very careful to keep their hands away from the blade.

3 Disconnect a direct-current electric instrument from its power source when not in use so that a team member cannot inadvertently activate it. Some electric saws and drills are activated by a foot pedal. As an added protection, set the instrument and attachments on a small sterile table, alone, when not in use. Air-powered instruments have fingertip controls. The safety slide should be set in position to prevent inadvertent activation until ready for use.

4 Always handle and store an electrical power cord or air hose with care. A broken cord can short-circuit the instrument. A broken hose under pressure can whip out of control, thereby possibly injuring the patient or personnel. Always inspect cord or hose prior to use.

5 Always be certain attachments and blades are completely seated and locked in the handle before activating power.

6 Always operate, clean, and sterilize power instruments according to the manufacturer's manual with directions for use and care. (Refer to general procedures for care of powered instruments in Chapter 11, p. 200.)

Implant-related Instruments Drivers, clamps, and retractors are used for inserting, securing, or removing fixation and prosthetic implants. Each type of implant requires its own instrumentation. As stated in Chapter 18, instruments used for insertion or extraction of metallic implants must be of the same metal as the implant to prevent galvanic reaction.

Items Used Frequently

Although not used in every orthopaedic procedure, the items discussed below are handled frequently.

Bone Grafts When necessary to remove a piece of bone from one part of the skeletal system to reinforce another bone, a separate small sterile table may be prepared for the instrumentation required for the donor site. If the recipient area is potentially contaminated, the donor site must be kept free from possible contamination from the recipient site. Autogenous cancellous and cortical bone is obtained from the crest of the ilium and cortical bone from the tibia. Free vascularized fibular grafts may be preferred to replace large segments of long bones following trauma or tumor resection.

Bone Bank Allografts Bone may be preserved for use as needed to fill a bone defect. This is especially useful when autogenous bone is not available in sufficient quantity, or the orthopaedist deems it undesirable to subject the patient to a secondary incision or the added operating time required to remove bone for an autogenous graft. Bone, such as a rib or femoral head, may be salvaged from patients free from malignancy or infection for a homogenous graft into another person. Autogenous bone may be preserved following operation by storage in the bone bank for subsequent grafting into the same patient.

Bone used for allografts must be clean and sterile. Immediately after removal, bone marrow, fat, and blood are rinsed out with sterile distilled water or normal saline. Bone may be put in sterile nested glass jars or double plastic or metal containers. If to be used for homogenous grafts, a small piece of bone is put into a sterile petri dish and sent to laboratory for culture tests. Bone should never be used until a negative culture report is received. Several methods are used to preserve bone.

1 *Freezing* is the most common method. Bone is quick-frozen in a freezer at -70°C (-94°F) or in liquid nitrogen. If bone will be used within six months, it can be stored in a refrigerator freezer at -15 to -20°C (-5 to -4°F). For prolonged storage of more than six months, freezer temperature must be maintained below -20°C (-4°F) to avoid damage from buildup of ice crystals. Bone frozen by liquid nitrogen is stored in vapor at about -150°C (-238°F). The container initially is placed on a shelf labeled "not ready for use." It is labeled "sterile" and moved to freezer compartment labeled "ready for use" when the negative culture report is recorded on the identification card.

2 *Freeze-drying* requires specialized equipment with a condenser and vacuum cycle.

3 *Ethylene oxide sterilization* ensures sterility of bone. It must be aerated for 72 hours prior to storage at room temperature or in a refrigerator. When protected from air and contamination, sterilized bone can be stored indefinitely, although a one-year expiration date is recommended if bone is placed in a heat-sealed peel-apart package. In lieu of ethylene oxide sterilization, packaged bone may be shipped in dry ice to a center equipped to sterilize it by irradiation.

4 *Formaldehyde solution,* 0.25 to 1% concentration, may have a bacteriostatic effect around graft site in repair of infected or contaminated wounds, such as in osteomyelitis. During storage, temperature is maintained at 2 to 4°C (35.6 to 39°F) in a refrigerator freezer.

5 *Antibiotics* in solution that do not denature bone morphogenetic protein can be used to preserve bone for grafting, but this method is least frequently used.

Fixation and Prosthetic Implants Fixation and prosthetic implants are used to temporarily stabilize or permanently replace bone, joints, or tendons. They are made of stainless steel 316L, cobalt or titanium alloys, silicone, polyester covered with silicone, polyethylene, or polytetrafluoroethylene. Owing to the high cost of these implants, the inventory is kept as low as possible, yet large enough to ensure their availability when needed. These expensive implants are usually patient-charge items. After measurements are taken in the operative field, the correct size, shape, and design is selected from the sets available to ensure handling only the one to be used without touching others. An infection around a fixation or prosthetic implant may require its removal, often resulting in permanent deformity or disability.

> NOTE. Hip measurements may be taken preoperatively from the patient's x-rays using templates. If these have not been taken, they must be taken at the operative field. The surgeon also takes trial measurement at site to verify correct selection of implant.

Bone Cement Methyl methacrylate powder and liquid components are mixed at the instrument table immediately prior to insertion into the intramedullary canal of a long bone, the shaft of a bone, or the socket of a joint. Bone cement is used to reinforce fixation of some prosthetic implants or to increase strength of fixation implants. Follow the manufacturer's instructions for handling this material and avoid excessive exposure to vapors (refer to Chap. 18, p. 353). Also avoid getting lipid solvent on gloves; it can diffuse through latex to cause an allergic dermatitis.

Bone Wax Used for hemostasis in bone, bone wax is put on the instrument table and opened as requested. Check the orthopaedist's preference card before opening packet.

Nerve Stimulator The nerve stimulator is used occasionally to verify neural tissue when doing a partial nerve resection to control spastic muscles. When the popliteal nerve, for example, is given a slight shock with it, the foot jerks. Both direct electric current and disposable battery-operated stimulators are available.

Sutures Ligaments, tendons, periosteum, and joint capsules are fibrous tissues. They are primarily tough, stringy collagen and contain few cells and blood vessels. As a result, they heal slower than do vascular tissues. Nonabsorbable materials are generally used to suture ligaments, tendons, and muscles involved in movement of bony skeleton. Absorbable suture is generally preferred to suture periosteum. Check surgeon's preference card before opening suture packets.

Casts and Braces A cast or brace is a means of obtaining external fixation of a fracture or a part following tendon repair, arthrodesis, or other type of operation. It is the means of putting a part at rest or attempting to correct an injury or abnormality. Cast application in the OR is discussed in detail later in this chapter (see p. 477).

Cast Room Casts are applied in the cast room, sometimes referred to as the *plaster room.* Many closed, noninvasive procedures are performed here, particularly those requiring general or regional anesthesia, when a cast room is located within the OR suite. This frees the OR for open, invasive operations. It also keeps plaster dust from the individual operating rooms, an important aspect of aseptic environmental control. Following open operation, the patient can be wheeled on the operating table into the cast room for application of a cast, if the patient is not endangered.

Clean-Air System Special care must be used to carry out strict asepsis. Infection is the most serious, dreaded, and costly complication of orthopaedic surgery. Many orthopaedists, therefore, prefer to operate within a clean-air system, especially for total joint replacement procedures. Laminar airflow, as described in Chapter 7, is probably used more frequently by orthopaedic surgeons than by any other surgical specialists.

Orthopaedic Table An orthopaedic table, often referred to as the *fracture table,* is used for many operations requiring traction, image intensification or conventional x-ray control, and/or cast application. The many available attachments make possible any desired position and traction on any part of the body. The table can be raised, tilted laterally, put into Trendelenburg's or reverse Trendelenburg's position. The attachments are designed not only for stabilizing patient in the desired position but also for exerting traction to help reduce a fracture, and for providing a means of evaluating the diagnosis or therapy by radiologic control. Bakelite or other material that does not interfere with radiographic studies is used for attachments that might otherwise obscure the findings.

Essential standard component attachments on all models of orthopaedic tables include three-section patient body supports, lateral body brace, sacral rest, and traction apparatus. Optional accessories are available to accommodate types of procedures performed and model of the table. When the orthopaedic table will be used:

1 Consult the surgeon's preference card, procedure book, and manufacturer's manual for attachments needed for each desired position.

2 Assemble the necessary attachments. Pad all parts of the table and attachments to prevent pressure on joints, sacrum, and perineum.

3 Attach the standard components and accessories to the table frame so that all is in readiness for positioning the patient when the orthopaedist arrives. The patient may be anesthetized before positioning is completed.

X-Ray Control Conventional x-ray equipment and image intensifiers frequently are used during orthopaedic procedures. Considerations for patient safety and personnel protection described in Chapter 11 apply to use of radiologic control for invasive or noninvasive orthopaedic procedures performed in the OR suite. Special positioning and draping techniques may be necessary, especially when an image intensifier is used.

Often both anterior-posterior (AP) and lateral views are necessary to assess the alignment of a bone or to determine the position of a fixation or prosthetic implant. X-rays or recorded fluoroscopic images document work of the orthopaedist.

Special Considerations

1 Although unit beds and wheeled equipment should not enter the OR suite, in the interest of the patient's comfort and safety this rule is relaxed for some orthopaedic patients, such as patients in traction apparatus. Beds, frames, and stretchers can be decontaminated in the exchange area.

2 A cast should be removed preoperatively in the cast room. If the OR suite does not have a cast room, a cast may be bivalved in the patient's room and then removed in the OR. Cover sterile tables with a large sterile sheet while cast is being completely removed to prevent airborne contamination from plaster dust.

3 Positioning on the orthopaedic table for some operations requires an extra amount of activity. When possible, it is well to position these patients in the cast room before transporting them into the OR, thereby avoiding dispersal of lint and microorganisms into the air that could settle on sterile tables.

EXTREMITIES

Although the instrumentation may vary by size of the structures involved, basic techniques apply to handling both upper and lower extremities.

General Considerations

1 A sterile irrigating pan is placed under an extremity to catch the solution if an open wound is to be cleansed, irrigated, and debrided, as for compound fracture (refer to Chap. 16, p. 311).

2 A pneumatic tourniquet is usually used for operation on or below the elbow and knee. This provides a field free of blood, and thus the surgeon can more readily see fine structures. (Refer to discussion of tourniquets in Chapter 17, p. 335.)

The tourniquet cuff is applied before the extremity is prepped. However, *it is not inflated* until draping is completed. Remember ischemia time is a critical factor in patient safety. Remind orthopaedist after the first hour and every 15 minutes thereafter, throughout tourniquet application.

An Esmarch's bandage may be applied before the pneumatic tourniquet is inflated to force blood from the extremity.

3 An extremity is always held up for skin preparation. See that the area under it is dry before draping (see Chap. 16). Prevent prep solution from running under tourniquet.

4 A self-adhering incise drape may be used as the first drape applied. It may be impossible to adequately drape with self-adhering plastic drapes or fenestrated sheets. If extremity must be manipulated during operation, the entire circumference must be draped. A limb or split sheet may be used.

5 Stockinet may be used over a self-adhering plastic drape or to cover skin. This is cut with nurses' scissors over the line of incision. The cut edges may be secured over skin edges with skin clips if a plastic drape is not used. A medicine cup is a handy receptacle for these clips after removal. The scrub nurse holds this at the field to receive clips as the orthopaedist removes them. They must be counted.

A self-adhering incise drape eliminates the need for either stockinet and metallic skin clips or towels and towel clips that might interfere with interpretation of x-rays or image intensification.

6 For operations on bone and/or implants, the orthopaedist may wear two pairs of sterile gloves to prevent contamination in event that a glove is torn by a bone fragment or hardware. Powder-free gloves should be worn by team members who handle prosthetic implants.

7 After operation on a knee joint, a pressure dressing is usually applied to prevent serum accumulation. This may be a Robert Jones dressing, which includes a soft cotton batting roll, sheet wadding, and cotton elastic bandage. A cotton roll, or other bulky material, may be placed on each side of the knee and held in place with sheet wadding. A four-ply, crinkled-gauze bandage or cotton elastic bandage over this provides even, gentle pressure. Depending on the operation, a plaster splint or other type of knee immobilizer may be preferred.

8 After operation on a shoulder, the arm may be bound against the side of the chest for immobilization. A large piece of cotton or sheet wadding is placed under the arm to keep skin surfaces from touching, as they may macerate. The arm is held in a shoulder immobilizer that supports the humerus and wrist, or it may be bound firmly to side of the chest with a cotton elastic bandage.

9 An extremity is elevated on a pillow.

Types of Procedures

Preoperative assessment of an acute or chronic disability affecting musculoskeletal system of an extremity includes evaluation of extent of bony or soft tissue involvement with or without concomitant neurovascular compromise. Because they are the essence of adult orthopaedic surgery, either due to trauma or a degenerative disease process, procedures on the following major anatomic classifications of structures will be discussed:

1 Fracture of bones
2 Reconstruction of joints
3 Repair of tendons and ligaments

FRACTURES

Intact bones are essential to stability and mobility of upper and lower extremities. A comminuted (splintered) or fractured (broken) bone can cause malfunction and pain. Fractures vary by etiology, location and type of fracture line, and extent of injury.

1 *Traumatic.* The impact, forced twisting, or bending of an accidental injury can break one or more bones in the body. Traumatic fractures are either simple or compound.
   a *Simple fracture.* Broken fragments do not protrude through underlying tissues to skin.
   b *Compound fracture.* Either the proximal or distal end of the bone, or both, protrudes from fracture site through underlying tissues and skin.
2 *Pathologic.* Primary or metastatic malignant bone disease can spontaneously fracture a diseased bone without undue stress. Although technically simple fractures, pathologic fractures require more than simple fixation of the bone fragments. Bone cement may be used as an adjunct to fill a bone defect and increase strength of a fixation implant.

Mechanical means are used to reduce a fracture and immobilize the parts, maintaining fragments in proper alignment. Fractures must be handled gently with support above and below site to prevent further trauma. A physician takes the responsibility for supporting and protecting the fracture site when moving a patient to or from a stretcher, bed, or table. Other personnel should be instructed about site of fracture and special care needed in transferring patient. The orthopaedist removes or directs removal of temporary splints or traction. Adequate personnel must be available so that patient can be lifted gently. All lifters should be on the affected side, since this helps support the fracture during transfer.

In treating a fracture, the orthopaedist seeks to accomplish a solid union of bone in perfect alignment, to return joints and muscles to normal position, to prevent or repair vascular trauma, and to rehabilitate the patient as early as possible. Treatment of fractures usually includes three distinct phases: reduction, immobilization, and rehabilitation. The methods of treating fractures include: (1) closed reduction with immobilization, (2) skeletal traction, (3) external fixation, (4) internal fixation, and (5) elcctrostimulation.

Closed Reduction

A fracture may be manipulated (set) to replace the bone in its proper alignment without opening the skin. This technique is referred to as a *closed reduction.* Many fractures of lower leg or arm can be treated by closed reduction. When both leg bones are fractured, fibula fractures are generally disregarded and attention is directed to the tibia.

Often performed in the emergency department, the patient may come to the cast room in the OR suite for closed reduction under anesthesia and application of a device for immobilization. A plaster, fiberglass, or other lightweight synthetic cast, cast-brace, or molded plastic fracture-brace may be used to hold the reduced fracture site in alignment during union.

Skeletal Traction

Traction is the pulling force exerted to maintain proper alignment or position. In skeletal traction, the force is applied directly on the bone following insertion of pins, wires, or tongs placed through or into the bone. A small sterile setup is required. Traction is applied by means of pulleys and weights. Weights provide a constant force; pulleys help establish and maintain constant direction until the fractured bone reunites.

Forearm or Lower Leg A Kirschner wire, either plain or threaded, or a Steinmann pin is drilled through bone (preferably cortical) distal to the fracture site. For forearm fractures the wire or pin must be strong enough to prevent side-to-side, angular, and rotary motion while the fracture is healing. A traction bow is attached to the protruding ends of the wire or pin. The pulleys are fastened to this bow. Cover ends of wire or pin with corks or plaster to protect patient and personnel from sharp ends.

Finger A fine Kirschner wire may be drilled through the distal phalanx, and ends attached to a banjo splint. Or a cast may be applied to the forearm with a loop of heavy wire incorporated in it that fans out beyond fingers. The Kirschner wire is fastened to this loop by a rubber band.

External Fixation

External fixation devices are used for treatment of selected types of skeletal injuries, especially to the pelvis and extremities, with marked soft tissue loss and instability. Skeletal pins and connecting bars permit rigid fixation, but with access to devitalized skin and soft tissue for wound management, especially for open injuries of tibia. Fixation devices used for unstable pelvic fractures allow early ambulation. Controlled fracture motion is not detrimental and may provoke an external callus response at the fracture site. External fixators can also be used for lengthening the femur and tibia following an osteotomy for limb-length discrepancy.

Internal Fixation

Open reduction and fixation are usually resorted to for those fractures not amendable to closed reduction, skeletal traction or external fixation methods of conservative treatment. If vascular structures have been traumatized, internal fixation followed by vascular repair may be necessary to restore arterial tissue perfusion and adequate venous drainage.

Excellent results can be obtained by internal fixation of fractures as soon as possible after they occur. This method gives firm immobilization and close approximation of fragments so that the gap between ends is not too great for the callus to bridge. It reduces to a minimum space between fragments and movement at fracture site. Healing seems to take place faster. The patient starts non-weight-bearing exercises and progresses to ambulation early, thus reducing joint stiffness and muscle atrophy, and avoids a long period of rehabilitation.

Many types of fixation implants are available. Each type serves its purpose well in the hands of those familiar with its use. Rigid internal fixation implants are made of a metal that is nonmagnetic and electrolytically inert. Only one kind of metal is used in a patient. An implant may be affixed to the cortex of bone or inserted into bone through the fracture site. Semirigid carbon-fiber-reinforced plastic plates are also used in some selected situations.

Screws, Plates, and Nails

Screws Screws alone may be used for fixation of an oblique or spiral fracture of a long bone. Screws must be long enough to penetrate both cortices. Hard cortical bone gives the best fixation and two cortices generally hold better than does one. Screws are available in various lengths and diameters. Not all screws have the same type head, e.g., single slot, cross slot, concave cross slot, hexagon, and Phillips head. The correct screwdriver must be used with each type screw.

Compression Plate and Screws Many fractures requiring open reduction are given rigid fixation through the compression method. Compression plates are heavy and strong. They are held in place by specially designed cortical lag screws. The threads of these screws are deeper than are those on other types of screws, and also farther apart, which allows a larger amount of bone between the threads. This construction gives maximum holding power and rigid fixation. A compression instrument may be used. It is connected to the end of the plate and then fastened to the bone with a short screw. By tightening the nut on the compression instrument, the bone fragments are brought tightly together. The rest of the screws are put into the plate and the fracture is fixed. Screws alone are used only in selected situations. A cast may or may not be applied.

Eggers Plate and Screws The plate is slotted, which permits the muscle tone of the extremity to keep the ends of the fragments pressed closely together. The pressure stimulates osteogenesis.

Sherman Plate and Screws The appropriate sized plate is fitted to the contour of the bone, by bending slightly if necessary, before applying the screws. Using a drill guide, holes for the screws are drilled with an electric or air-powered drill in the center of the screw hole and perpendicularly to the plate. The drill bit should be slightly smaller than the screws. The screws should pass through both cortices of the bone.

Nails An intertrochanteric fracture of the neck of the femur may be treated by inserting a nail, compression screw, or multiple pins through neck into the head of the femur. Many different types of nails are used. They are usually inserted over or alongside a guidewire. The nail may form a continuous angulated unit with a plate that fits on the outer lateral cortex of the femur. Or the plate may be attached and the nail, screws, or pins inserted separately. Screws secure the plate to the shaft of the femur before or after the nail is inserted, depending on design of the implant. Some of the more commonly used implants are:

1 Smith-Petersen cannulated nail with a McLaughlin adjustable plate.
2 Jewett cannulated nail and plate unit. A Jewett overlay plate may also be used with this implant.
3 Neufeld nail and plate unit.
4 Deyerle plate and multiple pins.
5 Lag screw with compression tube and plate.
6 Massie sliding nail and tube assembly.
7 Ken sliding nail.
8 I-Beam (Sarmenito) nail.

The patient is usually positioned on the orthopaedic table. The orthopaedist and assistants take the responsibility for moving and positioning the patient (see Fig. 24-1 for position for nailing left hip). If portable x-ray machines are used, one is on unaffected side for anterior-posterior view, and one is at foot of table for lateral view. Film for AP view is placed on cassette holder from unaffected side. Procedure may be performed with fluoroscopic image intensification rather than conventional x-rays. All sterile tables are positioned on the affected side. The orthopaedist may sit to operate.

Intramedullary Nailing An intramedullary nail, rod, or pin is driven into the medullary canal through site of the fracture. This brings ends together for union, splints fracture, and eases pain. It permits early return of function so that patient can be ambulatory. Intramedullary implants also provide a method of holding fragments in alignment in comminuted fractures. Rigid implants are usually used for pathologic fractures or impending fracture of diseased bone. Flexible intramedullary rods may be preferred for some traumatic fractures, particularly femoral fractures.

Intramedullary nailing may be done with fluoroscopic control following closed reduction when visualization of fracture site is unnecessary. Or fracture may be reduced by visual exposure of site and then the intramedullary implant inserted. In some situations, the medullary canal must be reshaped or enlarged before a nail is inserted. The length, size, and shape of nail or pin depend on the bone to be splinted. The most commonly used appliances include:

1 Kuntscher nail, for femur.
2 Hansen-Street pin, for femur.
3 Zickel intramedullary rod and hip nail, for femur. This is a particularly strong implant for stabilization of pathologic fractures.
4 Knowles pin, for femur.
5 Sampson rod, straight or curved, for femur.

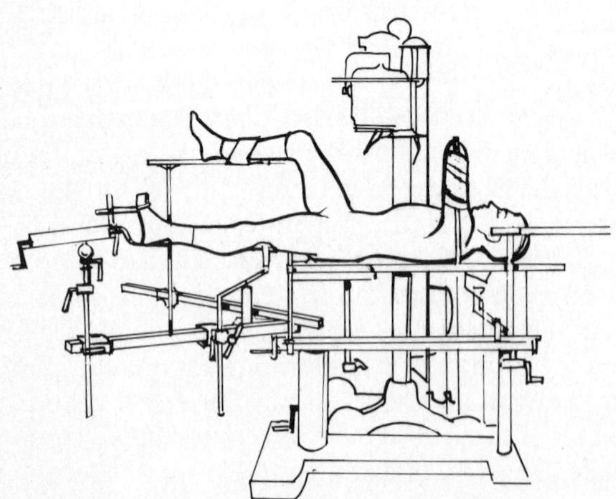

FIGURE 24-1
Position for nailing left hip. Note arm on affected side suspended from screen to remove it from operative field. Note traction on affected leg and support under knee. Elevated right leg permits x-ray tube to be adjusted under it for lateral view.

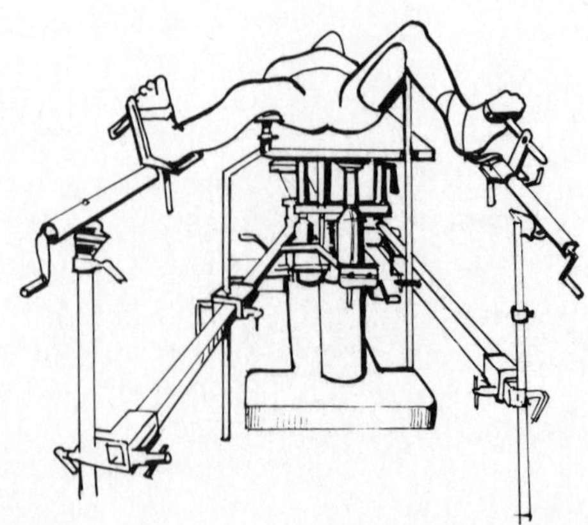

FIGURE 24-2
Position for intramedullary nailing left tibia. Note left foot anchored to footholder and knee resting on elevated curved knee rest. Right foot is anchored and knee rest adjusted for support of leg.

6 Enders nail, for femur, tibia, or humerus.

7 Schneider nail, for femur, tibia, fibula, ulna, or radius.

8 Lottes nail, for tibia.

9 Rush pin, for all long bones.

10 Steinmann pins, for clavicle, humerus, or ulna.

The implants may be removed after union at the fracture site has taken place.

The patient may be positioned on the orthopaedic table. This permits traction as needed. (See Fig. 24-2 for position of patient for intramedullary nailing of left tibia.)

Electrostimulation

Electrostimulation promotes cellular responses in bone and ligaments. Mechanically stressed (as by fracture) bone generates electric potentials related to patterns of bone regeneration. If stimulated, healing accelerates. Both internal and external techniques are used to stimulate bone and neural regeneration, revascularization, epiphyseal growth, and ligamental maturation. Electrostimulation is used most commonly at nonunion fracture sites.

Direct-Current Stimulation Constant direct current can be introduced through cathodes inserted across a nonunion fracture site. The patient is positioned on a radiographic table for fluoroscopy with image intensification. The cathodes are stainless steel K-wires, 1.2 mm in diameter, insulated with Teflon. They are inserted under local anesthesia with a hand drill or air-powered wire driver with a telescopic adaptor. The positioning and number of cathodes depends on fracture site and condition of surrounding skin and tissue. The protruding ends of the wires are bent parallel to the skin and attached to negative leads of the power pack. If on an extremity, the wires and power pack are enclosed in a cast. A self-adhesive disposable anode skin pad, connected to lead from the power pack, completes the battery circuit for constant electric current. This is placed close to the cast in an area of adequate soft tissue. The cathodes usually remain in place for a period of three months.

Pulsating Electromagnetic Field Electromagnetic fields of selected pulsating character can be generated from a coil placed directly over a nonunion site in a plaster cast or device worn by patient. Capacitatively coupling devices further enhance the electrostimulation of this noninvasive technique.

JOINT RECONSTRUCTION

Joint function depends on the quality of its structures. Articular cartilage covers the two ends of bone where they meet to form the joint. Bones are held securely in place at their articulation by ligaments and the joint capsule attached to both bone shafts. The synovial membrane lining the joint capsule secretes synovial fluid to lubricate the joint. When injured or altered by arthritis or other degenerative disease, normal joint motion is impaired and/or painful.

Dislocations

Dislocation of one or more bones at a joint may occur with or without an associated fracture. Tendons, ligaments, and muscles are deranged. The articular surface of the bone is displaced from the joint capsule. The force of displacement damages the capsule and tears ligaments and surrounding tissues. Blood vessel and nerve damage can occur, impeding circulation and causing changes in sensation and muscle strength. Closed reduction, with or without skeletal traction, may be necessary at time of acute injury. If closed reduction fails to stabilize joint and prevent recurrence, internal fixation may be necessary. Operations to stabilize chronic recurrent dislocations are most frequently performed on the shoulder.

Arthrodesis

Fusion of a joint may be achieved by removing the articular surfaces and securing bony union, or by inserting a fixation implant that inhibits motion. Arthrodesis may be performed following resection of a recurrent benign, potentially malignant, or malignant lesion that involves the ends of the bones and joint. After resection of the diseased portion of the bones, the joint may be stabilized with a bone graft or an intramedullary fixation implant. This procedure is performed most frequently for lesions in the distal femur and proximal tibia around or including the knee joint. Arthrodesis may also be performed to relieve osteoarthritic pain or to stabilize a joint that does not respond to other methods of treatment following injury, such as instability of the thumb. Because arthrodesis limits motion, other joint reconstructive procedures are usually attempted first.

Triple arthrodesis of the ankle is performed to correct deformity or muscle imbalance of the foot. The subtalar, calcaneocuboid, and talonavicular tarsal joints are fused. Staples are sometimes used to hold bones together.

Arthroplasty

Reconstruction of a joint may be necessary to restore or improve range of motion and stability, or to relieve pain. This may be done by resurfacing, reshaping, or replacing the articular surfaces of the bones.

Cup Arthroplasty of the Hip The hip joint is disarticulated by removing the head of the femur from the acetabulum. The femoral head is smoothed with a bone rasp to a spherical shape and the acetabulum is reamed to the configuration of a perfect hemisphere. A metallic cup is implanted into the acetabulum, to provide a smooth surface for joint movement, before the femoral head is placed back in the socket. Reamers must be correlated to the size of the cup to ensure proper articulation.

Femoral and Humeral Head Replacement A metal prosthetic implant can replace the femoral or humeral head and neck. These prostheses have a shaft that is driven into the medullary canal of the bone. The head of the bone is removed. The neck is shaped or removed as necessary for accurate placement of the prosthesis. A reamer may be used to enlarge the canal for insertion of the prosthesis. These prostheses are used:

1 To replace a comminuted fractured head when soft tissue attachments are destroyed

2 To replace the head if avascular necrosis or nonunion occurs following reduction of fractures

3 To mobilize the joint in arthritic patients

Femoral Head Surface Replacement As an alternative to femoral head replacement, a concentric metal shell is cemented over the femoral head. A high-density polyethylene shell is cemented into the acetabulum. Surface replacement is reserved for young adults with good femoral and acetabular bone stock to relieve severe hip pain and disability. Patients with sclerotic, well-vascularized subchrondral bone of hypertrophic osteoarthritis, for example, may be candidates for this procedure. The resurfacing procedure induces healing and reduces stress on the hip joint.

Total Joint Replacement Although prosthetic implants for some joints have not been as well-developed as are those for others, total joint replacement is an accepted therapeutic modality, especially for the hip, knee, and elbow joints. Usually performed to improve mobility and relieve pain of severe arthritic joints, total joint replacement may be indicated when other therapeutic measures have failed to correct a congenital defect, traumatic injury, or degenerative disease. A functional design for a prosthesis must consider a combination of load bearing, strain-stress, and kinetics in association with pathologic condition. Positioning of the prosthesis influences distribution of stress and rate of wear.

Charnley introduced a self-curing acrylic cement (see methyl methacrylate, Chap. 18, p. 353) for fixation of components of his low-friction torque arthroplasty of the hip joint. Three different preparations of polymethyl methacrylate, commonly referred to as *bone cement,* are available today. Following mixing of components, bone cement is injected in a state of low viscosity under pressure to fill interstices of bone and to provide long-term fixation. However, the major complication of total joint arthroplasty is loosening of weight-bearing prosthetic components over time, particularly in obese patients and active patients. Prostheses have been developed that do not require bone cement for fixation. Cementless prostheses require a precise fit in bones and must allow bone ingrowth into their porous surfaces for stability. These are particularly suited for young, active patients.

The bones on both sides of the joints are replaced or resurfaced. Both component parts must be solidly anchored to avoid movement of the prosthesis and wear on surrounding tissue. All movement must be between the two parts of the prosthesis. Metal to plastic joints are self-lubricating. Some joint fluids help to lubricate. Rate of wear on these parts is low, so that the prosthesis will remain functional over a period of many years (the exact number is not yet determined).

Total Hip Replacement Total hip prostheses have greatly reduced the number of arthroplasty procedures previously described, especially in patients over age 50 with degenerative hip disease.

With patient supine on the radiographic operating table, an incision about 10 in. (25 cm) long is made along lateral thigh to remove the greater trochanter. Removal of greater trochanter facilitates exposure to prepare sites for insertion of prosthesis. However, its removal can cause abductor muscle weakness, instability, and other complications. Therefore, some orthopaedists prefer an anterior approach to the hip joint with patient in supine position; others prefer a posterior approach with patient in lateral position. With all approaches, the femur is dislocated from the acetabulum. The femoral head is removed at the neck and replaced with a prosthesis. This may be a metal or ceramic head on a metallic stem that is seated into the medullary canal of the femur. Prior to inserting the femoral prosthesis, the acetabulum is reamed to the configuration of the cup-shaped acetabular component. This may be high-density polyethylene, metal, or ceramic with a smooth, rough, or porous outer surface. The inner surface is smooth to articulate with the smooth finish on head of the femoral prosthesis. The acetabular component is fixed in the socket. Then the femoral prosthesis is positioned. Several types and sizes of prostheses are available. Each has its own advantages and disadvantages. The surgeon must select the appropriate one for each patient's particular condition.

Total Knee Replacement Insertion of a total knee prosthesis may be indicated to provide for mechanical deficiencies in function of knee. Selection of the appropriate prosthesis from among the types available depends on deformity of the femorotibial articulation, patellofemoral articulation, and structure of the cruciate and collateral ligaments. To achieve stability, permanent bone ingrowth into a porous-coated or rough surface implant is desirable. Prostheses of this construction may not require bone cement for fixation.

Total Ankle Replacement Rheumatoid arthritis and posttraumatic osteoarthritis are the most common causes of ankle degeneration. Ankle joint replacement may be indicated as an alternative to arthrodesis in selected patients, usually over 60 years of age, to relieve pain and secondarily to increase motion and provide joint stability. An anterior incision is made between the anterior tibial and extensor hallucis longus tendons. Procedures vary depending on the type of prosthesis to be implanted. Two types have been developed: incongruent, which allows normal dorsiflexion, plantar flexion, and rotation of foot, but is inherently unstable; and congruent, which restricts motion to a single plane, but is inherently more stable. The tibial components of both types are high-density polyethylene and the talar components are metal. They are cemented in place.

Total Metatarsophalangeal Joint Replacement Hallux rigidus and hallux abductus valgus deformities can lead to pain and altered gait. By joint replacement, the deformity can be realigned with stability and motion. Several types of implants are available. The Silastic hinge toe, a double-stemmed silicone prosthesis with a hinge, is popular to restore motion of great toe and lesser metatarsophalangeal joints.

Hemi- and Total Shoulder Replacement Shoulder replacement may be indicated for severe destruction by disease or posttraumatic degeneration of humeral articular surface with resultant loss of motion, instability, and pain. The prosthesis replaces the humeral head and resurfaces the glenoid cavity, the articular surface of the scapula. The most commonly used prosthesis has a plastic component for the glenoid cavity and a metal humeral component. The patient is placed in a semi-Fowler's position for the operation.

Total Elbow Replacement Prosthetic replacement may be a necessity to correct interarticular problems within the elbow joint, especially those with severe joint surface damage. The prosthesis provides internal stability. A hinged or articulated type provides good functional range of motion of the humeroulnar prosthetic articulation. Surface replacement with a nonarticulating prosthesis may be indicated. Both the metallic humerus and ulnar components of these prostheses are cemented in place following shaping of the bones.

Metacarpophalangeal Joint Replacement Silicone rubber prosthetic implants are used to replace metacarpophalangeal joints in the hand. The implant bridges the excised joint and is secured to the adjacent bones by intramedullary stems. This type of prosthesis may also be used to replace small bones of the wrist.

Nursing Considerations in total joint replacement:

1 Prosthesis must be handled carefully.
  a High-density polyethylene components are susceptible to distortion. Avoid dents or scratches.
  b Metallic components must not be placed in contact with instruments, except those designed for their implantation.

c Open sterile packages just prior to use, after orthopaedist determines size and style.

2 Bone cement, if needed, must be mixed by scrub nurse prior to use.

a Fume evacuator, if used, may need to be recharged before and after use.

b Scrub nurse should know by feel and appearance when cement is correct consistency. A practice session is helpful before mixing for the first time during an actual operation.

c Room temperature can affect time necessary for cement to set.

d Pour cement into syringe as soon as it is mixed.

3 Air-powered drills must be properly connected with adequate pressure. Check pressure in tanks of compressed air or nitrogen before operation begins. It must be over 500 lb.

4 Suction tubing must be kept open and collection containers changed as necessary to maintain suction for irrigation during operation.

5 Exhaust system for personnel must be functioning properly if operation is performed within a clean air system (see p. 466).

6 Traffic through the operating room must be monitored and restricted to minimize air turbulence if laminar airflow is not installed. Infection is a major potential hazard of all bone and joint surgery. It can be disabling and financially costly.

Arthroscopy

Visualization within a joint through an arthroscope allows diagnosis and conservative treatment of some cartilagenous, ligamentous, synovial, and bony surface defects. Most frequently used for definitive treatment of meniscal, articular cartilage, and ligamentous defects in the knee, an arthroscope may be used in the shoulder, elbow, wrist, hip, and ankle. Fiberoptic arthroscopes have diameters ranging from 1.7 to 6 mm to accommodate to size of joint. Angles of the viewing lenses also vary from 30 to 90°.

Sterile irrigating solution, either normal saline or lactated Ringer's solution, at room temperature is necessary to distend the joint, although some arthroscopists prefer air or carbon dioxide. Solution is injected initially via needle and syringe. Then through a small stab wound, a cannula is inserted into the medial aspect of knee, for example, for inflow of irrigation. Outflow tubing is connected to the metal sheath of the arthroscope. It can be attached to suction or placed in a drainage bucket and allowed to drain by gravity.

The sheath (sleeve) over a sharp trocar is inserted through a stab wound in the skin at selected site of entry for the arthroscope. When the trocar penetrates the capsule, the capsule and synovium form a tight seal around the sheath. The sharp trocar is replaced with a blunt obturator to advance the sheath into the joint. The obturator is removed and the arthroscope inserted through the sheath. The inflow and outflow irrigating tubes are connected to the stopcocks on the sheath.

An operating arthroscope may have a channel for passage of long, thin, manually operated instruments such as probes, hooks, scissors, knives, punches, and grasping forceps. Or these instruments may be manipulated through separate puncture holes (portals) into the joint under visualization through the scope. Power-driven shavers are also used to smooth rough articular cartilage or bony surfaces. A carbon dioxide laser may be adapted to some arthroscopes. A video camera attached to the eyepiece allows projection of the view to a closed-circuit television monitor so that the surgeon can manipulate instruments more comfortably than by squinting through the eyepiece. Some cameras attach to the side of a beam splitter on the scope. Daylight film should be used with fiberoptic lighting.

Nursing Considerations for Arthroscopy

1 All metal components are steam sterilized. Some optical systems and fiberoptic cords can be steam sterilized; others require gas sterilization. Foam-lined sterilizing cases are recommended to protect the optics. If high-level disinfection in activated glutaraldehyde must be used, arthroscope must be rinsed in sterile distilled water before use. Follow manufacturer's recommendations for sterilization of arthroscope and its component attachments.

2 Scrub nurse checks all sterile equipment and instruments.

a Check arthroscope for clean lenses and unbroken optics.

b Check patency of inflow irrigation stopcocks.

c All component parts must be correct size, i.e., optics, trocar, and obturator must fit securely into sheath. Operating instruments must pass through channel. Fiberoptic cord must fit arthroscope and projection lamp.

3 Circulating nurse checks all nonsterile equipment, i.e., fiberoptic projection lamp, laser machine, video equipment.
4 Video camera and cable must be enclosed in a sterile cover unless camera has been gas sterilized. The scrub and circulating nurses coordinate the draping.
5 Tourniquet should be applied around patient's thigh for arthroscopy of the knee, but not inflated unless necessary to control bleeding.
6 Patient is prepped and draped as for any *sterile* procedure on the extremity (see Chap. 16), with extra precautions to provide waterproof barrier against contamination by irrigating solutions.
7 Circulating nurse hangs containers of irrigating solution on IV pole at least 3 ft (1 m) above joint to ensure adequate hydrostatic pressure to keep joint distended and to maintain flow of irrigating solution. Two to four 3000-ml containers may be needed. Extra containers should be available in the room. Solution is maintained at room temperature to avoid hyperemia from warm solution that may appear as inflammation of synovium, or blanching that produces avascular appearance from cold solution.
8 Equipment must be appropriately attached after patient is draped.
   a Scrub nurse secures drainage tubes, fiberoptic cord, suction, air-power cables, etc., to drapes in a location which will not impede movement of extremity.
   b Circulating nurse attaches tubings to irrigating and suction systems, cords to power sources, etc.

Arthrotomy

Incision into a joint may be necessary to biopsy synovium or cartilage, to remove bone or cartilage fragments, or to repair a defect in the synovium or joint capsule. Synovectomy may be the procedure of choice for relief of pain and control of inflammation in a rheumatoid arthritic joint.

Bunionectomy

Hallux valgus, a lateral deviation in position of great toe, increases prominence of the adjoining metatarsal head. Pressure at metatarsophalangeal joint causes inflammation that creates formation of an exostosis, bunion, beneath the bursa and joint capsule. A bunionectomy is done to remove the exostosis. One of several procedures may be selected to correct the deformity.

1 *Metatarsal osteotomy.* Metatarsal alignment is corrected by moving metatarsal head laterally.

2 *McBride operation.* Abductor tendon is fixed to lateral portion of metatarsal neck and sesamoid bone is excised.

3 *Keller arthroplasty.* Keller arthroplasty includes resection of the proximal third of the phalanx. A silicone implant may be placed in the intramedullary canal to stabilize the metatarsophalangeal joint.

NOTE. Bunionectomies are only one of the many procedures performed by podiatrists as well as orthopaedists in the treatment of foot-related disorders, including degenerative diseases and injuries of the foot and ankle.

REPAIR OF TENDONS AND LIGAMENTS

Tendons and ligaments may be severed, torn, or ruptured. These injuries are frequently seen in athletes. Total or partial avulsion of major ligaments and tendons torn from their attachments in or around an extremity joint requires repair to stabilize the joint.

Tendons can be lengthened, shortened, or transferred. When operation is indicated, tendon repair is a meticulous, but tedious, procedure. Close apposition of the cut ends of tendons, particularly extensor tendons, is imperative to successfully restore function. Tendons heal slowly. Stainless steel suture is widely used in tendon repair because of its durability and lack of elasticity. A tendon may be wrapped in a silicone membrane to prevent adhesions after repair. Artificial tendons are made of a polyester center covered with silicone rubber. A double velour polyester prosthesis is used for ligament repair of a shoulder separation.

Tendon surgery is within the realm of the orthopaedic surgeon; however, many plastic surgeons perform hand reconstruction, including tendon repair and transfer. Hand reconstruction has become a subspecialty of both orthopaedics and plastic surgery. The operating microscope is frequently used, especially when vascular and nerve repair are also involved in the reconstruction. (Refer to Chapter 34 for discussion of replantation of severed digits.)

Sports Medicine

Public interest in and orthopaedists' concern about athletic injuries have led to the development of sports medicine centers, which emphasize physical conditioning, injury prevention, and rehabilitation.

Ligaments in the knee are most prone to athletic injury. Arthroscopy is useful in diagnosis and treatment of some anterior cruciate ligament and meniscal tears (see p. 474). Other injuries require open operative reconstruction to obtain knee stability. Following rupture, the intraarticular anterior cruciate ligament may be transferred into the posterior aspect of the lateral femoral condyle. For chronic ligamentous instability, a bone-patellar, tendon-bone graft complex may be used for reconstruction. Artificial ligamentous substitutes may be preferred. Woven bovine collagen, a bovine and carbon fiber material, or a partially absorbable matrix of polylactic acid polymer and filamentous carbon may be used as a scaffold for new collagenous tissue ingrowth for disrupted ligaments.

VERTEBRAL COLUMN

Orthopaedic procedures on the back are usually performed to excise vertebral lesions, to relieve pressure on spinal cord, to stabilize vertebral column, or to correct gross deformities (refer to Chap. 33, p. 602, for discussion of scoliosis).

Primary neoplasms such as a giant cell bone tumor, bone cyst, hemangioma or osteoid osteoma, and metastatic tumors can occur in the vertebrae. Osteomyelitis, spondylolisthesis, and degenerative diseases are also indications for excision of bone from one or more vertebrae. Fracture, with or without dislocation of one or more vertebra, may be reduced by traction or excision of bony fragments. (Refer to Chapter 29, p. 557, for discussion of cervical traction.)

Laminectomy

Lumbar laminectomy is usually performed by the orthopaedist to remove a lumbar intervertebral disc that is exerting pressure on the spinal cord or nerve roots and causing low back pain. The spinous process and lamina on the affected side are removed. The herniated disc is removed from the intervertebral space. (Refer to Chapter 29, p. 556 for details of a laminectomy.)

Ligamentum Flavotomy

Some orthopaedists prefer a simple operation called *ligamentum flavotomy* with disc excision, rather than laminectomy, for some patients. The ligamentum flavum is the yellow elastic tissue that connects the lamina. It is incised and retracted laterally. The disc is removed. Then the ligamentum flavum is sutured back in place.

Chemonucleolysis

Chemonucleolysis, injection of chymopapain, may be procedure of choice to reduce size of a herniated lumbar disc rather than surgical discectomy. Chymopapain is a purified enzyme derived from the papaya plant. It hydrolyzes proteins, thus decreasing water-binding capacity when injected into the nucleus pulposus, inner disc material. The resultant reduction in size of the disc relieves pressure on the nerve root. Chymopapain must be refrigerated prior to use. Because alcohol can inactivate the enzyme, the vial top must air-dry after disinfection before drawing into syringe. Following dilution with sterile water, a test dose is injected into patient under fluoroscopy with image intensification to check alignment of spinal column and needle placement. The patient is observed for allergic reaction for 10 to 20 minutes before full dose is injected. Epinephrine 0.3 to 0.5 ml of 1:10,000 solution is administered as an IV bolus to treat anaphylaxis.

This technique is particularly effective for patients with sciatica, leg pain, and definite neurologic findings. The injected disc tends to reconstitute itself with normal tissue composition and within confines of intervertebral space.

Spinal Fusion

Spinal fusion may be indicated following spinal injury or excision of bone to stabilize the vertebral column. Bone grafts are placed in the intervertebral spaces or along the spinous processes to bridge over or to stabilize the defect. Either a posterior or anterior approach may be used to place the bone grafts. Homogenous cancellous bone from the bone bank may be preferred to provide a larger quantity of bone than can be obtained from an autogenous graft from the crest of the patient's ilium. Cancellous bone rather than cortical bone is usually preferred for spinal fusion.

Internal Fixation

Internal fixation may be preferred to stabilize a fracture or fracture-dislocation of the thoracic or lumbar spine. Harrington or Moe instrumentation with hooks or Luque rods (refer to Chap. 33, pp. 602 and 603) may be used to provide decompression of the spinal nerve roots following posterior spinal fusion. Dwyer or Dunn devices are used when an anterior approach is preferred. An internal spinal splint of stainless steel mesh filled with acrylic bone cement may be preferred to stabilize the spine initially, prior to a second-stage spinal fusion.

CAST APPLICATION

A *cast* is a rigid form of dressing used to encase a part of the body. It supports and immobilizes the part in optimum position until healing takes place. A cast usually includes the joints above and below the affected area. It may suffice as a conservative mode of treatment, as for fractures. It can be fitted to any body contour or position, and can be worn for months. Requisites of a cast are that:

1 It must fulfill its intended function of maintaining position of the desired parts.

2 It must not be too tight and must have no pressure areas, to permit adequate circulation. *Postapplication pain is an important symptom and must be promptly investigated.*

3 It must not be too loose. It must be as light as possible, yet strong enough to withstand usage.

4 It must be comfortable, with no binding or chafing.

Padding under Cast

Padding is usually put under casts and serves several functions.

1 It absorbs inevitable ooze from the wound following open operation. Sterile padding is put on over the dressing before applying the cast.

2 It protects the wound and the patient's skin.

3 It protects bony prominences.

Materials Used for Padding

Stockinet A knitted, seamless tubing of cotton 1 to 12 in. (2.5 to 30.4 cm) wide, stockinet stretches to fit any contour snugly.

Sheet Wadding A glazed cotton bandage 2 to 8 in. (5 to 20 cm) wide is available as a sheeting. It is used over stockinet or in place of it.

Soft Roll A soft roll of thin cotton batting has some stretch for smooth contour.

Felt Sheeting made of wool or blends of wool, cotton, or rayon available in thicknesses ranging from ⅛ to ½ in. (3 to 13 mm), felt is cut into desired sizes to fit bony prominences. Felt pads are applied over sheet wadding. Plaster adheres to them and prevents their slipping.

Foam Rubber Available as a sheeting ¼ to 1 in. (6.4 to 25 mm) in thickness, foam rubber may be used in place of felt.

Webril Webril is a soft lint-free cotton bandage. The surface is smooth but not glazed, so that each layer clings to the preceding one and the padding lies smoothly in place.

Plaster Casts

Plaster is gypsum or anhydrous calcium sulfate. It is finely ground to break up the crystals, and is then heated to drive out the water. When water is added again, recrystallization takes place and the plaster sets. It was first used as a method of splinting fractures in the nineteenth century.

Plaster bandages and splints are made of crinoline or other fabric with the plaster powder entrapped in the meshes. These are available in rolls or strips 2 to 8 in. (5 to 20 cm) wide. Plaster splints are either supplied precut or made from rolls as the need arises. Usually six or eight thicknesses of the desired length are used. Splints are applied over areas that may weaken from extra strain, to give added strength. Plaster bandages and splints are available with three types of plaster.

1 *Slow setting* requires up to 18 minutes to set. It is used in large casts requiring more time to apply and mold. It permits blending of the layers.

2 *Medium setting* requires up to 8 minutes to set. This type is used in average-size casts.

3 *Fast setting* requires 4 to 5 minutes to set. It is advantageous for small casts on children who are difficult to keep in position. Many orthopaedists prefer fast-setting type in all kinds of casts; it is the most universally used type of plaster.

Application of Plaster

1 Spread a disposable plastic or nonwoven fabric sheet on floor around table to catch drips.

2 Protect the table. If the orthopaedic table is used, spread a sheet over table parts, after patient is suspended.

3 Protect patient's hair with a cap.

4 Use a disposable plaster pail or a plastic liner bag in a plaster bucket.

5 Fill bucket with water at room temperature. Water warmer than 70 to 75°F (21 to 24°C) will speed setting time and may cause excessive loss of plaster from the fabric. More important, plaster will get even hotter than its normal exothermic reaction if dipped in hot water.

6 Don nonsterile disposable gloves to protect your skin from irritation by lime content.

7 Remove outer wrapping. Start soaking plaster only when surgeon is ready to apply it. Keep just ahead in soaking it. Have next roll ready when needed, but do not prepare several rolls ahead. They may harden and, if used, can produce an ineffective laminated cast. Avoid waste.

8 Hold bandage under water in vertical position to allow air bubbles to escape from the rolled end. When air bubbles stop rising, it is soaked through. Compress ends between fingers and palm of each hand to remove excess water. This procedure prevents telescoping during use.

9 Open the end about 1 in. (2.5 cm) and hand to the surgeon.

10 Fanfold a strip once toward the center, before soaking, leaving ends free to grasp. When soaking, grasp an end in each hand, press hands together and submerge strip in water for a few seconds; remove it and pull strip taut by the ends. It may seem drippy, but the layers blend together well when quite wet.

11 Ask the surgeon if another roll will be needed before soaking it when the cast appears near completion.

12 Handle the cast with care and support the patient in such a way that he or she cannot attempt to bend an incorporated joint. Wet plaster has only one-third to one-half its ultimate strength when dry. The person who supports an extremity while a cast is being applied takes care not to make finger-pressure areas in plaster that will damage tissue under it.

13 Elevate an extremity on a pillow until the cast hardens. If it is laid on a hard surface, flat pressure areas may be pressed onto it.

14 Clean up as much as possible while the cast is being applied. Wipe plaster off equipment as well as off the patient before it dries. It is easy to remove when still damp; after it dries it must be scraped off. Cast dryer, if used, hastens drying.

15 Avoid splashing plaster on furniture, walls, and floor.

16 Clean equipment and table thoroughly. If sink has a plaster trap, all plaster drip can be washed down the sink and contents of bucket poured into the sink. If there is no plaster trap, leave bucket until plaster in the bottom hardens; then empty water and throw plaster pail or plastic liner bag into the trash. Clean a reusable bucket as soon as finished with it.

Casts Commonly Used

Cylinder A circular cast, made by wrapping the plaster bandages around an extremity, is used after closed or open reductions of fractures, after some operations for immobilization, or for the purpose of resting a part of an extremity.

Walking Cast A rubber walking heel is applied to the sole of a cylinder cast for ambulation. Use of a lower extremity helps to maintain strength and muscle tone and to prevent atrophy.

Hanging Cast A cylinder is applied to arm with the elbow flexed. It extends from shoulder over the hand, leaving thumb and fingers free. A wire loop is incorporated at the wrist. A strap through this loop and around the neck suspends the arm. The weight of the cast provides needed traction on the humerus.

Shoulder Spica Applied to trunk, arm, and hand, leaving fingers and thumb free, a spica cast is used after some operations on the shoulder or humerus, or for fracture of the humerus. The orthopaedic table may be used for its application, or patient may sit on a stool with surgeon supporting arm in the desired position.

Hip Spica A hip spica cast is applied to trunk and one or both legs following some hip operations and fractures of the femur. The orthopaedic table is used. The sacrum rests on a sacral rest. The perineal post provides countertraction. Attachments may be used to support legs of an adult.

Minerva Jacket A Minerva jacket is applied from the hips to head. If head is to be completely immobilized, it is included in the jacket. The plaster is molded to fit around face and lower jaw. A part of the plaster at back of the head is cut out. It is used for fractures of cervical or upper thoracic vertebrae. The orthopaedic table is necessary.

Body Jacket A body jacket extends from axillae to hips to immobilize vertebrae. Application of this cast usually requires the orthopaedic or Risser table with the necessary attachments, although sometimes the patient may stand on floor. Traction may be applied by an overhead sling. If open operation is to be performed with patient in a body cast, a cast cutter must be at hand in case of respiratory difficulty. However, a body cast is usually bivalved before a patient is given an anesthetic.

NOTE. An opening is always made over the abdomen of a Minerva or body jacket to allow space for lung expansion and decompression of abdominal distention that normally occurs with ingestion of food. A folded towel may be placed over the abdomen before the stockinet is pulled over the body. This is removed when the opening is made in the cast to allow more space between the body and cast.

Plaster Shell A body jacket is cut along each side, into anterior and posterior parts. The parts may be fastened together by heavy straps with buckles, or the patient may rest in one while the other is temporarily removed.

Wedge Cast A wedge-shaped portion is cut from the cast. The edges are brought together and held with plaster reinforcement. It is used to overcome angulation in a fracture.

Plaster Splint Six or more thicknesses of plaster the desired width and length may be applied to posterior part of an extremity and bandaged with gauze or cotton elastic bandage. Excess water is pressed from plaster splint after it is immersed in water. A splint may be used for immobilization of a fracture of ulna or fibula.

Hairpin or Sugar-Tong Splint A splint twice as long as lower arm and hand is used for fracture of the ulna or radius. After plaster is soaked, it may be covered with stockinet. Starting with one end on back of the hand, the splint is placed around the flexed elbow. Palm of the hand and fingers rest on other end of it. It is secured with a bandage.

Abduction Hip Splint An abduction hip splint keeps hips in constant abduction. If desired for postoperative management, it is applied immediately after hip operation.

Plaster Rope Plaster rope may support arm in a shoulder spica or join legs in a bilateral hip spica. It is made by twisting a wet roll of plaster bandage into a rope as it is unwound, fanfolding to the desired length, and drawing it through cupped hand to blend the strands. A wooden splint may be incorporated into the rope for reinforcement.

Molds Molds are made as plaster patterns for removable metal or leather braces for the body, neck, or extremities.

Trimming, Removing, and Changing Casts Rough edges of plaster are trimmed off and edges of a cast are covered with stockinet or adhesive tape to protect the patient's skin. Instruments specifically designed for cutting through plaster must be used for trimming or removing casts. These include:

1 *Plaster knives,* which have short slightly curved blades.

2 *Plaster scissors,* which are heavy bandage scissors.

3 *Electric cast cutter,* which is an oscillating saw. It cuts the cast but not the stockinet or other padding under it, because the padding moves with the oscillations. The patient's skin also moves somewhat and is not injured if touched lightly, although care should always be taken not to touch the skin. One model has a vacuum attached to pick up the plaster dust created by the saw. A carbide steel blade is recommended for cutting fiberglass cast. A regular blade dulls quickly and can result in an inadvertent burn to patient.

4 *Cast spreader,* which is a long-handled instrument that has thin serrated jaws that can be inserted in the cutting line to pry open the cast.

5 *Cast bender,* which is a heavy forceps-type instrument used to bend a small portion of the edge of a cast away from an area, such as a portion of a jacket away from the mouth and chin, to give freer movement.

Sharp plaster knives or scissors are usually used to trim casts. For large casts the electric cast cutter may be used, for example, to cut an opening over the abdomen of a body jacket. In a hip spica, adequate space is provided for use of the bedpan without soiling. If it is necessary to cut a "window"—a small opening in a cast to remove sutures or to inspect an area—it is put back in place and secured with a few turns of plaster bandage. An opening in a cast encourages swelling of the tissues under it, known as *window edema.*

When edema in a wound under a cast recedes, the cast does not furnish as much immobilization as may be desired. The cast is usually changed at this stage.

Many times a change of cast also entails removal of skin sutures, if the cast has been applied following operation. A sterile suture removal tray should be ready for use when requested. Sterile sheet wadding may be needed to cover the wound after sutures are removed, before another cast is applied.

If patient has been in a cast for some time, the skin is apt to be oily, somewhat soiled, and rough. If surgeon wishes the skin cleansed before applying another cast, only superficial dirt can be removed. Scrubbing off oily scales may cause irritation. Usually skin is not washed but rubbed with cold cream or powdered with talc before applying sheet wadding and a new cast.

Provide a large empty cardboard carton or plastic-lined trash container in which to put the wrappings, trimming, removed cast, etc., during cast application and removal. (This can be taken directly to the incinerator for disposal with minimal environmental contamination.)

Wash off knives, scissors, cutter, spreader, and bender as soon as you are finished with them. Apply oil to all instrument joints before putting instruments away to avoid rust and corrosion.

Fiberglass Casts

A woven fiberglass tape impregnated with a water-activated or photosensitive resin can be used for casting or bracing. Polypropylene stockinet is applied over the patient's skin. Polypropylene web wrap may be used for extra padding over bony prominences and pressure points. The person applying the cast must wear gloves or coat hands with a silicone hand cream to facilitate smoothing and blending the layers of the fiberglass tape and to prevent resin pickup on the hands. The tape is applied in the same manner as is plaster; however, it does not become rigid until it is cured. Exposure to humidity or near ultraviolet light in the 3200- to 4000-angstrom (Å) range, commonly known as *black light,* cures the cast, depending on type of material used.

When cured, the cast is lighter, thinner, yet stronger and more porous for better ventilation than is a plaster cast. It can be immersed in water without deterioration. Because of the advantages they afford, these resin tapes are preferred by many orthopaedic surgeons for extremity casts.

ORTHOPAEDIC CART

For closed reduction of fractures, traction, and postoperative applications, many orthopaedic appliances must be available and at hand when needed. An orthopaedic cart can provide the necessary items for these situations. The items may vary somewhat at different hospitals but many will be universally used. The cart can be taken wherever needed in the OR suite. One shelf should be kept for sterile items.

1 Suture removal trays
2 Webril and soft roll
3 Assorted sponges, dressings, bandages
4 Skin antiseptic agents

Another shelf should contain nonsterile items.

1 Pulleys and attachments for beds
2 Ropes, weights, and carriers
3 Felt padding and foam rubber
4 Arm and shoulder immobilizers
5 Pelvic slings and rods
6 Assorted sizes of gauze and muslin bandages, stockinet, sheet wadding, soft rolls, etc.
7 Stapler
8 Safety pins
9 Cold cream and talcum powder
10 Disposable plaster pail or bucket with plastic liner bag
11 Plastic bag for trash
12 Assorted sizes of plaster rolls and splints
13 Cast cutters, knives, scissors, spreaders, and bender

Splints, overhead traction bars, shock blocks, foot-drop stops, and other bulky items are obtained from the cast room as needed.

CHAPTER **25**

OPHTHALMOLOGY

HISTORICAL INTRODUCTION

Disorders of the eye have plagued human beings since time immemorial. None has been as well-documented as has *cataract,* an opacification of the crystalline lens of the eye. The word *cataract,* originally derived from Greek, was translated in Arabic to mean "mist of a waterfall." Throughout history cataract has been called by various names, such as "pearl of the eye."

Awareness of cataract probably extends back at least 3000 years. The finding of Bronze Age (2000–1000 B.C.) instruments like those used for an ancient couching treatment helps substantiate this belief. Couching consisted of striking a blow to the front of the eye with a sharp instrument to spontaneously dislocate the opacified lens and push it back into the vitreous cavity. Light then entered the pupil. Couching was used by the Hindus, Greeks, Romans, and Arabs.

A treatise written many years before Christ by a reknowned Hindu surgeon, Súsruta, taught that cataract was an opacity of the lens due to a disorder of eye fluids. Hippocrates wrote that pupils of the eyes sometimes became distorted, taking on the color of the sea.

In the early Christian era, Celsus differentiated between incipient (beginning) and mature cataracts. Galen thought the white opacity to be partly in the lens and partly in the aqueous humor in the form of a membrane floating between the lens and the iris. That belief was held, and couching practiced sporadically, until the mid-eighteenth century when J. Daviel, a French surgeon, performed the first deliberate lens removal. The intracapsular technique, however, was not accepted and refined until the 1930s and 1940s, when it became a standard procedure of cataract removal.

The first corneal transplant in which a scarred cornea was replaced with a clear cornea was performed around 1817. It failed because heterograft tissue was used instead of homograft tissue. The first reported successful full-thickness graft of full corneal depth, that remained clear, was transplanted in 1905. Although attempted in the interval, corneal transplantation did not become an established technique until after World War II. Since then, technique has been refined to produce a high rate of favorable outcomes.

Fruitless attempts were made in the early eighteenth century to implant lenses. The modern era of implantation of plastic intraocular lens evolved from an incidental observation. Surgeons in England noted a lack of reactivity to fragments of plastic from shattered plane canopies that penetrated the eyes of fighter pilots in World War II. Posterior chamber lenses placed in the 1950s produced disappointing long-term results mainly because of dislocation. These lenses subsequently had to be removed because of inadequate fixation design. The first series of anterior chamber lenses placed in front of the iris sometimes produced delayed corneal damage. The iris-supported lenses were designed to avoid this complication, but are seldom used because of mechanical problems such as dislocation and corneal irritation. However, modifications of the anterior chamber lens of improved design to reduce complication are popular and successful. Also since the 1960s, attention has been redirected to posterior chamber placement with adequate fixation of the lens by means of loops called haptics.

The development of fluorescein angiography, visualization of the entire retinal vascular tree by injection of a fluorescing dye, has expanded knowledge of retinal and choroidal physiology and disease, resulting in improved therapy.

The advent of ophthalmic lasers that provide ablation of pathology with light energy was a great step forward for many patients. Laser therapy obviates the need for some operative procedures. Initially used primarily for vascular diseases such as diabetic retinopathy, laser use has expanded to include treatment of glaucoma and secondary cataract.

Ophthalmology pioneered the use of medical lasers and operating microscope.

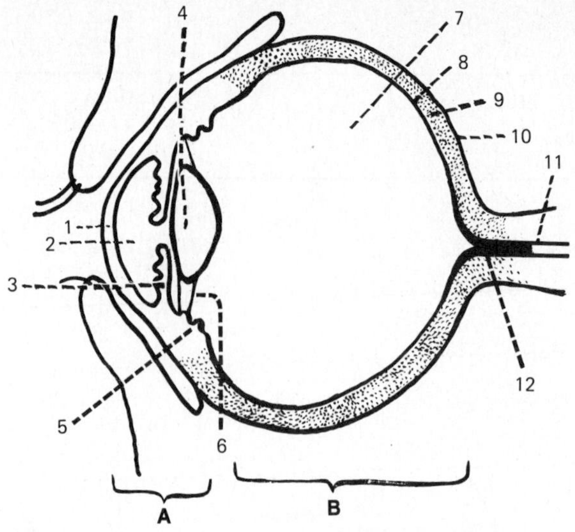

FIGURE 25-1
Anatomy of the eye. (**A**) Anterior segment: (1) cornea, (2) anterior chamber, (3) iris, (4) lens, (5) ciliary body, (6) zonule. (**B**) Posterior segment: (7) vitreous body, (8) retina, (9) choroid, (10) sclera, (11) optic nerve, (12) central retinal artery.

THE EYE

The main causes of blindness are retinal disorders, glaucoma, and cataract. A substitute system for vision in the eye, one of the most intricate organs in the body, does not exist, but modern ophthalmology can cure or greatly improve many types of impaired vision. Ocular disorders may be the initial manifestations of systemic disease. Early detection and referral on the part of an alert ophthalmologist can be life-preserving as well as sight-preserving.

Anatomy and Physiology

A thorough understanding of the anatomical structure and physiology of the eye is fundamental to comprehension of the operative procedures (see Fig. 25-1). The *globe,* or *eyeball,* is situated within the bony orbit surrounded by a padding of fatty tissue. Its position is maintained by extraocular muscles and fascial attachments. The outer wall of the globe is called the *sclera* (opaque white of eye), and is contiguous with the transparent avascular *cornea* anteriorly. The *conjunctiva* is the mucous membrane that lines the inner side of the eyelids and the exposed portion of the sclera except for the cornea.

The *anterior segment* of the eye includes the cornea, the anterior chamber filled with aqueous fluid (humor), the circular pigmented iris, and the lens. The lens consists of clear, transparent gelatinous protein encased in a capsule. It is supported by a series of suspensory ligaments called zonules. The portion of the eye lying beyind the lens is known as the *posterior segment.* This part contains the vitreous fluid, which must be clear for vision, the retina, and the choroid linings, which are the vascular nourishing layers.

The function of vision requires:

1 Visual apparatus
2 Source of light
3 Interpretation by the brain of what is seen

Basically the eye resembles a camera with a compound lens system. Light rays emanating from an object in the field of vision are transmitted to the eye, where they traverse the optical system to get to the retina. The retina corresponds to the film of the camera. The area of highest sensitivity for details is called the *macula,* which is located in the proximate center of the retina at the posterior pole.

The *optical system* is comprised of the transparent cornea, or window of the eye; the aqueous fluid behind the cornea; the pupil, or opening in the colored iris; and the lens. The naturally flexible lens focuses light rays by bending them to form an image on the retina, the innermost layer of the eye that contains the visual-nerve endings. These sensory cells translate patterns of light into nervous impulses, which are transmitted to the brain via the optic nerve. The cells are connected to nerve fibers, which converge toward the brain to become the optic nerve. The occipital portion of the brain interprets the light-ray images registered on the retina. The intensity of light is automatically determined by the size of the pupil, which is controlled by the iris muscles. The iris action functions like the shutter of a camera.

OCULAR OPERATIVE PROCEDURES

Operative treatment of the eye can be divided for convenience into two main classifications:

1 Extraocular, or conditions affecting the exterior surface of the eye or the orbit
2 Intraocular, or conditions pertaining to the interior contents of the eye

Extraocular Procedures

Eyelid

Plastic Repair of Lacerations Plastic repair involves approximation of anatomical layers. Penetrating wounds such as animal bites are debrided. If the laceration includes the lacrimal canaliculus or tear duct, special probes are used to identify the proximal portions for rejoining. Lacerations of the lacrimal canaliculus may be repaired by suturing over either of two types of stents. The Quickert-Dryden tubing consists of a length of flexible silicone with a malleable metal lacrimal probe swaged onto each end. One end of probe is inserted through the upper lid canaliculus, the passage leading to the tear duct. The other end is inserted correspondingly into the lower lid canaliculus. Both exit via the tear sac and nasolacrimal canal into the nose. The lacerated canaliculus is then sutured over the tubing, which is removed after healing takes place. Some surgeons prefer the rigid Veirs stainless steel rod. This is inserted into the lacerated canaliculus. A 4-0 silk suture swaged to one end permits withdrawal of the rod after healing.

Biopsy or Excision of Neoplasm of Lid Tissue may be excised with a knife, by electrodesiccation (high-frequency electric current), or by cryosurgery. An extremely common but benign tumor of the lid is the *chalazion,* a cystic alteration of one of the oil-secreting meibomian glands in the lid. The resulting accumulation of oil forms a hard tumor of the lid, requiring excision. This is usually an office or ambulatory operative procedure.

Plastic Repair of Defects Following removal of a lid malignancy, plastic repair employs the usual plastic procedures such as Z-plasty in addition to sliding flaps from adjacent areas and full- or partial-thickness flaps from the opposing lid to close the defect (see Chap. 27).

Correction of Ptosis (Drooping of Upper Lid) While more commonly congenital (see Chap. 33), ptosis may be acquired in adults. An incision on the front or back surface of the lid exposes the levator muscle. This is dissected free of its adjacent attachments and a variable amount is excised in proportion to the degree of ptosis. Fasanella-Servet is a popular operation for correcting a minor degree of ptosis.

Repair of Acquired Malformation of the Lid Conditions such as senile ectropion or entropion most commonly affect the lower lid. *Ectropion* is a condition in which either lid is *everted* (turned out) so as to expose the conjunctival surface of the lid. *Entropion* is the opposite condition in which the lid margin is *inverted* (turned in). Frequently the lashes then abrade the cornea. Various procedures may be employed with principles common to both conditions. A triangle of lid tissue is excised to erect the lid: in ectropion, the base of the triangle is up; in entropion, the base is down.

Blepharoplasty Common results of aging are stretching of the eyelid skin and bulging of orbital fat from between the muscle fibers of the lids. Both cause cosmetic disfigurement or "baggy lids," and in extreme cases may obstruct vision. Redundant fold(s) of skin and herniated pockets of fat are removed. Defects in the muscle layer are repaired. (Refer to Chapter 27, p. 528).

Lacrimal Apparatus

Lacimal-Duct Dilatation Lacrimal-duct dilatation is performed for excessive tearing. A series of probes, graduated in size, are introduced one by one into the duct system to permit freer drainage of tears.

Dacryocystectomy Extirpation or removal of the lacrimal sac is performed for chronic dacryocystitis. It does not reestablish the tear-drainage system.

Dacryocystorhinostomy Construction of a new opening into the nasal cavity from the lacrimal sac is done to correct congenital malformation or trauma to the nasolacrimal duct. A new tear-drainage system is constructed.

Extraocular Muscle Procedures Procedures on oculomotor muscles, those that control eye movement, are performed to correct misalignment that interferes with the ability of the two eyes to remain in simultaneous focus on a viewed object. The operations correct muscle imbalance by strengthening a weak muscle or by weakening an overactive one. While commonly performed on children (see Chap. 33), muscle procedures may be required in adult patients for:

1 Untreated childhood strabismus (squint)
2 Unsatisfactory result from childhood operation
3 Trauma to the brain stem or to the orbit with resultant muscle injury or paralysis
4 Systemic disease, such as thyroid exophthalmos, and muscle paralysis
5 Cerebrovascular accident (CVA) with resultant muscle paralysis

Orbital Procedures

Decompression Decompression is the operative treatment for severe exophthalmos that does not respond to medical treatment.

Exploration for Tumors Tumor exploration may be performed as indicated through a suitable approach such as the lateral wall or roof of the orbit, depending on location. The procedure may involve an interdisciplinary team of surgeons.

Procedures for Removal of Eye

Enucleation Enucleation is the complete removal of the eyeball and severing of its muscular attachments. The muscle stumps are preserved. The space between them forms a pocket into which a plastic spherical implant is usually inserted. The overlying fascia and conjunctiva are closed to contain the sphere in the socket. Contraction of the eye muscles cause the artificial eye (prosthesis) to move in the socket, simulating normal eye movements.

Evisceration In contrast to enucleation, evisceration consists of removal of the contents of the eyeball only, leaving the outer sclera and muscles intact. This procedure reduces the danger of transmission of intraocular infection to the orbit and brain. It provides points for attachment of a prosthesis. Predisposing factors include destruction of the eyeball by injury or disease, and absolute glaucoma (hard blind eye).

Exenteration Exenteration is removal of the entire eye and orbital contents (tendon, fatty, and fibrous tissues). It is done for malignant tumors of the lids or the eyeball that have extended into the orbit. Extensive plastic reconstruction is necessary before fitting an artificial eye.

Intraocular Procedures

Corneal Procedures Although resilient tissue, the continually exposed cornea is especially susceptible to injury and infection.

Repair of Laceration Repair of laceration is preferably accomplished by direct appositional suturing of the edges. Some irregular lacerations not easily closed by direct suturing may be closed and the leak stopped by application of cyanoacrylate glue. Usually a soft contact lens is placed as a bandage over the freshly glued eye. A conjunctival flap can be placed to achieve a similar seal, but it is used less frequently. A large laceration may require a penetrating keratoplasty as an emergency procedure to ensure the integrity of the eye.

Removal of Foreign Body A foreign object is removed very gently under aseptic technique to avoid secondary infection and further trauma.

Cauterization Cauterization with chemicals or heat is sometimes used for corneal ulceration that does not respond to antibiotics. This is most frequently performed for herpes simplex virus infections of the corneal epithelium. It is often used in conjunction with topical antiviral agents.

Pterygium Pterygium is a benign growth of conjunctival tissue over the corneal surface. Although usually slow growing, pterygia can become fairly aggressive, especially in southern climates. Significant decrease in visual acuity secondary to induced astigmatism and corneal scarring can result from the abnormal growth. One of many operative techniques devised for its eradication is the McReynolds transplant, which involves subconjunctival transplanting of the head of the pterygium. Beta radiation may be used as an adjunct to operative treatment.

Corneal Transplant (Keratoplasty) Diseased cornea may be removed and replaced with healthy human donor cornea. This procedure is indicated when scars or opacities on the cornea reduce or destroy vision by preventing transmission of a clear image. The front of the eye must be clear to permit light to enter and focus on the retina in the back of the eye. Corneal opacity may result from degenerative changes, scars from chemical burns, perforated corneal ulcers, trauma, or edema following cataract operation. In addition, ocular surgery such as phacoemulsification, vitrectomy, and intraocular lens implantation potentially can damage corneal epithelium. Keratoplasty is the most successful transplantation procedure, with considerably less rejection phenomenon than other tissues, except bone, since the cornea is avascular. The greatest advance in technique to reduce the rate of rejection and restriction of activity during convalescence has been the use of the operating microscope and microsutures. Continuous 10-0 nylon sutures can be left in situ for an extended period, even up to six months, with minimal tissue reaction. Two types of grafts are used:

1 Full-thickness, the common type, in which entire thickness of the cornea is replaced, usually 6.5 to 8 mm (penetrating keratoplasty)

2 Partial-thickness or lamellar, less popular, in which only the top layer of cornea, not its entire depth is replaced (lamellar keratoplasty)

An opaque cornea is an optically nonfunctioning one. The goal is to provide recipients with the highest quality corneal tissue. Fresh, healthy cornea cut from the promptly enucleated eye of a relatively young donor within four to six hours of death is considered the best for transplantation. It should be inserted in the recipient eye, which has a healthy retina and optic nerve, as soon as possible to preserve viability and to prevent opacity. However, the acceptable times for collection of tissue after death and transplantation are somewhat variable among eye banks. Generally, the sooner enucleated eyes are refrigerated or corneas removed from the eye globe, the better quality the donor tissue. An interval exceeding five hours from enucleation to storage is considered unsatisfactory by many corneal surgeons.

The cornea has five layers. The endothelium, the very sensitive inner single layer of corneal cells, must be kept intact for eventual transparency of the graft.

Donor tissue criteria include the following.

1 Medical information about potential donor should be carefully evaluated because of possible transmission of donor disease and unknown etiology of some diseases. Some conditions that preclude use of donor tissue are unknown cause of death, hepatitis, rabies, Reye's syndrome, and lymphosarcoma.

2 All donor information from acceptable donor must be documented on a donor screening form that accompanies the tissue. A copy should be filed at the eye bank.

3 Consent for enucleation should conform with state laws. Responsibility for documentation of legal consent rests with person performing enucleation.

4 Enucleation may be performed by a certified eye-bank technician. Important factors are use of sterile technique, removal of as much conjunctiva as possible from donor globe, avoidance of damage or contamination of removed eyes, use of appropriate transport jars and methods, and avoidance of donor disfigurement. Either whole donor globe is removed or cornea with scleral rim is excised for transplantation.

5 The sooner enucleated eyes are cooled, the less likelihood of deleterious effects. One of the most important factors in viability of donor tissue after death is prompt placement of ice bags over eyes to slow metabolism of corneal cells.

6 Enucleated eyes are placed in fixed environment at eye bank. Cornea is carefully evaluated for epithelial defects, clarity, presence of foreign body, or evidence of jaundice. Endothelial cells can be counted, which is a determining factor in estimating prognosis. The higher the count, the better the tissue. Evaluation form should be completed and accompany tissue. Transplant surgeon may also receive noncontact specular microscopy and photographs of endothelium.

Donor eye preservation: two major techniques are used for corneal tissue preservation and storage.

1 Refrigerated whole eyes. Moist chamber storage of whole globes at 39°F (4°C) preserves quality for 24 to 36 hours.

2 McCarey-Kaufman (M-K) medium. Allows longer storage, 72 to 96 hours, and is favored by many eye banks. At time of tissue preservation, antibiotics may be added to M-K medium, but this does not ensure sterility. *In OR,* surgeon should inspect container of M-K before using cornea. If there is any evidence of contamination such as a crack, or if the medium is turbid, cornea should not be used and eye bank should be notified. If M-K cornea is used, remaining corneoscleral rim should be placed in culture medium and sent to lab for culture. However, incidence of positive culture is low.

Other less common preservation methods are:

3 Tissue culture medium. This method has not become widespread because of problems with sterility which require strict observation by a lab technician and microbiologist. Donor epithelium must not be injured during the process.

4 Cryopreservation. Both cryopreserved corneal and scleral tissue can be used for transplantation or for patching purposes. Use generally is limited to emergency procedures when fresh tissue is not available. Usually this tissue is used less than six months after cryopreservation. Precise freezing and defrosting methods are of crucial importance in prevention of injury to the endothelium. When the solution is thawed, the team must work rapidly because of extreme time limitation, as corneal metabolism resumes with defrosting. Tissue must be placed immediately within its natural anatomical environment to enhance potential for successful grafting.

Regardless of storage method, tissue preferably is used as soon as practical after donation. In the OR, adequate preparation, teamwork, and standardized transplantation procedure are imperative. The recipient eye must be trephined to receive donor cornea. A separate sterile donor table is set for surgeon to use in preparing donor tissue to the exact measurement needed for the recipient eye. Also a tissue recipient information form is completed following operation. This form indicates how the tissue was utilized. It is mailed to the eye bank where it is kept on file. If the tissue is contaminated, the donor number and source can easily be traced. Forms include recipient medical information; previous keratoplasties; date, type, and details of current operation; and estimate of success.

Available corneal tissue is in limited supply, placing restraints on transplantation. Numerous eye banks in the United States constitute the Eye Bank Association of America, which is tangentially associated with the International Eye Bank. These groups are central clearinghouses for dispersion of accessible tissue. They follow a stringent code of ethics in their function to inform the public of the need for eye donations, procure donated eyes, assist in optimum use of donor corneas locally, or arrange for transportation to an area of greater need. Tissue procurement is facilitated by:

1 Distribution of donor forms from eye banks and organ donation societies.

2 Organ donation consent affixed to driver licenses.

3 Education of medical and paramedical personnel.

Refractive Keratoplasty (Corneal Reshaping) Refractive keratoplasty includes a group of operations which are designed to alter the shape and refractive power, i.e., focusing power, of the cornea to minimize the optical problems of myopia, aphakia, keratoconus, hyperopia, and astigmatism.

1 *Radical keratotomy* reduces myopia (nearsightedness) by making multiple small radial incisions in the cornea to approximately 90 percent of its depth. These incisions allow stretching and flattening of the anterior corneal surface to reduce corneal curvature and bring light to a focus closer to, or on, the retina. This flattening corrects the refractive error.

The procedure is performed on patients who have occupational requirements for a visual acuity level without use of glasses or contact lenses, such as selective airline, police, and firefighter positions. Less justifiable indication for operation is for purely cosmetic reasons. Potential complications include perforations of the cornea; permanent corneal scarring; glaring or variable vision; injury to the lens, causing cataract; and infection. Long-term results are somewhat unpredictable. The procedure should be limited to patients with healthy eyes.

2 *Keratomileusis and keratophakia* procedures modify corneal refractivity by inserting a lathed button of corneal tissue into the cornea, using a computerized technique. If the patient is the donor (*keratomileusis*), the anterior lamellae of the cornea are removed, reshaped by cryolathing, and then sutured in place. For *keratophakia,* the tissue is obtained from another donor and may be preserved. The lenticule is cryolathed at operation, inserted intralamellarly into the recipient cornea, and sutured in place.

These operations require a highly specialized experienced team and costly equipment, the cryolathe for shaping the button, and the computer. Research is ongoing to develop other materials that may be used in place of human tissue as a donor lenticule in keratophakia. Very high water content plastic similar to continuous-wear contact lens material has been utilized.

3 *Epikeratophakia* is performed to correct extreme refractive errors such as aphakia (absence of lens inducing extreme hyperopia), myopia, or keratoconus (cone-shaped cornea causing extreme astigmatism). The recipient corneal epithelium is removed and a previously cryolathed and preserved donor button of corneal tissue is sutured *onto* the recipient's corneal surface.

Iris Procedures

Excision of Prolapse Prolapse may follow eye laceration or an operation on the anterior segment. Fresh prolapses may be reduced mechanically at operation or pharmacologically with drugs. Older prolapses should be excised to avoid intraocular infection.

Procedures for Glaucoma Glaucoma is a disease characterized by an abnormally increased intraocular fluid pressure; it often involves the iris. If uncontrolled, glaucoma progresses to atrophy of the optic nerve, hardening of the eyeball, and blindness. The incidence of glaucoma in persons over 40 increases with each decade. There is a familial predisposition to the disease.

Intraocular pressure (IOP) is estimated in one of three ways:

1 *Schiotz mechanical tonometer* records the depth of indentation of the cornea by a plunger of known weight. The degree of indentation is calibrated on the tonometer to correspond to the intraocular pressure. Normal numerical value is 15 to 22. This tonometer can be sterilized for use in the OR for preoperative pressure measurement.

2 *Applanation tonometer* attached to the biomicroscope (slit lamp) records the force required to flatten a specified area of cornea. Normal value is 10 to 21. This is considered to be the most accurate method.

3 *Air puff device* measures the force of a reflected amount of air blown against the cornea.

Persons suspected of having glaucoma undergo additional testing. Tonography, using an electronic tonometer, measures rate of aqueous outflow. Visual fields detect diminished peripheral vision. Gonioscopy determines structure of the angle.

Two basic types of glaucoma are classified anatomically by size of the angle between the iris and the cornea: *narrow-angle or angle-closure glaucoma* and *wide-angle or open-angle glaucoma.* If the angle is narrow, the iris may mechanically obstruct outflow of aqueous. This will cause the pressure within the eye to rise and precipitate an attack of acute glaucoma, an emergency situation which is very painful. Operative intervention affords relief and is always necessary for this condition to open the angle and reduce pressure to avoid damage to the optic nerve. Intervention may be laser iridotomy or surgical iridectomy. Wide-angle or open-angle glaucoma, the most common, is a chronic type, often of insidious onset, which may cause permanent visual loss before it is detected. The obstruction is not mechanical but physiological, a lack of ability to filter aqueous. Operations for this type of disease are performed only if medical and/or laser therapy are unsuccessful. Optical lasers offer an alternative to conventional operation for many patients, with laser therapy to trabecular meshwork (trabeculoplasty) replacing surgery for some glaucoma patients (see optical lasers, p. 492). One of the following operations may be preferred.

1 *Iridectomy,* excising a sector of iris, or *iridotomy,* cutting a small opening in iris, is done to deflate the mechanical obstruction, thus increasing drainage by permitting normal outflow of aqueous from the posterior to the anterior chamber. Another use of iridectomy is to create a new pupillary opening to improve visual acuity in patients with corneal or lens opacity due to injury or cataract not associated with glaucoma.

2 *Filtering-type procedures,* of which there are many variations such as *trephining* and *trabeculectomy,* create an artificial fistula between the angle of the anterior chamber and the subconjunctival space, to bypass the usual blocked outflow channels. Iridectomy is usually performed as part of the procedure to eliminate blockage of the fistula by the underlying iris. The Nd:YAG laser may be used to reopen filtering sites that have scarred closed following previous surgery for glaucoma.

3 *Cyclodialysis, cyclodiathermy,* and *cyclocryotherapy* are performed to diminish aqueous secretion by the ciliary body. Cyclodialysis involves severing the blood supply of the ciliary body. Cyclodiathermy and cyclocryothermy utilize the application of heat or cold, respectively, for the same purpose.

Secondary glaucoma is often a complication of inflammation such as iritis, which usually responds best to medical treatment. On the other hand, neoplasm, vascular obstruction, trauma or hermorrhage, and other causes of obstruction to aqueous drainage may require operative intervention. Treatment is directed to the primary etiology.

Congenital glaucoma is manifested soon after birth (refer to Chap. 33 for discussion).

Cataract Procedures Cataract is an opacification of the crystalline lens, its capsule, or both. The more or less opaque lens does not transmit clear images to the retina. Symptoms are related to the location and configuration of opacity. Etiology may be a known factor, such as metabolic or systemic disease, toxic material, radiation, trauma, genetic factors, or an unknown factor. With advancing age, persons are more prone to develop cataracts, so the incidence is increasing. While often developing in both eyes, the two cataracts tend to mature at different rates. Usually only one eye is operated at a time. Many ophthalmologists perform cataract operations as ambulatory surgery procedures, but this is not a universal practice. Problems can easily arise because little control of the patient is exercised outside the hospital setting and emergency medical care may not be readily available if needed. Many cataract patients are elderly and benefit from an extra day of hospitalization and close observation.

Cataracts may be classified as:

1 Congenital
2 Senile or primary
3 Secondary, resulting from local or systemic disease, or eye injury

Operative removal, followed by appropriate optical rehabilitation, is the only treatment. The operative procedure is determined by the patient's age and type of cataract. Time of operation is planned according to visual requirements, general health, and potential for rehabilitation. Microsurgery has revolutionized cataract extraction, one of the most frequently performed operations in the United States.

Intracapsular Extraction The entire lens, intact within its capsule, is delivered through a moderately sized incision made in the region of the *limbus,* the junction of the cornea and the sclera. Prior to delivery, an iridectomy or multiple iridotomies are performed, chiefly to prevent iris prolapse and to preserve communication between the anterior and posterior chambers. The lens is grasped by the method of surgeon's preference, i.e., mechanical forceps, suction devices, or cryoextractor. A miniaturized cryoprobe freezes onto the surface of the cataract, thus obtaining very secure adherence. This efficient method facilitates removal of fragile or dislocated cataracts (see Figs. 25-2 and 25-3). Also, the freezing technique greatly reduces inadvertent rupture of the capsule during extraction. The scrub nurse should have a balanced salt solution irrigator available for use in case it is necessary to unfreeze unintentional attachment of the cryoextractor to the iris or cornea. The wound is closed watertight with multiple sutures, commonly 10-0 nylon.

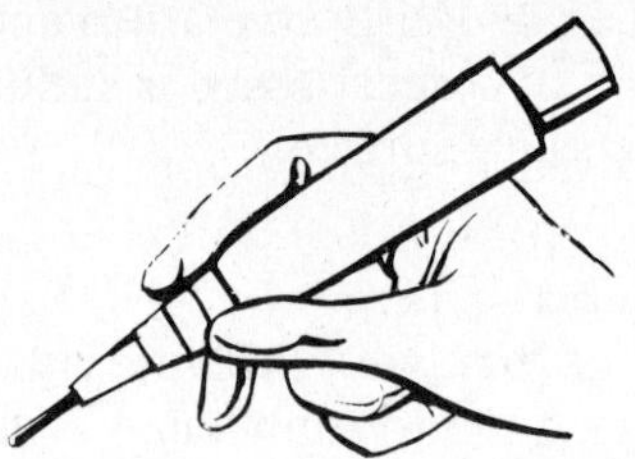

FIGURE 25-2
One type of sterile disposable cryoextractor used for cataract extraction.

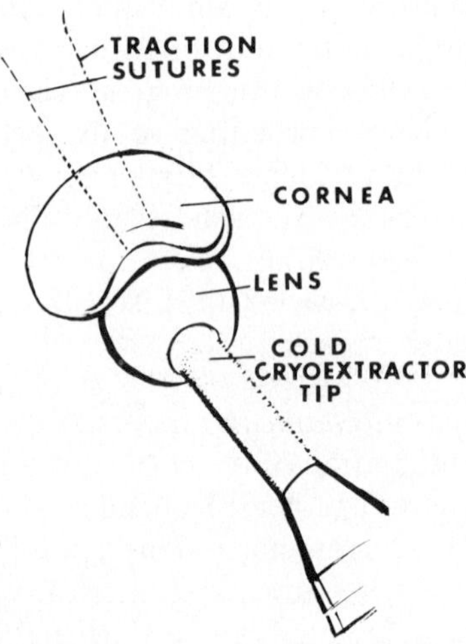

FIGURE 25-3
Refrigerated tip of cryoextractor adherent to anterior surface of lens while extracting lens. Two traction sutures elevate cornea.

With intracapsular lens extraction, no remnant remains in the visual axis that might proliferate or opacify to obstruct vision. Success rate for regaining vision is high. But the procedure's popularity waned somewhat when the development of fluorescein angiography brought attention to a number of patients who developed cystoid macular edema. This is a change in the macula resulting in marked loss of visual acuity. Intracapsular extraction may also be followed by retinal detachment, discussed later in this chapter.

Conventional Extracapsular Extraction Extracapsular extraction involves a similar but somewhat smaller incision than does intracapsular extraction. The anterior capsule is incised with a cystotome, a miniature hook-shaped knife, or with a bent 25-gauge needle, and then largely removed. The remaining cortex and nucleus are extracted by irrigation-aspiration, and expression from the posterior capsule, which is left in place. The wound is closed with a few sutures. The advantage of this procedure is protection of the vitreous and retina by the clear posterior lens capsule, which then serves as an anatomical barrier between posterior and anterior segments of the eye. Occasionally the posterior capsule will remain opaque, in which case discission (needling) is performed at a later date to provide an optically clear opening.

Linear Extraction Linear extraction is performed in young adults. A small incision is made through the limbus. The anterior capsule is incised and the major portion of it excised with a cystotome. The soft cataractous material is irrigated from the anterior chamber.

Phacoemulsification (Phacofragmentation) Although aspiration technique is commonly used in young persons, it was not successful in adults with senile cataracts until the late 1960s. At that time a sophisticated machine, the *phacoemulsifier,* was developed to break up and remove firm, insoluble lens nuclei. This machine, with components for ultrasonic vibration and irrigation-aspiration, permits extracapsular extraction through a very small incision in the limbus. All functions are controlled by foot pedal.

The handpiece of the phacoemulsifier consists of a 1-mm hollow titanium alloy needle surrounded by a silicone sleeve. The needle is inserted into the anterior chamber following removal of the anterior capsule with a cystotome and prolapse of the lens nucleus into the chamber through a widely dilated pupil. The activated needle breaks up the lens with ultrasonic vibrations. While the lens is thus emulsified, a constant flow of irrigating solution through the sleeve prevents heat buildup and dissolves the soluble lens. The irrigation-aspiration flow is automatically regulated to maintain anterior chamber depth. The aspirator removes the fragments. After the cortex (material surrounding lens nucleus) is removed by irrigation-aspiration, the posterior capsule may be polished with an instrument to remove any residual cortex. The posterior capsule is left intact unless an opacity remains, in which case it may be incised during operation or at a future time. The limbal incision is closed with one stitch.

Appropriate checks should be made before use of the various handpieces and for integrity of the vacuum and irrigating systems. The scrub and circulating nurses must work closely with the surgeon to monitor the various functions of the machine to avoid error. They must also observe the transparent tubes for flow of aspirate.

Phacoemulsification has certain *advantages:*

1 It dramatically shortens convalescence. The patient usually returns to full activity in one or two days.

2 It employs a small incision and minimal suture.

3 It retains the posterior capsule of the lens to preserve a more physiologically normal condition. The occurrence of post-lens extraction edema and retinal detachment is thereby diminished.

4 The posterior capsule supports an implanted intraocular lens.

The procedure also has *disadvantages:*

1 It is not suitable for many patients. Contraindications are corneal disease; dislocated lens; shallow anterior chamber; difficult-to-dilate pupils; completely hard, stonelike cataracts.

2 It requires special techniques which if not thoroughly mastered may precipitate operative complications, such as temporary or permanent corneal damage (opacification), prolapse of lens into the vitreous, vitreous loss.

3 It may injure the cells because of the necessary substantial amount of anterior chamber irrigation. Corneal cells are very sensitive to manipulation and can respond by loss of function.

4 It requires meticulous technical monitoring of the machine. Usual precautions for use of electrical equipment are also observed.

Rehabilitation Following Cataract Extraction Rehabilitation consists of substitution for the missing part, the lens, so that the optical system can function to focus incoming light on the retina. Patients with no optical substitute see only blurred objects of large size with no detail. Rehabilitation may be accomplished by spectacles, contact lens, or intraocular lens implantation.

Spectacle correction of *aphakia,* absence of the lens, provides focusing of light. However, because the *spectacle lens* is approximately 2 cm in front of the original lens, it magnifies images so that they are approximately 35 percent larger than those the patient saw before the development and extraction of the cataract. This magnification requires considerable readjustment to judge distances. Also, peripheral areas are distorted. Spectacle type of replacement is intolerable in patients who have good vision in the unoperated eye, because attempts to fuse the dissimilar images of the two eyes cause double vision.

A *contact lens* rests on the cornea only 2 to 3 mm from the original lens. Consequently it causes only 7 percent magnification and provides a full, undistorted field of vision. The better-tolerated contact lens is often used to replace the optical deficiency caused by cataract extraction, but it is difficult for many elderly persons to handle and care for because of lack of manual dexterity from infirmities or ocular defects in the unoperated eye. For such patients, an *implanted intraocular lens* (IOL) offers a feasible and popular substitute.

Implantation of Intraocular Lens An intraocular lens is implanted in almost the identical position of the original lens and therefore does not change the size of the retinal image. Spatial displacement as seen by the aphakic eye and narrowing and distortion of the visual field are eliminated, thereby producing early visual rehabilitation. With spatial displacement, orientation in space is changed. Objects are not where they appear to be. An intraocular lens is intended to remain in situ permanently. The implant is usually inserted through the same incision used to remove the cataractous lens. This is called *primary insertion.* Some surgeons prefer to implant the lens at a later time; this is referred to as *secondary insertion.* The type of IOL used is contingent on the type of cataract extraction the surgeon chooses. Anterior chamber lenses are inserted in conjunction with intracapsular cataract extraction. Posterior chamber lenses require extracapsular extraction. IOL implantation is a microsurgical procedure.

Prescription of the implanted lens (refractive power) involves complex preoperative calculations based on the patient's corneal curvature as determined by keratometer readings, anterior chamber depth, and eyeball axial length. Ultrasonography is helpful in making these determinations preoperatively. The information obtained is fed into a computer which automatically calculates refractive power of IOL to be selected.

Numerous intraocular lenses are under various stages of Federal Food and Drug Administration approval. The FDA requires that a special preoperative informed consent be signed by the patient for any IOL insertion.

The optical portion of the lens is made of an inert plastic, polymethyl methacrylate, well-tolerated by tissues. The fixation portion is made of plastic or synthetic nonabsorbable suture. Lenses differ in design and method of fixation. They can be classified according to placement or method of fixation.

Anterior Chamber (Angle Fixation) The lens of longest survival is the Choyce lens developed in England. It consists of a band of plastic of length sufficient to traverse the anterior chamber from one angle to the other. The optical portion is centrally located in the anterior chamber, in front of the pupil. The pupil remains mobile because iris adhesions are not required for fixation. Although anterior chamber lenses are commonly inserted primarily, they are the most popular lenses for secondary insertion. Many modifications of the Choyce lens are now in use, e.g., the Tennant, Leiske, Kelman. Other anterior chamber lenses employing fixation to the iris, anteriorly and posteriorly, have become unpopular because of complications.

Posterior Chamber (Capsular or Ciliary Body Fixation) Posterior chamber lenses are placed behind the iris and pupil where the patient's own lens had been. Placement of the IOL in the most normal physiological position results in stabilization of the iris; less irritation of uveal tract; reduced tendency to iritis, secondary glaucoma, and cystoid macular edema; stabilization of the optics. Posterior lenses permit safe dilation of the pupil if necessary to examine or treat posterior structures of the eye, such as the retina. The Simcoe, Shearing, Sinsky, and Kratz lenses, for example, are posterior lenses.

With capsular fixation, the lower loop of the haptic is inserted into a pocket of capsule created before extraction of the cataract. The lens does not touch the iris. The pupil is free to move.

With ciliary fixation, the haptics are placed between the iris and posterior capsule. They rest on the corona or inner rim of the ciliary body.

Dislocation of Lens For repair, the type of approach depends on amount of dislocation. With anterior approach, an anterior vitrectomy is performed to remove vitreous in front of the lens, followed by lensectomy, removal of the lens. With posterior approach, the vitrector is used to perform lensectomy through the pars plana (see p. 494).

Pros and Cons of IOL Implantation Final decision to implant an artificial lens rests with the surgeon, who must exercise good judgment to avoid serious complication. *Indications* for implantation are:

1 Elderly patients with disabling bilateral cataracts and others who cannot adapt to contact lens
2 Patients with occupations having specific visual requirements (airplane pilots) or difficult working environment (ranchers in a dusty area)
3 Children with traumatic cataract, to prevent amblyopia

Apparent *contraindications* are:

1 Impossible patient follow-up. An experienced implant surgeon should observe the patient for late complications.
2 Ocular conditions such as poorly controlled glaucoma or previous retinal detachment.
3 Diabetes.
4 Poor result in previous implant.
5 Patient anxiety in regard to the procedure.
6 Young patients with congenital cataracts.
7 Uniocular (one eye) patient.
8 Endothelial corneal dystrophy.
9 Cataracts associated with recurrent iritis.

Advantages are:

1 Superior spatial orientation and binocular vision
2 Permanent device unless complication develops
3 Additional option for postcataract refractive correction
4 Unrestricted pupillary dilation if necessary

Complications are:

1 Corneal damage or latent edema; corneal opacity
2 Dislocation or malposition of the lens, which can damage the cornea
3 Prolonged inflammation such as iritis or vitritis
4 Cystoid macular edema
5 Secondary cataract, opacification of the anterior vitreous, from recurrent iritis

Retinal Procedures

Repair of Detached Retina Repair is indicated when the retina becomes separated from its surrounding nourishing layer, the *choroid.* Separation (detachment) may occur in any region of the retina. The two types of detachment are *primary,* characterized by a hole in the retina, and *secondary,* characterized by fluid and/or tissue behind the retina. Serious visual disturbance results. Following accidental or operative trauma, or in some degenerative diseases, defects in continuity permit seepage of vitreous fluid into the potential space between the retina and the choroid, causing retina to become detached. Secondary detachment may be due to displacement of the retina by blood, fluid, or tumor. In the last instance, enucleation of the eye is usually indicated. Reattachment is effected only by operative intervention. The retinal defect is sealed off and, often, the subretinal fluid drained. The type of operation is determined by the type and location of the detachment.

1 The traditional procedure involves the application of *diathermy coagulation* to an area of the sclera overlying the region of the retinal defect. The resultant localized inflammation acts to seal off the break. Coagulation is delivered by a specialized short-wave diathermy unit.
2 Some surgeons prefer *cryosurgery* because of the type of adhesion obtained. Therapeutic applications of cryosurgery are basically similar to diathermy. Tissue reactions superficially resemble each other.
3 To achieve reattachment of the retina, internal elevation of the sclera may be increased by the *scleral-buckling procedure.* This technique involves implantation of a wedge of silicone epi- or intrasclerally. An encircling band of silicone may be used to keep constant external pressure on the buckle.
4 *Injection into the vitreous cavity* of air or slowly absorbable inert gas, such as sulfahexafluoride (SF6), is sometimes used to further approximate the retina to the choroid, i.e., flatten retina against choroid.
5 *Laser therapy* (see optical lasers, p. 492).

Two common complications in the immediate postoperative period are glaucoma or infection. Etiology of glaucoma may be congestion of the uvea by the buckle, increasing intraocular pressure, or movement of injected gas from desired site, causing blockage of outflow channels of aqueous humor. Infection is evident by swelling and purulent drainage.

Photocoagulation A retinal hole not surrounded by any detachment may be prophylactically sealed by photocoagulation or by laser burns. These therapeutic modalities, usually performed in an ophthalmic treatment area rather than the OR, were the outgrowth of a traumatic phenomenon. The idea of using intense heat for a beneficial burning effect to create a scar evolved from observation of numerous retinal burns caused by watching the eclipse of the sun. The origin of the photocoagulator concept was investigated by a physician using a mirror and series of lenses on a hospital roof to reflect the sun's rays.

The *xenon arc photocoagulator* utilizes an intense source of multiwavelength light furnished by a xenon tube. This is optically focused and concentrated into a delivering device that is basically a direct ophthalmoscope. The latter can also be used to view the area to be treated as well as to aim the light beam. The light may be directed to any of the various pigmented (light absorbing) layers of the eye, such as the iris or retina. These darker layers readily absorb the xenon tube's white light. The optical system of the eye is used in the process of focusing the light beam on the desired area. The amount of power and exposure time are completely controlled by the operating ophthalmologist. Vitreous shrinkage possibly leading to an inoperable detachment can be a complication. The pupil of the eye under therapy must be dilated to give maximum visibility to the surgeon, and the eye immobilized by local anesthesia to prevent undesired movement, which could result in burn to area other than the one desired. Also pain from intensity of the heat is prevented.

Optical Lasers Similar to the photocoagulator in principle and use, lasers are now preferred because of their advantages. In contrast to the monocular viewing of the photocoagulator, the laser delivery system employs the binocular microscope of the slit lamp, thus giving stereopsis and greater magnification. The nature of the laser beam permits extremely rapid delivery of radiant energy that produces a more sharply defined burn. The smaller lesion it produces can be placed close to the macula. Exposure can be as brief as one-hundredth of a second and the treated area as small as 50 μm (less than 2/1000 in.) in diameter. Because of this short exposure time, immobilization of the eye by drops is unnecessary unless the area for treatment is close to the macula, to avoid accidental macular burn. The macula is the central region of the retina, the point of clearest visual acuity. Injury to the macula may result in loss of central vision. Pupillary dilation is essential.

Use of an optical laser is often a safe alternative to conventional surgery. The development of these lasers provided new technology to ablate pathology with light energy (refer to Chap. 19). The color and wavelength of each laser determines which part of the eye it can best treat. Specific wavelengths destroy specific pathology in tissues whose pigments are capable of absorbing that wavelength (discriminating absorption). Conversely, the selected wavelength should be only minimally absorbed by vital adjacent tissues to be preserved. Lasers in use include the red-yellow krypton, blue-green and pure green argon, and the Nd:YAG. Each has selective use. The physician controls the power, intensity, and direction of the laser beam. The beam precisely cauterizes tissue and blood vessels, preventing bleeding encountered with other operative techniques.

The *argon laser* is effective in treating retinal holes or tears. In addition, one of its major uses is in treatment of diabetic retinopathy. Diabetes causes many bodily changes, which increase in frequency with duration of the disease. Diabetes can affect every part of the eye, causing lens changes (cataract), palsied extraocular muscles, glaucoma, or corneal problems. A person who has been a diabetic for over 15 years has significant likelihood of having some form of retinopathy, which generally occurs bilaterally. Severity may differ from one eye to the other. The dense network of capillary vessels in the retina makes the eyes vulnerable to microvascular disease. *Retinopathy* is classified as:

1 Background or nonproliferative. Bulges or microaneurysms form in retinal capillary walls, eventually permitting leakage and deposition of exudates. Intraretinal hemorrhages occur and are reabsorbed. Pathology is confined to retinal surface. Progressive changes in capillary membranes lead to blockage of capillaries, resulting in retinal ischemia. Deterioration then progresses to proliferative stage.

2 Proliferative. In an effort to relieve retinal anoxia, new blood vessels emerge from the retina and form in surrounding tissues. This is called neovascularization. These fragile vessels may rupture spontaneously, producing hemorrhage into the retina and/or vitreous humor (see vitrectomy). The eventual result may be partial or complete blindness. Panretinal photocoagulation (PRP) is one method of eliminating abnormal vascularization. PRP consists of the application of hundreds of laser burns to the peripheral retinal tissue to partially destroy it. Retinal metabolic need for oxygen is thereby reduced. After neovascularization has occurred, laser therapy is less effective in delaying or stopping the destructive process. Therefore, early diagnosis and treatment are crucial. In an effort to prevent new vessel formation, lasers are used to cauterize minute hypoxic areas of tissue before damage occurs.

The laser is also used for other retinopathies such as central serous retinopathy (swelling of macula); angiomas and hemangiomas; small tumors; bleeding (to seal vessel); and aneurysms.

Laser light is absorbed selectively by three pigments in the retina, namely, macular xanthophyll, hemoglobin in retinal and subretinal blood vessels, and melanin in retinal pigment epithelium. Clinical application for *selective uses of various optical lasers* include:

1 *Blue-green argon:* for diabetic retinopathy, macular neovascular lesions; laser trabeculoplasty, to lower intraocular pressure and facilitate aqueous outflow in selected patients with open-angle glaucoma; laser iridotomy, in place of iridectomy by incision, to create small opening in iris to allow aqueous to enter anterior chamber (angle-closure glaucoma). Laser use should reduce threat of endophthalmitis, inflammation of internal tissues of eyeball, a serious postoperative complication. Adherence of iris to laser burn sites (synechiae) is a complication of laser trabeculoplasty. A portable laser is available for intraoperative use. It permits surgeons to work inside the eye rather than through it while the patient is under general anesthesia.

2 *Red-yellow krypton:* for blood vessel aberrations of choroid, common to senile macular disease in which abnormal vessels damage adjacent nerve tissue; for lesions in perimacular region, laser burn passes through cloudy vitreous hemorrhage.

3 *Pulsed neodymium (Nd:YAG):* for preoperative anterior capsulotomy prior to extracapsular cataract extraction; capsulotomy (discission) of posterior capsule after extracapsular cataract extraction to make an opening in an opaque capsule to permit light to reach retina; lysis or severing of strands of vitreous and/or fibrous bands in vitreous that cause cystoid macular edema.

Visual problems not previously responsive to laser treatment are now treated with the Nd:YAG. In the eye, cloudy areas of tissue interfering with vision are painlessly pushed aside, resulting in immediate improvement in sight. Rather than producing effect by absorption, energy is released almost entirely at the point of focus. Problems in the front portion as well as in the posterior part of the eye are treatable. This laser does not require the target tissue to be pigmented for effectiveness as do the visible light lasers.

Advantages of laser therapy are:

1 Minimal possibility of infection. Treatment is noninvasive and sterile, a boon to diabetics and susceptible patients.

2 Minimal pain. Anesthesia, except topical, is eliminated.

3 Ambulatory surgery basis is possible.

4 Tremendous amount of energy is concentrated in very small area.

5 Highly flexible light. Seems to do little damage to the clear media it traverses.

6 Selective absorption. Ideally, only desired tissue is affected.

7 Useful in poor-risk operative patient or one who had previous unsuccessful operation.

Laser therapy is not effective in correcting severe retinal damage or detachment. In these patients operative intervention, often vitrectomy, is indicated.

Vitrectomy Vitrectomy is the deliberate removal of a portion of vitreous humor, also called vitreous body, that fills the area between the lens and the retina. Therapeutically, it is performed for vitreal opacities, vitreal hemorrhage, and certain types of retinal detachment. In addition to other mentioned causes, endophthalmitis and intraocular foreign body may result in vitreal opacity. Diagnostically, removal of a small amount of vitreous provides a sample for microbiological study in suspected endophthalmitis. The procedure also provides tissue for biopsy to establish diagnosis of intraocular tumors.

Whereas aqueous fluid is clear, the vitreous is normally a transparent, gelatinous, viscid material containing fibrils. The vitreous helps give shape to the eyeball, in addition to serving a refractive function. It permits light rays to pass through it to the retina after the rays have traversed the lens.

Alterations in vitreous can have serious consequences. Loss of vitreous during operative procedures has always been a dreaded complication, particularly of cataract extraction, because temporary deflation of the globe can lead to collapse. Subsequent to retinal hemorrhage, common in diabetic patients, bands of scar tissue may opacify the vitreous as well as insert into the retina near the original bleeding vessel. Traction on the retina by these bands or further cicatrization, scarring, can lead to retinal tears or detachment. Persistent hemorrhage, lasting over a year, is permanent. It will not absorb spontaneously.

For years the vitreous was considered an inaccessible inoperable area. Research and the advent of microsurgery changed this belief. Loss of vitreous from the posterior segment during operation is rendered relatively innocuous if the anterior segment is cleared of vitreous. Thus, no residual strands are present to block visual function. Also, the eye tolerates subtotal vitreal excision in the posterior segment if the vitreous body is proportionately replaced with balanced salt solution (BSS).

Vitrectomy is a microsurgical procedure that lasts two to three hours and requires a skilled retinal surgeon. It is performed with a vitrector, such as the Ocutome. This device, incorporating a micromotor, terminates in a needlelike tube that contains a cutting mechanism for severing abnormal adhesions and cutting obstructive tissue into small pieces. In addition, it has auxilliary connections for aspiration of vitreous, debris, or blood in the posterior segment, and replacement with BSS via an infusion catheter, to maintain adequate intraocular pressure. A fiberoptic light source or pic is inserted into vitreous to illuminate posterior portion of the globe. Various vitrectomy systems are available, but all have cutting, suction, infusion, and illumination systems. Two approaches to the vitreous body are:

1 Through the posterior segment, via the pars plana, the anterior attachment of the retina. Since the pars plana has no visual function, entry there is relatively nontraumatic, with least chance for retinal detachment. The anterior segment remains intact; intraocular pressure is maintained. Used to incise opacified vitreous, old hemorrhage, or bands of scar tissue, thereby giving a clear view of the retina and restoring visual function.

2 Through the anterior segment, via incision at the limbus, junction of cornea and sclera. A large corneal section is folded back and the vitreous exposed through the pupillary opening. Used for removal of vitreous inadvertently displaced into the anterior chamber during cataract removal, to avoid postoperative complications. The vitreous volume is replaced with BSS.

Generally vitrectomy patients have substantially impaired vision and complicated conditions preoperatively. Therefore, general anesthesia is used unless the patient's condition necessitates a local. The procedure is intricate, requiring a great deal of equipment. The surgeon may request bipolar cautery for vessels actively bleeding during operation. A special attachment (Charles clip) is required for intraocular cautery. Also a hand-held contact lens placed onto the cornea enhances view of the posterior chamber. Some lenses have a handle through which continuous infusion can be run to keep the cornea moist. Occasionally lensectomy is performed during vitrectomy to facilitate view of the posterior segment.

After removal of vitreous, before wound closure, and with the retina in clear view, the latter is inspected for defects such as holes or vascular abnormalities. If these are found, treatment is applied by means of endocryotherapy, a freezing application delivered by intraocular probe, or endophotocoagulation, photocoagulation delivered by an intraocular device. These maneuvers may be accompanied by injection of air or an inert gas such as SF6 to push the retina into physiological position.

Postoperatively these patients may experience considerable pain, requiring medication, ice packs, and steroid eye drops for inflammation. Postvitrectomy patients are usually aphakic and eventually need optical correction the same as that needed after cataract extraction. Vitrectomy can significantly improve vision, but only the surgeon should and can determine prognosis.

Complications of vitrectomy include iatrogenic retinal damage, vitreous hemorrhage, or cataract formation from damage to the lens. Secondary operation may be required to repair the retina, e.g., scleral buckling procedure or lensectomy. No present treatment for retinopathy is without danger. To save vision, some tissue must be destroyed or sacrificed.

Nursing duties. Scrub nurse and circulating nurse should assemble and check equipment before start of operation. Vitrectomy handpiece is attached to sterile tubing, which is connected to power console. While one activates various switches, the other tests suction vacuum and cutting function. Turn suction to maximum pressure to test. Place tip in sterile saline and activate until fluid reaches collection bottle. *Then lower pressure* to surgeon's preference. To assess cutting, activate switch and check tip visibly and audibly for movement. The infusion catheter is primed with solution of surgeon's choice to remove air bubbles that could disturb view in posterior segment. Consult manufacturer's manual.

TRAUMA TO THE EYE

Various forms and degrees of trauma may occur as a result of injury. *All types of injury require immediate appraisal by an ophthalmologist.* Delay of even minor ones may result in temporary or permanent loss of vision. Complications include hemorrhage; infection; iritis or tears of the iris; retinal tears or detachment; macular edema; and secondary cataract. Treatment may be immediate, or secondary, if delay is necessary because of life-threatening injuries. Improved operative management, such as vitrectomy and microsurgery, have reduced the loss of severely injured eyes. Optical result is especially crucial in patients with bilateral eye injuries. Patients with eye injuries should be kept supine if possible until seen by the ophthalmologist.

Evaluation of the injury may necessitate sedating or anesthetizing the patient to prevent further damage at examination. Pressure to the eye must be avoided, because bone fragments may be displaced or globe contents emptied.

Injuries may be simple, involving only the external layers, or compound, including inner structures. They may be nonpenetrating, usually caused by a blunt object, or penetrating, caused by a sharp object. The more structures involved, the more difficult it is to salvage an eye.

Treatment, determined by type or combination of injuries, aims to:

1 Promote healing and prevent anatomical distortion by reparative techniques
2 Preserve maximum vision and/or restore it
3 Control pain, by medication
4 Prevent infection and inflammation by antibiotic and steroid administration

Nonpenetrating Injuries

Lacerations of the Eyelid Lacerations are repaired according to anatomical principles.

Burns Burns may be caused by ultraviolet radiation, such as sunlamps or sunlight, or electric flash. These burns are basically self-limited but rarely operative. *A chemical burn constitutes an emergency.* Initial treatment consists of flooding the cornea with water. Alkali burns may be further neutralized by prompt irrigation of epithelium-denuded cornea with edathamil (EDTA). This is especially important if discrete particles of alkali are superficially imbedded within tissue. EDTA deactivates an enzyme, collagenase, and neutralizes soluble alkali such as sodium hydroxide (lye). Severe burns may be treated with specific amino acids, EDTA or acetylcysteine (Mucomist), to inhibit continuing destruction of cornea by collagenase, but they often progress to corneal opacity and blindness.

Contusions of the Globe Contusions may or may not be operative. If hemorrhage is present, treatment consists of bed rest and antiglaucoma therapy to keep intraocular pressure controlled. It is not unusual for a secondary hemorrhage to occur on the third or fourth day after injury. If the intraocular pressure remains high, blood staining of the cornea and damage to the optic nerve may result. It is then sometimes necessary to perform a *paracentesis,* an incision into the anterior chamber to drain the blood. If an organized clot is found, judicious irrigation may supplement incision.

Penetrating Injuries

Lacerations of the globe may occur with or without retained foreign body and with or without prolapse of ocular contents. In injuries to the globe, an ophthalmic surgeon should repair tissues adjacent to the eye, in addition to the eye wound.

With this type of injury there is the possibility of an eventual *sympathetic ophthalmia,* inflammation of the uninjured eye. Antitentanus therapy should be included in treatment of these injuries.

Vitrectomy and lensectomy have rendered some massive injuries salvageable that formerly were inoperable. Such injuries include extensive lacerations with cataract formation, vitreous hemorrhage, and retinal damage.

Without Foreign Body

Conjunctival Laceration Conjunctival laceration is usually debrided and, unless large, permitted to heal without suturing. If it is large, with loss of conjunctival tissue, sutures or rotating flaps of conjunctiva may be necessary for repair.

Corneal and Scleral Lacerations A small corneal laceration may be covered with a protective soft contact lens to seal it and hold the edges together. A larger wound requires accurate appositional sutures best placed under the operating microscope. The microscope is especially useful for irregular, complicated, or multiple tears. Adequate exploration, particularly of a scleral wound, is necessary to determine extent of injury as well as to ensure uncovering of the entire wound for repair. In instances of vitreous fluid presentation or loss, it is preferable to remove the fluid from the wound and the anterior chamber with the vitreotome before proceeding with repair. This is done to avoid undesirable vitreous adhesions postoperatively.

Prolapse of the Iris Prolapse of the iris or other uveal tissue is usually excised, except in very early clean wounds where repositioning it may be attempted.

Posterior Rupture of the Globe Rupture usually involves herniation of retinal and uveal tissue into the orbit. Although such injuries are self-healing, the eye is irreparably damaged. *Avulsion* (tearing) of the optic nerve produces permanent blindness even though the rest of the globe may be intact. This injury usually results in enucleation.

With Foreign Body

Extraocular Extraocular injuries are usually not extensive. A corneal foreign body is removed with a sharp probe (spud) and the surrounding rust ring is taken off with a rotating burr.

Intraocular The type, size, and position of a foreign body should be determined accurately before removal. Localization is accomplished by:

1 Direct vision with ophthalmoscope

2 Computerized axial tomography (CAT)—the most accurate method

3 Berman locator, a small but extremely sensitive version of a mine detector, which may indicate exact location of a ferrous metallic foreign body

4 X-ray, using a contact lens containing radiopaque landmarks (Sweet's localizer).

Fragments of ferrous metals can often be retrieved by utilizing the attraction of a strong electromagnet. In some cases these foreign bodies can be withdrawn along the path of entry. Nonmagnetic foreign objects present a more serious problem. Frequently they may be secured only by passing a delicate forceps into the globe. Such instrumentation is combined with partial vitrectomy, thus obtaining satisfactory results in formerly inoperable situations.

In summary, traumatic injuries may introduce infection or produce severe inflammatory reaction in greater degree than do elective operative procedures. Proper early treatment is indicated to save vision. Early reintervention, before scar formation, may be necessary in some patients.

GENERAL CONSIDERATIONS

The ophthalmic patient faces impaired or loss of vision if the outcome of operative intervention is unfavorable. Special features of ophthalmic surgery aim to prevent such a loss. Operation on the eye is extremely delicate, requiring precision instrumentation, a steady hand, and quiet surroundings.

1 Most ophthalmic surgeons use the operating microscope for intraocular procedures. The microscope, all special equipment, and microinstruments must be set up and checked before operation. Precision microinstrumentation is particularly critical in intraocular surgery. Outcome of operation is in great measure dependent on perfection of instruments used. The eye in particular tolerates *no* abuse. (Refer to Chapter 19.)

2 Eye patients have impaired vision that may produce prolonged severe stress and alter self-image. Many are aged. Reassure the patient, exercise patience, give directions clearly, anticipate needs, and check comfort level. Before positioning, offer bedpan if needed. Although patient should void before leaving unit, urgency can be a problem in elderly patients or those on diuretic medication. Severe urgency while the eye is operatively opened can incur strain. *Strain and gross movement are dangerous and to be avoided.*

3 The surgeon should verify the operative eye with patient as well as with office records. To avoid error, after confirmation some surgeons also place an indelible mark on side of patient's neck that corresponds to operative eye.

4 The patient is positioned supine on the operating table so that head and body are aligned. Top of head is in line with edge of table for accessibility. Head is stabilized. For intraocular procedures, patient's gown is untied at neck to prevent pressure. Also head must not be turned greatly in either direction. Any obstruction to venous circulation can cause undue pressure in the eye, which can produce loss of vitreous humor when eye is opened. Table is tilted so that head is elevated 5 to 10° to assist venous return from head. For long procedures, an egg-crate mattress may be placed on table.

5 Frequently mydriatic or miotic drops are administered to dilate or constrict the pupil. The *commonly used drops* are:

a *Mydriatic drops:* 2.5 or 10% phenylephrine to dilate pupil.

b *Mydriatic-cycloplegic drops:* 1% cyclopentolate (Cyclogyl), 1% atropine, 0.25% scopolamine to dilate pupil and paralyze ciliary body, diminish reaction to trauma, and prevent anterior synechiae, e.g., iris to lens. These are longer acting drugs than phenylephrine.

c *Miotic drops:* 2% pilocarpine to constrict pupil.

6 Circulating nurse instills medications, as well as anesthetic drops, as ordered, prior to skin prep. Common abbreviations are O.D., right eye; O.S., left eye; O.U., both eyes. *To instill eye drops:*

a Wash hands.

b Identify correct medication, eye, and patient.

c Explain procedure to patient.

d Tilt patient's head back. Tell patient to look up. While gently pulling down on the lower lid, instill the medication on the inner aspect of the lower lid, in the middle third. Release the lid while patient slowly closes the eye to retain the drop. Let patient close the eye between repeated drops. Gently blot excess fluid to prevent drainage into the tear duct, nose, and stomach. Some medications, such as atropine, may have a systemic effect. In small infants or young children, systemic absorption is avoided by applying finger pressure over the lacrimal sac region (inner canthus) of both eyes simultaneously for a minute. In a struggling child, have patient tilt head back and close both eyes. Instill medication at the inner canthus. The drop will roll into the eye as the patient reopens it.

e Only the specified number of drops, no more, no less, must be given.

f Read the label on the vial *each* time before instillation.

g Each patient should receive a fresh, single-use, disposable vial, discarded after use.

h Usually one drop of anesthetic is administered to the unoperative eye in case of inadvertent splash during the prep.

7 Refer to Chapter 16 for skin preparation and draping procedures. Sterile plastic drapes are often placed over textile drapes to prevent lint, especially in lens implantation. A patient with a drape over the face is often apprehensive and fearful of suffocation. Oxygen is delivered to the nostrils via nasal prongs or insufflated to facial area beneath the drape for comfort at 6 to 8 liters/minute.

8 Patient is instructed about importance of remaining still during operation. Patient could easily move out of field of vision under microscope or precipitate a complication.

9 Except for children and selected patients, local anesthesia is used. The patient is prepared as ordered. *Local anesthesia* consists of:

a Topical installation of anesthetic drops. Drugs used: 0.5% proparacaine hydrochloride (Ophthaine), 0.5% tetracaine (Pontocaine), 2% lidocaine (Xylocaine).

b Local infiltration of lids and tissue around eyes (Van Lint method) or O'Brien block of facial nerve, the seventh cranial nerve, for lid akinesia or paralysis of extraocular muscles. A 25-gauge needle, 1½ in. (3.8 cm) for Van Lint method or ½ in. (12.7 mm) for O'Brien block with 2-cc syringe are commonly used.

c Retrobulbar block. The needle is inserted behind the eyeball into the muscular cone, the common origin of the extraocular muscles, to obtain anesthesia of the globe and paralysis of the muscles. A 25-gauge needle, 1½ in. (3.8 cm), with sharp rounded point, e.g., Atkinson needle, and 5-cc syringe are usually used. Patient is asked to look up and away from injection site and is told that a slight burning sensation may accompany injection. Block may be followed by intermittent massage of eye to soften it, lower intraocular pressure (IOP), and facilitate operative manipulation during cataract extraction, especially when IOL insertion is contemplated. Massage is continued until IOP is lowered to satisfactory level, e.g., 10 to 12 scale reading on sterile Schiotz tonometer. Some surgeons apply the Honan balloon pressure device to eye after a retrobulbar block. This consists of a strap around the head with a small inflatable balloon placed directly over the closed eyelid. Balloon is inflated to 30 to 40 mm Hg for about 10 to 15 minutes. Purpose is to lower intravitreal pressure. An absolutely quiet eye is mandatory, especially at high magnifications with the microscope. Even when general anesthesia is used, most surgeons administer a retrobulbar block for immobility and lowering of intraocular pressure.

d Most operations are scheduled as *attended local.* An anesthesiologist is present to monitor the patient, administer oxygen, or supplement the local anesthetic if necessary. IV diazepam is often given to relax patient. Tolerance to procedures is increased because of minimal anesthesia. If general anesthesia is used, usual general anesthesia routines are followed.

10 Emphasis is placed on the need for extreme constant care with *ophthalmic solutions.* Nearly all are colorless and may be in similar receptacles. *Solutions must be immediately and individually labeled* by the scrub nurse. *Identity must not be confused,* because an error could result in total, irrevocable blindness for the patient. If identification is missing, discard the solution. *Solutions for intraocular use must be separated from all others* and ideally should be filtered with micropore filters. Medicine glasses may be properly inscribed or a sterile, metal labeling clip may be attached to the glass as soon as the solution is poured. This clip should hang outside the glass, because contact with the solution in some cases inactivates the solution. An example is alpha chymotrypsin. *Sterile solutions commonly used* include the following.

a On the Mayo stand, in medicine glasses in a rack:

1 Local anesthetic. Hyaluronidase (Zolyse) 1:5,000 or 1:10,000 is sometimes added to expedite spread of the anesthetic through the tissue and create more profound anesthesia.

2 Epinephrine hydrochloride 1:5,000 (1 to 2 ml) with an eye dropper, for hemostasis. After a drop is added to the local anesthetic, this glass is removed to the instrument table so that the medication is *never* inadvertently injected.

3 Alpha chymotrypsin (an enzyme solution) to soften the zonules holding the lens, prior to cataract extraction.

4 Small 30-ml sterile bottles of balanced salt solution (BSS) to which a convenient cannula may be attached are commercially available for irrigating anterior chamber and for keeping the cornea moist.

b On the instrument table, in a basin, distilled water for rinsing instruments.

c Other drugs on instrument table are:

1 Epinephrine 2 ml of 1:10,000 added to 50-ml balanced salt solution, used as irrigating solution to maintain pupil dilation intraoperatively, e.g., in vitrectomy and extracapsular cataract extraction. Dosage may vary among surgeons. Intracardiac solution has least amount of preservative.

2 Acetylcholine (Miochol) to irrigate anterior chamber during insertion of IOL to rapidly constrict pupil.

3 Steroids for topical application or subconjunctival injection of 1-ml methylprednisolone acetate suspension (Depo-Medrol 80 mg/ml or Depo-Kenalog) at conclusion of operation to diminish inflammatory response and to prevent corneal graft rejection.

4 Antibiotic for topical application or subconjunctival injection, e.g., 0.5-ml gentamicin sulfate solution, following intraocular procedures to prevent infection.

5 Mannitol 15%, 2 g/kg body weight IV, is an osmotic agent to draw fluid from eye to lower IOP.

The surgeon should check with the anesthesiologist before using medications intraoperatively. Epinephrine or other sympathomimetics may have side effects when used with some anesthetic agents. As the patient's advocate, the nurse shares this responsibility with the surgeon. Also, medications that may induce vomiting are avoided. Any straining or gross movement may cause intraocular hemorrhage, sudden rise in IOP resulting in loss of vitreous or expulsion of ocular contents through wound. All can cause blindness.

11 Prepare for emergencies by anticipating problems. Fast action can make the difference between a postoperative seeing or nonseeing eye. Rare but dreaded complications are:

a Systemic reaction to medication or local anesthetic drugs and cardiac arrest. Have cardiac arrest cart readily available.

b Loss of vitreous. Requires its removal from anterior chamber to prevent prolapse of wound, severe inflammation, updrawn pupil. Requires vitreous cutting device such as Ocutome or Kaufman disposable vitrector.

c Expulsive hemorrhage; expulsion of ocular contents. Requires sharp knife, such as Beaver blade or Wheeler knife, for fast cutdown into pars plana area, 18-gauge needle or cannula attached to aspirating syringe to aspirate mass and reduce pressure in effort to save eye and vision.

d Instrument failure. Hand aspiration devices and battery-operated cryoextractors should be available for immediate use.

12 A wide variety of fine-sized absorbable and nonabsorbable sutures is used. The scrub nurse follows the manufacturer's recommendations for handling these delicate materials and needles with appropriate needleholders. Special techniques are used in microsurgery.

13 Sponges are of precut compressed cellulose on sticks.

14 No foreign material should be introduced into the operative wound. In intraocular procedures, no portion of any instrument or item intended to enter the eye should be touched by a gloved hand. Intraocular lenses are soaked and rinsed in BSS before insertion to remove *any* debris or impurity.

15 Inflammation must be kept as minimal as possible, since even a slight infection may result in total functional loss. Steroids are often administered locally, subconjunctivally, and sometimes systemically. Antibiotic drops are often instilled topically for 24 hours pre- and postoperatively. The eye may respond violently to the slightest amount of trauma.

16 At the conclusion of operation, a sterile eye pad is applied. A protective shield is secured over it to guard against mechanical injury.

17 Patient must not be permitted to participate in move from operating table following intraocular procedures, to prevent sudden rise in IOP and/or dislocation of IOL.

18 Arm restraints are essential for infants and young children (see Chap. 33). Restraints are applied to adults only under extreme circumstances, such as disorientation. Use of siderails is usually standard procedure for patients over 65 and those having general anesthesia.

19 Outcome of ophthalmic procedures includes a cosmetic as well as a functional aspect.

20 Ideally, the ophthalmic patient should be physically separated, from admission to discharge, from patients of other services. Segregation not only minimizes cross infection but also provides for the specialized care required on the unit and in the OR.

21 The tendency is toward early ambulation and short hospitalization. A most important aspect of postoperative care is to inform the patient not to get out of bed alone. A fall or jar to the eye can nullify an otherwise successful operation. Patient must not do anything to increase IOP, e.g., bend over at the waist or lift heavy object. Deep breathing postoperatively is encouraged, but coughing is avoided, because it could rupture suture line. Patient should report any pain, swelling, redness, or discharge postoperatively.

22 Ophthalmic surgeons subspecialize in anterior chamber surgery, i.e., cataract extraction, or posterior chamber surgery, i.e., retinal procedures. Either type requires specialized instrumentation. Consult procedure book for setups.

CHAPTER **26**

OTOLARYNGOLOGY

Otorhinolaryngology has traditionally been concerned with research and surgical treatment of diseases of the ear (*oto*), nose (*rhino*), and throat (*laryngo*). Advances in scientific knowledge, diagnostic capabilities, and technology have broadened the scope of this field, which has led to subspecialization. General otorhinolaryngologists, commonly called *ENT surgeons,* practice within the total scope of this specialty. Other surgeons confine their practice to one of the subspecialties: otology, facial surgery, or head and neck oncology. The certifying body for this specialty is the American Board of Otolaryngology, Head and Neck Surgery.

HISTORICAL INTRODUCTION

Recognition of abnormal conditions of the ear, nose, and throat began in early times. Some of the first permanent records mentioning them, attributed to the Egyptians, date from 3500 B.C. Breathing was thought to occur through the ears via the eustachian tubes. Therefore, attempts were made to remedy deafness and ear discharges. Study of anatomy antedated the Christian era, leading to the practice of primitive procedures in India. For example, nasal fractures were splinted by insertion of a tube into the nostril.

Hippocrates realized that irregular teeth could cause various mouth and ear disorders. He also recognized otitis media as well as the fact that congenital deafness was incurable. He advocated immediate reduction of nasal fractures.

The early centuries of the Christian era brought attempts to devise mastoid operations. Tracheotomy, thought to have been known 2000 years ago, was described in detail by Antyllas, a surgeon of the second century. In the seventh century, physicians advocated its use to prevent suffocation in persons with laryngeal obstruction. Tracheotomy was performed frequently during a diphtheria epidemic in Europe in 1610. The lifesaving value of this procedure was further proved in later centuries when used for patients with severe croup or tuberculosis. The seventeenth century also saw removal of the tongue for tumor.

In 1855, tuning-fork tests, used in evaluating actual and residual hearing, were described by Rinné. European surgeons in the latter part of the nineteenth century attempted to restore hearing by operative incision of the eardrum and removal of the tympanic membrane and stapes. Eventually, operations such as fenestration and stapes mobilization were developed. Stapedectomy, devised in the 1960s, has largely replaced those procedures. Continued research in nerve deafness and in transplantation may well produce a cure for many persons now consigned to a world of silence.

Research resulting in refined equipment, techniques, and prostheses has brought the specialization of the present. One of the greatest advances in treatment was the development of antibiotics, which often eliminates the need for operation.

THE EAR

Anatomy and Physiology

The structures of the ear (see Fig. 26-1) are concerned with two functions:

1 Hearing, i.e., receiving sound, amplifying it, and transmitting it to the brain for interpretation
2 Maintaining bodily equilibrium

Anatomically, the ear is divided into three parts: the external, middle, and inner ear.

External Ear The outer ear consists of the *auricle,* or *pinna,* composed of cartilage and skin except for the lobe, and the *external auditory canal.* The meatus of the auricle leads via the ear canal to the *tympanic membrane,* or *eardrum.* This membrane separates the external and middle ear. Color change of the translucent eardrum, visible through a speculum, may be indicative of middle ear disease. The outermost lining of the tympanic membrane is derived from skin of the ear canal. The inner lining is continuous with middle ear mucosa. The eardrum protects the middle ear but may be perforated by injury or pressure built up in the middle ear by infection.

Middle Ear The middle ear consists of the *tympanic cavity,* a closed chamber that lies between the tympanic membrane and the inner ear. Within this cavity are the three smallest bones in the body, an *ossicular chain* comprised of the malleus, incus, and stapes. They resemble a hammer, anvil, and stirrups, respectively. The malleus, attached to the eardrum, joins the incus, the extremity of which articulates with the stapes, the innermost bone. The footplate of the stapes fits in the *oval,* or *vestibular, window,* an opening in the wall of the inner ear. The bones of the ossicular chain must be able to move mechanically in order to conduct sound from the eardrum to the inner ear. The *round,* or *cochlear, window,* also between the middle and the inner ear, equalizes pressure that enters through the oval window.

The middle ear opens into the nasopharynx by way of the *eustachian tube.* Normally closed during swallowing or yawning, the eustachian tube aerates the middle ear cavity. This mechanism is essential for adequate hearing.

Posteriorly the middle ear exits to the *mastoid process.* This inferior projection of the temporal bone is a honeycomb of air cells lined with mucous membrane. Since the antrum of the mastoid process connects with it, middle ear infection may produce mastoiditis. The middle ear is situated in the tympanic portion of the temporal bone, the inner ear in the petrous portion, which integrates with the base of the skull. The tympanic portion also forms part of the ear canal.

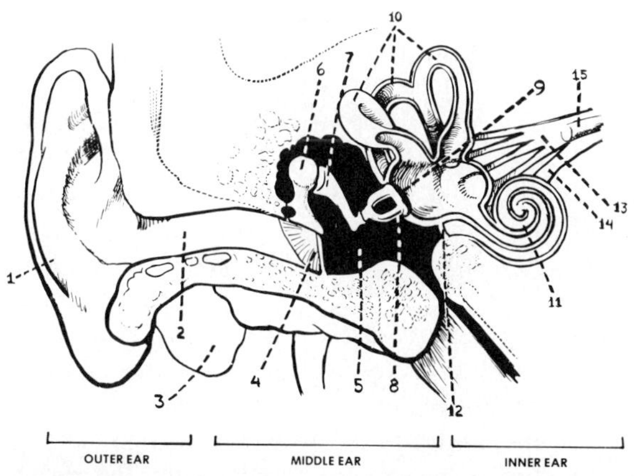

FIGURE 26-1
Anatomy of the ear: (1) pinna, (2) auditory canal, (3) mastoid process of temporal bone, (4) tympanic membrane, (5) tympanic cavity, (6) malleus, (7) incus, (8) stapes, (9) oval (vestibular) window, (10) semicircular canals, (11) cochlea, (12) round (cochlear) window, (13) vestibular nerve, (14) cochlear nerve, (15) facial nerve.

Inner Ear The end organs of hearing and equilibrium are situated in the inner ear. The two main sections, cochlear and vestibular, have precise functions, although coordinated. The *cochlea,* a bony spiral, relates to hearing. The *vestibular labyrinth,* composed of three semicircular canals, relates to equilibrium. These structures house two separate fluids, *endolymph* and *perilymph,* which nourish and protect the hearing receptors. Neuroepithelium of the *organ of Corti,* the end organ of hearing, holds thousands of minute hair cells, which respond to sound waves that enter the cochlea via the oval window. Neuroepithelium of the vestibular portion also contains hair cells. Rapid head motion produces current in the endolymph that may result in nausea or vertigo. The *vestibular nerve,* a portion of the acoustic nerve, governs reflexes to muscles to maintain equilibrium.

Proximal Structures The middle and the

inner ear are adjacent to many important structures. The seventh cranial or facial nerve is enclosed in a bony canal running through the tympanic cavity and mastoid bone. The meninges of the temporal lobe of the brain are also near the middle ear and the mastoid. Facial paralysis, meningitis, and intracranial infection such as brain abscess are potential complications of ear infection.

Significant blood vessels are the internal carotid artery and internal jugular vein as well as the lateral sinus. Thrombosis and infection of the lateral sinus of the dura mater is a potentially lethal complication of otitis media, with or without mastoiditis.

Auditory Process Sound or pressure waves enter the auricle. They pass along the ear canal to the tympanic membrane. The vibration of the waves is transmitted across the middle ear sequentially by the ossicles. Amplification of sound is effected to some extent by mechanical action of the ossicles but mainly by areal ratio. A large volume of sound-wave pressure from the tympanic membrane funnels to a small reactive area, the stapedial footplate, intensifying sound. At the footplate of the stapes, sound pressure is transferred to the inner ear via the oval window. The hair cells of the organ of Corti are set in motion by disturbance of the inner ear fluids as sound pressure moves from the oval to the round window. Mechanical energy is converted to electrical potential, which is delivered to the brain along auditory nerves that enter the inner ear. The brain interprets the sound as hearing.

Loss of Hearing Hearing affects the quality and quantity of interpersonal interactions. It is a major sense for communicating within one's environment. Loss of hearing, therefore, impacts on social relationships. The type of deafness or hearing loss in varying degrees may result from:

1 Disease, such as otosclerosis, in which changes in the bony capsule of the labyrinth occur. Otosclerotic bone invades the stapedial footplate, resulting in its fixation and ultimate inability to vibrate in the oval window. Hearing loss is gradual but progressive. This type of deficiency can be surgically corrected when auditory nerve endings are not destroyed.

2 Trauma, such as perforated eardrum, requiring repair to restore function and areal ratio.

3 Infection, usually controlled by antibiotics. While more common in children, infection may also occur in adults. It may cause accumulation of fluid in the middle ear. Mastoiditis results from extension of otitis media.

- **a** Serous otitis media may result from obstruction of the pharyngeal orifice of the eustachian tube. If blocked, for example, by hypertrophied adenoid tissue, infection, or allergic swelling, the tube is unable to equalize pressure because air cannot enter the middle ear from the pharynx. The vacuum or negative pressure thus created causes serum to be drawn into the tympanic cavity from blood vessels in the middle ear mucosa. Recurrent otitis media may require drainage of purulent exudate if conservative treatment fails.
- **b** Acute otitis media may require drainage of purulent exudate if conservative treatment fails.
- **c** Chronic otitis media with or without mastoiditis may follow recurrent otitis media with tympanic membrane perforation. It can produce a chronically draining ear.

Differential Diagnosis Measurements that compare bone conduction with air conduction are important in differential diagnosis. *Bone conduction* refers to hearing as transmitted through the skull; *air conduction* refers to transmission of sound waves from the tympanic membrane to the inner ear via air. Hearing loss caused by a defect in the external or the middle ear, referred to as *conductive loss,* is a mechanical obstruction of air conduction that usually can be helped by operative intervention. When the decrement is in the inner ear, referred to as *perceptive* or *sensorineural loss,* damage to nerve tissue and/or sensory paths to the brain is not benefited by operation.

Auditory acuity and function are measured by various tests. The audiogram is one measurement tool. Computer averaged tomography is used to measure and analyze electrical impulses, known as auditory brainstem responses, from the brain and cortical auditory pathway. An acoustic reflex latency test of the stapedius reflex provides information about hearing sensitivity.

OTOLOGIC OPERATIVE PROCEDURES

The advent of antibiotics greatly alleviated the necessity for operative intervention prevalent in previous decades. Emphasis was formerly on relief of infection and conversion of a draining ear to a dry one. Now infection is generally controlled pharmacologically. Attention has turned to operative measures to improve hearing following damage from chronic infection, and to restore hearing by reconstruction of the sound conduction pathways. Current techniques, instrumentation, and the operating microscope have enhanced the ability of otologists.

External Ear

Removal of a Foreign Body Removing a foreign body from the outer canal is performed most frequently in children. The object is washed out or removed to prevent purulent infection. A plant seed or vegetable foreign body such as a pea is not irrigated, because it may swell in the ear and increase the difficulty of removal. General anesthesia sometimes may be required. Trauma must be minimal during removal to prevent stenosis of the canal or perforation of the object through the eardrum.

Drainage of Hematoma Usually the result of injury, a hematoma is drained to avoid infection with subsequent chondritis and deformity of the auricle.

Excision of Tumor Extent of operation depends on size and type of tumor, either benign or malignant. The skin of the pinna is vulnerable to actinic (chemical) changes due to radiant energy of exposure to the sun. Basal-cell lesions do not metastasize, but squamous-cell carcinoma often does. Primary cancer may be excised by a wide or a wedge excision with primary closure, or a wide excision with skin graft. If lesion is extensive, partial or total pinnectomy may be necessary. The area can be skin grafted and reconstructed cosmetically with a prosthesis (refer to otoplasty, Chap. 27, p. 528). Radical temporal bone resection is indicated if the bone (canal) is involved. Neck dissection may be indicated if nodal metastases are present.

Middle Ear

Mastoidectomy Although rarely performed, eradication of the mastoid air cells may be indicated to treat mastoiditis (infection in mastoid).

1 *Simple mastoidectomy* is advocated for complications of acute mastoiditis. The mastoid is opened behind the ear and the air cells are removed without involving middle ear or external canal.

2 *Modified radical mastoidectomy* consists of simple mastoidectomy and removal of the posterior wall of the ear canal to provide drainage from the mastoid to the canal. It preserves the tympanic membrane and middle ear ossicles.

3 *Radical mastoidectomy* may be performed for chronic mastoiditis. In addition to simple mastoidectomy, the middle ear cavity and mastoid antrum are combined into a single cavity for easy inspection and cleaning. The ossicles and tympanic membrane are partially removed. The stapes and facial nerve are preserved.

Tympanoplasty Tympanoplasty, as a general term, refers to any procedure performed to repair defects in the eardrum and/or middle ear structures for the purpose of reconstructing sound conduction paths. The degree of hearing improvement following tympanoplasty is related to the degree of damage. Preferably the ear is uninfected at the time of operation. If not, infected tissue must be removed. As microsurgical procedures, tympanoplasties are classified into five types.

1 Type I, *myringoplasty,* is closure of a perforation in the tympanic membrane due to infection or trauma. The ossicular chain is normal. Autogenous fascia or vein is utilized to repair the perforation. Vein graft is taken from the patient's forearm or hand. Fascia, more commonly used as a patch over a perforation, is obtained from the temporalis muscle.

2 Type II is closure of a perforated tympanic membrane with erosion of the malleus. The graft is placed against the incus or remains of the malleus.

3 Type III replaces the tympanic membrane to provide protection for the stapes and round window. Due to disease, the tympanic membrane, malleus, and incus have been destroyed. The stapes is intact and mobile. A homograft of tympanic membrane with attached malleus and incus is placed in contact with the normal stapes, permitting transmission of sound.

4 Type IV is similar to Type III except that the head, neck, and crura of the stapes is missing. The mobile footplate may be left exposed with the graft placed around it. The air pocket between graft and round window provides sound protection for the round window. To conserve the middle ear hearing mechanism, homograft transplantation of tympanic membrane and ossicles may be used to rebuild the chain.

5 Type V is similar to Type IV except that the stapedial footplate is fixed due to otosclerosis (osteospongiosis). A fenestra (small opening) must be made in the horizontal semicircular canal. The homograft seals off the middle ear to provide sound protection for the round window.

Synthetic bioinert materials for reconstruction of the middle ear are available—for example, a combination of Teflon and vitreous carbon (Proplast) and a high-density polyethylene sponge (Plastipore). Fibrin glue is also used. Partial and total ossicular replacement prostheses have been developed, but complications following their use have been reported.

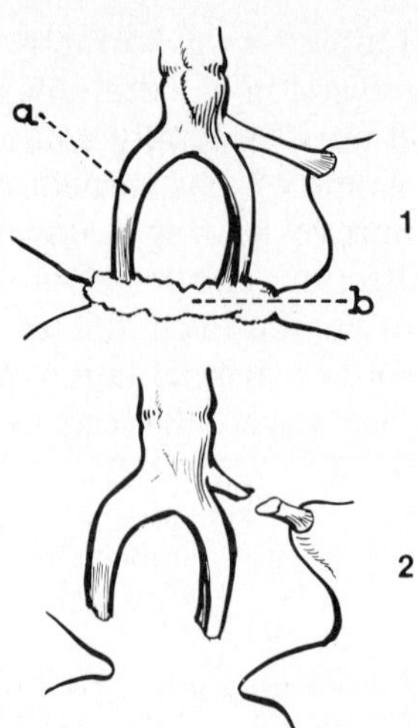

FIGURE 26-2
Partial stapedectomy. (1) Stapes superstructure (*a*) attached to fixed otosclerotic footplate (*b*); (2) footplate removed; superstructure remains.

Tympanomastoid Reconstruction Tympanoplasty may be combined with either simple or radical mastoidectomy. The mastoid is drained and cleaned prior to reconstruction of the eardrum or middle ear ossicles. Following incision behind the auricle, the tympanic membrane and tympanic cavity are inspected. The mastoid antrum is entered by drilling through mastoid bone.

Sometimes in chronic otitis media, the mucous membrane of the tympanic cavity is replaced by epithelium from the ear canal as it grows through a perforation in the eardrum. Desquamated skin cells then cannot escape and form a ball or cyst, known as a *cholesteatoma.* If present in the middle ear or mastoid, a cholesteatoma is removed during mastoidectomy and/or tympanoplasty.

Stapedectomy with Insertion of a Prosthesis To restore the conductive hearing loss of otosclerosis, the surgeon aims to restore vibration from the incus to the mobile oval window membrane to transmit sound. A partial stapedectomy involves removal of only the fixed footplate. The remaining superstructure is used to reconstruct the sound-conducting mechanism (see Fig. 26-2). More commonly, however, the entire stapes, including the footplate, is removed and replaced by a prosthesis.

Incision is made deep in the canal near but not in the eardrum. The eardrum is folded over, giving access to the middle ear. The stapes is disconnected from the incus, fractured by fine microinstruments, and removed. The oval window is

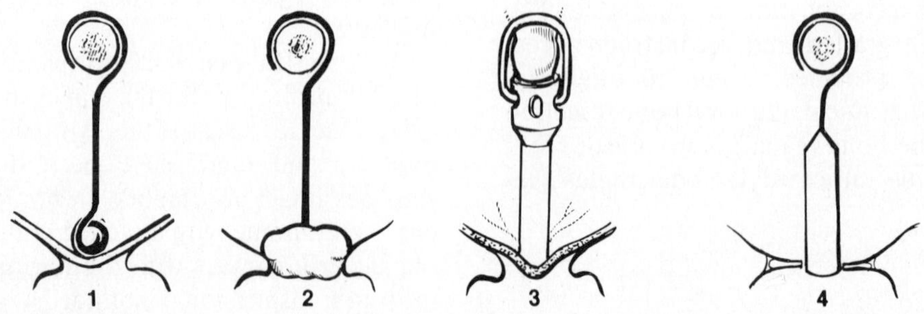

FIGURE 26-3
Stapedectomy prostheses and grafts: (1) wire-gelatin sponge, (2) wire-fat, (3) stainless steel piston-vein or fascia, (4) Teflon wire piston, without graft. End of wire loop is crimped over long process of incus. Opposite end of wire or piston is on center of graft covering oval window. Grafts become covered by mucous membrane or mucoperiosteum.

sealed by a graft of vein, perichondrium, fascia, fat, or Gelfoam over the oval window. A prosthesis is inserted and connected to the incus and to the graft, thus restoring sound conduction. Prostheses are made of various inert materials such as polyethylene, stainless steel, or tantalum (see Fig. 26-3).

By performing the microsurgical procedure under local anesthesia, the surgeon can reposition the eardrum and use voice to test if hearing is improved. Otosclerosis usually involves both ears, but stapedectomy is performed on only one ear at a time.

Stapes Mobilization The stapes is manipulated at the footplate to restore normal function. A break through an otosclerotic lesion is achieved by means of transcrural pressure or direct application of chisels and picks to the footplate. A mobile, noninvolved portion of a functioning stapes remains. Various techniques are used, with or without use of prosthetic devices. The advantage of the procedure is that the preserved stapedial footplate provides natural protection for the inner ear. The disadvantage is that frequently a continuing otosclerotic process causes the footplate to become refixed. Therefore, stapedectomy is more popular because it produces long-lasting results.

Stapes procedures are performed under direct vision with the operating microscope. The procedures do not disturb the integrity or position of the eardrum.

Middle Ear Vascular Tumors The argon laser is absorbed by red pigment. Therefore, it is suited for removal of small vascular tumors in the middle ear, such as glomus tympanicum tumors. The argon laser acts by photocoagulation (see Chap. 19, p. 364, and Chap. 25, p. 492).

Inner Ear

Endolymphatic Sac Shunt The endolymphatic sac is an appendage of the membranous inner ear located in the posterior fossa, anterior to lateral sinus and posterior to semicircular canals. An excessive accumulation of endolymph in this sac causes the episodic vertigo (dizziness), tinnitus (ear ringing), and sensorineural hearing loss of Ménière's disease. Through a simple mastoidectomy approach, the sac is opened and the inner ear drained into either the subarachnoid space or the mastoid. A shunt tube is inserted to maintain drainage.

Middle Fossa Vestibular Nerve Section The middle fossa approach to the internal auditory canal is a combined otologic and neurosurgical procedure. Through a middle fossa craniotomy, the superior portion of the internal auditory canal is exposed. The superior and inferior vestibular nerves, which control equilibrium, are sectioned to control intractable vertigo. The cochlear nerve, the hearing portion of the eighth cranial nerve, is not damaged, thus preserving hearing. A graft of temporalis muscle is placed over the exposed internal auditory canal to prevent leakage of cerebrospinal fluid.

Removal of Acoustic Neuroma Acoustic neuroma resection may be performed by an otologist and/or a neurosurgeon, depending on its location and extent of neurological involvement. An *acoustic neuroma* is a slow-growing encapsulated, benign tumor of the eighth cranial, the acoustic, nerve. It originates in the neural sheath in the internal auditory canal but grows to involve nerve fibers in the posterior fossa. Initially the patient experiences unilateral hearing loss and disturbances, especially tinnitus, and equilibrium problems such as mild vertigo. The syndrome may resemble Ménière's disease or an expanding intracranial tumor. Early differential diagnosis is enhanced by brainstem evoked response audiometry, vertebral angiography, and small-volume air-contrast computed tomography.

A small neuroma, confined to the internal auditory canal, may be resected by the otologist using microsurgical technique through a middle fossa approach to preserve hearing. If a translabyrinthine approach is used to gain access to the internal auditory canal posterior to the inner ear structures, the patient will have total hearing loss after operation. Acoustic neuromas extending into the cranial cavity are resected by the neurosurgeon (refer to Chap. 29, p. 552). The carbon dioxide laser has been used to excise acoustic neuromas through a transmastoid or craniotomy approach.

Implantation of Cochlear Prosthesis A cochlear implant can restore perception of sound to patients who have profound sensorineural deafness not responsive to external amplification (hearing aid). The implant has two major parts, the external and the internal. The external part has a microphone to receive sound waves, a stimulator/transducer to convert sound waves to electrical signals, and an external induction coil. The internal part has electrodes which are permanently implanted to bypass the damaged transduction system in the cochlea and to stimulate auditory nerve fibers.

Through a postauricular incision, the internal electrode coil is securely seated superficially in the mastoid cortex. To provide access to the inner ear, a mastoidectomy is performed. Under the operating microscope, the facial recess between the facial nerve and chorda tympani nerve is opened. The electrodes are placed from the mastoid cavity through this recess into the middle ear. The ground electrode is placed in the middle ear space, eustachian tube, or temporalis muscle. The active electrode is passed into the scala tympani of the cochlea through an opening made in the round window. A plug of fascia from the temporalis muscle or fat from the earlobe is placed around the electrode at the round window to prevent perilymph leakage.

The microphone, located in an external ear mold fitted to the auditory canal, transmits the sound waves converted in the stimulator/transducer to electric current via a wire to the external induction coil worn behind the ear directly over the internal coil. The electrical signal is transmitted through the skin to the internal electrodes by magnetic induction. The controls in the stimulator/transducer (power pack) allow the patient to adjust amplification of environmental sounds.

THE NOSE

Anatomy and Physiology

The supporting structures of the nose consist of two nasal bones and the nasal processes of the maxillary bones superiorly; lateral cartilages and connective tissue inferiorly; and the septum. The *septum,* composed of bone posteriorly and cartilage anteriorly, divides the nose into two chambers lined by mucous membrane. The *anterior portion,* or *vestibule,* holds the nasal hairs. The external anterior orifices are called *nares.*

The internal portion of the nose, the *nasal cavity,* extends to the *nasopharynx,* the space behind the *choanae,* or funnellike posterior nasal orifices. The nose communicates with the ear via the eustachian tube. The hard and soft palates divide the nasal and oral cavities. The nasal and cranial cavities are separated by the ethmoid bone.

The *paranasal sinuses* are the frontal, maxillary, ethmoid, and sphenoid. *Ostia* (openings from the sinuses and nasolacrimal ducts) are located in the nasal lateral walls. The ostia provide a drainage system for the sinuses as well as aerate them. Three turbinate bones (superior, middle, and inferior) are also situated in the lateral walls. These bones are covered with a vascular mucosa. Beneath each turbinate is a corresponding meatus. Tears drain into the nose through the nasolacrimal duct that enters the inferior meatus. Drainage from the paranasal sinuses is passed to the nose through the middle and superior meatuses.

External and internal carotid arteries and their branches supply blood to the nasal region. Because of the extensive vascularity, lymphatic supply, and proximity to the brain, infections on or about the face are potentially very dangerous. Microorganisms may readily be carried to or thrombi form in the cavernous sinus. The sensory nerve supply of the nasal area is associated with the trigeminal or fifth cranial nerve.

The *function of the nose* is twofold:

1 It provides filtered air to the respiratory system. Fine cilia in the mucous membrane propel mucus toward the nasopharynx. Air is warmed and moistened as it passes to the trachea and lower respiratory tract.

2 It contains the end organs for smell in the olfactory epithelium, which differs from other nasal epithelium. When nasal obstruction blocks off the olfactory epithelium, loss of smell (*anosmia*) results. The senses of smell and taste are closely related.

NASAL OPERATIVE PROCEDURES

Nasal operations are concerned with two factors: adequate ventilation to accessory spaces and adequate drainage from them. Abnormalities in structure, congenital or traumatic, and disease processes hinder function. Corrective procedures are done for several purposes as described below.

To Relieve Obstruction

Nasal obstruction may be due to allergies or nonoperative conditions. Operative intervention, however, can provide relief in certain instances.

Foreign Body or Abnormal Growth

Removal of Foreign Body Most frequent in children, often a foreign body is not suspect until discharge develops. After shrinkage of the mucosa with a vasoconstrictor and suctioning of secretions, the object is removed with a forceps. Usually local anesthesia suffices, but general anesthesia may be necessary if the child is uncooperative or the removal difficult.

Incision and Drainage of Nasal Abscess or Hematoma Infection is drained to relieve pressure. Accumulation of blood or pus separates *perichondrium,* connective tissue, from underlying cartilage. This may cause necrosis of cartilage with resultant deformity. Infection must be removed to avoid extension to the brain.

Polypectomy When the posterior choanae are obstructed by *polyps,* soft edematous masses project from the nasal or sinus mucosa. Polyps may be unilateral, bilateral, single, or multiple. In addition to impeding ventilation, they may obstruct the sense of smell if the olfactory epithelium is blocked. Multiple or large polyps are excised with a snare-type instrument. Packing, to control bleeding, is usually left in place two to three days. Since polyps frequently recur, persistent regrowth can be deterred by more extensive removal, i.e., by external or intranasal *ethmoidectomy,* removal of ethmoid sinuses, where most polyps originate.

Nasal Deformity

Reduction of Nasal Fracture Fracture of the septum or nasal bones often accompanies other trauma to the head. Intranasal manipulation under anesthesia is required to elevate depressed bone or cartilage that may be pushed into the paranasal sinuses. This should be performed as soon as possible to bring the parts in apposition. Delay of seven to ten days to permit edema to subside will not affect outcome, however. Bleeding from laceration must be immediately controlled and drained. Intranasal structure compatible with air passage must be preserved.

Septoplasty, Septal Reconstruction, Submucous Resection The terms septoplasty, septal reconstruction, and submucous resection are used interchangeably to describe correction of a deviated nasal septum. Often the result of injury, the condition interferes with breathing and drainage. Under local anesthesia, one side of the septum is incised its entire length. Membranous coverings are detached from cartilage and bone. The deformed part of the septum is removed, or straightened and replaced. Bilateral nasal packing is inserted to hold tissues in place and to prevent bleeding. The procedure creates a patent airway and straight septal line, thereby reducing sinus disease and polyp formation.

Rhinoplasty Rhinoplasty is a plastic procedure to correct deformity of the nose. It may be performed by a rhinologist or a plastic surgeon (refer to Chap. 27). It is a major procedure involving reconstruction and molding of the bones and cartilages. Septoplasty and rhinoplasty may be performed together; *septorhinoplasty* restores both function and cosmetic appearance. Local anesthesia is usually used. The skin is taped postoperatively to maintain nasal structures in alignment. A rigid shield is applied for protection. This must not be disturbed without specific order from the surgeon. Temporary ecchymosis from operative trauma surrounds the eyes postoperatively.

Repair of Perforated Septum Perforations occur most often in the anterior cartilage. If bleeding and crusting are severe, the perforation may be covered by rotated mucoperichondrial flaps. Or the mucosa of adjacent intact septum may be denuded and a skin graft applied to cover the perforation. Nasal packing is inserted.

To Ensure Drainage

The paranasal sinuses are air-filled spaces in the skull. Since the sinus mucous membrane lining is continuous with the mucous membrane lining of the nose, nasal infection may readily spread to the sinuses. Various procedures provide drainage for patients with chronic sinusitis that may result from repeated nasopharyngeal infection. Swelling of nasal mucosa can trap microorganisms within a sinus cavity. Abnormalities in walls of the nasal cavity also interfere with breathing and drainage. Sinus procedures are executed through an external or an intranasal approach.

Maxillary Sinus Operation The *maxillary sinuses* are located bilaterally between the upper teeth and the eyes.

Caldwell-Luc (Antrostomy) The maxillary sinus contents are approached through incision of the oral mucous membrane above the canine teeth. The flap is retracted. A section of maxillary bone is cut out to create a large nasoantral window for aeration and permanent drainage by gravity into the nasal fossa under the inferior turbinate. Polyps and diseased tissue are removed. At completion of operation, the sinus is packed with gauze impregnated with antibiotic ointment. One end of gauze is brought through the window and into the nose. The incision under the upper lip is sutured. The packing is eventually removed through the nose. Antrostomy is usually limited to adults because of unerupted teeth in children. Caldwell-Luc incision is also used for removal of a tumor in the maxillary sinus.

Ethmoid Sinus Operations The *ethmoid sinus* cells lie bilaterally between the nose and the orbits. The maxillary sinuses are below the ethmoid bones and the frontal sinuses are above them.

Ethmoidectomy Diseased tissue is removed from the ethmoid labyrinth, middle turbinate, and meatus. A large cavity is formed to facilitate aeration and drainage. Severe ethmoiditis can cause orbital abscess requiring drainage through intranasal or external (Lynch) incision that extends from the inner half of the eyebrow down along the side of the nose.

Turbinectomy Removal of portions of the inferior and middle turbinates increases aeration and drainage. The cavity is packed at completion of operation.

Frontal Sinus Operations The *frontal sinuses* are situated above the eyes. Usually approached through the external incision described for ethmoidectomy, a coronal incision may be made for exposure across the scalp from ear to ear.

Osteoplastic Flap Procedure The bone covering the frontal sinus is exposed and incised. Contents of the sinus, such as a *mucocele,* a cyst lined with mucous-secreting glands, are extracted. The lining of the mucocele sac is removed and the cavity packed with fat, from the abdominal wall, to obliterate the sinus with fibrous tissue that fills in the cavity. The incised bone flap is then repositioned and the incision sutured.

Killian Operation A frontal sinus cavity is reached by removal of the floor or anterior wall of the sinus through external incision above the eye. A large communication and drainage channel into the nose is formed.

Sphenoid Sinus Operation The *sphenoid sinus* is deep, almost in the center of the skull. It may be approached intranasally or via the external ethmoidectomy incision through the eyebrow.

Sphenoidotomy Sphenoidotomy involves the creation of an opening into the sphenoid sinus for drainage.

To Resect Tumors

Procedures for Carcinoma of Paranasal Sinuses Although rare, carcinoma does occur in the ethmoid sinuses and the maxillary antrum. The incidence increases with age. The sinuses are proximal to the orbits, oral cavity, and base of the skull. Tumor in the maxillary sinus may be associated with oral or nasal symptoms, such as loosening of the upper teeth, bleeding from the nose, or asymmetry of the face. Malignancy in the ethmoid sinus may be accompanied by displacement of the eye, disturbance of smell, and nasal obstruction. Chronic sinusitis is thought to play a role in etiology because of an associated replacement of respiratory epithelium by stratified squamous cells. Most sinus tumors are squamous-cell carcinoma. Often the bony walls are invaded and destroyed by the time symptoms appear, since the tumor tends to extend in all directions. Exploratory operation by Caldwell-Luc incision provides the best chance of early diagnosis. Radical craniofacial resection may be indicated (see Chap. 28).

To Control Epistaxis

Nasal bleeding may be spontaneous, as in patients with arteriosclerosis, hypertension, or blood dyscrasia, or may result from trauma. Bleeding is unilateral except in persons with systemic disease such as leukemia, or severe fracture. Dehumidified air may also cause changes in the mucosa and splitting of tiny vessels. Management consists of locating the precise bleeding site and promptly instituting appropriate therapy. Hypovolemia should be corrected preoperatively. A bleeding patient is in a precarious condition.

Placing an Anterior Pack An anterior pack will control the majority of nosebleeds. The vascular anterior portion of the nasal septum is a frequent site of bleeding (anterior epistaxis). Local vasoconstriction and pressure to the side of the nose are employed, and the bleeding point is cauterized if necessary. When bleeding is from the anterior ethmoid artery, inaccessible to cautery, packing is applied to the area of depression between the septum and the middle turbinate.

Placing a Posterior Pack A posterior pack may be necessary for constant pressure when bleeding in the posterior part of the nose is severe. Or operative intervention may be indicated. The pack consists of rolled gauze securely tied to the middle of a length of narrow tape or strong string. Commercial packs are available. The gauze is lubricated with antibiotic ointment before insertion to control infection and odor. After passing a catheter into the mouth via the nose, one end of tape is tied to the oral end of the catheter. The catheter and attached tape are then drawn back through the mouth and out one nostril, thereby pulling the pack up into the nasopharynx. Thus one end of tape comes out the nose, the other end out the mouth. These ends are secured to the patient's cheek with adhesive tape. The nasal end is taped to prevent the pack from slipping into the throat; the oral end facilitates removal of the pack. Some oozing may persist in spite of packing. The pack is left in place until bleeding is arrested, usually for at least 48 hours, but prolonged use can lead to otitis media or paranasal sinusitis.

Patients with postnasal packs are often apprehensive and uncomfortable. They must breathe through the mouth. Posterior packs tend to reduce arterial oxygen tension. All patients, especially the elderly or those with marginal pulmonary function, should be observed carefully for respiratory problems that may result from the pack dropping into the hypopharynx. Severe bleeding additionally may require anterior packing of the nose and correction of hypovolemia.

Artery Ligation A microsurgical procedure is performed to control persistent nasal hemorrhage by reducing the blood supply to the posterior portion of the nose. Some surgeons prefer this modality to packing, or it may be performed with a pack in place. Through a Caldwell-Luc incision, removal of the posterior wall exposes the maxillary sinus for transantral ligation. Terminal branches of the internal maxillary artery, a branch of the external carotid artery, are exposed, identified, and ligated with metallic clips. Electrocoagulation is employed to control intraoperative bleeding, but if it is excessive, creation of a nasoantral window establishes drainage. The replaced posterior mucosal flap is covered with absorbable gelatin sponge, and the incision is closed.

Incision along the left side of the nose and ligation of the anterior and posterior ethmoidal arteries is helpful in controlling bleeding in the superior aspect of the nose.

The argon laser may be used to control severe epistaxis.

THE ORAL CAVITY AND THROAT

Anatomy and Physiology

The *oral cavity* (mouth) is lined with thick mucous membrane (squamous mucosa) that connects with the nasopharynx above and the hypopharynx below. The *hard palate,* part of the maxillary bone, forms the floor of the nasal cavity and the anterior part of the roof of the mouth. The *soft palate,* a musculomembranous structure posterior to the hard palate, occludes the nasal cavity during phonation (speech) and deglutition (swallowing). These functions are aided by the *uvula,* a small conical appendage (tonguelike structure) that projects from the posterior free margin of the soft palate. It contains the uvular muscle covered by mucous membrane. The *tongue,* occupying much of the oral cavity, joins the soft palate and pharynx posteriorly by folds of mucous membrane.

The *throat* refers to space surrounded by the soft palate, the palatoglossal and palatopharyngeal arches, the base of the tongue, and the pharynx. The funnel-shaped *pharynx* is subdivided into the nasopharynx (above), oropharynx (middle), and hypopharynx (below). The *nasopharynx* communicates with the nasal cavity through the posterior choanae. The *oropharynx* includes the base of the tongue anteriorly, the tonsillar fossae laterally, and the oropharyngeal walls of the throat posteriorly. The *hypopharynx* leads from the oropharynx to the larynx, trachea, and esophagus. The pharynx, posterior to the larynx and the nasal and oral cavities, consists of constrictor muscles essential to swallowing. The proximity of food and air passages, and the joint function of the pharynx in their passage, contribute to the hazard of aspiration.

The nasopharynx and oropharynx contain masses of lymphoid tissue. The *adenoids* (pharyngeal tonsils) hang from the nasopharyngeal roof; the lingual tonsils are in mucosal crypts. The palatine tonsils lie on either side of the oropharynx. These, referred to as the *tonsils,* are supported in the tonsillar fossae by anterior and posterior pillars. A fibrous capsule adheres to each laterally.

OPERATIVE PROCEDURES OF THE ORAL CAVITY AND THROAT

The common operative procedures performed by ENT surgeons or laryngologists in these anatomic areas fall within two major classifications: those for infection and those for neoplasms or other life-threatening disorder. Additional operations in the oral cavity are discussed in Chapter 28. Those unique to infants and children are discussed in Chapter 33.

Palatopharyngoplasty Palatopharyngoplasty is performed to correct selective cases of obstructive sleep apnea (OSA). This disabling disorder causes oxygen desaturation during apneic episodes that occur during sleep. This can lead to life-threatening pulmonary hypertension and pulmonary heart disease (cor pulmonale) if untreated. Upper airway obstruction may be caused by nasal obstruction, deviated nasal septum, hypertrophied adenoids and/or tonsils, or mandibular retrognathism (overbite), which may be surgically corrected. To diagnose OSA in patients who do not have obvious abnormalities, airway obstruction can be viewed during sleep with fiberoptic nasopharyngoscopy and fluoroscopy. Some of the oropharyngeal muscles may become atonic and collapse inward, and the soft palate may drop down. Patients who have large drooping soft palate and at least moderately redundant lateral pharyngeal walls or large tonsils are good candidates for palatopharyngoplasty. These patients have moderate apnea but do not have severe cardiac arrhythmias.

The patient must be continuously monitored during induction of anesthesia. The surgeon must be present and an emergency tracheotomy tray available in case the patient obstructs.

The entire thickness of the posterior margin of soft palate, including uvula, and most of the anterior tonsillar pillar are resected. The lesser palatine artery is ligated. The tonsils or mucosa of the tonsillar fossae are resected. The remaining posterior tonsillar pillar is sutured to the resected anterior pillar. The palate is closed laterally.

Adenoidectomy Removal of hypertrophied adenoid tissue from the nasopharynx and behind the posterior choanae may be performed in adults to relieve upper airway obstruction. This is more commonly performed in children, often to prevent recurrent otitis media. Adenoid tissue usually atrophies after adolescence.

Tonsillectomy Chronically infected or hypertrophied tonsils are most frequently removed in childhood (refer to Chap. 33). However, even slightly enlarged tonsils can obstruct airflow to the lungs during sleep. Tonsillectomy may significantly improve the symptoms of sleep apnea in some adults. (Also refer to palatopharyngoplasty.)

The adult patient may be positioned in semi-Fowler's or sitting position on the operating table or may sit in a specifically designed chair, with the surgeon sitting in front of him or her. Local anesthesia is frequently used. The throat is anesthetized with a topical agent and local infiltration.

With sharp or blunt dissection, tonsil is separated from the pillars and capsule and removed from the fossa with a tonsil snare. Special attention is given to hemostasis so the operative area is clearly visible and aspiration prevented. Bleeding can be difficult to control and can occur postoperatively. Suture ligatures, free ties, and/or absorbable ligating clips may be used for hemostasis.

The scrub nurse assists by retracting the tongue, identifying the various colorless solutions used, and preparing sutures. Sponges are placed in forceps. In addition to monitoring the patient, the circulating nurse should observe how much blood is being drawn into the suction bottle and report an abnormal amount.

Incision and Drainage of Peritonsillar Abscess Less common since the advent of antibiotics, incision into anterior tonsillar pillar may be necessary to drain purulent material posterior to tonsillar capsule following acute tonsillitis.

Resection of Tonsillar Tumor A localized squamous-cell carcinoma of the tonsil may be resected by dissection or with cryosurgery. An en bloc resection includes the primary tumor and nodes. Metastatic nodes are common. Superior progression of tumor may reach the supratonsillar fossa, soft and hard palates, and uvula. Inferiorly, tumor may spread to the posterior and lateral walls of the larynx, base of tongue, and pyriform sinus. Neck dissection may be indicated for regional disease. Surgery may be combined with pre- or postoperative radiation therapy. The most common complications are fistula formation and delayed healing.

Removal of Tumors in Pharynx or Oral Cavity Small benign and early malignant tumors in oropharynx and oral cavity can be removed with carbon dioxide laser or local excision with primary closure. Extensive operations for oral carcinoma are discussed in Chapter 28.

Diverticulectomy Diverticulectomy, or removal of sacs or outpocketings of lower pharyngeal mucous membrane in which food collects, may be performed in extreme cases where regurgitation presents hazard of aspiration. The neck of the sac is dissected from the posterior pharyngeal wall and ligated. The stump of the excised sac is inverted into the pharyngeal wall. Diverticuli may be removed endoscopically, especially in high-risk patients.

THE NECK

Anatomy and Physiology

The *neck* connects the head and trunk of the body. It is supported by the cervical vertebrae posteriorly and muscles anteriorally and laterally. The larynx, leading to the trachea, and proximal end of the esophagus pass within the muscular structure. The vascular, nervous, and lymphatic systems leading to and from the head also pass through the neck.

The *larynx,* situated anteriorly between the hypopharynx superiorly and trachea inferiorly, consists of three major cartilages supported by ligaments and muscles: the thyroid cartilage, which protects the soft inner structures, the cricoid cartilage directly beneath it, and the paired arytenoid cartilages posterior to the thyroid and joined to the cricoid. The thyroid cartilage is incomplete posteriorly but the cricoid is a complete ring. The cricothyroid space lies between the thyroid and cricoid cartilages.

The larynx functions as an organ for speech and for closure of the glottis during swallowing to protect the respiratory passage and prevent aspiration. Extrinsic muscles open and close the *glottis,* the space between the true vocal cords. Intrinsic muscles regulate vocal cord tension. Movement of the paired arytenoid cartilages opens and closes the glottis. Folds of membrane covering muscle, the *true vocal cords* are attached to the arytenoid cartilages posteriorly and to the thyroid cartilage anteriorly. The cords are an integral part of phonation. They vibrate to produce sounds by rhythmically moving air particles. Production of vocal sound involves coordination of musculature of the lips, tongue, soft palate, pharynx, and larynx. The mouth and pharynx are the resonating cavities.

The tenth cranial or vagus nerve innervates the larynx. Its major branch to the larynx is the recurrent laryngeal nerve. Trauma to the nerve can result in laryngeal paralysis, devastating if both nerves are paralyzed.

The *trachea* is a tube composed of rings of cartilage anteriorly and membrane posteriorly. This membrane also forms the anterior wall of the *esophagus,* the musculomembranous canal between the pharynx and stomach. The trachea extends from the lower larynx to the carina in the chest, where it bifurcates to form the right and left main bronchi leading to the lungs.

OPERATIVE PROCEDURES OF THE LARYNX

Trauma or disease involving laryngeal cartilages, mucous membrane, or the vocal cords can obstruct respiration and/or speech. Operations are directed toward diagnosis of etiology and elimination of obstruction to maintain the larynx's dual functions in respiration and phonation.

Laryngoscopy

The mucous membrane lining of larynx and vocal cords can be examined with a lighted instrument, with or without the adjunct magnification of the operating microscope. Laryngoscopy is performed for diagnosis, biopsy, and/or treatment of laryngeal lesions including:

1 *Foreign body,* such as a coin or small toy.

2 *Papilloma of the vocal cords,* which prevent accurate cord approximation and normal voice.

3 *Laryngeal polyps,* with stripping of polypoid mucosa to alleviate recurrence.

4 *Juvenile papilloma,* multiple growths on the larynx, epiglottis, vocal cords, and trachea. These may be treated by cryosurgery or laser beam in lieu of excision.

5 *Leukoplakia,* a white thickening on the vocal cords, causing hoarseness. The lesion must be examined histologically for differentiation from carcinoma.

6 *Laryngeal web,* adherence of the anterior aspects of the vocal cords as a result of removal of mucous membrane, or following inflammation. After excision, a metal or plastic plate may be put between the cords until normal mucous membrane regenerates. The plate is then removed.

Preoperative preparation and endoscopic technique are similar for laryngoscopy, esophagoscopy, and bronchoscopy. General anesthesia is usually used, but local topical anesthesia may be preferred for some patients. The patient is supine with neck hyperextended and head supported. As following any anesthetization of throat, postoperative orders include nothing by mouth for a specific number of hours until throat reflexes have returned, to prevent aspiration.

Indirect Laryngoscopy A laryngeal mirror is inserted through the mouth to base of the tongue, with the patient in sitting position. Light is reflected to area by the surgeon's headlamp. During this simple diagnostic procedure, biopsy or polypectomy can be performed.

Direct Laryngoscopy A rigid hollow tubular laryngoscope is inserted into larynx for direct visualization. Suction tubes and grasping forceps are maneuvered through the hand-held laryngoscope. Fiberoptic light carriers must be connected to light source. Endoscopic principles as discussed in Chapter 19 are applicable.

Suspension Microlaryngoscopy The laryngoscope becomes self-retaining by suspension in a special appliance placed over the patient's chest. This gives the surgeon bimanual freedom in use of the operating microscope. The microscope provides binocular vision and magnification in critical inaccessible areas or areas difficult to visualize by direct laryngoscopy. A standard operating microscope with a 400-mm lens is used. Microlaryngeal instruments are added to the basic setup for direct laryngoscopy. Suspension microlaryngoscopy is used for most intralaryngeal operations.

Carbon Dioxide Laser Microlaryngoscopy The carbon dioxide (CO_2) laser was introduced in laryngology by Doctors Jako and Strong in 1971. It was initially used for removal of recurrent laryngeal papillomas. Now the CO_2 laser is used to remove a variety of other lesions in the respiratory tract, particularly in the larynx.

A micromanipulator, used to direct the laser beam, is coupled to the operating microscope. The invisible beam is focused by the microscope lens. It becomes visible by superimposing a red light beam from a helium-neon laser to facilitate aiming the CO_2 laser beam. Stainless steel mirrors are used for reflecting the laser beam into inaccessible areas.

Microlaryngeal instruments are used in addition to specific laser instruments. Anterior commissure vocal cord retractors with suction attachments are used to clear the smoke of tissue vaporization for visibility. A two-suction setup is necessary to rapidly clear the smoke during vaporization of a malignant tumor in the larynx.

The CO_2 laser is a safe instrument only when necessary precautions are taken.

1 The patient's eyes must be taped shut to prevent injury from inadvertent reflection of laser beam from a metal surface.

2 Only noncombustible anesthetic gases are used. Anesthetic gases exposed to area being treated by laser potentially can ignite.

3 A copper, stainless steel, or laminated silicone endotracheal tube or a ventilating bronchoscope avoids danger of ignition. Polyvinyl chloride and latex endotracheal tubes cannot be used because they are heat labile. Red rubber and silicone tubes may be wrapped with reflecting aluminum tape, but the tip is not always sufficiently protected if exposed to the laser beam. Ignition of endotracheal tubes has occurred. Moist gauze or cottonoid patties, attached to strings, are placed through the suspended laryngoscope to protect the endotracheal tube balloon (cuff) from rupture by stray or reflected laser beams. If this occurs, immediate replacement of the tube is necessary. A tracheotomy tray should be available for emergency use.

4 Combustible materials, such as gauze and drapes, must be kept moist. Water effectively inhibits penetration of laser energy into surrounding tissue and materials.

5 Division of a blood vessel larger than 0.5 mm requires ligation or electrocoagulation.

6 All other precautions for laser surgery must be taken (see Chap. 19, p. 367).

NOTE. The argon laser may be used for treatment of hereditary hemorrhagic telangiectasia (dilated groups of capillaries) in the larynx.

Laryngeal Injuries

Patients with abnormal laryngeal conditions bear close watching for respiratory distress. The anterior, unprotected location of the larynx predisposes it to trauma, such as crushing injury. Treatment is concerned primarily with maintenance of the airway, which may be occluded by edema, hematoma, torn mucosa, or cartilaginous fragments.

Tracheotomy may be necessary to prevent asphyxia. An intraluminal stent inserted into the larynx superiorly to the tracheotomy tube, and fixed to it for stabilization, may be worn for several months until the laryngeal laceration heals and an intralaryngeal airway re-forms. The stent is used to mold the tissues.

Preservation of voice is also a major concern. Severe laryngeal injury may result in permanent voice impairment. In unilateral vocal cord paralysis, because of muscle atrophy and muscle imbalance, a weak, hoarse ("air-spilling") voice is present. Inadequate glottic closure can be treated by injection of Polytef paste into the affected cord, to augment its size and thus help to bring the two cords into apposition. The injected material becomes firm and retains shape. A functioning cord and markedly improved voice quality result. This modality is used commonly when the recurrent laryngeal nerve is affected. It is not indicated, however, for acute glottic incompetence. A suspension of Gelfoam powder in saline can be used for temporary augmentation until compensation or need for permanent augmentation occurs.

Procedures for Carcinoma of the Larynx

Procedures vary depending on the size and location of the lesion, extent of invasion, presence of regional or distant metastasis, age, general condition, and rehabilitative capacity of the patient. Classification of malignancy by location includes *glottic* (true cords), *supraglottic* (above true cords), and *infraglottic* (below true cords). In the early stages, cancer of the larynx is one of the most curable of all malignancies because of the sparse lymphatic supply in the region of the vocal cords. Radiological examination of the lesion by various methods, such as contrast laryngography, is a valuable adjunct in selecting an appropriate therapeutic modality. Laryngograms can identify mucosal irregularity, vocal cord thickening or tumor, and outline the lesion, as well as portray functional alteration of laryngeal structures.

Symptoms vary as well. Hoarseness of over two weeks duration often signals origin of malignancy of the glottis, as a result of cord fixation by the lesion. Dysphagia is suggestive of tumor at the esophageal opening. Dyspnea from airway obstruction is a late manifestation.

Total Laryngectomy with/without Neck Dissection The entire larynx (epiglottis, false and true cords) and upper tracheal rings are removed, destroying connection between the pharynx and trachea, for advanced lesions of the true vocal cords or hypopharyngeal area. Pharyngeal walls and lower trachea are preserved. Thereafter the patient breathes and expels bronchial secretions through a permanent stoma in the anterior base of the neck. This is created by suturing the tracheal stump to the skin (*tracheostomy*). Size of the stoma should be recorded on the patient's record in event of emergency need for a tube at a later time. In patients with a permanent stoma, resuscitation always must be via stoma.

The nose no longer humidifies the air to the lungs. Sense of smell is also lost because the nasal olfactory epithelium is not stimulated by inhalation. Acclimatization to air intake through the neck constitutes a major adjustment for the patient.

A nasogastric tube is inserted at operation for temporary feeding. Although the laryngectomee no longer has normal voice, normal eating is resumed after healing takes place.

Formation of a salivary fistula is one complication of laryngectomy. Swallowed saliva leaks out through a weakness in the pharyngeal suture line and through the skin. Rupture of the carotid artery, especially in preirradiated patients, is another complication. This may occur if radical neck dissection was performed also, which places the artery in the operative area. (Refer to discussions of neck dissection in Chapter 28.)

Rehabilitation of the laryngectomee should begin preoperatively with diagnosis and include the family. It incorporates input from many professional disciplines, since major disability results from the operation. In working with the speech pathologist, some patients learn to develop esophageal speech. By intake of a bolus of air into the esophagus and vibration by cricopharyngeal muscles, sound is produced to articulate speech. Persons unable to perfect the technique may use an artificial larynx, an electronic device that includes pitch and volume.

Many patients are unable to acquire usable esophageal speech, with or without the artificial larynx. Some of these patients have undergone operative procedures to rebuild a functioning glottis, or to create a permanent tracheoesophageal fistula to shunt pulmonary airflow to the pharynx for phonation. Aspiration pneumonia due to leakage of saliva and food is a major problem following these procedures. Also pharyngeal constrictor muscle spasms or stenosis may inhibit speech rehabilitation. *Voice restoration* for these aphonic patients may be enhanced by a valved prosthesis. This is inserted through a tracheoesophageal fistula to allow free flow of air into the esophagus for phonation, to prevent aspiration, and to maintain patency of the fistula. Three types of one-way valve *voice prostheses* are used.

1 Blom-Singer duck bill prosthesis, so-named from shape of the slit valve, is a silicone tube with retention flanges (collarlike projections). The fistula for the prosthesis is created through an esophagoscope inserted into cervical esophagus. A needle is introduced to puncture posterior tracheal wall and anterior esophagus at the superior aspect of the laryngectomy stoma. A rubber catheter stent is inserted through the puncture to maintain patency during healing. When the prosthesis is fitted, the flanges are taped to the peristomal skin. The patient must occlude the stoma to produce a voice.

2 Blom-Singer tracheostoma valve and low-pressure prosthesis has a diaphragm that opens during normal respiration and closes in response to expiratory airflow for speech. The circular valve is recessed slightly into the tracheostoma with the polyvinyl chloride housing fixed to the peristomal skin with a hypoallergenic adhesive. The patient does not manually occlude the stoma during speech.

3 Panje Voice Prosthesis, commonly known as the voice button, is a biflanged silicone valve inserted into a simple tracheoesophageal stab wound. An insertion guide is used to place the prosthesis through the tracheostoma into the created fistula. The patient occludes the stoma to speak.

Practical help and moral support are offered the newly laryngectomized patient by others who are members of numerous groups, such as the International Association of Laryngectomees and the Lost Chord Club. The American Cancer Society is also a resource for assistance.

Total laryngectomy is a radical procedure. Whenever possible and for smaller lesions the surgeon instead will perform *conservative surgery of the larynx* or *partial laryngectomy.* These procedures yield the same rate of cure of selected malignancies as the radical procedure, without sacrificing phonation, deglutition, and respiratory function. Some natural voice is retained and a neck stoma may not be necessary for breathing.

Supraglottic Laryngectomy A conservative technique for carcinoma, the epiglottis and/or false cords are removed in addition to the hyoid bone. Horizontal incision is made above the true vocal cords, thus preserving the voice and normal airway. Neck dissection may be done simultaneously. A prophylactic tracheotomy is always part of the procedure because of the danger of aspiration. With the epiglottis removed, liquids in particular can easily spill into the trachea. Use of a cuffed tracheotomy tube (see p. 515) is a necessary precaution.

Vertical Hemilaryngectomy Also a conservative method, vertical hemilaryngectomy may be performed by several techniques. In hemilaryngectomy through a vertical incision, one true cord, false cord, arytenoid, and half the thyroid cartilage are removed. The epiglottis, cricoid, and opposite cord are preserved. Following healing, scar tissue that fills in the operative defect almost approximates the remaining vocal cord. Thus the patient has a usable although hoarse voice, satisfactory airway, and normal eating. Sometimes a muscle flap is used for glottic reconstruction to improve voice quality. A prophylactic tracheotomy may be done.

Subcutaneous emphysema, infiltration of air under the skin, is a potential complication.

OPERATIVE PROCEDURES OF THE TRACHEA

Upper respiratory tract obstruction and ventilatory failure may require operative intervention when the need for intubation or positive-pressure ventilation would be long-term or of indefinite duration, or when severe laryngeal obstruction is present. The obstruction is bypassed.

Tracheotomy

Tracheotomy is the formation of an opening into the trachea into which a tube is inserted, through which the patient breathes. It is performed in any age group to improve or maintain patency of the airway or relieve obstruction. The opening in the trachea provides easy accessibility for suctioning secretions from the tracheobronchial tree or administering anesthesia to patients with facial trauma or burns.

Airway crisis may result from mechanical obstruction due to a tumor, foreign body, infection, or secretions. It also results from congenital, neurologic, or traumatic conditions. Some of the many indications for the procedure are foreign body in the hypopharynx or larynx; acute laryngotracheal bronchitis or epiglottitis in infants and children; laryngeal edema; or any other condition that obstructs respiration.

Tracheotomy is commonly a controlled prophylactic procedure, but can be an acute emergency. An endotracheal tube may give temporary relief prior to and during tracheotomy.

Tracheotomy is often done under local anesthesia. The patient is supine with support under the shoulders to hyperextend the neck. A transverse incision is made, producing better cosmetic result, or a midline vertical incision is made between the cricoid cartilage and the suprasternal notch. The overlying isthmus of the thyroid gland is retracted or divided and the exposed third or fourth tracheal ring is incised. After tracheal aspiration to remove blood and secretions, a tracheotomy tube is inserted with the obturator in place. Immediately after insertion the obturator is removed to open the airway. (This remains with the patient constantly in case of future need.) The outer cannula is suctioned and the inner cannula fixed in place. The wound is closed with a few sutures, or superficial edges of the area above the tube may be sutured and the area below left with natural tissue approximation, for drainage. A smooth-edged dressing split around the tube protects the skin. Commercial tracheotomy dressings are available. Tapes tied to the ends of the outer cannula are secured around the neck. Proper tension allows insertion of one finger between the tape and skin. If tied too tightly, the tapes may compress the jugular vein; if too loosely, the tube can obtrude with coughing. The tube should not be removed in the first 24 to 48 hours by any person unable to perform tracheotomy, because the tract to the trachea may occlude and not be immediately located.

A sterile tube identical to the one inserted and a tracheotomy set must accompany the patient from the OR and constantly remain with him or her. The set is eventually released by surgeon's order.

A tracheotomy is an open wound. While rigid asepsis is not possible, every effort is made to keep contamination to a minimum. Only sterile equipment, with minimal handling, is used to prevent infection. Suctioning through a tracheotomy tube is done as a sterile procedure, with sterile catheter and gloves. Careful suctioning prevents trauma. Insert the catheter without application of suction, to protect tracheal walls and prevent suctioning out oxygen in the borderline patient. Apply suction as catheter is withdrawn. Run sterile solution through catheter after use to clean it and maintain patency. Disposable catheters are recommended; use once and dispose.

Some tracheotomized patients come to the OR for change of tube or other procedure. These patients may require suctioning while waiting in the holding area. Knowledge of and preparation for each patient is a prime responsibility of the circulating nurse.

Tracheotomized patients require humidified air, deliverable by various devices, to keep secretions liquefied and to prevent drying of tissues. Other needs are constant observation and special communication, e.g., pencil and paper.

Tracheotomy Tubes While an endotracheal tube may provide ventilation for short-term therapy, a tracheotomy tube is easier to suction and immobilize for extended use. It also reduces possibility of laryngeal injury.

Various materials such as plastic, nylon, and silicone have largely replaced silver tubes. The plastic tubes have certain advantages:

1 They can be left in situ during radiation therapy.
2 They are lighter in weight, softer, more pliable, less traumatic.
3 They can be cut to length.
4 They are bonded to the inflatable cuff.

The inside and outside diameters of some tubes are labeled in millimeters. French or Jackson scale is stated on others. All hospitals keep a variety of sizes and types of sterile tracheotomy tubes available in the OR suite, in the emergency department, and on emergency arrest/crash carts.

Most tubes have three parts—the outer cannula, inner cannula, and obturator. The inner cannula is periodically removed and cleaned to prevent blockage by crusting of secretions. *It always must be replaced immediately within the outer cannula* so that the latter remains free of crusting. The obturator provides a smooth tip during tube insertion to prevent trauma to the tracheal wall. Some plastic tubes do not require an inner cannula because they remain relatively free of crust. If crusts do form, the tube must be changed.

Some tubes have a built-in soft cuff that is inflated to eliminate any free space between the tube and the tracheal wall, thus preventing aspiration of drainage down the trachea. Cuffed tubes also facilitate function of any ventilatory apparatus. A pilot balloon in the inflation line, attached to the outer cannula, indicates cuff inflation or deflation. *Proper cuff inflation-deflation is highly important.* Irritation and pressure of the cuff against the tracheal wall can cause damage such as ulceration and necrosis of the mucosa, which can lead to infection, tracheobronchial fistula, erosion into the innominate artery, or stenosis from scarring. Precautionary measures include deflation at regular intervals, by written order, to increase blood flow to the cuff site; use of low-pressure or controlled-pressure cuff; constant monitoring of intracuff pressure; and minimum inflation to ensure a leak-free system. Overinflation can reduce tube diameter as well as cause the cuff to extend over the tip of the tube, thus obstructing ventilation. Or the tracheal wall may herniate over the tube end. Underinflation may cause subcutaneous emphysema. Cuffs also should inflate symmetrically. The amount of air needed for inflation varies with the size of the trachea and the tube. Understandably, less air is needed for larger tubes. Usually 2 to 5 ml of air provide a closed system.

Specific tubes have special variations, such as an opening in the wall opposite the bevel to permit ventilation in case of bevel occlusion. Others have a radiopaque tip that allows radiologic visualization of tube position. Many have connectors, some of which are a built-in swivel type permitting lightweight, flexible, easy connection to a ventilating system. These connectors reduce hazard of accidental disconnection. Still others have a fenestration in the outer cannula permitting air to flow through the larynx. These tubes are used in patients no longer requiring mechanical ventilation to allow assessment of spontaneous breathing and coughing in preparation for decannulation. With air passing through the larynx, the patient can speak with the proximal end of the cannula plugged. A so-called speaking tube permits introduction of humidified air and oxygen through a special line and, with upward flow of the gas through the larynx, the patient can speak.

Tracheotomy Set A tracheotomy set, with all essential equipment for performance of tracheotomy, should be in the operating room during any extensive operation on the face or neck, thyroidectomy, or radical neck dissection. If a tracheotomy tube is inserted during operation, the obturator must accompany the patient at all times. If a tube is not needed, the tracheotomy set accompanies the patient and remains at the bedside for a few days postoperatively, in case of development of respiratory obstruction due to edema. A set is kept at the bedside of a patient on a respirator. Sterile sets must *always* be available. Tubes are wrapped and sterilized individually to permit free selection.

OPERATIVE PROCEDURES OF THE ESOPHAGUS

Esophageal disorders may be congenital or acquired (refer to Chap. 33 for congenital). Abnormalities result from trauma, inflammation, or neoplasm. They may be studied by a gastroenterologist and/or laryngologist.

Esophagoscopy Endoscopic or direct visualization of the interior of the esophagus is performed to remove foreign bodies, obtain biopsy, brush cytologic or secretion specimens for diagnosis, and examine the esophagus and esophageal orifice of the stomach for organic disease. Inspection is made for diverticula, varices, strictures, lesions, or hiatus hernia, which may be manifested by symptoms of obstruction, regurgitation, or bleeding. (Refer to Chapter 19 for discussion of endoscopes, endoscopy, and care of endoscopic equipment.)

Esophagoscopes are rigid hollow metal tubes or the flexible fiberoptic type of scope that reduces discomfort and trauma. Accessory instruments, such as aspiration tubes and biopsy forceps, are similar for all endoscopes. Removal of an obstructing mass such as a steak bolus in the esophagus is better accomplished with the rigid metal scope. Various sizes of scopes are available to suit the individual patient's situation.

Patient is positioned with shoulders even with, or a little over, edge of body section of operating table. The head section is lowered. Patient's head is held by an assistant. Patient is encouraged to relax by breathing deeply if procedure is done with local topical anesthesia. The head is raised or lowered slowly, at the direction of the endoscopist as the esophagoscope is passed, until the neck is hyperextended. The esophagoscope is passed through the mouth and cricopharyngeal lumen to the cardiac sphincter at the esophagogastric junction. The entire area is carefully scrutinized. The esophagus may be distended by insufflation of air to assist in viewing in the presence of stenosis, or a lumen finder may be necessary. The scrub nurse introduces the tips of aspirating tubes, grasping forceps, bougies, and other long accessories into the rigid esophagoscope for the endoscopist.

Removal of Foreign Bodies Removal of foreign bodies from the pharynx and/or esophagus is relatively common. Persons who wear upper dentures are especially prone to swallowing sharp bones that cannot be felt against the covered palate. Pieces of meat or dental bridgework may lodge or impact in the food passage, occluding the airway by pressure. This is an emergency situation necessitating provision of a patent airway by endotracheal intubation or tracheotomy and endoscopic removal of the bolus or foreign object. Acute esophageal obstruction increases salivation, creating danger of tracheopulmonary aspiration.

Children frequently swallow objects such as coins, buttons, parts of toys, or safety pins that may remain in the throat. Metallic objects are visible on roentgenograms, but many others are not.

It is dangerous to attempt to push an object toward the stomach, because esophageal perforation can result. Esophagoscopy is the method of choice for removal, although the procedure is often difficult and painstaking. All effort is made to prevent trauma, with resultant mediastinitis.

Dilation of Stricture The esophageal lumen can narrow because of formation of scar tissue resulting from inflammation or burn at any level. Treatment consists of regular dilation with mercury-filled bougies of graduated sizes. Steroid administration is adjunctive therapy.

When an individual suffers a severe burn as from swallowing a caustic material, gastrostomy may be indicated to bypass the esophagus until it heals. Dilation of such strictures utilizes retrograde fusiform bougies with spindle-shaped shafts that are linked together. They are carried through the gastrostomy, up the esophagus, and out the mouth. The treatment must be continued for an extended period of time.

Dilation of stricture at the cardioesophageal junction may be necessary in patients with cardiospasm (*achalasia*). Gross dilatation above the stricture, often the result of muscular atrophy, leads to regurgitation. Diagnosis is made by roentgenography, esophagoscopy, or gastroscopy. If dilation is unsuccessful, a myotomy at the esophagogastric junction (Heller procedure) is performed to enlarge the opening into the stomach. Severe unyielding strictures may necessitate resection or esophageal replacement.

Neoplasms of the Esophagus Most often malignant, neoplasms of the esophagus are treated by resection or irradiation. Dysphagia or obstruction demands immediate investigation. Operative procedures fall under the classification of gastrointestinal surgery. Also refer to cervical esophageal reconstruction in Chapter 28.

OPERATIVE PROCEDURES OF THE BRONCHUS

Disorders of the bronchus are most commonly infection, presence of foreign body, trauma, or neoplasms. Diagnosis is made by radiologic study and endoscopy.

Bronchography A radiologic study of the tracheobronchial tree is frequently done in conjunction with bronchoscopy.

Bronchoscopy Direct visualization of the tracheobronchial tree through a bronchoscope is done for:

1 Diagnosis: securing uncontaminated secretion for culture, taking a biopsy, or finding the cause of cough or hemoptysis

2 Treatment: removing a foreign body, excising a small tumor, applying a medication, aspirating the bronchi, or providing an airway during performance of tracheotomy

Foreign bodies in the trachea and bronchi are very serious, requiring careful history and immediate bronchoscopy with preparation for potential tracheotomy. Maintaining a safe airway during extraction is a major risk. If the airway is not seriously obstructed, the aspirated foreign body may remain in the bronchus for months without producing symptoms until suppuration develops. Coughing and hemoptysis bring the patient to the physician.

Bronchoscopes are of two types: a rigid hollow metal tube or a flexible fiberoptic type. The rigid bronchoscope has a side channel incorporated into length of the instrument and perforations along sides of the tube to allow aeration of bronchi. Oxygen or anesthetic gases can be administered through side channel. The light carrier may have an incandescent bulb or may be fiberoptic. Aspirating tubes, foreign body or biopsy forceps, and argon and Nd:YAG laser beams are manipulated through the rigid bronchoscope. Tiny forceps at end of the flexible fiberoptic bronchoscope can be manipulated to obtain tissue biopsy. Because diameter is smaller, the flexible fiberoptic scope reaches into bronchi of upper, middle, and lower lobes for examination and/or biopsy.

Patient positioning, scrub nurse assistance, and

care of instrumentation are the same as previously described for other laryngological endoscopy (see pp. 511 and 512).

GENERAL CONSIDERATIONS IN ENT PROCEDURES

1 Preoperative explanations and postoperative instructions are vital to outcome. For example, following ear or nasal procedures the patient must avoid blowing the nose, which would force air up the eustachian tube potentially causing infection, force air through the incision, or dislodge a graft. To sneeze, both nose and mouth should be open.

2 Communication is a major problem for patients with loss of hearing or voice. Touch is an effective means of conveying concern and letting the patient know he or she is not abandoned. Pencil and paper or a magic slate board can be useful for the patient to communicate.

3 Care with prep solutions is necessary because they are very painful and irritating if allowed to touch a perforated eardrum. Disposable, lint-free drapes are often preferred for otologic operations. A patient may experience anxiety with drapes over the head. Air and oxygen (6 to 8 liters/minute) administered during the procedure afford relief.

4 It is mandatory in otologic surgery that gloves be powder- and lint-free. Formation of granuloma in the oval window can cause sensorineural (irreversible) hearing loss.

5 Although the operative area is often contaminated, such as the oral cavity, only sterile equipment and sterile technique are used to avoid introducing exogenous microorganisms.

6 Anesthesia is mainly local. It minimizes bleeding and postoperative discomfort in addition to affording the surgeon observation of patient response. It utilizes patient cooperation. Also, presence of an endotracheal tube, routine with general anesthesia, can distort features during operation.

   a The circulating nurse observes the usual precautions for local anesthesia, i.e., monitoring vital signs, ECG, in the absence of a standby anesthesiologist. She or he must record on the anesthesia record the amount of local anesthesia administered and write intraoperative nursing notes. A patient may be conscious of nausea, vertigo, or a sense of falling, from stimulation of the vestibular labyrinth in otologic operations.

   b If the patient experiences syncope, it must be differentiated rapidly from reaction to the local anesthetic (refer to Chap. 14). The patient may be in a fairly erect position for local tonsillectomy, for example, which may contribute to postural hypotension.

   c Patients for local anesthesia are permitted to wear pajama bottoms to the OR in some hospitals.

   Microsurgical laryngeal operations and endoscopies usually require general anesthesia.

7 Various colorless solutions are on the table. Each container must be accurately and clearly labeled for foolproof distinction between, for example, cocaine, lidocaine, and epinephrine. Preferably the surgeon draws the solution into the syringe to avoid potentially fatal error.

8 Illumination is provided by the overhead spotlight, the operating microscope, or the surgeon's reflective headlamp that enables him or her to see up and under surfaces. Some surgeons prefer a fiberoptic headlamp.

9 Instrumentation is varied to suit the area. It includes very delicate, small microsurgical implements in addition to bone instruments, because of the extensive involvement of cartilage and bone in facial structures and skull. These areas have relatively little soft tissue. Many instruments are angulated to permit insertion into areas of difficult access and curving passages.

10 Special care with electric appliances is indicated. Electrocoagulation is used to control oozing. Compressed air or nitrogen drills with foot-pedal control are used on bone, such as the mastoid area. A number of drills for the smaller extremely fine work, such as stapes sculpturing, are powered by small electric motors fitted into a handpiece.

11 Various types of endoscopes are used. The correct accessories must be used with each type. Light carriers must be the exact same length as the scope. Diameter of aspirating tubes and forceps must be small enough to pass through and length long enough to extend beyond end of scope. The lighting mechanism and all accessories should be checked for working order before an endoscopic procedure begins.

12 Cryosurgery is used to destroy tumorous tissue in accessible areas, especially those that bleed profoundly if incised.

13 Carbon dioxide lasers are used to vaporize tissue. Argon lasers coagulate tissue by heat generation. Appropriate instrumentation and at-

tachments must be available for each type of laser. Laser surgery is usually done in conjunction with the operating microscope. All safety precautions must be taken to avoid ignition and injury when a laser is used.

14 Microsurgical techniques are used for many ENT procedures because they facilitate distinction between normal and diseased tissue and allow more accurate dissection, e.g., in infinitely small areas such as the middle ear.

15 Sponges and cottonoid patties are relatively small and a distinct hazard when blood-soaked, because they can occlude an airway. They are easily controlled if a string or suture is attached to them.

16 One or two drops of blood can obscure a microsurgical field. The nurse must have hemostatic aids ready at all times. Gelfoam pledgets soaked in 1:1,000 epinephrine are used frequently. Handle tissue grafts and gelatin sponges with forceps, not the hands. Gelfilm, which is brittle, may be cut while in the primary wrap.

17 Irrigation equipment and solution at body temperature must be available to remove bone dust, clean burrs, and rinse suction apparatus. Very fine suction needles or cannulas must be irrigated constantly to avoid blockage.

18 Suction must be available at all times, including several patent cannulas. The degree of suction should be variable. A foot pedal may be used to interrupt wall suction so that the surgeon has control of it for grasping and releasing an object, e.g., in handling a prosthetic graft.

19 Tissue grafts must be kept from drying out prior to use. A convenient method is to place the graft on a moist cellulose sponge in a sterile, covered petri dish. Some surgeons intentionally dry a temporalis fascia graft to facilitate handling. This type of graft may also be flattened and thinned in a small press.

CHAPTER 27

PLASTIC AND RECONSTRUCTIVE SURGERY

Autografts, allografts, or prosthetic implants may be used to improve or restore contour defects or functional malformations due to congenital, developmental, or traumatic disfigurements. "Plastic surgery is surgery dealing with restoration of wounded, disfigured, or unsightly parts of the body. It includes cosmetic surgery or cosmetic corrections not necessarily related to the physical health or safety of the patient. The word 'plastic' in its classic sense means 'giving form or fashion to matter.' As used in plastic surgery, the word bears no relationship to the current concept of plastic materials and products."*

Elective operations desired by an individual in an attempt to improve appearance for psychological well-being are classified as aesthetic or cosmetic surgery. Thus the plastic surgeon's hand extends to alteration of cosmetically unacceptable body contours, as well as to repair and reconstruction of tissue injuries. Plastic surgeons have a philosophy about how tissues can be handled, and a technique for handling them that heals the patient's body and mind, limited only by the surgeon's ingenuity.

DEVELOPMENT OF PLASTIC SURGERY

Plastic surgery was probably the first form of surgery. Egyptian papyrus scrolls tell of skin grafts and pedicle flaps to replace deficiencies in tissue as early as 3500 years ago. Egyptian mummies have been found with artificial ears and noses. In India over 2000 years ago, the Hindus became skilled in transferring tissue to form noses for those who had lost them as a punishment. These ancient records verify attempts to improve people's appearance.

Two centuries ago, some plastic surgery was done in Europe. The beginning of the present interest and the great strides that have been made in plastic surgery began when Reverdin used pinch grafts. He reported his work with them in 1869. But the transplantation of skin met with mediocre success until World War I.

In the twilight of the nineteenth and the dawn of the twentieth centuries, descriptions of "featural surgery" were brazenly advertised by "cosmetic surgeons," often with unwarranted claims of success. Charles Conrad Miller (1880–1950) has been called both "the father of modern cosmetic surgery" and "an unabashed quack." Practicing in Chicago, Miller began around 1904 to improvise surgical procedures to alter facial features. He did them in his office under local anesthesia, employing a gentle technique of lifting structures by lenticular or crescent excisions and lowering tissues by excisions and vertical closures. He preferred to sew with fine needles and cautioned not to tie sutures tightly because this might cause suture marks. His text, first published in 1907 and expanded in 1925, described cosmetic

*The American Society of Plastic and Reconstructive Surgeons, Inc.

procedures for upper and lower lid blepharoplasty, subcutaneous sectioning of facial muscles, incisions to change lip posture, and a variety of rhinoplasties.

Vilray Papin Blair became a prominent plastic surgeon when he published in 1906 the results of closed ramisection of the mandible for micrognathia and prognathism. Within a short time, physicians from all over the United States and Europe sent patients to Blair in St. Louis for jaw reconstruction and other facial surgery.

Sir Arbuthnot Lane, a contemporary of Miller and Blair, was doing cleft lip, cleft palate, and some mandibular surgery in England. When Blair arrived in England in 1918 as Chief of Plastic and Oral Surgery for the American armed forces, he visited the center Lane had established for treating soldiers with facial injuries. The work being done there by Harold Gillies impressed Blair. The high quality of work done at this and other centers during World War I on facial injuries, burns, and reconstruction of other injured parts of the body did much to establish plastic surgery as a surgical specialty.

During World War II, the development of military plastic surgery centers led to rapid progress in the rehabilitation of casualties with maxillofacial and hand injuries. Plastic surgeons worked closely with other specialists in treating many types of war injuries. They found that by replacing lost skin with grafts, fractures under these areas healed better and more quickly and parts returned to normal function sooner.

Today's plastic surgery is largely the refinement of techniques developed during World Wars I and II to restore men disfigured by the ravages of war. These techniques are not only imaginative but precise. They are imaginative because plastic surgeons reshape and replant living tissue and augment tissue with prosthetic implants.

Plastic surgery has been called the "surgery of millimeters" because of the critical margin between good and poor cosmetic results. Each millimeter lack or excess of tissue can have an extreme psychological impact on the patient. If the patient thinks his or her appearance has improved, personality and self-image improve and others respond more positively to him or her.

Plastic surgery has been extended by increased knowledge of the principles and techniques of microvascular and microneural anastomoses for replantation and transplantation of tissue.

PSYCHOLOGICAL SUPPORT FOR PLASTIC SURGERY PATIENTS

Physical appearance psychologically affects self-image. Children can develop inferiority complexes and introverted personalities because of congenital malformations in body structure or deformity due to trauma. The defect may not affect physiological function but may predispose to psychological crippling if not corrected to the satisfaction of the patient.

Adults who are dissatisfied with their body image may believe that a change in personal appearance will solve their social, marital, or business problems. The plastic surgeon must assess the patient's psychological status, motivations, and expectations prior to scheduling an operation. Realistic goals must be set. The patient should be emotionally stable and aware of the potential outcomes. Psychiatric consultation is advisable for some patients preoperatively. Psychological preparation is essential prior to radical operations that will result in disfigurement, e.g., radical neck dissection.

Many extensive reconstructions for severe deformities are done in stages, often over a period of months or years. These patients require prolonged psychological support and encouragement.

SPECIAL FEATURES OF PLASTIC SURGERY

Scars are inevitable whenever skin is incised or excised, either intentionally by the surgeon's scalpel or accidentally by trauma. The plastic surgeon attempts to minimize scar formation by meticulous realignment and approximation of underlying tissues and wound edges. The plastic surgeon makes the incision along natural skin lines whenever possible. Many plastic procedures involve only the subcuticular tissues and skin. Reconstructive procedures, however, may include manipulation of underlying cartilage, bone, tendons, nerves, and blood vessels.

General Considerations

1 Colorless prep solution may be preferred so the plastic surgeon can observe the true skin color. Frequently this also is used for ambulatory surgical patients to avoid skin discoloration after minimal facial procedures.

2 Sterile dye, such as methylene blue or brilliant green, is often used to outline areas for incision. This can be done with a sterile marking pen after the skin is prepped.

3 Exposure of both sides for comparison is usually required for operations on the face, ears, and neck.

4 Draping often exposes much skin surface, which is unavoidable. A fenestrated sheet frequently cannot be used. The opening does not give adequate exposure, especially for skin grafting procedures. Use towels, self-adhering plastic sheeting, and minor and medium sheets under and around the areas, according to needs, to drape as much of the patient as possible. Drapes can be secured with towel clips or skin staples.

5 Local anesthesia is used for many operations on adults. Ephinephrine may be added to help localize the agent, prolong the anesthetic action, and provide hemostasis. Short 26- or 30-gauge needles are used for injection.

6 Number 15 and 11 scalpel blades are routinely used to cut small structures.

7 Instruments must be small for handling delicate tissues. Iris scissors, mosquito hemostats, fine-tipped tissue forceps, and other small-scale cutting, holding, clamping, and exposing instruments are part of the routine plastic surgery setup. Microinstruments are needed for microsurgical techniques (refer to Chap. 19, p. 379).

8 Nerve stimulator may be used to help identify nerves, especially in craniofacial, neck, and hand reconstruction procedures.

9 Bone, cartilage, or skin grafts may be needed. Homografts may be obtained from the tissue bank rather than the patient's own tissues.

10 Silicone or other prosthetic implants are used in plastic surgery to reconstruct soft tissue and cartilage defects. They cannot be used unless there is adequate soft tissue coverage. They cannot be used in an infected area. (Refer to Chapter 18, p. 356, for discussion of handling silicone implants.)

11 Suture sizes range from 2-0 through 7-0, depending on location and tissue, with sizes 8-0 through 11-0 sutures for microsurgery. The material varies according to the personal preference of the surgeon. Synthetic nonabsorbable and absorbable polymers are used more commonly than natural materials.

12 Swaged needles of small wire diameter with sharp cutting edges minimize trauma to superficial tissues. An appropriately fine-tipped needle-holder must be used with these delicate, curved needles.

13 Skin closure tapes may be used instead of skin sutures or as supplements to a subcuticular closure, if very close approximation of skin is required for good cosmetic results.

14 Many plastic surgeons prefer staples to close the skin or secure skin grafts.

15 Closed-wound suction drainage is frequently used to hold flaps against underlying tissue.

16 Fine mesh gauze may be used for the initial dressing. This may be impregnated with petrolatum or an oil emulsion, with or without medication, to cover denuded areas. Several types of sterile nonadhering dressings are commercially available. Dry gauze is not used on a denuded area because it adheres and acts as a foreign body; granulations grow through it.

17 Pressure dressings may be used following extensive operations to splint soft tissues and prevent contractures. The mild pressure keeps fluid formation in tissues or under a skin graft to a minimum. Commercial dressings for various body areas are preferred by some plastic surgeons. (Refer to Chapter 10, p. 168, for types of pressure dressings.)

18 Stent fixation is a method of obtaining pressure when it is impossible to bandage an area snugly, as the face or neck. A form-fitting mold may be taped over the nose. Long suture ends can be tied crisscrossed over a dressing to immobilize it and exert gentle pressure.

Categories of Plastic Surgery

Four main categories of problems are treated by plastic surgeons.

1 Congenital anomalies, especially in structure of the face and hands. The most commonly corrected anomalies are discussed in Chapter 33.

2 Cosmetic appearance, especially of the face and breasts.

3 Benign and malignant neoplasms, especially those leaving large soft tissue defects. Resection of extensive tumors other than those involving the skin or head and neck are not usually within the province of the plastic surgeon initially, but the patient may be referred for reconstructive surgery and rehabilitation. Frequently reconstructive procedures are done in conjunction with another specialty surgeon at the time of tumor resection.

4 Traumatically acquired disfigurements, especially facial lacerations, hand injuries, and burns. The objective of the plastic surgeon is to restore function as well as body image.

Tissue may be approximated, supplemented, excised, transferred, or transplanted. Many procedures are done in stages before complete reconstruction and restoration of function are achieved. Tissue flaps and grafts, prosthetic implants, and external prosthetic appliances may be required for functional and cosmetic restoration as a result of ablative surgery or trauma.

GRAFTING TECHNIQUES

Denuded areas of the body are resurfaced by transplanting or transferring segments of skin and other tissues from an uninjured area to the injured area. The plastic surgeon prefers to transfer tissues of compatible color and texture. Soft tissue autografts are used whenever possible. They are classified by the source of their vascular supply, essential for viability, as:

1 *Free graft.* Tissue is detached from the donor site and transplanted into the recipient site. It derives its vascular supply from the capillary ingrowth from the recipient site.

2 *Pedicle flap.* Tissue remains attached at one or both ends of the donor site during transfer to the recipient site. The vascular supply is maintained from the vessels preserved in the pedicle of the donor site.

3 *Free flap.* Tissue, including its vascular bundle, is detached from the donor site and transferred to recipient site. Microvascular anastomoses between arteries and veins in the flap or autograft and recipient site establishes vascularity necessary for viability.

Deformities caused by loss of soft tissue substance such as trauma of accidental injury, tumor resection, or radiation therapy may require a graft to fill in deficiencies in order to restore contours or to cover tendons and bones. Free grafts and pedicle flaps may be taken from various areas of the body to reconstruct soft tissue defects.

Free Skin Grafts

The epidermis including *corium,* the basal layer of the dermis that generates new skin, is transplanted from the donor site to a recipient site in which it becomes a part of the living tissue in that area. The depth of the graft will vary according to its purpose.

1 *Split-thickness graft.* The epidermis and half of the corium to a depth of 0.010 to 0.035 in. (0.3 to 1 mm) is removed. The donor site heals uneventfully unless it becomes infected. Split-thickness grafts are widely used to cover large denuded areas on the back, trunk, and legs.

2 *Full-thickness graft.* The epidermis, corium, and subcutaneous fat at a depth greater than 0.035 in. (1 mm) is removed or elevated. Full-thickness grafts inhibit wound contraction better than split-thickness grafts and generally are preferred on the face, neck, hands, elbows, axillae, knees, and feet.

The desired thickness of a free skin graft is predetermined by the plastic surgeon before the skin is incised. The appropriate cutting instrument is selected to obtain the graft.

Dermatomes A dermatome is a cutting instrument designed to excise split-thickness skin grafts. The thickness of the graft can be calibrated by adjusting the depth gauge. The width of the graft is determined by the width of the cutting blade. Blades are detachable and many are disposable, which always ensures a sharp new blade for every patient. The length of the graft may be limited by the type of dermatome used.

Oscillating-Blade Type Dermatomes may be electric or air-powered with compressed nitrogen or air. The length of the graft is limited only by the donor site. The surgeon checks the adjustable depth gauge before cutting the graft. The oscillating-blade dermatome is not usually used on the abdominal wall where underlying support is not firm. The oscillating blade, free of vibrations, takes an accurate graft from other donor sites.

> NOTE. Extreme care should be used in handling these precision dermatomes. If electric, the circulating nurse should remove the foot pedal as soon as the graft is taken. If air-powered, the scrub nurse and surgeon should place a thumb under the lever on the handle while preparing the instrument for use. These dermatomes *cannot be immersed in water* or put in a washer-sterilizer or ultrasonic cleaner. Follow manufacturer's instructions for use, care, and sterilization (see Chap. 11).

Drum Type Padgett and Reese dermatomes consist of one-half of a metal drum, which is one-half of a circle. A metal handle through the center of the drum has an arm on each end. These arms hold the bar that carries the blade. The bar swings around the drum to cut the graft. The size of the graft is limited by the width and length of the drum. An adhesive must be placed on both the skin surface and the drum to keep the skin in contact with the drum. The knife blade is moved from side to side as slight tension is exerted on the skin by rotating the drum. The drum-type dermatome is used on flat, open areas, because it is bulky. Its use is limited by body contour and amount of skin on the donor site.

Dermatome tape must be used with the Reese dermatome. Packaged sterile, the tape has an adhesive coating on each side covered with a paper backing. Remove the backing on one side and apply to the drum with care to line up the edges of the tape and the drum. After the backing paper is removed from the other side of the tape, the drum is placed on the skin, which adheres to it.

> NOTE. When handling a drum-type dermatome, *always* grasp the blade carrier to prevent its swinging around the drum and seriously injuring your hands. Leave the dermatome in the rack when not in use or until the blade is removed.

Kinds of Free Skin Grafts

Split-Thickness Thiersch Graft Removed with a skin-graft knife or dermatome, Thiersch grafts are used to cover superficial defects. The surgeon may use sutures or skin staples along the edges of the graft to hold it to underlying subcutaneous tissue. This prevents movement and helps obliterate dead space in the recipient site. The skin of the donor site regenerates rapidly and the same area can be used again in two or three weeks if necessary, or sooner if a thin graft is taken, from an infection-free donor site.

Split-Thickness Meshgraft Meshgraft makes it possible to obtain a greater area of coverage from a split-thickness skin graft. After removal with a dermatome, the graft is placed on a plastic derma-carrier, cut side down. This is a rigid base to keep the graft spread out flat while it is put through a mesh dermatome. This instrument cuts small parallel slits in the graft. When expanded, the slits become diamond-shaped openings. This permits expansion of the graft to cover three times as large an area as the original graft obtained from the donor site. The meshgraft can be placed over the recipient site with slight tension. The increased edge exposures are conducive to rapid epithelialization. The mesh minimizes serum accumulation.

Full-Thickness Wolfe Graft The Wolfe graft is cut exactly to size and shape of the recipient site with a skin-graft knife and sutured into place under normal skin tension. It is used on face, neck, or hands to fill in superficial denuded areas and over joints to prevent contractures. This graft does not become viable readily on granulated surfaces, and the amount that can be transferred is much more limited than in a Thiersch graft.

Free Composite Grafts

A composite graft usually includes skin, subcutaneous tissue and cartilage, bone, or other tissues. Hair transplants are composite grafts. Viability of the graft depends on ingrowth of vascular system from the recipient site.

Free Omental Grafts

Omentum, grafted to provide vascularity, can be resected from the peritoneal cavity and transplanted to an avascular area if sufficient recipient blood vessels are available for anastomoses to the right or left gastroepiploic artery and vein. An omental graft can be used, for example, to resurface the scalp. The gastroepiploic vessels can be anastomosed to the temporalis artery and vein. Split-thickness skin grafts are placed over the omental graft.

Pedical Flaps

Creation of a pedicle flap may be the procedure of choice to reconstruct deformities of soft tissue loss that will create, or have created, an obvious aesthetic or functional disability for the patient. The *pedicle,* which is the attachment of elevated tissue to the donor site, must contain a vascular bundle to maintain blood supply to the tissue. Pedicle flaps are constructed from several types of tissues and sources of the vascular bundles.

Arterialized Skin Flap A full-thickness skin graft contains a vascular bundle within subcutaneous tissue and skin. Arterialized flaps may be:

1 Those with axial vasculature from axial vessels that supply a fairly definite area of skin and subcutaneous tissue. A direct cutaneous artery flows through the length of the flap.

2 Those with random or local vasculature from the subdermal plexus of musculocutaneous arteries.

3 Those with both axial and random vasculature. A deltopectoral flap, for example, has axial vessels from the sternal region and random vessels in the deltoid area.

Depending on the proximity of the recipient site to the donor site, the pedicle flap will be one of the following types.

Rotational Flap One end of the flap is rotated and sutured to the recipient site to cover a denuded area. The flap tissue is obtained from an area near the recipient site. Arterialized skin pedicle flaps with axial vasculature are rotated in a one-stage procedure.

Cross-Finger, -Thigh, or -Calf Flap Tissue at the donor site is undermined and rotated to cover the defect in an adjacent extremity site. For example, a flap can be sutured between two adjacent digits. Or an ankle can be covered by a flap from the thigh or calf of the opposite leg.

Bipedicle Flap A full-thickness skin flap is elevated on the abdomen or anterior surface of the thigh. Both ends are left attached. A denuded hand or wrist is placed under the flap and sutured along the edges of the flap. It remains under the flap until the blood supply becomes established. The flap is then divided along each side of the resurfaced extremity, and the donor area is covered with a split-thickness skin graft.

Distant Tubular Flap Both ends of an elevated skin flap are attached to the donor site. The skin edges are approximated and sutured together into the form of a cylinder. A Thiersch graft covers the tissue under the tube. After vascularity is well-established by delay, one end of the flap is freed and transferred to an intermediate site. Again after vascularity is established, the other end is freed from the original donor site and transferred to the intended recipient site. For example, the tubular flap may be elevated on the abdomen: one end transferred to an arm; the other end attached to the face. In this way, a pedicle flap may be migrated from the abdomen to arm to face, and it is kept viable by its vascular attachment at each stage of the procedure.

Delayed Skin Flap In the delayed skin flap procedure, which is done in several stages, the blood supply in the flap is permitted to become established between stages. A tubular flap is one process of delay. Sometimes, preliminary to making a tube, the plastic surgeon elevates the tissue for the flap, leaving the ends attached, and then sutures it back to its original site. This stimulates the random vasculature in the tissue to increase size of blood vessels, and thus increases the viability of the flap when it is rotated or migrated to the recipient site.

Tissue Expansion Flap Epidermal surface area can be increased by implanting a tissue expander device subcutaneously. An expandable silicone shell or bag filled with isotonic saline (sodium chloride), or other similar inert device, is inserted under a raised skin flap. Natural physiological skin stretching occurs. Vascularity also increases. After a period of weeks, the stretched skin can be used for an arterialized pedicle skin flap.

Myocutaneous (Musculocutaneous) Flap A myocutaneous flap incorporates the muscle, overlying fascia, subcutaneous tissue, and skin. It receives a vigorous blood supply from the vascular pedicle that supplies the underlying muscle. It may include a neurovascular bundle with nerve fibers to innervate the muscle in the flap. Usually done as a one-stage procedure, myocutaneous flaps can be created from the following and other muscles:

1 Trapezius
2 Sternocleidomastoid
3 Platysma
4 Latissimus dorsi
5 Pectoralis major
6 Rectus abdominis
7 Gracilis
8 Gluteus maximus
9 Tensor fascia lata
10 Biceps femoris

Pedicle myocutaneous flaps allow safe and rapid transfer of tissue over long distances to cover large defects and vital structures. They are used, for example, to close soft tissue defects in the lower extremities, to cover pressure sores on paraplegics, to reconstruct contour following head and neck resection and mastectomy, and to provide cervical esophageal reconstruction. Myocutaneous flaps have literally revolutionized reconstructive surgery and stimulated the imagination of plastic surgeons.

Flap survival seems to depend on a reduction in vascular resistance or an increase in arterial perfusion pressure, or both. Several techniques are used to monitor circulation in the flap. These include:

1 Ultraviolet light (Woods lamp) to evaluate perfusion of 5% fluorescein sodium after IV injection of 20 ml. The room must be darkened to see the fluorescence.

2 Fluorometer for perfusion measurement of a fluorescing dye.

3 Reflection photoplethysmography for skin transillumination. A pulsative change in blood volume in tissue produces a corresponding change in amount of light reflected.

4 Thermocouple probe for microvascular patency.

5 Photomultiplier to amplify skin fluorescent emission.

Fascial Cutaneous Flap Mobilized fascia, subcutaneous tissue, and skin are transferred as pedicle flaps similarly as myocutaneous flaps are transferred.

Muscle Flap Divided section of a muscle with its proximal blood supply intact can be rotated over a soft tissue defect, such as an ulcer on the leg or buttock. The muscle flap may be covered with a split-thickness skin graft.

Omental Flap Omentum is mobilized from the peritoneal cavity, without compromise of the vascular pedicle, to cover the defect in the chest wall following resection for irradiation necrosis or neoplasm. The vascularity of the donor omentum revascularizes the reconstructed chest-wall recipient site. Split-thickness skin grafts, which may be meshgrafts, cover the omental flap. If additional rigidity is needed to restore the chest wall, polypropylene mesh may be sutured inside the rib cage to supplement the strength of the omental flap.

Free Flaps (Microsurgical Free Flap Transfer)

Composite free flaps or grafts of tissue are resected and transplanted from one area of the body to another to cover a denuded area, to restore function, or to restore body contour. Microsurgical techniques allow one-stage transfer of the tissues. The main artery and vein supplying donor tissues must be anastomosed to vessels in recipient site under the operating microscope. Often two teams work simultaneously at the donor and recipient sites.

Microvascular Free Myocutaneous (Musculocutaneous) Flap Free island grafts of skin, subcutaneous fat, and muscle are resected and transplanted in a distant recipient site. The iliofemoral area (groin flap) is a common donor site, using the superficial circumflex iliac artery and vein or the superficial epigastrics to maintain the vascular supply. After resection, the defect in the groin is partially closed primarily. The rest of the area is covered with a split-thickness skin graft. The gluteal, deltoid, and scapular regions may also be donor sites. The recipient site may be the cheek, scalp, neck, leg, foot, or arm.

Free Muscle Graft Free island grafts of functional muscle can be resected and transplanted to replace motor function in another area. Although a small percentage of the graft survives, significant regeneration of muscle occurs. Free muscle, transferred by microvascular techniques, then covered with a split-thickness skin graft promotes healing of infected wounds.

Neurovascular Free Flap Fascicles of nerves must be anastomosed to restore sensation, as well as microvascular anastomoses of arteries and veins to maintain viability of the donor tissue. A neurovascular free flap, also known as a sensate flap, may be taken from the scapular region. Many surgeons use the scapular flap because it is easy to dissect, has a long vascular pedicle, and creates a minimal donor site deformity. Other donor sites include the medial and lateral thigh and the lateral aspect of the upper arm.

Digital Replantation or Transfer Traumatically amputated digits are replanted using microneurovascular techniques (see Chap. 34, p. 618). Less common is the toe-to-thumb transfer, called the free wraparound neurovascular flap, performed when an amputated thumb cannot be salvaged. Skin from the dorsum of the foot, the great toe including tendons and bone, and the second toe web space as a sensory flap are transferred to the hand. After bone fixation and tendon anastomoses, arterial and venous circulation is established under the microscope. Then digital nerves are anastomosed to reinnervate sensation and function. Other toes can be similarly transferred for finger reconstruction.

Free Autogenous Bone Graft Vascularized autografts of bone are superior in strength and cause less osteoporosis (deossification, structural weakness) than do conventional bone grafts (see Chap. 18, p. 355). Anastomosis of the vascular bundle with a free rib, for example, may increase the chance of survival of the donor bone graft in a poorly vascularized recipient site such as the jaw following partial mandibulectomy.

Compound Osseocutaneous Free Flap Skin and iliac crest on a vascular pedicle from the deep circumflex iliac artery is useful in one-stage reconstruction of compound defects of the head and neck when skin, soft tissue, and mandibular reconstructions are necessary.

Free Revascularized Intestinal Autograft A segment of the small intestine, usually jejunum, can be mobilized and transferred into the neck to reconstruct the cervical esophagus (see Chap. 28, p. 543). An experienced microvascular team is essential to revascularize free intestinal autografts.

General Considerations for All Tissue Autografts

1 Hyperthermia blanket or a water mattress is placed on the operating table to keep the patient warm. Room temperature should be increased to 75 to 80°F (24 to 27°C).

2 Skin may be prepped with a colorless antiseptic agent so the plastic surgeon can see true skin color and assess vascularity of the donor graft.

3 Donor and recipient sites are prepped and draped separately, but concurrently, care being taken that cross contamination does not occur from the one site to the other.

4 Recipient site is covered with a sterile towel or sheet until ready to apply free graft or pedicle flap, if preparation of this will be the first procedure. If the recipient site must be prepared to receive the donor graft or flap, the donor site is covered.

5 Separate sterile instrument table is prepared for the donor site. This includes appropriate instruments for obtaining the graft or flap and dressings for the donor site.

NOTE. *Always* put a dermatome on a separate, small sterile table, never on the recipient instrument table. Handle dermatomes carefully so that the depth gauge is not disturbed.

6 Graft must be kept moist by covering with a sponge wet with normal saline. A free flap should be kept in iced saline slush until the recipient site is prepared.

7 Hemostasis is obtained during operation by warm saline packs, pressure, or thrombin.

8 Dressings over grafts vary by surgeon preference. Stent fixation to obtain pressure on the grafted area may be preferred. Some plastic surgeons omit pressure dressings and use the exposure technique on grafts for selected areas so that they can watch the graft and incise a hematoma if necessary. The graft is kept covered with sterile, moist saline sponges to keep the skin moist until revascularization occurs. A plaster cast is frequently applied to immobilize extremities during migration or transfer of pedicle flaps.

HEAD AND NECK RECONSTRUCTION

Craniofacial Operations

The plastic surgeon usually heads the multidisciplinary team that performs the complex craniofacial procedures discussed in Chapter 28. Many of the concepts developed for these procedures are applied in less-complicated operations. A variety of extracranial osteotomies, with or without bone grafts, reshape the bony framework. These maneuvers, plus reconstruction of soft tissues, contour facial deformities. The desired aesthetic and functional results can be obtained only by painstakingly careful dissection and repositioning with the utmost patience and cooperation of all OR team members.

Maxillofacial and Oral Operations

Plastic surgeons reconstruct *soft tissue* defects around and in the mouth that are caused by trauma or operative resection. Those maxillofacial operations involving bony structures that may also be performed by plastic surgeons are discussed in Chapter 28. Congenital deformities are discussed in Chapter 33.

Transfacial Nerve Grafting Restoration of the quality of facial expressions in a patient with severe facial nerve paralysis can be accomplished by transfacial nerve grafting. Segments of nerve grafts are brought through tunnels across the lips from the normal side of the face to the paralyzed side. These are anastomosed to the distal facial nerve on the normal side and then to the proximal branches of the injured nerve on the paralyzed side. The overpull of the mouth and lower face toward the normal side is balanced when the nerve graft is anastomosed between fascicles of the intact facial nerve innervating the facial muscles to the same fascicles on the denervated side.

Repair of Lacerations of Lip or Mouth Wound edges of lip(s) and/or mucosa in the mouth are carefully sutured to repair lacerations.

Excision of Leukoplakia Dissection or carbon dioxide laser is used to resect a precancerous lesion. Chronic irritation can result in an abnormal whitening of the mucous membrane of the lip and tongue, a lesion primarily seen in heavy smokers.

Excision of Tumor of Lip Excision of a lip tumor may be minor, with V-wedge excision, or extensive, depending on the stage of malignancy. Extensive lesions require a flap procedure for reconstruction.

Lip Reconstruction Lips can be adequately reconstructed by a variety of techniques to restore sensation and motor function following trauma or surgical resection. Lip cancer is the most common type of cancer in the upper respiratory and digestive tracts. Operations to reconstruct lips may be classified as:

1 Those amendable to repair by primary closure of the remaining lip segments.
2 Those that can be closed with a full-thickness cross-lip flap from the opposite lip.
3 Those that utilize arterialized or myocutaneous flaps from adjacent cheek or nasolabial tissue.
4 Those that employ distant flaps. Arterialized and innervated myocutaneous flaps from the forehead or deltopectoral region may be used. These require staged procedures. Free composite grafts are done in one stage.

The ideal repair yields a lip that is not tight and has a good vermilion border, an adequate sulcus, good sensation, and good muscle tone.

Aesthetic Procedures

Blepharoplasty Redundant skin and/or protruding orbital fat is excised to correct deformities of the upper or lower eyelids of one or both eyes. *Blepharochalasis,* loss of elasticity of the skin of the eyelids, can occur at any age and usually is of unknown etiology. *Dermatochalasis* primarily involves hypertrophy of the skin of the upper lids. Resection of the excessive redundant skin removes the mechanical visual obstruction caused by these two conditions. *Protrusion of intraorbital fat* into the lids is the most common eyelid deformity. It is often familial, sometimes seen in patients as young as in their twenties. This fat must be removed from the compartments in the upper and/or lower lids to correct the deformity. This may be associated with dermatochalasis. A free graft of cartilage and mucosa from the nasal septum may be necessary to reconstruct lower eyelid defects following excision for tumor. *Hypertrophy of the orbicularis muscle* appears as a horizontal bulge below the lower lid margin. A skin-muscle flap resection may be performed. An operation for lifting the eyebrows will secondarily correct a hooding deformity of the upper lids caused by ptosis of the eyebrows.

These procedures are usually performed under local anesthesia. The patient should wear dentures to the OR, because facial contour is distorted without them and the surgeon could remove too much or too little redundant skin. Because of proximity to the eye, these oculoplastic procedures may be performed by an ophthalmologist, as mentioned in Chapter 25.

Otoplasty Deformities of one or both external ears of an adult are usually the result of traumatic avulsion. A segment of the external ear that is partially or completely amputated often can be reattached to the remaining segment and buried beneath a flap of postauricular skin. The area over a completely severed auricular cartilage, which cannot be sutured back in place, is covered with a split-thickness skin graft initially. Later reconstruction may include insertion of cartilage taken from the rib cage or a silicone prosthetic implant.

Rhinoplasty An operation for reshaping the nose, although usually performed for cosmetic appearance desired by the patient, may be necessary to correct defects caused by trauma or surgical resection of neoplasms. Subtle changes with limited nasal reduction, preservation of the normal physiology and anatomy, and augmentation of the nasal tip with the patient's own nasal cartilage can result in aesthetically attractive and physiologically normal noses in most patients. A free composite graft or pedicle flap may be necessary to close a large tissue defect. Bone or cartilage grafts may be needed for skeletal support. Prosthetic reconstruction for partial or total loss of the nose may be the procedure of chioce.

Rhytidoplasty Commonly referred to as a "face lift," rhytidoplasty involves extensive dissection from above the ear downward along the jaw line and upper neck. The skin is freed from underlying fascia. Wrinkles and folds of the normal aging process smooth out as the skin is lifted up and sutured in place. Dissection beneath the platysma muscle, referred to as the SMAS (submuscular aponeurotic system) procedure, minimizes the amount of skin undermined. The platysma is sutured back to the mastoid. Redundant skin is trimmed away. Frequently other procedures, such as blepharoplasty or rhinoplasty, accompany this operation. Meticulous hemostasis is essential to prevent hematoma formation, the foremost complication of rhytidoplasty. Hypotensive anesthesia may be used to help reduce this incidence. Closed-wound suction drainage is frequently used with or without a pressure dressing applied after operation.

Neck Dissection

Dissections for tumors originating in the head or neck regions are discussed in Chapters 25 and 27. Following primary resection by a laryngologist or oral surgeon, the plastic surgeon may be called upon to reconstruct the resultant defect. Or the plastic surgeon may be the primary surgeon who resects a tumor or lesion approached through the oral cavity or neck, followed by an immediate reconstruction. Some plastic surgeons subspecialize in head and neck oncology and reconstruction.

RECONSTRUCTION OF OTHER BODY AREAS

Adipose Tissue

Lipectomy is an excision of excessive fat and redundant skin from the upper arms, abdomen, buttocks, or thighs.

Suction-assisted lipectomy removes rather extensive localized fat deposits to alter body contour. Placed into the area through a small incision, a suction curettage instrument removes fat quickly, with negligible scar deformity.

Breast

Augmentation Mammoplasty A bilateral mammoplasty is often performed for aesthetic effect on women who desire larger breasts. Unilateral augmentation is sometimes performed to correct asymmetry of a congenital small breast.

Silastic implants are inserted under either breast tissue or underlying muscle. Two types of implants are available: a contoured silicone sac containing a soft silicone gel and an inflatable silicone sac. The inflatable type is implanted and then filled with sterile saline or dextran through a self-sealing valve. Some implants are supplied sterile by the manufacturer. Manufacturers' instruction for sterilization of nonsterile implants must be followed. Refer to Chapter 18, p. 357, for precautions in handling silicone implants. Sterile packages should not be opened by the circulating nurse until the surgeon selects the appropriate-sized implants. Silastic sizers are frequently used to make this determination. The implant identification card should be put in the patient's chart and each implant's catalog and lot number recorded.

The breast implant can be inserted through a periareolar, transaxillary, or inframammary approach. The *periareolar* incision, made around the outside border of the lower half of the areola, is the most difficult for insertion of the implant, but it leaves the most inconspicuous scar. The *transaxillary* incision in the axilla does not scar the breast. The *inframammary* incision, the most common, is made transversely along the submammary fold. The implant is inserted into a pocket formed between the mammary gland and pectoralis muscle or under the muscle.

Hematoma, infection, capsular contraction, and skin necrosis are potential complications following prosthetic implantation for breast augmentation performed either unilaterally or bilaterally.

Reconstructive Mammoplasty Breast reconstruction following mastectomy psychologically helps the patient deal with altered body image. The type and timing of reconstruction are influenced by the patient's psychological response to mastectomy, the type of mastectomy, and the patient's diagnosis and prognosis. Technical maneuvers of the general surgeon at the time of mastectomy will influence the possibility of an aesthetically acceptable result following breast reconstruction by the plastic surgeon.

To reconstruct breast contour, a silicone implant may be inserted at the time of subcutaneous mastectomy. Following modified radical or radical mastectomy, the wound should be well-healed, the scar mature, and the skin well-vascularized prior to implantation. A prosthesis can be implanted only when reliable skin is available to cover it. Skin flaps should be cut as thickly as consistent with a curative mastectomy. If sufficient skin flaps are not available, the plastic surgeon may transfer a pedicle skin flap from the abdomen or back to the chest wall.

Immediate breast reconstruction, or a delay of only a few days, after a modified radical mastectomy can be psychologically advantageous in women who have small lesions and no metastases. A latissimus dorsi myocutaneous flap may be used with a silicone implant. A transverse rectus abdominus island myocutaneous flap with the vascular bundle from the superior epigastric vessels can be used without an implant. Either of these flaps can also be used weeks to months postmastectomy for reconstruction. Aesthetically the end result is a semblance of a breast. An areola and nipple complex may be constructed in a second-stage operation.

Reduction Mammoplasty Reduction mammoplasty is usually performed for comfort as well as aesthetic improvement in body image. Hyperplasia of the breasts is reduced by resection of skin and glandular tissue. The nipple-areola complexes may be placed as free grafts. If this is not done, several other procedures have been developed which allow the nipple-areola complexes to be transferred intact with the underlying breast tissue, maintaining the blood and nerve supply. In younger patients, these are preferred to procedures involving amputation of the breast tissue with a free nipple graft.

Hand

The plastic surgeon is dedicated to salvaging injured tissues whenever possible. Therefore, it is not surprising that those who subspecialize in hand reconstruction have turned to the operating microscope. Microsurgical revascularization and primary nerve repair salvage many traumatized hands that have lost their blood supply and sensation. Neurovascular island flaps also reinnervate and revascularize digits. Other traumatic hand injuries can be repaired by resurfacing with free skin grafts or pedicle flaps. Lacerated tendons are sutured or grafted. Hand reconstruction is also performed to correct joint deformities of degenerative diseases or for secondary release of contractures. Silicone rubber prosthetic implants may be used to replace metacarpophalangeal joints. (Refer to Chapter 24, p. 467, for general considerations pertaining to operations on an extremity.)

Scars

Dermabrasion Dirt and cinders can become embedded in the dermis from a brush-burn injury. The plastic surgeon uses a wire brush or sandpapers out dirt and irrigates it from the area with warm saline solution. Sandpapering is also done to improve acne scars. This procedure is not always satisfactory if many pitted scars are too deep to reach or there are changes in pigment of scars. Some plastic surgeons prefer chemical dermabrasion in selected patients for face peeling.

Sandpaper, in the form of narrow abrasive bands, is mounted on a hollow core attachment to an electric, air-powered, or battery-operated drill. This is used for small areas of deeply embedded dirt and cinders or acne scars. For more superficial areas, sandpaper may be cut into 1-, 2-, or 3-in. (2.5-, 5-, or 7.5-cm) widths and wrapped around a gauze bandage. Waterproof sandpaper can be steam sterilized.

Scar Revision The plastic surgeon attempts to make a scar as fine a line, as level, and as smooth as possible at the time of primary wound closure or as a secondary scar revision. Scar formation, the body's mechanism for healing wounds, is inevitable whenever skin is incised. The plastic surgeon can excise an aesthetically displeasing scar, realign wound edges, and resuture or close them with anticipation of a better cosmetic result. The direction of a scar can be changed to be less conspicuous in the natural skin lines. Scars are frequently revised following extensive reconstructive procedures or following a laceration with or without soft tissue trauma, particularly a facial scar. Z-plasty, W-plasty, Lazy-S, Y-V-plasty, and other techniques are used to improve the appearance of a hypertrophied or prominent scar.

BURNS

Skin and underlying tissues can be destroyed by thermal, chemical, or electrical injury. Burns are open wounds. As in other injuries, initial treatment is aimed at saving the patient's life. Then the treatment is directed toward preserving or restoring to normal, or as near normal as possible, the patient's bodily functions and appearance as rapidly as possible. Depending on the depth, extent, and location of the burn, reconstruction may extend over long periods of time: months to years. The patient must be helped to accept the disfigurement; thus rehabilitation from a psychological standpoint is important. Psychotherapy as well as surgery and physiotherapy may be necessary to promote as early a return to normalcy and usefulness as possible.

Classification of Burn

The severity of injury is determined by individual factors such as pretrauma medical history; other injuries sustained; and location and etiology of the burn. The Abbreviated Burn Severity Index (ABSI) is a five-variable scale used to evaluate burn injury severity and probability of survival. The five variables are sex, age, presence of inhalation injury, presence of full-thickness burn, and percentage of total body surface burned. An ABSI score of 2 to 18 is calculated by summation of coded values for each variable. Burns are classified by depth and extent as soon after injury as possible. The depth of a burn is classified by degree of tissue involvement.

First-Degree Superficial Burn Only the outer layer of the epidermis is involved in first-degree burn. Superficial erythema, redness of the skin, and tissue destruction occur, but healing takes place rapidly.

Second-Degree Partial-Thickness Burn All epidermis and varying depths of the corium are destroyed in second-degree burn. This is usually characterized by blister formation, pain, and a moist, mottled red or pink appearance. Hair folicles and sebaceous glands may be destroyed. Reepithelialization can occur provided the deepest layer of the epithelium is viable. However, superimposed infection can interfere with healing.

Third-Degree Full-Thickness Burn The skin with all its epithelial structures and subcutaneous tissue is destroyed in third-degree burn. This is characterized by a dry, pearly-white, or charred-appearing surface void of sensation. The destroyed skin forms a parchmentlike *eschar* over the burned area. If removed or left to slough off, eschar leaves a denuded surface that can extend to the fascia. Third-degree burns require skin grafts for healing to occur unless the area is small enough for closure by reepithelialization.

Fourth-Degree Burn Sometimes referred to as *char burns,* fourth-degree burns may damage bones, tendons, muscles, blood vessels, and peripheral nerves. An electrical burn, for example, causes damage much deeper than is apparent on the skin surface. Often muscle and bone necrosis must be excised.

Estimation of Burn Damage

Two methods are used to estimate the total percentage of body surface burned and the percentage of each degree of burn.

Lund and Brower Chart The percentage sizes of the head and lower extremities differ between infancy, childhood, and adulthood. Per guidelines of this chart, percent of burn is estimated on the basis of age in addition to anatomic location of the burn.

Rule of Nines The body surface of an adult can be divided into areas equal to multiples of 9 percent of the total body surface.

1 Head and neck—9 percent
2 Anterior and posterior trunk—18 percent each
3 Upper extremities—9 percent each
4 Lower extremities—18 percent each
5 Perineum—1 percent

Initial Care of Burn Patient

1 *Stop the burning process.* All clothing, jewelry, metal, and synthetic objects in contact with patient's skin are removed.

2 *Ensure a patent airway.* The respiratory system may be damaged from inhalation of superheated air or toxic gases. Endotracheal intubation is attempted initially. Tracheotomy may be re-

quired several days later for prolonged respiratory assistance if burn includes head and neck or respiratory tract injury.

3 *Establish intravenous fluid therapy.* Blood samples are drawn for laboratory analysis and type and cross match when a venipuncture or cutdown is performed to establish an intravenous route for fluid and nutritional administration. Fluid and electrolyte balance must be restored as quickly as possible. An electrolyte, usually lactated Ringer's solution, is infused initially. Plasma or other nutrients may be infused later.

4 *Insert a retention catheter.* Urine specimens are sent for analysis and then checked for pH and specific gravity at frequent intervals. Hourly output is recorded.

5 *Cleanse the wound.* All burns are treated aseptically. A mild cleansing agent, such as povidone-iodine, and *warm* saline or water are used to gently remove debris and loose devitalized tissue. Areas surrounding the burn should be shaved. Copious amounts of water, along with appropriate neutralizing agents, are used to cleanse and irrigate chemical burns. After cleansing, wet sheets under and around the patient must be removed and dry sterile ones applied. Nonwoven sheets specifically designed for burn care are commercially available.

6 *Estimate percent and depth of burn.* Definitive treatment may be completed in the emergency department, or the patient may be transported to an immersion tank for further cleansing and debridement, or to the operating room for initiation of further therapy as indicated by assessment of the burn. The burned area is covered with sterile or clean linen for transfer of the patient from the emergency department.

Methods of Operative Treatment

Prevention of infection and promotion of healing are of utmost concern in the treatment of burned patients. The probability of infection developing increases in greater proportion to the percentage of body surface burned. Colonization may begin as early as 24 hours postburn.

Excisional Therapy Primary excision of necrotic tissue from deep second-degree and all full-thickness third-degree burned areas, followed immediately by skin grafting, is performed beginning as soon as possible after injury. Debridement can be accomplished with a scalpel, free-hand skin-graft knife, dermatone, electrosurgical knife, or laser beam. The surgeon selects the most appropriate instrument for the particular burned area to be excised. Hypotensive anesthesia may be used to help control massive blood loss during extensive excisions.

Tangential Excision Burned tissue is excised until normal dermal tissue is reached below the depth of the wound. The wound base, containing some viable dermal structures necessary for regeneration, is covered with a split-thickness autograft. A homograft may be used when sufficient autografts cannot be harvested from the patient, or to cover the area temporarily as regeneration proceeds. If neither an autograft nor homograft is available, a heterograft may be applied. Homografts and heterografts are used as biological dressings (see p. 553) until autografts are available. Meshgrafts are frequently used to expand available autografts.

Tangential excision is usually the procedure of choice for deep partial-thickness burns of the dorsum of the hand or on the arms or legs. It is advantageous to minimize contractures. Early tangential excision and grafting in one procedure for body-surface burns can reduce mortality and septic complications and shorten hospitalization.

Escharectomy Full-thickness eschar is excised down to the fascia when viable tissues in more superficial layers are not evident, except on hands, neck, or face. All denuded areas created by excision are covered with a biological dressing for three to five days. They are then grafted with full-thickness autografts. Frequently split-thickness meshgrafts must be used to spread over large areas and allow seepage of serous fluids. These are not placed on the face and neck or over joints. If sufficient skin is not available for autografting, homografts or heterografts continue to be used as biological dressings for short periods of time. They are changed every three to five days.

Other Operative Procedures During the course of hospitalization a burned patient may come to the operating room for one or many procedures.

Escharotomy Shrinkage of eschar may occur and cause a tourniquet effect in circumferential burns of the extremities or thorax. Bilateral incisions through the eschar, not including the fascia, are made to improve circulation to an extremity. Multiple incisions on the chest wall relieve respiratory distress. Site of incisions avoid major peripheral nerves to prevent irreversible neurological complications.

Fasciotomy If adequate decompression does not occur following escharotomy, incision may be extended into underlying fascia.

Amputation of Digits Amputation may be necessary to control infection in the extremity and septicemia.

Debridement Debridement of underlying tissues helps prevent extension of tissue loss. Nonviable tendons, cartilage, or bone may be excised, as from the hand, ear, or skull.

Full-Thickness Skin Grafts With or without tarsorrhaphy, full-thickness skin grafts are used to prevent contracture of the eyelids. The cornea must be protected from exposure.

Split-Thickness Skin Grafts Autografts are applied to debrided areas as rapidly as possible. Hands and face are first priority to restore function; joints and flexion creases are second to prevent contractures; extremities and trunk are lowest priority. Skin from donor sites is cut thin if the site will be used again. Meshgrafts are frequently used to cover very large surfaces or irregular areas such as the perineum.

Biological Dressing Changes Instead of leaving a biological dressing in place until rejection, with attendant inflammatory reaction, a biological dressing is usually replaced every few days until the area is ready for autograft or skin for autograft is available. Biological dressings may be homografts of human skin from a living or cadaver donor, placenta or amniotic membranes, or a heterograft of porcine skin. Porcine dressings are frequently applied initially on second-degree burns as a temporary dressing, or used in conjunction with extensive excisional therapy. Synthetic "artificial" skin may be used. A biological dressing is used for several reasons.

1 It helps to control infection by covering denuded areas.

2 It prevents loss of serum.

3 It decreases pain.

4 It seems to stimulate formation of epithelium in dermis under it.

5 It promotes growth of granulation tissue.

Dressing Changes Occlusive dressings, if used, must be changed frequently to control infection harboring under them. An antimicrobial or chemotherapeutic agent may be applied as an integral part of the dressing.

1 Silver sulfadiazine (Silvadene) cream may be applied directly onto the burned area. This makes removal of a dressing less painful and does not disturb the healing process as it is removed. Fresh cream is applied after cleansing and debridement. A layer of fine mesh gauze is laid over it (unless the open-exposure method will be used for further healing). Then soft, absorbent material, such as fluffed gauze, and a preformed splint may be used. These are held in place by a cotton elastic bandage. An occlusive dressing may be used to hold a hand, foot, or joint in functional position.

2 Mafenide acetate (Sulfamylon) cream penetrates rapidly and is quite successful in reducing bacterial counts to optimal levels for skin grafting. However, application directly on the burned area is painful for the patient after cleansing and debridement. It may cause maceration under the dressing. Absorption may result in metabolic acidosis, so acid-base balance must be closely monitored.

3 Silver nitrate solution may be preferred. After cleansing and debridement, multiple-thickness dressings are applied to the area. These are kept saturated with 0.5% silver nitrate solution and changed every 12 hours. When doing a debridement, sterile distilled water is used for irrigation because saline may cause the precipitation of silver salts.

> NOTE. Care is taken to avoid splashing silver nitrate solution on walls and floors because staining can occur. If disposable drapes and gowns are not used, stained linen must be laundered separately from other linen.

Serial Biopsy Cultures Through two linear incisions, a biopsy of tissue including subcutaneous fat is excised for culturing. This is done every two or three days, until the eschar begins to separate, to monitor the colonization of microorganisms in the wound. The results of serial biopsy culture enable the surgeon to make decisions specific to the therapeutic needs of the patient. An antimicrobial or chemotherapeutic topical agent is selected or changed according to these results.

Curling's Ulcer Gastrointestinal complications may occur anytime from the early postinjury period through rehabilitation. Complaints must be carefully evaluated. The patient who develops massive bleeding from a Curling's or stress ulcer in the stomach and duodenum must be operated on. Vagotomy with antrectomy is most frequently performed by a general surgeon.

Marjolin's Ulcer An ulceration due to malignant changes can develop in the surface area of a burn scar. As long as 20 years postburn, a prolonged ulceration can lead to squamous-cell carcinoma of the skin. A Marjolin's ulcer should be excised.

Environmental Considerations for Burn Patients

1 Environmental control is perhaps the essence of burn therapy. The environment must protect the wound from further injury and microbial invasion. *A burn wound is always potentially contaminated until epithelialization occurs.* Open exposure of the wound to room air may be the choice of the plastic surgeon for selected patients. Regardless of method of treatment, the following adjuncts are used, if the equipment is available, in the care of burned patients in addition to strict adherence to all the principles of aseptic technique.
   a *Reverse isolation technique* may be practiced to protect the patient, whose resistance is low, from cross infection from personnel. Caps, masks, shoe covers, and sterile gowns and gloves are worn by all personnel attending the patient. This may be referred to as *protective isolation.*
   b *Laminar,* or downward unidirectional, *airflow* away from the wound helps minimize airborne contamination.
   c *Plastic isolator* protects the patient. Personnel do not directly enter this isolation unit. Nursing and medical care is given through clear plastic access walls. The environment around the patient inside the isolator is controlled at 90°F (32°C) and 94 percent relative humidity to conserve heat loss by evaporation.
2 Patients with extensive burns may be placed on a Stryker frame or a circle electric bed specially designed to facilitate handling and turning. They are transported to the OR on these frames or beds. Patients must be turned slowly and gently, because they are often hypovolemic postinjury.
3 Hypothermia must be prevented. The patient's thermoregulatory mechanism is altered by the destruction of skin that normally acts as an insulator. Heat loss is the greatest single problem the burn patient faces in the OR. Room temperature should be increased to between 80 and 90°F (27 and 32°C) with low relative humidity of about 30 percent. Warm hyperthermia blankets can cover the operating table. Solutions should be warmed prior to irrigation or infusion.
4 Operating during nighttime hours is advantageous for the patient:
   a Normal schedule for oral intake is not interrupted.
   b The OR can be preheated to above-normal temperature.
5 Hypnosis and biofeedback techniques can reduce potential postanesthetic complications when many operative procedures are necessary to achieve acceptable functional and cosmetic results postburn. The OR environment must be quiet to be conducive to hypnotic suggestions given to the patient.

CHAPTER **28**

MULTIDISCIPLINARY TEAM APPROACH TO HEAD AND NECK SURGERY

Reconstruction of the skeletal framework and all the structures of the head and neck region is not within the province of any one surgical specialty. Subspecialists from many disciplines, most notably plastic surgeons, otolaryngologists, and dentists, limit their surgical practice to specific types of problems involving areas of the head and/or neck. Training in these subspecialties is included in specialty postgraduate programs. For example, endoscopy of the head and neck area (discussed in Chap. 26) is essential for residency approval by the American Board of Plastic Surgery. The American Board of Otolaryngology pursued changing its name to American Board of Otolaryngology—Head and Neck Surgery. Oral surgery, orthodontics, prosthodontics, and periodontics are specialties within dentistry.

Dental and skeletal deformities of alignment and function coexist with aesthetic appearance. These deformities may be congenital or they may be due to trauma or disease. They may interfere with breathing, eating, swallowing, speaking, seeing, or hearing. A *multidisciplinary team* of surgical specialists is often required to reconstruct complex deformities. This team may be as all-inclusive as a plastic surgeon, neurosurgeon, oral surgeon, orthodontist or prosthodontist, otolaryngologist, ophthalmologist, and general surgeon; or it may be limited to two or three specialists. The team may also include a radiologist, anesthesiologist, psychiatrist, speech pathologist, and social worker, plus, of course, the nursing staff. A team must include all the specialties needed for complete preoperative assessment, intraoperative care, and postoperative rehabilitation of the individual patient.

HISTORICAL INTRODUCTION

Trauma has historically been a major source of facial disfigurement. Repair of mandibular fractures dates back to 600 B.C. Intermaxillary wiring was documented in 1835. In 1901, René LeFort identified and classified patterns of midfacial and maxillary fractures. His classifications are still used.

Evidence of prosthetic restoration of facial disfigurement has been found in Egyptian mummies with artifical eyes, ears, and noses. Lacquered-wood nasal prostheses were made in India and China in the second century A.D. Gold, silver, and metal alloy replacement parts were developed by the sixteenth century. Ceramic-like materials and rubber were fashioned into facial prostheses in the nineteenth century. After World War I, methyl methacrylate was used to make artificial eyes and dentures. Silicone elastomer has replaced other materials for nasal and ear prostheses, either implanted or affixed externally, following traumatic amputation or surgical resection.

Attempts to remove malignant tumors of the head and neck by pioneers at the Mayo Clinic early in the 1900s and others, such as Hayes Martin at Memorial Hospital in New York City, introduced radical surgery as a modality of treatment.

During the 1950s surgeons recognized that major ablative surgery could not be successfully accomplished without regional tissue pedicle flaps. This concept was not new, however. The first regional flap recorded in the literature was a forehead myocutaneous flap reported in *Sushutra,* published in 700 B.C. Unfortunately the concept was lost for over 2000 years. The reintroduction of regional myocutaneous flaps in the 1970s, plus microvascularized free flaps and other types of grafts and flaps, has led to their being an important part of reconstruction for head and neck oncology and facial deformity. They reduce gross deformity, protect essential structures, improve physiologic function and appearance, and facilitate psychologic rehabilitation.

The well-established fundamentals of excisional surgery in the head and neck have increasingly become more sophisticated to include use of microvascular and microneural techniques, cryosurgery, and laser surgery. Computerized axial tomography, cephalometric tracings, radiographs, photographs, and dental models enhance diagnosis, evaluation, and planning to achieve successful outcomes of surgical intervention. The potential for altering alignment, function, and appearance is limited only by the imagination of the surgeons.

One of the most imaginative surgeons of modern times is Paul L. Tessier of Paris. In 1967, he reported his work to surgically correct gross facial and skull deformities of children with Crouzon's and Apert's syndromes. Tessier's results have had a monumental impact on the development of craniofacial surgery as a new surgical subspecialty. Surgeons are able to systematically dismantle, rearrange, and reconstruct the entire musculoskeletal system between the top of the head and the oral cavity. This requires a multidisciplinary team. Special craniofacial centers have been established for these complex procedures.

PATIENT'S SELF-IMAGE

Psychologic feelings one has about self are inherent in behavior of a social human being. Physical appearance contributes to these feelings. Facial beauty is prized in our society. Therefore, facial configuration may be perceived by the patient as a deformity, and hence the source of personal discomfort reinforced by ridicule or lack of familial or social acceptance. The psychological trauma of a negative self-image can lead to asocial behavior.

The degree, duration, and impairment of facial disfigurement, as perceived by the patient, will influence desire for surgical correction. Patients with recently acquired deformities as the result of trauma are usually more concerned with appearance than individuals who grew up with cosmetically displeasing facial features. Impairment of function due to deformity or disease may offer the patient no alternative other than surgical intervention.

Patients must be psychologically prepared for and supported following ablative surgery. Extensive, or even minimal, excision of the structures and soft tissue of the face or neck can cause severe psychological trauma. Patients must be thoroughly evaluated preoperatively. A psychiatric consultation may be advisable.

Family members must also be prepared to accept the permanent or temporary disfigurement of a loved one following ablative surgery. Reconstruction frequently is performed in stages. The patient and family must cope with the physical limitations between operations, for example, of speaking and eating, as well as physical appearance. The patient's willingness to care for the wound may be the first sign of acceptance. The home situation should be assessed to ascertain whether or not the patient will receive adequate home care and support after discharge.

THE FACE

Anatomy and Physiology

The *face* is the anterior part of the head, including the forehead, cheeks, nose, lips, and chin, but not the ears. The eyes, situated in the bony orbits (see Chap. 25, p. 482), contribute to the features of the face, although they are not technically a part of the face. The structure and function of the nose, the prominent organ in the center of the face, are discussed in Chapter 26 (see p. 506).

The skeletal structure of the face includes the *frontal bone* of the forehead. It forms the upper part of the orbits. Divided by sutures, the lines of union between bones, the frontal bone joins the sphenoid and ethmoid, and the paired nasal, lacrimal, maxilla, and zygoma. The posterior orbits are formed by the *sphenoid bone,* which is shaped like a butterfly with extended wings, and the palatal bones. The medial walls are formed by the ethmoid, lacrimal, nasal bones, and maxilla. The lateral aspect is formed by the *zygoma* (malar bone), the cheekbone. The irregular-shaped *eth-*

moid bone also forms the roof and posterior lateral wall of each nasal cavity. The *nasal bones* form the bridge of the nose between the orbits.

The *maxilla,* the upper jaw that holds the palate, extends laterally to the zygoma and temporal bone, under the orbit, and along the anterior nasal cavity. The maxillary bones are paired and join in the midline between the nose and oral cavity. The alveoli that hold the teeth are along the alveolar processes of the maxillae.

The ramus of the *mandible,* the arch-shaped bone of the lower jaw, articulates with temporal bones at the temporomandibular joints in front of the ears. The alveoli, the tooth-bearing bodies, meet at the alveolar process to form the chin (mental region).

The bony structure of the face is covered with muscles, superficial blood vessels and nerves; epidermis, and dermis. Other structures, i.e., ducts and sinuses (air spaces), are also in the soft tissues or bony structure of the face (refer to paranasal sinuses in Chap. 26, pp. 506, 507, and 508).

OPERATIVE PROCEDURES OF THE FACE

Craniofacial Operations

Craniofacial refers to the cranium and face. Craniofacial surgery of increasing complexity has been performed since World War II. However, the approach developed by Tessier has led to previously inaccessible anatomical areas. Exposure for dissection of soft tissues and bone to restore contour and symmetry in practically every type of facial deformity, whether congenital, neoplastic, or traumatic in origin, can be accomplished by a multidisciplinary team of surgeons. This team may include a plastic surgeon, neurosurgeon, anesthesiologist, ophthalmologist, oral surgeon, and otorhinolaryngologist. Some operations require over 100 separate maneuvers and may take as long as 14 to 16 hours to complete.

Many of the concepts developed for these very complex procedures are applied in the more common and less complicated operations to reshape sections of the skill or reconstruct soft tissues. Craniofacial reconstruction should be performed as soon as indicated by the physiological and psychological impacts of the deformity upon the patient, regardless of age. Early operation not only decreases psychological trauma, but may also prevent craniofacial distortion due to brain and nerve damage of a disease process or traumatic injury.

Analysis of cephalometric tracings accurately superimposed on transparent photographs of the patient preoperatively is essential to determine the extent of facial deformity and the plan for skeletal rearrangement. The exact size of the defects that will need bone grafts can be determined.

Many procedures involve correction of malocclusion of the mandible at the same time the orbitocranial skeleton is restructured. Dental models are cut and mounted on an articular for reference.

Hypotensive anesthesia reduces blood loss during these extensive procedures. The patient must be continuously monitored throughout the procedure to estimate blood loss. A preoperative tracheotomy may be necessary to maintain an adequate airway postoperatively.

Midface Advancement The base of the anterior cranial fossae can be exposed through a bifrontal incision to elevate a frontal bone flap (see Chap. 29). While the neurosurgeon is raising the flap, the plastic surgeon takes donor bone from the iliac crest, if autogenous bone grafts will be needed.

The facial skeleton is separated from the cranial base. The plastic surgeon raises the periorbita, orbital contents, and soft tissue over the dorsum of the nose. The subperiosteum of the anterior maxillae is elevated. Osteotomies are cut in the supraorbital region to mobilize the lateral walls. Anterior maxillary osteotomy, through an infraorbital approach, extends across and below the frontal processes of the maxillae. Osteotomies of the anterior cranial fossae, and the medial and lateral orbital walls and floors are completed. The mobilized bones can be functionally advanced in three dimensions as desired. They are then wired into position. Bone grafts are wired into place in the resulting defects to maintain stability. Decalcified bone or bone dust may be preferred to bone grafts to induce osteogenesis. The frontal bone flap is replaced and the incision is closed.

Mandibular osteotomies may be done before closure to correct alignment of the jaws. Whether or not this is necessary, the mandible is stabilized after closure with intermaxillary wires and suspension wires to the zygomatic arch.

Depending on the deformity, variations of the intracranial and extracranial osteotomies are done to advance, align, or reposition the facial bones and reconstruct soft tissues. Many patients return to the OR for additional corrective procedures:

eyelid ptosis and/or extraocular muscle surgery performed by the ophthalmologist; dacryocystorhinostomy and/or nasal reconstruction performed by the rhinologist; and bone augmentation or resection of the maxillae and/or mandible for repositioning by the plastic surgeon or oral surgeon. During all procedures, the surgeons must avoid injury to facial nerves, arteries, and veins.

Orbital Hypertelorism and Orbital Dystopia Procedures An abnormally wide distance between or malposition of the orbits is usually secondary to other craniofacial malformations. Only the medial orbital walls may be moved to correct minimal hypertelorism. Advancement of superior and lateral walls, rather than total orbit advancement, may suffice to correct a dystopia.

Resection of Tumors Radical craniofacial resection may be indicated to remove gigantic benign nasal dermoid tumors and malignant tumors of the paranasal sinuses. In a one-stage procedure, all involved soft tissue is excised with simultaneous correction of the underlying skeletal structure.

Basal-cell carcinoma is a common type of nasal tumor. Operation alone may be used, or combined therapy. Immediate repair by skin graft or pedicle flap accompanies excision of well-defined lesions. Reconstruction is postponed in multicentric (many-centered) cancer or doubtful extension of the tumor. More advanced lesions require replacement of the nose by prosthesis.

Erosion of a growth in one of the sinuses into an adjacent nasal wall can occlude the air passage. Resection may include partial or total maxillectomy and removal of surrounding tissues. The cavity usually is covered by skin graft. Unilateral enucleation of the eye may be necessary. Radical operation for ethmoid tumor also may involve removal of part of the base of the skull and excision of the maxillary antrum and the palate on the affected side.

In providing maxillofacial prostheses to replace facial structure following various procedures, the prosthodontist works closely with the surgeon and radiation therapist. Splints or stents hold tissue grafts in place, seal cavities from each other, or unite bony segments. A dental prosthesis to close the defect in the upper jaw and eye prosthesis following enucleation contribute to the patient's rehabilitation following extensive operation.

Midfacial Fractures The facial bones provide a shield for the brain, but they also protect the senses of sight, smell, hearing, and taste. Although midfacial fractures and soft tissue injuries are seldom fatal, inadequate treatment can result in disfigurement and sensory impairment. For example, virtually all blindness secondary to trauma is permanent.

Facial fractures should be suspected when the patient complains of pain, malocclusion of the jaws, or diplopia (double vision). Swelling and asymmetry of the face may be obvious. Diagnosis is confirmed by x-ray to identify the bone(s) involved. The LeFort classification of fractures is useful in determining appropriate method of reduction and stabilization.

1 LeFort I is a transverse fracture of the maxilla, fragmenting the upper alveoli and palate.
2 LeFort II is a pyramidal fracture of the frontal processes of the maxillae, the nasal bones, and the orbital floor. The maxillae are freely movable.
3 LeFort III fracture includes both zygomas, maxillae and nasal bones, and the ethmoid, sphenoid, and other orbital bones. This creates a craniofacial dysjunction (separation).

Facial fractures must be reduced, stabilized, and immobilized. Priorities of initial treatment following injury, however, concern airway obstruction, possible cervical spine injury, and hemorrhage. Treatment of the fracture may be delayed. The surgeon follows the principles of approaching fractures from "inside out, downward up." This means that bony structures are repaired first, then the soft tissues; the mandible, or most distal fracture, is reduced first before working upward toward the cranium.

Reduction of Orbital Fractures The injury may involve the rim or the floor of the orbit, or both. If orbital contents are depressed into the maxillary sinus, operative exploration through an orbital or a transsinal approach is indicated. Extent of the trauma should indicate the most appropriate operative management.

1 *Fractures of the orbital rim,* frequently associated with fractures of the zygoma, are usually detected by deformity. The fracture is reduced by appropriate means. Fragments are wired into place as necessary.
2 *Blowout fracture of the orbit* may result from a direct blow to the eyeball, which is, in turn, transmitted to the very thin floor of the orbit. A typical fracture is in the medial third of the floor with dislocation of floor fragments into the maxillary sinus. The fracture may occasionally extend

into the ethmoid plate. Consequently orbital contents, which may include the inferior extraocular muscles, are usually herniated into the antrum. This produces limitation of upward gaze and some degree of enophthalmos or recession of the eyeball into the orbit. The herniated orbital contents must be reduced from the antrum back into the orbit with special attention to freeing the entrapped muscles. Plastic or silicone sheeting may be used to close the defect in the floor. Or the fragments may be elevated by packing the antrum through a Caldwell-Luc (sinus) approach. Diagnosis may be overlooked unless a laminogram is taken.

Reduction of Nasal Fractures As stated in Chapter 26 (see p. 507), fracture of the nasal bones and septum often accompanies other trauma to the head, such as a blowout fracture of the orbit (discussed above). If the zygoma or maxilla is involved, reduction may be done through a small incision anterior to the ear and superior to the zygomatic arch. Periosteal elevators are used to raise depressed bone and cartilage fragments. Nasal fractures are splinted with nasal packs and external splint.

Reduction of Zygomatic (Malar) Fractures Dislocations of the zygoma are more common than fractures. Zygomatic fractures always involve the orbital bones. Those of the zygomatic arch are particularly unstable and require intraosseous or transosseous wire fixation following internal reduction with counterpressure from underneath the arch. Transantral Steinmann pinning may be necessary to maintain reduction of fragments in severely fragmented fractures.

Maxillofacial Operations

Maxillofacial pertains to the part of face formed by the upper and lower jaws. Most maxillofacial operations are designed to reconstruct defects in the lips, the buccal sulcus, maxilla, alveolar ridge, floor of the mouth, mandible, and/or chin. These defects may be the result of trauma or resection of tumor. Whenever feasible, intraoral incisions are used to minimize facial scarring. Soft tissue reconstructions of the lips are discussed in Chapter 27. Congenital deformities are discussed in Chapter 33.

Intermaxillary Fixation of Fractures Following closed or open reduction, fractures of maxilla and mandible are usually immobilized by interdental wiring if the patient has upper and lower teeth. If the patient is edentulous (without teeth), open reduction and skeletal fixation by circumferential wiring over an intraoral splint or screws and connecting bars may be necessary.

Erich arch bars are shaped along the dental arches. Wires are passed between the teeth to anchor the splints on the upper and lower jaws. Each splint contains a series of small lugs. Tiny rubber bands, placed around opposing lugs, hold the teeth in occlusion. Splints frequently are not used for fixation of these fractures. The teeth may be held in occlusion by wires passed around opposing teeth.

> NOTE. Following fixation of the mandible or maxilla, a pair of wire scissors must accompany the patient from the OR and remain at the bedside as long as wires or rubber bands are in place. If the patient experiences respiratory difficulty, the wires may have to be cut to prevent aspiration. Fluids may be difficult to swallow.

Mentoplasty The chin can be reshaped by removing sections from or adding to the mandible for aesthetics and/or functional bite disorders. Classification of occlusion (closure) of the teeth is based on the anteroposterior relationship of the upper and lower jaws. Malocclusion occurs when the teeth do not close together properly. Psychologically debilitating facial deformity and bite disorders can be caused by malocclusion of any one of four types:

1 *Prognathism.* The lower jaw projects too far forward.

2 *Micrognathia.* The dental arch, usually of the mandible, is too small to accommodate the teeth. Teeth are pushed out of alignment because they are crowded together.

3 *Open bite.* The front teeth do not close because the back teeth come together first.

4 *Rotation.* A tooth or teeth shift out of proper position.

Mentoplasty is usually performed in combination with orthodontic treatment. Preoperative orthodontia may be required to align and level the teeth. Surgical correction may include extraction of one or more teeth, maxillary and/or mandibular osteotomies with repositioning of bone segments to change shape of the facial structure, and/or repositioning of alveoli. *Prognathism,* forward jutting of the jaw, is corrected by removing bone or by recessing the lower jaw. *Micrognathia,* abnormally small jaws, is augmented with bone or cartilage grafts or silicone implants, or by advancing the jaw. Mobilized bony structures are stabilized by intermaxillary fixation.

Postoperative orthodontia may be required to complete the closure of the spaces around the osteotomies to stabilize occlusal function. Bands may be applied to the teeth when the upper or lower jaws are moved for correction of malocclusion.

Temporomandibular Joint Replacement Although rare, degenerative disease can impair function of the temporomandibular joint. Trauma can also impair this joint. Silicone elastomer implants and, more recently, a titanium alloy prosthesis are used to reconstruct the joint.

Alveolar Ridge Reconstruction The alveolar ridge is the bony remains of the alveolar process of the maxilla or mandible that formerly contained the teeth. Some edentulous patients have atrophic maxillae and/or mandibles or bony defects due to trauma or tumor resection that will not support artificial dentures. The alveolar ridges can be augmented or reconstructucted.

Inlay Bone Grafts Bone grafts are used for augmentation of the maxillae and/or mandible. A prevascularized autogenous rib graft may be transplanted into a maxillary defect using microvascular anastomosis. Composite grafts of freeze-dried cadaver rib with autogenous particulate cancellous bone and marrow may be preferred in the maxilla and used to augment the mandible.

Mandibular Staple The staple fastener prosthesis is implanted as an alternative to bone grafting to restore the ability of the mandible to support a denture. The titanium alloy (Tivanium) device has two transosteal pins with a set of fasteners and lock nuts between them on the curved cross-arch connecting plate. The staple must be inserted using the drill guide and twist drills specifically designed for it. The staple is evenly seated in the holes drilled in the mandible to the point of contact with the inferior border.

A scratch or bend may weaken the staple and may result in a fracture of the device. A deformed staple will not fit into the drill holes properly. The prosthesis must be carefully protected and handled prior to implantation.

Dentofacial Operations

Just as the scope of many of the surgical specialties has broadened, such as otolaryngology—head and neck surgery, so has dentistry. Likewise subspecialization within dentistry, through extensive specialized postgraduate education, has given operating room practice privileges to dentists who perform operative procedures in and around the oral cavity. Among these are:

1 *Oral surgeon.* Oral surgery may be limited to exodontia (extraction of teeth) and minor surgery in the oral cavity. It may also include correction of dentofacial deformities, i.e., oral and maxillofacial surgery. A qualified oral surgeon is competent to complete a history and physical examination to determine the patient's ability to undergo the proposed operative procedure.

2 *Orthodontist.* Orthodontics focuses on irregularities of the teeth, malocclusion, and associated facial problems.

3 *Prosthodontist.* Prosthodontics is concerned with artificial restoration of intraoral and external facial structures.

4 *Periodontist.* Periodontics is the treatment and prevention of disease in the gingiva (gum), underlying soft tissues, and alveoli surrounding the teeth.

Patients with medical problems admitted to the hospital by oral surgeons and all patients admitted for dental care must have an admission history, physical examination, and evaluation of their overall medical risk by a physician preoperatively. This physician is responsible for care of a preexisting condition and any medical problem that arises during hospitalization.

Just as physicians from various specialties function as members of a multidisciplinary team, so do oral surgeons and dentists, each contributing to the dental health of the patient. Frequently they also function as collegial members of the teams involved in craniofacial or maxillofacial surgery. They assist with reconstruction of the face, correction of jaw deformities, and establishment of optimum dental occlusion. For example, the orthodontist may move teeth prior to the maxillofacial or oral surgeon repositioning the jaws to correct malocclusion. Many patients undergo both pre- and postoperative orthodontia. Prosthodontics may be necessary to replace missing teeth. Prosthodontists also may fit an artificial nose postoperatively following rhinectomy for tumor or trauma.

Patients seeking dentofacial treatment usually have functional problems. These may include difficulty with mastication (chewing), deglutition (swallowing), speech, abnormal tongue posture, or lip incompetence.

Treatment of periodontal disease is usually done in the periodontist's office. However, patients who have medical problems, such as hemophilia or other blood dyscrasia, severe diabetes, or heart disease, are admitted to the hospital for periodontal surgery. The most common operations include:

1 *Gingivectomy:* excision of portion(s) of the gingiva (gum), the mucous membrane and underlying soft tissue that covers the alveolar process and surrounds the teeth, to remove deep pockets of plaque, calculus, and inflamed soft tissue.

2 *Gingivoplasty:* excision of excessive gum tissue to contour or reshape gingiva for improved physiologic form.

3 *Flap procedures:* retraction of gingiva from teeth to remove underlying inflamed tissue and calculus. The alveoli may be reconstructed to change their shape. Gingival flaps or free grafts from the palate may be used to cover receded areas and to augment inadequate zones of masticatory gingiva. Gingival onlay grafts are also used to enhance ridges where trauma or extraction has resulted in a reduced ridge, thus creating an aesthetic problem.

4 *Root amputation:* removal of one root from a multirooted tooth, a molar for example, after advanced destruction from disease around the tooth.

5 *Bone grafts:* rebuilding of alveolar defects with autogenous grafts, ceramic bone, or freeze-dried homografts, or some combination of grafting materials. A combination of freeze-dried cadaver bone with autogenous bone has the highest rate of success.

THE ORAL CAVITY

Anatomy and Physiology

Anatomy and physiology of the oral cavity and throat is presented in Chapter 26. In addition to the hard and soft palates, pharynx, and tongue, the *salivary glands* are located in the soft tissue walls of the oral cavity. The six major paired glands are the submandibular, sublingual, and parotid. The parotids are the largest. The ducts of these major glands, in addition to lesser glands, secrete saliva into the mouth. Saliva functions to moisten and lubricate food to aid in swallowing, to dissolve some substances and enzymatically digest starches, and to facilitate tasting. Structures in the oral cavity are associated with both respiration and deglutition (the act of swallowing). Pathology may affect any of the structures: the lip, tongue, floor of the mouth, palates, salivary glands, or pharynx. Abnormalities result from infection, trauma, congenital malformation, improper occlusion or jaggedness of teeth, or tumors.

OPERATIVE PROCEDURES OF THE ORAL CAVITY

The common procedures in these anatomic areas fall within two major classifications: those for trauma and those for neoplasms.

Many of the craniofacial, maxillofacial, and dentofacial procedures previously described in this chapter are performed through intraoral incisions. Other procedures done orally are described in Chapters 26, 27, and 33. The following procedures may be performed by plastic surgeons, oral surgeons, laryngologists, or a multidisciplinary team through intra- and extraoral incisions.

Excision of Tumors of Salivary Gland

Benign mixed tumors of the salivary glands are more common than are malignant tumors, and most frequently are located in a parotid gland. Most tumors can be removed by dissection and some by cryosurgery. The incision must be adequate to expose the entire gland and the facial nerve. A nerve stimulator is used to identify the nerve and its branches. Injury to the nerve results in postoperative facial paralysis.

Parotidectomy Parotidectomy is performed through an incision in the neck below the angle of the mandible and extending upward to one or both sides of the ear. A swelling beneath the skin in the area in front of or below the ear is almost invariably within the substance of the parotid gland. This may be a benign, mixed, or malignant tumor. Benign lesions localized superficially may be excised by superficial subtotal parotidectomy. Lesions deep within the gland, extending under the mandible, frequently present in the oral cavity by displacing the soft palate. Radical neck dissection or hemimandibulectomy may be indicated to remove a highly invasive malignant tumor. For most parotid tumors, the facial nerve can be isolated and preserved during total parotidectomy, unless the nerve is inextricably involved by the tumor. If the facial nerve must be sacrificed, the nerve may be primarily grafted to prevent total facial nerve paralysis, using the great auricular nerve as a graft.

Excision of Oral Carcinoma

Primary malignant lesions may be in the lower lip, tongue, or floor of the mouth. Because of the proximity of cervical lymph nodes, metastasis occurs early. A painful bleeding ulcer should be suspect. However, oral cancer in its earliest stages may be asymptomatic and painless. Small tumors may be treated with only irradiation, local excision with primary closure, or vaporization with laser beam. Larger lesions compel more extensive procedures.

Subtotal or Hemiglossectomy Part or half of the tongue is removed. Extent of resection will determine type of reconstruction to resurface the oral cavity.

Total Glossectomy All of the tongue and often the floor of the mouth are resected. A pectoralis major myocutaneous island flap is more advantageous than are the cervical, pectoral, or forehead flaps also used to restore intraoral lining. Respiratory embarassment and chronic aspiration are significant problems after glossectomy. Cricopharyngeal myotomy may be performed to facilitate swallowing and reduce aspiration. The tip of the epiglottis is often sutured to the pharyngeal wall (epiglottopexy) to decrease aspiration. Unless involved directly with tumor, the larynx is preserved. Laryngeal suspension, by placing a heavy suture around the mandibular ramus, holds the larynx laterally. Extension into the larynx and cervical metastases are indications for uni- or bilateral neck dissection, usually with laryngectomy (refer to Chap. 26, p. 513). A tracheotomy is always performed with a total glossectomy to maintain an airway. A nasogastric tube is inserted before closing the pharynx for postoperative alimentation.

Mandibulectomy Partial or total removal of the lower jaw is performed for extension of tumor into bone of the floor of the mouth. It may be performed with glossectomy and radical neck dissection for wide excision. Mandibular replacement combines bone graft and synthetic materials for restoration of speech and appearance. A compound osseocutaneous flap from the illiac crest, with microvascular anastomosis of the deep circumflex iliac artery vascular pedicle, may be transferred for reconstruction. If the patient is dentulous, relationship of the opposing teeth is maintained; if edentulous, the patient wears a denture. Whenever possible, mandibular tissue is preserved.

OPERATIVE PROCEDURES OF THE NECK

Anatomy of the neck region is described in Chapter 26. Operative procedures performed primarily by laryngologists are also discussed in that chaper. Many laryngologists and plastic surgeons, and some oral surgeons, perform neck dissections when cervical lymph nodes are involved in head and neck oncology. General surgeons may join the multidisciplinary team to assist in reconstructive surgery or perform some procedures, such as excision of a thyroglossal duct cyst.

Neck Dissections

Tumors, benign and malignant, occur in the head and neck regions. Although the origin of many of these neoplasms is technically in the head, the cervical lymph nodes are frequently involved secondarily by metastases from a primary head or neck malignant tumor. Treatment is directed toward definitive management for eradication of the tumor and metastases, with consideration for rehabilitation. In an attempt to eradicate all cancer foci, neck dissection may be performed at a time later than removal of a primary lesion of, for example, the parotid gland or tongue, or simultaneously as a one-stage procedure. This composite resection removes primary tumor and metastatic lesions at the same time en masse. Sometimes, however, metastasis occurs before a primary lesion is discovered.

Various reconstructive techniques provide immediate restoration to improve speech, reestablish oral function, or prevent airway obstruction. Others involve delayed reconstruction. The method of repair depends on the type of defect resulting from excision of the lesion. Preoperatively, the patient's emotional stability is analyzed if the operation will result in cosmetic deformity. Reconstruction is planned prior to or at the time of the operation so that local tissue can be used whenever feasible, and normal function preserved whenever possible. The aim of reconstruction is to restore function and appearance.

Radical Neck Dissection Malignant tumors of the oral or pharyngeal cavities, cutaneous malignant melanoma, and skin cancer in the head and neck region often require wide resection of the primary lesion and excision of all the cervical lymph nodes on one or both sides of the neck. This procedure gives the patient with cancer of the cervical lymphatic chain a chance for cure and arrest of spread. When metastasis is known to be present or is highly suspect because of location or stage of the malignancy, the operation is predicated on the assumption that metastases are regional and not distant.

The head and neck surgeon must plan the operation with reconstruction in mind, so that the incisions will allow good exposure but provide as much local flap tissue as possible for reconstruction. Incisions used for the tumor resection will necessarily vary according to the type of reconstruction planned. Thus, no single operative procedure can be used to treat all lesions. However, certain basic features remain common to all neck dissections.

All lymph-bearing tissue from the midline anteriorly to the trapezius muscle posteriorly and from the mandible superiorly to the clavicle inferiorly is removed. All tissue between the deep cervical fascia and the platysma muscle externally is removed except the carotid artery system, the vagus, phrenic, and hypoglossal nerves, and the brachial plexus.

The massive tissue resection, removal en bloc, includes all nonvital structures of the neck on the side of the tumor. These are the jugular vein, eleventh cranial (spinal accessory) nerve, sternocleidomastoid muscle, and submandibular salivary gland. Elimination of the motor nerve to the trapezius muscle contributes to muscular atrophy, subsequent shoulder drop on the affected side, and possibly decreased strength in raising the arm.

Various techniques are used to close the large defect in the anterior neck. When the occipital, posterior auricular, facial, and superior thyroid arteries can be preserved, arterialized skin flaps designed to incorporate branches from these vessels can be constructed with length up to three or four times the width. Otherwise the length of a flap should not exceed twice the width. A deltopectoral pedical flap or a pectoralis major myocutaneous free flap may be needed. An exposed carotid artery must be covered. Cervical flaps carrying their own blood supply may be used for this, and to restore the oral pharyngeal lining intraorally.

The mandible is preserved, unless involved by direct extension of tumor into the bone. Access through a mandibular osteotomy or partial mandibulectomy is usually required for effective resection in the posterior oral cavity. Solid bony continuity and realignment of the dental arches must be established for functional restoration of speech and chewing. A bone graft from the rib or iliac crest, cancellous bone chips, or a composite graft may be used to stabilize the mandible.

Effective drainage of the wound is important to healing. This is accomplished by application of continuous negative pressure to catheters inserted through stab wounds below the clavicle. Drainage protects viability of the thin skin flaps and facilitates approximation of wound surfaces.

A prophylactic tracheotomy may be performed to protect the patient from respiratory distress in neck dissection alone. A tracheostomy is always done in a composite radical neck resection.

A feeding esophagostomy tube or cervical pharyngostomy tube is inserted for anticipated extended extraoral feeding. This permits suction to avoid aspiration and gastric distention in addition to providing a feeding route. The tube is usually inserted in the OR.

Potential complications of neck dissection are numerous, depending on the tumor itself, irradiation therapy, or necessary sacrifice of vital structures. Intraoperatively, hemorrhage may occur from injury to a major vessel or the thoracic duct. Postoperatively, invasion of overlying skin necrosis into a major vessel wall, such as the carotid artery, can cause an often fatal blowout of the vessel. Slight previous bleeding may be forewarning.

Although reconstruction begins at the time of primary neck dissection, the patient usually requires considerable postoperative rehabilitation, psychologically, and staged operations before cosmetic and functional reconstruction is complete.

Cervical Esophageal Reconstruction Restoration of continuity of the alimentary tract is a major challenge following ablative surgery of the neck, particularly after cervical esophagectomy or circumferential pharyngectomy. Location of the primary tumor and its extension, and the extent of resection are contributing factors in determining the most satisfactory reconstruction. A pectoralis major myocutaneous flap or a free revascularized intestinal autograft (see Chap. 27, p. 527) will satisfactorily restore continuity in some situations.

Transposition of the mobilized stomach into the neck may be performed when the entire esophagus is resected. Two teams working simultaneously perform this gastric pull-up procedure. The team of general surgeons performs the abdominal dissection to mobilize the stomach while the other team resects the primary tumor in the neck. The tumor may arise from the hypopharynx, cervical esophagus, or thyroid gland. Radical neck dissection is carried out for extension into the cervical lymph nodes. Anastomosis of the stomach to an esophageal remnant may be accomplished with a circular intraluminal stapler if the primary esophageal tumor is above the level of the thoracic inlet. Primary pharyngogastric anastomosis may be required for high transsection of the pharynx.

Thyroglossal Duct Cyst During fetal development, the thyroid gland descends through the thyroglossal duct from the foramen cecum near the base of the tongue to the neck below the larynx. In adulthood, remnants of this embryonic duct may form a cyst in the anterior midline of the neck. Excision of the cyst includes removal of the hyoid bone, because this surrounds the duct.

GENERAL CONSIDERATIONS IN HEAD AND NECK SURGERY

1 Tape eyes shut before prepping skin to prevent solution from getting into eyes and to prevent corneal abrasion after patient is draped.

2 Eyelid edema due to facial trauma may expose the conjunctiva. Lubricate with ophthalmic ointment or artificial tears to minimize corneal damage.

3 Monitoring during extensive operations includes at least arterial and venous pressure lines, Foley catheter for keeping accurate output record, and rectal temperature probe.

4 Instrumentation may include bone and dental power saws and drills, bone instruments, nasal instruments, oral retractors, and soft tissue instruments.

5 Electrosurgical and cryosurgical units, laser beam, and the operating microscope may be used. All equipment must be checked for proper working order and operated correctly.

6 The surgeon(s) often wear headlights to supplement overhead lighting.

7 Wire cutter must accompany patient who has had intermaxillary wiring of the jaws. Nursing personnel in the recovery room and on the patient units must know which wires to cut in an emergency.

8 If the patient did not have a tracheotomy in the OR, a sterile tracheotomy tray should accompany any patient who has a potential risk of airway obstruction postoperatively.

CHAPTER 29

NEUROSURGERY

Neurosurgeons specialize in surgery associated with dysfunction, disease, or injury of the nervous system. The nervous system includes the brain and spinal cord (*central nervous system,* CNS) and the cranial, spinal, and autonomic peripheral nerves (*peripheral nervous system,* PNS). Neural tissues control motor and sensory functions throughout the body. Generalized cerebral function is manifested in overall behavior, level of consciousness, orientation, and intellectual performance. These functions may be altered by a metabolic disorder, a chromosomal defect, a disease process, or a traumatic injury. Assessment of neurological deficits or changes in functional activity establishes the indications for neurosurgical intervention. The scope of neurosurgery is broad to include: removal of pathological lesions; relief of pain, spasm, or other neurophysiological conditions; and repair of nerve injuries and tissue defects.

HISTORICAL DEVELOPMENT

The earliest time when operative procedures were done is not known, but evidence exists in trephined skulls from prehistoric burial sites. It is possible that these trephines were done to let out evil spirits. This may be considered the forerunner of psychosurgery to treat mental illness by frontal leukotomy or topectomy, procedures rarely performed since the advent of tranquilizing drugs.

The Smith Papyrus from Egypt, from the seventeenth century B.C., describes treatment of head and vertebral column injuries as well as methods of holding wound edges together. Ancient Greeks and Romans used cranial instruments. Hippocrates described the use of a trephine to treat headache. He also treated skull fractures, epilepsy, and blindness.

Surgery of the nervous system advanced slowly through the centuries. Cranial surgery, for example, was limited until the 1880s to treating trauma or trephining to evacuate pus or blood. The first brain tumor was removed in England in 1884 by Sir Rickman Goodlee. In 1887, W. W. Keen of Philadelphia was the first surgeon in the United States to excise a tumor from the brain.

Sir Charles Sherrington (1857–1952) was a pioneer in the study of the physiology of the spinal cord. In 1887, Sir Victor Horsley (1857–1916) removed a spinal cord tumor. Subsequently Horsley attempted operations on the brain. He was the first to approach the pituitary gland. He may be considered the first neurosurgeon.

The recognized father of modern neurosurgery, however, is Harvey W. Cushing (1869–1939). Among his many accomplishments, Cushing described the relation of intracranial pressure to blood pressure in 1900 and, in 1932, pituitary basophilism, commonly known as *Cushing's disease.* He established at Harvard the first school of neurosurgery, which led to development of a discipline recognized throughout the world.

Application of increasing knowledge of neurophysiology and advances in diagnostic methods, such as those of W. E. Dandy and A. E. Moniz prior to impact of computerized axial tomography, led to success of intracranial and intraspinal operations. Stereotaxis led to development of less-destructive techniques to replace some extensive invasive procedures and to treatment of some otherwise inoperable lesions. Use of lasers has further enhanced neurosurgery. The operating microscope opened up a new field of microneurosurgery that has created interest in cerebral revascularization techniques previously unattempted, and offers advantages in operative management of many other pathological lesions. Sophistication in physiologic monitoring has advanced these therapeutic modalities.

DIAGNOSTIC PROCEDURES

Computerized tomography (CT scanning) provides safe and accurate diagnoses of many disorders in the central nervous system. Several forms of scanning are used. Water-soluble contrast agents are injected into subarachnoid space to define intracranial and intraspinal cerebrospinal fluid pathways. Positron-emission tomography assists with morphologic study of brain metabolism and cerebral blood flow. Single-photon tomography provides a simple study of cerebral biochemistry.

Cerebral angiography has been an important diagnostic tool since its introduction in 1927. Newer techniques include digital subtraction angiography for visualizing and evaluating vascular disorders.

Developments in technology of CT scanning have obviated the need in some patients for invasive x-ray studies, such as pneumoencephalogram, ventriculogram, myelogram, and arteriogram. Nuclear magnetic resonance (NMR) imaging provides views of brain and skull similar to CT scans but without radiation. (Refer to Chapter 20 for discussion of these diagnostic procedures.)

SPECIAL CONSIDERATIONS IN NEUROSURGERY

Neurosurgical procedures are classified according to anatomic location of the nervous system involved: brain and cranial nerves; spinal cord and nerve roots; and autonomic and somatic peripheral nerves. Regardless of location of operative site, neural tissue must be handled gently to minimize functional disability of surgical trauma. Hemostasis is a critical factor to sustain vital functions of circulation and respiration. Visibility of structures in the operative site must also be assured.

Hemostatic Agents

Refer to Chapter 17 for a complete description of the methods of hemostasis. The hemostatic agents commonly used by the neurosurgeon for most procedures include the following.

Bone Wax Victor Horsley discovered the value of beeswax to seal bleeders in bone during his animal experiments in 1885. Now supplied as a refined blend of beeswax and a synthetic ester, bone wax is used on cranial and vertebral bones.

Compressed Absorbent Patties Made of rayon, cotton, or polyester, patties rather than mesh gauze sponges are used on fragile, delicate neural tissues to absorb blood and fluids. They also are used for protection of wound edges and for hemostasis. An assortment of sizes are moistened with saline and pressed out flat on a solid surface easily accessible to the neurosurgeon. Although they have no loose fibers, they could pick up lint if placed on a towel. Moisture must not soak through drapes.

Policy for sponge counts may include counting these patties. They must be retrieved before the operative site is closed. Some neurosurgeons use only patties with a thread securely attached to each one. This reminds surgeon that they are in the wound and facilitates their removal. They should be x-ray detectable.

Gelatin Sponge or Microfibrillar Collagen Chemical hemostatic agents may be used following resection to control bleeding from large vessels, sinuses, or surface of a tumor bed. The scrub nurse must moisten gelatin sponge with normal saline or thrombin before handing it to the neurosurgeon. Microfibrillar collagen is applied dry. Tips of tissue forceps should be dry to prevent this substance from adhering to them.

Ligating Clips Clips are applied on larger vessels where electrocoagulation would be insufficient or its thermal effect would be hazardous. Some clips, such as intracranial aneurysm clips, are specifically designed only for neurosurgical use. Each type and size clip requires a specific applier.

Electrosurgery Small vessels are coagulated. Current frequently is conducted through hemostatic forceps, fine smooth-tipped tissue forceps, or metal suction tip to bleeding vessels. A combination of suction-fulguration tip may be used.

Lasers Argon, carbon dioxide, and Nd:YAG lasers are selectively used in neurosurgery in conjunction with the operating microscope and stereotaxis (see p. 553). Each type has benefits, but all have definite limitations. Depending on the type of laser (see Chap. 19) and the location and type of tumor or vascular lesion, the laser may vaporize, shrink, or coagulate tissue. Precise hemostasis, minimal damage to contiguous structures, and visualization of effects are definite advantages of laser surgery for removal of brain and spinal cord tumors. Lasers are also used to assist in microvascular anastomoses.

Cryosurgery Some brain tumors may be frozen with a cryoprobe and then removed by dissection, although this is done infrequently. Cryohypophysectomy is most common cryosurgical procedure (see p. 554).

Ultrasonic Aspirator Although not technically a method of hemostasis, ultrasonic emulsification and aspiration devices divide and remove tissue with minimal bleeding. The emulsification process assists in hemostasis of small vessels. The technique can be used to debulk or remove benign tumors in relatively inaccessible areas of the brain and intramedullary spinal cord. The high-frequency sound waves of the ultrasonic probe, commonly called a Cavitron, virtually sweep tumor from adjacent structures, such as nerves and blood vessels. The tumor is emulsified and removed by suction. Various settings on the instrument allow the surgeon to adjust for removal of firm or calcified tumor or soft masses. Ultrasonic probes are also used on exposed dura mater to localize small intracranial tumors.

Interventional Neuroradiology Under fluoroscopy, a team of neurosurgeon and neuroradiologist may insert a percutaneous transfemoral catheter into a strategic point in the intracranial circulation feeding an arteriovenous malformation, an aneurysm, or a vascular occlusion. A substance, such as silicone or isobutyl 2-cyanoacrylate, or a detachable microballoon is injected to effectively embolize the lesion or its major deep-feeding arteries. This facilitates surgical resection of the lesion by minimizing potential hemorrhage. The intravascular procedure may be done preoperatively or intraoperatively.

Adjuncts to Visibility

Neural tissues must be as clean, dry, and visible as possible without damaging them. Visibility is enhanced by the following procedures.

Irrigation Most wounds are irrigated frequently with normal saline or lactated Ringer's solution. The scrub nurse should keep a bulb syringe filled ready for use. The solution must be maintained at room to body temperature. A thermometer in the basin of solution helps provide a safety check.

Suction Suction is necessary to evacuate blood, cerebrospinal fluid, and irrigating fluid from the operative site so that the neurosurgeon can identify structures. Necrotic tissue, pus, or cystic matter may also be aspirated. Usually a Ferguson-Frazier tip is used. Caution is taken to avoid applying vacuum directly on normal neural tissue, especially brain tissue. This tissue is protected by compressed absorbent patties. Suction must be available for all neurosurgical operations.

Retractors A variety of self-retaining retractors are used to retract scalp or skin and muscles. Dura mater is usually retracted with traction sutures. Blunt spatulas are used to retract brain tissue. Because visibility of structures is critical, retractors with a lighting system incorporated into them may be used, especially for intracranial operations.

Headlight A fiberoptic headlight is used by some neurosurgeons for supplemental lighting in the operative site.

Endoscope An endoscope with a fiberopic sideviewing telescope may be used to enhance visibility at obscure angles in otherwise visually inaccessible areas. This endoscope is particularly useful to identify lesions in the sella turcica, cerebral aneurysms, and intervertebral discs, for example. An endoscope may be used for placement of electrodes for stimulators. The argon laser can be used through ventriculoscope for intraventricular obliteration of choroid plexus and intravascular treatment of lesions and neoplasms.

Operating Microscope The operating microscope provides an intense light as well as magnification for visualization of intracranial structures. Microsurgery (see Chap. 19) permits removal of tumors and vascular lesions inaccessible or inoperable by heretofore standard operative approaches. Although it is indirect, projection of operative site via video camera, attached to the microscope, onto a television screen provides a clear view for the assistant and scrub nurse.

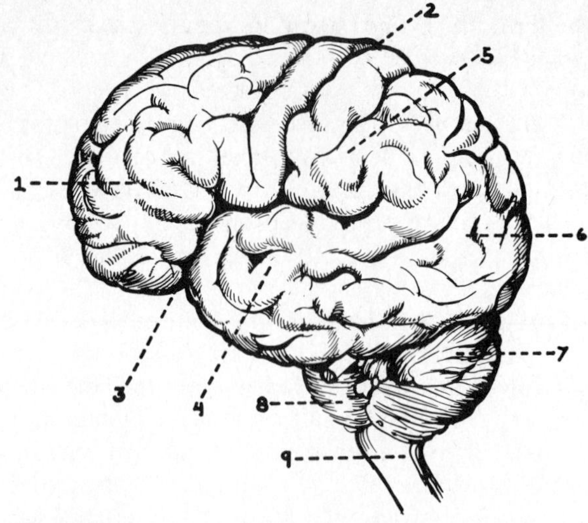

FIGURE 29-1
Left lateral view of cerebral hemisphere: (1) frontal lobe, (2) central fissure of Rolando, (3) lateral fissure of Sylvius, (4) temporal lobe, (5) parietal lobe, (6) occipital lobe, (7) cerebellum, (8) pons, (9) medulla oblongata.

CRANIAL SURGERY

Anatomic Approaches

An understanding of basic anatomy and physiology is essential for preparing for the approach the neurosurgeon will use to reach desired section of brain or a cranial nerve. The brain must be approached through the skull. Although several bones are fused together to protect and support the brain, the *skull* is described as divided into three areas: the anterior, middle, and posterior fossae. *Galea,* tough fascialike tissue over the skull, connects muscles of temples, forehead, and base of skull. The *scalp* (skin) covers the muscles and extracranial vessels and nerves in subcutaneous tissue.

The *meninges,* fibrous membranes, lying between the skull and brain are the dura mater, arachnoid, and pia mater. Cranial *dura mater,* firmly attached to the skull, has two layers that separate in planes to form venous sinuses. The *arachnoid,* which lies next to dura mater, has threadlike connections with the *pia mater,* which closely adheres to the brain. The *subarachnoid space* is formed between the arachnoid and pia mater. The *cortex* is the superficial outer layer of gray matter of the brain, often referred to as cerebral cortex or cerebellar cortex, depending on location. The *brain* has three distinct anatomical units that consist of several subdivisions, as shown in Fig. 29-1.

Cerebrum Consisting of two hemispheres, right and left, the cerebrum occupies most of the area within the skull. The brain in each hemisphere is divided into four lobes.

1 The *frontal lobe* lies within the anterior fossa.

2 The *parietal lobe* lies in the superior and anterior portion of the middle fossa.

3 The *temporal lobe* lies inferior to the frontal and parietal lobes within the middle fossa.

4 The *occipital lobe* lies posteriorly within the middle fossa.

The *hypothalmus* and *thalmus* also lie within the cerebrum. Although it lies in the sella turcica outside the cerebrum, the pituitary body attaches to the hypothalmus.

Cerebellum Also consisting of two hemispheres, the cerebellum lies below occipital lobes, posterior to brainstem, within the posterior fossa. It is about one-fifth the size of cerebrum.

Brainstem Including the midbrain, pons, and medulla oblongata, the brainstem lies anteriorly within the posterior fossa. It extends from the cerebral hemisphere to the base of the skull, where it merges with the spinal cord. It also contains the nuclei of 10 of the 12 pairs of cranial nerves, all except the olfactory (I) and optic (II) nerves.

Ventricles The lateral ventricles, one lying in each hemisphere, are within the cerebrum. These open into a central cavity, the third ventricle, which is connected by the aqueduct of Sylvius with the fourth ventricle lying anterior to the cerebellum and posterior to the brainstem. *Cerebrospinal fluid* produced in the choroid plexuses lining the ventricles circulates, through the subarachnoid space, around the meninges covering the brain and spinal cord to cushion these structures. Obstruction to flow of cerebrospinal fluid causes intracranial pressure.

General Considerations

1 Preparation of the patient in the OR usually begins with clipping hair. Hair usually can be removed from a male patient with electric clippers. A female head is shaved after initial hair removal with clippers. The neurosurgeon or assistant usually removes it. Hair on the head is considered the patient's personal property. When all of it must be removed, it is saved unless permission is granted by the patient to destroy it.

2 Location of the intended line of incision determines the headrest that will be needed to position patient. The basic unit of a neurosurgical headrest attaches in place of the head piece on the standard operating table. The headrest stabilizes and supports the head. If the patient will be in supine position, the configuration of the headrest contours to the back of the head. For prone position, the padded headrest equalizes weight distribution around the face.

Fowler's or sitting position may be desired. The headrest is attached at the head end of the operating table to support the back of the head for a unilateral or nasal approach. For a posterior fossa approach, the headrest is attached to a cross-bar attachment placed in the stirrup holders on the table. The forehead is supported. A special neurosurgical chair may be used.

The circulating nurse must be familiar with the neurosurgical headrest attachments for each desired position. The supine position is used most commonly for approaches to the frontal, parietal, and temporal lobes within the anterior and middle fossae. Lateral position may be preferred for some operations. Prone position is used to reach the occipital lobe. It may also be used for a suboccipital approach, but most neurosurgeons prefer the sitting position to approach the posterior fossa.

3 Infiltration of a local anesthetic agent beneath the scalp is desirable for many intracranial procedures. The scalp, extracranial arteries, and portions of the dura mater are the only structures covering the brain that are sensitive to pain. Epinephrine may be added to the agent to prolong its effectiveness and to constrict superficial blood vessels. The anesthetic may be injected before the patient is prepped and draped.

4 Administration of general anesthetic agents via endotracheal tube may be preferred for extensive intracranial operations, although the skull and brain are insensitive to pain. The patient is positioned after he or she is anesthetized, before prepping and draping.

5 Anticipation of difficulty in achieving hemostasis by the methods previously discussed is not unusual for some operations to remove vascular intracranial lesions. Controlled hypotension may be initiated by the anesthesiologist, with the concurrence of the neurosurgeon, to lower blood pressure (refer to Chap. 13). Hypothermia with elective circulatory arrest, via femoral artery cannulation, is an alternative when conventional approaches to control of blood loss would be unsatisfactory. Hypothermia decreases cellular metabolism and therefore oxygen consumption of the brain and heart during interruption of circulation.

6 Prevention of cerebral edema during repair of cranial injuries may be accomplished with hypothermia. Hypothermia may also be used to decrease cerebral blood flow and venous pressure, and to decrease brain volume and intracranial pressure (refer to Chap. 13). Patients are cooled either by surface-induced hypothermia, bloodstream cooling, or a combination of both.

7 Prevention of potential air embolism in patients in Fowler's or sitting position must be considered. The brain is higher than the heart in these positions. Venous pressure may be lower than atmospheric and can allow for entry of air into the heart via an open venous channel. An antigravity suit may be used (refer to Chap. 17, p. 335). This extends from the patient's rib margin to the ankles, and is inflated if the patient becomes hypotensive. In lieu of a G-suit, antiembolic stockings are worn. If the Gardner-Wells frame with pin fixation is used, antibiotic ointment is applied around each fixation pin to form an airtight seal. This reduces risk of air embolism and infection.

8 Reduction of intracranial pressure and brain volume may be accomplished by withdrawing spinal fluid. An intrathecal catheter or Tuohy needle is inserted, before prepping and draping, for the anesthesiologist to remove cerebrospinal fluid during operation as desired by the neurosurgeon.

9 Demarcation of the desired outline for the incision may be made on the scalp after the skin prep, prior to draping. A sterile disposable skin marker is available.

10 Instrumentation is usually arranged on a large table over the patient in supine or prone position. The scrub nurse must stand on a tiered platform to easily set up and reach the instruments for the neurosurgeon. The drapes over the head are attached to the table drapes (refer to Chap. 16, p. 319 for procedure). A one-piece sheet that provides a combined sterile table cover and the patient's cranial drape with a self-adhering incise area is available.

A double Mayo stand setup is usually preferred if the patient will be in Fowler's or sitting position. These Mayo stands are placed above and lateral to drapes over the patient. Mayo stands are also used for microneurosurgical procedures.

11 Armamentarium may include air-powered instruments for cutting through the skull. For cranial surgery, a dura guard attachment must be used to protect the dura mater.

12 Prevention of sudden movement around the surgeon and bumping the operating table or microscope is crucial. A slip of the surgeon's hand under the operating microscope or in the cranial cavity could be fatal for the patient.

Physiologic Monitoring

Cerebral edema (brain swelling), cerebral arterial perfusion, and intracranial pressure can be safely controlled before, during, and after operation. These parameters must be continously monitored, however. Function or organic activity of the brain may be monitored by *electroencephalogram* periodically throughout operation (see Chap. 14, p. 272). Sterile subdermal needle electrodes may be used, if surface scalp electrodes cannot be used.

A *Doppler ultrasound* transducer is secured over the precordium to continuously monitor patient in sitting position for gas entrapment or air embolism. An altered ultrasound response results if air is present in right atrium.

Evoked Responses *Somatosensory evoked potentials* guide anesthesiologist in handling arterial blood pressure, ventilation, inspired oxygen concentration, or patient positioning. Changes in cortical evoked potentials can indicate cerebral ischemia and systemic hypoxia. Both cortical and subcortical sensory evoked potentials can show operative invasion of spinal cord, peripheral nerve, nerve plexus, brainstem, or midbrain. The surgeon may adjust retractors, alter approach to a tumor, or perform subtotal tumor resection based on changes in evoked potentials to avert permanent injury. The anesthesiologist may adjust depth of anesthesia.

Auditory brainstem evoked potentials, with stimulus to the ear, may be used to monitor the eighth cranial nerve and brainstem during operative procedures in the posterior fossa, if performed under local anesthesia.

Intracranial Pressure Intracranial pressure (ICP) rises with an increase in volume of the brain, cerebrospinal fluid (CSF), and/or cerebral blood supply, or with decompensation, the inability to compensate for pressure changes. In adults, normal ICP ranges from 10 to 20 mm Hg (or 13 to 27 cm H_2O). When an abnormal elevation is sustained, intracranial pressure prevents adequate perfusion of cerebral cortex. The brain is deprived of blood supply. Pressure monitoring is the only exact method to determine rise in ICP and impending neurologic crisis during cranial operations or following head injury. ICP monitoring is accomplished by implanting a ventricular catheter, subarachnoid screw, or epidural sensor.

A ventricular catheter is the most-invasive but most-accurate method of *intracranial pressure monitoring.* The cannula and reservoir are inserted into ventricle through a twist drill hole in the skull. Proper positioning of stopcocks is important as incorrect placement may result in excessive CSF drainage with sudden drop in ICP and possible brain herniation. This method evaluates volume/pressure responses and permits drainage of large amounts of CSF and installation of contrast media and antibiotics. Catheter patency must be checked frequently and patient observed for signs of infection, such as meningitis or ventriculitis.

A hollow steel subarachnoid screw is placed in subdural space via a twist drill hole in skull and a small incision in dura mater. While measuring ICP accurately and directly from CSF, this method cannot drain large amounts of fluid, but provides access for CSF sampling. The screw may become occluded with blood or tissue. It must be checked frequently for patency.

A small epidural sensor is implanted in epidural space of brain through a small burr hole in the skull. The sensor is attached to a transducer, which converts CSF pressure to electrical impulses. The sensor cable is plugged into a monitor, from which a continuous readout is observed. This is the least-invasive method of ICP monitoring, but it is of questionable accuracy.

Craniectomy

Craniectomy is removal (*-ectomy*) of a portion of the bones of the skull (*cranium*). Bone must be perforated or removed to approach the brain. This may be accomplished through one or more burr holes or twist drill holes. Each hole is drilled manually with a Hudson brace and burr or with an electric or air-powered instrument. *Burr holes* are approximately ½ in. (13 mm) in diameter. Some diagnostic and therapeutic procedures are performed through them. Additional bone may be removed with a rongeur to increase exposure of the brain for more extensive procedures, such as an approach to the cranial nerves or tumors in the posterior fossa or suboccipital region.

Bone may be cut between the burr holes with a flexible multifilament wire (Gigli saw) or air-powered craniotome. This is performed to raise a large area of bone for temporary or permanent removal. Attached to the muscle, which acts as a hinge, the bone may be turned back to expose the underlying dura. This is referred to as raising a *bone flap.*

Burr holes may be plugged with a soft, pliable silicone, disc-shaped cover, with or without a channel for introduction of a hypodermic needle. The cover may be used to eliminate a cosmetically undesirable indentation of scalp into the created bone defect. Postoperative access to the cranial cavity through the hole or channel in the cover can be used for drainage of fluid or installation of chemotherapeutic drugs. Intracranial pressure monitoring devices can also be attached.

Electrode plates of a brain pacemaker or cerebellar stimulator are implanted through small occipital and suboccipital craniectomies. Silicone-coated polyester fiber mesh plates, each with four pairs of platinum-disc electrodes, are applied to the anterior and posterior surfaces of the cerebellum. One or two receivers, implanted just below the clavicle prior to the craniectomies, are attached to the electrodes on the cerebellum by subcutaneously placed leads. Stimulation of the pacemaker electrodes is controlled by an external transmitter through an antenna placed on the skin over the subdermal receiver. This device is used to control muscular hypertonia and seizures related to cerebral palsy, epilepsy, stroke, or brain injury.

Craniotomy

Scalp, bone, and dural flaps are raised to expose a large area of the cerebrum for exploration, definitive treatment, or excision of lesions within the brain. The three semicircular or U-shaped flaps are turned in opposite directions. Hemostatic forceps or compression clips designed to control bleeding from the scalp are applied to the galea and over the edge of the skin flap. The bone flap is turned as described for craniectomy. Moistened sponges protect both the scalp and bone flaps. The dural flap is protected with large compressed patties. For wound closure, the thin but tough fibrous dural flap is laid over the brain. Usually it is sutured with many interrupted stitches to provide a tight seal that prevents leakage of cerebrospinal fluid. The bone flap may be anchored with stainless steel suture or silicone burr hole buttons. The galea is closed with interrupted sutures before the scalp is sutured or approximated with staples.

A silicone rubber suction drain may be placed in the subdural space to drain residual fluid from a subdural hematoma or the bed of a brain tumor, or to remove red blood cells in cerebrospinal fluid after craniotomy.

Intracranial tumors can originate from the neural tissues of the brain itself, the meninges, glandular tissue, choroid plexuses, cranial nerves, blood vessels, embryonal defects, or metastatic lesions. A craniotomy may be performed to remove a circumscribed, encapsulated, slow-growing, benign brain tumor. Some of these tumors, such as a meningioma, are highly vascular. Primary or metastatic malignant tumors are broadly classified as *gliomas.* These have an unregulated cellular proliferation of rapidly growing cells, which invade surrounding brain tissue. *Glioblastoma multiforme* is the most common and most malignant type of brain tumor. Due to the hemorrhagic and edematous effects of a rapidly growing tumor, a lobectomy may be performed to give the brain area for expansion and to impede mortality. The rigid characteristics of the skull prevent its expansion or contraction; however, the brain can expand or contract. Subdural decompression by craniectomy to reduce intracranial pressure and papilledema may be the palliative procedure of choice. By anatomic location, some benign tumors are considered malignant because they cannot be safely removed without severe neurological deficits or threat to life-sustaining functions. Microneurosurgery and stereotaxis (see p. 553) provide access to tumors in some anatomic locations that are otherwise impossible to reach, such as in third ventricle and pineal regions.

Cranioplasty

Traumatic or surgically created skull defects are corrected with autogenous bone grafts or a synthetic or metallic prosthesis. Large defects in the anterior or middle fossae are covered for protection of the brain and cosmetic effect. The bone flap may be removed following intracranial operation to allow cerebral decompression postoperatively. It is stored under sterile conditions in the bone bank until it can be positioned in the skull.

Bone removed because of an extensively comminuted fracture or bone disease may be replaced with methyl methacrylate. This material contours better than preformed metal plates. The resin powder is mixed with the liquid polymer to form a doughy mass. This is placed in a sterile plastic bag and rolled to the thickness of the skull with a roller. While still pliable, it is molded to the contour of the head and the size of the defect. When hardened, it can be trimmed with a rongeur and the edges smoothed with a special small emery wheel mounted on the electric bone saw. The prosthesis is wired to the skull in several places. The brain expands to meet it and leaves no dead space between it and the dura.

> NOTE. The outside of the ampuls of resin powder and liquid polymer and the mixing bag must be sterile. They can be sterilized in ethylene oxide gas or immersed for ten hours in glutaraldehyde solution. The roller and emery wheel can be steam sterilized.

Dural defects can be closed with autogenous fascia graft, fibrin film, polyethylene film, synthetic absorbable mesh, or freeze-dried human cadaver dura mater grafts. A trimmed and measured piece of dura mater is freeze-dried, sterilized by exposure to ethylene oxide, and stored in a vacuum container. This may be stored at room temperature indefinitely provided vacuum is maintained. The graft is reconstituted by the addition of saline to the container for a minimum of 30 minutes. The majority of these grafts are used for closure of dural defects, but may also be used to repair abdominal and thoracic wall defects.

Intracranial Microneurosurgery

The magnification and lighting afforded by the operating microscope have refined techniques and made possible approaches to many neurologic problems. Refer to Chapter 19 for discussion of the operating microscope. A laser may be adapted to the microscope for ablation of benign or malignant intracranial tumors. Some other microneurosurgical procedures include the following.

Excision of Acoustic Neuroma Middle fossa or translabyrinthine approaches may be used by otologists for removal of small acoustic neuromas confined in the internal auditory canal (refer to Chap. 26, p. 505). A neurosurgeon resects an acoustic neuroma that more commonly extends into the cranial cavity. An acoustic neuroma can grow progressively into the trigeminal, facial, and abducens nerves, and into the cerebellopontine angle (the area between the pons, medulla oblongata, and cerebellum). Potentially life-threatening, symptoms of these involvements are manifested by facial weakness, paresthesia, and dysphagia.

The suboccipital retrolabyrinthine approach is preferred by most neurosurgeons. The patient is placed in semi-Fowler's or sitting position, using the Gardner-Wells frame with pin fixation. This position provides good exposure but has the potential risk of air embolism. The operating microscope offers the potential for preservation of functional hearing. Particular caution must be taken to obtain meticulous hemostasis, spare the auditory artery if hearing is to be preserved, and avoid trauma to or resection of the facial nerve. It is impossible, however, to salvage facial nerve function in a percentage of patients. If the facial nerve is sacrificed, the patient may return for a facial-hypoglossal or facial-accessory nerve anastomosis four to six weeks postoperatively.

Transtemporal approaches or a transtentorial (subtemporal) approach may be preferred. The patient remains in a supine position for the latter procedure. The surgeon's decision to preserve or sacrifice the facial nerve and/or hearing will influence approach to an acoustic neuroma.

Decompression of Cranial Nerves Microsurgical exploration of cranial nerves with definitive decompression relieves the severe and disabling symptoms of some cranial nerve disorders such as trigeminal or glossopharyngeal neuralgia, acoustic nerve dysfunction, and hemifacial spasm. Initial symptoms of hyperactivity in a cranial nerve can progress to loss of function. Some disorders are due to mechanical cross-compression, usually vascular, of the nerve root at the brainstem. Symptoms are dependent on the sensory and/or motor functions of the nerve.

With the patient in sitting position, a retromastoid craniectomy is performed to explore the cerebellopontine angle. A supracerebellar exposure is used for the trigeminal nerve, and an infracerebellar exposure for the remainder of the cranial nerves. An artery or vein compressing the nerve root may be mobilized away from the nerve. A tiny piece of Silastic sponge may be placed between the vessel and nerve to relieve the pulsating pressure on the nerve. A tissue sling may be created to lift the vessel off the nerve. Preoperatively undiagnosed tumors are excised. If vascular decompression or other pathology is not evident, the nerve may be sectioned to relieve pain.

Cerebral Revascularization Anastomosis of an extracranial artery to an intracranial artery for bypass of stenotic or occlusive vascular disease distal to bifurcation of the common carotid provides an additional and significant source of blood to the cerebral circulation. An artery in the scalp such as the superficial temporal, occipital, or another branch of the external carotid artery is anastomosed to a branch of the middle cerebral artery or a cortical branch of the cerebral. Vessels must be 1 mm in diameter or larger. The procedure is primarily prophylactic to prevent development of a major stroke in patients who have had transient ischemic attacks or minor strokes with temporary disruption of brain function due to blockage of the cerebral vascular system.

The patient is positioned supine with head turned or laterally with head stabilized flat on operating table for an approach through a temporal craniectomy. The anastomosis is made on surface of the brain either end-to-end, side-to-side, or end-to-side of arteries.

In some patients, plaque can be removed from the middle cerebral artery rather than bypassing the occlusion. Cerebral embolectomy with detachable balloon, or other intravascular technique may be done to obliterate carotid-cavernous fistula or arteriovenous malformation in conjunction with extracranial-intracranial arterial bypass. Because these operations take seven to ten hours or longer to complete, the circulating nurse must check pressure points on patient's body to prevent peripheral nerve and circulatory damage.

Occlusion of Aneurysms Aneurysms of the cerebral and vertebral arteries vary from the size of a pea to the size of an orange. Most intracranial aneurysms are located near the basilar surface of the skull and arise from the internal carotid or middle cerebral arteries. Cerebral artery (berry) aneurysms are usually located on the circle of Willis at the base of the brain between the hemispheres of the cerebrum. Most aneurysms are associated with a congenital defect of the media of the intracranial vessel wall. Hemodynamic forces of pulsatile pressure cause enlargement, outpouching, and thinning of the arterial wall, which eventually ruptures. This is the most common source of subarachnoid hemorrhage. The majority of aneurysms seal spontaneously, but operation may be indicated to prevent rebleed. If diagnosed, an unruptured asymptomatic aneurysm may be operated prior to rupture.

With the patient in sitting position for suboccipital or subfrontal craniectomy, the aneurysm is exposed for occlusion. The neck (base) is occluded with low-pressure aneurysm clip or ligated if it can be isolated. If it cannot be isolated, the aneurysm and parent vessel may be wrapped in fine mesh gauze and coated with methyl methacrylate, isobutyl 2-cyanoacrylate, or other epoxy resin to reinforce the wall. More commonly the aneurysm is coagulated with bipolar electrosurgery or laser. Induced hypotension may be used to decrease blood flow in the artery feeding the aneurysm. This aids in dissection and occlusion. The operating microscope is used for delicate dissection of the arteries at the base of the brain.

Stereotaxis

Stereotaxis is the accurate location of a definite circumscribed area within the brain from external points or landmarks on the skull. It defines three-dimensional coordinates (planes) to approach deep structures without damaging overlying structures. The technique is used to create or ablate a lesion in otherwise inaccessible parts of the brain. By determining specific reference points on CT scan and x-ray, the exact area for target site of the lesion is calculated. A lesion may be made by laser; high-frequency or radio-frequency electrocoagulation; freezing (cryosurgery); ultrasound; injection of a chemical or radioactive substance;

or mechanical curettage. Operations are performed under local anesthesia when patient cooperation to test motor or sensory function may be needed during operation.

A *stereoencephalotome,* a specially designed mechanical apparatus, is attached to the skull. After this is in place, computerized tomograph (CT scan) shows localizers of the apparatus in relation to intracranial structures. The ventricular system provides the internal landmarks, verified by ventriculogram (x-ray). Of the many models available, three basic types of stereoencephalotomes are used. Nursing personnel must know how to sterilize and assemble the apparatus, and must prepare necessary instrumentation. The patient is in sitting position for fixation of stereoencephalotome.

1 *Semicircle arc system.* Steel screws are tapped through each of four burr holes for fixation of head to a ring supported from a pedestal on the floor. The ring is secured to arc plates. The head rather than the apparatus is moved.

2 *Rectilinear system.* Apparatus is securely applied to skull by attachment to burr holes. It can be moved back and forth and side to side around head to make adjustments.

3 *Single arc system.* An arc over the head is securely attached to burr holes. Angular adjustments can be made.

A burr hole is made for positioning the instrument that will be used at the target site. Another burr hole may be needed for a Scott ventricular cannula for ventriculogram. The CT scanner can be used with a stereoencephalotome or apparatus built into the scanner.

Thalamotomy The forerunner of other stereotactic procedures, thalamotomy may be done to relieve involuntary tremor or rigidity of muscles, to reduce intractable pain, or to control functional psychotic behavior.

Cingulotomy Cingulotomies are appropriate treatment for relief of pain of benign etiology that has not responded to other methods of treatment. The *cingulum* is a bundle of connecting fibers in medial aspect of each cerebral hemisphere, between the frontal and temporal lobes. Bilaterally symmetrical radio-frequency lesions are placed to disrupt pathways.

Electrostimulation Intermittent electrostimulation of brain by stereotactically implanted electrodes can control a variety of intractable pain problems. One electrode is placed in the somatosensory system to evaluate pain of central origin, and another in the paraventricular gray matter for pain of peripheral origin. Following postoperative evaluation of the effectiveness of electric stimulation of each electrode, the patient returns to the OR to have a receiver placed under skin on the anterior chest wall. A connecting wire is tunneled from receiver to electrode. An external transmitter and antenna placed over the receiver stimulate the electrode as desired by patient.

Radio-Frequency Retrogasserian Rhizotomy Radio-frequency retrogasserian rhizotomy relieves the pain of trigeminal neuralgia, also known as *tic douloureux.* The fifth cranial nerve, the trigeminal, carries sensory impulses for touch, pain, and external temperature from the face, scalp, and mucous membranes in the head. Trigeminal neuralgia is an intense paroxysmal pain in one side of the face. It can be controlled by damaging the gasserian (trigeminal) ganglion.

The patient lies in supine position. Using x-rays for control, an insulated cannula with an uninsulated tip is placed through the cheek and foramen ovale and is advanced to the gasserian ganglion. The ganglion is coagulated when a radio-frequency generator activates the tip of the cannula. Several lesions can be made to achieve the desired extent of paresthesia.

Cryohypophysectomy The cryosurgical probe is introduced into the sella turcica through a frontal burr hole. Cryogenic lesions may be the procedure of choice for treating growth-hormone-producing pituitary adenomas with no suprasellar extension. During creation of lesion, ocular movements and visual acuity are carefully monitored.

Intracranial Neoplasms Using CT scan for stereotactic guidance, a tumorscope is introduced through brain tissue to margin of a deep-seated intracranial tumor. A forceps may be inserted to obtain a biopsy. Then a laser beam can be directed through scope to destroy tumor while preserving normal cerebral tissue. The debris is evacuated through the tumorscope.

Interstitial Radiation Radioactive substances may be stereotactically implanted into malignant brain tumors. A computerized tomograph assists in directing stereotactic instrument to center of tumor. Radioactive iodine 125 or an activated hematoporphyrin derivative may be used. The latter is activated by argon or tunable laser to create a cytotoxic photochemical reaction in tumor cells.

Intracranial Vascular Lesions Thrombosis of a cerebral aneurysm can be accomplished by a stereotactic magnetic-metallic technique. Tiny particles of iron are injected through a magnetic field into the aneurysm. The purpose is to reinforce the wall of the aneurysm by forming a firm scar that will not grow.

Embolization of arteriovenous malformations are also performed for large dural and many otherwise inoperable cerebral arteriovenous malformations. Some aneurysms or arteriovenous malformations can be electrocoagulated, coagulated with argon laser, vaporized with carbon dioxide laser, or clipped through stereotactic instruments.

Extracranial Operations

The cranial procedures previously discussed include access to the operative site through the skull. A few cranial neurosurgical procedures do not require craniectomy or intracranial incision.

External Occlusion of Carotid Artery When an internal carotid or middle cerebral artery aneurysm cannot be reached or controlled by other operative techniques, a carotid clamp can be applied extracranially in the neck. Progressive turns on the clamp over several days cause it to occlude the carotid artery gradually until compete occlusion of blood supply to the aneurysm is accomplished.

Transsphenoidal Operations As a palliative operation, *hypophysectomy,* the enucleation of the pituitary gland, may be performed for pain relief and endocrine ablation in patients with disseminated metastatic carcinoma of the breast or prostate gland, or to relieve intractable pain from other types of disseminated carcinoma. The microsurgical transsphenoidal approach also is used for removal of intrapituitary tumors or other lesions within the region of the sella turcica, a cavity of the sphenoid bone. Visual loss and endocrinopathy are the main symptoms of pituitary tumor. Tumor tissue in the sella turcica is distinguished both by color and texture from the normal firm, yellowish anterior and red-gray posterior lobes of the pituitary.

Patient is placed in semi-Fowler's position with head slightly flexed and tilted so that patient's body is out of the way when the neurosurgeon sits in front of face to work in median sagittal plane. The image intensifier is positioned lateral to patient's head with horizontal beam centered on the sella turcica. A television monitor is placed behind and just above patient's head, so that surgeon can look at screen in line with binocular of the microscope. Televised radio-fluoroscopy is used as an aid in placing instruments and resecting tissue. The image intensifier is switched on and off, as needed, to minimize exposure to radiation.

The floor of the sella turcica is exposed through the sphenoid sinus. A horizontal incision is made under upper lip, at junction of gingiva, and carried deep to bone of the maxilla. Soft tissues are elevated; bone and nasal cartilage are resected. The resected nasal cartilage is preserved on instrument table for possible replacement. A specially designed nasal speculum is inserted in the oral incision to visualize the sphenoid sinus. This is opened widely until floor of sella turcica can be identified. The floor is opened with an air-powered drill. The microscope is brought into position for visualization of pituitary and other structures and lesions inside and around the sella turcica.

Head Injuries

A patient with severe head injury requires *first* a patent airway. Relaxed jaw and tongue should be raised; if necessary, suction through the mouth. An endotracheal tube may be inserted. Ultimately a tracheotomy may be necessary.

Vital signs, blood pressure, dilatation of pupils, and level of consciousness are checked frequently. Osmotic dehydrating IV solution, such as mannitol, may be ordered to reduce cerebral edema if there is no evidence of intracranial hemorrhage. After these supportive measures have been carried out, definitive treatments are initiated.

1 Scalp lacerations are thoroughly cleansed, debrided, and sutured. The scalp is very vascular, so lacerations bleed profusely. Hypovolemic shock is rare, but possible.
2 Simple linear or comminuted fractures usually require no treatment. A depressed skull fracture must be elevated when bone is pressed 5 mm or more into any part of the brain.
3 A compound fracture requires debridement. The extent of operation will depend upon the specific extent of injury. Dura may need to be sutured. Some macerated brain tissue may have to be excised.

4 Intracranial hematoma may be present. Depending on location, intracranial hemorrhage may require immediate, emergency operation.

a *Epidural hematoma.* Bleeding due to rupture or tear of the middle meningeal artery, or its branches, forms a hematoma between the skull and dura. Usually associated with a skull fracture, symptoms of increased intracranial pressure due to rapid compression of the brain may occur immediately or within a few hours. When hemorrhage is arterial, the patient presents an extreme surgical emergency to evacuate the clot and clip or electrocoagulate the bleeding vessel through a burr hole or small craniectomy.

b *Subdural hematoma.* Bleeding between dura mater and arachnoid is usually caused by laceration of veins that cross the subdural space. A large encapsulated collection of blood over one or both cerebral hemispheres produces increased intracranial pressure and other neurologic changes. Onset and extent of these changes depends on cause, size, and rapidity of growth of the hematoma. Treatment may necessitate a burr hole. A bone flap may be raised if more extensive exploration is indicated. Subdural hematoma may be:

1 Acute. Usually due to arterial bleeding, symptoms occur rapidly. The vessel must be ligated with clips or electrocoagulated.

2 Subacute. Usually due to venous bleeding, symptoms appear within 24 to 48 hours to five days after injury.

3 Chronic. Symptoms do not appear until six or more months postinjury.

c *Intracerebral hematoma.* Tears in brain substance at the point of greatest impact most commonly occur in the anterior temporal and frontal lobes. Although usually absorbed, hematoma may require evacuation and debridement of necrotic tissue.

SPINAL SURGERY

The bony structure of the vertebral column extends from the foramen magnum at the base of the skull to the coccyx. The 33 vertebrae, which provide support for the body, vary in size and are classified according to location: the 7 cervical vertebrae are in the neck; the 12 thoracic vertebrae articulate with the ribs; the 5 lumbar vertebrae are posterior to the retroperitoneal cavity; the 5 sacral vertebrae are fused to form the sacrum; and the 4 fused coccygeal vertebrae form the coccyx. The spinal cord passes through a canal in the cervical and thoracic vertebrae to a level of the second or third lumbar vertebra. It terminates in a fibrous band that extends through the lumbar vertebrae and sacrum and attaches to the coccyx. Pairs of spinal nerve roots branch off to each side of the body from 31 segments of the spinal cord as it passes through the vertebrae. They carry sensory and motor impulses between the central nervous system and the peripheral nervous system.

Because of proximity of the vertebral column to the spinal cord, both neurosurgeons and orthopaedic surgeons perform operations in this area. They may work together as a multidisciplinary team. For example, the neurosurgeon may remove a herniated lumbar intervertebral disc and the orthopaedist will do the spinal fusion (refer to Chap. 24, p. 476). Only the most common operations for spinal lesions performed by the neurosurgeon will be described.

Laminectomy

Removal of the spinous process(es) and lamina from one of more vertebra is performed to expose an intervertebral or spinal cord lesion. A laminectomy is usually carried out through a vertical midline skin incision with patient in prone or lateral position. However, some neurosurgeons prefer a transverse skin incision with patient in modified prone position. Patient may be positioned on a Hastings frame to hyperextend the spine, to reduce epidural blood loss by lowering blood pressure in vena cava, and to reduce pressure on abdomen.

The extent of the incision will depend on the number of laminae to be removed. The fascia and muscles are retracted to expose spinous processes and laminae. These are cut off with a rongeur, as necessary for exposure of spinal cord dura, spinal nerve roots, or interlaminar lesion. An intervertebral disc, spinal cord tumor, bone fragments, and extradural or intradural foreign bodies may be removed after the laminectomy is completed.

Discectomy Herniated or ruptured intervertebral discs are the most common spinal problems seen by neurosurgeons. Most of these occur in the lower lumbar and lumbosacral regions and are traumatic in origin. Displaced intervertebral discs are rare in the thoracic area but do occur in the cervical spine. Normally intervertebral discs are held between each vertebral body by the annulus fibrosis and posterior longitudinal ligament. The disc itself is a fibrocartilaginous substance known as *nucleus pulposus.* Under stress of lifting or twisting, the nucleus pulposus can protrude through a tear in the annulus fibrosis and posterior ligament. The protrusion compresses the spinal nerve roots within the spinal canal against the vertebrae. This causes pain from the lumbar or sacral region to the lower back and radiating down the sciatic nerve pathway to one leg, or from the cervical region of the neck to an arm. At operation, the herniated nucleus pulposus or ruptured portion of the annulus fibrosis is excised.

A unilateral, one-level *microdiscectomy* may be performed under the operating microscope. This technique permits exposure of herniated nucleus pulposus without extensive manipulation of paraspinal muscles or removal of large section of lamina.

NOTE. As alternatives to surgical excision, chymopapain may be injected percutaneously into disc spaces (see Chap. 24, p. 476) or a percutaneous lumbar discectomy may be performed to treat selected patients. These procedures are done under fluoroscopy. In the latter, the herniated or protruding lumbar disc is removed through a small cannula placed in the disc capsule via a percutaneous channel.

Excision of Spinal Cord Tumor Primary tumors of the spinal cord include ependymoma, lipoma, meningioma, and neurofibroma. The posterior segment of the vertebral arch must be removed to expose dura over involved section of the spinal cord. The dura is incised and retracted with sutures. The tumor is excised and dura closed tightly to prevent leakage of cerebrospinal fluid. Both intrinsic and extrinsic spinal cord tumors can be removed by laser with decreased tissue trauma. The laser is especially useful in areas difficult to reach by dissection, such as the foramen magnum or anterior spinal cord.

Rhizotomy Anterior motor roots of spinal nerves can be divided to control the involuntary muscle contractions associated with torticollis and spastic paralysis. Cutting roots of cervical spinal nerves controlling the neck muscles, for example, relieves the muscular imbalance that causes the head to rotate intermittently and tilt significantly in patients with torticollis.

Treatment of Spinal Injuries Vertebral fractures, with or without dislocation, can cause spinal cord compression that denervates nerve tracts below the injury. Resultant paralysis may be relieved if operation is done within a very short time after injury. Results are frequently discouraging. Damage to the cord may be too extensive for return of function or, at best, only an incomplete return. Care must be taken in moving patient to avoid further paralysis.

A lumbar puncture with pressure readings may be done. If a block in flow of spinal fluid is present, a laminectomy is done to decompress the spinal cord in a patient with complete paralysis or partial paralysis that is becoming progressively worse. Laminectomy may also be done to remove bone fragments. Internal fixation may be combined with decompression for thoracic lumbar fractures.

Anterior Cervical and Thoracic Operations

The anterior cervical spine can be exposed through a transverse skin incision in the neck and dissection through the cleavage plane between the carotid artery and esophagus. The spinous processes and laminae remain intact. A ruptured intervertebral disc and/or a fracture-dislocation with bone fragments compressing the cervical spinal cord or nerve roots can be completely explored. Removal of the posterior margins of the vertebral bodies may be indicated to decompress the nerve root. The operating microscope is a valuable adjunct to anterior cervical intervertebral discectomy and for an anterior approach to other cervical spinal lesions. A bone graft may be placed between the vertebral bodies for interbody fusion, usually by an orthopaedic surgeon.

An anterior approach is also procedure of choice for thoracic vertebral disc herniations, spinal cord tumors, or fractures. A thoracic surgeon assists with a transthoracic approach. Fractured bone fragments can be stabilized by anterior spinal fusion or placement of posterior rods by costotransversectomy in thoracic region.

Cervical Traction

To stabilize the head and neck of a patient with cervical spine injury, traction is applied by means of a Sayre sling as an emergency measure. A Sayre sling is a canvas or leather halter that buckles around the neck and chin. The patient lies with head at the foot of the bed, to permit traction appliances to be attached to the footboard. Countertraction is accomplished by the weight of the patient, who rests in bed in semi-Fowler's position.

If patient has a cervical fracture and/or dislocation, the Sayre sling may be replaced, in the OR, by an appliance, such as Vinke or Crutchfield tongs, for skeletal traction. A sterile table setup with a dissecting set of instruments and a drill is necessary. Through a small incision over lateral parietal bones on each side of the head, holes are drilled in the skull for positioning the mechanical apparatus. Pins of Crutchfield tongs, when tightened, are controlled by a locking and positioning mechanism that forces points medially and upward away from the inner table of the skull. Traction is then transferred from Sayre sling to the tongs, giving the patient free movement of the jaw. The amount of weight applied to the tongs will depend on extent of injury and weight of patient. Halo traction allows patient to be ambulatory.

Relief of Intractable Pain

Many patients suffer intractable pain in advanced stages of some illnesses such as cancer, occlusive arterial disease, myelinating or degenerative diseases, or from some benign lesions. Intractable pain cannot be relieved satisfactorily by drugs without hazard of narcotic addiction or incapacitating sedation. Implantation of a continuous infusion pump for intraspinal administration of low doses of morphine may be procedure of choice, however, for chronic pain of malignant tumor origin. Other operative techniques may be indicated to interrupt the sensory fibers carrying pain sensations through the spinal cord to the brain.

Anterior Cervical Chordotomy Exposure of the cervical spinal cord, through an anterior approach, can be used to sever sensory fibers at the base of the brainstem. A microsurgical technique may be used for this procedure. Good relief from severe pain of advanced carcinoma may be achieved.

Commissural Myelotomy Commissural or sagittal midline myelotomy may be preferred to relieve intractable midline or bilateral pain in the lower half of the body. The sensory nerve fibers of the cervical or thoracic spinal cord are exposed and severed. The operating microscope is a valuable aid to the neurosurgeon in identifying the nerve tracts to be cut or resected.

Percutaneous Cervical Chordotomy To avoid an open operation, a percutaneous approach may be used to destroy sensory fibers. Under local anesthesia, a spinal needle is introduced just below the ear into a cervical interspace. The neurosurgeon avoids the pyramidal tract that carries motor impulses. The position of the needle is checked on x-ray or image intensifier. An electrode wire, inserted through the needle, is connected to a radio-frequency lesion generator. The fibers are destroyed when the positive charge is activated through the electrode. The patient retains sense of touch but not pain.

Electrostimulation Chronic intractable pain of organic origin may be relieved by electrostimulation in some selected patients. Fibers of the peripheral nerves conduct pain impulses to the spinal cord. These pain impulses can be blocked by induced electrostimulation that modifies the impulses transmitted from peripheral nerve receptors through the spinal cord to the brain. Electrodes to transmit an electric current to the spinal cord or peripheral nerve are placed transcutaneously or percutaneously or implanted.

Transcutaneous Electric Nerve Stimulation (TENS) TENS is applied to the surface of the skin over the spinal cord or a peripheral nerve. These devices are used for many types of chronic pain problems.

Percutaneous Stimulation Percutaneous stimulation is done by inserting an electrode into the spinal canal or subcutaneous tissue adjacent to the peripheral nerve. This is performed in the OR or radiology department under local anesthesia, fluoroscopic control, and sterile conditions. The patient is prepped and draped as for an invasive procedure. For spinal cord stimulation, two platinum-tipped electrodes are threaded cephalad through needles placed in the epidural space. After the electrodes are connected to a percutaneous transmitter, they are manipulated until the patient feels paresthesia in the desired area. When in the correct position, the electrodes are secured to the lumbodorsal fascia by Silastic patches. The distal ends are attached to a lead wire brought through the skin. This connects to an external transmitter for temporary stimulation. When conversion is to be made from temporary to permanent stimulation, the electrodes are attached to a receiver implanted in the lateral chest wall, usually on the left side midway between the axilla and waistline. An antenna, placed on the skin over the implanted receiver, connects to the external transmitter.

Dorsal Column Stimulator (DCS) DCS operates on the same principle as the percutaneous stimulator. However, a laminectomy must be performed to suture the electrode over the dorsal column of the spinal cord. For permanent peripheral nerve stimulation, the electrode is attached to a major sensory nerve. The receivers for these stimulators are implanted in subcutaneous tissues.

PERIPHERAL NERVE SURGERY

The peripheral nervous system includes the cranial nerves, spinal nerves, and autonomic nervous system located outside the central nervous system. *Ganglions,* a group of nerve cell bodies also located outside the CNS, can transmit either *autonomic* (involuntary) or *somatic* (both reflex and voluntary) impulses. *Somatic nerves* supply voluntary muscles, skin, tendons, joints, and other structures controlling the musculoskeletal system. *Afferent nerve fibers* carry sensory impulses from the organs and muscles to the CNS. *Efferent fibers* transmit motor impulses from the CNS back to them. Peripheral nerve operations are performed on both the autonomic and somatic nervous systems. The neurosurgeon may identify nerves and test function with a nerve stimulator before or after dissection or repair.

Autonomic Nervous System

The autonomic nervous system is an aggregation of ganglions, nerves, and plexuses through which the viscera, heart, blood vessels, smooth muscles, and glands receive motor innervation to function involuntarily. This system is divided into:

1 *Sympathetic nervous system.* This thoracolumbar division arising from the thoracic and first three lumbar segments of the spinal cord includes the ganglionated trunk near the spinal cord, plexuses, and the associated preganglionic and postganglionic nerve fibers. The efferent fibers transmit impulses that stimulate involuntary activity in the heart, blood vessels, smooth muscle of the viscera, and all glands in the body.

2 *Parasympathetic nervous system.* This craniosacral division includes the preganglionic fibers that leave the CNS with cranial nerves III (oculomotor), VII (facial), IX (glossopharyngeal), and X (vagus), and the first three sacral nerves, outlying ganglions near the viscera, and postganglionic fibers. In general, this system innervates the same structures but has a regulatory function opposite to that of the sympathetic nervous system. These efferent fibers act to restore stability for quieter activity.

Operations most frequently performed on the autonomic nervous system are discussed.

Sympathectomy Resection or division of the sympathetic ganglions and nerve fibers of the autonomic nervous system is performed in an attempt to increase peripheral circulation or to decrease pain of peripheral vascular disease or intractable pain of other organic origin. It may be an emergency procedure to relieve severe vasospasm following arterial embolism or freezing of an extremity. The paravertebral ganglionic chains and/or nerve fibers that innervate the affected area are resected or divided. The procedure may be termed *sympathetic ganglionectomy* or *splanchnicectomy,* but usually the operation is specified by the location of the ganglions and nerves. (General surgeons also perform some of the following operations.)

Upper Cervical Sympathectomy Upper cervical sympathectomy is done to increase blood supply in the internal carotid arteries. Through an anterior cervical approach in the neck, the superior cervical ganglion is resected. Ptosis of the eyelid may occur postoperatively because this ganglion innervates eyelid retraction.

Cervicothoracic Sympathectomy Cervicothoracic sympathectomy may aid the patient with Raynaud's disease of the upper extremities by relieving the chronic vasoconstrictive process. It may also be done to relieve angina pectoris or causalgia. Through a transaxillary-transpleural incision, the stellate ganglion of the middle cervical ganglionic chain is hemisected and the lower half resected along with the second through fifth thoracic nerve ganglions.

Thoracic Sympathectomy Thoracic sympathectomy is usually done for the relief of chronic intractable pain of biliary and pancreatic disease. Through a posterior paravertebral incision over the transverse processes of the thoracic vertebrae, the ganglions of the sixth through twelfth thoracic nerves are resected and the splanchnic nerves divided.

Thoracolumbar Sympathectomy Thoracolumbar sympathectomy is performed for the treatment of essential hypertension. Usually done in two stages, bilateral resection is necessary to reduce blood pressure by altering vascular tone and denervating the viscera. With the patient in prone or lateral position, a paravertebral incision parallel to the vertebral column extends from the ninth rib downward and then curves anteriorly toward the iliac crest. The lower half of the thoracic and the first through third lumbar chains with the ganglions and splanchnic nerves are resected.

Lumbar Sympathectomy Lumbar sympathectomy may be of some value in the treatment of vasospastic disease, such as Buerger's disease, ischemic ulcers of the lower extremities due to vasospasm of the peripheral vessels, and some types of causalgia. Usually through a flank incision, the lumbar chain and ganglions located in the retroperitoneal space between the vertebral column and the psoas muscle are resected from above the second to below the third ganglions.

Presacral Neurectomy The hypogastric nerve plexus may be resected for relief of idiopathic intractable dysmenorrhea.

Somatic Nervous System

As the cranial and spinal nerves extend out from the CNS into plexuses and peripheral nerve branches through the body, the somatic nervous system provides involuntary control over sensations and both voluntary and involuntary control over muscles. Loss of sensation and muscular control occurs distal to the site of severed or compressed nerve fibers. Sensation and function will be restored only if regeneration of the nerve axons takes place distally from an unobstructed axis cylinder proximal to the site of disruption.

Most peripheral nerve surgery is performed to repair traumatic nerve injury in an extremity. However, dissection is also done to remove tumors or relieve pain. Etiology determines the location and length of the skin incision.

Neurorrhaphy The suturing of a divided nerve must provide precise approximation of the nerve ends if function is to be restored. Primary repair may be accomplished by suturing the *epineurium,* the outer sheath. Under magnification of the operating microscope, accurate fascicular alignment and epineural end-to-end suturing of larger nerve bundles are the desired technique to enhance regeneration of function. For a successful result, however, nerves must not be repaired under tension. Primary repair soon after injury may be advantageous to align the fascicles.

A tumor, such as a neurofibroma or posttraumatic neuroma, is excised. If the nerve ends can be brought together without tension, they are anastomosed. Silastic membrane may be wrapped around the anastomosis to prevent adhesions with the surrounding tissue.

Neurolysis Freeing of a nerve from adhesions relieves pain and restores function. Carpal tunnel syndrome, for example, a neuropathy caused by entrapment of the median nerve, produces tingling and numbness over all or part of the hand and compromises hand functions. Release of the transverse carpal ligament overriding the nerve affords relief of this syndrome.

Neurotomy, Neurectomy, and Neurexeresis Neurotomy is the division or dissection of nerve fibers; neurectomy is excision of part of a nerve; neurexeresis is extraction or avulsion of a nerve. These procedures may be performed to relieve localized peripheral pain.

CHAPTER **30**

THORACIC SURGERY

Thoracic surgery concerns disorders of the lungs, mediastinum, thoracic esophagus, diaphragm, and chest wall. Operative intervention is most frequently indicated for neoplasms, traumatic injuries, and disease processes such as tuberculosis. Inclusion of vital organs of respiration and circulation within the thoracic cavity mandates special attention to sustaining an oxygenated blood supply to body tissues, especially the brain, during and after operation.

HISTORICAL DEVELOPMENT

Interest in the thorax and lungs dates back to ancient times. The brutal practice of dissecting live criminals was related by Celsus who noted that when the *diaphragma,* or transverse septum, was cut, the thorax was widely opened and the person expired. Vesalius used animals to demonstrate to his students the transparent pleura and motion of the lungs beneath it. As exposure was widened and the pleural cavity entered, the lung was seen to collapse. Experimental animals were revived by tracheotomy with a reed pipe used as a tracheotomy tube. Invention of the stethoscope by René Laennec in the eighteenth century facilitated study of thoracic disease.

Learning safe access to the pleural cavity and lungs was a difficult step in the development of thoracic surgery. Thoracentesis with needle and trocar, for open drainage of acute empyema, was performed in the United States in the mid-nineteenth century. Sporadic attempts at thoracic surgery in the nineteenth century, e.g., pulmonary resection, were accompanied by unacceptable mortality rates.

In 1913, F. Torek, a pioneer in chest surgery, successfully removed a carcinoma of the esophagus, resecting ribs but not the scapula, as was the mode. Sucking wounds of the chest, created by shell fragments during World War I, drew new interest in thoracic problems. In 1920, Evarts Graham brought attention to the significance of the relaxation of vital capacity to the size of an opening in the thorax and in 1923 presented a staged procedure: cautery pneumonotomy and partial excision of the lung. The first successful pneumonectomy, using exposure by rib resection, took place in 1931.

Development of thoracic surgery paralleled advances in endoscopy, endotracheal anesthesia, mechanical ventilation, closed chest-drainage systems, and respiratory care techniques.

CHEST AND THORACIC CAVITY

An essential balance must be maintained between atmospheric pressure outside the chest and internal pressures within the thoracic cavity to sustain the vital function of respiration. Knowledge of the anatomy and physiology of the chest and thoracic cavity is necessary for an understanding of thoracic surgery.

Anatomy and Physiology

Thorax The thorax, or chest, is the part of the trunk between the neck and abdomen. It holds the chief organs of respiration and circulation, the lungs and heart, and the great vessels. These vital organs function under the protection of a bony framework consisting of the sternum, 12 pairs of ribs, and 12 thoracic vertebrae, all encased with soft tissue. The framework is bounded superiorly by structures of the lower part of the neck and inferiorly by the diaphragm. External and internal intercostal muscles, which lie between the ribs, have a corresponding artery, vein, and nerve, which require meticulous dissection to avoid inadvertent injury.

The ribs articulate posteriorly with the thoracic vertebrae. The first seven ribs articulate anteriorly in the midline with the sternum composed of three parts—the manubrium, gladiolus, and xiphoid process. The eighth, ninth, and tenth ribs are joined anteriorly to the cartilage of the rib above each; the eleventh and twelfth ribs have no anterior fixation. The esophagus, trachea, and great vessels leading to and from the neck and arms pass through the small space between the manubrium and vertebrae. Any structure pushing into this narrow opening, e.g., a mediastinal tumor, may obstruct breathing, venous return from the neck and arms, and swallowing.

The chest cavity is divided into right and left compartments by the *mediastinum,* the space and vertical loose connective tissue wall between the two pleural cavities. The mediastinum has superior, anterior, middle, and posterior sections, each containing structures: the thymus lies within the anterior and superior sections, the thoracic aorta within the posterior, the heart and great vessels in the middle, and esophagus and trachea in the superior section. Organs are surrounded and suspended by the loose tissue diffused throughout the mediastinum. Division of the pleural cavities is flexible and alterations in pressure affecting one cavity are felt in the other.

Lungs The lungs lie in the right and left pleural cavities (see Fig. 30-1). The main function of these porous, spongy, conical organs is oxygenation of blood with inspired air and expiration of carbon dioxide. The apex of each extends to the neck; the base rests on the diaphragm. The lungs are enveloped by serous membrane, the visceral or pulmonary pleura. Parietal pleura lines the internal surface of the thoracic cavity.

The trachea divides at the *carina* into two main branches, the *bronchi,* leading to the right and left lungs. The right lung, with three lobes, is larger than the left lung, which has only two lobes. The left lung is narrower and shares the space in the left chest with the heart.

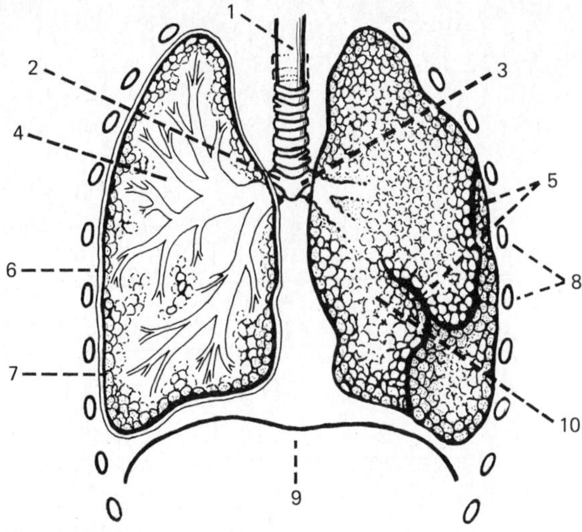

FIGURE 30-1
Respiratory system within thoracic cavity: (1) trachea, (2) right main stem bronchus, (3) left main stem bronchus, (4) right lung (cross section of bronchi), (5) lobe divisions, (6) parietal pleura, (7) visceral pleura, (8) ribs, (9) diaphragm, (10) left lung surface.

The *bronchopulmonary segments* within each lung are wedges of tissue separated by veins and thin connective membrane. Although configuration of the segments differs and variations in the bronchi and blood vessels exist between the right and left lungs, it is generally accepted that both lungs normally have ten bronchopulmonary segments. (Some nomenclatures refer only to eight or nine segments in the left lung.) Although not demarcated by surface fissures as are the lobes, these segments represent zones of distribution of the secondary bronchi and may be excised individually when the segment contains a small lesion, thus preserving the uninvolved portion. Each segmental bronchus subdivides into numerous increasingly smaller branches that eventually end in terminal *bronchioles.* These fine tubules invested by smooth muscles can constrict to close off the air passage, as in asthma. The terminal bronchioles give rise to respiratory bronchioles from which arise the *alveoli.* The approximately 300,000,000 alveoli are the functional units wherein oxygenation takes place at the capillary level.

The *hilus* of the lung, on the mediastinal surface, is the point of entry for the primary bronchus, nerves, and vessels. The right primary bronchus is a more direct continuation of the trachea. The pulmonary veins and arteries to and from the heart provide pulmonary circulation. Organs of respiration are innervated by the autonomic nervous system.

Size of the thorax varies with the bellows action of the thoracic wall and diaphragm, increasing with inspiration and decreasing with expiration. A partial vacuum between parietal and visceral pleurae expands the lungs. A negative (subatmospheric) pressure normally within the thorax is essential to life. Alterations of intrapleural pressure are of major concern because an uncontrolled opening in the thoracic wall and pressure change can be fatal. The uncontrolled increased positive pressure in one side causes a collapse of the lung on the other side. Referred to as *mediastinal shift,* this reaction attends entrance of either air or fluid to the pleural cavity, compressing opposite lung and causing dyspnea. When the mediastinum has moved its limit, it can no longer accommodate a great pressure change; the lung on affected side collapses. Air in the pleural space between parietal and visceral pleura constitutes *pneumothorax.* Blood in pleural space is *hemothorax.*

Mediastinal shift disturbs heart action and circulation. Changes in pressure balance within the thorax reduce *vital capacity,* the greatest amount of air that can be exchanged in one breath. Many diseases and conditions alter vital capacity, for example, anesthesia, thoracic tumors, or injury.

Operative entry into the thoracic cavity can be accompanied by pulmonary distress. However, administration of endotracheal anesthesia under controlled positive pressure prevents physiologic imbalance and prevents lung collapse in the presence of controlled pneumothorax. This is essential for entry into the chest for intrathoracic procedures. An airtight pleural cavity must be restored and negative pressure maintained for maximum pulmonary function postoperatively.

SPECIAL FEATURES OF THORACIC SURGERY

1 Sterile closed water-seal drainage system is essential when the chest has been opened by operation or trauma, except after a few specific procedures. Chest tube(s) are inserted through a 1- or 2-cm (½ to 1-in.) incision and are anchored to the chest wall with suture and tape. Two tubes are sometimes inserted into the pleural space and connected to separate drainage systems. The tube at the base of the pleural space is usually inserted at the seventh costal interspace, near the anterior axillary line, to evacuate fluid. An upper tube, if indicated, is inserted at the apex through the anterior chest wall at the third costal interspace to evacuate air leaking from the lung. (Review chest drainage in Chapter 17, p. 332.) Tubes may be connected to suction at 15- to 20-cm water pressure to ensure better evacuation of air and fluid.

- **a** Connections must be taped for tight seal. The system must be kept intact.
- **b** System components must be kept below the level of the patient's body to prevent reentry of air or fluid from the drainage collection system into the pleural cavity.
- **c** Depending on the surgeon's preference, tubes may be clamped prior to insertion and connection to the system, and during transportation, to avoid introduction of air.

2 Portable chest x-rays are taken immediately and 24 hours after the procedure to assess status of the operative area, pleural cavities, and lung reexpansion.

3 Operating rooms for thoracic surgery should be provided with electrocardiographic and pressure monitors. Equipment for bronchoscopy, esophagoscopy, and mediastinoscopy must be readily available. Team members especially skilled in meeting emergency situations are essential. These patients require very close observation because changes may occur rapidly. Laboratory facilities must be available on a 24-hour basis to monitor blood gases.

4 Endotracheal anesthesia permits the lungs to expand and function even when subjected to atmospheric pressure. At conclusion of operation, the operated lung is reexpanded by the anesthesiologist and negative pressure in the chest is restored.

5 Properly cross-matched blood for transfusion should be available at all times. Hemorrhage is a major threat intra- and postoperatively.

6 Instrumentation includes basic laparotomy setup with addition of thoracic instruments. These include bone instruments and power saws; rib stripper, spreaders, and approximator; large self-retaining chest retractor; bronchus and lung clamps; and long instruments for work in a deep incision.

7 A large variety of sutures may be used for

bone, soft tissues, and vessels. The bronchus usually is closed with staples.

8 Sponges for hemostasis or blunt dissection are placed on long ring-handled forceps. Periosteal bleeding may be controlled by electrocoagulation. Bone wax may be needed for bone marrow oozing.

9 The field is potentially contaminated by secretions and contact with open air passages when a bronchus is opened and sutured. Used items and instruments are isolated in a discard basin. Maintenance of a dry field is important to prevent aspiration of blood and fluid, predisposing patient to postoperative pneumonia.

10 Major complications of thoracic surgery are hemorrhage, atelectasis, persistent undrained fluid or air pockets in pleural space, empyema, bronchopleural fistula, retained tracheobronchial secretions, pulmonary shunting.

THORACIC INCISIONS AND CLOSURES

Factors Influencing Choice of Incision

1 Adequate exposure into thoracic cavity.

2 Physiologic intrapleural pressure changes and constant movement of chest.

3 Maintenance of integrity of the chest wall and diaphragm. Because of continuity of thoracic cavity with the neck and abdominal structures, the cavity may be entered for neck and upper abdominal procedures as well as thoracic procedures.

Access to Thorax

Surgeon preference and the procedure determine method of entrance into the thorax. Access may be gained by anterior, lateral, or posterior approaches, or a combination of these. Entrance through the rib cage may be intercostal between the ribs, through the periosteal bed of an unresected rib, or by rib resection. By incising near top of a rib, the surgeon protects nerves and vessels that lie in the intercostal spaces. Intercostal approach may be used to drain an empyema pocket or mediastinal abscess, or to biopsy lymph nodes or lung. To enter via the periosteal bed, periosteum of rib is incised and removed from unresected rib, and incision is made through the bed. For entrance via rib resection, periosteum is incised and removed superiorly and inferiorly with a periosteal elevator, and the rib is divided. Rib spreaders increase exposure but if it is inadequate, the rib above or below the incision may be resected.

Commonly Used Thoracic Incisions

Posterolateral Thoracotomy The classic incision for exploration of the thoracic cavity, a posterolateral incision permits maximum exposure to lung, esophagus, diaphragm, and descending aorta. Beginning anteriorly in the submammary fold, about at nipple level, a curved incision is made, extending below scapular tip, following course of underlying ribs. Then curving upward and posteriorly, it may be carried as high as spine of scapula. Subcutaneous tissue is incised, latissimus dorsi, lower margin of trapezius, rhomboideus, and serratus muscles are divided, and bleeders are ligated. In dividing the serratus, special precaution is taken to avoid neurovascular bundle on the surface.

In closure, ribs are reapproximated with a rib approximator and sutures, intercostal muscles are sutured, and incision in periosteal bed and pleura is closed. Muscles are reapproximated anatomically and sutured; subcutaneous tissue and skin are closed. Uses: pulmonary resections, some cardiac operations, repair of hiatus hernia, procedures on thoracic esophagus or posterior mediastinum.

Anterolateral Thoracotomy With patient supine, sandbags are placed under the operative side to tilt shoulder 20 to 45° for extension of incision posteriorly. A pad behind the buttocks may rotate hips slightly. Submammary incision, immediately below breast but above costal margin, extends from the anterior midline to mid- or posterior axillary line. To avoid the axillary apex and painful scar, the posterior end of incision is curved downward. Superiorly, access is desired at about the fourth interspace. Further anterior exposure can be gained if desired by transecting sternum and continuing the incision to contralateral interspace. Pectoralis muscles are divided, serratus anterior fibers separated, intercostal muscles divided, and thorax entered through an intercostal space. When anterior incision extends to sternal border, internal mammary arteries and veins are ligated and divided. If incision is carried far laterally or posteriorly, injury to long thoracic nerve must be avoided to prevent a "winged" scapula.

In closure, sternum is reapproximated with heavy suture, ribs are approximated with pericostal sutures, and muscles, subcutaneous tissue and skin are closed. Uses: resection of pulmonary cyst or local lesion.

Thoracoabdominal The thoracoabdominal incision extends from posterior axillary line to abdominal midline, paralleling the selected interspace (usually the seventh or eighth). Following insertion of a rib spreader, incision in intercostal muscles and pleura may be extended posteriorly from within for added exposure. The diaphragm may be divided peripherally. This incision exposes upper abdomen, retroperitoneal area, and lower aspect of chest (see Fig. 30-2).

In closure, the diaphragm is closed with interrupted sutures. Costal margin is secured by approximating the margins of divided costal cartilages with suture. Tissue layers are closed in reverse order of incision. Uses: repair of hiatus hernia, esophagectomy; also used in general surgery for retroperitoneal tumor and cardioesophageal lesions.

Other Less Common Incisions Less common incisions may be used, such as:

1 Cervical mediastinotomy, for drainage high in the mediastinum, e.g., following esophageal perforation

2 Anterior approach, for upper dorsal sympathectomy, exposing upper thoracic ganglia

3 Supraclavicular (scalene approach), for phrenic nerve section, cervicothoracic sympathectomy

4 Axillary approach, for upper mediastinal or lung biopsy, or exposure of second to fifth thoracic ganglia

5 Median sternotomy, for mediastinal neoplasms or trauma, exposure for simultaneous bilateral pulmonary operations, or for cardiac and aortic operations

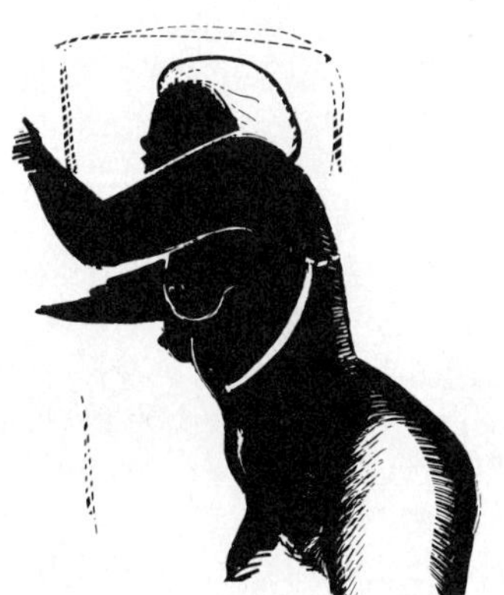

FIGURE 30-2
Left thoracoabdominal incision with patient in lateral position.

THORACIC OPERATIVE PROCEDURES

Elective surgery depends on accurate diagnosis by radiologic, endoscopic, physiologic pulmonary function studies, biochemical, cytological, and histological determinations and evaluations.

Endoscopy

Bronchoscopy In addition to its use in preoperative diagnosis, endoscopic examination of the bronchi may be performed to ascertain patency of the tracheobronchial tree (refer to Chap. 26, p. 517, for indications) and to treat some bronchial lesions as with a laser. Both rigid and flexible fiberoptic bronchoscopes are used for diagnostic and treatment procedures.

Mediastinoscopy Mediastinoscopy may immediately follow bronchoscopy. To prevent needless thoracotomy, it is performed for assessment of resectability in patients with suspected bronchogenic carcinoma and for diagnosis of mediastinal lesions. Mediastinoscopy uncovers mediastinal lymph nodes for direct visualization and biopsy. Subaortic nodes draining the left lobe of the lung may be out of reach for biopsy with this technique. With the scope, the mediastinoscopist can see down to the carina and about 4 cm distal to it along each bronchus. If more than one biopsy specimen is obtained, each should be placed in a separate container and identified by location. The procedure gives a high percentage of accurate diagnoses and information in staging extent of a lesion and determining operability for curative resection. Sometimes a frozen section is done while the patient is in the OR and resection is done immediately following the report.

General endotracheal anesthesia is used. The patient is supine with the neck hyperextended and the head turned slightly to the right. A small transverse incision is made in or about 2 cm above the suprasternal notch between borders of sternocleidomastoid muscle. Dissection is carried down to pretracheal fascia. After blunt dissection, the scope is passed behind suprasternal notch and advanced behind arch of the aorta into superior mediastinum to level of the carina. Care is exercised because of proximity to the great vessels. Bleeding is controlled by coagulation with an insulated electrosurgical suction tip. Usually performed without complication, mediastinoscopy may be accompanied by major bleeding, requiring immediate thoracotomy. A chest x-ray is frequently obtained after the procedure.

Mediastinotomy

Anterior mediastinotomy may be indicated when x-ray studies show hilar or mediastinal nodal involvement inaccessible to mediastinoscopy. With patient supine under general anesthesia, incision is made over right or left third costal cartilage. The cartilage bed is incised and extrapleural dissection is carried toward hilus of lung, and biopsy is taken. If desired nodes are deep, a mediastinoscope may be inserted through the incision to obtain a biopsy. Or, the pleural space may be entered for lung biopsy. If this space is entered, closed water-seal chest drainage is required. If not entered, the incision is closed in layers without drainage. Mediastinotomy allows assessment of extent of lesion involvement.

Excision of Lesions A median sternotomy, vertical sternal splitting procedure (see Chap. 31, p. 576), may be necessary to resect a cyst, benign or malignant tumor in the upper anterior mediastinum. Cutting instruments are needed to divide the sternum. Heavy-gauge stainless steel sutures are used to close the sternum.

Through a posterolateral thoracotomy incision, tumor may be resected or an abscess drained in the posterior mediastinum.

Correction of Pectus Excavatum (Funnel Chest) Although congenital deformities of the chest wall are usually corrected in childhood (refer to Chap. 33, p. 606), correction of pectus excavatum is sometimes delayed until adolescence or adult years. A depression deformity of the chest wall, the sternum is pushed back toward the spine. The converse, *pectus carinatum* (pigeon chest), is forward projection or keel of the sternum. *Pectus excavatum* (funnel chest), the more common, is due to elongation of the costal cartilages. Operation is performed for cosmetic improvement or correction of mediastinal compression, to relieve respiratory distress or pressure on the heart.

Various techniques may be employed. Usually, with patient supine and upper chest slightly hyperextended, costal cartilages are exposed by muscle splitting and/or division through anterior midline or horizontal inframammary incision. Involved costal cartilages and deformed rib ends are freed from sternal attachments and resected or straightened. The sternum is mobilized and restored to normal position and its corrected position maintained by fixation. An alternative method corrects the contour deformity with a silicone prosthesis introduced through inframammary incision. Dacron patches on posterior surface stabilize the prosthesis.

Thoracotomy

Incision through the thoracic wall is indicated for drainage of pleural spaces, exploration of thoracic cavity, or cardiac and pulmonary operations. Thoracic operations, exclusive of cardiac procedures, include the following.

Closed Thoracostomy Closed thoracostomy is performed to establish continuous drainage of fluid from the chest (usually purulent from sepsis) or to aid in restoring negative pressure in the thoracic cavity. It involves insertion of a tube through an intercostal space via trocar and cannula.

Open Thoracotomy Open thoracotomy may be employed for spontaneous pneumothorax, for large air leaks that prevent reexpansion of the lung, or for persistent leaks and incomplete lung reexpansion. This type of pneumothorax usually occurs from rupture of a bleb on the lung surface. By posterolateral incision through fourth interspace, an apical bleb may be ligated or the involved segmental area of lung resected. Abrasion or cauterization of the parietal pleura effects adhesion to visceral pleura, thereby eliminating future rupture of blebs. Open chest drainage is also used to eliminate an empyema cavity, which accompanies chronic disease and lung adherence to the chest wall. With this procedure, portions of one or two ribs are removed to aid establishment of drainage.

Exploratory Thoracotomy Exploratory thoracotomy is usually performed to confirm diagnosis and extent of involvement of bronchogenic carcinoma or other chest disease, such as mediastinal lesion. Posterolateral intercostal or anterior approach may be used. Lung and hemithorax are exposed after ribs are spread and pleura is opened. Biopsy is taken. Etiology of bleeding or detection of injury after trauma are other indications for exploration. Postoperative pain is due to continuous movement of the chest.

Lung Resection All or part of a diseased or traumatized lung may be resected. Generally, the indications are neoplasms; emphysematous blebs; and fungal infection, localized residual lung abscess, tuberculosis and/or bronchiectasis resistant to nonoperative treatment. Neoplasms are the predominant indication. Anterior intercostal incision with division of costal cartilages above and below the incision may be used for excision of pulmonary nodules or lung biopsy. Posterolateral incision is commonly employed for lobectomy and pneumonectomy. Endotracheal anesthesia is used. Special precautions in pulmonary resection include meticulous hemostasis and closure of the bronchus, as well as continual attention to cardiopulmonary function pre-, intra-, and postoperatively. Particular hazards are hemorrhage, which is difficult to control because of size and friability of major pulmonary vessels and proximity to the heart; cardiopulmonary insufficiency; risk of injury to other intrathoracic structures such as the vagus, phrenic, and left recurrent nerves and the esophagus. Specific resections include the following.

Segmental Resection Removal of individual bronchovascular segments of a lobe is preferred when wide excision is not necessary, as for pathology distributed segmentally or for acute hemorrhage. Arteries, veins, and bronchus to the involved segment are ligated and divided. The segment is separated from surrounding lung tissue and removed. The proximal bronchial stump is closed with sutures or staples.

Wedge Resection Wedge resection is a conservative procedure performed when a lesion is thought to be benign. With adequate margin of normal lung tissue, the diseased peripheral portion of a lobe is removed and the lung tissue is sutured. A stapler may expedite removal and closure. Frozen section is done. If benign diagnosis is confirmed, the wound is closed in layers, and water-seal drainage is used. If the lesion proves to be malignant, lobectomy or other appropriate procedure may be done. Advantage of wedge resection is its simplicity with minimal blood loss and operating time.

Lobectomy One or more lobes of a lung are excised when disease or neoplasm is confined to the lobe. The remaining portion of lung expands to fill space formerly occupied by the removed lobe. Through a posterolateral incision, entrance to the chest may be intercostal or by rib resection. The pulmonary pleura is incised and freed from hilus of the lobe. Arteries and veins to pulmonary tissue being resected are ligated and divided. The bronchus of the lobe is identified by lung inflation while bronchus to be resected is clamped prior to its resection. Suction of blood and secretions from the open bronchus may precede closure of bronchus by sutures or staples. A suture line in the bronchus is covered with a flap of parietal pleura to prevent leakage. Dissection is completed, specimen is removed, and chest is closed.

Bronchoplastic Reconstruction Extensive partial pulmonary resection may be followed by bronchoplastic reconstruction to ensure maximum preservation of residual pulmonary tissue. These techniques require successful bronchial anastomoses to retain a patent airway to the bronchioles.

Pneumonectomy Major indications for excision of an entire lung are malignant neoplasms or extensive unilateral pulmonary disease. The chest wall is opened by posterolateral incision, pleura incised, lung exposed, and pleural cavity examined. Following immobilization of the lung, hilus is dissected free on all sides. The pulmonary artery and veins are ligated and divided. Bronchus is clamped, divided, and closed with sutures or staples. Bronchus is checked for air leaks by instillation of saline solution and the bronchial stump is covered with surrounding pleura. After wound closure, intrathoracic pressure is measured and residual air aspirated from hemithorax until desired pressure is reached. Use of chest drainage is governed by surgeon preference, but usually no chest tube is inserted.

Sacrifice of one lung places entire respiratory and circulatory function on the remaining lung. Potential complications are respiratory insufficiency, cardiac arrhythmia, and infection, the latter predisposed by the amount of dead space. The empty hemithorax gradually fills with fluid and eventually consolidates, thus preventing mediastinal shift. Dehiscence of the bronchial closure may produce bronchopleural fistula.

Thoracoplasty Usually done extrapleurally, the chest wall is mobilized to obliterate the pleural cavity or reduce thoracic space by resection of one or more ribs. Indications are inadequate expansion of lung to fill pleural space after resection, persistent shift of mediastinum to the empty space after pneumonectomy, or chronic empyema. Tissue fibroses, contracts, and eventually obliterates the space. Thoracoplasty is reserved for patients in whom excessive space in the chest cannot be eliminated satisfactorily by other means to maintain mediastinum in midline.

Pulmonary Decortication In patients with empyema, a fibrinous thickening or peel on the visceral pleura may restrict pulmonary ventilation. A pleural procedure, removal of the restrictive layer or membrane over the lung permits the entrapped lung to reexpand and fill space remaining after drainage of an empyema cavity. Minimum damage to rib cage by thoracotomy incision is desired to permit motion of chest wall that is as normal as possible. Intercostal incision is usually preferred, but in some patients resection of a rib may facilitate access to intrapleural space. Adequate postoperative drainage via chest tube(s) is essential.

Transplantation Lung allografts and combined heart-lung transplants are discussed in Chapter 34.

Repair of Hiatus Hernia

Repair of herniation of stomach through the diaphragm may be performed by a general surgeon (refer to Chap. 21) or by a thoracic surgeon utilizing thoracic routines, such as chest tube insertion with underwater-seal drainage. The thoracic approach is preferred when:

1 Exposure from an abdominal approach would be difficult, as with an obese patient.

2 Hernia is incarcerated into the thoracic cavity and would be difficult to reduce through diaphragm into abdomen.

3 Hernia is recurrent and direct visualization will facilitate procedure.

CHEST TRAUMA

Trauma to the chest varies in severity and may result in injury to the thoracic wall or intrathoracic organs such as the heart and lungs. If severe, the patient is plunged into critical condition. Rapid initial evaluation of extent of injury is necessary to save life, with priority needs met first. These include resuscitation with relief of airway obstruction, treatment of shock and blood loss, and restoration of as nearly as normal cardiorespiratory dynamics. Impairment of these dynamics may be due to various factors such as disturbance of lung expansion.

Trauma is categorized as *blunt* or *penetrating*. Blunt trauma usually results from a fall, blow, severe cough, blast, or deceleration injury. The patient may have little overt evidence of chest injury, even though he or she may be bleeding internally. Penetrating wounds are usually caused by low- or high-velocity missile, such as knife stab or bullet. Operative exploration may be required.

Blunt Trauma

Treatment of Fractured Ribs Rib fracture is the most common injury to the chest wall, the fourth to the eighth ribs being the ones mainly involved. Pain may be relieved by intercostal nerve block. Operative treatment is usually not required unless sharp edges or displaced bone fragments puncture the pleura or lung. Extensive pneumothorax requires immediate reexpansion.

Multiple rib or sternal fractures often produce an unstable chest wall, resulting in flail chest. Normal respiration changes to paradoxic motion of the chest wall. The chest wall collapses on inspiration and expands on expiration. This results in ineffective respiration and coughing. As the chest wall expands, the free-floating sternum is sucked inward, thus impairing ventilation and producing hypoxia. The following measures are used to stabilize the chest wall.

1 *Internal stabilization* is achieved by controlled respiration through a tracheotomy tube (refer to Chap. 26, p. 515). Frequent aspiration maintains a free airway; paradoxical motion and dead air space decrease.

2 *Operative stabilization* is achieved by insertion of pins.

Penetrating Wounds

Anatomical visualization of the path of the projectile or instrument producing injury is important. A knife, for example, should not be removed except under direction of a physician, because it may be penetrating the heart or a major vessel.

An open chest wound must be converted to a closed chest wound. Air rushes in an open wound, building up atmospheric positive pressure inside the pleural space. Pneumothorax followed by mediastinal shift ensues.

Thoracentesis Air or blood in the pleural cavity may be detected and aspirated by needle and syringe. If bleeding persists, the chest is opened and closed thoracotomy drainage may be instituted or the chest is opened and vessels are ligated or repaired.

Closure of Sucking Wound Pneumothorax is relieved and further air prevented from entering the chest by suture of the wound and insertion of chest tube(s).

INTRATHORACIC ESOPHAGEAL PROCEDURES

Esophageal disorders may be congenital or they may be acquired by trauma or disease, as discussed in Chapters 21, 26, 28, and 33. Thoracic surgeons may perform esophageal resections for lesions, usually malignant tumors, in the thoracic esophagus. Early detection of esophageal carcinoma, by the brush biopsy technique for example, increases rate of cure by operative resection. Unfortunately, symptoms are not usually apparent in early stages, so that carcinoma of the esophagus generally presents a poor prognosis. Most operative procedures provide palliation rather than cure. Radical en bloc mediastinectomy may become the procedure of choice, but esophagectomy is more commonly performed.

Esophagectomy

With patient in lateral position, a posterolateral thoracotomy or thoracoabdominal incision extends across chest wall to expose the affected segment of esophagus, i.e., upper, middle, or lower third. The thoracic cavity is opened and the mediastinal pleura is incised. The esophagus is dissected away from the aorta and transected above and below the lesion.

For combined thoracoabdominal exposure of lesion in the lower third of esophagus, the diaphragm is opened and the stomach mobilized for transection and intrathoracic esophagogastrostomy. In some patients, resection and anastomosis may be performed without thoracotomy by means of a substernal resection to avoid morbidity associated with thoracoabdominal exposure.

High esophageal resection followed by hypopharyngeal reconstruction may be procedure of choice for tumors in the upper third of esophagus. Reconstruction of cervical esophagus is discussed in Chapter 28. Total esophagectomy for tumors in the middle third may be carried out through abdominal and cervical incisions, without thoracotomy. The stomach is mobilized for esophagogastric anastomosis in the neck.

CHAPTER **31**

CARDIOVASCULAR SURGERY

Cardiovascular surgery encompasses the spectrum of clinical pathology associated with congenital anomalies and acquired diseases of the circulatory system. The often complex operations involving the heart, great vessels, and peripheral blood vessels mandate experienced operating teams with special education and training. The goal of cardiovascular surgeons is to restore or preserve adequate cardiac output and circulation of blood to the brain and tissues throughout the body. Technological advancements in diagnosis, anesthesia, hemodynamic monitoring, extracorporeal circulation, myocardial preservation, prosthetic devices, and transplantation have made possible the correction of many defects and treatment of cardiovascular diseases.

HISTORICAL DEVELOPMENT

Whereas experiments with transfusion using animal blood flourished during and after the seventeenth century, the most noteworthy disclosure prior to the twentieth century was the discovery of circulation of the blood by William Harvey, an English physician, who published his famous treatise in 1628. Harvey derived much knowledge of comparative anatomy from lengthy dissections and experiments on the heart chambers, arteries, and veins. Then in 1791 Galvani, a physiologist and surgeon, discovered fundamentals of electric stimulation of the heart.

Stephen Paget published the first textbook of thoracic surgery in 1896. In the chapter on the heart he stated, "Surgery of the heart has probably reached the limits set by nature to all surgery; no new method, and no new discovery, can overcome the natural difficulties that attend a wound of the heart." His successors in the twentieth century have expunged this contention. The advances in cardiac surgery are to medicine what aerospace is to aviation.

Cutler, in 1924, utilized a sternum-splitting incision to open the chest for exposure of the heart. Early procedures on the heart and vessels included correction of coarctation of the aorta and patent ductus arteriosus, both congenital anomalies. In the late 1940s, Bailey placed his finger into the heart to open a mitral valve stenosis. This *closed* mitral commissurotomy began the evolution of modern cardiovascular surgery, which has accelerated rapidly since about 1950.

Development of the heart-lung machine, which permits safe direct vision for *open-heart* operations, is credited to John Gibbon. In 1953 he performed intracardiac surgery using the first successful pump oxygenator. Since then many complex operations have been developed, made possible only with the aid of cardiopulmonary bypass.

Heart catheterization and angiography provide evaluation of hemodynamics in intracardiac and intravascular function. Revascularization of ischemic myocardium to increase blood supply has progressed from abrasion of epicardium with asbestos in the 1950s to internal mammary artery implantation and coronary bypass procedures developed in the 1960s. Electronic devices provide cardiac pacing for an irregular heart. Care of cardiac patients immediately following operation has improved markedly, reducing mortality, due in no small measure to sophisticated monitoring modalities.

The greatest challenge to cardiac surgeons continues to be the physiologic problems associated with cardiac transplantation and development of mechanical devices as substitutes for organs beyond repair. Since the first successful heart transplant in South Africa in 1967, cardiac transplantation has become an accepted modality in some medical centers. The advent in 1981 of a combined heart-lung transplant and the implantation of a mechanical artificial heart in 1982 may provide hope in the future for patients with end-stage cardiopulmonary diseases.

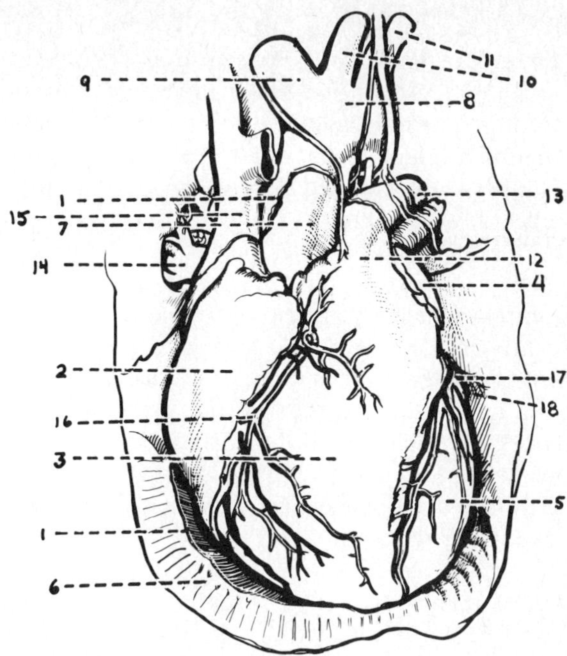

FIGURE 31-1
Anterior view of the heart and great vessels: (1) pericardium (parietal), (2) right atrium, (3) right ventricle, (4) left atrium, (5) left ventricle, (6) diaphragm, (7) ascending aorta, (8) aortic arch, (9) brachiocephalic trunk, (10) left common carotid artery, (11) left subclavian artery, (12) pulmonary trunk, (13) left pulmonary artery, (14) right pulmonary artery, (15) superior vena cava, (16) right coronary artery, (17) left coronary artery, (18) circumflex branch of left coronary artery.

HEART AND GREAT VESSELS

Cardiac operations involve the heart and associated great vessels. Congenital malformations corrected in infancy or early childhood are discussed in Chapter 33. This chapter focuses on operations performed for acquired heart diseases. To understand diagnostic procedures, hemodynamic monitoring, myocardial preservation techniques, and cardiopulmonary bypass used in conjunction with cardiac surgery requires knowledge of normal anatomy and physiology of the heart.

Anatomy and Physiology

The cardiovascular system supplies oxygen and nutrients to body cells and carries waste away from cells by flow of blood through the system. The heart, blood, and lymph vessels constitute this circulatory system. The heart, the hollow muscular organ located in the thorax, maintains circulation of blood throughout the body.

Heart The *heart* is located in middle mediastinum slightly left of midline. The heart is a muscular "pump" enveloped by a closed, double-walled, fibroserous sac, the *pericardium.* Normally the sac contains a small amount of clear serous fluid that lubricates the heart's moving surfaces. The base of the pericardium is attached to the diaphragm; the apex surrounds the great vessels arising from the base of the heart. (See Figs. 31-1 and 31-2.)

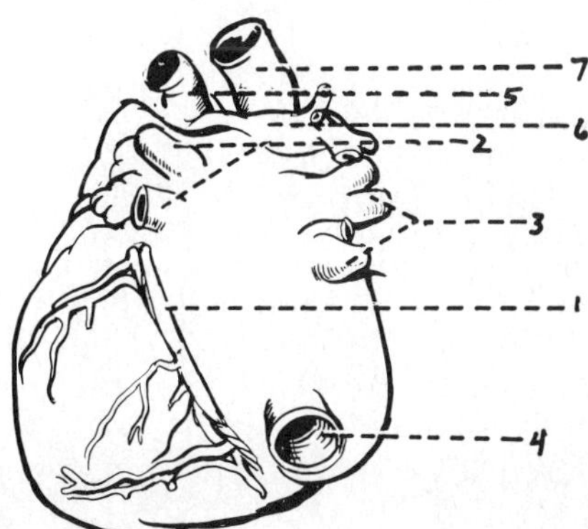

FIGURE 31-2
Posterior view of heart and great vessels: (1) coronary sinus, (2) left pulmonary veins, (3) right pulmonary veins, (4) inferior vena cava, (5) left pulmonary artery, (6) right pulmonary artery, (7) ascending aorta.

The layers of the heart are the *outer epicardium* (visceral pericardium), *myocardium* (muscle fibers), and *endocardium* (inner membrane lining). Divided into right and left halves by an oblique longitudinal septum, each half of the heart has two chambers, a thin-walled upper *atrium* and a thick-walled lower *ventricle.* The atria receive blood from veins; the ventricles pump blood into and along the arteries. The heart's rounded apex, formed by the left ventricle, is behind the sixth rib slightly to the left of the sternum. The base is formed by the atria and great vessels. The atria, lying mainly behind the ventricles, continue anteriorly on each side of the aorta to form the auricular appendages. The long axis of the heart extends from base to apex, i.e., from behind forward, downward, and to the left.

Coronary circulation is predominantly right or predominantly left. The coronary arteries arise from the aorta and, with their branches, supply oxygen and nutrients to the heart muscle. The left coronary artery divides shortly after origin into two main trunks:

1 The anterior descending or interventricular branch courses toward the apex of the heart. Its branches distribute over the anterolateral wall of the left ventricle. Septal branches supply the anterior interventricular septum.

2 The circumflex branch passes posteriorly. Following the atrioventricular groove and passing under the left atrial appendage, it meets the right coronary artery at the base of the junction of both ventricles. The right coronary artery is directed to the right, passing to the posterior aspect of the heart and eventually running between the two ventricles. Its branches supply the posterior interventricular septum.

The vagus nerve (parasympathetic) and cardiac branches of the cervical and upper thoracic ganglia (sympathetic) innervate the heart.

Four *heart valves* promote unobstructed unidirectional blood flow. They are the right tricuspid and left mitral atrioventricular (AV) valves, the pulmonary valve between the right ventricle and pulmonary trunk, and the aortic valve between the left ventricle and aorta. The latter two are referred to as *semilunar valves.* The mitral has two cusps, or endocardial leaflets; the other valves have three. Bases of the cusps of the AV valves attach to the fibrous ring that surrounds the opening. When the ventricle begins to contract, the cusps float up to close the opening, preventing backflow. Sequential heart sounds are heard by stethoscope as the valves open and close.

Conducting System The heart's conducting system permits synchronous contraction of the atria followed by contraction of the ventricles. Right and left sides of the heart function simultaneously but independently. Muscular contractions of the atria and ventricles are controlled by an electric impulse that originates in the *sinoatrial (SA) node.* This "pacemaker" is a dense network of specialized Purkinje fibers situated at the junction of the right atrium and superior vena cava. These fibers become continuous with muscle fibers of the atrium at the node's periphery. The stimulus is passed to the smaller *atrioventricular (AV) node* beneath the endocardium in the interatrial septum. A mass of interwoven conductive tissue, this node's specialized fibers are continuous with atrial muscle fibers and the atrioventricular bundle of His. The *bundle of His* provides conduction relay between atria and ventricles. Arising from the atrioventricular node, the band of conducting tissue passes on both sides of the interventricular septum, its branches dividing and subdividing to penetrate every area of ventricular muscle and to transmit contraction impulses to the ventricles. Thus, expansions of conducting tissue, providing coordinated excitation of muscle areas, spread through both atria and ventricles. Each atrial contraction (depolarization) is followed by a period of recharging (repolarization) during which the ventricles contract. Ventricular contraction is followed by a period of recovery while the chambers fill with blood as the atria contract due to higher pressure.

Cardiac Cycle (Circulation) Myocardial contraction is referred to as *systole,* relaxation as *diastole.* Venous blood from the entire body enters the right atrium via the *vena cavae* and passes through the tricuspid valve to the right ventricle from which it is ejected through the pumonary valve into the pulmonary arterial trunk. Right and left *pulmonary arteries* originating from the trunk carry blood to the lungs, where it takes up oxygen and gives off carbon dioxide. Oxygenated blood is transported from the lungs to the left atrium by the *pulmonary veins* and enters the left ventricle through the mitral valve. Contraction of the left ventricle propels blood through the aortic valve into the *aorta* from which it is carried to all parts of body by arterial branches. The highest pressure reached during left ventricular systole is the *systolic blood pressure.* Following contraction the ventricle relaxes, during which time systemic intraarterial pressure falls to its lowest level, *diastolic blood pressure.* Each contraction of the right ventricle forces blood through the pulmonary valve into the pulmonary arteries to the lungs. In summary, there are two circulations:

1 *Pulmonary,* from right ventricle to lungs and back to left atrium
2 *Systemic,* from left ventricle to aorta, to body tissues and organs and back to right atrium

Interference in any part of the circulatory system can jeopardize survival.

Diagnostic Procedures

Operation is preceded by extensive cardiovascular assessment utilizing noninvasive and invasive studies that dictate subsequent treatment.

Noninvasive Routine examination and electrocardiography are augmented by determination of venous pressure, cardiac output, circulation time, and blood chemistry studies. Chest x-ray reveals heart size, position, and outline. Screening or functional capacity testing, such as stress testing, is informative. Pulmonary function tests may detect left ventricular failure. Echocardiography by ultrasound reveals heart structure and gives information pertinent to congenital heart disease and valvular disease. Radionuclide imaging may be used to detect regional reductions in myocardial blood flow and thus help to confirm or deny the diagnosis of myocardial infarction.

Invasive Radiographic visualization following injection of a nontoxic radiopaque substance permits study of heart chambers, great vessels, and coronary circulation.

Angiography *Angiocardiography,* by intravascular injection of a radiopaque substance, permits radiographs of the heart chambers, thoracic vessels, and coronary arteries. Rapid serial radiographs or motion pictures on an enlarged fluoroscopic screen show heart outline and passage of contrast materials in the great vessels. *Selective angiocardiography* or *coronary angiography* is done in association with cardiac catheterization to evaluate coronary artery disease and determine extent of obstructive disease in the coronary vessels. Aneurysms may also be diagnosed by angiography. (Refer to Chapter 20, p. 389, for more complete discussion of angiography.)

Cardiac Catheterization Under image intensification fluoroscopy, using sterile technique, a sterile catheter is introduced through cutdown into a brachial vessel in the arm or percutaneously into a femoral vessel in the groin and passed into the heart or a coronary artery. The procedure permits precise:

1 Evaluation of heart function
2 Measurements of intracardiac pressure
3 Visualization of heart chambers

Catheterization is utilized to diagnose coronory artery disease, valvular heart disease, or congenital anomalies. It is the ultimate tool for diagnosis of ischemic heart disease.

For study of the coronary arteries, a single catheter is passed and its tip inserted into the ostia of the arteries for injection of dye and trace of solution flow. Cinefluorograms record findings. After catheter removal, the incision is closed and pressure dressings are applied.

Electrocardiography is monitored continuously by oscilloscope, as cardiac arrhythmias may occur.

SPECIAL FEATURES OF CARDIAC SURGERY

1 The principles of general and thoracic surgery apply to cardiac surgery, but several factors require emphasis:
  a Extra minutes are not available; seconds save lives.
  b The team concept is of utmost importance. An experienced team working together can handle emergencies expeditiously.
  c Comprehensive physical and psychological preparation of the patient precedes operation. Postoperatively the patient is taken to an intensive care unit. The patient is monitored constantly intra- and postoperatively.

2 Operating room for cardiovascular surgery must be equipped with:
  a Cardiac defibrillator, pacemaker, and intraaortic counterpulsation devices.
  b Cardioplegic (to induce cardiac arrest) and inotropic (to modify cardiac muscle contractibility) drugs, to include but not limited to:
    1 Calcium channel-blocking agents
    2 Dopamine
    3 Dobutamine

4 Epinephrine
5 Intravenous nitroglycerin

c Laboratory facilities for blood gas and acid-base balance determinations. Modern analyzers have electronic computers to determine values.

3 Basic thoracic setup is used with the addition of cardiovascular instruments, e.g., various noncrushing vascular and anastomosis clamps, cardiotomy suction tips and sump tubes, and cardiovascular sutures.

4 Local and/or systemic hypothermia may be used intraoperatively to reduce the body's need for oxygen (refer to Chap. 13, p. 249).

5 Properly cross-matched blood for transfusion must be available. Intraoperative autotransfusion may be used for blood volume replacement (see Chap. 10, p. 173). Blood substitutes such as hetastarch, an albumin substitute for plasma expansion, may be administered.

6 Closed water-seal drainage or suction drainage is used postoperatively to drain the chest or mediastinum.

Invasive Hemodynamic Monitoring

Although placement of invasive pressure monitoring lines is not their responsibility, OR nurses should be aware of implications of data and potential for complications, e.g., infection or thrombus. To assess tissue perfusion, invasive hemodynamic monitoring is used to determine blood pressures in major arteries, veins, and heart chambers. Indwelling catheter lines are inserted to measure:

1 Radial and femoral artery pressures.

2 Central venous pressure (CVP).

3 Pulmonary artery pressures. The Swan-Ganz catheter line also determines right atrial, right ventricular, and pulmonary capillary wedge pressures of left ventricular function.

These invasive monitoring techniques are discussed in detail in Chapter 14, pp. 260 to 272. Indwelling catheters are inserted preoperatively. During operation they provide information relative to effects of anesthetic agents, operative manipulation of heart, hypothermia, extracorporeal circulation, induced ischemia, and cardiac arrest. The circulating nurse may draw blood samples from the pressure lines at intervals during cardiopulmonary bypass perfusion for blood gas analysis (refer to technique on p. 262). Catheter patency is maintained with heparinized flush solutions.

In addition to artery and CVP pressure lines, during open-heart operation the surgeon may insert a small plastic catheter directly into the left atrium to assess *left atrial pressure.* Postoperatively this catheter is connected to a transducer and monitor. The transducer balancing port must be level with right atrium. The catheter is flushed with heparinized 5% dextrose in water, because inadvertent overload with this solution is less dangerous than is overload with normal saline. Also, an air filter is attached to end of pressure tubing as a precaution against fatal air embolism. Every part of the line and filter must be flushed and free of air or the pressure bag could force a bubble into left atrium, causing embolus. In absence of mitral valve disease, left atrial pressure at end of atrial diastole, just before mitral valve opens, indicates left ventricular end-diastolic pressure and, therefore, left ventricular filling pressure and function.

Postoperatively, hemodynamic monitoring detects arrhythmias due to impaired myocardial perfusion, transient reduction in cardiac output with subsequent hypotension, hypovolemia secondary to hemorrhage, and tamponade. Circulating blood volume, pulmonary volume overload leading to pulmonary edema, and reactions to titrated pressor agents can also be identified.

Cardiopulmonary Bypass (Extracorporeal Circulation)

Cardiopulmonary bypass is the technique of oxygenating and perfusing blood by means of a mechanical pump-oxygenator system. Referred to as the *heart-lung machine,* this apparatus temporarily substitutes for function of patient's heart and lungs during cardiac surgery. Cardiopulmonary bypass is used for most intracardiac (open-heart) and coronary artery procedures. Venous blood is diverted from the body to the machine for oxygenation and pumped back to the patient.

During bypass the lungs are kept inflated and immobilized. In preparation for bypass, the patient is heparinized to prevent clot formation. Catheters are inserted, for venous diversion, into inferior and superior vena cavae through small incisions in the right atrium. A catheter for return of oxygenated blood to arterial circulation is placed in ascending aorta or femoral artery. Catheters are connected to the machine by sterile tubing before institution of bypass.

Components of the Bypass System

Oxygenator Oxygen is taken up and carbon dioxide is removed from the blood. Types of oxygenators include:

1 *Bubble.* Bubbles of oxygen are supplied to the blood by direct blood/gas contact.

2 *Membrane.* Oxygen and carbon dioxide diffuse through a permeable Teflon or polyethylene membrane that contains the blood. This method diminishes blood/gas interface. Several types of disposable membrane oxygenators are available.

3 *Microporous membrane.* Blood film is separated from ventilating gas by a microporous polypropylene membrane folded like an accordian and operated like a bubble oxygenator. Blood pressure in oxygenator exceeds gas pressure at all times, thus precluding gas bubbles passing through the microporous membrane.

Heat Exchanger Incorporated in the circuit, a heat exchanger regulates blood temperature. Water at thermostatically controlled temperature circulates through exchanger, which can rapidly produce, control, or correct systemic hypothermia. Hypothermia is often used in conjunction with bypass to reduce oxygen demands of tissues, and to protect myocardium during arrest.

Pump Rollers turning over sterile plastic tubing propel reheated oxygenated blood in a relatively nonpulsatile flow through a blood filter and bubble trap to the arterial cannula for recirculation through the body. Rate of flow can be varied. It is calculated according to patient weight or body surface area. Reduced flow accompanies hypothermia.

Perfusion Immediately before operation the machine is primed (filled) with a balanced salt solution, frequently lactated or acetated Ringer's solution, and a cardiopreservative solution including sodium bicarbonate and heparinized plasma volume expander. For a hemodilution technique of priming, the system is filled with fluid that will replace blood diverted to the pump-oxygenator system and is recirculated through the circuit to remove air bubbles. The priming solution should be of sufficient volume and of a suitable hematocrit so that when mixed with patient's blood the resultant buffered plasma will be capable of achieving adequate perfusion and preventing myocardial acidosis. Blood is added as needed to maintain adequate oxygen-carrying capacity and perfusion rate.

Bypass may be partial or total. In *partial,* only a portion of venous return is routed to the pump-oxygenator circuitry, the remaining portion following normal systemic circulation. In *total* bypass, all venous return is diverted to the machine for total body perfusion. Cord tapes placed around the caval catheters when inserted are tightened to drain all venous return to the machine, and the heart is arrested.

During perfusion the patient is intensely monitored, i.e., arterial and venous pressures, body and blood temperatures, blood gases and electrolytes, and urinary output. General anesthesia may be maintained by an anesthetic vaporizer that adds vapor to the oxygenating mixture, or by intravenous anesthesia.

At conclusion of defect repair, air is removed from the heart, heartbeat is restored, ventilation is reestablished by respirator, the patient is rewarmed, and perfusion is gradually decreased to wean patient from the machine. After discontinuance of bypass, cannulas are removed and purse-string sutures around insertion sites are tied. Protamine sulfate is injected to reverse the effect of the heparin previously administered.

Cardiopulmonary bypass may also be employed in conjunction with deep hypothermia during neurosurgical operations, in major organ transplantation, and for the perfusion of an isolated segment of the body in cancer chemotherapy.

Myocardial Preservation Although excellent results are obtained with most procedures, significant derangements can occur following cardiopulmonary bypass, which are most obvious in infants or after prolonged operations in adults. Refer to Chapter 36, p. 635, for a discussion of complications associated with cardiopulmonary bypass. During bypass, the perfusionist is in control of the patient's body temperature and preservation of body and brain. The surgeon must assume responsibility for preservation of the heart. Bypass time is kept to a minimum because ischemia causes myocardial injury of time-related severity.

A dry, motionless field allows direct vision of heart and its interior for repair of coronary circulation or intracardiac defects. Cardiopulmonary bypass permits purposely induced cardiac arrest. Deliberate arrest may be effected by one or a combination of methods.

Aortic Cross-clamping The aorta is occluded with a vascular clamp to block systemic circulation. Ischemic (anoxic) cardiac arrest occurs as the blocked systemic blood within the heart becomes deoxygenated and cardiac metabolic needs are depleted. This technique can be maintained for a limited period, however, because myocardial damage and necrosis will occur when oxygen supply and energy required to maintain subcellular system are depleted.

Ventricular Fibrillation Electrical shock to produce ventricular fibrillation induces cardiac arrest by failure of the heart to perfuse blood into systemic circulation.

Hypothermia Hypothermia reduces systemic metabolic needs. Local hypothermia can be induced by topical application of iced saline slush around heart or iced Ringer's solution to heart externally and/or internally. Cardiac arrest can also be induced by deliberately lowering body temperature below 26°C (78.8°F).

Cardioplegia Modern, safe cardiac surgery is based on the use of cardioplegic solutions used alone or in combination with the techniques discussed above. These are preparations of a small amount of potassium in crystalloid, blood, or other solution. When injected into the coronary artery system, hyperkalemia immediately induces complete electromechanical cardiac arrest. Composition and temperature of solution and infusion techniques can be determined for each patient's disease process. Some solutions have a calcium antagonist, such as verapamil or nifedipine, to help prevent myocardial ischemia. Some are infused warm, others cold. Infusion may be continuous or intermittent. When solution is flushed out of collateral circulation at end of operation, the heartbeat may resume spontaneously. If not, the ventricular fibrillation is treated with countershock.

CARDIAC OPERATIONS

The purposes of heart surgery are to correct anatomical abnormalities, repair or replace defective heart valves, excise ventricular aneurysm, or revascularize ischemic myocardium. The procedures may be performed with or without cardiopulmonary bypass. (Refer to Chapter 33 for pediatric operations.)

Commonly Used Thoracic Incisions

Median Sternotomy (Vertical Sternal Splitting) With patient supine, incision extends through midline from suprasternal notch to below xiphoid, which is resected. Retrosternal tissue is dissected and sternum is divided. Caution is used to avoid injury to underlying mediastinal structures.

At closure, heavy-gauge stainless steel sutures are placed around or through the sternum, tightly pulled together, twisted, and the ends buried in the sternum. Other nonabsorable sutures may be used to provide firm fixation. The linea alba, subcutaneous tissue, and skin are sutured. Complications are brachial plexus injury, costochondrial separation from too vigorous sternal retraction during operation, and keloid formation. Uses: open-heart procedures, pericardiectomy.

Transsternal Bilateral Thoracotomy Bilateral submammary incision is made with patient supine. In the midline the incision curves superiorly to cross sternum at fourth intercostal space level. Lateral extension is to the midaxillary line. The pleural cavity is entered via the interspace after division of pectoralis muscles. The internal mammary arteries and veins are ligated and divided, and the sternum is divided horizontally.

At closure, sternum is reapproximated securely, ribs are approximated with pericostal sutures, and remaining tissue layers are closed. Uses: resection of ventricular aneurysm, aortic arch grafts, complicated pericardiectomies. This incision is less common and causes more discomfort.

Other Thoracotomy Incisions Left anterolateral or posterolateral thoracotomy incisions may be preferred for some cardiac operations. Refer to descriptions of these incisions in Chapter 30, p. 564.

Valvular Heart Disease

Valvular disease may arise from a congenital abnormality or be acquired. Abnormal vibrations or heart murmurs may be congenital or the end result of disease such as rheumatic fever or degenerative change. Valves can become thickened and calcified, resulting in loss of valve substance, narrowing of the orifice, and immobility. They then develop *insufficiency,* failure to close completely, and permit blood leakage or regurgitation. Failure to open completely is caused by *stenosis,* which impedes flow. A defective valve is reconstructed if possible. To prevent heart failure, prosthetic valves are inserted in patients who have return of symptoms after reconstruction or have a valve that cannot be reconstructed.

Closed Mitral Commissurotomy An example of closed-heart surgery, the breaking apart of fused stenosed leaflets of the mitral (left AV) valve reduces left atrial and right ventricular pressures that decrease lung function. The thorax is entered by left anterolateral incision. To provide hemostasis, purse-string sutures are placed around the left auricular appendage prior to opening it. The surgeon frees fused leaflets by inserting a finger, valvulotome (knife), or transventricular dilator into the valve. After this is accomplished, purse-string sutures are tied and the auricular appendage is sutured. Lungs are reexpanded, a chest tube is inserted, the incision is closed, and the tube is connected to water-seal drainage.

Open Mitral Commissurotomy Fused leaflet commissures in a mitral valve which have not become thickened and calcified may be incised under direct vision during cardiopulmonary bypass. *Open mitral commissurotomy* and other plastic repairs, such as *valvuloplasty* and *annuloplasty,* improve leaflet function and protect against thromboembolism. A potential hazard of the open method is air embolism by expulsion of air from left ventricle into aorta. Residual air must be vented to avoid this complication.

Valve Replacement A diseased mitral or aortic valve may be excised and replaced. Several types of prosthetic heart valves are available. They may be mechanical or biological. With disc- or ball-type synthetic mechanical valves, disc or ball freely opens and closes according to flow of blood. One type consists of a cage in which a spherical ball is enclosed. Other models are constructed with discs resembling leaflets of human valves. The discs of some are tilted. The metal ring at base of the cage may be covered with polyester fabric to facilitate suturing. It also encourages tissue ingrowth, an aid to long-term fixation. Biological valves have also been developed from homograft or heterograft (porcine bioprosthesis or bovine pericardial xenograft) donor material. Formaldehyde storage solution must be rinsed from heterografts prior to use. An effective prosthesis is nontoxic, nonthrombogenic, and nondeteriorating. The surgeon selects the most suitable type and size for defect to be repaired. Contamination of a valve can be cause of a serious postoperative endocarditis. Sterility must be maintained prior to and during insertion.

Mitral Valve Replacement Cardiopulmonary bypass is used for mitral valve replacement, an open-heart procedure. Through median sternotomy or left thoracotomy incision, the pericardium is incised and retracted. When bypass catheters are placed, the left ventricle may be vented with a plastic tube to decompress the heart and prevent overdistention of the ventricle at unclamping of the aorta after anoxic arrest. The left atrium is opened. The mitral valve is exposed, inspected, and removed by circumferential excision and severance of muscular attachments to the ventricular wall. The fibrous ring or annulus surrounding the valvular opening remains intact. A sterile prosthetic valve is inserted and sutured in place, and the atrium is sutured. Teflon felt pledgets are commonly used as a buttress under sutures to prevent the annulus from tearing when the prosthetic valve is seated and sutures are tied.

The probability of thromboembolic complications is sufficient in a patient with chronic atrial fibrillation and an enlarged left atrium to warrant postoperative anticoagulant therapy. Therefore, a durable synthetic mechanical prosthetic device may be the valve of choice for this procedure.

Postoperatively, temporary pacing may be required (see p. 579). Pacing wires are implanted in the wall of the right or left ventricle during operation. If sequential pacing will be necessary, additional wires are placed in the right atrium. Then the pericardium is closed. Blood is returned to heart and air removed from it. Partial cardiopulmonary bypass is resumed as patient is being weaned from the machine. Cannula incisions are closed. Thoracic wound closure is carried out and water-seal chest drainage is used.

Aortic Valve Replacement Operation for aortic valve replacement is basically the same as that described for mitral valve replacement, except that the aortic valve is exposed through a transverse incision in the aorta. Either a mechanical valve or bioprosthesis may be used. Biological prostheses offer the advantage of low embolic rate and obviate the need for prolonged anticoagulation therapy.

Ischemic Heart Disease

Coronary arteries supplying the heart muscle (myocardium) may become stenosed or obstructed, which is referred to as *occlusive coronary artery disease.* Resultant myocardial ischemia may result in angina or myocardial infarction. Myocardial revascularization to improve blood supply to the affected myocardium is possible by operative intervention in selected patients. The operation relieves anginal pain. *Ventricular arrhythmias* also are a major problem associated with ischemic heart disease. These may be treated by interrupting reentry pathways by endocardial resection. Results of these operations depend on numerous factors, including the patient's preoperative cardiovascular status.

Coronary Artery Bypass Graft Segment(s) of saphenous vein and/or internal mammary artery are used to bypass coronary artery obstruction. The right coronary, left anterior descending, and circumflex arteries are most commonly involved. Single or multiple bypasses are done depending on the number of vessels affected and degree of obstruction present. Techniques of cardiopulmonary bypass are influenced by the surgeon's preferred procedure and extent of grafting.

Saphenous Vein Bypass Graft The procedure for saphenous vein bypass graft is expedited by two teams; one harvests the saphenous vein for graft while the other opens the chest and prepares for cardiopulmonary bypass. (A cephalic vein may be used if the saphenous vein is diseased or has been previously stripped.) Adequate vein is removed for sufficient graft material. The distal end of each vein segment removed is identified and the graft is placed in heparinized normal saline after harvest. It is handled gently to avoid trauma to the intima.

The chest is opened by median sternotomy and the pericardium is incised. Cardiopulmonary bypass is established. After a small opening is created in the aorta, the reversed vein is sutured to the aperture. It is important to position graft with distal end of the vein at the aortic anastomosis site to permit normal direction of blood flow through venous valves. The coronary artery is opened distal to obstruction; the free end of the graft is anastomosed to artery end-to-side. Cardiopulmonary bypass is discontinued and all incisions are closed. Chest drainage is used. After removal from extracorporeal circulation and stabilization of blood pressure, flow may be measured in each graft with an electromagnetic flowmeter.

Internal Mammary Artery Anastomosis The internal mammary artery is dissected up to its origin from the subclavian artery. After mobilization, end-to-side anastomosis is performed primarily between internal mammary and left anterior descending artery, distal to the obstruction. It may also be used as a graft to other diseased coronary arteries. The pericardium is not sutured to provide adequate drainage. The wound is closed in usual manner for sternotomy with water-seal drainage.

Endarterectomy of Coronary Arteries Removal of an organized thrombus and attached endothelium or atherosclerotic fatty plaques from an arterial wall is performed infrequently. Endarterectomy may be combined with venous bypass grafting. Small endarterectomy spatulas and wire loops are used to remove segments of obstructing core to increase blood flow through the graft, especially to the right coronary artery.

Percutaneous Transluminal Coronary Angioplasty Performed under fluoroscopy with image intensification, balloon dilation of coronary arteries may be procedure of choice for selected patients with significant atherosclerotic narrowing in a major coronary artery. The coronary arteries are approached by either percutaneous femoral artery entry or brachial artery cutdown. A balloon-tipped catheter is passed through a guiding catheter into area of coronary artery with atherosclerotic material (plaque). The balloon is inflated by a hydraulic pump to compress plaque against the arterial lining and dilate the arterial wall, thus enlarging the lumen. This procedure is performed in the cardiac catheterization laboratory or special procedures room in x-ray department. However, a standby OR team must be available for emergency coronary artery bypass in the event that acute coronary obstruction occurs.

Endocardial Resection Severe ventricular arrhythmias associated with ischemic heart disease and malignant ventricular tachyarrhythmias can be surgically treated by ablating areas of myocardial damage. With epicardial and endocardial mapping techniques, the surgeon is able to identify and then excise specific sites of arrhythmias, thus interrupting reentry pathways. This procedure may be done in conjunction with aneurysm repair.

Excision of Ventricular Aneurysm Atherosclerotic coronary disease predisposes an individual to myocardial infarction. Ventricular aneurysm, a segmental dilatation of predominantly the left ventricular wall, may develop any time from a few weeks but mainly to a few years postinfarction. The thin-walled fibrous aneurysm, result of ventricular force on an area of nonfunctioning scar tissue, often contains clots within it. Left ventricular aneurysm usually produces hemodynamic instability manifested by congestive heart failure and ventricular arrhythmia. Utilizing cardiopulmonary bypass, the surgeon can excise the aneurysm and reconstruct the ventricle.

The chest is opened by median sternotomy and cardiopulmonary bypass established before adhesion between the aneurysm and pericardium is detached. The ascending aorta is cross-clamped and cardioplegic solution is injected. The aneurysmal sac, entered by stab wound, collapses with suctioning when the heart is empty. Viable myocardium retains shape. The apex is opened with vertical incision and fibrotic myocardium is excised circumferentially with a rim of fibrous tissue left to hold the sutures used to close the left ventricle. Pledgets may be employed to reinforce sutures. All air is removed from the ventricle by suction before completion of closure. Heartbeat is restored, the patient is decannulated, and all other incisions are closed in the usual manner.

Aneurysmectomy may be done as a single procedure or in conjunction with coronary artery bypass or valve replacement procedure.

Cardiac Transplantation

Cardiac transplantation may be the only alternative for patients with end-stage cardiac disease who are incapacitated by chronic heart failure. Refer to Chapter 34 for discussion of organ transplantation.

Mechanical Devices

Mechanical assist devices may be indicated for patients with cardiac dysfunction. These devices may be implanted in conjunction with other cardiac operations or to provide long-term assistance for life-sustaining cardiac function.

Cardiac Pacemaker The conducting system of the heart may be altered or interrupted at any point by degenerative disease, drugs, or operative trauma. This may cause syncope, diminished cardiac output, hypotension, arrhythmias, partial or complete heart block, or sinus bradycardia (sick-sinus syndrome). Patients with these conditions may be treated by artificial pacing, i.e., delivery of electric impulse by a pacemaker, to correct atrial and ventricular arrhythmias and to interrupt ventricular fibrillation.

A pacemaker consists of a pulse generator to produce electric impulses and leads to carry impulses to stimulating electrodes placed in contact with the heart. A pacing system must include electromyocardial conduction. Lithium batteries supply power for years to the microprocessor of the pulse generator. Platinum alloy or stainless steel electrodes, with leads encased in plastic, may be unipolar or bipolar. With bipolar systems, electric current flows between two electrodes during pacing; it flows between electrode tip and pulse generator in unipolar systems.

A pacemaker may be either a standby *ventricular demand* type or the *physiologic* type. Both types are intermittent and noncompetitive with the patient's own pacing system. They monitor the heart's normal activity. The impulse to stimulate the heart is not emitted unless rate of heartbeat falls below a preset level. Also known as the R-wave-inhibited or QRS-inhibited pacemaker, electrodes of the ventricular demand pacemaker are placed in the ventricle. Stimulating electrodes are placed in atrium, ventricle, or both, depending on type of physiologic pacemaker to be used.

Effective external pacing for ventricular standstill led to development of partially implanted electrode leads connected to an external stimulator for long-term pacing for other conditions. Fully implantable pacemaker systems for long-term use have been available since 1960. An implantable microprocessor generator is hermetically sealed in a metallic container impermeable to body fluids. Selection of system depends on specific pacing requirements of the individual patient. Pacemakers may be temporary or permanent. Endocardial (transvenous) or myocardial (epicardial) electrode leads may be used. Most of these units are programmable to alter pacing function. Temporary pacing is often necessary prior to and during permanent-system implantation. Systemic complete heart block and sinus bradycardia are the most frequent indications for permanent implantation. Permanent pacing may be initiated by the following.

Insertion of Endocardial Pacemaker A transvenous electrode lead is placed in the endocardium and attached to a pulse generator. Under local anesthesia, an incision is made just beneath the clavicle on either side of the chest. The lead may be placed by incision in the cephalic vein or by the Seldinger technique in the subclavian vein. Under fluoroscopy, an endocardial electrode catheter (lead) is advanced via the superior vena cava into the apex of right ventricle, where it is wedged against the endocardium. Atrial leads are directed into right atrial appendage. The lead is connected to the pulse generator which, in turn, is placed into a previously prepared subcutaneous pocket. Incision is closed with or without suction drainage.

Placement of Myocardial Electrodes Myocardial electrodes are placed under general anesthesia via a transthoracic approach to the heart. For an extrapleural parasternal approach, the pericardium is entered by subperichondrial resection of fifth costal cartilage. Two sew-on or screw-in type myocardial electrodes are implanted 1 cm apart in epicardium (outside myocardium) of right or left ventricle and/or atrium. After the pacing thresholds are measured from an external source, electrode leads are tunneled under costal margin to the pulse generator implanted in a subcutaneous pocket in left upper quadrant of abdominal wall. Water-seal chest drainage is necessary only if pleura has been opened.

Precautions with Pacemakers Use of electrosurgical unit is usually avoided during placement of pacemaker or when a patient with a pacemaker is operated on. Electromagnetic interference may affect the pulse generator, depending on type of pacemaker. If necessary, the electrosurgical generator should be kept as far away from pulse generator as possible. An inactive electrode ground pad or plate should be placed in buttocks or thigh area, not near chest.

A pacing system analyzer measures the amount of energy in milliamperes (mA) needed to stimulate the heart. It is used to locate area of myocardium where least amount of energy will be needed, generally 0.4 to 0.8 mA, and to test function of electrode and pulse generator prior to placement. Telemetric communication capabilities of some pacemakers allow surgeon to obtain direct evidence of battery output.

Patient with a pacemaker requires adequate follow-up and should carry identification containing serial number, model, rate, manufacturer's name, and date of insertion. *The circulating nurse must record this information in patient's chart, along with time of insertion.* Patients with demand or radio-frequency units should be warned to avoid proximity to radar devices, since electrical interference may stimulate heart activity. Newer models have metallic shielding to minimize this concern.

Defibrillator-Cardioverter Implantable antiarrhythmic devices are available for patients who have episodes of life-threatening ventricular tachyarrhythmias or fibrillation. The device delivers a synchronized shock when the sensor recognizes changes in patient's heart rate and cardiac cycle length. The electric conduction pattern of the heart is converted to a more normal pattern. Placement of devices is similar to procedures described for implantation of cardiac pacemakers.

Intraaortic Balloon Pump An intraaortic balloon pump (IABP) is a supportive device used to assist a patient with prolonged myocardial ischemia, reversible left ventricular failure, cardiogenic shock, or for temporary support following cardiac surgery. It often is inserted in the OR in conjunction with open-heart operation to reduce left ventricular workload and increase delivery of oxygen to myocardium, thereby increasing cardiac output and systemic perfusion.

The cylinder-shaped balloon is inserted into the descending thoracic aorta, just below the left subclavian artery, by way of a femoral artery. The balloon catheter may be inserted percutaneously or by direct vision, or inserted via a prosthetic arterial graft anastomosed end-to-side to the femoral artery. After insertion, the balloon catheter is connected to a pump console.

IABP utilizes principles of counterpulsation. In contrast to systemic arteries, coronary arteries are constricted during systole and fill during diastole. Therefore, inflating the balloon during diastole increases coronary perfusion, aiding contractility and oxygen transport. When the balloon is inflated, the blood volume displaced increases coronary arterial pressure. When the balloon deflates during systole, resistance that the ventricle must pump against is decreased. Balloons vary in size to provide 20-, 30-, or 40-ml volume displacement, thus giving maximum assist without total aortic occlusion. When balloon is placed and position is verified by chest x-ray, the complete system is vented of air and filled with either helium or carbon dioxide, for balloon inflation, depending on type of counterpulsator. The ratio of ventricular assist is determined by the individual patient's hemodynamic status. The pump can be regulated automatically, triggered by an electrocardiogram signal, or operated manually. To prevent potential thrombi, pumping should be continuous. Intraaortic balloons are made of antithrombic material. Manufacturer's instructions for use must be followed. Pumps are equipped with sensors, e.g., an alarm and an automatic shut-off, to minimize danger. Weaning from IABP is usually gradual in accordance with the patient's tolerance.

Left Ventricular Assist Pumps Powered left ventricular assist devices, partial artificial hearts, can provide short- or long-term mechanical support of failing heart or circulation when IABP is inadequate. A *short-term abdominal left ventricular assist device* (ALVAD) may be interposed between apex of left ventricle and infrarenal abdominal aorta. It augments cardiac output and coronary perfusion and supports circulation during episodes of ventricular standstill or fibrillation. ALVAD is connected to an external pneumatic power source. It is used to wean patients from cardiopulmonary bypass, to support circulation following postinfarction cardiogenic shock, and as a temporary bridge prior to heart transplantation. Left atrial to aortic bypass may also be used during recovery following myocardial infarction.

A totally implantable *long-term left ventricular assist system* (LVAS) provides circulatory support by synchronous counterpulsation for patient with profound cardiac failure. The electrically actuated pump, implanted in the abdomen, receives blood from the apex of left ventricle and ejects it into the abdominal aorta. The internal battery pack and control unit are connected to an external battery pack.

Artificial Heart The ventricles are removed and replaced with mechanical devices. The devices may be made of molded polyurethane (Biomer), supported on metallic bases, with tilting-disc valves in the inflow and outflow ports of the pumping chamber. Connector cuffs are sutured to the remaining atria, pulmonary artery and aorta. These cuffs attach to the artificial ventricles, which are connected to an external battery-powered pneumatic or electronic drive system. The system has safety alarms and a backup mechanism in event of mechanical or electric failure. An artificial heart ultimately may be used as an alternative to heart transplantation in patient with chronic end-stage progressive congestive heart failure, or as temporary support while patient is awaiting a transplant.

CHAPTER **32**

PERIPHERAL VASCULAR SURGERY

Circulation within the peripheral vascular system affects the brain, internal organs, and the extremities. An expanding body of knowledge relating to vascular physiology and development of the art of vascular surgery has improved the quality of life for many patients with peripheral vascular diseases.

HISTORICAL DEVELOPMENT

For centuries human beings have been plagued with peripheral vascular disease and its complications, such as pain, loss of an extremity or life. Longevity has increased the number of people suffering from diseases of the vascular system, atherosclerosis being the most common, producing arterial stenosis or occlusion. An endarterectomy was first performed in 1946 to treat localized disease. In 1948 the first bypass graft was implanted to treat diffuse disease. The decades of the 1960s and 1970s marked advancement in the development of many new operations utilizing improved instrumentation, sutures, synthetic grafts, angiography, and microvascular techniques.

In 1983 the American Board of Surgery began a certification program in general vascular surgery. To qualify, candidates must have specialized training and practice in peripheral vascular surgery and be a Diplomate of the American Board of Surgery and/or the American Board of Thoracic Surgery. Peripheral vascular surgery is the newest subspecialty with accredited residency programs. Approved programs may be combined with general surgery or cardiothoracic training.

PERIPHERAL VASCULAR SYSTEM

Circulatory problems may affect any part of the body, but this discussion focuses on the most common pathology amenable to vascular operations performed by vascular surgeons.

Anatomy and Physiology

Vessels in the thorax, abdomen, extremities, and extracranial cerebrovascular area constitute the *circulatory system.* The ascending aorta, originating from the left ventricle, carries oxygenated blood from the heart to the arteries. The major arteries leading to the head and upper extremities branch off from the aortic arch in the middle mediastinum above the heart. These are the brachiocephalic trunk, left common carotid, and subclavian arteries. The thoracic aorta then descends through the posterior mediastinum at left side of vertebral column. Passing through the diaphragm, the abdominal aorta descends to level of fourth lumbar vertebra where it bifurcates, divides, to form the common iliac arteries leading to the lower extremities. Arteries from the abdominal aorta carry blood to the kidneys and the abdominal and pelvic organs. The femoral artery, originating from the iliac, is the main artery in each leg.

Blood flows from the arterial system through the capillary network and returns to the heart via the venous system. The vena cavae enter the right atrium—the superior vena cava formed by the major veins from the head and upper extremities and the inferior vena cava formed by the major veins from the lower extremities and abdomen.

Related diseases that cause occlusion or stenosis, such as atherosclerosis, are usually acquired. Inadequate blood supply causes ischemia in tissues. If untreated, this can lead to thrombus, embolus, ulceration, necrosis, or gangrene. Obstructions to venous return, venous stasis disease, can cause hemodynamic imbalances. Through vascular surgery, vessels are repaired, reconstructed, or replaced to improve peripheral (systemic) circulation. Infection is a devastating postoperative complication that must be avoided through strict adherence to aseptic and sterile techniques.

Diagnostic Procedures

Peripheral arterial and venous diseases are assessed prior to and following operative intervention. Peripheral vascular laboratories have been established in many centers to perform noninvasive studies.

Noninvasive A Doppler *ultrasound* velocity detection device measures segmental arterial pressures and venous patency in extremities. Sonography is a major diagnostic tool for abdominal circulation as well. *Ocular plethysmography* and *carotid phonoangiography* are techniques used to obtain blood-flow measurements to localize obstructions in vessels of head and neck. A *pulse volume* recorder is also used to localize segmental obstructions in the vascular system.

Invasive *Aortography* is radiographic visualization of aorta by injection of a nontoxic radiopaque substance. Selective *arteriography* permits study of a particular artery or branch of the aorta. These are angiographic procedures as previously described (see Chap. 20, p. 389).

Iatrogenic Arterial Injuries

Vascular injury can occur during invasive diagnostic, monitoring, or therapeutic procedures. Iatrogenic arterial injuries, those resulting from an unexpected outcome of a procedure, can cause loss of function or even death due to ischemia, hemorrhage, or embolus. The patient must be carefully observed and monitored for signs of complications during and following these procedures.

SPECIAL FEATURES OF PERIPHERAL VASCULAR SURGERY

1 A thorough understanding of principles of general surgery should be combined with special training in vascular operative techniques. An experienced operating team is essential because of the tendency of blood to clot. Speed and accuracy are imperative.

2 A hypo-hyperthermia blanket or mattress is put on operating table before patient arrives, in the event that it is needed. Temperature regulation may be a problem during long procedures or when multiple blood transfusions are given.

3 Local or attended local anesthesia is usually preferred for most angiographic studies. General anesthesia or regional block is used for the operative procedure.

4 Meticulous care is exercised in anastomosing vessels to avoid danger of postoperative thrombosis.

5 To prevent undue trauma to vessels, an assortment of scissors, noncrushing vascular clamps, and forceps specifically designed for vascular surgery are included in the instrument setup. Umbilical tape or synthetic loops are used for retraction and vascular control.

6 The operating microscope may be used for anastomosing vessels. Appropriate instrumentation for microsurgery must be available.

7 Synthetic nonabsorbable suture materials are preferred because they are strong and pass through vessel walls and grafts easily with minimal trauma and tissue reaction. Swaged needles also minimize trauma. Double-armed needle sutures are frequently employed for vessel anastomosis.

8 Heparinized solution must be available for use as an anticoagulant. If given IV for immediate systemic effect, the average dose is 100 units per kilogram of body weight. At end of procedure before closure, protamine sulfate in equivalent dose may be given to reverse anticoagulant effect.

9 Blood must be available at time of operation, since it is lost by flushing of clots and debris. It may be warmed prior to transfusion. Blood loss should be calculated.

10 The most serious immediate postoperative complications are thrombosis and hemorrhage. The patient may need to return to the operating room for *immediate* correction of these problems.

Doppler ultrasound is frequently used intraoperatively as well as pre- and postoperatively to assess blood flow.

Vascular Prostheses

Biological or synthetic prosthetic grafts are required to bypass vascular obstruction or to reconstruct vessels. These substitute conduits for blood flow vary in length, diameter, and configuration to meet requirements of each situation. A graft may be straight or bifurcated into a Y shape. Pieces of synthetic material may be cut to size for use as patch grafts. Grafts are sterilized in see-through containers or packages to permit surgeon to select the appropriate size after exposure of the operative site.

Biological Vascular Grafts Autografts, homografts and heterografts may be used for arterial or venous grafting.

Saphenous Vein An autogenous graft is taken from the patient's saphenous vein. When placed in arterial system, the vein is reversed from normal anatomic position so that the valves will not obstruct arterial blood flow.

When a saphenous vein graft will be used, two surgeons may work simultaneously, one exposing the operative site while the other prepares the vein for grafting. A separate sterile table, supplied with fine vascular instruments and basin of heparinized saline for flushing the vein, is used for vein preparation. The surgeon may use magnification loupes to check for imperfections while preparing the vein.

Venous Allograft Veins harvested for grafting may be treated with cyclosporine and be cryopreserved. The resultant altered immunologic reaction improves late patency of the graft. Fresh venous allografts are also used. The recipient patient receives immunosuppression when these grafts are used.

Modified Human Umbilical Vein Graft A special glutaraldehyde tanning process converts an umbilical vein into an inert biopolymer. Fine mesh polyester is applied to outer surface for added strength. The antithrombogenic nature of this graft with no ingrowth or intimal hyperplasia makes this an effective graft. The glutaraldehyde must be thoroughly irrigated from the graft with sterile heparinized saline or Ringer's solution before implantation. After rinsing, the graft should remain in sterile heparinized saline solution to keep it moist until implanted. Only noncrushing clamps should be used to avoid damage to the graft during handling.

Bovine Carotid Artery Enzymatically treated bovine carotid artery heterografts may be used to create arteriovenous vascular shunts or fistulas (see p. 588).

Synthetic Vascular Prostheses Various forms of synthetic materials are used to construct arterial vascular prostheses. Some materials are more suitable for specific applications than are others. The surgeon selects the most appropriate graft for each patient.

Knitted Polyester Knitted polyester (Dacron) grafts are porous enough to allow ingrowth of fibrous tissue into interstices. However, they are also porous enough to allow seepage of blood through the material. Therefore they must be preclotted before insertion. For the *preclotting process,* the surgeon withdraws blood from patient at the operative site prior to anticoagulation therapy. The blood is transferred to scrub nurse, who may inject it into lumen of the graft and/or soak graft in the blood in a sterile basin. The prime goal in preclotting is to make the wall of graft impervious to blood by filling the interstices with fibrin. The fabric-fibrin conduit later becomes firmly placed in tissue and provides a hypothrombogenic flow surface.

Filamentous Velour Knitted velour construction of these polyester grafts has uniform porosity for easy preclotting and ensures rapid tissue ingrowth. They may be crimped or noncrimped, with velour inside and/or outside. One type, the exoskeleton (EXS) prosthesis, has a spiral polypropylene support fused to the outer surface of noncrimped velour. This graft was developed specifically for use across the knee joint. Another type, with amikacin bonded to knitted filamentous velour polyester with a collagen matrix, provides an antibiotic in the prosthetic wall. This construction also renders the porous graft impervious to leaks, obviating the need for preclotting. Bonded albumin also reduces porosity and potential thrombosis. This can be achieved by "baking-on" autologous plasma. The graft is soaked in patient's plasma and then autoclaved.

Woven Polyester The weave of woven polyester (Dacron) grafts is tight enough to be leakproof.

Therefore, these grafts do not require preclotting. The more inflexible construction limits their use, however, to aortic replacement or bypass of large-caliber arteries.

Polytetrafluorethylene (PTFE) The microporous wall of PTFE serves as a lattice framework into which cells grow to become surface for contact with blood. These prostheses do not require preclotting. They are usually used for small- or medium-sized vessels.

CONSERVATIVE THERAPY

Percutaneous Transluminal Angioplasty

Severe ischemia due to segmental stenosis or occlusive disease in the femoral and iliac arteries can be conservatively treated by dilation. *Percutaneous transluminal angioplasty* is performed under local anesthesia and fluoroscopy, frequently in the x-ray department by a radiologist. The artery is punctured percutaneously and a guide wire is advanced through the stenotic or occluded segment. A Gruntzig balloon catheter is passed over the guide wire. Catheters of several diameters with balloons of various widths and lengths are available. The polyvinyl chloride balloon can be inflated to a preselected cylindrical shape. When inflated, atheromatous material is compressed against the arterial wall. There may be actual splitting of the plaque and intima and stretching of the media, thus dilating lumen of a stenosis or recanalizing an occlusion.

Thrombectomy and Embolectomy

A Fogarty catheter, inserted proximally, may be advanced into a vessel distally beyond an obstruction. The balloon on the tip is inflated. Thrombotic or embolic material is removed as catheter is withdrawn. This procedure is performed under local anesthesia to restore blood flow usually to an extremity. If this conservative attempt is unsuccessful, a graft to replace or bypass the occluded segment of the vessel may be necessary.

PERIPHERAL VASCULAR OPERATIONS

Arterial Bypass

Blockage of an artery may be due to occlusive vascular disease or trauma. Arterial injury may indirectly occur near the site of fractures. The vessel lumina above and below the lesion is usually normal. Vascular reconstruction is performed in an attempt to restore normal circulation. The surgeon selects an appropriate method to bypass the obstruction.

1 The involved segment may be excised and the ends anastomosed if they can be approximated without tension.

2 If direct suture is impossible, the involved segment is excised and an autograft or synthetic prosthetic graft is used as replacement.

3 The lesion can be bypassed using the long saphenous vein from one thigh as a vein graft, or a synthetic prosthetic graft may be used. Ends of the graft are anastomosed to the artery proximal and distal to the lesion. The obstructed segment of the artery is not resected.

4 The lesion can be bypassed by interposing a prosthetic graft between a patent artery and the artery distal to lesion, an extra-anatomical bypass. For example, in femoral-femoral bypass, graft is placed from femoral artery of unaffected leg to femoral artery of ischemic leg. In axillofemoral bypass, graft is placed from axillary artery to femoral artery of ischemic leg.

Femoropopliteal Artery Bypass The femoral artery is most prone to obstruction by occlusive vascular disease in a lower extremity. A femoropopliteal bypass may be procedure of choice for severe ischemic disease and limb salvage. It is the most frequently performed bypass operation in an extremity. The patient is positioned supine on operating table with thigh of affected leg slightly abducted and knee flexed and supported. The entire extremity is prepped and draped to allow adequate exposure. Incisions are made over femoral and popliteal arteries to expose arteries and explore area before bypassing the obstruction in the femoral artery. An autogenous saphenous vein graft, PTFE graft, or externally supported non-crimped velour graft may be used. During operation, pulsations of proximal and distal popliteal artery are checked as well as pulsations in the foot. Postoperatively, the distal pulsations may be checked with a Doppler pulse detector, an instrument that detects blood flow through arteries by means of ultrasound.

Endarterectomy

Atherosclerotic plaques may cause localized stenosis in major arteries such as the femorals and carotids. A loosely attached plaque is removed by dissection in the media utilizing vascular wire loops, spatulas, and/or catheters. Plaque can be vaporized with laser beam.

Carotid Endarterectomy Carotid endarterectomy is done to prevent stroke in patient with severe carotid artery insufficiency. Atherosclerotic plaques at the carotid bifurcation cause localized stenosis or ulceration. Endarterectomy is indicated when there is significant narrowing causing transient ischemic attacks (TIA). Patient is positioned supine with head turned away from operative side. Care must be taken not to place undue extension on neck, because this may occlude vertebral blood flow. An oblique incision about 4 in. (10 cm) long in neck is carried through subcutaneous tissue, platysma muscle, and anterior border of sternocleidomastoid muscle. Retraction of sternocleidomastoid muscle and jugular vein allows exposure of carotid artery and its branches. After systemic heparinization, special vascular instruments are used to clamp above and below occluded area. In certain instances a shunt will be inserted in the artery to maintain blood flow to brain while the plaque is removed. Many surgeons use a shunt routinely; others use alternative means of cerebral protection, such as deliberately producing mild to moderate hypertension or hypercapnea. In any event, prolonged delay of the procedure at this time may cause serious neurological complications. The carotid is incised and plaque is removed. Reconstructive procedures may include patch-graft angioplasty or bypass grafting. Bilateral endarterectomies may be indicated for severe bilateral occlusion, but operations are performed at least a week apart.

Laser Surgery Atherosclerotic plaques can be vaporized with laser beam from femoral and carotid arteries. Subsequent inflammation and fibrosis is minimal and healing is rapid.

Aneurysmectomy

An *aneurysm* is a localized abnormal dilatation of an artery with formation of a sac due to mechanical pressure of blood on a vessel wall weakened by biochemical alterations. Atherosclerosis is the most common cause but trauma may be an etiologic factor. Cystic medial necrosis causes dissecting aneurysm, usually of the thoracic aorta. Loss of structural integrity is implicit in every aneurysm. Abdominal aorta, thoracic aorta, and popliteal arteries are vessels usually affected. Diagnostic evaluation combines physical examination, laboratory findings, ultrasound, aorto- or arteriography, and NMR (see Chap. 20). Location and extent of lesion determine operability and type of reconstruction. However, a ruptured aneurysm precludes further evaluation and operation must be performed *immediately.*

Resection of Abdominal Aortic Aneurysm Abdominal aneurysmectomy may be a lifesaving operation. However, serious hazards, including massive hemorrhage and injury to ureters and other nearby structures, are associated with it. Renal failure is a potential complication. Modern techniques have greatly reduced mortality rate. Survivors of the operation enjoy the same life expectancy as do other patients with comparable atherosclerotic disease.

Constant monitoring of cardiac function with a Swan Ganz pulmonary artery catheter (see Chap. 14, p. 266) may be used in high-risk patients. Unstable patients may require frequent blood gas determinations. Central venous pressure monitoring is a guide for regulating fluid replacement. Blood must be available for transfusion. Autotransfusion may be used if massive hemorrhage is encountered, as with a ruptured aortic aneurysm. Urinary output must be recorded. A Foley catheter is inserted preoperatively. Mannitol can be infused to prevent ischemic renal failure. Blood flow in extremities should be checked immediately pre- and postoperatively to detect embolic problems. A Doppler device may be used.

The patient is in supine position. The abdomen from nipple line to pubis, groins, and upper thighs are prepped and draped. A long midline incision from xiphoid process to pubis usually is used. The abdomen is thoroughly explored, the small intestinal mesentery mobilized, and the posterior peritoneum overlying the aorta incised to expose the aneurysm. A self-retaining abdominal wall retractor helps give needed exposure. The small intestine and ascending colon are delivered outside the abdomen to increase exposure and to prevent injury. Warm moist tapes, plastic sheeting, or a Lahey bag may be used to protect these structures.

Before occlusion of aorta, blood is withdrawn if needed for preclotting in the graft. Heparin is injected for anticoagulation. Appropriate-sized aortic clamps are placed proximal to aneurysm and iliac arteries are clamped distally. The distal aortic stump or iliac arteries may be closed with staples. The aneurysmal wall is opened. The clot and loose intraluminal debris are removed. A tube graft is used if aneurysm is confined to aorta. More commonly, a bifurcated graft is sutured into place above the aneurysm and to the common iliac or appropriate arteries distally. Living tissue, for example, posterior portion of aneurysm sac or mesentery, must cover the prosthesis to prevent contact of prosthesis with intestines. Failure to accomplish this may result in fistula formation. The long abdominal incision is usually closed with nonabsorbable sutures placed in the midline fascia. Retention sutures are frequently used.

Embolectomy

An *embolus* is a mass of undissolved matter carried by the bloodstream until it lodges in a blood vessel and occludes it. An embolus may be an air bubble, a fat globule, a clump of bacteria, a piece of tissue, or a foreign body. The occlusion of a blood vessel by an embolus causes various symptoms, depending on size and location of occluded vessel. Occlusion of a vessel in the brain, lungs, or heart can cause rapid and sudden death. Surgical intervention is the primary treatment for embolus unless operation is contraindicated. Selected patients may be treated with heparin, vasodilators, and perhaps sympathetic blocks. Renal or mesenteric emboli are usually treated by embolectomy or bypass grafting. To perform an embolectomy, the affected blood vessel is incised and the embolus is removed.

Pulmonary Embolus Occlusion of pulmonary artery or one of its branches usually occurs from emboli originating from veins in lower extremities or pelvis. Emboli pass up the inferior vena cava to right side of the heart and are ejected from right ventricle into pulmonary artery. Pulmonary embolism may be diagnosed by lung scans, pulmonary angiograms, and phlebograms. Operation may be indicated when anticoagulant therapy fails or is contraindicated, to prevent passage of emboli to the lungs. Blood flow may be partially interrupted with plastic serrated clips or filter blocks. The inferior vena cava may be ligated to prevent passage of septic emboli arising from infected pelvic veins.

Mobbin-Udden Filter Procedure The Mobbin-Uddin filter procedure is one effective technique for partial interruption of the inferior vena cava. A long applicator with stylet and loading cone is assembled with the collapsed umbrellalike filter inside. Under fluoroscopy with television amplification, the applicator is inserted through a right internal jugular venotomy. The filter is ejected and fixed in position below the renal veins and above the point of juncture of the iliac veins. The procedure may be performed on poor-risk patients under local anesthesia with an anesthesiologist in attendance.

Vena Caval Ligation or Plication Vena caval ligation or plication may be performed by abdominal approach in patients who are reasonable risks for general anesthesia. The surgeon may choose midline transabdominal, retroperitoneal, or subcostal intraperitoneal approach, depending on the exposure needed. After inferior vena cava is exposed and freed, a clip is passed around vein and secured with a plicating suture, or the vein may be ligated. This allows blood to return to the right ventricle of the heart without passage of emboli. Thighs and legs frequently are wrapped with elastic bandages and elevated before patient leaves the OR to prevent postoperative edema, the main complication.

Venous Stasis Disease

When valves of veins fail to function normally, increased back pressure of blood causes veins to become dilated, tortuous, or elongated. These are known as *varicose veins.* Pain and secondary complications, such as thrombophlebitis and varicose ulcers from venous stasis, may follow. It is believed that there is a familial tendency toward varicosities, which afflict both men and women. Habitual long periods of standing, repeated pregnancies, and obesity are other predisposing factors.

A procedure may be performed to bypass a venous obstruction, such as iliac-venous occlusion or femoropopliteal occlusion. Newer techniques are used for venous valve repair or venous valve transposition to correct femoral valvular incompetence and severe venous stasis.

Ligation and Stripping of Veins The most common operative treatment of varicose veins consists of ligating the great saphenous vein at the femoral junction. The vein is then excised in toto with the aid of a stripping device. Additional incisions are made along its course from groin to ankle as required to excise affected tributaries. Preoperatively, the surgeon may wish to mark with an indelible marker areas of varicosity for incision.

Following closure of incisions and application of dressings, full length of the leg is wrapped in cotton elastic bandages for compression. Postoperatively, it is important to stimulate circulation and prevent venous thrombosis by early ambulation.

Vascular Shunts

Normal circulation can be altered to increase or decrease blood flow to a specific organ. Vascular clamps, hemostatic agents, and blood products for blood volume replacement must be available for portosystemic shunt procedures requiring vascular anastomoses. A prosthetic vascular shunt may be inserted to establish an external route for diversion of blood flow through a mechanical device.

Arteriovenous Shunts and Fistulas Access to the vascular system through an arteriovenous shunt or fistula can be a lifesaving technique for patients suffering from chronic uremia who need renal dialysis, or for patients requiring a series of exchange blood transfusions. Insertion of a shunt or creation of an internal or external fistula requires attention to detail, since longevity is an important consideration. The most frequent complications are thrombosis and infection. (Refer to Chapter 23, p. 451, for discussion of renal hemodialysis procedures.)

Portacaval Shunt Portacaval shunting is definitive therapy in selected patients with gastrointestinal bleeding due to esophageal varices when bleeding is not controlled by conservative methods. The purpose of the operation is to reduce portal venous hypertension and/or portal venous blood flow. Hypertension, increase in portal pressure, is caused by intrahepatic blood-flow obstruction as a result of cirrhosis, hepatitis, or thrombosis. The increased pressure thus produced results in venous dilatation. The patient may have ascites.

Anastomosis of the portal vein to the inferior vena cava relieves hypertension by bypassing obstruction and diverting return flow of blood to liver from portal vein. Shunting does not repair an already damaged liver but, if successful, prevents further hemorrhage. A portacaval shunt may be performed with end-to-side anastomosis of end of portal vein to side of inferior vena cava, with side-to-side anastomosis between portal vein and inferior vena cava, or with a graft inserted between portal vein and inferior vena cava. In the latter technique, the graft may be obtained from patient's internal jugular or saphenous vein, or a prosthetic graft may be used.

Subcostal, transabdominal, or thoracoabdominal incision may be used. Two suction setups should be available to evacuate the copious amounts of ascitic fluid that may be anticipated when peritoneum is opened. Abdominal, vascular, and thoracic setups are prepared. Pressure within the portal vein is measured with a manometer, via a cannulated branch of the superior mesenteric vein, at beginning and conclusion of operation. Because of venous distention and vascularity of operative area, hemorrhage is a major intraoperative hazard. Care is taken to avoid injury to adjacent structures, including hepatic artery and common duct. After a thoracoabdominal operation, chest drainage must be established.

Splenorenal Shunt Splenorenal shunt is generally employed when the portal vein is not available for shunting because of obstruction in the hepatic portal venous system. It involves anastomosis between the splenic vein tributary to the portal vein and the renal vein. A PTFE graft may be interposed when technical difficulties preclude a tension-free anastomosis. A splenectomy is usually performed, however, some surgeons advocate a selective splenorenal shunt, leaving the spleen in situ.

Superior Mesenteric-Inferior Vena Caval Shunt A mesocaval shunt may be employed when previous shunts for portal decompression have failed, or if a splenic vein is too small for a successful shunt. Superior mesenteric-inferior vena caval shunt is well-tolerated by young patients. If surgeon elects a mesocaval shunt, the superior mesenteric vein located between a major tributary of the portal vein is anastomosed to the inferior vena cava.

Microvascular Anastomosis

The operating microscope may be needed for anastomosis of small vessels to revascularize tissues. Patency of the anastomosis depends on factors related to surgeon's technical skill, blood flow and coagulation, and vessel spasm. Vessels must be approximated without trapping adventitia in lumen. Collagen fibers, tissue thromboplastin, and other thrombogenic factors in adventitia predispose to rapid platelet aggregation that may cause thrombus formation. Interrupted sutures are placed through full thickness of vessel wall, i.e., adventitia, media, and intima. Veins are technically more difficult to anastomose than arteries, because their walls are thinner and have less substantial muscularis. Anastomoses may be end-to-end or side-to-side. An interpositional vein graft may be needed to add length or bridge gap between ends of either an artery or vein. A patent artery should pulsate distal to anastomosis. Although most frequently employed with tissue transplants, for example, vascularized free flaps, or replants such as severed digits, the peripheral vascular surgeon may be called upon to assist with vascular problems requiring microvascular techniques.

CHAPTER **33**

PEDIATRIC SURGERY

The surgical problems peculiar to children from birth to maturity are not limited to any one area of the body or to any one surgical specialty. Malformations and diseases affect all body parts and therefore may require the skills of any of the surgical specialties. However, pediatric surgery is a specialty in itself and is not adult surgery scaled down to infant or child size. Skill is required in performing pediatric operations, and specialists in all fields must develop it as a refinement of their specialties. Surgeons who perform pediatric surgery must have knowledge of the physiological, embryological, and pathological problems peculiar to the newborn, infant, and child.

PEDIATRIC STAGES OF DEVELOPMENT

1 Fetus: in utero.
2 Newborn infant, referred to as a neonate:
  a True premature. Gestational age is less than 37 weeks; birth weight is 2500 g or less.
  b Large premature. Gestational age is less than 37 weeks; birth weight is more than 2500 g.
  c Term neonate. Gestional age is 37 weeks or more; birth weight is appropriate for gestational age, usually over 2500 g. If less than 2500 g, the neonate is considered dysmaturely small for date.
3 Infant: birth to 18 months.
4 Toddler: 18 to 30 months.
5 Preschool: 2½ to 5 years.
6 School age: 6 to 12 years.
7 Adolescent: 12 through 16 years.

CLASSIFICATIONS OF PEDIATRIC SURGERY

Pediatric surgery in all specialties can be divided into three classifications.

Congenital Anomalies

A congenital anomaly is a deviation from normal structure or location in any organ or part of the body. It can alter function or appearance. Multiple anomalies are often present at birth. If the anomaly does not involve sustaining life functions, surgical intervention may be postponed until the results can be maximized and the risks of operation are minimized by growth and development of body systems. If the newborn has a poor chance of survival without operation, the risk is taken within hours or days after birth. Defects in the alimentary tract are the most common indication for emergency operation during the newborn period, followed in frequency by cardiac and respiratory system defects. Mortality rates in the newborn are influenced by three uncontrollable factors: the multiplicity of anomalies, prematurity, and birth weight.

Acquired Disease Processes

Appendicitis is the most common surgically corrected childhood disease process. Malignant tumors do occur in infants and children, but the frequency in comparison to adults is minimal. Benign lesions are surgically excised, usually without further difficulty to the child.

Trauma

Accidental injury is the leading cause of death in children. Injury can occur during the birth process and anytime thereafter to any part of the body. Trauma can be cause of physical deformity, prolonged hospitalization with multiple operations, and emotional problems. The margin for error in diagnosis and treatment of a child is less than that for an adult with a similar injury. A child's blood volume is small and even a small loss of blood can be critical. The comparatively large skin area causes rapid heat loss. The child's chest cavity is small, so abdominal or chest injury can be critical. Fatal collapse can result rapidly. It is imperative that diagnosis be made quickly, the patient sent to the operating room if indicated, and lifesaving measures taken immediately.

GENERAL CONSIDERATIONS

Knowledge has advanced pediatric surgery so that many anomalies, diseases, and traumatic injuries formerly considered fatal or inoperable now yield to successful surgical intervention. This is due to:

1 Recognition of differences between newborns, infants, and children and adults.

2 Accurate diagnosis, especially in the fetus, premature, and term neonate. Many defects can be repaired if diagnosis is made early.

3 Understanding of preoperative preparation of the total patient.

4 Availability of total parenteral alimentation for management of many neonatal surgical problems.

5 Advances in anesthesiology: new agents, perfection of techniques of administration, and understanding of responses of infants and children to anesthetic agents.

6 Refinements in operative procedures and instrumentation.

7 Understanding of postoperative care.

Differences by Age Factor

Newborns, infants, and children through adolescence differ from each other according to age. All differ from adults. Infants, for example, have great vitality beyond that indicated by their size, but their reactions are different than are those of adults.

Metabolism Infants have relatively greater nutritional requirements than adults to minimize loss of body protein; thus they develop disturbances more rapidly than adults. Complications increase proportionately with increase in time of fluid restriction. Procedures on infants and small children should have priority on the operative schedule so as to deprive them of food and fluid for as short a time as possible, and to return them to normal routine as quickly as possible.

1 Infants are given regular formula or a varied diet up to 12 hours before anesthesia and clear liquids, usually dextrose in water, up to four hours prior to operation. A good state of hydration is maintained and curds are absent from stomach. Infants may be breast-fed up to four hours before operation. Breast milk has less or no curd and empties faster from stomach than formula. Infants should not miss more than one or two feedings. Oral intake is resumed promptly after the infant recovers from anesthesia, except following an abdominal operation.

2 Toddlers and preschool children usually are permitted clear liquids up to six hours preoperatively.

3 Children over five years of age may have nothing by mouth (NPO) after midnight or eight hours prior to induction of anesthesia. Exceptions may be necessary for children with fever, diabetes, or other special problems. For them clear liquids with supplemental glucose may be ordered to be given up to six hours preoperatively.

4 Older children may require slower progression of oral dietary intake postoperatively and are maintained with supplemental intravenous therapy that includes protein and vitamins. Vitamins K and C may be given to any age group.

Fluid and Electrolyte Balance The newborn is not dehydrated and withstands major operative procedures within the first four days of life without extensive fluid and electrolyte replacement. The renal system can be easily overloaded with the administration of intravenous fluids. The newborn has a lower glomerular filtration rate and less efficient renal tubular function than does an adult. (Renal function improves during the first two months of life and approaches adult levels by two years.) During the time of an average operation on a newborn, 10 to 30 ml of fluid may be administered. Blood loss, in most cases, is small, but it must be measured. Blood volume of the average newborn is 250 ml, approximately 75 to 80 ml per kilogram of body weight. Significant blood loss requires replacement. Blood is typed and cross matched in readiness.

Infants become dehydrated rapidly. They have a relatively larger body-surface area to body-mass ratio than do adults. When the body becomes dehydrated, body functions are disturbed, as is the acid-base balance. Plasma proteins differ in concentration from those of an adult. Fluid and electrolyte replacement are necessary, as is significant blood loss. Hemoglobin level is lowest at two to three months of age. A loss of 30 ml may represent 10 to 20 percent of circulating blood volume in an infant. The small margin of safety demands replacement of losses exceeding 10 percent of circulating blood volume. When replacement exceeds 50 percent of the estimated blood volume, sodium bicarbonate is infused to minimize acidosis.

1 Dehydration is avoided. Therapy for metabolic acidosis, should it develop, is guided by measurement of pH, blood gases, and serum electrolytes. Blood-volume loss is measured and promptly replaced.

2 Rapid transfusion of blood may produce transient but severe metabolic acidosis in an infant.

3 Intravenous fluids and blood are infused through pediatric-size cannulated needles or catheters connected to drip-chamber adaptors and small solution containers. Scalp veins are used frequently on infants. A cutdown on an extremity vein, usually the saphenous, may be necessary for toddlers and older children. An extremity should be splinted to immobilize it. An extra length of tubing may be needed between the cannula and the solution container so that the tubing will reach under the drapes and the container can be elevated high enough for the solution to drip. Remember that the tubing lies on the operating table under the drapes. Take care that instruments are not placed on it to obstruct the flow. A cardboard box, with ends cut out, can be placed over the tubing as a protection. A 250-ml solution container is used to help avoid the danger of overhydration. Adaptors are set for accurate control of the desired flow rate.

Body Temperature Newborns, especially prematures, infants, and children have wider average body temperature variations than do adults. This can vary with environmental changes. Body temperature in the newborn tends to range from as low as 97 to 100°F (36 to 37.7°C). Temperature begins to stabilize within this range 12 to 24 hours after birth if the environment is controlled. The relatively high rate of heat loss in proportion to heat production in the infant results from an incompletely developed thermoregulatory mechanism and from body-mass ratio with a thin layer of subcutaneous fat for insulation. Extensive superficial circulation also causes rapid dissipation of heat from the body. Oxygen consumption is at a minimum when abdominal skin temperature is 97°F (36°C). A room temperature 5° cooler than that of abdominal skin produces a 50 percent increase in oxygen consumption, creating hazard of acidosis. These factors account for the infant's susceptibility to environmental changes. Heat loss can occur in infants by:

1 *Evaporation.* When skin becomes wet, evaporative heat loss can occur.

2 *Radiation.* When heat transfers from body surface to surfaces such as walls of the room that are not in direct contact with the body, radiation heat loss can result.

3 *Conduction.* When air currents pass over skin, heat loss by convection results; cold diapers and blankets can cause heat loss by conduction.

Newborns, infants, and children must be kept warm during operation to minimize heat loss and to prevent undesired hypothermia. Body temperature tends to fall in the operating room because of air conditioning, open body cavities, etc. Room temperature should be maintained as warm as 85°F (29°C). Other precautions should be taken.

1 Hyperthermia blanket or a water mattress is placed on operating table and warmed before the infant or child is laid on it. It is covered with double thickness of linen. Temperature is maintained at 100°F (37.7°C) to avoid skin burns and elevation of temperature above normal range. Excessive hyperthermia can cause dehydration and convulsions under anesthesia.

2 Radiant heat lamp should be placed over newborns prior to draping. Wrapping head (except face) and extremities of infants and small children in plastic, such as Saran wrap, or Webril helps prevent heat loss. An aluminum warming suit may be used for toddlers and older children.

3 Telethermometer monitors the body temperature throughout the operation. A *telethermometer* is an electronic instrument that when connected to a probe provides direct temperature readouts on the dial. Rectal, esophageal, axillary, or tympanic probes are used. A probe placed into the rectum must not be inserted more than 2 or 3 cm (an inch), because severe trauma to an infant through perforation of the rectum or colon can occur.

4 Drapes must permit some evaporative heat loss to maintain equalization of body temperature. Excessive drapes that can retain heat and put a weight on the body are avoided.

5 Solutions should be warm when applied to tissues to minimize heat loss by evaporation and conduction. The circulating nurse should pour warm skin preparation solutions immediately prior to use. The scrub nurse dampens sponges in warm saline before handing them to the surgeon.

6 Blood can be warmed prior to transfusion by running the tubing through a blood warmer or basin of warm water. Intravenous solutions should also be warmed.

7 Blankets should be warmed to place over infant or child immediately after dressings are applied and drapes are removed. Keep infant covered whenever possible before and after operation to prevent chilling from the air conditioning.

Hyperthermia, core temperature of the body over 104°F (40°C), during operation presents a hazard. Causes are fever, dehydration, decrease in sweating from atropine administration, excessive drapes, and drugs that disturb temperature regulation such as general anesthetics and barbiturates. Dire consequences ensue. Operation should be delayed if the patient is febrile preoperatively to allow reduction in temperature and to permit fluid administration. If immediate operation is necessary and fever persists, anesthesia is induced and external cooling employed.

Cardiopulmonary Response The heart rate is unstable and fluctuates widely in infants, toddlers, and preschool children. After age five, cardiopulmonary response to stress resembles that of a young adult. Cardiac and respiratory sounds are continuously monitored in all age groups by precordial or esophageal stethoscope. Blood pressure, vital signs, ECG, and other parameters as indicated are also monitored throughout the operation.

Infants and toddlers are particularly susceptible to respiratory obstruction because of anatomic structure. They have small nares, relatively large tongue, presence of lymphoid tissue, and small diameter of trachea, causing disproportionate narrowing of airway. Cylindrical thorax, poorly developed accessory respiratory muscles, and increased volume of abdominal contents limit diaphragmatic movement.

Infection Newborns and infants are susceptible to nosocomial infection and show less resistance to overcoming it than do adults. Many premature infants suffering from respiratory distress and circulatory problems survive because of the advances in perinatal medicine. This has increased the population of high-risk and debilitated infants with reduced humoral and cellular defenses to infection. Aseptic technique is essential in handling these and all other pediatric patients.

Elective operation should be delayed in the presence of respiratory infection because of the risk of airway obstruction. Intubation of inflamed tissues may cause laryngeal edema. *Coryza,* inflammation of mucous membranes of the nose, is often a premonitory sign of an infectious respiratory disease.

Pain Infants and children differ greatly from adults in their sensitivity to pain. Pain may be intense, but infants, toddlers, and preschool children are unable to describe its location and nature. School-age children may refer pain to a part of the body not involved in the disease process. Insecurity and fear in an older child may be more traumatic than is the pain itself. Children must be observed for signs of pain. Children also differ from adults in their response to pharmacological agents; their tolerance to analgesic drugs is altered.

Preparation of the Total Patient

Preoperative visits are made by an OR nurse to see and talk to the infant or child and/or parents. The pediatric surgical patient must be considered as a whole person with individual physical and psychosocial needs assessed in relation to natural stages of development. Equally important to the patient are the adjustment and attitude of the parents toward the child, the illness, and the hospital experience. Parents' anxiety about the impending operation may be transferred to the child. Emotional support of both patient and parents, as well as parent and child teaching, are important aspects of preoperative preparation. Most adults face stress with more control when fear of the unknown is eliminated; children do not differ in this respect. Understanding does, however, vary with age.

1 Psychologically it is better for the infant as well as the parents if a congenital anomaly is repaired as soon after birth as possible. The infant under one year of age will not remember the experience. Parents will gain confidence in learning to cope with a residual deformity as the infant learns to compensate for it.

2 Separation from mother or parental equivalent is traumatic for infant over one year, toddler, and preschool child. Infants require cuddling and bonding. Toddlers are only reaching the autonomy stage when hospitalization forces them into passive behavior. Separation anxiety is greatest in them. Such young children may fear strangers. The mother's presence is mandatory for the toddler. She should be encouraged to stay with hospitalized child as much as possible. The child should be permitted to bring a toy or other security object to the OR suite, where mother cannot be present. In some hospitals a parent is permitted to rejoin child in the recovery room, if condition permits.

> NOTE. Ambulatory surgery, if feasible, is an advantage, because the child enters the hospital an hour or two before the operation and returns home following recovery from anesthesia. This minimizes the trauma of separation.

3 Fear of body mutilation or punishment may be of paramount importance to a preschool or young school-age child. Children from two to five years of age have great sensitivity and a tenuous sense of reality. They live in a world of magic, monsters, and retribution, yet are aggressive. School-age children, with an enhanced sense of reality, value honesty and fairness. Their natural interest and curiosity aid communication. These children need reassurances and explanations in vocabulary compatible with developmental level. Choose words wisely. Avoid negative connotations. Stress positive aspects. Talk on child's level about his or her interests and concerns.

4 Anxiety in the school-age child may be stimulated by remembrance of a previous experience. Many children undergo two or more staged operations before the deformity of a congenital anomaly or traumatic injury is cosmetically reconstructed or functionally restored. Familiarity with the nursing staff reassures the child. Ideally, the OR nurse who circulated for the first operation should visit preoperatively and be with the child during subsequent operations.

5 Fear of the unknown about being put to sleep may become exaggerated into extreme anxiety with fantasies of death. The school-age child and adolescent need facts and reassurances. Do not refer to anesthesia as "putting you to sleep." Child may equate this phrase with former euthanasia of a pet who never returned home. Rather say, "You will sleep for a little while," or "take a nap." In lieu of "recovery room," tell child about the "nice nurses" who will be in the "wake-up room after your nap." Encourage parents to also display confidence and cheerfulness, to avoid transmitting anxiety. Parents must be honest with their child, but maintain a confident manner. The OR nurse must do the same. However, do not give a school-age child information not asked for; answer questions and correct misunderstandings. Be especially alert to silent, stoic, noncommunicative children. Many have difficult induction and emergence from anesthesia.

> NOTE. Some hospitals hold "parties" for children and their parents prior to hospital admission or after admission prior to operation to explain hospital routines and procedures. Others take children to the OR suite so that they can see the different attire, lights, tables, anesthesia machine, and other equipment that might interest them. A child-sized anesthesia mask becomes a play toy and not something to be feared. A plastic mask, like those which pilots wear in an airplane, is less psychologically traumatic to a child than is an opaque black rubber mask. An effective method of explaining to children is to use a doll and dress it as the child will look postoperatively. For example, show a plaster hip spica cast on the doll to explain the cast if the child will have one postoperatively.

PEDIATRIC ANESTHESIA

Pediatric anesthesia has become increasingly specialized as the many variables in the management of infants and children have become better understood. The anesthesiologist recognizes and respects the small margin for error and the uniqueness of the physiology and responses to drugs of pediatric patients. For example, the high metabolic rate of children causes rapid oxygen consumption. Changes occur rapidly in infants and children.

Preoperative Assessment

A preoperative visit by the anesthesiologist to establish rapport and assess the patient is also a vital part of preparation of the total patient. This visit is preferably made in the presence of parents so that the child will consider the anesthesiologist as a trustworthy and caring friend. During physical assessment, special attention is given to heart, lungs, and upper airways. Loose teeth are noted. Possible difficulties are anticipated. Preoperative care includes correction of dehydration, reduction of excessive fever, compensation for acidosis, and restoration of depleted blood volume. An ASA physical status classification is assigned the pediatric patient (see Chap. 3, p. 55). Consideration is given to age, developmental stage, personality makeup, and past history to determine the patient's probable response to the anesthetic experience.

Premedication

Crying greatly increases mucus in the respiratory tract. Premedication may be ordered to produce serenity, at discretion of the anesthesiologist. Some prefer children to be well-medicated; others favor minimal or no sedation. Children over seven years of age may not require premedication if prudently prepared. Tailored to the individual, premedication varies considerably by age and weight. Preanesthetic sedation should allow the patient to be taken to the OR lightly asleep and induced without awakening. It should also provide some analgesia during the recovery period.

Timing of administration is extremely important. To be effective, drugs should be given at least 45 to 60 minutes prior to the time child is sent for. An order to "premedicate and send to OR" is unacceptable. A terrified child will thus be rushed off to the unknown, just before induction. *The circulating nurse should check with the anesthesiologist before sending for the patient.* If ample time is not available for appropriate effect of premedication, the anesthesiologist may prefer to omit the medication to avoid precipitation of psychic trauma.

No ideal premedicant exists, but the following drugs are commonly used.

1 *Atropine sulfate* given to inhibit secretions, especially in a child with severe airway problem, or to counteract bradycardia. Cardiac effects last about one hour. This may be given to an infant under six months of age. It is given IM preoperatively or IV at induction. It is not given in presence of fever.

2 *Glycopyrrolate,* an alternative to atropine, also lowers gastric acidity.

3 *Meperidine hydrochloride* given IM.

4 *Diazepam* given orally for relaxation.

Anesthesia Equipment

Simple lightweight equipment is used. Disposable equipment is popular. Face masks, designed for minimal dead space, are available to closely fit a child's relatively flat face. Nonrebreathing circuits provide less resistance and valves for fresh flow of gas at higher flow rates relative to a child's metabolism and ventilation. High gas flows require scavenging equipment. To avoid hypothermia, anesthesic gases are warmed and humidified. Neonates are especially at risk for fluctuations in temperature regulation.

Induction

Induction is facilitated by a quiet atmosphere, soft voice, and reassuring touch. Children should be told what to expect without precipitating fear. The induction experience can be described as "getting on a merry-go-round. Noises will seem louder." It is best for child to listen to one person speak at this time to avoid confusion. The circulating nurse should remain at patient's side and maintain gentle touch, and be alert to patient's needs and condition.

1 Restraints should be loose. Minimal pressure should be applied. If the patient is a newborn, infant, or toddler, restraint straps are omitted while the circulating nurse holds the patient during induction. A toddler or preschool-age child is less frightened holding onto someone's hands. Restraints can be applied after the patient is asleep.

2 A few drops of food extract of child's choosing, e.g., mint, banana, strawberry, can be placed in face mask. This makes the anesthetic gas more acceptable and gives patient a sense of control.

3 If the child is awake, crying, or struggling, apprehension during induction can be avoided by distraction and rapport. It is not easy to establish rapport with young children. Their cooperation may be solicited by counting out loud, singing the alphabet song, blowing up a balloon, taking a "space trip," or discussing a favorite plaything or television character. The face mask can be held slightly above the face, permitting anesthetic gas to flow by gravity, and lowered gently as the child becomes drowsy. Some anesthesiologists permit the child to hold the mask.

4 Induction may be accompanied by regurgitation and aspiration of gastric contents in infants with pyloric stenosis, tracheoesophageal fistula, intestinal obstruction, or food in the stomach. The hazard is minimized by aspirating gastric contents by sterile catheter prior to induction, and leaving the tube in place for drainage during operation. Or, *rapid-sequence induction* is used. This consists of thiopental sodium, muscle relaxant, and intubation with cricoid pressure (Sellick's maneuver) applied to close esophagus and avoid silent regurgitation of food from stomach.

Types of Induction

Inhalation If asleep from medication upon arrival in OR, child can be put to sleep fast. Or induction may be pleasant with high-flow nitrous oxide and oxygen, with gradual addition of halothane.

Rectal Given by enema, methohexital sodium (Brevital) produces sleep in four to eight minutes and lasts 45 to 60 minutes. This is a painless method used in presence of parents for preschoolers or toddlers. The parent may hold the child. It is good for short diagnostic procedures. Anesthesiologist remains with patient.

Intramuscular Ketamine, given IM or IV, is useful in combative, burned, or hypovolemic patient.

Intravenous IV infusion is often preferred by patients over nine or ten years of age. It is rapid.

Intubation

1 Endotracheal intubation is used by some anesthesiologists for all procedures in infants under one year of age. It is mandatory for intraabdominal, intrathoracic, neurosurgical procedures, and those about the head or neck areas, and for emergency procedures with uncertainty about contents of stomach.

2 Airway obstruction in infants and children usually occurs early during anesthesia administration. When anesthesia deepens, airway insertion is essential after prior assisted ventilation. Assisted or controlled ventilation reduces the labor of breathing and therefore metabolism. Intubation and suctioning are preceded and followed by oxygen administration.

3 Sterile equipment and gentle manipulation to avoid soft tissue injury are essential for intubation and suctioning. Nasotracheal tubes may inadvertently dislodge adenoid tissue and carry it into the trachea. Endotracheal tubes for children under eight years old are not cuffed.

4 A newborn's head must be maintained in a neutral position midway between full extension and full flexion, while an endotracheal tube is in place. The tip of the tube should be placed at the mid-trachea position. The average distance between the vocal cords and the carina, where the trachea separates into two branches, is only 4 or 5 cm (about 2 in.) in a term neonate and much less in a premature. If the head shifts, the tube can slip up or down and lead to disastrous consequences. Awake intubation is used in neonates.

Anesthetic Agents and Maintenance

1 Topical agents are generally avoided because of the hazard of overdose.

2 Inhalation anesthesia, especially halothane, is popular. Nitrous oxide-oxygen-halothane is most commonly used. Few cases of hepatotoxicity have been reported in preadolescent school-age groups. Induction is smooth, fast, and pleasant. Forane is irritating, necessitating slow and more difficult induction to prevent laryngospasm, but it offers the advantage of circulatory support. It is not useful in short procedures.

Alveolar concentrations of inhaled anesthetics rise much more rapidly in pediatric patients than in adults because of relatively greater blood flow and smaller functional residual capacity. Children therefore have higher anesthetic requirements than do adults. To produce the same level of anesthesia, neonates require about 40 percent more halothane than adults. Increased anesthetic requirement and more rapid induction can cause hypotension and reduced cardiac output in infants and children.

3 Ketamine provides sedation for younger children, e.g., for invasive diagnostic procedures. While useful in asthmatics, it is not advised for teenagers. Diazepam counteracts possible emergence delirium.

4 Narcotics are used in situations similar to adult indications (see Chap. 13, p. 224). Nitrous oxide-narcotic-relaxant provides stable anesthesia for the very ill. Fentanyl has minimal cardiovascular effect.

5 Critically ill neonate does not tolerate anesthesia well. Adequate ventilation and oxygenation are vital, but care must be taken to avoid oxygen toxicity with resultant retrolental fibroplasia. This is neovascularization of the retina, which can produce blindness. Neonates and premature infants under 34 weeks gestation, when the retina is developing, are at risk. Adequate blood-gas tension is ensured only by measurement.

6 Neuromuscular blockers are used judiciously. Infants under one year exhibit lesser degree of blockade from succinylcholine than older children. Bradycardia and intraocular tension rise are more conspicuous in infants. Response decreases with age. Dosage varies. A peripheral nerve stimulator should be used to assess blockage to avoid overdosage. Blockers seldom are required in infants because of poorly developed abdominal musculature.

7 Consideration is given for postoperative analgesia. When halothane is reduced near end of operation, narcotic may be given. Or regional or local infiltration will provide relief of pain, for example, following circumcision or cleft lip repair.

8 *Malignant hyperthermia* is a potentially severe intraoperative complication (refer to Chap. 14, p. 276). Placing surgical gloves filled with ice directly over major arteries, including femoral, carotid, and axillary, is a rapid method to cool infants and small children.

Emergence and Extubation

Airway problems are the most common concern on emergence and immediately postoperatively. At conclusion of operation, the oropharynx and stomach are suctioned. All monitors are left in place until the patient is fully awake and extubated.

Extubation of an infant or child is a treacherous time. It is preceded and followed by oxygen administration and performed either under deep anesthesia or on return of spontaneous respiration since laryngospasm is possible between these periods. Heart and breath sounds are monitored following extubation. If spasm occurs, oxygen is given by positive pressure. Airway obstruction, aspiration, and hypothermia are hazards of the recovery period. Children, particularly in the two to five age group, may develop hoarseness and a croupy cough following removal of an endotracheal tube. Racemic epinephrine (Vapanefrin) provides relief; 0.5 ml of 2.25% diluted in 3 ml of sterile water can be delivered through a face mask and nebulizer. Constant observation following extubation is required.

Postoperative Care

The patient should not be taken from the OR if body temperature is below 95°F (35°C). Below this crucial level, high incidence occurs of acidosis, hypoglycemia, bradycardia, hypotension, and apnea. This depression and delayed return of activity set the stage for possible sudden cardiac arrest. Dehydration and low humidity increase viscosity of secretions. Pediatric patients require *close* watching for development of laryngeal edema noted by croupy cough, sobbing inspiration, intercostal retraction, tachypnea, or tachycardia. Laryngeal edema greatly reduces the small diameter of the airway of an infant or toddler. Controlled humidity and oxygen are vital.

O.R. NURSING PROCEDURES

Basic principles of nursing care and operating room techniques discussed in preceding chapters apply to pediatric surgery. A few points specific to pediatric surgery are mentioned to differentiate this specialty from care of adult patients.

1. Hair is not removed with a depilatory or shaved, except for cranial operations and as ordered by the surgeon for an adolescent.
2. Diagnostic studies may be done in the OR under local anesthesia prior to induction of general anesthesia for an open operative procedure. An infant may be swaddled on a padded board to restrain him or her from moving while x-rays are taken and to permit easy change of position. A sugar nipple will help comfort and keep the infant quiet.
3. Patient must be protected from injury. An infant or child should *never* be left alone anywhere in the OR suite, including the holding area. Preparation for induction should be made before the child's arrival.
   - **a** Guard against fall from a crib or stretcher. Siderails must be up at all times. An overbed cage on a crib helps confine a toddler without restraint. Children must be restrained on a stretcher or in a specially designed pediatric cart.

b Do not place a crib where the patient can reach an electric outlet or any article that can be picked up and cause injury.

c Pad wrists and ankles after infant is asleep with several turns of sheet wadding. Restrain with muslin or roller gauze and pin straps to sheet on the operating table. Sheet wadding prevents possible abrasion of delicate skin by the restraint straps. Care must be taken not to restrict circulation.

d Safety pins, open or closed, must not be left within reach of an infant or child.

4 Catheters as small as size 8 French are available for use as needed in newborns and infants. A plain tip or whistle tip catheter is used for a stomach tube. For urinary retention, a Foley catheter with a 3-cc bag is used. Small, calibrated drainage containers are connected to permit accurate determination of output.

5 Positioning principles are essentially the same as those described in Chapter 15. Correspondingly smaller towel rolls, pillows, and sandbags are used to protect pressure points and to stabilize anesthetized infants and children. Size of the child or adolescent determines appropriate supports to maintain desired position. A small towel roll at each side of body takes weight of drapes off the small body of an infant or keeps patient in lateral position.

6 Disposable drape sheet without a fenestration is often advantageous: the surgeon can cut an opening of desired size to expose site of intended incision. Small towels and towel clips are used with a laparotomy sheet if self-adhering and disposable drapes are not used. A standard opening 3 by 5 in. (7.6 by 12.7 cm) in a pediatric lap sheet is frequently too large for a newborn or infant. Part of the fenestration must be covered with a towel.

7 Sponges are weighed while still wet; blood loss through suction is measured and estimated in drapes. The surgeon and anesthesiologist will determine if blood replacement is necessary, volume for volume, as it is lost.

8 Adhesive tape is abrasive to tender skin and should be avoided when possible. An adhesive spray or collodion is adequate over a small incision with a subcuticular closure and is especially desirable under diapers, unless dressings are needed to absorb drainage. Care must be taken that clothing or blanket does not touch this substance until dry. Skin closure strips may be used instead of a liquid adhesive.

9 Dressings on the face or neck must be protected from vomitus and food soil as well as from an infant's or toddler's hands. Elbows must be splinted when patient potentially may disturb the incision, dressings, or a tube. This is particularly important following eye surgery or cleft lip or palate surgery, and when a tracheotomy tube is inserted.

10 Stockinet pulled over dressings on an extremity protects them from soil and helps keep them in place. This can be changed easily if soiled, leaving the dressings in place.

Instrumentation

Gentleness and precision in handling small structures and fragile tissues are essential. Basic or standard instrument sets, sutures, needles, and other items used for operations on adults must be duplicated in miniature to take care of infants and children in each surgical specialty. The OR nurse and technologist must be informed about their patient and then use good judgment in preparing supplies for pediatric surgery.

1 Size and weight are more critical factors than age in the selection of instruments, sutures, needles, and equipment.

2 Small instruments must be used on delicate tissues of a newborn, infant, or small child.

3 Hemostats should have fine points. A mosquito hemostat will clamp a superficial vessel but not a major artery.

4 Noncrushing vascular clamps permit occlusion of major blood vessels. They also can be placed across the intestine of a newborn or infant rather than a large, heavy intestinal clamp.

5 Lightweight instruments will not inhibit respiration. Instruments not in use on tissues must *never* be laid on patient, especially not on the chest. An instrument's weight could restrict respiration or circulation or cause bruises. Return instruments to Mayo stand or instrument table immediately after use.

6 Umbilical tape is used frequently to retract blood vessels and small structures, thereby giving the surgeon greater visibility in a small operative site and eliminating the weight of retractors.

7 Needleholders must have fine-pointed jaws to hold small, delicate needles.

8 Operation on an adolescent will require adult-size instruments.

9 An efficient scrub nurse will closely watch the

tissue being dissected and select the instruments to hand the surgeon accordingly.

COMMON OPERATIONS

General Surgery

Endoscopy Gastroscopy, colonoscopy, and laparoscopy are performed for diagnosis of complaints of abdominal pain or symptoms of intestinal obstruction. Procedures, such as insertion of a gastrostomy tube, polypectomy, sphincterotomy, can be done in lieu of laparotomy. Endoscopic injection of sodium morrhuate is an alternative to portosystemic shunt in children with bleeding esophageal varices.

Anastomosis within Alimentary Tract Alimentary tract obstruction is the most frequent cause for emergency operation of the newborn or young infant. The common sites of obstruction are in the esophagus, duodenum, ileum, colon, and anus. *Atresia,* an imperforation or closure of a normal opening, and *stenosis,* a constriction or narrowing, are the common causes of obstruction. The obstructive lesion is usually resected and the viable segments of the viscera are anastomosed. A temporary gastrostomy, ileostomy, or colostomy may be necessary. Intestinal obstruction can develop in infants and children months to years after the newborn period from a predisposing or associated congenital anomaly or acquired disease process. Inflammatory diseases such as necrotizing enterocolitis, ulcerative colitis, Meckel's diverticulitis or Crohn's disease, and other intestinal conditions such as Hirschsprung's disease or familial polyposis require intestinal resection and anastomosis. An endorectal pull-through may be procedure of choice to preserve the rectum.

Biliary Atresia A form of intrauterine cholangitis that results in progressive fibrotic obliteration of bile ducts, biliary atresia may cause jaundice in the newborn. Excision of extrahepatic ducts or hilar dissection with a portoenterostomy procedure, such as portal hepatojejunostomy, is performed before infant is two months old to relieve jaundice by improving bile drainage. If liver function becomes progressively impaired, liver transplantation may ultimately be necessary for survival.

Tracheoesophageal Fistula Esophageal atresia, with or without tracheoesophageal fistula, is an acute congenital problem in the newborn. Primary repair is performed by division of the fistula and anastomosis of the trachea and esophagus. Submucosal myotomies and lengthening of upper pouch permit primary anastomosis to establish alimentary tract continuity.

Imperforate Anus If the anus remains closed during fetal development, the intestinal tract must be opened surgically soon after birth. A posterior sagittal anorectoplasty or an abdominoperineal pull-through operation may be done for primary management. Many children endure fecal incontinence or chronic constipation as they grow into their teens following these procedures in infancy. Various secondary operations are performed, most frequently an endorectal pull-through procedure or gracilis muscle transplant for reconstruction of rectal sphincter.

Pyloromyotomy *Pyloric stenosis,* a congenital obstructive lesion in the area of the pylorus of the stomach, is relieved by cutting through the serosa and dividing the muscle layers of the pylorus. Onset of symptoms usually occurs between the third and eighth weeks of life.

Herniorrhaphy Hernia repair is the most frequently performed elective operation in infants and children by general surgeons. Of the four types of hernias seen in pediatrics, indirect inguinal hernia is the most common; it occurs much more frequently in males than females and appears during the first ten years of life. Although frequently seen, most umbilical hernias do not require surgical intervention. Hiatus (diaphragmatic) hernia and femoral hernias require surgical correction but are rarely acute problems in childhood. A hiatus hernia is a surgical emergency in the newborn if abdominal contents are in the chest, causing acute respiratory distress. Extracorporeal membrane oxygenation may be used for management of respiratory diseases in these newborns. Hernias seen in infants and children are caused by congenital weakness in the fascia, abdominal wall, or diaphragm.

Omphalocele Failure of the intestines to become encapsulated within the peritoneal cavity during fetal development results in herniation through a midline defect in the abdominal wall at the umbilicus. The intestinal contents of the omphalocele are reduced back into the peritoneal cavity. A Silastic chimney or silicone pouch may be used temporarily in conjunction with total parenteral nutrition for this. Then primary closure of fascia and skin is attempted. For large defects, synthetic mesh or sheeting may be used with primary skin closure. Delayed secondary fascia closure may be necessary.

Appendectomy *Appendicitis,* an acute inflammation of the appendix requiring removal of the organ, is the most common cause for abdominal operation in the school-age child. Gangrene or rupture may occur prior to diagnosis or operation.

Splenectomy Removal of the spleen may be indicated to correct hypersplenic disease, either congenital or acquired. Emergency splenectomy is necessary following rupture of the spleen, usually from blunt trauma. An attempt is made to salvage as much of the organ as is possible to minimize future susceptibility to infection.

Urology

Pediatric urology concerns itself basically with the diagnosis and treatment of infections and congenital anomalies within the genitourinary tract. Some type of anomaly of the genitourinary system may be found in 10 to 15 percent of newborns. Secondary infections are frequently associated with congenital anomalies; chronic diseases are frequently associated with infections. The following operative procedures include those most commonly performed by pediatric urologists.

Cystoscopy Diagnostic evaluation and therapeutic removal of obstructions within the structures of the genitourinary tract may be performed through an infant- or child-size cystoscope. Cystoscopes from 9½ through 16 French are used for infants and children. A size 3 Fr ureteral catheter can be introduced through the smallest-size cystoscope.

Nephrectomy, Nephrostomy, or Pyeloureteroplasty Hydronephrosis, congenital or acquired, may necessitate operation. Nephrectomy is indicated only if severe disease is unilateral with contralateral kidney capable of life-sustaining function. More conservative nephrostomy or pyeloureteroplasty is indicated for bilateral or moderate to mild kidney disease. Nephrectomy is necessary to resect *Wilms's tumor,* a sarcoma of the kidney that develops rapidly in a child usually under five years of age.

Exstrophy of the Bladder In exstrophy of the bladder, a congenital anomaly, the bladder herniates through lower abdominal wall in the suprapubic region. Repair requires reconstruction of lower abdominal wall and external genitalia as well as provision for passage of urine. This can usually be accomplished in one operation on a female infant but requires two or more staged operations in a male infant. If urinary continence cannot be established, urinary diversion through ureteral reimplantation may become necessary.

Ureteral Reimplantation Repositioning of the ureters may be performed to correct either congenital or acquired total urinary incontinence or vesicoureteral reflux.

Incontinence, involuntary leakage of urine from the bladder, causes parents to seek help for an infant or child. Incontinence is usually not due to a single factor, so the urologist must plan the operation on basis of an accurate assessment of anatomic and physiologic etiology. Creation of a tubularized trigonal muscle, when reconstructed into a new bladder neck, acts as a sphincter to maintain continence. With ureters in normal position, this muscular tube in the bladder wall cannot be constructed. Therefore, the ureters must be reimplanted superiorly into the bladder using a tunnel technique. Care must be taken so that the ureters are not hooked or angled but follow a smooth curve into the bladder.

Vesicoureteral reflux is the most common reason for reimplanting ureters in pediatric patients. Chronic reflux, regurgitation of urine from the bladder into the ureters, can lead to pyelonephritis and hydronephrosis. Ureteral reimplantation may be required to prevent kidney damage. The objective of the operation is to position a segment of the ureters at a higher level within the bladder wall so that the urine lies below the orifices and intravesical pressure prevents reflux.

When ureters cannot be reimplanted in the bladder, a urinary diversion procedure may be necessary. Ureters are usually anastomosed to a nonrefluxing colon conduit.

Urethral Repair The external opening of the urethra may be displaced at birth. *Hypospadias* is an anomaly in the male in which the urethra terminates on the underside of the penis or on the perineum; in the female, the urethra opens into the vagina. With *epispadias* in the male, the urethra terminates on the dorsum of the penis; in the female, it terminates above the clitoris. Multistage procedures are usually necessary to correct these anomalies. The goal is to center meatus at tip of glans penis of male. This may be accomplished in a one-stage procedure by an island flap derived from prepuce or by a vertical-incision/horizontal-closure technique for distal coronal or subglandular hypospadias. This is usually performed between ages two and four.

Orchiopexy One or both testicles that failed to descend during fetal development can be brought into the scrotum and stabilized with a traction suture until healing takes place. Frequently done as a two-stage Torek orchiopexy, the testicle and supporting structures are dissected free from the inguinal region. Adequate length of the spermatic vessels must be obtained to permit the testicle to reach the scrotal sac. After it is pulled down through the scrotum, the testicle is sutured to the fascia of the thigh. Two to three months later at the second-stage operation, the testicle is freed from the fascia and embedded into the scrotum.

If one or both testicles are absent, silicone prostheses may be inserted into the scrotum for cosmetic appearance. Psychologically for child and parents, undescended (*cryptorchism*) or absence (*agenesis*) of testicles are usually repaired at age five or six, before the boy begins school.

Circumcision Excision of the foreskin of the penis may be done to prevent *phimosis,* in which the foreskin becomes tightly wrapped around the tip of the glans penis, or to remove redundant foreskin. Circumcision is the most commonly performed pediatric operation.

Orthopaedic Surgery

Pediatric orthopaedic surgery is principally elective and reconstructive in nature to correct deformities of the musculoskeletal system. These may be congenital, idiopathic, pathologic, or traumatic in origin. The extensiveness of the anomalies and functional disorders often involve prolonged immobilization and hospitalization. Many patients require a series of corrective procedures. Some of the conditions most commonly seen in the operating room include the following.

Fractures Fractures occur in infants and children and are treated generally as in adults, as described in Chapter 24. However, fixation devices are not well-tolerated by children and often prevent uniting of fracture. Closed reduction of long bone fractures is preferable.

Tendon Repair Tendons may be lengthened, shortened, or transferred to correct congenital deformities of the hand or foot. Lacerated tendons must be repaired to restore function. A tourniquet is always used to control bleeding. Tourniquet cuff size must be appropriate for size of infant or child. Padding under cuff must be applied smoothly. Sheet wadding may be used under an infant cuff to protect delicate skin. The cuff must be tight but without restricting circulation before inflation. Time of inflation must be closely watched to prevent ischemia. The surgeon may ask the circulating nurse to release the pressure every 30 minutes on an infant; up to one to two hours, depending on age of older child. Tendon procedures are often lengthy.

Congenital Dislocated Hip Displacement of the femoral head from its normal position in the acetabulum can be present at birth, either unilaterally or bilaterally. If diagnosed early in infancy, closed reduction with immobilization usually corrects the dislocation without residual deformity. If not diagnosed until after child has begun to walk, open reduction of the hip with an osteotomy to stabilize the joint may be necessary.

Leg-Length Discrepancies The epiphyseal cartilaginous growth lines progressively close as the child matures. Bones lengthen from the activity of the epiphysis. The absolute physiologic criterion for completion of childhood is when this cartilage becomes a part of bone. A discrepancy in activity of an epiphyseal line may retard or overstimulate growth of a bone in one extremity and not its contralateral counterpart. When this occurs in one femur, legs become unequal in length. The orthopaedic surgeon may correct leg-length discrepancies, usually in excess of 1 in. (2.5 cm), by epiphyseal arrest—stopping growth of the bone. This is done in the contralateral leg to let the shorter extremity catch up. The longer leg may be shortened by a closed intramedullary procedure. Under fluoroscopy, a reamer is inserted into medullary canal of femur through a small incision high on the hip. After the reamer widens the canal, a rotating saw is manipulated to cut a section from the bone. The bone ends are aligned and fixed with a flexible intramedullary rod.

Slipping of the upper femoral epiphysis causes displacement of the femoral head, which can occur as a result of traumatic injury or as a chronic disability usually seen in obese adolescents. Fusion of the epiphysis to the femoral neck may be necessary to prevent slipping and shortening of the leg.

Talipes Deformities Combinations of various types of deformities of the foot, especially those of congenital origin, are referred to as *talipes* plus the medical term to describe whether the forefoot is inverted (*varus*) or everted (*valgus*) and whether the calcaneal tendon is shortened or lengthened.

Talipes varus, the condition known as *clubfoot,* is the most common of these deformities. Either unilateral or bilateral, the forefoot is inverted and rotated, accompanied by shortening of calcaneal tendon and contracture of plantar fascia. Conservative treatment by casting during infancy usually corrects deformity before the infant bears weight on the foot. A wedge cast with turnbuckles may be applied to an older child to allow gradual manipulation. If conservative treatment is unsuccessful, arthrodesis or other open operative procedure may be necessary.

Scoliosis Scoliosis is a lateral curvature and rotation of the spine, most frequently seen in rapidly growing school-age children or adolescents. Treatment depends on degree and flexibility of the curvature, chronological and skeletal age of the child, and preference of the surgeon. The child may be fitted with a Milwaukee brace, immobilized in a cast, or stretched by traction. As an alternative to these techniques, an electrical device may be applied with an underarm brace to stimulate muscle contraction on convex side of curvature. If untreated at an early stage, scoliosis produces secondary changes in vertebral bodies and in the rib cage. Spinal fusion must ultimately be performed if the curvature has become severe or must be stabilized following corrections. Government-mandated screening programs have reduced the need for surgical correction in many children.

1 A wedge body jacket or Minerva jacket (see Chap. 24, p. 478) may be applied. Turnbuckles may be incorporated. These are adjustable metal rods placed along the edges of the wedge of the cast. Gradual opening of the turnbuckles by the surgeon as tolerated by the patient corrects the lateral curvature of the spine.

A Sayre sling, an appliance used for head traction, is used sometimes when applying a body jacket to correct slight scoliosis. Traction is obtained by means of pulleys and a rope suspended from the ceiling or an arm of the fracture table.

2 Halo traction is used to stretch the spine in some patients in whom the spine is too rigid to be straightened in a cast. A metal band is applied to the skull by means of four pins inserted into the cortex of the skull. A Steinmann pin is inserted into the distal end of each femur. A traction bow is put on each one. Weights, usually equal, are put on the Halo and Steinmann pins and gradually increased as tolerated. When x-rays show maximum correction, a spinal fusion is done. Traction may be continued until healing has taken place to the degree that there will be no loss of correction; a plaster jacket is then applied.

3 Risser jacket is applied a few days preceding posterior spinal fusion to gain as much correction as possible. The orthopaedic table is used. Traction is applied by a chin strap, similar to a Sayre sling, and countertraction is applied by a pelvic girdle. The spine is straightened as much as possible and the body and head are encased in plaster.

4 Posterior spinal fusion may be performed as a two-stage procedure: vertebral body wedge resection at first stage and insertion of Harrington rods with fusion at second stage. Bone fragments removed during the first stage may be saved for the second-stage fusion or sent to the bone bank. Harrington rods and hooks are stainless steel. Harrington instruments are required to insert them. Two rods are inserted, one on either side of the curvature. These are secured to the spine and force it into a more nearly normal position. Implanted on outside of vertebral column, these rods apply a longitudinal force on the spine. The spine is then fused.

The operation may be done through a window in the Risser jacket, but usually the cast is bivalved and patient lies in anterior section. If operation is done through a window, an electric cast cutter should be at hand to bivalve cast if the patient has any respiratory difficulties. After operation the bivalved posterior part is put in place and jacket is fastened together by several rounds of plaster or by webbing straps with buckles. The patient is in the Risser jacket for a year. Progress is checked by x-ray.

5 Segmental spinal fixation with Luque rods may be procedure of choice to stabilize spine following fusion. Two L-shaped rods are placed next to the spinous processes and held by wires threaded under lamina of each vertebra to be fused. Transverse traction internally on each vertebra stabilizes spine without need for a postoperative cast.

6 Anterior spinal fusion through a transthoracic approach is performed as a one-stage operation to correct severe curvatures in patients who have malformed vertebral bodies. Using Dwyer instruments, titanium staples are fitted over vertebral bodies on convex side of curve. Each staple is held in place by two titanium screws. A multistrand titanium cable, threaded through heads of the screws, is tightened to compress vertebrae and straighten curve. A series of staples and screws are secured the full extent of the curvature. A plaster body jacket may be applied after operation to immobilize the back until the fusion is healed. The patient then is ambulatory.

Ophthalmology

Congenital Obstruction of Nasolacrimal Duct An obstruction, usually at lower end of nasolacrimal duct, that enters the inferior meatus of the nose often results in dilatation and infection of the lacrimal sac. Treatment consists of passing a malleable probe from the lid punctum through the nasolacrimal passages to push out the obstructing plug of tissue.

Oculoplastic Procedures on Eyelids Congenital malformations such as *ptosis* (drooping of upper or lower eyelid) are corrected by extraocular procedures. Ptosis repair is indicated when the levator is inadequate. In the levator resection procedure, which shortens the muscle and gives a more physiologic result, the levator muscle may be approached through the skin (Berke method) or the conjunctiva (Iliff method). Fascial sling operation to support the lid consists of attaching the upper lid margin to the frontalis muscle. Materials used include autogenous fascia from the thigh, homograft fascia, or synthetic nonabsorbable suture material. The Fasanello-Servat is a simpler operation for obtaining only a small amount of lid elevation.

Extraocular Muscle Operations Operations on muscles to correct stabismus or squint are the third most commonly performed pediatric operations between ages six months and six years. The trend is to correct the congenital type during infancy and the acquired type in preschool years. Patterns of using two eyes together are more flexible and adaptable in a young child. These operations on extraocular muscles are done to correct muscle imbalance and promote coordination either by strengthening a weak muscle or by weakening an overactive one. The mechanical strength of a weak muscle can be increased by:

1 *Tucking.* Tuck is sutured in muscle to shorten it, thereby increasing its effective power.

2 *Advancement.* Attachment point of muscle is freed and reattached closer to cornea, thereby increasing its leverage.

3 *Resection.* Part of muscle is removed to shorten it, and cut ends are sutured together.

An overactive muscle can be weakened by:

1 *Tenotomy.* Point of attachment of muscle is severed and muscle is dropped back, held by ligaments only.

2 *Recession.* Muscle is detached from eyeball and reattached farther back to decrease its action.

3 *Myotomy.* Fibers of a section of muscle are divided in order to diminish muscle action.

4 *Myectomy.* Section of muscle belly is excised.

5 *Fadin operation.* Muscle belly is sutured to posterior sclera, thereby restricting muscle action considerably, producing a super-weakening effect.

Intraocular Procedures

Congenital Cataract Extraction Under the operating microscope, using irrigating and suction/cutting instruments, cataract and often the posterior capsule and a portion of the anterior vitreous are removed at one time. This procedure obtains a clear optical zone so that a contact lens can be fitted on the infant's eye within a few days postoperatively. The goal is to avoid intractable amblyopia (lazy eye) by operating during the first few weeks of life.

Goniotomy Although rare, goniotomy, the early operative intervention for congenital glaucoma, is urgent to prevent blindness. This microsurgical procedure involves dividing a congenital layer of abnormal tissue covering the drainage angle of anterior chamber. It is performed by use of a special operative contact lens placed on the eye that permits visualization of the angle. Incision is made through an opening in the contact lens.

Otolaryngology

Myringotomy Secretory otitis media is the most common chronic condition of childhood. Fluid accumulates in the middle ear from eustachian tube obstruction. This condition is corrected by myringotomy, incision in eardrum for drainage. By aspiration of fluid and pus, pressure is released, pain relieved, and hearing restored and preserved. Myringotomy is done to prevent perforation of the eardrum and possible erosion of middle ear ossicles. When the exudate is especially viscid, the patient has "glue ear" or mucoid otitis media.

Myringotomy is most commonly performed in association with tympanotomy. A self-cleaning plastic ventilating tube is placed in the incision, bypassing eustachian tube, to facilitate continued aeration of the middle ear space and prevent the reformation of serous otitis media. Premature extrusion of the tube before normal eustachian tube function resumes may necessitate repeated operation.

Middle Ear Tympanoplasty Congenital deafness may occur in varying degrees; no cure has been found for the nerve type. Congenital or acquired conductive deafness may be helped by tympanoplastic operative techniques (refer to Chap. 26, p. 503).

Correction of Choanal Atresia When bone or fibrous tissue blocks the posterior choanae, excision of the obstructive tissue, usually via a transseptal approach, corrects the problem. The carbon dioxide laser may be used to develop appropriate apertures. Newborns are obligate nose breathers and may die at birth if choanal atresia is undiagnosed. They are unable to breathe and feed properly without adequate nasal airway.

Adenoidectomy A patient should preferably be at least two years old before having adenoid tissue in the nasopharynx removed, but it can be removed earlier. The procedure is usually done in conjunction with a tonsillectomy.

Tonsillectomy Excision of hypertrophied or chronically infected tonsils is not generally advised before three years of age. General anesthesia is used for patients up to about 14 years of age. Tonsillectomy and adenoidectomy are frequently performed together, appearing on operating schedule as *T&A*. Sterile technique is carried out throughout the operation. Precautions during operation include control of bleeding and prevention of aspiration of blood or tissue.

Esophageal Dilation Children, usually of preschool age, may ingest caustic agents that cause chemical burns of the mouth, lips, pharynx, and corrosive esophagitis. Long-term gradual esophageal dilation with bougies may be necessary to restore adequate oral intake of food after acute phase of traumatic injury. When all attempts at dilation fail, the esophagus must be replaced. The most satisfactory source of esophageal replacement is the colon.

Tracheal or Laryngeal Stenosis Some accidental injuries result in a narrowing of the trachea or larynx. Of greater concern are the injuries that result from therapy for respiratory problems, especially in newborns. Prolonged endotracheal intubation can lead to injury from tubes that are too large for the lumen, are too long, or move too much. These injuries may require dilation and/or endoscopic resection of the stenotic area. Most infants then require an intraluminal stent to maintain patency of their airways.

Tracheotomy Tracheotomy is advisable in situations of severe inflammatory glottic diseases, when endotracheal intubation would be required longer than 72 hours, and when respiratory support is necessary for longer than 24 to 48 hours to treat respiratory problems. Appropriate sizes and types of tracheotomy tubes for infants and children must be available. Tubes that are too large, too rigid, or too long, or have an improper curve can produce ulceration and scarring at pressure points. Strictures that develop at the site of tracheotomy may require resection to relieve airway obstruction after decannulation.

Plastic and Reconstructive Surgery

With the exception of burns and other traumatic tissue injuries, most plastic and reconstructive surgery performed on infants and children is done to correct congenital anomalies. The most common of these include the following.

Cleft Lip Lack of fusion of the soft tissues of the upper lip creates a cleft or fissure. Cleft lips vary in degree from simple notching of lip to extension into floor of the nose. They may be unilateral or bilateral. The number of operations required for correction depends on severity of deformity. Some plastic surgeons do a primary *cheiloplasty,* closure of cleft lip, within the first few days after birth to facilitate feeding and to minimize psychological trauma of parents. Surgeons who prefer to wait until the infant is older follow the "rule of 10": 10 weeks, 10 g of hemoglobin, 10 lb of body weight. Regardless of preferred timing, infiltration of local anesthetic agent with epinephrine is usually anesthesia of choice.

To relieve tension on the incision postoperatively, a Logan bow (a small curved metal frame) may be applied over area of incision and held in place by narrow adhesive strips, to splint the lip. Skin closure strips may be used. Arm or elbow restraints are imperative to prevent infant from removing bow or strips and injuring the lip. These restraints are applied in the OR.

Cleft Palate Failure of tissues of the palate to fuse creates a fissure through roof of the mouth. Palatal clefts may be a defect only in the soft palate or may extend through both hard and soft palates into the nose and include the alveolar ridge of the maxilla. Cleft palate is often associated with cleft lip; however, the two deformities are closed separately. *Palatoplasty,* closure of the soft palate, is done before speech begins to avoid speech defects. A mouth gag must be used during operation to permit access to the palate without obstructing the airway. General anesthesia is administered via endotracheal tube. This may be supplemented by infiltration of local anesthetic agent. When epinephrine is used by the surgeon to minimize bleeding, the anesthesiologist must be informed.

In patients with bilateral and frequently unilateral clefts, an additional operation will be performed before the age of four to elevate tip of the nose and correct asymmetry.

Hemangioma Hemangiomas are the most common of all human congenital anomalies. An angioma that is made up of blood vessels is a hemangioma that may pigment or appear as a growth on the skin. All hemangiomas have abnormal patterns of hemodynamics, which is the effect of blood flow through tissues. But variations in vessel size distinguish the different types of these tumors. Argon laser or surgical excision in combination with skin graft or pedicle flap repair are treatments of choice for intradermal capillary hemangiomas (port-wine stain). Cryosurgery, surgical excision, or steroid therapy may be used for some other cavernous-type tumors.

Otoplasty Abnormally small or absent external ears can be reconstructed in several operative stages. Autogenous rib cartilage graft or silicone prosthesis is used for the supporting framework to produce anatomic contour. Usually necessitated by microtia, a congenital anomaly, reconstruction of external ear, can follow traumatic injury with loss of all or part of the pinna. Free flaps of temporal parietal fascia may be used to cover a carved cartilage armature for secondary reconstruction.

Otoplasty procedures to correct protruding or excessively large ears are performed more frequently than are procedures for microtia. These often are done on preschool-age children, usually boys, to prevent psychological harm from teasing.

Syndactylism Webbing between fingers is the most common congenital hand deformity. Tissue holding digits together must be cut to separate fingers. Separation of webbed digits almost always requires skin grafts to achieve good functional results. Syndactyly may occur in the foot also.

Neurosurgery

Children of all ages sustain head injuries with hematomas that must be evacuated (refer to Chap. 29, p. 556). Brain tumors do occur in children; however, the more frequently performed pediatric neurosurgical procedures are related to correction of congenital anomalies.

Craniosynostosis If one or more of the suture lines in the skull, normally open in infancy, fuses prematurely, the skull cannot expand during normal brain growth. The surgeon removes the fused bone, a *craniectomy,* to reopen the suture line. A strip of polyethylene or Silastic film may be inserted to cover bone edges on each side, or the newly formed suture lines may be cauterized with Zinker's solution to prevent refusion. More extensive freeing of other bones may be necessary to achieve decompression of frontal lobes and orbital contents. For example, the craniofacial dysostosis of Apert's syndrome and Crouzon's disease are associated with multiple skull and facial deformities. These must be corrected by craniofacial surgery performed by a multidiciplinary team (see Chap. 28. p. 537). If bone grafts are required, the infant's skull provides a donor site without creating a deformity.

Encephalocele Brain and neural tissue can herniate through a defect in the skull. This is present at birth as a sac of tissue on the head. Usually these lesions can be removed 6 to 12 weeks after birth, unless complicated by hydrocephalus.

Hydrocephalus Usually congenital, dilatation of the ventricles by obstruction, excessive formation of cerebrospinal fluid, or failure of the absorptive mechanisms produces impairment in the normal circulation of cerebrospinal fluid. Fluid accumulates in the ventricles. Pressure thus created causes enlargement of infant's head, if it develops prior to fusion of the cranial bones, and often causes brain damage. Hydrocephalus may be diagnosed in utero by cephalocentesis and a ventriculoamniotic shunt may be inserted to drain the ventricles. After birth, operative treatment involves establishment of a mechanism for transporting excess fluid from the ventricles to maintain a close-to-normal ventricular pressure. This may be done by implantation of a shunt, which carries fluid from lateral ventricle to the peritoneal cavity (*ventriculoperitoneal shunt*) or to right atrium of the heart (*ventriculoatrial shunt*). Other types of shunts are used, but less commonly, to bypass localized obstructions.

One end of the shunt catheter is put into the ventricle; the other end may connect to a one-way valve, which in turn is connected to the catheter that drains fluid distally from head. An endoscopic technique may be used for catheter placement in the ventricle. Shunt malfunction is usually caused by obstruction by the choroid plexus or debris. This complication can be reduced by positioning shunt catheter tip opposite the foramen of Monro visually via a miniature fiberoptic pediatric endoscope.

Catheters are silicone rubber. An antithrombotic coating may be incorporated into distal end. Some valves are regulated to open for drainage when predetermined pressure in the ventricle is reached. Other valves are designed as flushing devices to keep the distal catheter patent; skin over the device is manually depressed to flush the system. The surgeon chooses shunt mechanism for each patient that will be safest for the particular type of hydrocephalus being treated. Follow-up minor revisions are sometimes necessary, generally due to growth of the child.

Myelomeningocele A saclike protrusion bulges through a defect in a portion of the vertebral column that failed to fuse in fetal development. If the nerves of spinal cord remain within vertebral column and only the meninges protrude into the sac, the congenital anomaly is a *meningocele.* However, if sac also contains a portion of the spinal cord, it is a *myelomeningocele* with associated permanent nerve damage. Degree of impairment depends on level and extent of defect. Clubfeet, dislocated hips, hydrocephalus, neurogenic bladder, paralysis, and other congenital disorders often accompany myelomeningocele. Each patient must be evaluated and treated individually according to priorities of needs. In general, it is best to delay operating to repair a myelomeningocele until danger of hydrocephalus developing is passed or cerebrospinal fluid has been shunted. If sac is covered with a thin membrane, *meningitis* (infection of meninges) is an imminent danger unless defect is repaired soon after birth, usually within the first 48 hours, to close cutaneous, muscular, and dural defects.

Spina Bifida Incomplete closure of the paired vertebral arches in midline of vertebral column may occur without herniation of the meninges. A spina bifida may be covered by intact skin. Laminectomy may be indicated to repair the underlying defect.

Thoracic Surgery

Pectus Excavatum A congenital malformation of the chest wall, pectus excavatum, is characterized by a pronounced funnel-shaped depression over the lower end of the sternum. The deformity is corrected by resecting the lower intercostal cartilages and substernal ligaments to free up the sternum. The sternum is elevated and the cartilages are fitted to the sides of it. The operation is done primarily for cosmetic purposes, but occasionally it is necessary to establish normal respiratory and circulatory function.

Cardiovascular Surgery

Congenital cardiovascular defects are the result of abnormal embryological development of the heart or major vessels. Most are diagnosed in infancy, often when symptoms of congestive heart failure develop within the first few days or months after birth. Corrective or palliative operations are necessary to sustain or prolong life of these infants. Many of the operations are enhanced by or possible only with profound hypothermia and cardiopulmonary bypass (refer to Chap. 31). However, significant brain damage may be associated with cardiopulmonary bypass in infants. Bypass perfusion time should not exceed 40 minutes between periods of temporary normal circulatory perfusion. Congenital defects in infants or children amendable to surgical intervention include the following.

Anomalous Venous Return Failure of any one or combination of the pulmonary veins to return blood to the left atrium precludes the full complement of oxygenated blood from entering the systemic circulation. The anomalous pulmonary vein(s) must be transferred and anastomosed to the left atrium.

Coarctation of the Aorta A *coarctation* is a narrowing or stricture in a vessel. This is one of the more common congenital cardiovascular defects, usually occurring in the aortic arch. It may cause hypertension in the upper extremities above the obstruction and hypotension in the lower extremities from slowed circulation below the coarctation. To correct the defect, the coarctation is resected and the aorta may be anastomosed end-to-end. An aortic graft may be necessary when length of the coarctation prevents anastomosis. A subclavian flap angioplasty capable of growth in length and width is operation of choice in infants.

Patent Ductus Arteriosus During fetal life the ductus arteriosus carries blood from the pulmonary artery to the aorta to bypass the lungs. Normally this vessel closes in the first hours after birth to prevent recirculation of arterial blood through the body. If closure does not occur, blood flow may be reversed by aortic pressure, causing respiratory distress. Surgical intervention is indicated, in lieu of prolonged ventilatory support, to prevent development of chronic pulmonary changes. The patent ductus arteriosus is clamped and ligated.

Septal Defects Open-heart operation with cardiopulmonary bypass is necessary to close abnormal openings in the walls separating the chambers within the heart.

Atrial Septal Defect An opening in the wall between right and left atria may be sufficiently large to allow oxygenated blood to shunt from left to right and return to the lungs. This can increase pulmonary blood flow with eventual pulmonary hypertension if defect is not closed. If defect cannot be closed with sutures, a patch graft is inserted.

Ventricular Septal Defect A ventricular septal defect is usually located in the membranous portion of the septum between the right and left ventricles. It is the most common of the congenital heart anomalies. Patients with small defects are relatively asymptomatic and repair may be unnecessary. Large defects with left-to-right shunting of oxygenated blood back to the lungs, thus increasing pulmonary hypertension, are closed. A patch graft may be required to close the defect.

Atrioventricular Canal Defect Also referred to as an *endocardial cushion defect,* the atrioventricular canal of connective tissue that normally divides the heart into four chambers has failed to develop. Deficiencies are present in lower portion of interatrial septum, upper portion of interventricular septum, and tricuspid and mitral valves. The result is a large central canal which permits blood flow between any of the four chambers of heart. Pulmonary artery banding, constriction to reduce diameter of artery, is an alternative to primary repair in infants less than one year of age to decrease pulmonary blood flow, thus relieving pulmonary hypertension. Corrective operation involves repair of mitral and tricuspid valves and patch grafts to close septal defects.

Tetralogy of Fallot Tetralogy of Fallot is a combination of four defects:

1 Ventricular septal defect

2 Stenosis of pulmonary valve and/or outflow tract into pulmonary artery

3 Hypertrophy of right ventricle

4 Displacement of aorta to right so that it receives blood from both ventricles

Often referred to as "blue babies," these infants are cyanotic because insufficient oxygen circulates to body tissues. Total correction of the multiple anomalies is difficult. Assessment of the technical ease of correction is generally the dominant consideration. If cyanosis is severe, a palliative shunt operation may be performed during infancy to increase pulmonary blood flow.

1 *Blalock-Taussig operation:* end-to-side anastomosis of right subclavian artery to corresponding pulmonary artery. Mixed arterial-venous blood from aorta flows through the shunt to pulmonary artery and into lungs for oxygenation.
2 *Potts-Smith-Gibson operation:* side-to-side anastomosis of aorta and left pulmonary artery. The shunt enlarges as child grows but is more difficult to reconstruct than is a Blalock shunt at a later time when corrective operation is performed.
3 *Waterston operation:* anastomosis of aorta and right pulmonary artery. The anastomosis is placed on posterior aspect of aorta to provide perfusion to both pulmonary arteries.

With cardiopulmonary bypass and hypothermia, the ventricular septal defect is closed with a patch graft that also corrects the abnormal communication between right ventricle and aorta. Then the obstruction to pulmonary blood flow is relieved. This may include enlarging the pulmonary valve and/or widening the outflow tract. Resection of obstructing cardiac muscle may be necessary with insertion of prosthetic outflow patch. An aortic allograft containing the aortic valve with the septal leaflet of the mitral valve and the ascending aorta attached may be inserted. The septal leaflet of mitral valve is used as a portion of the right ventricular outflow patch. All or part of the aortic valve and ascending aorta is used as a new conduit with the pulmonary artery or as a patch graft.

Transposition of the Great Vessels In a transposition, the aorta rises from right ventricle and the pulmonary artery from left ventricle. This essentially creates two separate circulatory systems: one systemic and the other pulmonary, but not interconnected as in normal anatomy. Life depends on presence or creation of associated defects to permit exchange of blood between the two systems. These defects may include a patent foramen ovale, patent ductus arteriosus, atrial septal defect, or ventricular septal defect. A palliative operation is performed in newborn, usually to enlarge atrial septal defect by balloon catheter septostomy to sustain life until the infant grows enough to tolerate a corrective procedure that may include partial transposition of the pulmonary veins.

Tricuspid Atresia Absence of a tricuspid valve between right atrium and ventricle prevents normal blood flow through chambers of the heart. Blood flows through an atrial septal defect, into an enlarged left ventricle, through a small right ventricle to the pulmonary artery. Anastomosis of superior vena cava to right pulmonary artery, or other type of aorta-pulmonary artery shunt may be created as a palliative procedure to increase pulmonary blood flow. Fontan-type and Bjork direct anastomosis of right atrium to infundibulum of right ventricle are reconstructive procedures.

Truncus Arteriosus A single artery carries blood directly from heart with a large associated ventricular septal defect, to coronary, pulmonary, and systemic circulatory systems. Initial palliative banding of the pulmonary arteries, as close to their origins off the truncus as possible, decreases pulmonary blood flow in infant in congestive heart failure. At a later stage a corrective procedure can be performed to close the ventricular septal defect and insert a conduit with an ascending aortic graft and aortic valve. Correction in infancy requires replacement of conduit as child grows.

Valvular Obstructive Lesions Congenital aortic and pulmonary valve stenosis require valvulotomy.

FETAL SURGERY

Maternal prenatal testing after 12 weeks of gestation (see Chap. 22, p. 442) makes possible prenatal diagnosis of some malformations in the fetus. An abnormal amount of fluid in cystic structures, such as myelomeningocele, is detected, as are some congenital anomalies in the abdomen and intestinal tract. Diagnosis of cleft lip and palate is possible. Obstructive uropathy, including renal parenchymal loss and obstructive hydronephrosis, is most commonly diagnosed. Prenatal diagnosis allows choice of elective cesarean section of mother to avoid further compromise during delivery and to promote immediate postnatal care of neonate.

Some selective lesions are amendable to surgery in utero, fetal surgery. Among these are hydronephrosis, hydrocephalus, and diaphragmatic hernia. Decompression of the obstruction may repair the malformation to reduce anticipated mortality. In considering fetal therapy, the following criteria are used.

1 Pregnancy has a single fetus.

2 Parents are fully counseled about risks and benefits to mother and fetus.

3 Multidisciplinary team experienced in fetal diagnosis and anomalies will manage the infant after birth. This team includes an obstetrician, neonatalogist, and pediatric surgeon.

4 High-risk obstetrical unit and neonatal intensive care unit are available.

CHAPTER **34**

TRANSPLANTATION AND REPLANTATION

Transplantation biology is the science of transplantation of living tissues. Concentrated efforts continue in search of compensation for or suitable replacement of deficient tissues and organs. One modality is transplantation or graft, the application to or insertion into the body of tissues or organs taken from another part of the same body or from another body. Indication for transplant is irreversible functional failure of the organ.

DEVELOPMENT OF TRANSPLANTATION

Interest in transplantation is many centuries old. Celsus wrote that tissues could survive after grafting from one part of the body to another. Galen attempted reconstruction of facial defects. Centuries later it was observed that full-thickness autografts survived whereas allografts failed, although the reason was not understood.

Darwin's theory of evolution and Mendel's laws of heredity shed new light in the nineteenth century, spurring researchers to pursue the study of regenerative capacity in animals. In the early twentieth century, A. Carrel and R. Guthrie performed blood vessel anastomoses, an essential component of organ transplantation. Performing heterotopic heart transplants in animals, they demonstrated that a heart could be removed, transplanted and resume beating.

In the 1930s, the maintenance of organs in vitro opened the way to organ preservation. Expanded information concerning patient response to operation during the decade of the 1940s marked advances in operative therapy. Open-heart surgery, as well as acquisition of basic knowledge required for clinical transplantation, evolved in the 1950s. Pioneers in transplantation biology, Peter Medawar and Frank M. Burnet, received the Nobel prize in 1960 for their work on immunologic tolerance in tissue transplantation in animals.

Many scientific disciplines contribute to and fuse information to aid progress in clinical transplantation. Foremost among these are physiology, genetics, immunology, and pathology. Practical application of clinical transplantation became possible in the 1960s after investigative efforts led to development of supportive techniques such as cardiopulmonary bypass and immunosuppressive drug therapy.

Although kidney transplantation preceded it by more than a decade, the first successful heart transplant, performed by Dr. Christian Barnard in 1967 in South Africa, expanded the era of clinical organ transplantation.

TYPES OF TRANSPLANTS

Some tissues and whole organs can be transplanted and grafted to restore bodily function. The type of transplant selected will depend on purpose of graft, anatomic function, and availability of tissue or organ. The types of biologic transplants include the following.

Allografts (Homografts) Tissue grafted between different or genetically dissimilar individuals of same species.

Autografts Tissues grafted in same person from one part of body to another. The donor is also the recipient.

Isografts Tissues grafted between genetically identical donor and recipient, as between identical twins.

Xenografts (Heterografts) Tissues grafted between two dissimilar species. Heterografts may be used when allograft material is unavailable or temporary replacement is necessary.

Orthotopic Transplant Transplant to an anatomically natural or normal recipient site.

Heterotopic Transplant Transplant to an anatomically abnormal location in the host. Heterotopic grafts may function normally in the unnatural site.

TISSUE TRANSPLANTATION

Some tissues such as skin can function normally even though moved to a different area of the body.

1 Skin grafts provide a protective surface covering, initially acquiring then eventually losing vascular connection with the host.

2 Corneal grafts replace nonfunctioning corneal tissue.

3 Bone grafts afford temporary structural supports and a pattern for regrowth of the host's bone, the graft then being resorbed.

4 Blood vessel grafts are used to bypass or replace diseased or obstructed segments of vessels.

ORGAN TRANSPLANTATION

While tissue grafts are commonplace, transplantation of whole vital organs designed to remain as permanent functional units presents ethical and philosophical dilemmas in addition to technical factors. A supply of donor tissue from the living involves a real sacrifice. Therefore, primarily cadaver sources are used. Transplantation can potentially restore the recipient to normal or near-normal physiological status.

Transplant of kidneys has been the most successful and principal clinical application of organ transplantation. If the graft fails, the patient may survive by returning to hemodialysis and receiving another transplant. Transplantation of the heart and liver, although becoming increasingly successful, has not equaled that of kidneys. Transplantation of pancreas, lung, and intestines is far less successful. In addition, no practical prolonged artificial support exists for these organs in the event of allograft failure.

Transplantation of each organ involves unique technical and physiologic problems, but the major barriers and causes of failure of all transplants are infection and immunologic rejection, treated by appropriate use of antibiotics and manipulation of immunologic agents. Transplant patients are similar to other critical patients with severe chronic illness. They are prone to sepsis because of combined lowered host-resistance factors. In addition, defense mechanisms are further depressed by immunosuppressive agents. Reverse isolation may be used to protect patient although endogenous infection may occur.

Immunologic Rejection

The technical aspects of transplantation have been largely solved. However, the body possesses an innate tendency to reject and destroy any foreign material introduced into it except tissue from an identical twin. Transplanted cells from donors even slightly dissimilar to the recipient may be rejected.

Organ rejection involves the patient's immunologic system. Both cellular and humoral immune systems seem to be involved in responses to transplanted cells. Activation of the immune system is a response to antigens introduced by donor graft. An immunologic reaction usually is accompanied by a febrile systemic reaction, local inflammation, and deteriorating function of the graft. A knowledge of antigens, individual-specific and species-specific, and their genetic transmission is important for avoidance of violent reactions. Many factors influence the strength and rate of a rejection reaction. Some of these are acquired immunologic tolerance, lymphatic depression, or previous sensitization by blood transfusions, pregnancies, or transplants. Rejection may be reversible with intensive therapy or progressive with cessation of transplant function.

Combating Rejection Attempts must be made to find compatible donors and to minimize rejection.

Preoperative Matching of Donor to Recipient Tissue typing and matching are essential prerequisites of transplantation to determine genetic disparity between donor and recipient. Histocompatibility implies acceptability by an individual of tissue from another. Histocompatibility tests, although not infallible, result in improved organ survival from both related and cadaver sources. They assist in donor-recipient selection. The better the histocompatibility match and degree of genetic similarity between donor and recipient, the less serious is the rejection. Histocompatibility testing, *tissue typing,* is based on detection of cell-surface antigens known to affect rejection. Favorable results are expected when few histocompatibility antigens are detected. Preformed antibodies appear to have a harmful effect on graft survival. Testing employs serological techniques, methods for in vitro analysis for study of cell-to-cell interaction and identification of the mediator of the interaction, as well as cell-culture techniques. Complex assay techniques measure effects of antibodies and lymphocytes against donor tissue in a culture setup. *Cross matching* between recipient's serum and donor's peripheral blood target cells is accomplished by multiple serologic reagents or flow cytometry using fluorescent-labeled monoclonal antibodies.

Immunosuppressive Therapy in the Recipient Specific alterations in immune responses are produced by inactivating or destroying lymphoid cells potentially capable of responding to the antigens. The goal is to selectively suppress antigenic reactions to the transplant without impairing body's defense against pathogenic organisms. An attempt is made to neutralize or modify the body's protective antigenic mechanisms by use of various immunosuppressive agents to allow the transplant to remain and function. This barrier can be pierced at least temporarily by creating an increase in transplant tolerance or paralyzing the recipient's immunologic system. Since lymphocytes and globulins seem to be mainly responsible for rejection, an attempt is made to vary their synthesis. Antibody formation and immune reaction can be suppressed by certain factors. Protocol is fairly standard in all transplant centers.

1 Cyclosporine (Sandimmune), a soil fungus derivative, is a potent immunosuppressant that acts mainly on thymus-derived lymphocytes, the cells primarily responsible for rejection. This drug reduces rejection, especially in early or inductive phase, without suppressing entire immune system. It may be given orally or intravenously. It is always used with low doses of adrenal corticosteroids, but not usually with other immunosuppressive agents. Its absorption rate is variable, and it has toxic effects on kidneys and liver that must be monitored.

2 Corticosteroids, such as prednisone, have an anti-inflammatory effect useful in reversing early rejection reaction. There is an inverse relationship between steroids and lymphocytes.

3 Polyvalent antithymus globulin is as effective as are steroids in reversing rejection, and reverses some steroid-resistant rejections.

4 Agents cytostatic or cytotoxic to lymphatic tissue, such as azathioprine (Imuran), suppress the entire immune system and have serious side effects on other systems. Extracorporeal perfusion with these drugs and localized radiation to the transplant may be used, either separately or concurrently.

5 Heterologous horse or rabbit antithymocyte globulin or antilymphocytic globulin or serum act against circulating lymphocyte T cells and induce suppressor cells.

6 Monoclonal antibodies have ability to reverse initial episode of rejection by binding to specific precisely targeted surface antigens on mature T lymphocytes. These antibodies are also used for immunologic monitoring posttransplant.

7 Drainage of thoracic duct or common lymph trunk, splenectomy, and thymectomy are performed occasionally.

Employment of immunosuppressive measures is not without complication. Leukopenia and susceptibility to infection are common sequelae. Therapy may not totally abolish rejection by the host but may delay onset and decrease incidence of rejection episodes during the crucial first month or two following transplantation.

Pretransplant Transfusions Blood transfusions from donor expose the recipient to a limited number of leukocyte antigens that seem to reduce risk of sensitization to prospective donor transplant and to increase graft survival. Different blood products, including platelets, and pharmacologic conditioning may be part of a pretransplant transfusion protocol to induce specific immune modification in the recipient. However, random preoperative blood transfusions prior to a cadaveric organ transplant may increase risk of sensitization, although this may improve allograft survival.

Availability of Organ Allografts

The goal is selection of a donor-recipient pair with adequate histocompatibility to permit a functioning organ without complications and to use the lowest possible safe doses of immunologic drugs.

Cadaver Sources Cadaver sources are used except for bone marrow and some kidney transplants. Most kidneys are procured, harvested, from nonliving individuals because of an inadequate supply of living donors. Since written informed consent is required to obtain donor organs, many persons carry a signed "Uniform Donor Card" or other identification stating that in case of death certain or all organs may be removed for transplant. This card is legal under the Uniform Anatomical Gift Act enacted by all 50 states.

Ideal cadaver donors are young persons with confirmed brain death, often the result of automobile accident, where the organ can be preserved in vivo. All donors must be without sepsis or malignancy, preferably under 50 years of age, and with previous good function of the donor organ. *Organ banks* exchange organs, collect organs from donors, and register patients in need of a transplant as well as information about their blood grouping and tissue typing. Less is known concerning potential transmissible disease when cadaver organs are used.

Organs from cadaver sources must be removed under sterile conditions, and preserved and transported to the recipient. A brain-dead individual may be maintained for organ procurement on mechanical ventilation and/or cardiopulmonary bypass to prevent ischemic damage to vital organs. Time is paramount when critical organs are involved, for their value depends on preserving maximum functional viability. The time factor is less urgent with less critical tissue.

Living Sources In patients for kidney or marrow transplantation, the use of an organ or marrow from a biologically related living donor has distinct advantages: results are better than are those with cadaver organs because donor-recipient matches are usually good (identical twin sources are ideal for compatibility); waiting time is reduced; lengthy dialysis is avoided; and the procedure is planned. Many patients die while awaiting a compatible cadaver organ. Use of living donors involves special protocol.

1 Adults, preferred over adolescents or children, must be able to give informed consent voluntarily without coercion. Children are used as donors only for a twin or for a patient with predictable results. If the donor is a minor, court (legal) as well as parental or guardian consent is required to avoid bias. The donor must fully comprehend the sacrifice; if the physician deems it advisable, psychiatric examination is included along with intelligence testing.

2 The donor must be in excellent health. The *donor's* physician confers with him or her and performs the preoperative physical examination to permit a rational decision. Renal arteriograms are done to confirm bilateral kidneys and identify renal vasculature prior to a nephrectomy.

3 The donor should have no psychiatric complications. Donor reactive depressions may follow organ removal if adequate gratitude is not shown by all concerned.

Preservation of Organ Allografts

Successful use of donor tissue depends on rapid organ resection and cooling, since the period of ischemia must be kept to a minimum. Long-term preservation of tissue remains a problem; current techniques utilize a variety of cryoprotective agents. Controlled freezing may produce lethal cell injury. This technique is used for skin, and sperm or blood suspensions, but not for whole organs. Hypothermia above freezing (4 to 8°C, 39 to 46°F) with or without perfusion with cold solutions reduces general metabolic demands, thereby providing a safety margin. Methods of hypothermia include the following.

1 Simple flush techniques with cold electrolyte solutions and storage by immersion in electrolyte or flush-out solution in a plastic container kept at a hypothermic temperature

2 Hypothermic continuous pulsatile perfusion with oxygenated electrolyte solution.

Human Kidney Allotransplantation

Begun in 1951, kidney transplantation is an accepted clinical modality. Combined hemodialysis and transplantation have significantly changed the outlook and notably improved the quality of life of many patients with terminal renal disease. Patients may choose to accept transplantation rather than undergo chronic dialysis for the rest of their lives. Indication for transplantation is end-stage renal disease, most often glomerulonephritis, pyelonephritis, polycystic disease, or nephrosclerosis. Ideal recipients are 5 to 40 years of age without severe extrarenal disease, malignancy, or active sepsis. Pretransplant bilateral nephrectomy may be performed in patients with uncontrollable hypertension. Patients with detected presensitization states have to wait longer for a suitably matched donor and statistically have a lower one-year graft survival rate than do unsensitized patients.

Recipients are carefully prepared preoperatively with kidney dialysis, fluid and electrolyte intake regulation, pretransplant transfusions, and control of hypertension. Proper donor-recipient matching is performed.

Donor preparation is equally important. Removal of a kidney is associated with low morbidity, although a living donor must guard against bruising or rupturing the remaining kidney for the rest of his or her life. The donor is therefore advised to avoid body-contact sports.

Transplantation Unless a transported cadaver donor organ is used, two adjoining operating rooms and teams are employed. One team procures and preserves donor kidney while the other prepares recipient site and transplants the kidney.

Donor Nephrectomy In a living donor the kidney is removed through a flank incision. Adequate renal perfusion and urinary output, maintenance of adequate blood pressure and ureteral blood supply, as well as gentleness in manipulation, are extremely important intraoperatively. As soon as excised, the kidney is flushed with cold heparinized solution to remove red blood cells. Total ischemia time is usually less than an hour. The donor's incision is closed per routine technique.

Recipient Procedure The iliac fossa is the standard site for transplantation in an adult patient. The hypogastric artery is anastomosed to the renal artery and the common iliac vein to the renal vein. Reconstruction of urinary tract is the main technical problem. Implantation of donor ureter into the bladder, ureteroneocystostomy, is the preferred technique for urinary drainage. Alternative methods include ureteroureterostomy and ureteropyelostomy.

Complications of Renal Allotransplantation Complications may be renal-related or extrarenal. The most common renal-related include rejection (the dominant cause of graft loss), recurrent nephritis, acute tubular necrosis, or technical failure from genitourinary or vascular problems. Postoperative management is similar to that of other surgical patients with emphasis on initial adequacy of renal function, prevention of hazardous effects of immunosuppressive therapy, and observation for allograft rejection. Possible *types of rejection* are:

1 *Hyperacute,* due to presensitization. This is an immediate acute rejection that occurs right after anastomosis of blood vessels or within 24 hours. It includes thrombosis and extensive destruction of allograft vasculature.

2 *Accelerated,* due to presensitization. The graft may function for up to five days, followed by rapid loss of renal function. Treatment for both hyperacute and accelerated rejection is immediate removal of the transplant.

3 *Acute.* This usually occurs one week to four months following transplantation and is often reversible unless immune response is severe. Systemic and local symptoms, as well as reduced urinary output and abnormal laboratory findings, are present.

4 *Chronic.* Antibodies developing long after transplantation produce insidious onset with mild hypertension and diminishing renal function. This rejection is not reversible. Acute and chronic rejection may be diagnosed by renal biopsy.

Extrarenal complications, usually caused by immunosuppressive or corticosteroid therapy, include infection (the leading cause of death on a long-term basis), pneumonitis, hepatitis, gastrointestinal bleeding, and psychological problems from perpetual fear of rejection. Immunosuppressive therapy must be used with caution.

Results of kidney transplantation are gratifying; life can be significantly prolonged. Causes for concern are chronic liver failure and vascular disease, a major cause of death in dialysis patients, which may occur in the long-term transplant patient. The incidence of malignant neoplasm in patients surviving renal transplantation more than a year exceeds that expected in the general population.

Heart Allotransplantation

Heart transplantation may be performed in selected patients with terminal cardiac disease such as irreversible extensive myocardial failure and widespread atherosclerotic deterioration. These are patients with very limited life expectancy for whom no alternative therapy remains to sustain life. A brain-dead donor with the heart preserved in vivo may be used. Optimum preservation of the donor heart is necessary because it must resume full activity after transplantation. As with renal transplantation, two teams operate in adjoining rooms; one procures donor organ at precisely the time it is needed. Thus ischemia time is kept to a minimum, and must be less than three hours. After removal, the donor heart is rapidly cooled and immediately implanted in the recipient. The operative procedure and postoperative care are similar to open-heart surgery, with anticoagulation therapy and cardiopulmonary bypass utilized during operation. Two operative modalities are available: total orthotopic heart replacement, or heterotopic insertion of a transplanted heart as an assist device without removal of the recipient's heart.

Most mortalities occur in the first two postoperative months, the crucial period of immunologic rejection. Electrocardiogram changes such as drop in voltage, reduced cardiac output, arteritis, myocardial ischemia, and myocardial necrosis occur during rejection. Diagnosis and monitoring of acute rejection may be facilitated by serial transvenous endomyocardial biopsies, which also may confirm effectiveness of therapy. Under fluoroscopy, a forceps is passed through a catheter into apex of right ventricle via the right internal jugular vein. A small sample of myocardium is removed for histologic study. A major obstacle to long-term survival is the development of obliterative coronary artery disease in the transplanted heart. The rejection process accelerates atherosclerosis. Improvement in survival rates is attributed to more accurate early diagnosis of rejection and vigorous measures to prevent atherosclerosis, thought to be due to immunologic injury to intima of the coronary vessels. An increase in malignant neoplasms in heart transplant patients has been observed. These patients need psychological support to maintain a will to live and to adjust to problems that may arise at any time.

Combined Heart-Lung Allotransplantation

The organs of the cardiopulmonary system can be transplanted as a unit. The operative technique preserves the recipient's phrenic nerves on tissue pedicles, a portion of the right atrium and vena cava, and the aortic arch. The trachea is transected above the carina, and the heart and lungs are removed as a unit. Cyclosporine given postoperatively enhances successful healing of the tracheal anastomosis and combats cellular mediated rejection. Patients with congenital or acquired heart disease with associated untreated or chronic end-stage pulmonary disease may be candidates for heart-lung transplantation.

Lung Allotransplantation

Lung transplant may be performed in patients with terminal respiratory failure such as insufficiency from emphysema. Patient selection is difficult, since other organ systems, especially the heart, are often damaged by pulmonary failure.

Optimum preservation of the donor organ is vitally important, because most recipients have inadequate pulmonary reserve. Moreover, the transplanted lung must assume oxygenation immediately, with respirator aid. Adequate preservation of donor lungs, more difficult than is preservation of other organs, remains a problem. Brain-dead cadaver donors afford minimum ischemia time.

Many special problems affect the success of clinical lung transplantation.

1 Recipients usually have some degree of pulmonary infection at the time of operation. The recipient's remaining lung, if diseased, may be a source of infection.

2 Ventilation-perfusion imbalance between the transplanted lung and the remaining lung may result in reduced function in the transplant.

3 Imminent rejection is not recognized easily.

4 Vascular and fibrotic changes produced by rejection create ischemia and anoxia.

5 Healing at site of bronchial anastomosis is a problem, but less so with cyclosporine.

6 Procedure is technically difficult. Size of donor lung, hilar structures, and bronchus must approximate those of recipient.

Liver Allotransplantation

Hepatic transplantation may be performed in selected patients with end-stage liver disease, either malignant or nonmalignant. Ideal recipients are patients with primary liver disease. Successful liver transplantation is performed on infants and children with biliary atresia who develop chronic liver failure or those with other liver or biliary problems. Preexisting infection in any part of the body is a distinct contraindication, since patients' preoperative status is poor and they lack protective proteins normally produced by the liver. Postoperative infection is always a marked danger.

Organ preservation presents a problem as hepatic tissue is very susceptible to damage from ischemia. Even though the liver can be preserved up to eight hours outside the body, a brain-dead cadaver donor with intact circulation is preferred. Donor and recipient hepatectomies ideally can be synchronized so the orthotopic recipient site is ready before circulation to donor liver is arrested.

Complexity and friability of the liver contribute to technical hazards. Extensive dissection is required as well as ligation of vessels to avoid postoperative hemorrhage. The vena cava must be mobilized. After it is divided, the liver is removed and the donor organ anastomosed to upper then lower vena cava as quickly as possible. During this critical period, venous return from lower half of the body must be decompressed via Portex pump from iliac to axillary arteries. Following anastomoses of portal vein and hepatic artery, any bleeding must be controlled prior to bile duct reconstruction.

Rejection may be noted by changes in laboratory findings, such as alterations in serum enzyme levels and elevated serum bilirubin. Cellular infiltration of the graft causes impairment of clotting factors, liver-cell necrosis, and impaired function. Complications from reconstruction of the biliary tract may lead to graft failure.

Pancreas Allotransplantation

A variety of techniques have been used in clinical endocrine transplantation in the treatment of patients with severe diabetes with associated systemic complications. These techniques require exocrine drainage. The goal is to provide physiological islet function to achieve more satisfactory carbohydrate metabolism and to restore normal glucose homeostasis, and to prevent or halt secondary complications associated with diabetes mellitus. Either the whole pancreas, distal segment, or isolated islets may be transplanted.

Bone Marrow Transplantation

A tissue rather than an organ transplantation, bone marrow harvest follows the protocol for organ transplant since it is also fraught with hazards. It is performed only after conventional methods of treatment have failed to reconstitute hematologic and immunologic functions. Indications are severe combined immune deficiency disease, acute leukemia or chronic myelogenous leukemia in blastic phase, and aplastic anemia. Contraindications are renal or cardiac disease, or previous maximum radiation dosage. Blood-typing and antigen-compatibility testing are essential. An allogenetic donor is usually a sibling, with an identical twin preferred. Autologous stem cells may be collected from leukemic patients in remission, cryopreserved, and stored to be given back to them during subsequent relapse.

Prior to transplantation, which consists of marrow infusion, the recipient is given a high-dose regimen of immunosuppressive chemotherapy to eradicate leukemic, lymphoid, and bone marrow cells, thereby inducing marrow depression. The recipient also receives total body irradiation (TBI) to penetrate areas resistant to the drugs. During this period of pretransplant preparation, the patient is placed in reverse isolation, preferably in a laminar airflow clean or sterile (germ-free) environment. Patient is closely monitored for side effects of immunosuppressive chemotherapy and TBI.

When pretransplant protocols are completed, the donor is hospitalized prior to the scheduled transplant. In the operating room under general or spinal anesthesia, 500 to 700 ml of bone marrow are aspirated at multiple sites from iliac crests. The marrow is filtered, heparinized, and placed in sterile containers for infusion. The donor is watched for bleeding and may need blood and fluid replacement.

Marrow is infused into the recipient intravenously, or via a Hickman or Broviac catheter, over several hours. Patient is constantly attended and closely monitored for adverse reaction during this time. By an unknown process, the marrow migrates into the marrow cavities of the bones. For 10 to 30 days after transplant the recipient may receive daily transfusions of lymphocytes, platelets, and granulocytes, preferably taken from the donor to counteract the predictable side effects (mainly hemorrhage and infection) of pretransplant immunosuppressive therapy. If it is not from an identical twin, blood is irradiated before transfusion to destroy lymphocytes. Mature blood cells and platelets are unaffected. Daily marrow aspirations and complete blood counts are done on the host. Success or failure of transplantation is usually decided 10 to 20 days afterward when the new marrow begins to function.

Complications include leukemic relapse or graft versus host disease, the rejection of the host by transplanted tissue. This does not occur in an identical twin, but it may occur when genetically different cells are introduced into a host unable to reject foreign material.

Transplantation Societies and Registries

The American Society of Transplant Surgeons and the International Society of Transplantation meet regularly to exchange ideas and information among persons of different scientific backgrounds. The aim is to achieve the best possible patient survival rather than merely transplant survival.

The Organ Transplant Registry of the American College of Surgeons in conjunction with the National Institutes of Health collects data on transplant operations and approves and funds various registries. The Human Kidney Transplant Registry collects information on worldwide renal transplantation.

The Federal Organ Transplantation and Procurement Act of 1983 provided financial grants for initial development of regional organ procurement centers and a transplant registry. The initiation of the United Network for Organ Sharing was an important step for sharing and transporting organs throughout the United States. A national task force has also been established to analyze medical, legal, ethical, economic, and social issues of concern in organ procurement and transplantation.

Future Hope in Transplantation

Important areas of clinical transplantation investigation include:

1 Identification of host responses on an immune level and ability to identify posttransplant immune status on a daily basis.

2 Improvement in donor-recipient matching.

3 Increase in supply of good cadaver organs that would provide better tissue matching. Improvements in procedures for arranging during lifetime for organ gifts by potential donors.

4 Long-term storage of organs in a viable state.

Immunologic rejection and shortage of donor organs remain the principal deterrents in transplantation.

REPLANTATION OF AMPUTATED PARTS

Replantation may be attempted to salvage a traumatically amputated digit, hand, or entire upper extremity. Severing of a foot or lower extremity presents more formidable problems because of the functional necessity for weight bearing. The victim of amputation of scalp, nose, or penis is also a candidate for replantation. Using microsurgical techniques, replanted parts can survive with varying degrees of effectiveness. Functional recovery, up to 80 percent of normal in some patients, may take up to a year or longer, since it takes time for nerves to regenerate. A team of specialists in hand surgery or plastic and orthopaedic surgeons with microvascular skill is vital to success in these arduous procedures. Experienced teams are on call in replantation centers.

Correct care and preservation of the severed part for transport with the patient are also vital to success. The amputated part should be placed dry into a plastic bag, which is then sealed and immersed in crushed ice inside an insulated container (e.g. styrofoam) to retard melting of ice during travel. *The part should not be warmed, frozen, or packed in dry ice.* Rapid transport and cooling with ice buys time.

Initial treatment involves assessment of the total patient while the severed part is cleansed with isotonic solution under sterile technique. Ringer's lactate or saline is used; water will lyse cells. The injured extremity should be elevated. The patient and family should be supported emotionally but not given definitive promises in regard to outcome.

In judging whether or not to perform replantation, the surgeon considers numerous factors: need for the part, associated disease and injuries, economic and psychological factors, and age. Two criteria are of special significance.

1 The replanted part must have potential for being useful.

2 There should be no undue risk to the general safety of the patient if the procedure is performed.

Replantation is more successful in young patients than in older patients. Also, incomplete amputations are more successful because they have intact subcutaneous venous circulation in the skin bridges. Restoration is much more difficult in crush injuries than in sharp, clean amputations. Contraindications to replantation include prolonged warm ischemia, severe bruising or crushing injury, multiple fractures or injury at different levels in the same digit, or associated injuries that preclude the effort.

Supportive therapy following injury includes tetanus toxoid, intravenous antibiotics and fluids or blood products, and judicious administration of anticoagulants.

Preoperative patient preparation is in anticipation of a long procedure. Operation may take from 4 to 16 hours. The patient is placed on an air or water mattress. The head, scapulae, sacrum, and heels are padded. A footboard may be used and antiembolic stockings applied. An indwelling catheter is inserted. Most replants of the hand are done under preoperative sedation and axillary or supraclavicular block with a long-acting agent, such as Marcaine, without epinephrine. General anesthesia is used for children and may be needed for adults for a long procedure.

These operations usually involve a two-team approach; one team prepares the recipient site and the other prepares the severed or distal part. In the OR, debridement of crushed tissue is carried out. Vessels are isolated for repair, and vessel patency is ensured. The basic steps of replantation of digits or extremities include:

1 Identifying proximal and distal tendons, nerves, and vessels.

2 Shortening bone within acceptable limit necessary for tension-free repair of blood vessels, nerves, and soft tissues.

3 Stabilizing skeletal structure such as with internal wire-fixation techniques to maintain joint continuity and fusion in functional position.

4 Suturing tendons and ligaments, both extensors and flexors, appropriately to lessen the junctional scar process that can inhibit motion.

5 Reanastomosing veins. A general rule is that more veins are reanastomosed than are arteries to provide sufficient venous return and thereby minimize edema. Swelling creates pressure that impedes circulation, leading to necrosis.

6 Reanastomosing arteries. The vessels may be flushed with heparin solution, and systemic anticoagulants may be given. Antispasmotic agents may be needed.

7 Repairing nerves and soft tissues.

8 Skin grafting or tissue flap or transfer if necessary.

NOTE. 1. Microsurgical techniques are necessary for nerve, artery, and vein repairs of structures that have an external diameter of 1 mm or less.

2. Backup replantation teams must be available for lengthy procedures. This is especially important when the patient has multiple amputations or requires repeat of replantation soon after initial operation.

To avoid constriction, a circular bandage is not applied. Instead, foam bandage is used and the extremity suspended from a bedside IV pole with stockinet wrapped around the arm. The dressing is padded to prevent pressure sores and nerve damage. The original dressing is not changed for ten days unless indicated.

Postoperative care is extremely important. Dressings must be checked carefully, since even slight manipulation can cause great damage. Checking only the tip of the digit for circulation is not adequate. Circulation is verified by *cautiously* going into the dressing to check capillary refill, color, temperature, and drainage. A Doppler flow meter and a temperature probe may be used to evaluate circulation. Patients are not permitted to smoke, because tobacco is a vasoconstrictor. Constriction of vessels may reduce circulation.

The many hours expended by the OR team initially to achieve a successful repair of all structures can relieve the patient of subsequent operations. The objective is to obtain maximal return of function by minimizing permanent disability. Physical and occupational therapy are important in rehabilitation.

CHAPTER **35**

ONCOLOGY

Oncology is the study of scientific control over neoplastic growth. It concerns the etiology, diagnosis, treatment, and rehabilitation of patients with known or potential neoplasms. Clarification of terminology is essential to an understanding of oncology.

DEFINITIONS

Neoplasm An atypical new growth of abnormal cells or tissues.

Tumor Any neoplasm in which cells are permanently altered but have the capability of growth and reproduction. A tumor consists of two elements—the tumor cells themselves and a supporting framework of connective tissue and vascular supply.

Benign Tumor An aggregation of cells closely resembling those of the parent tissue of origin. The tumor usually grows slowly by expansion, is localized, and is surrounded by a capsule of fibrous tissue.

Malignant Tumor A progressively growing tumor originating from a specialized organ such as the lung, breast, or brain, or a tumor localized to a specific body system such as bone, skin, lymph nodes, or blood vessels. Four characteristics differentiate malignant from benign tumors. A malignant tumor:

1. Is anaplastic. Cells, resembling embryonic cell forms, are morphologically and functionally differentiated from normal tissue of origin. They vary in size, shape, and texture.
2. Infiltrates and destroys adjacent normal tissue.
3. Grows in a disorganized, uncontrolled, and irregular manner, usually rapidly increasing in size perceptibly within weeks or months.
4. Has power to metastasize. Tumor cells migrate from primary focus to another single focus or multiple foci in distant tissues or organs via lymphatic or vascular channels.

Cancer A broad term that describes any malignant tumor within a large class of diseases. More than 100 different forms of cancer are known, each with histologic variations. Cancerous tumors are divided into two broad groups:

1. *Carcinoma* is a malignant tumor of epithelial origin affecting glandular organs, viscera, and skin.
2. *Sarcoma* is a malignant tumor of mesenchymal origin affecting bones and muscles.

-oma A suffix denoting a tumor or neoplasm.

Oncologist A specialist in study and treatment of neoplastic growths.

TREATMENT AND PROGNOSIS OF CANCER

Treatment and prognosis of cancer are based on extent of the disease. Each type of cancer differs in its symptoms, behavior, and response to treatment. Cancer is a potentially curable disease, but it is the second leading cause of disease-related death in the United States.

Clinical Signs and Symptoms

The clinical signs and symptoms of cancer are:

1 Palpable tumor
2 Abnormal bleeding
3 Steady decrease in weight, appetite, and energy
4 Chronic cough or change in bowel habits

High-Risk Related Factors

With respect to cancer the high-risk factors are:

1 Exposure to *carcinogens*—cancer-producing agents such as coal tar, chemicals, radiation
2 Age, sex, or racial predisposition
3 Predisposition to cancer due to specific environmental conditions, genetics, hereditary or acquired conditions, or diseases

Extent of Disease

Carcinoma in situ Normal cells are replaced by anaplastic cells but the growth disturbance of epithelial surfaces shows no behavioral evidence of invasion and metastasis in carcinoma in situ.

Localized Cancer A localized cancer is a malignant tumor contained within the organ of its origin.

Regional Cancer The invaded area of regional cancer extends from the periphery of the organ or tissue of origin to include tumor cells in adjacent organs or tissues, e.g., the regional lymph nodes.

Metastatic Cancer In metastatic cancer, tumor has extended by way of lymphatic or vascular channels to tissues or organs beyond the regional area.

Disseminated Cancer Multiple foci of tumor cells are dispersed throughout the body in disseminated cancer.

Curative versus Palliative Therapy

Cancer is basically a systemic disease. Therapy is *curative* if the disease process can be totally eradicated, but success depends largely on early diagnosis. When a cure is not possible, *palliative* therapy relieves symptoms, but does not cure the disease. Tumors are classified to determine most effective therapy.

Tumor Identification System

A standardized tumor identification system, which includes classification and staging, is essential for establishing treatment protocols and evaluating the end result of therapy. Hospitals maintain a tumor registry of patients to evaluate therapeutic approaches to specific types of tumors.

Classification includes the anatomical and histological description of a tumor. *Staging* refers to the extent of tumor. Three basic categories of the system are:

T: primary tumor
N: regional nodes
M: distant metastases

The TNM categories are identified by pretherapy clinical diagnosis, tissue biopsy, and/or histopathological examination following operative resection of tumor. Subscripts are used to describe the findings, e.g., bronchogenic carcinoma$_T$ meaning primary tumor in the lung without regional nodes or distant metastases. Older staging systems are referred to in literature as stages I, II, III and IV.

Adjunctive Therapy

Operative resection, endocrine therapy, radiation therapy, chemotherapy, immunotherapy, hyperthermia, or combinations of these procedures are used in treatment of cancer. The surgeon or oncologist must determine the most appropriate therapy for each patient. Consideration is given to:

1 Type, site, and extent of the tumor, and whether lymph nodes are involved
2 Type of surrounding normal tissue
3 Age and general condition of the patient, including nutritional status, and whether other diseases are present
4 Whether curative or palliative therapy is possible

OPERATIVE RESECTION

Operative resection is the modality of choice to remove solid tumors. Resection of a malignant tumor is, however, localized therapy for what may be a systemic disease. Each patient must be evaluated and treated individually, and the operative procedure must be planned appropriately for the identified stage of disease. The surgeon selects either a radical curative operation or a salvage palliative operation, depending on localization, regionalization, and dissemination of tumor. In planning operation, the surgeon considers length of expected survival, prognosis of surgical intervention, and effect of concurrent diseases on the postoperative result.

Accessible, well-differentiated primary tumors are frequently treated by excision. Extremely wide resection may be necessary to avoid recurrence of tumor. The pathologist is able to make judgments about questionable margins by making rapid frozen sections while operation is in progress. Pathologist's findings guide surgeon to determine extent of resection needed so residual tumor is not left in the patient.

Many of the operations described in previous chapters are performed for ablation of tumors by primary resection. In addition, *lymphadenectomy* may be performed as a prophylactic measure to inhibit metastatic spread of tumor cells via lymphatic channels. Other modalities of therapy may be administered pre-, intra-, and/or postoperatively to reduce or prevent recurrence or metastases.

Specific Considerations

Malignant tumor cells can be disseminated by manipulation of tissue. Because of their altered nutritional and physiological status, patients with cancer may be highly susceptible to the complications of postoperative infection. To minimize these risks, specific precautions are taken in the operative management of these patients.

1 Skin over the site of a soft tissue tumor should be handled gently during hair removal and antisepsis. Vigorous scrubbing could dislodge underlying tumor cells.

2 Gowns, gloves, drapes, and instruments are changed following a biopsy, e.g., a breast biopsy, before incision for a radical resection, e.g., a mastectomy. The tumor is deliberately incised to obtain a biopsy for diagnosis. However, margins of healthy tissue surrounding a radical resection must not be inoculated with tumor cells.

3 Instruments placed in direct contact with tumor cells are discarded immediately after use. Even when the tumor appears to be localized, most cancers have disseminated to some degree. Therefore, some surgeons prefer to use each instrument once and then discard it.

4 Antibiotics are administered pre-, intra-, and postoperatively as a prophylactic measure to provide an adequate antibacterial level to prevent wound infection.

5 Time-honored precautions such as handling tissue gently, keeping blood loss to a minimum, and avoiding an unduly prolonged operation influence outcome for the patient.

6 Messages should be conveyed periodically during a long radical operation to the patient's anxiously awaiting family members or significant others, to reassure them that their loved one is receiving care from a concerned OR team.

ENDOCRINE THERAPY

Tumors arising in organs that are usually under hormonal influence, such as breast and uterus in a female and prostate in a male, may be stimulated by hormones produced in the endocrine glands. Cellular metabolism is affected by presence of specific hormone receptors in tumor cells: estrogen and/or progesterone in a female and androgens in a male. Some breast, endometrial, and prostatic cancers depend on these hormones for growth and maintenance. Recurrence or spread of disease may be retarded by therapeutic hormonal manipulation. Endocrine manipulation does not cure, but it can control dissemination of disease if the tumor progresses beyond the limits of effective operative resection or radiation therapy. Cancer of the breast or prostate may metastasize to soft tissues or to the brain, lung, liver, and bone.

Hormonal Receptor Site Studies

Identifying hormonal dependence of the primary tumor by receptor site studies is a fairly reliable way of selecting patients who will benefit postoperatively from endocrine manipulation. Following a positive diagnosis of cancer, either by a frozen section biopsy or by pathologic permanent sections, the surgeon will probably request receptor site evaluation of a primary breast, uterine, or prostatic tumor. The tissue specimen removed by operative resection should *not* be placed in Formalin preservative solution, since this will alter the receptor cells enough to negate hormonal study.

Endocrine Ablation

Since 1896, surgeons have described positive clinical responses in patients with metastatic breast cancer treated by *endocrine ablation,* the surgical removal of endocrine glands. If the surgeon plans to eliminate endocrine stimulation surgically in a patient with a known hormone-dependent tumor, all sources of the hormone should be ablated.

Bilateral Adrenaloophorectomy Both adrenal glands and ovaries may be resected to prevent recurrence, control soft tissue metastases, or relieve bone pain from metastatic breast cancer. These may be removed as a one-stage operation. If two separate operations are preferred, bilateral oophorectomy precedes bilateral adrenalectomy, except in menopausal women in whom only the latter operation may be indicated. (See Chapter 22, p. 436, for discussion of oophorectomy and Chapter 23, p. 458, for discussion of adrenalectomy.)

Bilateral Orchiectomy and Adrenalectomy Both testes may be removed following prostatectomy for advanced carcinoma of the prostate to eliminate androgens of testicular origin. Bilateral adrenalectomy may also be indicated. (See Chapter 23 for discussion of these operations.)

Hypophysectomy Enucleation of pituitary gland may be indicated in patients with recurrent or progressive breast or prostatic cancer to eliminate stimulating hormones produced by the pituitary. (See Chapter 29, p. 555, for discussion of operation.)

Hormonal Therapy

Hormones administered orally or intramuscularly can alter cell metabolism by changing the systemic hormonal environment of the body. To be effective, tumor cells must contain receptors. Hormones must bind to these receptors before they can exert an effect on cells.

Androgens A male sex hormone is given to women with cancer of the breast to inhibit estrogen action following oophorectomy or during the normal postmenopausal life cycle. Preparations of testosterone are most commonly used.

Corticosteroids When bilateral adrenalectomy or hypophysectomy is contraindicated, corticosteroids may be administered to suppress estrogen production. Prednisone, cortisone, hydrocortisone, or some other preparation of corticosteroids may be administered as an anti-inflammatory agent along with chemotherapeutic agents given for control of disseminated disease.

Estrogens A female sex hormone is given to both men with prostatic carcinoma and women with breast cancer. Diethylstilbestrol is one of the most common estrogens for both sexes.

Progesterones Progesterone inhibits proliferation of endometrium and will retard the growth of some endometrial carcinomas. It also is given to retard renal cell and breast cancers.

Antiestrogen Therapy

Patients with medical contraindications to endocrine ablation may receive antiestrogen therapy. An estrogen antagonist deprives an estrogen-dependent tumor of estrogen necessary for its growth. Nafoxidine hydrochloride, a synthetic nonsteroidal drug, inhibits normal intake of estrogen at the estrogen receptor sites. It is given orally.

PHOTORADIATION

Hematoporphyrin derivative (HpD), an artificial porphyrin made from hemoglobin, photosensitizes malignant and reticular endothelial cells. An IV injection of HpD selectively localizes in many types of malignant tumors and makes cells fluorescent. When exposed to 631 nanometer light from an argon laser-pumped rhodamine-B laser (tunable dye laser), HpD absorbs light, causing a photochemical reaction. This reaction produces singlet oxygen which destroys tumor cells. The HpD is injected approximately three days prior to the photoradiation treatment. The laser can be administered interstitially, externally, or endoscopically, depending on tumor site.

RADIATION THERAPY

Treatment of malignant disease with radiation, referred to as *radiation therapy* or *radiotherapy,* includes the use of high-voltage irradiation and other radioactive elements to injure or destroy cells. Like operative resection, radiation is localized therapy applicable for a limited number of specific tumors. Radiation is the emission of electromagnetic waves or atomic particles from the disintegration of nuclei of unstable or radioactive elements. Ionizing radiation is used for therapy.

Ionizing Radiation

Ionization is a physical production of positive and negative ions capable of conducting electricity. Radiation of sufficient energy to disrupt the electronic balance of the atom is called *ionizing radiation.* When this takes place in tissue cells or extracellular fluids, the effect can range from minor changes to profound disturbances. Radiation may come from particles of the nuclei of disintegrating atoms or from electromagnetic waves that have no mass. Types of ionizing radiation include the following.

Alpha Particles Alpha particles are relatively large particles that have a very slight penetrating power. They are stopped by a thin sheet of paper. They have dense ionization, but can produce tremendous tissue destruction within a short distance.

Beta Particles Beta particles, relatively small, are electrical and travel with the speed of light. They have greater penetrating properties than do alpha particles. Their emissions cause tissue necrosis. They produce ionization, which has destructive properties.

Gamma Rays and X-Rays Electromagnetic radiation of short wavelength but high energy, gamma rays and x-rays are capable of completely penetrating the body. They affect tumor tissue more rapidly than normal tissue. Rays are stopped by a thick lead shield. Protons ranging in energy from 30 kilovolts (kV) to 35 million electron volts (eV) are available for treatment of various cancers. Gamma rays are emitted spontaneously from nucleus of the atom of a radioactive element.

Effects of Radiation on Cells

Cancer cells multiply out of normal body control. They are in a state of active, uncontrolled mitosis, the nuclear division of the cytoplasm and nucleus. Radiation affects the metabolic activity of cells. Cells in an active state of mitosis are most susceptible. However, effects of radiation also depend to a large extent on tissue oxygenation. As a tumor grows, the periphery is well-oxygenated, but the central portion becomes necrotic and poorly oxygenated. The cells killed by radiation are directly related to both amount of tissue and oxygen within tumor. Therefore, hypoxic effect is a factor in determining therapeutic radiation dose. Gamma rays and x-rays, acting over a period of time, cause a cessation of cell growth and a regression of the tumor mass. The cells die and are replaced by fibrous tissue.

Sensitivity to radiation varies. Some tumors can be destroyed by a small amount of radiation; others require a large amount. The sensitivity of the normal cells from which the tumor cells are derived determines the sensitivity of the tumor cells. Cells originating from bone marrow and lymphoid tissue are especially susceptible to radiation. Tumors in bone are resistant.

Dosage of radiation cannot be limited solely to the area to be treated. Danger of injuring normal surrounding tissue is a limiting factor in dosage and selection of the most appropriate type of radiation therapy. A factor in dosage is the ratio of tumor tissue to the surrounding normal tissue. Dosage is computed in rads. A *rad* (roentgen absorbed dose) is the unit used to measure the absorbed dose of radiation. One rad is the amount of radiation required to deposit 100 ergs of energy per gram of tissue. Dosage of irradiation delivered to a specific tissue site is measured by distance from source and duration of exposure by radiophysics or by instruments such as Geiger counters or scintillation probes. Doses are measured in rads to determine if dosage is adequate for therapy and not so excessive that it would cause damage to normal tissues.

Radiation energy penetration is calculated from the rate of decay or disintegration, known as half-life. *Half-life* is the time required for half the radioactive element to disintegrate and to lose one-half its activity by decay.

Sources of Radiation

Alhough effects are similar, sources and their application for radiation therapy differ. Some sources are implanted into body in direct contact with tumor tissue; others are passed through body to the tumor from an external beam.

Radium Radium is a radioactive metal. Mme. Curie, a research chemist, and her husband, a physicist, discovered and named it in 1898. Several years earlier, Mme. Curie had been given the task of finding out why pitchblende would record its image on a photographic plate. She and her husband knew that pitchblende emitted more radiation than the known minerals in it justified. It took six years of painstaking, difficult work for the Curies to isolate radium as a pure element and learn of its radioactive properties. Their research eventually led to use of radium in treatment of malignant tumors.

Metallic radium is unstable in air. Radium chloride or bromide salts emit fluorescence and heat. One gram gives off 134 calories per hour. Alpha and beta particles and gamma rays are products of its disintegration. The half-life of radium is about 1620 years; half the remaining life is lost in another 1620 years, and so on. The final product is lead.

Radon Radon is a dense radioactive gas liberated as the first byproduct from the disintegration of radium. Mme. Curie discovered this gas and first named it "emanation." Radon is collected by an intricate process in gold capillary tubing. Seeds for implantation are then cut and sealed. Dosage is computed for the hour of insertion into tissue. It is measured in millicurie-hours. The half-life of radon is four days; its total life is about 30 days.

Radionuclides A radionuclide is an element that has been bombarded in a nuclear reactor with radioactive particles. It shows radioactive disintegration and emits either alpha and beta particles or gamma rays. Those emitting alpha and beta particles are used primarily for treating malignant tumors. (See Chapter 20 for use of radionuclides in diagnostic procedures.) Therapeutic radionuclides may also be referred to as *radiopharmaceuticals.* Historically they were known as *radioactive isotopes,* or *radioisotopes,* and these terms are still found in the literature. Cesium, cobalt, iodine, iridium, and yttrium are the most commonly used elements for therapy. *Brachytherapy,* internal application with sealed sources of radionuclides, has almost totally supplanted the use of radium and radon. The gamma rays of cesium 137, for example, have greater penetrating power than do those of radium.

Radionuclides are controlled by the Atomic Energy Commission and are released only to individuals trained and licensed to use them. Available in liquid or solid forms, they may be ingested orally, infused intravenously, instilled into a body cavity, injected or implanted into tumor, or applied to skin externally. The ionizing radiation emitted has an action on tissue similar to that of radium, but radionuclides differ from radium in the following ways:

1 Half-life is short. Radionuclides disintegrate at varying rates depending upon their type. Each element has a specific half-life, but each one is different. They vary from a few hours, such as the 6 hours of technetium 99, to the 8 days of iodine 131 or the 5.3 years of cobalt 60.

2 Irradiation does not spread so much into adjoining tissue, therefore a stronger dose can be used in a malignant tumor. Radiation is not absorbed by bone and other normal body tissues.

3 Irradiation can be more easily shielded. The surgeon and other personnel get less radiation exposure in placing or removing radionuclides.

Exposure to radionuclides, like exposure to radium and radon, is always potentially dangerous. Radiation may treat cancer, but it can also cause a malignancy.

Implantation of Radiation Sources

All radiation sources for implantation are prepared in the desired therapeutic dosages by the nuclear medicine department. Many types of sources are used to deliver maximum radiation to the primary tumor. No single type is ideal for every tumor or anatomic site.

Interstitial Needles Interstitial needles are hollow sheaths, usually made of platinum or Monel metal. Radium salts or radionuclides are encased in platinum or platinum-iridium short units or cells, which in turn are sealed in the metal sheath of the needle for implantation into tumor tissue. A needle may contain one or several short units or cells of the radiation source, depending on length of needle to be used. Needles vary in length from 10 to 60 mm, with a diameter of 1 to 2 mm. The choice of length depends on area involved as well as dosage. Dosage is measured in milligram hours, which can be converted to rads.

Needles, usually containing cesium 137, are implanted in tumors near body surface or in tissue accessible enough to permit their use, such as in the vagina, cervix, tongue, mouth, or neck. In the OR, these needles are inserted at the periphery of and within the tumor. One end of the needle is pointed and the other has an eye for a heavy (size 2) suture. Needles are threaded to prevent loss while in use and to aid in removal. After surgeon inserts needles, the ends of sutures are tied or taped together and taped to the skin in an adjoining area. Needles are usually left in place for four to seven days depending on planned dosage to the tumor bed.

Interstitial Seeds Sealed seeds containing cesium 137, iridium 192, or iodine 125 may be implanted directly into tumor tissue. These radionuclide seeds are removed after desired exposure. Seeds are useful in body-cavity tumors, localized areas, and tumors that are not resectable because they are located near major vessels or the spinal cord. Seeds can be inserted with or without an invasive operation. Because they are small, seeds can be placed to fit a curved area without immobilization. However, they may move about if there is much motion.

Seeds are 7 mm or less in length, 0.75 mm in diameter, with a wall 0.3 mm thick. Length depends on desired dosage. Seeds may be strung on a strand of suture material or placed in a hollow plastic tube. With a needle attached, the strand or tube is woven or pulled through the tumor. Seeds in a hollow plastic tube may be inserted like a catheter through a trocar.

Intracavitary Capsules A sealed capsule of radium, cesium 137, iodine 125, yttrium 192, or cobalt 60 may be placed into a body cavity or orifice. Usually used to treat tumors in the cervix or endometrium of the uterus, a capsule is inserted via the vagina. The capsule may be a single tube of radioactive pins fixed in a tandem loading or a group of individual capsules each containing one radioactive pin. These methods are used for treating cancer of the uterine corpus.

In a patient with cervical cancer, an instrument such as an Ernst applicator is employed. A metal or plastic tube with radioactive pins is inserted in the uterus. Metal pins are used in conjunction with hyperthermia. The tube is attached to two vaginal ovoids, each containing a radioactive pin, that are placed in cul-de-sacs around the cervix. This type of application delivers the desired dosage in a pear-shaped volume of tissue, which includes the cervix, corpus, and tissue around the cervix, but spares the bladder and rectum from high doses of irradiation.

A blunt intracavitary applicator is utilized to position the parts. The applicator must be held securely and remain fixed to ensure proper dosage to tumor without injury to normal surrounding structures. The surgeon may suture the applicator to the cervix for stabilization. Vaginal packing is used. Two different methods of application are employed to insert the radiation source.

Afterloading Techniques Afterloading techniques afford the greatest safety for OR personnel. A "cold," unloaded, hollow plastic or metal applicator, such as the Fletcher afterloader, is inserted into or adjacent to tissues to receive radiation. This is done in the OR. After verification by x-ray of correct placement, the radiation source is loaded into the applicator at the patient's bedside.

Preloading Techniques Preloading techniques require insertion of the "hot" radiation capsule in the OR. Nurses and technologists should not be permitted in the room during this procedure. To deliver a uniform dose to the desired area, the surgeon inserts an adjustable device, such as the Ernst applicator, designed to hold the radiation source in proper position in the tissues. The bladder and rectum are held away from the area with packs to avoid undesired radiation. The surgeon checks the position of the radiation source on x-ray films of the pelvis to measure distances from critical sites to calculate dosage.

NOTE. *All* preparations for insertion are made by the nursing team members before they leave the room. (They wait in substerile room during insertion.) Preparations include: setting sterile table with vaginal packing, antibiotic cream for packing, radiopaque solutions for x-ray studies, basin of sterile water, etc.; placing x-ray cassette on operating table and notifying x-ray technician; obtaining radiation source; positioning patient; and putting radiation sheet on patient's chart and card on stretcher.

Intracavitary Colloidal Suspensions Sterile radioactive colloidal suspensions of gold or phosphorus are used as palliative therapy to limit growth of metastatic tumors in the pleural or peritoneal cavities. The effect is due to the emission of beta particles, which penetrate tissue so slightly that radioactivity is limited to the immediate area in which the colloidal suspension is placed. A trocar and cannula are introduced into the pleural or peritoneal cavity. The colloidal suspension is injected through the cannula from a lead-shielded syringe. These instruments must be stored in a remote area until decay of radioactivity is complete. Radioactive colloidal gold 198 is most commonly used; it has a half-life of 2.7 days. It may also be instilled within the bladder.

Safety Rules for Handling Radiation Sources

The principles of radiation safety for both personnel and patients listed below apply to handling all types of radioactive materials. The cardinal factors of protection are *distance, time, and shielding.*

1 Radiation intensity varies inversely with square of the distance from it; double distance equals one-quarter intensity, etc. Personnel must stay as far from the source as is feasibly practicable.

2 Radiation sources, i.e.. needles, seeds, capsules, and suspensions, are prepared by personnel in the nuclear medicine department from behind a lead screen with hands protected by lead-lined gloves, if possible, or special forceps during handling.

3 Radiation sources are transported in a long-handled lead carrier so that they are as close to floor and as far away from body of the transporter as possible. The lead carrier should be stored away from personnel and patient traffic areas while it is in the OR suite.

4 Each needle, seed, or capsule is counted by the surgeon with the radiation therapist when radiation sources are delivered to the OR. The number is recorded.

5 Glutaraldehyde solution is poured into lead carrier to completely submerge the radiation sources. When ready to use, lead carrier is transported into the OR. Needles, seeds, or capsules are removed from lead container with sterile long-handled instruments and *rinsed thoroughly* with sterile water.

6 All radiation sources are handled with special, long, ring-handled forceps from behind a lead protection shield. *Never touch radiation sources with bare hands or gloves.* Radiation sources are never handled with a crushing forceps, since the seal of hollow containers can be broken. A groove-tipped forceps, designed for this purpose, is used.

7 Radiation sources are handled as quickly as possible to limit time personnel are exposed to radiation.

8 Account for all radiation sources before and after use. Report any loss at once to supervisor. Do not remove anything from room. Call a radiation therapist or nuclear medicine department technician to bring a Geiger counter. This instrument, which is used to locate a lost radiation source, is constructed so that an indicator moves when near radioactive substances.

9 A *radiation sheet* is completed and put in the patient's chart. The surgeon fills in amount and exact time of insertion and time source is to be removed. Each nurse who cares for the patient on the unit signs this sheet in turn just before going off duty, thereby passing responsibility for checking patient and radiation source to the nurse who relieves. To check needles, sutures attached to each needle are counted.

10 Patient's bed and door of the room are conspicuously labeled with a "radiation in use" card.

11 Radiation source is removed by the surgeon at the exact time indicated so the patient will not be overexposed.

12 Be careful—observe rules. Radiation is not seen or felt. Potential dangers from excessive exposure to personnel are anemia, sterility, and burns. Refer to Chapter 11, p. 207, for procedures to monitor and minimize exposure.

External Beam Radiation Therapy

Ionizing radiations of gamma or x-rays generated from machines are used externally to alter tumor cells within the body. This type of radiation therapy is noninvasive.

A maximum dose of radiation is concentrated on the malignant tumor, with a minimum dose to the surrounding tissue. The angle of approach is changed a number of times during treatment to spread amount of radiation to normal tissue over as wide an area as possible. *Orthovoltage,* low-voltage equipment producing 200 to 500 kV, and *megavoltage* equipment, such as the cobalt 60 beams and linear accelerators or betatrons, are in use for external beam radiation therapy.

External radiation may be the only therapeutic modality used to cure some cancers. The dosage of radiation that will provide the optimal cure with an acceptable balance of complications is difficult to determine. With the advent of the megavoltage equipment, intense rays can deliver cancercidal doses without permanently injuring normal tissue and causing skin irritation. Even so, most oncologists recommend a combination of radiation therapy and operative resection for many tumors. Radiation therapy may be administered pre- and/or postoperatively, or intraoperatively. External radiation therapy may also be combined with internal sources such as intracavitary radiation capsules to build up dosage to large tumor areas.

Intraoperative Radiation Therapy Delivery of a single high dose of radiation directly to an intraabdominal or intrapelvic tumor or tumor bed during operation may provide an additional palliative or localized means of control. Normal organs or tissues can be shielded from exposure. Radiation may be used following resection of bulk of the tumor. An orthovoltage unit may be installed in the OR. The cone is placed directly over tumor site. All team members must leave the room during treatment. The room must be lead-lined. In other hospitals, the patient is geographically transported from the OR to the radiation therapy department. Following exposure to a megavoltage electron beam, the wound may be closed in the treatment area.

CHEMOTHERAPY

In 1854, the first drug used for cancer chemotherapy was synthesized. However, this type of therapy did not attract much attention until after World War II when reports were published purporting that tumor cells circulate in the venous blood of patients undergoing operation. Administration of chemotherapeutic agents during and shortly after operation, in the hope of destroying these cells, seemed justified in selected patients. Nitrogen mustard was first used in 1942. A cooperative clinical study involving 23 medical centers was begun in 1958 to evaluate the efficacy of triethylenephosphoramide following radical mastectomy. Since then, many researchers have investigated over a quarter of a million compounds in search of systemic antineoplastic substances that would kill tumor cells without excessive toxicity or damage to normal cells.

A variety of chemotherapeutic agents are capable, either alone or in combination, of providing measurable palliative remission or regression of primary and metastatic disease with decrease in size of tumor and no new metastases. In some instances, a complete response with disappearance of all clinical evidence of tumor is achieved. The trend is toward earlier and greater use of adjuvant chemotherapy. More than one agent may be administered to enhance the action of another cytotoxic or antigenic substance. Adjuvant therapy is designed to maximize the benefits of each agent in the combination, while avoiding overlapping toxicities. The following factors are important in determining the ability of tumor cells to respond to chemotherapy:

1 Size and location of tumor. The smaller the tumor, the easier it will be to reach cells. The mechanism for passage of drugs into the brain differs from that for other body organs.

2 Type of tumor. Cells of solid tumors in lung, stomach, colon, and breast may be more resistant than cells in lymphatic system, for example.

3 Combinations of adjunctive and adjuvant therapy. Chemotherapy may be used as an adjunct to all other types of therapy in selected patients. Precise scheduling of dosages is necessary to attain effective results.

4 Specific biochemical requirements of the tumor. Agents are selected according to the appropriateness of their structure and function. More than one agent is usually given.

5 State of cancer cell life cycle. An understanding of this phenomenon is necessary for understanding chemotherapy. Cancer cells go through the same life-cycle phases as do normal cells.

Cell Life Cycle

Deoxyribonucleic acid (DNA) is a double molecule in the cell nucleus that contains its genetic code. DNA is capable of reproducing itself and also of producing ribonucleic acid (RNA), which in turn synthesizes protein. Protein is essential for cellular function. Therefore, DNA is vital to cell viability. It regulates the processes of growth, rate of mitosis, differentiation, specialization, and death of cells. Cell division requires assimilation of nutrients in the cell, their incorporation into DNA, synthesis of new DNA, and splitting of DNA to form two new cells. RNA is synthesized in the rest intervals between phases of DNA replication. Duration of the rest interval is related to the proliferative activity of the tissue cells. Malignant tumor cells may proliferate more rapidly than normal cells.

Action of Chemotherapeutic Agents

Antineoplastic cytotoxic agents are destructive to rapidly dividing cells. However, each dose will kill only a fractional portion of the tumor cells present. The action of these agents takes place within the cell, but each agent acts differently to interrupt the cell life cycle. Antineoplastic agents are classified according to their structure and function. Only a few of the many agents in use are mentioned as examples of each classification. Cytotoxic action may be:

1 *Cell-cycle specific.* Agent may affect cell during one or more phases and have no adverse effect during other phases. Some interfere with DNA synthesis; others inhibit mitosis when cell is most susceptible; still others prolong rest intervals.
 a *Antimetabolites* affect cells as they enter the DNA synthesis phase, thus interfering with RNA synthesis. This causes death of cell by inhibiting the DNA cycle. These agents include floxuridine (FUDR), fluorouracil (5-FU), and methotrexate.
 b *Mitotic inhibitors* prevent cell division in a subphase of mitosis. They may be plant al-

kaloids such as vinblastine sulfate and vincristine sulfate or enzymes such as L-asparaginase.

2 *Cell-cycle nonspecific.* Agents affect cell throughout the entire life cycle. They have a more prolonged action that is independent of the phases of the life cycle.

   a *Alkylating agents* denature or inhibit DNA to interfere with mitosis and synthesis, thereby preventing rapid cell growth. Their action is similar to that of radiation therapy. These agents include cyclophosphamide (Cytoxan), melphalan (L-phenylalanine mustard, L-PAM), mechlorethamine nitrogen mustard (Mustargen), chlorambucil (Leukeran), and CIS-platin (Platinol).

   b *Antibiotics* bind with DNA to block RNA production, thus disrupting cellular metabolism. Those used as antineoplastic agents include dactinomycin, actinomycin-D (Cosmegen), bleomycin sulfate (Blenoxane), and doxorubicin hydrochloride (Adriamycin).

Indications for Chemotherapy

Patients with systemic signs of advanced or disseminated disease, generally indicated by extranodal involvement, may be candidates for chemotherapy pre- or postoperatively.

Preoperative Therapy The objective may be to shrink the tumor sufficiently to permit radical operative resection. Tumor regression with tumor necrosis may occur with or without adjunctive radiation therapy. Agents may eliminate subclinical microscopic metastatic disease.

Postoperative Therapy Operative resection followed by regional chemotherapy often can control local disease to keep a tumor in remission. Residual metastatic disease may be treated with systemic chemotherapy to cure the patient or prolong life. Multiple doses may be given over a long period of time (several months to a year or more) to delay recurrence of tumor.

Administration of Agents

The method of administration depends on how disseminated or localized the tumor cells are and on the agent, or combination of agents, selected. Agents can be instilled locally into a target site by continuous infusion, injected intramuscularly or intrathecally, infused by intravenous push or drip, or ingested orally. A patient with widely disseminated metastatic cells usually receives systemic therapy via IV, IM, or oral route.

Regional intraarterial or intravenous infusion may be used for patients whose tumor cannot be removed because of its location, e.g., a primary or metastatic tumor in the liver. An infusion catheter may be placed percutaneously or directly into an artery leading to tumor site, into a vein, or both. Continuous or intermittent infusion of the chemotherapeutic agent is maintained by means of a pump attached to the catheter. Both portable and implantable infusion units are available.

An implantable infusion pump device (Infusaid) is implanted in a subcutaneous pocket created in the abdominal wall, beneath the clavicle or under the scalp. The titanium, stainless steel, and silicone rubber device resembles a hockey puck. The inner reservoir is filled with chemotherapeutic agent, such as FUDR. When the reservoir is collapsed by pressure, the agent is infused into an outlet catheter inserted into an artery, vein, body space, or ventricle. The pump must be warmed to 30 to 40°C (86 to 104°F) to initially activate the fluorocarbon propellant in chamber around the reservoir. It is placed over a body prominence for support when refilling. The drug is replenished periodically by percutaneous injection. These infusion devices are used primarily for localized liver, head and neck, and brain tumors. They are also used for control of severe systemic conditions, such as diabetes, thromboembolic disease, or pain from malignant disease. Insulin, heparin, or morphine is infused, respectively, for these diseases.

Toxic Side Effects

Cytotoxic agents are destructive to rapidly dividing cancer cells, but they also affect rapidly dividing normal cells such as hematopoietic cells of bone marrow, epithelial cells of oral cavity and gastrointestinal tract, and hair follicles. Patients must be informed of the toxic side effects to be expected from the specific agents they are receiving. These can include:

1 *Alopecia.* Loss of hair can occur suddenly or gradually. This can be devastating to the patient's self-image. It is most often caused by the alkylating and plant alkaloid agents, and by some antibiotics. Hair grows back after therapy is discontinued.

2 *Bone marrow suppression.* Suppression of bone marrow function is the most hazardous toxic effect from cytotoxic agents. Therapy may have to be discontinued to allow for bone marrow recovery. Suppression increases patient's susceptibility to:
  a Leukopenia. White blood cell count is lowered below normal number of leukocytes in the peripheral blood. Leukocytes protect body against invasion of microorganisms. The patient with leukopenia is therefore highly vulnerable to spread of infection from one part of body to another, or to acquiring a nosocomial infection from the environment.
  b Thrombocytopenia. The number of platelets in blood decreases below normal with variable consequences. Spontaneous hemorrhage into skin, sclera, joints, or brain may occur. Normal blood clotting time can be prolonged. Patient may require platelet transfusion.
3 *Gastrointestinal disturbances.* Anorexia, nausea, vomiting, and/or diarrhea are common complaints. Usually these subside within a few hours or days after each dose is administered.
4 *Neurotoxicity.* Symptoms of neurotoxicity to the plant alkaloids usually begin with constipation. Toxicity can progress to impaired sensation, ataxia, and an unsteady gait. The effects are cumulative during course of therapy but reversible when therapy is discontinued.
5 *Stomatitis.* Ulcerative lesions in mouth and oropharynx are often early signs of severe toxicity from antimetabolite and antibiotic agents. These can be very painful and may lead to secondary infection.
6 *Vein hyperpigmentation.* A dark discoloration of a vein may occur over length of arm during prolonged infusion of some agents. A vesicular rash around injection site may develop from use of some other agents. Although unsightly, these effects are not uncomfortable for the patient.

IMMUNOTHERAPY

Immunization against disease is a well-established concept. Ancient Chinese and Arabic writings describe stimulation of the body's immune system to combat infectious diseases. Immunization against smallpox was practiced in Turkey long before Edward Jenner developed a vaccine in England in the late sixteenth century. The concept developed by Jenner, Pasteur, Salk, and Sabin, to mention a few historic names, of using vaccinations and immunizations to prevent or treat infectious diseases forms the basis of modern immunotherapy.

Immunotherapy utilizes agents that stimulate or activate the body's own host defense immune system to combat disease. This is the same immune system that normally wards off microorganisms which cause infection. Cancer may become clinically apparent only when the immune system ceases to function properly. Immune response may be defective, or become compromised, as disease progresses. Immunosuppression can stimulate tumor growth and prolong wound healing. If patient can be helped to regain partial or complete immunocompetence, the immune system can be utilized against the "foreignness" of tumor cells.

Attempts to treat cancer by immunization date back to 1895. However, it was not until 1957 that antigens specific for tumors were conclusively demonstrated in animals by R. J. Prehn and J. M. Main. Although intensive experimental research was conducted during the 1960s to investigate the applications of immunotherapy as a therapeutic modality, its use in selective types of cancer was not validated by clinical research until the 1970s. Monoclonal antibodies are major sources in the 1980s for identifying tumor-associated antigens and biologic response modifiers, and on a limited scale for treating selective cancer cells by IV administration.

Types and Agents

Tumor antigen evokes an immune response either by an antibody (*humoral response*) or a specifically reactive lymphocyte (*cell-mediated immunity*). Patients are initially tested for a delayed cutaneous hypersensitivity response to establish an index of immune function. The type of immunotherapy is selected that will most effectively strengthen the immune response.

Active Immunotherapy Antigens are injected to stimulate development of antibodies against tumor cells by patient's own humoral immune response.

1 *Active specific immunotherapy.* A vaccine of specific tumor antigen stimulates the immune response. A series of small doses are administered intradermally.

a *Autologous vaccine* is prepared from patient's own tumor cells and reinoculated.
b *Allogenic vaccine* is prepared from tumor cells of the same type obtained from a donor. This introduces antigens new to the patient's immune system.
c *Modified tumor cell vaccine* is treated to increase antigenicity.

2 *Active nonspecific immunotherapy.* Vaccine containing antigens other than tumor cells causes increased antibody and lymphocyte production.

a *BCG* (bacillus Calmette-Guerin) is accentuated bovine tubercle bacillus. Most widely used, it is a potent stimulant of the defensive mechanism of the reticuloendothelial system. It is usually administered intradermally by scarification, the time grid technique, or by injection gun. It may also be injected intralesionally or intrapleurally.
b *MER* is methanol extractable residue of BCG.
c *Corynebacterium parvum* is a gram-positive anaerobic bacillus.
d *Levamisol* is an antihelminthic given to stimulate host defense.

Passive Immunotherapy Antitumor antibodies can be transferred from one person to another to establish transient, acquired, cell-mediated immunity. Antisera from a cured patient with the same type of tumor or from a family member with natural or acquired immunity may be injected subcutaneously or infused intravenously. The patient's own lymphocytes may be sensitized in the laboratory and reinfused to increase lymphocyte-to-tumor cell ratio. Passive immunotherapy is transient because lymphocytes in antisera are continually made and destroyed by the body.

Adoptive Immunotherapy The patient accepts passive immunity from systemic transfer of immunocompetent cells and then actively maintains cell-mediated immunity. This is maintained by administration of immunostimulant extracts from human white cells, called *transfer factor,* or of lymphoid extracts from animals, called *immune RNA.* These extracts are highly specific, rapid in action, and long-lasting in effect. Transfer of this delayed-type hypersensitivity depends upon dosage used and duration of therapy necessary to develop sufficient lymphocytes to inhibit tumor growth.

Advantages of Immunotherapy

Immunotherapeutic agents have a relatively weak killing capacity but no limitation on the kinds of cells that they can destroy. Although highly specific, they can destroy small numbers of tumor cells but are not effective against large numbers. They can regress or eradicate a small tumor mass or eliminate cells resistant to chemotherapy. Combining these agents may accomplish what neither can do alone, either with or without operative resection—delay recurrence and prolong survival. An immunotherapeutic agent:

1 Attacks only cancer cells
2 Does not damage normal cells
3 Can be continued for long periods with fewer hazardous side effects than chemotherapy
4 Can be injected subcutaneously, infused intravenously, or applied topically or intradermally as for skin cancer and melanomas

HYPERTHERMIA

Hyperthermia at temperatures of 41.5°C (106.7°F) or above has a regressive tumoricidal effect with necrosis proportional to thermal dose. Thermal energy inhibits DNA synthesis. Increasing temperature of tumor cells sensitizes them to effects of radiation therapy or chemotherapy. Therefore, hyperthermia is used as an adjunct to these therapeutic modalities for some tumors. Since drug action is greater at higher temperatures, perfusate is warmed before regional infusion of cytotoxic agents. An extremity also is warmed externally during regional perfusion. Systemic total-body hyperthermia may be applied externally by placing patient on a hyperthermia blanket or mattress. Systemic hyperthermia can also be produced with extracorporeal circulation via a shunt placed in the thigh.

For localized palliative management of some solid tumors, a surface or interstitial hyperthermia device applies microwave energy. Temperature is measured by probes in target and surrounding normal tissue and controlled by computer adjustment of power. When tissue absorbs microwave radiation, energy converts into heat that dissipates by blood perfusion. Solid tumors with less blood perfusion dissipate heat slowly and hence retain heat longer than normal surrounding tissue.

HYPERALIMENTATION

Cancer can produce weight loss and lead to malnutrition if sufficient nutrients are not supplied to meet protein demands of body and tumor. Tumor cells extract nutrients at a rapid rate at expense of body mass. Malnutrition depresses established cell-mediated immunity to infection and immunologic reactivity to the tumor. The only hope of cure or palliation of cancer in a malnourished patient may be a treatment that itself produces malnutrition. Healing may be delayed following operative resection in poorly nourished tissues of patients who have some degree of malabsorption of nutrients. This can deter resumption of oral intake after head and neck or gastrointestinal operations. Radiation therapy, chemotherapy, and immunotherapy can cause loss of appetite due to nausea, and often produce vomiting or diarrhea that may necessitate delay in therapy. Adequate nutrition can be maintained before and during treatment with total parenteral hyperalimentation (TPN, see Chap. 3, pp. 45–47). Any patient who cannot be nutritionally maintained by other means is a candidate for TPN.

Long-term indwelling catheters are inserted through the internal or external jugular, cephalic, or subclavian vein into the superior vena cava or right atrium. Either a single-lumen Broviac or Hickman catheter or a double-lumen catheter is used. These catheters are polymeric silicone with a polyester fiber cuff. Under fluoroscopy, the tip of the catheter is threaded into the vein through a venotomy to the desired position. The external end is brought through a subcutaneous tunnel with an exit point between the right nipple and the sternum. The cuff anchors the catheter in the tunnel. The *Broviac catheter* is slightly smaller (1.0 mm inside diameter) than the Hickman catheter (1.6 mm inside diameter). Therefore, the *Hickman catheter* may be used intermittently for infusion of chemotherapeutic agents, antibiotics, and/or blood products or for withdrawal of blood samples. A double-lumen catheter affords advantages of both: the Broviac port is used for continuous TPN and the Hickman port for other needs. For example, patients with acute leukemia or those who receive bone marrow transplants may require massive doses of antibiotics and blood products in addition to TPN. The external end of the catheter, with an adaptor, is connected to administration set(s). Hyperalimentation solutions are usually viscous. A positive pressure pump device may be needed to ensure infusion. Volume also may need to be regulated over a specified time with a volumetric control device.

Patients are usually started on hyperalimentation prior to oncologic therapy and supported postoperatively or throughout other therapy. If the tumor responds to therapy, appetite returns, weight gain is maintained, and immunocompetent cells return as a defense mechanism against tumor cells. During this period, patients who manage their TPN at home must be taught signs and symptoms of hyperglycemia and hypoglycemia, to test urine for sugar and acetone, and to manage a volumetric infusion pump.

FUTURE OF ONCOLOGY

As described, many therapeutic modalities are used, and researchers are constantly seeking others, to improve survival chances and quality of life for patients with neoplasms. The complex nature of the disease makes adjuvant therapy and cancer research a multidisciplinary effort. Early diagnosis, while disease is still localized, is crucial for selection of appropriate curative therapy. In poor-risk patients with extensive tumors and advanced disease, only palliative therapy may be possible.

Oncologists study the cause (epidemiology) of cancer, as well as the diagnosis, treatment, and rehabilitation of cancer patients. Moreover, patients are demanding that their surgeons give attention to reconstruction of body image and rehabilitation to a useful life. Management of cancer patients must, therefore, be through the efforts of a multidisciplinary team of surgeons in conjunction with pathologists, radiation therapists, pharmacists, immunologists, oncologists, and others. Nurses in all patient care settings must provide, in addition to physical care, psychological support for cancer patients and their families.

Development of *hospice care* helps terminally ill cancer patients and their families cope with physical, emotional, and spiritual needs. The roots of hospice can be traced back to the Middle Ages, but the modern team concept of care was influenced by a British physician in the 1960s. Hospice teams of doctors, nurses, social workers, and clergy provide a network of support that makes home care for the dying feasible.

CHAPTER **36**

POTENTIAL COMPLICATIONS IN SURGICAL PATIENTS

INTRODUCTION

No operative procedure, even the most simple, is without risk. The patient faces potential complications from the moment he or she is premedicated. For example, the patient may experience an anaphylactic reaction to a preoperative medication. A bowel obstruction secondary to adhesions may occur months to years after bowel surgery. However, pulmonary embolism is the major cause of death during operation and in the immediate postoperative period. Wound infections occur all too frequently. By being aware of possible complications, the operating room nurse must watch for and help prevent them.

PULMONARY COMPLICATIONS

One of the primary areas of postoperative complications is the respiratory tract. Potential for developing pulmonary problems depends on several factors. Any preexisting lung disease such as emphysema, infection, or asthma predisposes the patient. Heavy smokers have highest risk of succumbing to postoperative pulmonary problems, due to chronic irritation of the respiratory tract with consequent production of excess mucus. Chest wall deformities, obesity, and extremes of age are other pertinent preoperative influences. *Intraoperative factors* include:

1 Type of preoperative medications
2 Type and duration of anesthesia
3 Type and duration of assisted ventilation
4 Position of patient during operation
5 Extent of operation

Postoperatively, one of the most critical factors is the patient's ability to mobilize secretions by deep breathing, coughing, and ambulation. Patients undergoing chest and abdominal surgery are likely to breathe shallowly, due to pain, and not adequately raise accumulated secretions. Development of one pulmonary complication frequently predisposes patient to development of another.

Airway Obstruction

Airway obstruction is the most frequent cause of respiratory embarrassment in the immediate postoperative period. This serious complication may lead to cardiac arrest if not relieved in seconds. The tongue may block the oral airway in a patient who is semiconscious, weak from muscle relaxants, or experiencing a convulsion. If airway is totally obstructed, breath sounds will be absent; if partially obstructed, a snoring sound will be elicited. The patient may exhibit paradoxical respiration—downward movement of the diaphragm occurring with contraction rather than expansion of the chest. Use of accessory muscles for breathing may also be evident. Pulse is rapid and thready. As condition worsens, the patient becomes restless, confused, delirious, diaphoretic, cyanotic, and finally unconscious.

To relieve obstruction, gently hyperextend neck and elevate chin. If obstruction is still present, ventilate the patient with an Ambu bag and suction any obstructing blood, mucus, or emesis. Nasal airway or endotracheal intubation may be necessary.

Hypoventilation

Inadequate or reduced alveolar ventilation can lead to hypoxemia. Hypoventilation also produces hypercarbia, an elevation in the level of carbon dioxide, often associated with a flushed or reddened appearance. Pain, a faulty position, a short thick neck, or a full bladder are contributing factors. Hypoventilated patients have an increased pulse rate, often are restless, or have an anxious facial grimace. Acid-base balance can be affected. Retention of carbon dioxide also leads to acidosis. Treatment consists of alleviating cause, if possible, encouraging coughing and deep breathing, and administering oxygen therapy as indicated. An endotracheal tube may be left in place postoperatively to supprt assisted ventilation.

NOTE. 1. Oxygen is a medication requiring proper dosage. Patients with chronic obstructive pulmonary disease (COPD) cannot tolerate large oxygen concentrations; therefore, to prevent cardiac arrest, a 2- to 3-liter flow is recommended for them.

2. Patients who received Narcan need close watching. They may awaken too rapidly, cough, and inadvertently extubate.

Atelectasis or Pulmonary Collapse

Partial collapse of lung is one of the most common postoperative problems. If mucus obstructs a bronchus, air in alveoli distal to the obstruction is resorbed. That segment of lung then collapses and consolidates. Retained mucus, although initially sterile, becomes contaminated by inhaled bacteria; patient may develop bronchopneumonia. Factors that promote increased production of mucus, e.g., certain irritating anesthetics, and decreased mobilization of mucus, e.g., a tight abdominal dressing, predispose to pulmonary collapse. Furthermore, normal respiration includes a deep sigh several times an hour to help keep lungs expanded. This natural sigh is inhibited by anesthetics, narcotics, and sedatives.

Atelectasis increases temperature, pulse and respiratory rate. Patient may appear cyanotic and uncomfortable, with shallow respirations and pain upon coughing. Breath sounds are diminished, with fine rales. Chest x-ray reveals collapsed areas of lung as patch opacities, generally involving the lung bases.

Measures to help prevent or treat atelectasis are abstention from smoking, a regimen of coughing and deep breathing, and early ambulation. An upright position allows for better lung expansion. Medication for pain, when appropriate, before breathing exercises or ambulation improves ability to breathe deeply and cough effectively. Splinting chest or abdominal incisions with a pillow also aids in decreasing pain of coughing. Repeated vigorous coughing is contraindicated in some patients, e.g., following cataract extraction, craniotomy, or herniorrhaphy.

Pulmonary Embolism

Pulmonary embolism is an obstruction of the pulmonary artery or one of its branches by an embolus, most often a blood clot. The most important factor leading to *pulmonary emboli* is stasis of blood, particularly in deep veins of the legs and pelvis where the majority of thrombi arise. These become detached and are carried to the lungs. Changes in vessel wall and coagulative changes in blood are also important factors. Bed rest may decrease blood flow to lower extremities by more than 50 percent. Blood flow is impaired further if knees are raised on a pillow, putting pressure on vessels. Venous stasis is also correlated with obesity, congestive heart failure, and atrial fibrillation. Local trauma to a vein or venous disease enhances the chance of thrombus formation. Hypercoagulability may coexist with conditions such as pregnancy, fever, myocardial infarction, and some malignancies, and after abrupt cessation of anticoagulant therapy.

Prevention consists of a regimen of prophylactic anticoagulants or antiplatelets for high-risk patients and routine measures to prevent venous stasis, such as elevation of the foot of bed and antiembolic stockings. Because of the origin of thrombi in deep veins, it is important to observe for thrombophlebitis, evidenced by heat, edema, redness, pain in the calf, or a positive Homan's sign, which is pain in calf upon forceful dorsiflexion of foot.

Nonspecific symptoms depend on whether the embolism is mild or massive. The patient may have dyspnea, pleural pain, hemoptysis, tachypnea, rales, tachycardia, mild fever, or persistent cough. Patients with massive emboli have air hunger, hypotension, shock, and cyanosis. Treatment of pulmonary emboli consists of bed rest, oxygen, anticoagulant therapy, thrombolytic agents, and sometimes operation to remove emboli or prevent their recurrence.

Fat embolism occurs primarily following fracture of a long bone, pelvis, and ribs. However, it sometimes occurs after blood transfusion, cardiopulmonary bypass, or renal transplant. Fat globules enter bloodstream. Patient becomes symptomatic when globules block pulmonary capillaries, causing interstitial edema and hemorrhage. Frequently, *adult respiratory distress syndrome* ensues 24 to 48 hours after injury, with hypoxia and decreased surfactant production, resulting in collapse of alveolar membrane and microatelectasis. The syndrome develops most frequently in patients over age ten, especially those who have traveled long distances with an immobilized fracture. Symptoms include disorientation, increased pulse and temperature, tachypnea, dyspnea, rales, and pleuritic chest pain. Other significant signs are fat in sputum and urine and a petechial rash on anterior chest. Treatment is supportive. Mortality rate is high.

Air embolism may follow injection of air into a body cavity, or a bolus of air in an intravenous or intraarterial infusion. Another portal of entry is transection of large veins with patient in a sitting position. The pull of gravity on the blood column exerts a significant negative pressure that sucks air down the veins and into the heart.

Intrauterine fetal death or placenta previa may precipitate an *embolism of amniotic fluid.* Also, tumors may cause emboli from primary or metastatic sites.

Pulmonary Edema

Pulmonary edema may result from congestive heart failure or fluid overload. Blood stagnates in the pulmonary circulation, with fluid exuding from the pulmonary capillaries into the alveoli. When this mixes with air, frothy pink sputum is produced. Reduction of capillary membrane perfusion leads to hypoxia. Bounding rapid pulse, rales, dyspnea, apprehension, and engorged peripheral veins should alert nurse to possibility of pulmonary edema. Treatment includes digitalization, diuretics, upright position, oxygen, and rotating tourniquets to extremities to decrease circulatory overload.

Other Pulmonary Complications

Adult respiratory distress syndrome, also known as *progressive pulmonary insufficiency* or *shock lung,* may develop in the first 24 to 48 hours following a traumatic injury. Beginning with dyspnea, grunting respirations, and tachycardia, signs progress to cyanosis, hypoxemia, and alveolar infiltration. The mortality rate is high.

Other potential pulmonary complications are pneumothorax, hemothorax, and pleural effusion. Aspiration of emesis may cause aspiration pneumonia and lung abscess with necrosis of the pulmonary parenchyma.

CARDIOVASCULAR COMPLICATIONS

The emotional and physical stresses to which a surgical patient is subjected may lead to cardiovascular complications. These include cardiac arrest, congestive heart failure, myocardial infarction, thromboembolism and/or thrombophlebitis, hypotension, and various arrhythmias. Patients with a history of cardiac problems or those undergoing cardiovascular surgery are prone to develop these complications. Cerebral thrombosis or embolism may result in prolonged coma. Patients who receive blood transfusions should be watched closely for transfusion reactions. Other problems may occur, including the following.

Venous Stasis

The venous stasis that develops in lower extremities during operation can be effectively counteracted in most patients. This is especially important in patients with thromboembolic disease to prevent thrombophlebitis and pulmonary embolism postoperatively. Methods of augmenting venous flow from legs during operation include:

1 *Elevation of legs.* An elevation of 15° above horizontal is effective in preventing venous stasis. Surgeons frequently order this position for potentially susceptible patients postoperatively.

2 *Intermittent pneumatic compression.* Inflatable, double-walled vinyl boots use alternating compression and relaxation to reduce risk of deep vein clotting in legs of high-risk patients undergoing general anesthesia. Pressure between 40 and

50 mm of mercury applied quickly for 12 seconds and then released for 48 seconds empties blood from deep leg veins.

Postoperatively, flexion and extension of legs and feet, frequent turning, and early ambulation, unless contraindicated, aid circulation.

Hypertension

Abnormal elevation of blood pressure may occur, especially in a hypertensive or arteriosclerotic patient. Hypertension, if not controlled, may precipitate a cerebrovascular accident (CVA) or bleeding from surgical site, or may threaten the integrity of vascular bypasses. Etiologic factors include pain, shivering, hypoxia, hypercapnia, effects of vasopressor drugs, or hypervolemia from overreplacement of fluid losses. Treatment consists of administration of oxygen, diuretics, and antihypertensive drugs as indicated.

Hypotension

Some narcotics and anesthetic agents, operative trauma, anoxia, and blood loss combined can lead to postoperative hypotension by interfering with the complex physiologic mechanisms that support blood pressure. Peripheral vessels dilate. A degree of cardiovascular collapse ensues. Kidney function may decrease or fail due to vasoconstriction that reduces renal blood flow. Patients must be monitored postoperatively for sudden drops in blood pressure and other signs of shock. Vasoactive drugs, such as ephedrine or methoxamine, and oxygen may be administered. Fluid management is critical during recovery phase of renal function following restoration of systemic blood pressure to avoid hypertension.

Following Cardiopulmonary Bypass

Although the incidence of complications following cardiopulmonary bypass has been reduced, the patient may encounter serious problems. Alterations in clotting may occur due to heparinization of blood, mechanical damage to platelets and clotting factors, and direct exposure of blood to oxygen. When red blood cells are hemolyzed due to trauma or transfusion reaction, viscosity in the renal tubules may cause tubular necrosis and renal failure.

Inadequate or extended perfusion and oxygenation may promote tissue anoxia and metabolic acidosis. Fluid and electrolyte balance merit close watching, particularly for hypervolemia. When nonblood fluids are used to prime the pump, they may diffuse into interstitial spaces. As this fluid returns to circulation postoperatively, hypervolemia may result. Furthermore, increased levels of aldosterone and antidiuretic hormone induced by the stress of surgery cause retention of sodium and water. Fluids are restricted for 24 hours postoperatively. Cerebral edema and brain damage at times ensue, for unknown reasons. However, these developments are generally temporary.

"Post-pump psychosis" consists of visual and auditory hallucinations and paranoid delusions. This often terminates when patient is transferred from the intensive care unit.

The most severe pulmonary complication of extracorporeal circulation is postperfusion lung syndrome. Etiology is unknown. It is often fatal, due to development of atelectasis, pulmonary edema, and hemorrhage. Metabolic acidosis during bypass may lead to "low cardiac output" syndrome postoperatively. This occurs most frequently in patients with long histories of cardiac disease. Finally, cardiac tamponade is another potential complication, reflected by a drop of more than 10 mm of mercury in systolic blood pressure upon inspiration (pulsus paradoxus).

SHOCK

Shock is a state of inadequate blood perfusion to parts of the body. If untreated, it will become irreversible and result in death. All forms of shock carry high mortality rates. The best treatment is prevention. The five main classifications of shock are the following.

Hypovolemic or Hemorrhagic Shock

Decrease in circulating blood volume is due to loss of blood, plasma, or extracellular fluid. Fluid loss is excessive when it is greater than the compensatory absorption of interstitial fluid into the circulation. Shock resulting from hemorrhage or inadequate blood volume replacement, often seen in the OR and recovery room, usually is reversed by prompt restoration of circulating blood volume.

Cardiogenic Shock

The pumping action of the left ventricle is insufficient to pump enough blood to vital organs. It may be precipitated by congestive heart failure, myocardial contusion or infarction, coronary air embolism, mechanical venous obstruction, or hypothermia. In addition to drugs, various mechanical devices may be used, such as an auxiliary ventricle or counterpulsation with the intraaortic balloon to temporarily increase left ventricular function.

Neurogenic Shock

Loss of neurogenic tone in peripheral blood vessels leads to sudden vasodilatation and pooling of blood. Peripheral resistance is too great for compensation by increased cardiac output. Causes may be brain damage, deep anesthesia, emotional trauma, vagal reflex from pain or operative manipulation, or spinal cord injury.

Traumatic Shock

Damage to the capillaries due to soft tissue trauma causes increased capillary permeability, with loss of volume into the tissues. This state is aggravated by pain, which inhibits the vasomotor center, leading to vasodilatation and toxic factors associated with intravascular coagulation.

Vasogenic Shock

The two most common forms of vasogenic shock are anaphylaxis and septic shock.

Anaphylaxis A *severe allergic reaction* in which cells release histamine or a histaminelike substance, anaphylaxis causes vasodilatation, hypotension, and bronchiolar constriction. Within seconds after introduction of an antigenic substance, the patient will exhibit edema and itching around site of injection or contact, and sneezing, followed by edema of hands and face, wheezing, cyanosis, and dyspnea. Treatment includes epinephrine and antihistamines to control bronchospasm. Isoproterenol, vasopressors, corticosteroids, and aminophylline may also be administered.

Septic Shock Septic shock is a state of widely disseminated infection, often borne in the bloodstream. Early septic shock may begin with fever, restlessness, sudden unexplained hypotension, a cloudy sensorium, hypoxia, tachycardia, rapid breathing, and/or oliguria. One or more of these possible symptoms may be present. Toxic or metabolic by-products increase capillary permeability, permitting loss of circulating fluid into the interstitial fluid. Endotoxins released by bacteria promote vasodilatation and hypotension.

Septic shock differs from most other types in its abrupt onset and high cardiac output. As shock progresses, the patient develops cold clammy skin, sharply diminished urinary output, respiratory insufficiency, cardiac decompensation, disseminated intravascular coagulation, and metabolic acidosis. The high-risk category comprises patients with severe infection (e.g., peritonitis), trauma, burns, impaired immunological state, diabetes mellitus, age-extreme patients, or patients who have undergone an invasive procedure.

Treatment consists of control of the infectious process, early administraton of antibiotics, fluid-volume replacement, and oxygen. Diuretics, sodium bicarbonate, vasoconstrictors, vasodilators, inotropic agents, or heparin may also be indicated. Corticosteroids may be used, but their use is controversial.

HEMORRHAGE

Severe bleeding into or from a wound is a major contributing factor to operative and postoperative morbidity and mortality. If uncontrolled, the patient can exsanguinate. Massive hemorrhage may cause hypovolemic shock, ventricular fibrillation, or death due to marked decrease in cardiac output. Common symptoms are arterial hypotension, pale or cyanotic moist skin, oliguria, bradycardia from hypoxia, or tachycardia after moderate to marked blood loss, restlessness, and thirst in the conscious patient.

In the operating room, hemorrhage is readily visible. Meticulous hemostasis during every step of operation and good nutritional status of patient preoperatively are crucial to prevention. Preoperative evaluation of clotting time and history of bleeding (personal and familial), type and cross match of blood, and insertion of an intravenous line prior to incision are necessary precautions.

In treating hemorrhage, the surgeon locates the source of bleeding and applies digital compression to severed or traumatized vessels until noncrushing vascular clamps can be placed to occlude vessel proximally and distally to site of bleeding. The vessel is then ligated, electrocoagulated, or sutured. Circulating blood volume must be restored promptly. If much blood is transfused, it must be fresh and warmed to limit electrolytic changes. Sodium bicarbonate may be given intravenously to reduce acidosis. Multiple intravenous infusion routes can be utilized, by cutdown if necessary, to infuse blood under pressure. Lactated Ringer's solution or plasma expanders are used when blood is contraindicated, e.g., for religious reasons. Oxygen is administered to combat hypoxia. Accurate measurement of blood and fluid losses intraoperatively, followed by adequate replacement, will help prevent hypovolemic shock.

Hemorrhage can be detected postoperatively by observation of blood-soaked dressings. The patient must be checked frequently for both observable and nonobservable symptoms of hemorrhage. Internal bleeding can be caused by slipping or sloughing of a ligature or by the blowout of clots from ligated or coagulated vessels.

DISSEMINATED INTRAVASCULAR COAGULATION

Disseminated intravascular coagulation (DIC) is a life-threatening syndrome. It can follow many conditions, for example, hemorrhagic or septic shock, extracorporeal circulation, certain complications of pregnancy such as abruptio placentae, severe infection, and massive soft tissue damage of extensive trauma or burns. Coagulation is initiated throughout the bloodstream, especially in the microcirculation. Vital organs become ischemic. The body's supply of platelets and major clotting factors is exhausted. As blood becomes depleted of these factors, massive hemorrhaging ensues throughout the body. Cutaneous petechiae appear, and bleeding may be noted from various sites, such as through a nasogastric tube. The patient may also have hypotension, nausea and vomiting, severe muscular pain, convulsions, oliguria, and coma. Diagnosis is based on blood laboratory studies.

Treatment begins with control of the primary condition. If given early, heparin may help prevent coagulation and thus prevent depletion of clotting factors. Blood, plasma, dextran, and clotting factors can be administered intravenously.

POSTOPERATIVE WOUND INFECTIONS

Patients most prone to develop wound infections are listed under septic shock. Compromised patients are highly likely to develop endogenous infection. Operations on potentially contaminated areas, such as gastrointestinal tract, are more apt to result in postoperative infections. (Refer to Chapter 7 for detailed discussion of predisposing factors and infection control.) The following measures, in addition to those discussed under infection control, may help prevent wound infections.

1 Some surgeons prefer to irrigate potentially contaminated wounds with topical antibiotics intraoperatively.

2 Cultures obtained during operation, rather than those obtained postoperatively, should be used for antibiotic sensitivity testing.

3 Indwelling catheters should be discontinued as soon as possible to prevent urinary tract infection, which increases in incidence the longer the catheter is in the patient.

4 Special precautions must be taken when prostheses such as porcine heart valves, total hip prostheses, or intraocular lenses are implanted. Infection can have disastrous effects.

Gram-negative bacteria are the primary contaminants in wound infection. They are the predominant flora in gastrointestinal tract and the primary pathogens in urinary tract, abdominal, and intravenous catheter infections, as well as in pneumonia. These infections carry a high risk of bacteremia and therefore require prompt intervention.

Nonbacterial opportunists such as fungi and viruses are a particular hazard to trauma or burn patients. Likelihood of infection is related to severity of injury. Initial gram-positive infection is frequently followed by a virulent gram-negative or fungal infection. Candida is a common fungal colonizer and invader.

Staphylococci species of gram-positive cocci are common pathogens that may occur as normal flora of the skin, hair, and upper respiratory tract. Staphylococci wound infections acquired in the operating room are characterized by pus deep beneath a cleanly healed wound. A red wound accompanied by pus and fever within seven days after operation may indicate such an infection. Infections appearing more than seven days postoperatively usually are acquired on the unit.

Streptococci species of gram-positive cocci are found primarily in the upper respiratory tract. Beta-hemolytic streptococci are the pathogenic strain of this group.

Pseudomonas aeruginosa is an aerobic gram-negative bacillus found in water, soil, and intestinal tracts. It has the ability to survive in plain water. It is readily recognized by a bluish-green fluorescent color and characteristic odor.

Difficult to eradicate, these infections often progress to septicemia and multiple-abscess formation in the viscera or body areas, resulting in fatality.

Isolation precautions may be required for staphylococcal, streptococcal, or gram-negative wound infections (see Chap. 7, p. 111).

Enteric organisms are normally found in the intestinal tract. Gram-negative bacilli are often resistant to long-established antibiotics. Peritoneal contamination can result from visceral manipulation without mechanically entering the gastrointestinal tract in patients with cancerous lesions. A bowel wall can erode, permitting intestinal organisms to escape into the peritoneal cavity.

Anaerobic organisms thrive in unoxygenated tissues. They outnumber aerobic organisms in the intestinal tract and are less susceptible to antibiotics than are aerobes. Often present in the lower genital tract of females, they cause severe pelvic infection. Anaerobic infections are caused by:

1 Peptostreptococcus and peptococcus.

2 *Bacteroides* species and fusobacteria which are the most frequently isolated microorganisms from blood cultures. They are common in the colon.

3 *Clostridium perfringens, C. welchii,* which is found in the colon. This is a species of highly resistant gas-producing spore formers, contributing to a high mortality rate.

Investigation of Postoperative Wound Infections

A special form is used to record specific data. Investigation, usually by the infection control coordinator, includes:

1 Analysis of each infection to seek cause

2 Consultation with all persons who cared for patient

3 Review of any problem encountered intraoperatively, such as a break in sterile technique

4 Review of possible contributory factors

5 Evaluation of procedures relating to patient

6 Review of chart, symptoms, cultures

7 Review of postoperative dressing changes

WOUND DISRUPTION

Failure of a wound to heal or closure material to secure it during the healing process leads to wound disruption, a separation of wound edges. Disruption usually occurs from fifth to tenth postoperative day. This is the lag period in healing, the time when wound is not yet strong. Wound disruption is caused not by a single factor but by a combination of predisposing factors that influence healing.

Although it may occur in any body area, acute wound disruption most frequently follows abdominal operations. It starts with a small opening in the peritoneum, allowing a wedge of omentum to slip into it. This omentum becomes edematous and extends the opening along line of incision and upward through other layers of abdominal wall. Disruption is usually precipitated by distention or a sudden strain, such as vomiting, coughing, or sneezing. Terms used to describe abdominal wound disruption include:

1 *Dehiscence.* Partial or total splitting open or separation of layers of wound. "Cutting out" of sutures is the most important cause of dehiscence. Strength of tissues and extent of separation determine whether or not wound must be reclosed.

2 *Evisceration.* Protrusion of viscera through abdominal incision. While wound disruption of any degree calls for emergency care, *an evisceration is a catastrophe requiring immediate replacement of viscera and reclosure of incision.*

Symptoms

Patients who disrupt frequently do not present a smooth immediate postoperative course. They may have undue pain, discomfort, nausea, drainage, slight fever, vomiting, or hiccups. Acute symptoms include:

1 Tachycardia.

2 Vomiting.

3 Abnormal serosanguineous discharge.

4 Change in contour of wound.

5 Sudden pulling pain during straining. The patient feels something give. Suspect any seepage of serosanguineous fluid after a sudden sharp pain that lasts only momentarily after an effort. Send some of this fluid for culture and smear.

Any of these symptoms should be investigated at once. Examination of wound may show it gaping somewhat, or viscera may appear at skin surface.

Treatment at Bedside

1 Put in an emergency call for surgeon. Have a

nasogastric tube ready for insertion to relieve distention.

2 Reassure patient.

3 Apply sterile, moist saline dressings over wound and a loose binder.

4 Give drugs according to surgeon's order.

5 Do not give patient anything by mouth.

6 Prepare patient for return to the operating room. Treatment in the OR consists of secondary wound closure.

Prevention of Wound Disruption

Factors that may contribute to wound disruption are eliminated to the extent possible preoperatively.

1 Malnutrition and avitaminosis are corrected.

2 Obesity is reduced.

3 Anemia is corrected.

4 Operation is postponed, if possible, if patient has a transient illness, such as cold or influenza.

5 Antibiotics may be given prophylactically. While antibiotics cannot supplant sterile technique, some can render the operative field more free of microorganisms than it normally would be, as in operation on gastrointestinal tract.

Precautions during Operation

1 The surgeon gives meticulous attention to sterile technique, hemostasis, tissue handling and approximation, and selection of wound closure materials.

2 The entire OR team carefully carries out strict aseptic and sterile techniques to prevent infection.

COMPLICATIONS OF ABDOMINAL SURGERY

Patients are particularly prone to *pulmonary complications* following abdominal surgery. They are also subject to a variety of *fluid and electrolyte imbalances* for several reasons. For example, they are generally on nothing by mouth postoperatively. They may lose sodium, potassium, chloride, and water through nasogastric suction. If great quantities of alkalotic pancreatic secretions are lost through decompression of small bowel, metabolic acidosis may result. Loss of acidic stomach secretions may lead to metabolic alkalosis.

Peritonitis and wound infection are more common after gastrointestinal surgery because of spillage of contaminants from lumen of the GI tract. Another complication that may occur months to years postoperatively is *adhesions.* These may cause no problem, or may cause a mechanical bowel obstruction. Formation of this scar tissue is enhanced by peritonitis or postoperative radiation therapy. Increased intraabdominal pressure even years postoperatively may induce an *incisional hernia* through an old weakened scar.

RENAL COMPLICATIONS

Oliguria is frequently seen postoperatively. Water and sodium are conserved by antidiuretic hormone, aldosterone, epinephrine, and norepinephrine secreted during stress. This decreases urinary output. Dehydration, shock, cardiac failure, renal failure, or third-space loss such as edema or ascites may contribute to oliguria. Because prolonged oliguria may result in renal failure, urinary output of less than 30 ml an hour should be reported to surgeon. Treatment depends on cause.

The patient should be watched for infection following all urinary tract procedures because of the introduction of instruments and catheter. Cloudy urine, dysuria, frequency, urgency, and pain or burning upon urination are symptoms of urinary tract infections. Damage to bladder sphincters from instrumentation or urethral infection may lead to incontinence. Sharp abdominal pain following cystoscopy or manipulation of a ureter to remove calculi may suggest peritonitis from bladder or ureteral perforation. Particular susceptibility to infection accompanies urinary diversion.

ELECTROLYTE IMBALANCES

Fluid and electrolyte imbalances may be caused by many different factors. They may be manifested by numerous symptoms, e.g., disorientation. Maintenance of correct balance is a very relevant aspect of postoperative care, which greatly influences outcome of operative intervention.

WITHDRAWAL SYMPTOMS

Symptoms of withdrawal from either alcohol or drugs may appear postoperatively in habitual users. Unexplained agitation, disorientation, and/or hallucinations may be symptomatic of the body's reaction to deprivation of accustomed intake of chemical substances. An altered response, i.e., either increased or decreased effectiveness, is likely following administration of anesthesia, narcotics, and/or sedatives in chemically dependent patients.

CHAPTER **37**

REALITIES OF CLINICAL PRACTICE

When a formal educational experience is completed, a learner is eager to apply skills and knowledge in an employment setting. However, of necessity, a transition period from dependent learner to independent practitioner occurs. The realities of the work environment and the ethical dilemmas of some situations must be faced as basic competencies are developed. It can take six months to one year to feel fully confident as a functioning operating room team member.

REALITY SHOCK

Reality is a sense of actuality, a feeling that this is what the real world is all about. One must learn the rules and accepted behaviors and assume responsibilities for one's own behavior. Reality shock sets in as you make the transition from being a beginning learner to becoming an employed graduate professional nurse or surgical technologist. The familiar instructor and peer learners are no longer at your side to give counsel, advice, and moral support. As you attempt to adapt to the new demands placed on you, remember :

1 Learning never ends with basic education. It is an ongoing process throughout your career for improving skills and mastering new technologies.

2 Everyone you are working with has stood in your shoes. They have all experienced the feelings and frustrations of being the newest staff member.

3 Rely on the principles you have learned to make sound judgments and appropriate decisions.

4 Ask questions. Acknowledge when you do not know how to do something. Seek help. To promote your professional growth, use human and material resources.

Everyone wants and needs to become an accepted member of both social and work groups. The OR nursing staff collectively is a social group. The OR team, including the surgeon and anesthesiologist, is a work group. You will have ambivalent feelings as you enter these groups. You will feel pleasure functioning as a staff and team member. But you will also feel uncertain about your ability to perform well and about your new interpersonal relations.

Initially your goals will probably be skill-oriented as you learn the policies, procedures, and routines. Eventually you will replace insecurity with self-confidence. This will earn you trust, respect, and recognition from others as well as the personal satisfaction of accomplishment.

As you get acquainted with the surgeons, anesthesiologists, nursing supervisors, peers, and subordinates, you will learn the expected norms of behavior both from them and yourself.

EUSTRESS VS. DISTRESS

Physical and emotional stresses are part of daily life. In fact, Selye has said, "complete freedom from stress is death."* Stress is the nonspecific reaction of the body, physiologically and/or psychologically, to any demand. The demand may be pleasant or unpleasant, conscious or unconscious. The intensity of the stressor will dictate adaptation. Your own individual perception of a situation will influence your reaction to it.

Stress is not only an essential part of life but a useful stimulant. Positive stress, referred to as *eustress,* motivates you to be productive and efficient. It forces you to adapt to the ever-present changes in the OR environment. You must respond quickly, for example, when a trauma victim arrives or a patient has a cardiac arrest. To expect the unexpected is part of OR nursing. Eustress fosters a sense of achievement, satisfaction, and contentment.

Stress that becomes overwhelming and uncomfortable is referred to as *distress.* In the OR, behavior of others may be perceived as cause for distress. Hospital policies, or lack of them, can also be a source of distress if they are in conflict with your expectations. Through your adaptive mechanisms you cope with the tensions, conflicts, and demands of the OR environment either in a collaborative way or in an unproductive manner. Even though perceived as distress, some conflict is necessary to stimulate change in work methods and solve organizational problems.

Nursing personnel may be distressed by conduct of other team members. For example, it is uncomfortable to be harshly criticized by a surgeon. Keep in mind that much that is said is not personally directed. Often the surgeon is reacting to his or her distress caused by unanticipated circumstances presented by the patient during the operation. Your reactions will be influenced by your own attitudes, mood, cultural and religious backgrounds, values and ethics, experiences, and concerns of the moment. Outbursts of anger are inappropriate at the operating table at any time. However, constant frustration and inner conflict create the distresses that can lead to job dissatisfaction.

While the ideological differences of personnel in the OR may at times be a source of conflict, teamwork and the task at hand must overcome any disparities. Other distresses that arise as a result of many complex procedures, heavy operating schedules, shortages of available staff, etc., must not interfere with the delivery of efficient, individualized patient care.

*H Selye: *The Stress of Life,* 2d ed, New York: McGraw-Hill, 1976.

ETHICAL DILEMMAS

Some situations that arise in the OR environment may be contrary to your personal morals, values, beliefs, or religion. Nursing personnel assume legal and ethical rights, duties, and obligations by vitrue of the relation with patients, the employing institution, and other health care professionals. Both personal and professional values and attitudes enter into these relations. Legal and ethical considerations can cause conflicts. You must establish priorities and decide for yourself the appropriate course of action to take in handling these conflicts. When does life begin? When does it end? What is the quality of life between conception and death? What is your role in health care? If you decide not to participate, discuss the issue with your supervisor prior to being put in a compromising position. You have a right to refuse to participate, but not at the expense of a patient's safety and welfare. The patient cannot be harmed by acts of commission or omission.

A few of the ethical dilemmas facing physicians and OR nursing personnel are mentioned for personal consideration.

Reproductive Sterilization

Voluntary nontherapeutic sterilization as a contraceptive method may be contrary to a nurse's or surgical technologist's moral, ethical, or religious beliefs. A few states have statutes regulating this practice; most do not.

Therapeutic (to preserve life or health) and eugenic (to prevent procreation by mentally retarded, habitual criminals, and sexual deviates) sterilizations are regulated in many states. Nursing personnel should be familiar with statutes in the state in which they practice regarding participation and right to refrain on basis of personal beliefs.

Abortion

State statutes have legalized abortion, the deliberate termination of pregnancy. In the 1973 decision of *Roe v. Wade,* the United States Supreme Court ruled that any licensed physician can terminate pregnancy during the first trimester with the consent of the woman. During the second trimester, the Court requires that a state statute regulate abortion on the basis of preservation and protection of maternal health. During the third trimester, legal abortion must consider meaningful life of the fetus outside the womb and endangerment to the mother's life and health.

By law, health care facilities may or may not be required to admit patients for abortion. In hospitals and ambulatory care facilities where abortions are performed, employees have the right to refrain from participation because of moral, ethical, and/or religious beliefs except in a maternal life-threatening emergency. These beliefs must be made known to the employer. Some states have a protection statute for employees and employers regulating good-faith efforts to accommodate employees' beliefs.

Human Experimentation

Intrauterine fetal surgery, vital organ transplantation, mechanical or prosthetic device implantation, and other procedures still in developmental stages are performed in clinical research-oriented hospitals. Those willing to be pioneers in human experimentation have given, or will give, hope to many patients with poor prognoses. Can you ethically be a team member in experimental surgery? If not, seek employment in an OR where only established therapeutic or palliative procedures are performed.

Organ Donation and Transplantation

Under the Uniform Anatomical Gift Act of 1968, many adults carry cards stating that upon death they wish to donate body organs or parts for transplantation, therapy, medical research, or education. Most states provide this card as part of a driver's license. If this legal authority is not available, the family may consent to operation to harvest one or more organs or parts of the deceased after death has been pronounced.

Transplant surgeons rely on the OR teams who procure donor organs, eyes, bone, and/or skin. Organ transplantation has complicated the issue of time of death. Perfusion of oxygenated blood through tissues must be sustained by artificial means to harvest vital organs with functional viability. Therefore, the accepted definition of irreversible coma for potential donors includes unreceptivity and unresponsivity, no spontaneous movements of respiration, no reflexes, and flat electroencephalogram. When brain death is determined by two physicians not part of the transplant team, the donor will be taken to the operating room with artificial support systems functioning to perfuse organs. Some nurses and surgical technologists have difficulty assisting with removal of viable organs from seemingly living bodies.

Quality of Life and Its Relation to Euthanasia

Surgeons must often make critical decisions before or during surgical intervention regarding the quality of the patient's life following operation. Palliative procedures may relieve pain. Life-support systems may sustain vital functions. Life-sustaining therapy may prolong the dying process. But many questions are raised regarding the care of terminally ill, severely debilitated or injured, and comatose patients. What will be the outcome in terms of mental or physical competence? When should cardiopulmonary resuscitation be discontinued? The surgeon decides, but all team members are affected by this decision. How do you define euthanasia? Is mercy killing ethical, legal, or justified? Does the patient, family or guardian, physicians, or courts have the right to decide to abandon heroic measures to sustain life? The patient who is informed of the options, and whose decision-making capacity is competent, has the right of self-determination. This rarely is feasible in the OR.

Death and Dying

Death is inevitable. Intellectually we know this. But for the health care team, a patient's stages of dying and ultimate death can be a difficult burden to bear because our education, experience, and philosophy are dedicated to survival. Regardless of religious or cultural beliefs, death is a mystery we do not understand. It is a passing from the known to the unknown.

Terminally ill patients, and fleetingly even fatal or nearly fatal trauma victims, pass through stages of dying. These include denial and isolation, anger, bargaining, depression, and acceptance. A therapeutic relation with the dying patient must be open and caring. Truth as it is perceived by physicians and nurses is most important in maintaining the patient's trust. Trust is more important than are efforts to relieve fears associated with death and dying. Tell the patient what he or she wants to know with sensitivity to minimize psychic trauma. Acknowledge the patient's feelings in a supportive manner that lets the patient know it is all right to feel and behave the way he or she does. The patient should choose how he or she wishes to live while dying. The right to death with dignity should be respected to the extent possible. Facing the reality of death can help one to understand the meaning of life. Patients fear abandonment. Reassure the patient that he or she is not alone.

CLINICAL COMPETENCE

Performance can be identified as novice, competent, proficient, and expert. The novice lacks experience in situations in which he or she is expected to perform. Assistance must be available. As experience is gained, competence develops from a minimal level to an advanced level of expertise. Most employers provide a formal orientation program for newly graduated registered nurses and surgical technologists that lasts from 6 to 12 months. Within this time, the necessary knowledge, skills, and abilities should be developed to function at a basic competency level.

In 1982, AORN published statements of basic competencies for perioperative nurses. These statements are intended to serve as guidelines for a nurse to reasonably expect to achieve by the end of the first year of employment in the OR. They are written in broad terms to be applicable in any practice setting. Although the written job descriptions for perioperative or OR nurses and surgical technologists will not be the same, these statements are included as a summation of this text.* They incorporate the many principles, procedures, and practices elaborated throughout this text. Functions are identified in the following categories:

1 Physiological and psychosocial: nursing actions directed toward meeting the physical, emotional, and spiritual needs of patient receiving nursing care in the OR.
- **a** Assess the health status of patient experiencing surgical intervention by collecting pertinent health data through:
  - **1** Patient interview
  - **2** Observation
  - **3** Review of records
  - **4** Consultation with other members of health care team
- **b** Assess the physical status of patient experiencing surgical intervention by collecting pertinent health data about patient in the following areas:
  - **1** Respiratory, circulatory, and renal status
  - **2** Condition of skin and mucous membranes
  - **3** Results of diagnostic studies
  - **4** Allergies
  - **5** Sensory perceptions
  - **6** Nutritional status
  - **7** Motor ability
- **c** Assess the psychosocial status of patient experiencing surgical intervention by being aware of:
  - **1** Patient's perception of surgery
  - **2** Patient's expectations of care during hospitalization
  - **3** Patient's fears and anxieties
  - **4** Patient's level of understanding
  - **5** Patient's philosophical, cultural, and religious beliefs
- **d** Develop a plan of nursing care that reflects use of:
  - **1** Current knowledge
  - **2** Available resources
  - **3** Patient rights
  - **4** Communication with the individual, family, and health care personnel
- **e** Implement the psychosocial aspects of the nursing care plan for patient experiencing surgical intervention through:
  - **1** Providing support
  - **2** Using touch in communication when appropriate
  - **3** Explaining events and giving information to patient, family, and other health care team members

2 Skills: ability to use knowledge in clinical performance by applying technical, interpersonal, teaching, leadership, and communication concepts.
- **a** Demonstrate ability in assessing the physical status of patients by checking:
  - **1** Anticipated incision area
  - **2** General condition of skin
  - **3** General mobility of body parts

*AORN ad hoc Committee on Basic Competencies in Operating Room Nursing, *Developing Basic Competencies for Perioperative Nursing,* Denver: Association of Operating Room Nurses, Inc., 1982. Adapted with permission.

    4 Vital signs
    5 Absence or presence of motor or sensory impairments
    6 Obvious signs of abnormalities
    7 Presence or absence of prostheses
    8 Impairments involving cardiovascular and respiratory systems
  b Demonstrate ability to identify and anticipate patient care needs.
  c Maintain patient safety by applying principles of body alignment and adapting them to varying situations during positioning.
  d Know and apply principles of aseptic practice and recognize necessity for following established procedures and adapting them according to varying situations. Adaptation is almost always appropriate for the situation.
  e Cooperate in team planning and execution of plan to care for patient effectively.
  f Organize nursing activities in an efficient manner.
  g Demonstrate tact and understanding when dealing with patients, team members, members of other disciplines, and the public.
  h Convey ideas, concepts, and facts related to patient care in a logical and concise manner.
  i Report and/or record information relative to patient.

3 Professional characteristics: attributes that affect professional performance.
  a Demonstrate integrity in aseptic practice and call attention to and suggest measures to correct breaks in technique by all team members.
  b Use judgment in determining nursing actions that are in the best interest of patient and make decisions based upon scientific knowledge, nursing experience, and patient information.
  c Preserve patient privacy through:
    1 Maintenance of confidentiality in communication and documentation
    2 Physical protection of patients during interviews, examinations, transportation, positioning, and draping.
  d Exhibit professional behavior when interacting with other members of health care team.
  e Exhibit flexibility and adaptability to changes in nursing practice.
  f Accept constructive criticism and respond appropriately in relation to nursing practice by implementing corrective actions.

4 Accountability: being responsible and answerable to self, patients, profession, and institution for nursing care given in the OR.
  a Maintain a safe environment by implementing technical and aseptic practices.
  b Deliver care to surgical patients by:
    1 Checking patient identification
    2 Proper handling of surgical specimens, completing incident reports, and documenting care
  c Respect patients' rights by:
    1 Providing privacy
    2 Maintaining confidentiality of patient information
    3 Ensuring the right to ethnic and spiritual beliefs and by recognizing each person's individuality
  d Collaborate with others to provide nursing care that requires additional skill.
  e Seek opportunities for continued learning.

The four categories of the statements above have relevance to all nursing personnel who have contact with patients. Physiological and psychosocial concerns for patients, skills, professional (or paraprofessional) characteristics, and accountability are the essence of patient care in the operating room.

After achievement of basic competency, you should strive to progress along the continuum to proficient to expert achievement in practice. Certification should also be one of your professional career goals.

Demonstrated skills and observable behaviors are continually evaluated in the work setting. Established criteria provide a means for evaluating the development of nurses and surgical technologists.

Surgical Conscience

Development of a surgical conscience to carry out all functions in the best interests of every surgical patient is a matter of self-discipline. Novices tend to emulate peers who are proficient and expert. Therefore, every nurse and surgical technologist should, *by exemplary dedication to the highest level of moral conduct,* serve as a worthy role model. Eligibility to progress up the clinical ladder will be determined by personal performance. Recognition for expertise in clinical practice is the prime contributor to job satisfaction.

BIBLIOGRAPHY

The references included in the bibliography represent the most recent and relevant content when the manuscript was written. Medical technology and research change rapidly. References in the bibliography are cited in the form adopted by the National Library of Medicine for its indexes including the official abbreviations for periodicals.

MULTIPLE SOURCES—BOOKS

American College of Surgeons, Pre- and Postoperative Care Committee: *Manual of Preoperative and Postoperative Care,* 3d ed, Philadelphia: Saunders, 1983.

American College of Surgeons, Subcommittee on Control of Surgical Infections: *Manual on Control of Infection in Surgical Patients,* 2d ed, Philadelphia: Saunders, 1984.

Anderson RM, Romfh RF: *Technique in the Use of Surgical Tools,* New York: Appleton-Century-Crofts, 1980.

Anthony CP, Kolthoff NJ: *Textbook of Anatomy and Physiology,* 11th ed, St. Louis: Mosby, 1983.

AORN Standards and Recommended Practices for Perioperative Nursing, Denver: Association of Operating Room Nurses, Inc., 1985.

Blakiston's Gould Medical Dictionary, 4th ed, New York: McGraw-Hill, 1979.

Brunner LS, Suddarth DS: *Textbook of Medical-Surgical Nursing,* 5th ed, Philadelphia: Lippincott, 1984.

Cordner JW: *Logic of Operating Room Nursing,* 3d ed, Oradell, N.J.: Medical Economics Books, 1984.

Drain CB, Shipley SB: *The Recovery Room,* Philadelphia: Saunders, 1979.

Ethicon, Inc.: *Wound Closure Manual,* Somerville, N.J.: 1985.

Fuller JR: *Surgical Technology: Principles and Practice,* Philadelphia: Saunders, 1981.

Groah LK: *Operating Room Nursing: The Perioperative Role,* Reston, Va.: Reston Publishing, 1983.

Gruendemann BJ, Meeker MH: *Alexander's Care of the Patient in Surgery,* 7th ed, St. Louis: Mosby, 1983.

Hejna WF, Gutmann CM: *Management of Surgical Facilities,* Rockville, Md.: Aspen, 1984.

Isselbacher KJ et al (ed): *Harrison's Principles of Internal Medicine,* 9th ed, New York: McGraw-Hill, 1980.

Joint Commission on Accreditation of Hospitals: *AMH/85 Accreditation Manual for Hospitals,* Chicago: 1984.

LeMaitre GD, Finnegan JA: *The Patient in Surgery: A Guide for Nurses,* 4th ed, Philadelphia: Saunders, 1980.

Long B, Phipps W: *Essentials of Medical-Surgical Nursing,* St. Louis: Mosby, 1985.

Luckmann J, Sorensen KC: *Medical-Surgical Nursing: A Psychophysiologic Approach,* Philadelphia: Saunders, 1980.

McCaughan JS: *Lasers in Medicine and Surgery,* Columbus, Ohio: Laser Medical Research Foundation, 1983.

McVay CB: *Anson and McVay Surgical Anatomy,* Vol 1 & 2, 6th ed, Philadelphia: Saunders, 1984.

Miller B, Keane CB: *Encyclopedia and Dictionary of Medicine, Nursing and Allied Health,* 3d ed, Philadelphia: Saunders, 1983.

National Fire Protection Association: *National Fire Codes,* Vol 4, Quincy, Ma.: 1981.

Nora PF (ed): *Operative Surgery: Principles and Techniques,* 2d ed, Philadelphia: Lea & Febiger, 1980.

Phipps WJ et al: *Medical-Surgical Nursing,* 2d ed, St. Louis: Mosby, 1983.

Sabiston DC Jr (ed): *Davis-Christopher Textbook of Surgery: The Biological Basis of Modern Surgical Practice,* 12th ed, Philadelphia: Saunders, 1981.

Schwartz SI et al (ed): *Principles of Surgery,* 4th ed, New York: McGraw-Hill, 1984.

Trott A: *Principles and Techniques of Minor Wound Care,* New Hyde Park, N.Y.: Med Exam Publishing, 1985.

Weiner MB, Pepper GA: *Clinical Pharmacology and Therapeutics in Nursing,* 2d ed, New York: McGraw-Hill, 1985.

Wind GC, Rich NH: *Principles of Surgical Technique: The Art of Surgery,* Baltimore: Urban & Schwarzenberg, 1983.

MULTIPLE SOURCES—JOURNALS

Bartley J, Chamberlin DA: The barriers to infection, Todays OR Nurse 5(7):26–29, 32–34, Sep 1983.

Belkin NL: Evaluating surgical gowning, draping fabrics, AORN J 34(3):499, 502, 506, 510–511, Sep 1981.

Berry MS et al: Task analysis of surgical technology occupations, Surg Technol 13(6):15–18, Nov–Dec 1981.

Christman NJ: Surgical implants: Psychological responses, AORN J 37 (7): 1292–1295, June 1983.

Cichlar, PG: Troubleshooting power equipment in arthroscopic surgery, Todays OR Nurse 6(10):21–24, Oct 1984.

Communication and cooperation stressed at OR symposium, Bull Am Coll Surg 68(10):28–30, Oct 1983.

Craig CP: Infection surveillance for ambulatory surgery patients: An overview, QRB 9(4):107–111, Apr 1983.

Cruse PJE: Preparing the patient for operation, Bull Am Coll Surg 66(5):16–18, 22–25, May 1981.

Curtin L: Wound management: Care and cost—An overview, Nurs Manage 15(2):22–25, Feb 1984.

Deckert B et al: Clinical ladders, Nurs Manage 15(3):54–55, Mar 1984.

Dixon JA: Surgical applications of lasers, Bull Am Coll Surg 67(1):4–9, Nov 1982.

Evanoff J: The debate continues . . . Laminar airflow in surgery, Todays OR Nurse 6(7):21–24, 28, July 1984.

Furnas DW: Reconstructive microsurgery: An overview, Bull Am Coll Surg (69)6:21–29, June 1984.

Gelfant BB: Mental health attitudes in the OR, Todays OR Nurse 4(10):17–19, 48, Dec 1982.

Groah L, Reed EA: Your responsibility in documenting care, AORN J 37(6):1174, 1176–1177, 1180, 1182, 1184–1185, 1188, Mar 1983.

Hagan B: Infection: "A convenient myth?", Nurs Manage 13(1):26–27, Jan 1982.

Hargest TS: A clinical engineer's view of medical instrumentation, Med Instrumentation 14(4):215–217, July–Aug 1980.

James SM, Smith S: Breaking the chain of infection, Nurs Manage 12(10):29–31, Oct 1981.

Klann SS, Palmer PN: What's new in surgery: The ACS clinical congress, AORN J 39(2):194–206, 208–209, Feb 1984.

Kleinert HE: Microsurgery in trauma: Its evolution and future, Bull Am Coll Surg 67(6):10–19, June 1982.

Koerner M et al: Communicating in the OR: Part II: Listening, AORN J 40(6):858–866, Dec 1984.

Laufman H: Infection control: A moral issue, Todays OR Nurse 5(7):38–41, 44, 46, Sep 1983.

LoCicero J, Nichols RL: Environmental health hazards in the operating room, Bull Am Coll Surg 67(5):2–5, May 1982.

McLain NB: Risk management in the operating room, AORN J 31(5):873–874, 876–877, Apr 1980.

Palmer PN, Poland V: What's new in surgery: The ACS clinical congress, AORN J 41(2):436, 438–439, 441, 443, 445, 447, 449, 451, 453, 455, Feb 1985.

Patterson P, Schrader ES: Surgeons review what's new, AORN J 35(1):74–75, 78–79, 82–83, 86, 90–91, 94–95, 98–99, 104, 106, 108, 110, 112, Jan 1982.

Poland V, Schrader ES: Surgeons review new technology at ACS meeting, AORN J 37(2):259–261, 264–265, 268–270, 272–273, 276–277, Feb 1983.

Proposed recommended practices: Radiation safety in the operating room (including lasers), AORN J 40(6):881–886, Dec 1984.

Recommended practices for documentation of perioperative nursing care, AORN J 35(4):744, 746, 748, Mar 1982.

Recommended practices: Monitoring the patient receiving local anesthesia, AORN J 39(6):1080, 1082–1083, May 1984.

Recommended practices: Storing, preserving, and maintaining skin, bone, cartilage, and blood vessel tissue, AORN J 40(3):392–396, Sep 1984.

Schrader ES, Patterson P: Surgeons summarize progress, AORN J 33(1):73, 77–78, 80, 82, 86, 88, 92–93, 96–97, Jan 1981.

Spencer FC: Observations on the teaching of operative technique, Bull Am Coll Surg 68(3):3–6, Mar 1983.

Steven DL: Use of the carbon dioxide laser in your operating room, J Oper Rm Res Inst 2(7):7–11, July 1982.

Surgical sepsis a delicate balance, AORN J 35(4):786, 788, 790, Mar 1982.

Terrion J: Documentation of nursing care in the operating room, Point View 21(2):10–11, 1984.

Tish Knobf MK et al: Breast cancer: For CE credit, Am J Nurs 84(9):1109–1128, Sep 1984.

Viers VM: Introducing nurses to computer world, Nurs Manage 14(7):24–25, July 1983.

Warfield CA: Intraspinal narcotics: A new method of pain management, AORN 41(5):910–912, 914, May 1985.

Wells P: Teaching aseptic technique, Todays OR Nurse 5(7):20–24, 57, Sep 1983.

Wilson DC: Efficient OR management, Nurs Manage 15(4):42A, 42D–42F, 42H, Apr 1984.

Zeller JM: Surgical implants: Physiological response, AORN J 37(7):1284–1291, June 1983.

CHAPTER 1
INTRODUCTION FOR THE LEARNER

Berglund S: Berglund addresses purposes of LCC, Surg Technol 16(4):15–17, July–Aug 1984.

Burger M: Surgical technologists—professional or not?, Surg Technol 15(2):25, Mar–Apr 1983.

Conner MV: A vital link in reaching for recognition: An in-depth study of licensure and certification, Surg Technol 15(2):12–14, 16, Mar–Apr 1983.

Girard NL: Putting the OR back in nursing education, Todays OR Nurse 6(5):25–27, May 1984.

Gough FA: The perioperative elective, AORN J 39(6):1009, 1012–1013, 1016–1017, 1020, 1024, May 1984.

Gulack R: "I'm a professional," RN 46(9):28–35, Sep 1983.

Hedrick HL: Allied health education and accreditation, JAMA 248(24):24–31, Dec 1982.

Hercules PR, Kneedler JA: *Certification Series Unit I: Certification Process, Unit II: Assessment of Professional Practice,* Denver: Association of Operating Room Nurses, Inc., 1979.

Holder L: Allied health perspectives in the 1980's, Surg Technol 14(2):22–27, Mar–Apr 1982.

Kingsinger RE: Allied health education: Challenges for a new decade, Surg Technol 14(4):32–36, July–Aug 1982.

Knowles MS: *The Modern Practice of Adult Education,* New York: Associated Press, 1972.

Knowles MS: *Self-Directed Learning,* Chicago: Associated Press, 1975.

LaMontagne C: OR students are people too, Todays OR Nurse 4(9):32–33, 36–37, Nov 1982.

May M: Licensure vs. certification, Surg Technol 15(4):43–45, July–Aug 1983.

Pick J: Specialization in nursing: Will we find a way to meet the need?, Can Nurse 80(5):22–23, May 1984.

Sparks SM: AVLINE for nursing education and research, Nurs Outlook 27(11):733–737, Nov 1979.

Thompson R: How can nurses be attracted to theatre work? Why did I choose theatre nursing and did I achieve my goals?, NATNews 20(3):10–12, Mar 1983.

Weisfield N, Falk D: Professional credentials required, Hospitals 57(3):74–79, Feb 1, 1983.

CHAPTER 2
THE HEALTH CARE TEAM

Altman BJ: BMET: New member on the OR team, AORN J 30(3):435–441, Sep 1979.

Bachman DJ, Ridley JM: Using preceptors for the new OR nurse, Todays OR Nurse 6(7):14–18, July 1984.

Ball JR: Credentialing versus performance: A new look at old problems, QRB 10(3):75–80, Mar 1984.

Bartilotta K, Rzasa CB: Quality assurance utilizing a computerized patient information system, QRB 8(3):17–22, Mar 1982.

Brzezicki MJ: Surgery case carts do work, Point View 19(3):20, July 1982.

Coppage D: Reality and accountability of hospital environmental control, Point View 22(1):4–5, Jan 1985.

Dwelle CA: Expanded roles promote patient advocacy, Point View 18(2):7–9, April 1981.

Faulconer DR, Reeves DM: Clinical ladders and specialty teams, AORN J 35(4):669–678, Mar 1982.

Gelfant BB: Postanesthesia recovery: A life saver, Point View 21(3):18–19, Sep 1984.

Gilbert B: Relating quality assurance to credentials and privileges, QRB 10(5):130–135, May 1984.

Hardy JD: The resident's responsibility, Bull Am Coll Surg 65(3):16–18, Mar 1980.

Isaac DN: Suggestions for organizing a quality assurance program, QRB 9(3):68–72, Mar 1983.

Lynch BL: Team building: Will it work in health care?, Surg Technol 14(5):24–26, 28–29, Sep–Oct 1982.

Maihot C, Slezak L: Nurse-physician committee eases tension in OR, AORN J 38(3):411–415, Sep 1983.

Murphy EK: OR nursing law: When is the RN first assistant practicing within the scope of nursing?, AORN J 40(2):256–257, 260, Aug 1984.

Murphy EK: OR nursing law: When is the RN first assistant protected by institutional policy?, AORN J 40(3):436, 438, 440, Sep 1984.

Nora PF: Ethics in housestaff training, Bull Am Coll Surg 69(5):3–5, May 1984.

Parks P: Competition between physicians and limited licensed practitioners: Some issues and implications, Bull Am Coll Surg 69(4):9–13, Apr 1984.

Parmer MA: Ethics of a professional surgeon, Bull Am Coll Surg 67(7):2–5, July 1982.

Plasse NJ, Lederer JR: Preceptors: A resource for new nurses, Superv Nurse 12(6):35–36, 40–41, June 1981.

Reeves DM, Faulconer DR: Reorganizing an operating room, Todays OR Nurse 3(7):17–22, Sep 1981.

Schrader ES: RN as circulator gets backing in new Medicare regs, AORN J 37(2):181–182, Feb 1983.

Standards of administrative nursing practice: OR, *AORN Standards and Recommended Practices for Perioperative Nursing,* Denver: Association of Operating Room Nurses, Inc., 1985.

Task force defines first assisting, AORN J 39(3):403–405, Feb 1984.

Tenzer I: The RN circulator, Todays OR Nurse 5(3):26, 31–32, 34–35, May 1983.

Terrion JM: O.R. nurses' role perception, Point View 18(2):4–6, Apr 1981.

Wyers MEA et al: Clinical nurse specialist: In search of

the right role, Nurs & Health Care 6(4):203–207, Apr 1985.

CHAPTER 3 THE PATIENT: THE REASON FOR YOUR EXISTENCE

AORN official statement on RN first assistants, AORN J 40(3):441, 443, Sep 1984.

Bender JM, Faubion JM: Total parenteral nutrition: Nursing implications, AORN J 40(3):354–359, Sep 1984.

Brock AM: How do the aged cope with surgery?, Todays OR Nurse 6(9):16, 20–22, 25, Sep 1984.

Castillo P: Consumer's surgery preparation, Point View 19(3):4–6, 1982.

Danner D: Patients rights emphasized in informed consent ruling, Malpractice Digest 10(4):1–2, Dec 1983.

Davis J et al: Sure-fire asepsis for your TPN patients, RN 45(12):39–41, 91, Dec 1982.

Giordano C, Conly D: Taking the worry out of hyperal, Part I, RN 44(6):42–48, June 1981.

Heinecke CD, Gibson JF Jr: Sickle cell trait and cardiopulmonary bypass, Anesthesiology Rev 7(9):18–21, Sep 1980.

Janik J, Seeler RA: Perioperative management of children with sickle hemoglobinopathy, J Pediatr Surg 15(2):117–120, Apr 1980.

Juliani LM: Trouble-free administration of hetastarch and TPN, RN 44(8):64–65, Aug 1981.

Linehan MS: Sickle cell anemia—the painful crisis, J Emerg Nurs 4(6):12–19, Nov–Dec 1978.

Macklin R: Dilemmas of informed consent for surgery, Bull Am Coll Surg 67(7):6–9, July 1982.

McConnell EA: Be prepared for double trouble if your surgical patient's a diabetic, Nursing (Horsham) 11(11):118–123, Nov 1981.

McFadden EA et al: Hypocalcemia: A medical emergency, Am J Nurs 83(2):227–230, Feb 1983.

Meckes PF: Perioperative care of the elderly patient, Todays OR Nurse 6(9):8–11, 14–15, Sep 1984.

Metheny N: Preoperative fluid balance assessment, AORN J 33(1):51–56, Jan 1981.

Miller VG: The sickle cell anemia patient in surgery, AORN J 30(6):1083–1090, Dec 1979.

Nemchik R: Diabetes today: Facing up to the long-term complications, RN 46(7):38–44, July 1983.

Palmer PN: Malnutrition: Reversing the trend in the surgical patient, AORN J 40(3):347–352, Sep 1984.

Pool MK: One hospital's approach to developing standards of care, QRB 8(8):19–22, Aug 1982.

Reeder JM: Understanding von Willebrand's disease, AORN J 35(7):1310, 1314–1315, 1318–1319, June 1982.

Robertson E, Stevenson E: Loss, stress and the diabetic surgical patient, Can Nurse 79(5):30–33, May 1983.

Shaukat M, Dalton BA: A scoring system to assess preoperative anesthetic preparation, QRB 7(3):17–20, Mar 1981.

Shipley SB: The obese patient in surgery: Implications for nursing care, Point View 17(2):12–14, Apr 1980.

Silva MC: Ethics, informed consent and the OR nurse, Todays OR Nurse 4(1):21–22, 24, 62–63, Mar 1982.

Smith CL: Implication of malnutrition in the surgical patient, Point View 18(3):6–7, July 1981.

Starker PM et al: The response to TPN: A form of nutritional assessment, Ann Surg 198(6):720–724, Dec 1983.

Steinmiller AM: The surgical patient with hemophilia, Surg Technol 15(6):46–48, Nov–Dec 1983.

Stotts N: Nutritional assessment before surgery, AORN J 35(2):207–214, Feb 1982.

Walts LF: Managing diabetics during surgery, AORN J 37(5):928, 930, 939–941, Apr 1983.

Watson S, Hickey P: Help for the family in waiting, Am J Nurs 84(5):604–607, May 1984.

Winters B: Promoting wound healing in diabetic patient, AORN J 35(6):1083–1087, May 1982.

CHAPTER 4 PERIOPERATIVE NURSING

American Nurses' Association Division on Medical-Surgical Nursing Practice and Association of Operating Room Nurses: *Standards of Perioperative Nursing Practice,* Kansas City, Mo.: ANA, 1981.

Ammon KB, Fowler LM: A perioperative elective for baccalaureate students, AORN J 37(4):754, 756, 758, 760–761, 764, Mar 1983.

Barness SK, Long CS: Perioperative nursing: A special project, AORN J 39(4):609–615, Mar 1984.

Botsford J: Implementing outcome standards: A planning strategy, AORN J 40(4):572–575, Oct 1984.

Brennan PE: Preoperative visits: Controlling the stress, Todays OR Nurse 4(10):9–13, Dec 1982.

Case BA, Rooney DS: Patient care planning strategies, Nurs Manage 13(4):23–26, Apr 1982.

Chansky ER: Reducing patients' anxieties: Techniques for dealing with crises, AORN J 40(3):375–377, Sep 1984.

Committee on Nursing Practices: Standards of perioperative nursing practice: Using the revised standards, AORN J 36(3):363–365, 371–377, Sep 1982.

Edwards BJ, Brilhart JK: *Communications in Nursing Practice,* St. Louis: Mosby, 1981.

Elfman P: A practical format for care planning, AORN J 37(6):1190, 1192–1194, 1196, May 1983.

Fraulini KE: Coping mechanisms and recovery from surgery, AORN J 37(6):1198, 1200–1201, 1204–1205, 1208, May 1983.

Gelfant BB, Doyle ED: The perioperative nurse, Nurs Manage 14(11):34B–34D, Nov 1983.

Hamer BA: Managing OR patients' fears, Todays OR Nurse 7(5):28–30, May 1985.

Keithley JK, Tasie PW: A unified approach to assessment of the surgical patient, Am J Nurs 82(4):612–614, Apr 1982.

Kleinbeck SVM: SOAPing the preoperative interview, AORN J 28(6):1031–1035, Dec 1978.

Kneedler JA, Dodge GH: *Perioperative Patient Care,* Boston: Blackwell Scientific Pub, 1983.

Lancaster J: Communication: The anatomy of messages, Nurs Manage 14(9):42–45, Sep 1983.

Lunney M: Nursing diagnosis: Refining the system, Am J Nurs 82(3):456–459, Mar 1982.

Mackie R et al: Perioperative care plan guides, AORN J 40(2):192–201, Aug 1984.

Mallick MJ: Nursing diagnosis and the novice student, Nurs & Health Care 4(8):455–459, Oct 1983.

Manuel BJ: *Reporting and Documenting Patient Care: OR,* Modular Independent Learning Systems, Denver: Association of Operating Room Nurses, Inc., 1980.

Manuel BJ: *The Nursing Process Series 1: An Overview,* Modular Independent Learning Systems, Denver: Association of Operating Room Nurses, Inc., 1979.

McConnell E: How nursing care plans help you, Nurs Life 2(1):55–59, Jan–Feb 1982.

Nodhturft VL, MacMullen JA: Standardized nursing care plans, Nurs Manage 13(10):33–36, 40–42, Oct 1982.

Nursing Practice Committee: A model for perioperative nursing practice, AORN J 41(1):188, 190, 192–194, Jan 1985.

Palmateer L: Surgical-psychological crisis: Awake and paralyzed, Todays OR Nurse 4(10):22–25, 27, 39, Dec 1982.

Patient outcome standards for perioperative nursing, AORN J 39(3):400–402, Feb 1984; AORN J 40(4):578–580, Oct 1984.

Petty C: Opinion: A physician's perspective on allaying patients' fears, AORN J 41(3):537, 540, 542, Mar 1985.

Phippen MK: Nursing assessment of preoperative anxiety, AORN J 31(6):1019–1026, May 1980.

Project 25 Task Force: Operating room nursing: Perioperative role, AORN J 27(6):1156, 1160–1162, 1164–1165, 1168, 1170, 1175, May 1978.

Ryan J: The neglected crisis, Am J Nurs 84(10):1257–1258, Oct 1984.

Shaw H: What aspects of the nursing process are applicable in theatre nursing and how can they be implemented?, NATNews 20(5):11–13, May 1983.

Shaw L: Apply standards? You do it every day, AORN J 36(3):366–370, Sep 1982.

Shaw LM: The patient as an adult learner, AORN J 33(2):233–239, Feb 1981.

Smitherman C: Dealing with the patient's denial: What should you do?, Nursing (Horsham) 11(12):70–71, Dec 1981.

Smitherman C: Your patient's anxious: What should you do?, Nursing (Horsham) 11(10):72–73, Oct 1981.

Thompson R: Implementing the nursing process in operating theatres, NATNews 18(10):18–19, 22, 24, Oct 1981.

Vernon J: Getting in touch, Todays OR Nurse 5(9):30–32, Nov 1983.

Wardell B: A standard care plan for the operating room, AORN J 36(2):279–287, Aug 1982.

Yoder ME: Nursing diagnosis: Applications in perioperative practice, AORN J 40(2):183–188, Aug 1984.

CHAPTER 5
AMBULATORY SURGERY

Ambulatory surgery: When and what procedures, Bull Am Coll Surg 67(11):21–23, 30, Nov 1982.

Becker A: Same day surgery: A psychological approach, Todays OR Nurse 5(5):8–11, 43, July 1983.

Burns LA: Ambulatory surgery growing at rapid pace, AORN J 35(2):260, 263–264, 266, 268, 270, Feb 1982.

Conner MV: Why ambulatory surgery deserves greater esteem, Surg Technol 14(4):12–15, July–Aug 1982.

Cox SA: Perioperative nursing in the ambulatory setting, Point View 18(4):4–7, Oct 1981.

Curtin LL: Ambulatory surgery: Organization, finance, and regulation, Nurs Manage 15(6):22–24, June 1984.

Hoffmann GL: Quality control in ambulatory surgery, Bull Am Coll Surg 66(11):6–8, Nov 1981.

Horwitz R: Ambulatory surgery: Care of the patient under local anesthesia, Point View 22(2):14–15, May 1985.

Levinski B: A satellite OR: One hospital's answer, Todays OR Nurse 5(5):18–21, July 1983.

Maudlin BC (ed): *Ambulatory Surgery: A Guide to Perioperative Nursing Care,* New York: Grune & Stratton, 1983.

Palmer PN: Ambulatory surgery means business, AORN J 38(3):470, 472–473, Sep 1983.

Schneck LH: Ambulatory surgery: Its origin, its present state, and its future direction, AORN J 40(2):248–250, Aug 1984.

Stump D: An outpatient/same-day surgery program based on peer review, QRB 9(4):112–115, Apr 1983.

Thee KG, Obrecht W: Using a patient routing list to document preoperative instruction, QRB 10(5):149–150, May 1984.

Wetchler BV: Anesthesia for outpatient surgery, AORN J 34(2):282, 284, 286, 288, 290, 292, 294–296, Aug 1981.

Wetchler BV: Postanesthesia scoring system: Discharging ambulatory surgery patients, AORN J 41(2):382–384, Feb 1985.

Wetchler BV: The role of anesthesia in outpatient surgery, Todays OR Nurse 4(7):18–23, 62, Sep 1982.

Wright G et al: Utilization review to increase ambulatory-based surgery, QRB 9(4):100–106, Apr 1983.

Williams S: How can computers be used in the operating department?, Br J Theatre Nurs 21(4):6, 8–9, Apr 1984.

CHAPTER 6
PHYSICAL FACILITIES

Beck WC: Operating room illumination: The current state-of-the-art, Bull Am Coll Surg 66(5):10–15, May 1981.

Cook M: Selecting the right computer system, Nurs Manage 13(8):26–28, Aug 1982.

DeVera F et al: Using computers in the OR, AORN J 38(3):438, 440–441, 444–445, Sep 1983.

Edmunds L: Computer-assisted nursing care, Am J Nurs 82(7):1076–1079, July 1982.

Foley ER: OR design shows nurses' touch, AORN J 36(2):288–293, Aug 1982.

Hatridge L: Holding room in the O.R. a must, Point View 21(3):15, Sep 1984.

Heyes CC, Smith KF: A computer information system for the OR suite, AORN J 33(4):672–676, Mar 1981.

Hinshaw JR: The art and science of OR management, Bull Am Coll Surg 66(5):6–9, May 1981.

Klebanoff G: Operating-room design: An introduction, Bull Am Coll Surg 64(11):6–10, Nov 1979.

Laufman H (ed): *Hospital Special Care Facilities—Planning for User Needs,* New York: Academic Press 1981.

Lee AA: What computers can do for you . . . and what they're already doing for the lucky few, RN 45(9):43–44, 121–122, 124, 126–127, Sep 1982.

LoCicero J, Nichols RL: Environmental health hazards in the operating room, Bull Am Coll Surg 67(5):2–5, May 1982.

McGuire HP: Computerizing an OR, AORN J 39(2):184–189, Feb 1984.

McNeal A: Making case carts work, Todays OR Nurse 6(7):8–10, 12, July 1984.

Minimum Requirements of Construction and Equipment for Hospitals and Medical Facilities, Rockville, Md.: HHS Publication HRS-M-HF-84-1, 1984.

OR lights, J Oper Rm Res Inst 2(8):8–12, 21–23, 38–41, Aug 1982.

Paquet JB: OR computers: The future is today, Todays OR Nurse 4(9):10–16, Nov 1982.

Radziewicz KM: Programming for success, Todays OR Nurse 5(10):16–17, 20–22, Dec 1983.

Recommended practices for traffic patterns in the surgical suite, AORN J 35(4):750, 754–755, 758, Mar 1982.

Reilly D: A computerized patient information system, Nurs Manage 13(8):32–36, Aug 1982.

Thomas R: Unidirectional flow vs traditional system, AORN J 31(4):722, 724, 726, 728, 730, 732–733, 736, Mar 1980.

Weeks J: The planning of operating theatre suites, NATNews 19(7):9–12, July 1982.

CHAPTER 7
ASEPSIS, INFECTION CONTROL, AND PRINCIPLES OF STERILE TECHNIQUE

Allen JR: Wound infection: Identifying the source, Todays OR Nurse 6(9):10–17, Sep 1983.

Beck WC: Aseptic barriers in surgery: Their present status, Arch Surg 116(2):240–244, Feb 1981.

Brown P et al: Sodium hydroxide decontamination of Creutzfeldt-Jakob disease virus, N Engl J Med 310(11):727, Mar 15, 1984.

Conte JE Jr et al: Infection control guidelines for patients with AIDS: Special report, Hosp Top 62(2):44–48, Mar–Apr 1984.

Coppage D: Reality and accountability of hospital environmental control, Point view 22(1):4–5, Jan 1985.

Crow S, Greene VW: Aseptic transgressions among surgeons and anesthesiologists: A quantitative study, Arch Surg 117(8):1012–1016, Aug 1982.

Crow S, Taylor E: Nurses' compliance with aseptic technique, AORN J 37(6):1066–1072, May 1983.

Cruse PJE, Foord R: The epidemiology of wound infection: A ten-year prospective study of 62,939 wounds, Surg Clin North Am, 60(1):27–40, Feb 1980.

Devorene et al: Torch infections, Am J Nurs 83(12): 1660–1665, Dec 1983.

Engelhard LA: AIDS: A killer confined, Todays OR Nurse 5(10):26–30, 34, Dec 1983.

Fernsebner B: Antimicrobial therapy for surgical patients, AORN J 36(3):479–486, Sep 1982.

Fernsebner B: Patients at risk for nosocomial infections, AORN J 38(4):613–617, 620, Oct 1983.

Freeman BA (ed): *Burrows Textbook of Microbiology,* 22d ed, Philadelphia: Saunders, 1984.

Garner JS et al: Epidemic infections in surgical patients, AORN J 34(4):700–701, 704–705, 708–709, 712–713, 716, 721, 724, Oct 1981.

Garner JS, Simmons BP: CDC guideline for isolation precautions in hospitals, Infect Control 4(4):249–325, July–Aug 1983.

Gurevich I: For CE credit: Viral hepatitis, Am J Nurs 83(4):571–586, Apr 1983.

Harvey CK et al: The experts research: Q&A: AIDS: A frightening disease in the OR, AORN J 37(6):1036, 1038, May 1983.

Harvey CK: The experts research: Q&A: Rare virus requires "overkill" cleanup despite some damage, AORN J 37(2):169–170, Feb 1983.

Harvey EL, Middaugh SE: Discipline without punishment, AORN J 37(5):914, 916–917, 920, 922, 924, Apr 1983.

Jackson MM, Lynch P: Infection control: Too much or too little, Am J Nurs 84(2):208–211, Feb 1984.

Jarvis WR: Precautions for Creutzfeldt-Jakob disease, Infect Control 3(3):238–239, May–June 1982.

Killion A: Reducing the risk of infection from indwelling urethral catheters, Nursing (Horsham) 12(5):84–88, May 1982.

Kirkman-Liff BL, Dandoy S: Hepatitis B exposures: A study of the risks and costs, AORN J 40(3):366–367, 369–370, Sep 1984.

Landsman S et al: Special report: The AIDS epidemic, N Engl J Med 312(8):521–525, Feb 21, 1985.

Laufman H et al: Scanning electron microscopy of moist bacterial strike-through of surgical materials, Surg Gynecol Obstet 150(2):165–170, Feb 1980.

Lucey J, Baroni M: Herpetic whitlow, Am J Nurs 84(1):60–61, Jan 1984.

Mathieu A, Burke JF: *Infection and the Perioperative Period,* New York: Grune & Stratton, 1982.

Mauldin BC: Need for basic aseptic technic, Point View 19(3):10–11, 1982.

Nelson JP: Effectiveness, costs of clean rooms, helmet aspirators, AORN J 27(4):718, 720, 722, 724, 726, 728, 730, 732, 734, Mar 1978.

Platt R et al: Mortality associated with nosocomial urinary-tract infection, N Engl J Med 307(11):637–642, Sep 9, 1982.

Poland V: What high-risk personnel need to know about the hepatitis B vaccine, AORN J 40(3):372–373, Sep 1984.

Popkin B et al: Nursing grand rounds: Caring for the AIDS patient—fearlessly, Nursing (Horsham) 13(9):50–55, Sep 1983.

Questions and answers: Acquired immune deficiency syndrome, JAMA 250(4):539, July 22/29, 1983.

Quraishi ZA: Movement of personnel and wound contamination, AORN J 38(1):146–147, 150, 152, 154, 156, July 1983.

Recommended practices for basic aseptic technique, *AORN Standards and Recommended Practices for Perioperative Nursing:* Part III, section 2-1-4, Denver: Association of Operating Room Nurses, Inc., 1985.

Simmons BP: CDC guidelines for prevention of surgical wound infections, AORN J 37(3):556, 560–562, 564–565, 568–569, 572–574, Feb 1983.

Simmons BP et al: CDC guidelines for the prevention and control of nosocomial infections: Guideline for hospital environmental control, Am J Infect Control 11(3):97–120, June 1983.

Stratton CW (ed): Topics in clinical microbiology: Creutzfeldt-Jakob disease: Procedures for handling diagnostic and research materials, Infect Control 5(1):48–50, Jan–Feb 1984.

West KH: Infection control: Communicable diseases in the OR: When are you at risk?, J Oper Rm Res Inst 3(7):14–15, 18, 20, July 1983.

Whettam J: Update on toxic shock: How to spot it and treat it, RN 47(2):55–56, 58, 60, Feb 1984.

Williams WW: CDC guideline for infection control in hospital personnel, Infect Control 4(4):326–349, July–Aug 1983.

Williams WW: CDC guidelines for the prevention and control of nosocomial infections: Guideline for infection control in hospital personnel, Am J Infect Control 12(1):34–63, Feb 1984.

Wroblewski SS: Toxic shock syndrome, Am J Nurs 81(1):82–85, Jan 1981.

CHAPTER 8
STERILIZATION AND DISINFECTION

Association for the Advancement of Medical Instrumentation Steam Sterilization Subcommittee: *Good Hospital Practice: Steam Sterilization and Sterility Assurance,* Arlington, Va.: AAMI, 1980.

Association for the Advancement of Medical Instrumentation Sterilization Committee: *Good Hospital Practice: Ethylene Oxide Gas—Ventilation Recommendations and Safe Use,* Arlington, Va.: AAMI, 1981.

AORN recommended practices for inhospital sterilization, AORN J 32(2):222, 224–225, 228, 230, 238–239, 243–244, 246, Aug 1980.

AORN recommended practices: Recommended practices for inhospital packaging materials, AORN J 37(2):255–256, 258, Feb 1983.

Greene VW et al: Effects of patching on sterilization of surgical textiles, AORN J 33(7):1249–1261, June 1981.

Karle DA, Ryan P: Guidelines for evaluating wet packs, AORN J 38(2):244–245, 248, 250, 252, 254, 256, Aug 1983.

Kralovic R: Powered surgical instruments: HIMA guidelines and implications, AORN J 41(1):264, 266, 268, Jan 1985.

Leach ED: A new synergized glutaraldehydephenate sterilizing solution and concentrated disinfectant, Infect Control 2(1):26–30, 1981.

Litsky BY: Microbiology of sterilization, AORN J 26(2):334, 337, 339–340, 342, 344, 346, 348, 350, Aug 1977.

Mattia MA: Hazards in the hospital environment: The sterilants: Ethylene oxide and formaldehyde, Am J Nurs 83(2):240–243, Feb 1983.

Occupational Safety and Health Administration: Ethylene oxide standard, Federal Register 49: Rules and Regulations 25734–25809, June 22, 1984.

Pepper RE: Comparison of the activities and stabilities of alkaline glutaraldehyde sterilizing solutions, Infect Control 1(2):90–92, 1980.

Perkins JJ: *Principles and Methods of Sterilization in Health Sciences,* 2d ed., Springfield, Ill.: Chas. C Thomas, 1980.

Phillips GB: Industrial sterilization of medical devices,

AORN J 37(6):1225–1226, 1228, 1230, 1232, 1234, May 1983.

Samuels TM: Occupational exposure to ethylene oxide: OSHA's new proposed rule—a document whose time has come!, Hosp Top 61(4):35–37, July–Aug 1983.

Schneider PM: Powered surgical instruments: Microbiological considerations in sterilization, AORN J 41(1):254, 256, 258, 260, 262, Jan 1985.

Smith RF: Microbiological safety index, AORN J 36(2):311, 314–316, Aug 1982.

Sparks BJ: Product sterilization: Why industry uses radiation, AORN J 40(3):388–390, Sep 1984.

CHAPTER 9
SURGICAL SCRUB, GOWNING, AND GLOVING

AORN recommended practices: Recommended practices for aseptic barrier materials for surgical gowns, AORN J 37(2):253–255, Feb 1983.

Barry RF: The evolution of face masks, J Oper Rm Res Inst 2(8):26–31, Aug 1982.

Fay MF: Glove powders on trial, Todays OR Nurse 5(9):9–12, Nov 1983.

Fay MF: The threat of talc on surgical gloves, Todays OR Nurse 4(9):27–29, 31, Nov 1982.

Jensen KME et al: The role of surgical face masks in preventing infection, Asepsis 4(2):10–15, Mar–Apr 1982.

Kaul AF, Jewett JF: Agents and techniques for disinfection of the skin, Surg Gynecol Obstet 152(5):677–685, May 1981.

Moylan JA: Clinical evaluation of gown-and-drape barrier performance, Bull Am Coll Surg 67(5):8–12, May 1982.

Moylan JA, Kennedy BV: The importance of gown and drape barriers in the prevention of wound infections, Surg Gynecol Obstet 151(4):465–470, Oct 1980.

Recommended practices: OR attire, AORN J 39(4):710, 713–714, 718, 720, Mar 1984.

Recommended practices: Surgical scrubs, AORN J 39(6):1084, 1086, 1088, May 1984.

Roth RA, Whitbourne J: A pilot study of open and closed surgical gloving, AORN J 36(4):571–576, Oct 1982.

Schwartz JT, Saunders DE: Microbial penetration of surgical gown materials, Surg Gynecol Obstet 150(4):507–512, Apr 1980.

CHAPTER 10
DIVISION OF DUTIES: SETUP, PROCEDURE, CLEANUP

Bahu GAB: Administering blood safely, AORN J 37(6):1073–1077, 1080–1081, 1084–1087, 1090–1091, 1094–1096, 1100, May 1983.

Cozad J: Autologous blood recovery, Point View 22(2):20, May 1985.

Darden ML: Blood loss determination, AORN J 33(7):1367–1368, 1372, 1374, 1378, 1380, June 1981.

Duff L: Intraoperative autotransfusion, AORN J 37(6):1102, 1104, 1106, 1108–1109, 1112, May 1983.

Greaves J: Implementing counts in the operating room, NATNews 18(7):19–22, July 1981.

Kirkis J, Ettorre DM: Seven sticky problems (and their solutions) in blood transfusions, RN 46(4):59–62, 94, Apr 1983.

Laufman H: Operating room cleanup techniques, J Surg Pract 8(1):65–67, 69–70, Jan–Feb 1979.

Leser DR: Synthetic blood: A future alternative, Am J Nurs 82(3):452–455, Mar 1982.

Levine AH, Imai PK: Hypothermia and hemodilution with autologous transfusion, AORN J 37(6):1060–1065, May 1983.

Litsky BY: A universal infection control problem: Clean up in the operating room, Surg Technol 15(1):42–43, Jan–Feb 1983.

Masoorli ST, Piercy S: A lifesaving guide to blood products, RN 47(9):32–37, Sep 1984.

Masoorli ST, Piercy S: A step-by-step guide to trouble-free transfusions, RN 47(5):34–38, May 1984.

Petty C: Assisting the patient receiving a regional anesthetic, Point View 21(3):16–17, Sep 1984.

Querin JJ: 12 simple, sensible steps for successful blood transfusions, Nursing (Horsham) 13(11):34–45, Nov 1983.

Ravitch MM: The incision, Surg Technol 15(1):27–28, Jan–Feb 1983.

Recommended practices: OR sanitation, AORN J 39(5):838–840, 843, 844, Apr 1984.

Recommended practices: Sponge, sharp and instrument counts, AORN J 39(4):699, 702–703, 706, Mar 1984.

Schwarz T: It's not artificial blood—but it can do the work of RBCs, RN 45(10):38–41, Oct 1982.

Sheridan D: EBL study, Surg Technol 13(4):18, 20–21, July–Aug 1981.

Steel J: Too fast or too slow—the erratic IV, Am J Nurs 83(6):898–901, June 1983.

Warren M: The total care of a patient within the operating department, NATNews 18(4):13–15, Apr 1981.

CHAPTER 11
ECONOMY, WORK SIMPLIFICATION, AND SAFETY

Bird S, Mailhot C: DRGs: A new way to reimburse hospital costs, AORN J 38(5):773–777, Nov 1983.

Clark D et al: The care and use of surgical instruments, Surg Technol 15(5):32–33, Sep–Oct 1983.

Dowd SB: Radiation exposure to the surgical technologist, Surg Technol 16(4):26–29, July–Aug 1984.

Handy DA: When time is money, A study in cost effectiveness, Todays OR Nurse 6(4):16–18, Apr 1984.

Hirsh JH: Across the table, Todays OR Nurse 4(10):28–30, Dec 1982.

Keelan JA, Stokoe SJ: Taking the stress out of OR communication, AORN J 37(5):847–853, Apr 1983.

Koch F et al: Four experts talk about: Reprocessing disposable items, AORN J 38(3):427–429, 432, 434, 436, Sep 1983.

Koerner M et al: Communicating in the OR, AORN J 39(7):1158–1162, June 1984.

MacClelland DC: Therapeutic communication through music, Point View 19(1):4–5, Jan 1982.

McCluskey FJ: Music in the operating suite, NATNews 20(9):33, 35, 38, 40, Sep 1983.

Swanberg G, Fahey B: More operating rooms or better use of resources?, Nurs Manage 14(5):16–19, May 1983.

The Care and Handling of Surgical Instruments, Randolph, Ma.: Codman & Shurtleff, 1981.

Thompson LF: The role of the surgical technologist, Surg Technol 14(4):22–23, July–Aug 1982.

Thro E: Surgical instruments: Their care and characteristics, J Oper Rm Res Inst 3(9):3–8, Sep 1983.

Voetz GL: Ionizing radiation, Occup Health Safety 51(7):34–37, July 1982.

Wilson DC: Efficient OR management, Nurs Manage 15(5):38A–38D, 38H–38J, 38L–38N, May 1984.

Wilson E: Nursing care in a technological age, Superv Nurse 12(6):59, 62, June 1981.

Young R, Walsh P: Sterilization of powered surgical instruments, AORN J 37(5):945–946, 948, 950, 952–953, 957, Apr 1983.

CHAPTER 12
LIABILITY AND ACCOUNTABILITY

Buckingham WB, Gardner K: An inside look at malpractice by an expert witness, QRB 8(1):7–10, Jan 1982.

Cushing M: The legal side: A matter of judgment, Am J Nurs 82(6):990, 992, June 1982.

Cushing M: The legal side: Expanding the meaning of accountability, Am J Nurs 83(8):1202–1203, Aug 1983.

Cushing M: The legal side: Informed consent—An MD responsibility?, Am J Nurs 84(4):437, 439–440, Apr 1984.

Cushing M: The legal side: Malpractice: Are you covered?, Am J Nurs 84(8):985–986, Aug 1984.

Gebhard PG: The surgeon's liability in endoscopy, Bull Am Coll Surg 69(6):33–35, June 1984.

Geldbach PL et al: Quality control circles solving OR problems, AORN J 34(6):1029–1035, Dec 1981.

Lomando K, Faulconer DR: A workable plan for OR quality assurance, AORN J 35(7):1291–1295, June 1982.

Randall JP: Nursing law at your fingertips, Nurs Life 2(1):61–68, Jan–Feb 1982.

Reed EA: Quality assurance: The JCAH standard, AORN J 35(7):1287–1290, June 1982.

Reed ME: A hospital's liability for negligence, Bull Am Coll Surg 68(5):18–20, May 1983.

Reed ME: Liability under the extension doctrine, Bull Am Coll Surg 68(11):14–15, Nov 1983.

Reed ME: Operating surgeon's liability for the negligence of an assisting nurse, Bull Am Coll Surg 67(11):19–20, Nov 1982.

Sandroff S: Why you really ought to have your own malpractice policy, RN 46(6):28–33, June 1983.

Spaulding JA: Risk management: A hospital-wide approach, Nurs Manage 13(4):29–31, Apr 1982.

Tilbury MS, Ganley S: The perioperative role: New avenue for risk management, Todays OR Nurse 4(4):16–19, June 1982.

Wrenn AJ: The incidence report as a risk management tool, Superv Nurse 12(1):34–35, Jan 1981.

CHAPTER 13
ANESTHESIA: CONCEPTS, TECHNIQUES, AND AGENTS

Abouleish E: Epidural blood patch for the treatment of chronic post-lumbar-puncture cephalgia, Anesthesiology 49(4):291–292, Oct 1978.

American Society of Anesthesiologists: *Annual Refresher Course Lectures, 1982,* Park Ridge, Ill.: 1982.

Bailey CJ et al: Epidural morphine infusion: Continuous pain relief, AORN J 39(6):997, 1000, 1002, 1004–1005, 1008, May 1984.

Brodsky JB: Exposure to anesthetic gases: A controversy, AORN J 38(1):132, 134, 136–137, 140–141, 144, July 1983.

Brown DG et al: Anesthetic gas exposure, AORN J 41(3):590, 591, 594, 596, 598–599, 602–603, 606–608, Mar 1985.

Dripps RD et al: *Introduction to Anesthesia: The Principles of Safe Practice,* 6th ed, Philadelphia: Saunders, 1982.

Duberman S, Wald A: An integrated quality control program for anesthesia equipment, QRB 9(11):328–336, Nov 1983.

Etomidate for induction of anesthesia, Med Lett Drugs Ther 25(640):71–72, Aug 5, 1983.

Gever LN: Naloxone: Administering this narcotic antagonist safely, Nursing (Horsham) 13(5):102, May 1983.

Greene NM: Neurologic complications associated with regional anesthesia, Current Reviews Clin Anesthesia 2(26):202–208, 1982.

Hess J: What are the sounds of success in the OR?, Todays OR Nurse 7(2):28–30, 33, Feb 1985.

Hudson MF: Safeguard your elderly patient's health through accurate physical assessment, Nursing (Horsham) 13(11):58–64, Nov 1983.

Hussar DA: New drugs, Nursing (Horsham) 15(6):33–39, June 1985.

Luedtke M: Taking the chill out of surgery, Todays OR Nurse 5(10):32–33, Dec 1983.

Mattia MA: Hazards in the hospital environment: Anesthesia gases and methyl methacrylate, Am J Nurs 83(1):72–77, Jan 1983.

Moore DC et al: Long-acting local anesthetic drugs and convulsions with hypoxia and acidosis, Anesthesiology 56(3):230–232, Mar 1982.

Moree N et al: Great expectations: How do the new drugs measure up?, Am J Nurs 84(7):906, July 1984.

Nursing update: Narcotic and opioid analgesics, Nursing (Horsham) 13(10):64a, Oct 1983.

Petty C: Assisting the patient receiving a regional anesthetic, Point View 21(3):16–17, Sep 1984.

Recommended practices: Cleaning and processing anesthesia equipment, AORN J 41(3):625, 627, 629, 631, Mar 1985.

Rodman M: New drugs of the year, Part 2, RN 46(5):69, May 1983.

Rogers AG: What to expect from the most common analgesics, RN 46(5):44–46, May 1983.

Tinker JH: Deliberate hypotension: How and when, Current Reviews Clin Anesthesia, 2(23):178–184, 1982.

Tobias R: Circulator, you can help your anesthetist, Point View 17(3):4–5, July 1980.

Wade JG, Stevens WC: Isoflurane: An anesthetic for the eighties?, Anesth Analg (Cleve) 60(9):666–682, Sep 1981.

Walts LF: Trace anesthetic gases: An unproven health hazard, AORN J 37(4):728, 729, 732, 736, 737, 740, Mar 1983.

Wlody GS: Isoflurane: The newest anesthetic agent, AORN J 40(4):568–571, Oct 1984.

Yaksh TL: Spinal opiate analgesia: Characteristics and principles of action, Pain 11(3):293–346, Dec 1981.

CHAPTER 14 PATIENT MONITORING, POTENTIAL COMPLICATIONS UNDER ANESTHESIA, AND CARDIOPULMONARY RESUSCITATION

Adelman EM, Thornton SR: Cardiac crisis: Are you *sure* you know what to do?, RN 46(8):22–29, Aug 1983.

American Society of Anesthesiologists: Technical bulletin for malignant hyperthermia, ASA Newsletter, Anesthesia Technical Bulletin 1:5, Nov 1982.

Balloon flotation catheters: What they can tell you now, RN 46(9):36–41, Sep 1983.

Beal JM: *Critical Care for Surgical Patients,* New York: Macmillan, 1982.

Borchardt AC, Fraulini KE: Hypothermia in the postanesthetic patient, AORN J 36(4):648, 652–653, 656–657, 660–661, 664–665, 668–669, Oct 1982.

Brantigan CO: Hemodynamic monitoring: Interpreting values, Am J Nurs 82(1):86–89, Jan 1982.

Burkhardt SS: Patient monitoring in the operating room: An introduction and overview, J Oper Rm Res Inst 3(4):10, 14, 16, 18–19, 22, Apr 1983.

Computers assist anesthesia monitoring, AORN J 37(3):588, Feb 1983.

Darovic G et al: New protocols for the Swan-Ganz, RN 46(10):54–59, Oct 1983.

Fassi, AJ Jr, Wurm WH: Local anesthesia toxicity, Current Reviews Clin Anesthesia 2(11):82–88, 1981.

Fay MF, Delyanis VR: Intraoperative monitoring: The EEG monitor can be a window to the brain, AORN J 41(6):1046–1049, June 1985.

Fernsebner B: A protocol for malignant hyperthermia, AORN J 31(5):814–818, Apr 1980.

Galin R, Jaeger VG: What's wrong? An inservice for cardiac arrests, AORN J 35(5):956, 958, 960, 962, 964, 966, Apr 1982.

Gatch G: Cardiac arrest in the OR, AORN J 32(6):983–993, Dec 1980.

Gever LN: Administering epinephrine in an emergency, Nursing (Horsham) 15(6):65, June 1985.

Grundy BL et al: Intraoperative hypoxia detected by evoked potential monitoring, Anesth Analg (Cleve) 60(6):437–439, June, 1981.

Jones S: New IV catheters that can do it all, RN 48(2):20–23, Feb 1985.

Jones S: What to do after CPR: Use ABGs to fine-tune resuscitation, RN 48(5):35–41, May 1985.

Kaye W, Paraskos JA (eds): *Instructors Manual for Advanced Cardiac Life Support,* Dallas: American Heart Association, 1982.

Lalli SM: The complete Swan-Ganz, RN 41(9):64–78, Sep 1978.

Marchildon MB: Malignant hyperthermia: Current concepts, Arch Surg 117(3):349–351, Mar 1982.

Matheny LG: Defibrillation: When and how to use it, Nursing (Horsham) 11(6):69–72, June 1981.

McIntyre KM, Lewis AJ (eds): *Textbook of Advanced Cardiac Life Support,* Dallas: American Heart Association, 1983.

Niemczura J: 8 rules to remember when caring for a Swan-Ganz catheter, Nursing (Horsham) 15(3):38–41, Mar 1985.

Noback CR, Tinker JH: Hypothermia after cardiopulmonary bypass in man, Anesthesiology 53(4):277–280, Oct 1980.

Norsen LH, Fox GB: Understanding cardiac output and the drugs that affect it, Nursing (Horsham) 15(4):34–41, Apr 1985.

Nurses' drug alert: Elderly patients need smaller doses of morphine, Am J Nurs 82(5):842, May 1982.

Purcell JA: Shock drugs: Standardized guidelines, Am J Nurs 82(6):965–973, June 1982.

Recommended practices: Monitoring the patient receiving local anesthesia, AORN J 39(6):1080, 1082–1083, May 1984.

Rogers AL, Sturgeon CL Jr: Malignant hyperthermia: A perioperative emergency, AORN J 41(2):369–374, Feb 1985.

Rosenberg H: Malignant hyperpyrexia, Am J Nurs 81(8):1484–1486, Aug 1981.

Santolla A, Weckel C: A new closed system for arterial lines, RN 46(6):49–52, June 1983.

Scordo KA: Taming the cardiac monitor, Part 1, Nursing (Horsham) 12(8):58–63, Aug 1982.

Scordo KA: Understanding what the monitor's telling you: Taming the cardiac monitor, Part 2, Nursing (Horsham) 12(9):60–68, Sep 1982.

Seifert PC: Invasive hemodynamic monitoring, AORN J 38(3):416–425, Sep 1983.

Sigg LV, Fallucca LL: Recognizing hypoventilation in the recovery room, AORN J 38(2):270, 272, 274, 276–277, 280, 282, 284–285, Aug 1983.

Standards and guidelines for cardiopulmonary resuscitation (CPR) and emergency cardiac care (ECC), JAMA 244(5):453–509, Aug 1, 1980.

Stanford JL et al: Antiarrhythmic drug therapy, Am J Nurs 80(7):1288–1295, July 1980.

Sweeney SS: OR observations: Key to postop pain, AORN J 32(3):391–400, Sep 1980.

Technology today: Pick of the new products: Monitor checks urine output, RN 46(11):75, Nov 1983.

Using Monitors: Nursing Photobook, Horsham, Pa.: Intermed Communications, 1981.

Visalli F, Evans P: The Swan-Ganz catheter, a program for teaching safe, effective use, Nursing (Horsham) 11(1):42–47, Jan 1981.

Wells P: A teaching plan for emergency procedures, AORN J 37(5):989, 992, 994, 996–997, Apr 1983.

Yanick CB, Lavery S: Intraoperative cardiac arrest: Nursing implications, AORN J 41(2):404, 406, 408, 410–411, 413, 416, 418–419, 421, Feb 1985.

CHAPTER 15
POSITIONS

Foster CG et al: Effects of surgical positioning, AORN J 30(2):219–232, Aug 1979.

Martin JT: *Positioning in Anesthesia and Surgery,* Philadelphia: Saunders, 1978.

Merrill S: A teaching plan for positioning, AORN J 35(1):63–66, Jan 1982.

Phippen ML: OR nurses guide to preventing pressure sores, AORN J 36(2):205–212, Aug 1982.

Tobias R: Circulating responsibilities: An anesthetist's view, Surg Technol 13(3):12–14, 16–18, 20–22, May–June 1981.

CHAPTER 16
PREPARATION OF THE OPERATIVE SITE AND DRAPING

Alexander JW et al: The influence of hair-removal methods on wound infections, Arch Surg 118(3):347–352, Mar 1983.

AORN recommended practices: Recommended practices for aseptic barrier materials for surgical drapes, AORN J 37(2):249–250, Feb 1983.

AORN recommended practices: Recommended practices for preoperative skin preparation of patients, AORN J 37(2):244–245, 248, Feb 1983.

Beck WG: Benefits of alcohol rediscovered, AORN J 40(2):172, 174, 176, Aug 1984.

Bernard HR: Experiences with reusable barrier materials, 1976–1980, Bull Am Coll Surg 67(5):18–21, May 1982.

Brown TR et al: A clinical evaluation of chlorhexidine gluconate spray as compared with iodophor scrub for preoperative skin preparation, Surg Gynecol Obstet 158(4):363–366, Apr 1984.

Fay MF: Aseptic surgery in a bubble prevents postop infections, Todays OR Nurse 7(3):25–26, 28–29, Mar 1985.

Friedman FB: Why not use a Foley?, RN 45(11):71–72, 74, 76, Nov 1982.

Geelhoed GW et al: A comparative study of surgical skin preparation methods, Surg Gynecol Obstet 157(3):265–268, Sep 1983.

Geelhoed GW, Sharpe K: The rationale and ritual of preoperative skin preparation, Contemp Surg 23(9):31–36, Sep 1983.

Janoff K et al: Foreign body reactions secondary to cellulose lint fibers, Am J Surg 147(5):598–600, May 1984.

Laufman H: Surgical barrier materials: Product promotion vs controlled evidence, Bull Am Coll Surg 67(5):13–17, May 1982.

Masterson TM et al: Bacteriologic evaluation of electric clippers for surgical hair removal, Am J Surg 148(3):301–302, Sep 1984.

CHAPTER 17
WOUND HEALING AND METHODS OF HEMOSTASIS

Bolton ME: Hyperbaric oxygen therapy, Am J Nurs 81(6):1199–1201, June 1981.

Bremer C: Promoting healing of trauma wounds, AORN J 35(6):1150, 1154, 1156, 1160–1161, 1164, 1166, 1168, 1170, May 1982.

Bricker PL: Chest tubes: The crucial points you mustn't forget, RN 43(11):20–26, Nov 1980.

Collins PA: Hemostatic agents, J Oper Rm Res Inst 3(8):8–12, Aug 1983.

Ducey DY: The phases of wound healing and wound irrigation, Point View 20(4):4–7, Oct 1983.

Erickson R: Chest tubes: They're really not that complicated, Nursing (Horsham) 11(5):34–43, May 1981.

Flynn ME, Rovee DT: Wound healing mechanisms, Am J Nurs 82(10):1544–1558, Oct 1982.

Frogge MH: Promoting wound healing in the irradiated patient, AORN J 35(6):1088–1092, May 1982.

Fuller BF: Hemostasis: A balanced system, AORN J 34(2):225–230, Aug 1981.

Groszek DM: Promoting wound healing in the obese patient, AORN J 35(6):1132, 1134–1135, 1138, May 1982.

Keenan KM et al: Surgical cautery revisited, Am J Surg 147(6):818–821, June 1984.

Keithley JK: Wound healing in malnourished patients, AORN J 35(6):1094–1098, May 1982.

Kirschenbaum HL, Rosenberg JM: Coumarin, RN 45(1):54–56, Oct 1982.

Kloch SM, Kloch GM: Oral medications affecting blood coagulation, Plast Surg Nurs 4(2):52–55, Summer 1984.

Kottra CJ: Wound healing in immunosuppressed host, AORN J 35(6):1142, 1144–1145, 1148, May 1982.

McEwen JA: Complications of and improvements used in surgery, Surg Technol 14(1):23–28, Jan–Feb 1982.

McEwen JA, Auchinleck GF: Advances in surgical tourniquets, AORN J 36(5):889–896, Nov 1982.

Neuberger GB, Reckling JB: A new look at wound care, Nursing (Horsham) 15(2):34–41, Feb 1985.

Powanda MC: Plasma proteins and wound healing, Surg Gynecol Obstet 153(5):749–755, Nov 1981.

Recommended practices: Preparation, utilization, and maintenance of the pneumatic tourniquet, AORN J 39(2):808, 810, 812, Apr 1984.

Rosenberg JM, Kirschenbaum HL: Heparin, RN 44(9):50–52, Sep 1981.

Saum M: Taking the mystery out of chest tubes, AORN J 32(1):86, 88, 90, 92, 94, 96, 98–100, July 1980.

Schumann D: The nature of wound healing, AORN J 35(6):1068–1077, May 1982.

Schwartz SI et al: Symposium: Hemostasis, Contemp Surg 19(10):135–139, 142–143, 146–147, 151, 154–157, Oct 1981.

Strange JM: An expert's guide to tubes and drains, RN 46(4):34–42, Apr 1983.

Taylor DL: Clinical insights: Wound healing, Nursing (Horsham) 13(5):44–45, May 1983.

Yordan EL, Bernhard LA: The surgeon's role in wound healing, AORN J 35(6):1078–1082, May 1982.

CHAPTER 18
WOUND CLOSURE MATERIALS

Bonier P: An unusual alternative: Preparing the amniotic membrane dressing, Am J Nurs 85(4):418–419, Apr 1985.

Bright RN, Green WT: Freeze-dried fascia lata allografts: A review of 47 cases, J Pediatr Orthop 1(1):13–22, 1981.

Clark DE: Surgical suture material, Contemp Surg 17(1):33–35, 38–40, 42–43, 46–48, July 1980.

Dolph JL et al: Amnion: A useful biological dressing, Contemp Surg 17(2):65–66, Aug 1980.

Fielden HL: Surgical implants: Consumer aspects, AORN J 37(7):1315–1316, 1320–1321, June 1983.

Jasinkowski NL, Cullum JL: Human amniotic membrane, AORN J 39(5):894–895, 898–899, Apr 1984.

Johnson A et al: Automatic disposable stapling devices for wound closure, Ann Emerg Med 10(12):631–635, Dec 1981.

Kline SN, Rimer SR: Reconstruction of osseous defects with freeze-dried allogeneic and autogenous bone, Am J Surg 146(4):471–473, Oct 1983.

Medical device regs: Are they doing the job?, AORN J 33(5):946, 949–950, 952, 954, 956, 958, 960, Apr 1981.

Scott M: 32,000 years of sutures, NATNews 20(5):15–17, May 1983.

Trier WC: Considerations in the choice of surgical needles, Surg Gynecol Obstet 149(7):84–94, July 1979.

CHAPTER 19
STATE OF THE ART TECHNOLOGY: SPECIALIZED SURGICAL TOOLS

Ad hoc committee: Guidelines for preparation of laparoscopic instrumentation, AORN J 32(1):65–66, 70, 74, 76, July 1980.

Burkhardt SS: Lasers in medicine: An update, J Oper Rm Res Inst 3(7):6–7, 10–12, July 1983.

Crow S et al: Disinfection or sterilization? Four views on arthroscopes, AORN J 37(5):854–859, 862, 864, 866, 868, Apr 1983.

Fay MF: Harnessing light for lasers, Todays OR Nurse 6(5):8–11, May 1984.

Gray FN: CO_2 lasers: Everything you wanted to know about lasers ... and more, Todays OR Nurse 6(5):14–17, 20–21, May 1984.

Gray R: The cleaning and disinfection of flexible endoscopes and their accessories, NATNews 19(9):30–32, Sep 1982.

Harvey CK: The experts research: Q & A, AORN J 38(2):196, 198, Aug 1983.

Hausner K: Electrosurgery and patient monitoring, Med Electronics, No 85:110–113, Feb 1984.

Huether SE: How lasers work, AORN J 38(2):207–215, Aug 1983.

Larrow L, Noe JM: Port wine stain hemangiomas, Am J Nurs 82(5):786–790, May 1982.

Lundergan D, Smith S: Nurses' administrative responsibilities for lasers, AORN J 38(2):217–222, Aug 1983.

MacDonald E: Rigid endoscopes, Part I, AORN J 39(7):1236–1237, 1240, 1242, 1244, June 1984; Part II, AORN J 40(1):46, 58, 60, 62, 63, July 1984; Part III, AORN J 40(2):230, 232, 236, 238, 240, Aug 1984.

Pfister J, Kneedler JA: *A Guide to Lasers in the OR,* Aurora, Colo.: Education Design, 1983.

Pilcher L: Carbon dioxide lasers in laryngeal surgery, AORN J 33(7):1402–1407, June 1981.

Recommended practices: Electrosurgery, AORN J 41(3):633, 635, 637, 639, 641, Mar 1985.

Rogers P et al: *Laser Safety in Surgery and Medicine,* Cincinnati: Rockwell Associates, 1984.

Serafin D, Georgiade NC: *A Laboratory Manual of Microsurgery*, Durham, N.C.: Duke University Medical Center, 1983.

Superior disinfection of endoscopes, Infectious Diseases, 11(9):17, Sep 1981.

Thiele B: Electrosurgery is 'cool,' Surg Technol 12(4): 6–10, July–Aug 1980.

CHAPTER 20 DIAGNOSTIC PROCEDURES

Balch CM: Cancer surgery, Bull Am Coll Surg 69(1):3–7, Jan 1984.

Bastarache MM et al: Assessing peripheral vascular disease: Noninvasive testing, Am J Nurs 83(11):1552–1556, Nov 1983.

Berger ME, Hübner KF: Hospital hazards: Diagnostic radiation, Am J Nurs 83(8):1155–1159, Aug 1983.

Cook CV, Cook BA: Nuclear magnetic resonance scanning: New wave imaging modality, Can Nurse 80(6):36–38, June 1984.

Criss E: Digital subtraction angioplasty, Am J Nurs 82(11):1706–1707, Nov 1982.

Haughey CW: What to say . . . and do . . . when your patient asks about CT scans, Nursing (Horsham) 11(12):72–77, Dec 1981.

Hurwitz M: Intraoperative ultrasound, AORN J 38(6):979–984, Dec 1983.

Kindschi GW: Frozen sections: Their use and abuse, JAMA 251(19):2559–2560, May 18, 1984.

Little JR et al: Intravenous digital substraction angiography in brain ischemia, JAMA 247(23):3213–3216, June 18, 1982.

Marinelli-Miller D: What your patient wants to know about angiography—but may not ask, RN 46(11):52–54, Nov 1983.

Mason K: Safer lumbar myelograms—the search continues, Can Nurse 79(6):28, June 1983.

Moosa AR: The impact of computed tomography and ultrasonography on surgical practice, Bull Am Coll Surg 67(11):10–14, Nov 1982.

Nuclear magnetic resonance devices approved, FDA Bull 14(2):18, Aug 1984.

Osbakken M: Nuclear magnetic resonance imaging: Surgical applications, Bull Am Coll Surg 69(6):3–11, June 1984.

Schneck LH: Nuclear magnetic resonance, AORN J 39(7):1182, 1184–1185, 1188, 1190, 1192–1193, June 1984.

CHAPTER 21 GENERAL SURGERY

Abcarian H: Anorectal disorders: When is conservative care enough?, Modern Med 48(1):37–41, 44, Jan 1980.

Atkinson LJ: Trends in gastrointestinal surgery, Point View 18(3):4–5, July 1981.

Beck ML: Preparing your patient physically for an esophagogastroduodenoscopy, Nursing (Horsham) 11(2):88, 90–91, 94, 96, Feb 1981.

Brogberg M: Surgical management of breast cancer, Surg Technol 14(4):16–20, July–Aug 1982.

Brooks P: Duodenal ulcer operation: Billroth I & II gastro-enterostomy, Surg Technol 17(1):14–19, Jan–Feb 1985.

Busuttil RW: Selective and nonselective shunts for variceal bleeding, Am J Surg 148(1):27–35, July 1984.

Carey LC: Gastrointestinal and biliary conditions, Bull Am Coll Surg 67(1):15–17, Jan 1982.

Crooks L (ed): *Operating Room Techniques for the Surgical Team,* Boston: Little Brown, 1979.

D'Agostino R: Abdominal gunshot wounds: Exploratory laparotomy, Surg Technol 15(4):33–40, July–Aug 1983.

Dam C: From jejunoileal bypass to gastroplasty, Surg Technol 14(5):10–14, 16–19, Sep–Oct 1982.

Danzi JT: Endoscopy and the surgeon, Bull Am Coll Surg 69(6):30–32, June 1984.

Fisher B et al: Five-year results of a randomized clinical trial comparing total mastectomy and segmental mastectomy with or without radiation in the treatment of breast carcinoma, N Engl J Med 312(11): 665–673, Mar 14, 1985.

Gebhart EM: Perioperative care of the ostomy patient, AORN J 36(2):296, 298–299, 302–303, 306–307, 310, Aug 1982.

Gruber M, Nuwer N: Treating esophageal varices with injection sclerotherapy, Am J Nurs 82(8):1214–1216, Aug 1982.

Halverson JD: The aftermath of intestinal bypass, Bull Am Coll Surg 67(6):8–9, June 1982.

Hambrick E: Colon and rectal surgery, Bull Am Coll Surg 69(1):12–14, Jan 1984.

Herrington JL: Proximal gastric vagotomy, JAMA 249(18):2553, May 13, 1983.

Hymphreys JW Jr: General surgery redefined in the era of specialization, Bull Am Coll Surg 69(7):4–6, July 1984.

Jones RS: Gastrointestinal, biliary, and pancreatic surgery, Bull Am Coll Surg 68(1):13–17, Jan 1983.

Kostiak PE: The splenic mystique: An anatomical & physiological review of the spleen, Surg Technol 15(4):31–32, July–Aug 1983.

Little L: Vagotomy and antrectomy, Surg Technol 15(4):17–20, July–Aug 1983.

McCarver L: Cholecystitis: Cholecystectomy with x-ray, Surg Technol 15(5):28–30, Sep–Oct 1983.

Peternel E: A high-tech approach to a GI problem, RN 48(6):44–47, June 1985.

Rossi RL, Braasch JW: Surgery of biliary cancer: When to do what, Surg Technol 15(2):31–32, 34–38, Mar–Apr 1983.

Russell TR et al: Percutaneous gastrostomy, Am J Surg 148(1):132–137, July 1984.

Sabina S: Carcinoma of the thyroid, Surg Technol 15(4):12–14, July–Aug 1983.

Saik RP et al: Pros and cons of parietal cell versus truncal vagotomy, Am J Surg 148(1):93–98, July 1984.

Silen W: Gastrointestinal and biliary conditions, Bull Am Coll Surg 69(1):15–18, Jan 1984.

Simmons S, Given B: Nissen fundoplication for hiatus hernia repair, AORN J 34(1):35–46, July 1981.

Sproat C: Gastric stapling for morbid obesity, Surg Technol 13(4):14, 16–17, July–Aug 1981.

Terry BE: Surgical management of morbid obesity, Bull Am Coll Surg 67(6):3–5, June 1982.

Thompson C: Cholecystitis: Cholecystectomy, Surg Technol 13(3):28–29, 31, May–June 1981.

CHAPTER 22
GYNECOLOGY AND OBSTETRICS

Affonso DD, Stichler JF: Cesarean birth: Women's reactions, Am J Nurs 80(3):468–470, Mar 1980.

Baggish MS: High-power-density carbon dioxide laser therapy for early cervical neoplasia, Am J Obstet Gynecol 136(1):117–125, Jan 1, 1980.

Brengman SL, Burns MK: Vaginal delivery after C-section, Am J Nurs 83(11):1544–1547, Nov 1983.

Dingle RE et al: Continuous transcutaneous O_2 monitoring in the neonate, Am J Nurs 80(5):890–893, May 1980.

Dugan KK: The bleak outlook on ovarian cancer, Am J Nurs 85(2):144–147, Feb 1985.

Evans C, Shapiro P: Gynecologic microsurgery, Todays OR Nurse 5(9):16–20, Nov 1983.

Faulconer DR et al: Decentralizing cesarean births to labor and delivery, Todays OR Nurse 5(3):10–15, May 1983.

Fleming C, Jenks AD: Microscopic tubal reversal, AORN J 37(2):199–204, Feb 1983.

Gelfant BB: Preoperative teaching of gynecological patients, Point View 21(1):4–7, Jan 1984.

Griffin ME: Resolving infertility: An emotional crisis, AORN J 38(4):597–601, Oct 1983.

Guidelines for preparation of laparoscopic instrumentation, AORN J 32(1):65–66, 70, 74, 76, July 1980.

Hallmark G, Findlay M: Cesarean birth in the operating room, AORN J 36(6):978–984, Dec 1982.

Hedahl KJ: Cesarean birth, a real family affair, Am J Nurs 80(3):471–472, Mar 1980.

Holden LS: Helping your patient through her hysterectomy, RN 46(9):42–46, Sep 1983.

Jackson SH et al: Effects of fathers at cesarean birth on postpartum infection rates, AORN J 36(6):973–977, Dec 1982.

Kovacs RR: When your patient is also pregnant, AORN J 36(4):559–565, Oct 1982.

Lagasse LD: Obstetrics and gynecology, Bull Am Coll Surg 70(1):22–25, Jan 1985.

Levine AH, Imai PK: Intrauterine treatment of fetal hydronephrosis, AORN J 35(4):655–662, Mar 1982.

Loughlin, Sister N: Cesarean childbirth: Current perspectives, Todays OR Nurse, 4(6):8–13, 46, 49, Aug 1982.

Manzagol KA: Gynecologic surgery using the CO_2 laser, Point View 21(1):14–16, Jan 1984.

Patterson P: Fetal therapy: Issues we face, AORN J 35(4):663–668, Mar 1982.

Pritchard J et al (eds): *Williams Obstetrics,* 17th ed, Norwalk, Ct.: Appleton-Century-Crofts, 1985.

Puls KS: Abruptio placentae, Nursing (Horsham) 12(9):69, Sep 1982.

Reedy NJ et al: Intrauterine fetal surgery: A nursing challenge, J Obstet Gynecol Neonatal Nurs 13(5):291–295, Sep–Oct 1984.

Robusto N: Advising patients on sex after surgery, AORN J 32(1):55–61, July 1980.

Rogers SF, Moore J: Variations in vaginal surgery: Severe uterine prolapse and vaginal wall defects, Point View 21(1):8–10, Jan 1984.

Romney SL et al (ed): *Gynecology and Obstetrics: The Health Care of Women,* 2d ed, New York: McGraw-Hill, 1981.

Sachs BP et al: Cesarean section: Risks and benefits for mother and fetus, JAMA 250(16):2157–2159, Oct 28, 1983.

Wells MP: In vitro fertilization: Hope for childless couples, AORN J 38(4):591–596, Oct 1983.

Winer WK: Laser treatment of cervical neoplasia, Am J Nurs 82(9):1384–1387, Sep 1982.

Youngstrom PC et al: Pain relief and plasma concentrations from epidural and intramuscular morphine in post-cesarean patients, Anesthesiology 57(5):404–409, Nov 1982.

Zinn SE et al: Opinions: Should cesarean sections be done in OR or OB?, AORN J 31(5):936, 938, 940, 942, Apr 1980.

CHAPTER 23
UROLOGY

Barrett N: Ileal loop and body image, AORN J 36(4):712, 716, 718, 720, 722, Oct 1982.

Blume E: Sound, shock waves shatter kidney stones, JAMA 249(18):2434–2435, May 13, 1983.

Bushey J: An introduction to cysto, Todays OR Nurse 5(3):16–19, 22, 54, May 1983.

Cain L, Bigongiari LR: The percutaneous nephrostomy tube, Am J Nurs 82(2):296, 298, Feb 1982.

Clayman RV et al: Percutaneous nephrolithotomy: An approach to branched and staghorn renal calculi, JAMA 250(1):73–75, July 1, 1983.

Cozad J: Penile implants: The surgical treatment for impotence, Point View 21(1):20–21, Jan 1984.

Cozad J: Permanent urinary diversion, Point View 18(3):19, July 1981.

Dillon MJ: Coagulum pyelolithotomy to remove multiple stones, AORN J 36(4):680, 684–685, 688–689, Oct 1982.

Doyle JE: Treating renovascular hypertension: Bypass

graft surgery, Am J Nurs 82(10):1559–1562, Oct 1982.

Doyle JE, Sequeira JC: Treating renovascular hypertension: Renal artery dilation, Am J Nurs 82(10):1563–1564, Oct 1982.

Flechner SM et al: Screening for transplant renal artery stenosis in hypertensive recipients using digital subtraction angiography, J Urol 130(3):440–443, Sep 1983.

Glenn JF (ed): *Urologic Surgery,* 3rd ed, Philadelphia: Lippincott, 1983.

Googe MCS, Mook TM: The inflatable penile prosthesis: New developments, Am J Nurs 83(7):1044–1047, July 1983.

Gould DE: Vascular access procedures for hemodialysis, AORN J 36(4):704, 706, 708, 710, Oct 1982.

Hager T: New surgical techniques ease incontinence, JAMA 249(24):3284, 3286–3287, June 24, 1983.

Hoffman DJ et al: Treatment for impotence: Penile implants, Todays OR Nurse 6(8):16–21, Aug 1984.

Huffman JL et al: Transurethral removal of large ureteral and renal pelvic calculi using uteroscopic ultrasonic lithotripsy, J Urol 130(1):31–34, July 1983.

Jones AG, Hoeft RT: Cancer of the prostate, Am J Nurs 82(5):826–828, May 1982.

LaFollette SS: A continent urostomy, AORN J 40(2):207–209, 212–215, Aug 1984.

LaFollette SS: Effective treatment: Testicular cancer, AORN J 38(4):622, 624, 633–636, Oct 1983.

Lancaster LE: Renal failure: Pathophysiology, assessment and intervention, Nephrol Nurse 5(2):38–44, Mar–Apr 1983.

Lawler PE: Benign prostatic hyperplasia: Knowing pathophysiology aids assessment, AORN J 40(5):745–748, 750, Nov 1984.

Libertino JA, Zinman L: Renal revascularization using aortorenal saphenous vein bypass grafting, Surg Technol 14(3):31–39, May–June 1982.

Maree, SM: Assessing the excretory system, AORN J 33(4):734–735, 738, 742–743, 746–747, 750, 752, 754, 756, Mar 1981.

McConnell EA, Zimmerman MF: *Care of Patients with Urologic Problems,* Philadelphia: Lippincott, 1983.

Palmer JM: Role of partial nephrectomy in solitary or bilateral renal tumors, JAMA 249(17):2357–2361, May 6, 1983.

Parker C: Ambulatory surgery for a penile prosthesis, AORN J 36(3):487–494, Sep 1982.

Parker CB: Alternative to urinary diversion, AORN J 39(6):968–972, May 1984.

Scott FB et al: Implantation of an artificial sphincter for urinary incontinence, Contemp Surg 18(2):11–14, 16, 25–27, 30–31, 34, Feb 1981.

Sheldon CA, Smith AD: Chemolysis of calculi, Urol Clin North Am 9(1):121–130, Feb 1982.

Sos TA et al: Percutaneous transluminal renal angioplasty in renovascular hypertension due to atheroma or fibromuscular dysplasia, N Engl J Med 309(5):274–279, Aug 4, 1983.

Stano D: Treatment of prostatism, Surg Technol 15(4):15–17, July–Aug 1983.

Stone L: Percutaneous nephrolithotripsy: An advancement in kidney stone extraction, AORN J 39(5):779–781, Apr 1984.

Volkmann-Jones S: A new method of kidney stone retrieval, Todays OR Nurse 6(8):8–10, 14–15, Aug 1984.

CHAPTER 24
ORTHOPAEDICS

Alexander A, Wall T: NATN workshop: Orthopaedics, NATNews 20(9):20–21, 23, Sep 1983.

Apfelbach H: Technique for chemonucleolysis, Todays OR Nurse 6(1):21, 24–25, Jan 1984.

Brantley P: Orthopedic innovations: Porous coated hip implants, Todays OR Nurse 6(10):8–11, Oct 1984.

Brown SL: Avoiding postop pitfalls with hip fracture patients, RN 45(5):48–54, May 1982.

Burn ED: Promoting healing of bone tissue, AORN J 35(6):1186, 1188, 1190–1191, May 1982.

Chymopapain administration procedures modified, FDA Bull 14(2):14–15, Aug 1984.

Connolly JF: Orthopaedic surgery, Bull Am Coll Surg 69(1):30–33, Jan 1984.

Cozad J: Chemonucleolysis: An alternative to laminectomy, Point View 21(3):4–5, Sep 1984.

Crawford-Gamble P: The treatment of nonunions with stimulation, Todays OR Nurse 4(11):23–25, 27, 56, Jan 1983.

D'Aquila LC: The surgical technologist during arthroscopic menisectomies, Surg Technol 14(4):26–29, July–Aug 1982.

Drucker MM: Arthroscopic surgery of the knee joint, AORN J 36(4):585–593, Oct 1982.

Evanoff J: Sterilizing and preserving human bone, AORN J 37(5):972–973, 976, 978, 980, Apr 1983.

Fryer J: Fixation of an inter-trochanteric fracture by intermedullary nails of the Ender type, NATNews 18(5):18, 20–21, May 1981.

Fuss M: Disk therapy without surgery: Nursing responsibilities, Todays OR Nurse 6(1):18–20, Jan 1984.

Gill KP, Laflamme D: External fixation: The erector sets of orthopedic nursing, Can Nurse 80(5):29–31, May 1984.

Greer RB: Orthopaedic surgery, Bull Am Coll Surg 68(1):37–39, Jan 1983.

Jackson RW: *The Scope of Arthroscopy,* Warsaw, Ind.: Zimmer, 1982.

Kanes G: The history and development of the arthroscope, NATNews 18(9):45–48, Sep 1981.

Kapela AJ: The Bechtol total hip implant, Surg Technol 13(2):7–11, Mar–Apr 1981.

Krempen JF et al: Ligamentum flavotomy—Alterna-

tive to laminectomy in herniated disc, Surg Technol 14(6):32–34, 36, Nov–Dec 1982.
Lahde RE: Luque rod instrumentation, AORN J 38(1):35–43, July 1983.
Lane PL, Lee MM: Special care for special casts, Nursing (Horsham) 13(7):50–51, July 1983.
Laskin RS, Varrichio DM: Total knee replacement, AORN J 36(4):577–584, Oct 1982.
Lonergan RP: Arthroscopic meniscectomy using the transpatellar tendon approach, Surg Technol 13(2):25–30, Mar–Apr 1981.
Macek C: Bony ingrowth holds new "joints" in place, JAMA 247(12):1680–1681, 1685, Mar 26, 1982.
Moss V: Chemonucleolysis: Enzyme eases back pain, AORN J 38(6):965–973, Dec 1983.
Musolf J: Chemonucleolysis: A new approach for patients with herniated intervertebral disks, Am J Nurs 83(6):882–885, June 1983.
Parks S: Total joint revision surgery, Todays OR Nurse 4(11):16–18, 20, 57, 61, Jan 1983.
Prendergast S: Thompson's hemi arthroplasty, NAT-News 19(12):8–12, Dec 1982.
Sampson WA: L-5 laminectomy, Surg Technol 15(5):34–35, 37–38, Sep–Oct 1983.
Shahriaree H (ed): *O'Connor's Textbook of Arthroscopic Surgery,* Philadelphia: Lippincott, 1984.
Skinner HB: Porous coatings in total-joint arthroplasty: The wave of the future, Bull Am Coll Surg 70(5):14–15, May 1985.
Specialty supplement: Orthopaedic surgery, Br J Theatre Nurs, Feb 1985.
Steinberg ME: Orthopaedic surgery, Bull Am Coll Surg 67(1):36–39, Jan 1982.
Stinchfield FE: The evolution of total hip replacement, Surg Technol 15(3):16–18, May–June 1983.
Thompson MB: An overview of arthroscopy, Todays OR Nurse 4(11):9–13, Jan 1983.
Voluz JM: Surgical implants: Orthopedic devices, AORN J 37(7):1341, 1344–1345, 1348–1349, 1352, June 1983.
Weil LS (ed): *Clinics in Podiatry: Symposium on Implants in Foot Surgery,* Philadelphia: Saunders, 1984.

CHAPTER 25
OPHTHALMOLOGY

Alcantara NT et al: A holistic approach to extracapsular lens extraction, Todays OR Nurse 6(3):16–18, 20, 22, 40, Mar 1984.
Aron-Rosa D: *Pulsed Yag Laser Surgery,* Thorofare, NJ: Slack, 1983.
Blodi FC: Ophthalmology, JAMA 247(21):2970–2971, June 4, 1982.
Boyd-Monk H: A fortunate accident—radial keratotomy, Todays OR Nurse 6(3):25–26, 31, Mar 1984.
Clayman HM et al: *Intraocular Lens Implantation: Techniques and Complications,* St. Louis: Mosby, 1983.
Easterlin MN, Schneider HA: Acute angle closure glaucoma following surgery, AORN J 39(6):992, 994–995, May 1984.
Eye Bank Association of America: *Medical Standards for Member Eye Banks,* San Diego, June 1980, Sep 1980.
Girard LJ: *Corneal Surgery,* Vol 2, St. Louis: Mosby, 1981.
Hussey LCT: Intraocular lens implant, AORN J 39(5):880, 882, 884, 886, 890–891, Apr 1984.
Interview: Mary Gowarty, RN, OR nurse/manager, Scheie Eye Institute, Todays OR Nurse 5(1):32–34, Mar 1983.
Jennings B: Combined ophthalmic implant and transplant, AORN J 28(1):41–46, July 1978.
MacFadyen JS: Caring for the patient with a primary retinal detachment, Am J Nurs 80(5):920–921, May 1980.
Marta M: A guide to the posterior vitrectomy, Todays OR Nurse 5(1):26–29, 69, Mar 1983.
Moore CR: Scleral buckling for retinal detachment, AORN J 36(3):495, 498, 500, 502–503, 506, Sep 1982.
Nemchik R: Diabetic retinopathy: The current status of therapy, RN 46(6):34–37, 40, 63, June 1983.
Quigley HA: Long-term follow-up of laser iridotomy, Ophthalmology 88(3):218–224, Mar 1981.
Resler MM, Tumulty G: Glaucoma update, Am J Nurs 83(5):752–756, May 1983.
Schneeman YT, Taylor JA: A technical look at vitrectomy, AORN J 33(5):867–872, Apr 1981.
Sperduto RD et al: Lens opacities and senile maculopathy, Arch Ophthalmol 99(6):1004–1008, June 1981.
Stamper RL: What's new in ophthalmic surgery, Bull Am Coll Surg 70(1):26–30, Jan 1985.
Stark LA: Treating vision loss, Todays OR Nurse 6(3):8–10, 13, 44, Mar 1984.
Sugar J: Ophthalmic surgery, Bull Am Coll Surg 69(1):28–29, Jan 1984.
Symposium: Argon-laser surgery for treating glaucoma, Todays OR Nurse 6(3):34–35, 38–40, Mar 1984.
Troutman, RC: *Microsurgery of the Anterior Segment of the Eye,* Vol 2, St. Louis: Mosby, 1977.
Whitton S: Penetrating keratoplasty: The gift of sight, Todays OR Nurse 5(1):20–21, 24, 72, Mar 1983.
Zack PL, Smirnow IH: IOL implantation, Todays OR Nurse 5(1):12–16, 18, 68–69, Mar 1983.

CHAPTER 26
OTOLARYNGOLOGY

Adornato SG: Tonsillar hemostasis: A new approach, Otolaryngol, Head Neck Surg 91:24, Apr 1983.
Babin RW: Recent advances in otolaryngologic—head and neck surgery, Surg Technol 13(6):7–10, Nov–Dec 1981.

Balkany TJ et al: The cochlear implant, Surg Technol 13(3):25, 27, May–June 1981.
Brown I: Trach care? Take care—infection's on the prowl, Nursing (Horsham) 12(5):44–49, May 1982.
Byers R et al: Squamous carcinoma of the external ear, Am J Surg 146(4):447–450, Oct 1983.
Carrell BL: Laser treatment of laryngeal polyps, AORN J 38(2):232–234, 236, Aug 1983.
Chasse PS: Hope of hearing, Todays OR Nurse 5(8):14–17, Oct 1983.
Garrett PG et al: Cancer of the tonsil: Results of radical radiation therapy with surgery in reserve, Am J Surg 146(4):432–435, Oct 1983.
Hybels RL: Selected new techniques in laryngeal surgery, Surg Technol 14(5):30, 32–34, 36–37, 40–41, Sep–Oct 1982.
Ingram NM: Stanching nosebleeds: Your guide to all the measures available, RN 45(9):50–53, 115, Sep 1982.
Knapp BA, Panje WR: A voice button for laryngectomees, AORN J 36(2):183–192, Aug 1982.
Lyons RJ: Surgical implants: Voice prostheses, AORN J 37(7):1369, 1372–1373, 1376, 1378, 1380, June 1983.
Matz GJ: Otolaryngology—head-and-neck surgery, Bull Am Coll Surg 68(1):40–42, Jan 1983.
McGuirt WF: Otolaryngology—head-and-neck surgery, Bull Am Coll Surg 67(1):40–43, Jan 1982.
Nimmo M: Palatopharyngoplasty, Todays OR Nurse 5(8):8–12, Oct 1983.
Saunders WH et al: *Nursing Care in Eye, Ear, Nose and Throat Disorders,* 4th ed, St. Louis: Mosby, 1979.
Sproat C: Tracheal resection, Surg Technol 17(2):29–31, Mar–Apr 1985.
Tucker HM: What's new in otolaryngology, Bull Am Coll Surg 69(1):34–36, Jan 1984.
Weaver TE: Bronchoscopy, laryngography, and their potential complications, RN 45(12):64, Dec 1982.
Wong ML: Recent advances in ear surgery, Surg Technol 13(6):10–13, Nov–Dec 1981.

CHAPTER 27
PLASTIC AND RECONSTRUCTIVE SURGERY

Acres C, Kraft ER: Skin transplantation, Am J Nurs 81(8):1466–1467, Aug 1981.
Baj P: Lipo-suction: 'New wave' plastic surgery, Am J Nurs 84(7):892–893, July 1984.
Cherskov M: Tissue expansion: 'Future of plastic surgery for next 20 years', JAMA 247(22):3039–3040, June 11, 1982.
Cohen BE, Aaronson S: Microvascular reconstructive surgery: Free tissue transfer, AORN J 38(4):602–609, Oct 1983.
Cohen IK: What's new in surgery: Plastic surgery and burns, Bull Am Coll Surg 67(1):50–51, Jan 1982.
Engeman SA: The burned patient, AORN J 40(1):36–41, July 1984.
Frazier TG, Noone RB: Immediate reconstruction in the treatment of primary carcinoma of the breast, Surg Gynecol Obstet 157(5):413–414, Nov 1983.
Hyland WT, Schreiber M: Subcutaneous mastectomy, Surg Technol 15(2):26–30, Mar–Apr 1983.
Kaiser TL et al: Burns of the hand: What can nurses do?, Todays OR Nurse 5(4):14–15, 18, 20, 22–23, June 1983.
Kraft E et al: Skin banking: A new field fulfills a vital need, Surg Technol 12(3):6–12, May–June 1980.
Lyon RJ: Promoting healing of skin flaps and grafts, AORN J 35(6):1174, 1176, 1178–1179, 1182–1183, May 1982.
Moore BG: OR nurse's role during flap transfer, AORN J 38(4):610–612, Oct 1983.
Pruitt BA, McManus WF: Surgical management of burns, Contemp Surg 16(5):11–16, May 1980.
Seaton C et al: Suction lipolysis: A personal perspective, Plast Surg Nurs 4(2):47–49, Summer 1984.
Serafin D: What's new in plastic surgery and burns, Bull Am Coll Surg 69(1):45–49, Jan 1984.
Smith D: Augmentation mammoplasty, Surg Technol 15(5):16–17, 19, Sep–Oct 1983.
Spira M: What's new in surgery: Plastic surgery, Bull Am Coll Surg 68(1):49–52, Jan 1983.
Vasconez LO et al: Reconstruction of the breast: Where do we fall short?, Am J Surg 148(1):103–110, July 1984.
Walsh MH, Stefanski DM: Surgical implants: Breast prostheses, AORN J 37(7):1381, 1384–1385, 1388–1389, 1392, June 1983.
Yates BW: Toe to finger transfer, Point View 17(4):4–5, Oct 1980.

CHAPTER 28
MULTIDISCIPLINARY TEAM APPROACH TO HEAD AND NECK SURGERY

Angelini C, Schmidt M: Putting the bite on mandibular deficiency, Todays OR Nurse 6(6):14–17, June 1984.
Black JM, Arnold PG: Facial fractures, Am J Nurs 82(7):1086–1088, July 1982.
Conley J: Changes in head and neck surgery, Am J Surg 146(4):425–428, Oct 1983.
Hopkins J: Mid-face advancement, Todays OR Nurse 5(4):9–13, June 1983.
Hutton B, Hutton J: Living with a facial prosthesis: A guide to patient care, Am J Nurs 84(1):50–52, Jan 1984.
Jacoby ZI: When cancer strikes: Nursing strategy for partial glossectomy, Todays OR Nurse 6(6):8–10, June 1984.
Krespi YP, Sisson GA: Reconstruction after total or subtotal glossectomy, Am J Surg 146(4):488–491, Oct 1983.
Liss G: Malformation of the mandible, NATNews 20(1):13–15, Jan 1983.
McConnell P et al: Surgery for dental function: The

team approach to LeForte I ostectomy, Todays OR Nurse 6(6):19–21, 24–25, June 1984.

Piliero CR: Surgical treatment of orbital hypertelorism, Surg Technol 13(2):12–19, Mar–Apr 1981.

Razack MS et al: Total glossectomy, Am J Surg 146(4):509–511, Oct 1983.

Rusch FJ: Fractures of the mandible, Surg Technol 15(4):23–26, July–Aug 1983.

Spiro RH et al: Gastric transposition in head and neck surgery, Am J Surg 146(4):483–487, Oct 1983.

Warden LS, Robinson MK: Osteotomy with intermaxillary fixation, AORN J 33(7):1304, 1306, 1308, 1310, 1312, 1314, June 1981.

Yanachek MP: Growing role for the nurse in oral surgery, AORN J 30(2):314, 318–319, 322–323, 326, Aug 1979.

CHAPTER 29 NEUROSURGERY

Berry PR: Cerebral occlusion: Extracranial-intracranial anastomosis, AORN J 41(5):901–902, 904–905, 907, 909, May 1985.

Bray CA: Benign but fatal: Acoustic neuroma, Todays OR Nurse 6(1):8–11, 14–15, Jan 1984.

Conway-Rutkowski BL: *Carini and Owens' Neurological and Neurosurgical Nursing,* 8th ed, St. Louis: Mosby, 1982.

England EF: Outcome standards at work: A neurosurgical case study, AORN J 40(4):582–583, 586–587, 590–591, Oct 1984.

Fay, MF: Controlling pain, Todays OR Nurse 5(10):10–13, Dec 1983.

Flamm ES: Neurosurgery, Bull Am Coll Surg 68(1):21–25, Jan 1983.

Gary RA: Caring for patients with cerebral aneurysms, AORN J 37(4):631–642, Mar 1983.

Grey D: Intrathecal morphine: Relief from intractable pain, Can Nurse 79(1):50–52, Jan 1983.

Hickey JV: *The Clinical Practice of Neurological and Neurosurgical Nursing,* Philadelphia: Lippincott, 1981.

Houston C: Giant aneurysm surgery, AORN J 37(4):643–651, Mar 1983.

Houston C: Transsphenoidal pituitary microsurgery, Todays OR Nurse 5(9):23–25, 28, Nov 1983.

Leatherland JE et al: Cerebellar implant, AORN J 39(7):1143–1149, June 1984.

MacClelland DC, The glossopharyngeal neuralgia patient, AORN J 31(4):589–598, Mar 1980.

Mauldin BC: The hypophysectomy patient in the OR, AORN J 33(2):253–255, Feb 1981.

McCash AM: Meeting the challenge of craniotomy care, RN 48(6):26–33, June 1985.

Medina J: Percutaneous lumbar diskectomy: An alternative to laminectomy, Surg Technol 15(1):30–34, Jan–Feb 1983.

Meyer TM: Tens—Relieving pain through electricity, Nursing (Horsham) 12(9):57–59, Sep 1982.

Mulford EF: Degenerative disease or 'slipped' disc? The clues are clear-cut, RN 44(2):44–49, Feb 1981.

Norman SE: Surgical treatment of epilepsy, Am J Nurs 81(5):994–996, May 1981.

Perdue P: Life-threatening head and spinal injuries, RN 44(6):36–41, 102, June 1981.

Riley JM: Intracranial pressure monitoring made easy, RN 44(9):53–57, Sep 1981.

Savoy SM: The craniotomy patient: Identifying the patient's neurological status, AORN J 40(5):716–724, Nov 1984.

Stein BM: Neurosurgery, Bull Am Coll Surg 69(1):22–27, Jan 1984.

Temple AP: Stereotactic surgery: An alternative to craniotomy, AORN J 40(4):543–550, Oct 1984.

Thompson L: The pituitary: The master gland, Surg Technol 15(4):27–28, July–Aug 1983.

Tindall GT, Mauldin BC: Transsphenoidal hypophysectomy, AORN J 33(2):246–252, Feb 1981.

Walker ML: Using lasers in neurosurgery, AORN J 38(2):238–241, Aug 1983.

Wilkins RH: Neurosurgery, Bull Am Coll Surg 67(1):22–25, Jan 1982.

CHAPTER 30 THORACIC SURGERY

Baue AE: Surgery, JAMA 247(21):2987–2989, June 4, 1982.

Cameron TJ: Fiberoptic bronchoscopy, Am J Nurs 81(8):1462–1464, Aug 1981.

Collins JJ Jr: Cardiothoracic surgery, Bull Am Coll Surg 67(1):8–9, Jan 1982.

Eren EE, Ott DA: Transverse sternotomy for concomitant cardiac and pulmonary surgery, Texas Heart Institute J 11(2):192–196, June 1984.

Gatch G: Thoracoscopy in children, Todays OR Nurse 3(11):16–18, 61, Jan 1982.

Hopkins RA et al: Stapled esophagogastric anastomosis, Am J Surg 147(2):283–287, Feb 1984.

Hoyt KS: Chest trauma, Nursing (Horsham) 13(5):34–41, May 1983.

Kildea J Jr: Mediastinoscopy in bronchogenic carcinoma, AORN J 33(1):57–63, Jan 1981.

Wilcox BR: Cardiothoracic surgery, Bull Am Coll Surg 68(1):6, Jan 1983.

CHAPTER 31 CARDIOVASCULAR SURGERY

Armour D: The pacemaker: Function and malfunction, Surg Technol 13(5):7–14, Sep–Oct 1981.

Bigelow WG: Cold hearts and vital lessons, Bull Am Coll Surg 69(6):12–19, June 1984.

Blaszkowski J: Aortic valve replacement, Surg Technol 15(6):36–39, Nov–Dec 1983.

Cooley DA: Results with Björk-Shiley tilting disc and Ionescu-Shiley bioprosthesis, Texas Heart Institute J 9(4):467–469, Dec 1982.

Cooley DA: *Techniques in Cardiac Surgery,* 2d ed, Philadelphia: Saunders, 1984.

Corsaro MC: Balloon catheters: Rising to the occasion, J Oper Rm Res Inst 3(4):42–45, Apr 1983.

Corsaro MC: Intraaortic balloon counterpulsation: Saving more lives with technology, J Oper Rm Res Inst 3(6):14–17, June 1983.

Cozad J: Intra-aortic balloon pump: Hope for the failing heart, Point View 22(3):8–9, Sep 1985.

DeGeorge D: Cardioplegic drugs: An alternative myocardial preservation technic, Point View 17(4):8–9, Oct 1980.

Frazier OH: Cardiac assist devices, Texas Heart Institute J 9(4):442–446, Dec 1982.

Gimelson P: A pioneering effort: The artificial heart, Todays OR Nurse 5(2):10–13, 50, 53, Apr 1983.

Hall RJ et al: Percutaneous transluminal coronary angioplasty update, Texas Heart Institute J 11(1):10–16, Mar 1984.

Hastings SM: Surgical implants: Pacemakers, AORN J 37(7):1324, 1326, 1328, 1330, 1332–1333, 1336–1337, 1340, June 1983.

Hauser RG: Multiprogrammable cardiac pacemakers, Am J Surg 145(6):740–745, June 1983.

Hurst JW (ed): *The Heart, Arteries and Veins,* 5th ed, New York: McGraw-Hill, 1982.

Kabbani SS et al: Surgical experience following percutaneous transluminal coronary angioplasty, Texas Heart Institute J 11(2):112–116, June 1984.

Kafrouni G: Intraaortic balloon counterpulsation, Am J Surg 147(6):731–734, June 1984.

Karlson KE et al: Initial clinical experience with a low pressure drop membrane oxygenator for cardiopulmonary bypass in adult patients, Am J Surg 147(4):447–450, Apr 1984.

Kleehammer P et al: Pumps that bolster a failing heart, RN 48(5):44–50, May 1985.

Krumbach B, Maran JN: Pacemaker insertion: The perioperative role, Todays OR Nurse 6(11):8–12, 15, Nov 1984.

Maurice J: Medical news: First three patients for new type of implantable cardioverter, JAMA 250(14): 1809–1811, Oct 14, 1983.

Ott DA et al: Surgical treatment of cardiac dysrhythmias, Surg Technol 15(1):44–48, 50–53, Jan–Feb 1983.

Pairitz DM: Surgical implants: Valvular prostheses, AORN J 37(7):1394, 1396–1397, 1400, June 1983.

Patterson P: Replacing a human heart, AORN J 37(2):183–186, 189–194, Feb 1983.

Pierce WS: Cardiothoracic surgery, Bull Am Coll Surg 69(1):8–11, Jan 1984.

Purcell JA: Coronary angioplasty, AORN J 35(2):199–206, Feb 1982.

Purcell JA, Burrows SG: A pacemaker primer, Am J Nurs 85(5):553–568, May 1985.

Purcell JA et al: Intra-aortic balloon pump therapy, Am J Nurs 83(5):775–790, May 1983.

Reddy SB et al: Left ventricular aneurysm: Twenty-year surgical experience with 1572 patients at the Texas Heart Institute, Cardiovasc Dis 8(2):165–186, June 1981.

Rossi LP, Antman EM: Calcium channel blockers: New treatment for cardiovascular disease, Am J Nurs 83(3):382–387, Mar 1983.

Seifert PC: An OR nurse's guide to coronary artery bypass, AORN J 33(6):1049–1057, May 1981.

Seifert PC: Hemodynamic monitoring: A many-faceted tool, Cardiothoracic Nurse 2(1):10–12, Jan 1984.

Seifert PC: Mitral valve replacement, AORN J 36(6):959–972, Dec 1982.

Seifert PC, Lefrak EA: Aortic valve replacement: A team effort, Todays OR Nurse 5(2):26–29, 32–34, 54, Apr 1983.

Senning A: Cardiac pacing in retrospect, Am J Surg 145(6):733–739, June 1983.

Shaw LM: A teaching plan for coronary artery bypass, AORN J 33(6):1058–1066, May 1981.

Simmons K: Implantable assist pump—final heart option?, JAMA 251(6):700–701, Feb 10, 1984.

Swan H: The importance of acid-base management for cardiac and cerebral preservation during open heart operations, Surg Gynecol Obstet 158(4):391–414, Apr 1984.

Underhill SL et al: *Cardiac Nursing,* Philadelphia: Lippincott, 1982.

Ventura B: What you need to know about cardiac catheterization, RN 47(9):24–30, Sep 1984.

Willard PD: Percutaneous transluminal angioplasty, Point View 22(3):4–7, Sep 1985.

Zoll PM: Cardiac pacemakers: Present and future, Texas Heart Institute J 9(4):447–448, Dec 1982.

CHAPTER 32
PERIPHERAL VASCULAR SURGERY

Adamson J: Intraoperative nursing care of the patient with ruptured abdominal aortic aneurysm, Point View 19(4):4–7, Oct 1, 1982.

Barman AA et al: Use of interposed polytetrafluorethylene (PTFE) graft in distal splenorenal shunt, Cardiovasc Dis 8(4):555–557, Dec 1981.

Baum PL: Abdominal aortic aneurysm? This patient takes AAA care, Nursing (Horsham) 12(12):34–41, Dec 1982.

Baum PL: Carotid endarterectomy, Nursing (Horsham) 13(3):50–61, Mar 1983.

Blumenberg RM, Gelfand ML: Application of intestinal

staples to aortoiliac surgery, Am J Surg 144(8):198–202, Aug 1982.

Butler S: Carotid endarterectomy: Care in the OR, AORN J 32(1):42–47, July 1980.

Connett MC et al: Peripheral arterial emboli, Am J Surg 148(1):14–19, July 1984.

Czapinski N et al: Nursing plan for abdominal aortic aneurysms, AORN J 37(2):205–208, 210, Feb 1983.

Fahey VA, Bergan JJ: Venous reconstruction: Surgery for severe venous stasis, AORN J 41(2):423–424, 426, 428–429, 431–432, 434, Feb 1985.

Fahey VA, Finkelmeier BA: Iatrogenic arterial injuries, Am J Nurs 84(4):448–451, Apr 1984.

Fry WJ: Peripheral vascular surgery, Bull Am Coll Surg 67(1):47–49, Jan 1982.

Goldfarb D, Nelson S: Arterial vascular prostheses: A primer on grafts, Surg Armarium 3:5–7, 10–12, Summer 1983.

Haimovici H: *Vascular Surgery: Principles and Techniques,* 2d ed, Norwalk, Ct.: Appleton-Century-Crofts, 1984.

Hessler K, Kenny M: Using human umbilical vein grafts, AORN J 33(5):862–866, Apr 1981.

Hinnant JR, Stallworth JM: Simplified surgery for varicose veins, AORN J 34(1):135, 138–139, 142–143, 147, 150, July 1981.

Jasinowski N: The unique needs of a distal bypass patient, RN 45(3):44–47, 122, Mar 1982.

Kukich E: Rinse procedure simplifies graft preparation, AORN J 35(5):899–902, Apr 1982.

Jones C: The total care of a patient in the operating theatre, NATNews 19(3):16, 18–20, 22, Mar 1982.

King DE: Portal shunts: A fighting chance for your patient, RN 46(7):31–37, July 1983.

King SL: Patient care in vascular surgery, AORN J 33(5):843–848, Apr 1981.

Logan J, Ziebell E: Axillofemoral artery bypass for lower limb ischemia, Can Nurse 78(8):25–29, Sep 1982.

Moore WS: Vascular surgery, Bull Am Coll Surg 68(1):65–68, Jan 1983.

Persson AV et al: Femoral-to-femoral bypass graft, Surg Technol 14(2):10–14, Mar–Apr 1982.

Persson AV, Griffey SP: Carotid endarterectomy, Surg Technol 14(1):7–12, Jan–Feb 1982.

Persson AV, Griffey SP: Common femoral artery-to-proximal popliteal artery bypass and common femoral artery-to-tibial artery bypass, Surg Technol 14(2):15–20, Mar–Apr 1982.

Raab D: Peripheral vascular disease: How to recognize it, how to treat it, Can Nurse 78(8):30–33, Sep 1982.

Salzano T: Abdominal aortic aneurysms, Surg Technol 16(1):14–21, Jan–Feb 1984.

Sauvage LR: Porous fabric arterial prosthesis, AORN J 33(5):854–861, Apr 1981.

Schulmeister L: Vascular access grafts in cancer chemotherapy, Am J Nurs 82(9):1388–1389, Sep 1982.

Sigley DP: Nursing roles in vascular access surgery, AORN J 38(5):811, 814–815, 818, 820, 822, Nov 1983.

Silver D: Peripheral vascular surgery, Bull Am Coll Surg 69(1):42–44, Jan 1984.

Sprayregen S: Percutaneous transluminal angioplasty, Contemp Surg 16(4):53–55, 58–59, 62–63, Apr 1980.

Winston TR et al: Surgery for peripheral vascular disease, AORN J 33(5):849–853, Apr 1981.

CHAPTER 33
PEDIATRIC SURGERY

Allard JL, Dibble SL: A look at Luque rods, Am J Nurs 84(5):609–611, May 1984.

Allard JL, Northrop WA: Nursing care: Segmental spinal instrumentation, AORN J 38(1):45–50, July 1983.

Bailey CR, Miller NK: Routine circumcision of the male neonate, Can Nurse 79(1):28–31, Jan 1983.

Brown C: The pediatric patient undergoing surgical intervention, Point View 19(1):18–19, Jan 1982.

Brown D, Peake J: Presurgical education, AORN J 39(7):1163–1170, June 1984.

Campbell DN et al: Congenital heart surgery: A five year study, Surg Technol 15(1):14–19, Jan–Feb 1983.

Committee on Practice: *OGN Nursing Practice Resource No 12: Neonatal Skin Care,* Washington, D.C.: NAACOG, 1985.

Coran AG: Pediatric surgery, Bull Am Coll Surg 69(1):37–41, Jan 1984.

Damron C, Stetson P: A preoperative teaching program: Preparing a child for ambulatory surgery, AORN J 41(2): 352–354, Feb 1985.

Diniaco MJ, Ingoldsby BB: Parental presence in the recovery room, AORN J 38(4):685, 688–689, 692–693, Oct 1983.

Gatch G: Caring for children needing anesthesia, AORN J 35(2):218–226, Feb 1982.

Heaman DJ, Mattle LF: Adolescent emergence excitement, AORN J 35(2):230, 234–235, 242, Feb 1982.

Heyman S: Correcting transposition of the great arteries, AORN J 36(1):35–44, July 1982.

Kuhn PL: Surgical correction of neonatal PDA, Point View 22(3):10–11, Sep 1985.

Levine AH, Imai PK: Intrauterine treatment of fetal hydronephrosis, AORN J 35(4):655–662, Mar 1982.

Marshall JG, Ross JL: Hydrocephalus: Ventriculoperitoneal shunting in infants and children, AORN J 40(6):842–846, Dec 1984.

Minx SM, Stellwagen G: Pediatric airway obstruction, AORN J 40(3):338–343, Sep 1984.

Pleasants DG: Managing hydrocephalus with a ventricular shunt, AORN J 35(5):885–892, Apr 1982.

Sataloff RT, Colton CM: Otitis media: A common childhood infection, Am J Nurs 81(8):1480–1483, Aug 1981.

Shipley SB: Perioperative care of the pediatric orthopedic patient, Todays OR Nurse, 3(11):9–15, 60, Jan 1982.

Sieber WK: Pediatric surgery, Bull Am Coll Surg 66(1):40–42, Jan 1981.

Steinbacher C: Congenital heart defects, Surg Technol 13(2):20–24, Mar–Apr 1981.

Stout JA, Gibbs KB: The child undergoing a leg-lengthening procedure, Am J Nurs 81(6):1152–1155, June 1981.

Timmerman RR: Preoperative fears of older children, AORN J 38(5):827, 830–831, 834, Nov 1983.

Value of tonsillectomy vs recurrent throat infection is short & slight, Infectious Diseases 14(6):1, 3, June 1984.

Vile J: Scoliosis and spinal fusion, Surg Technol 13(4):9–12, July–Aug 1981.

Vries JK: Endoscopy as an adjunct to shunting for hydrocephalus, Surg Neurol 13(1):69–72, Jan 1980.

CHAPTER 34 TRANSPLANTATION AND REPLANTATION

Benson J et al: Saving sight, Nurs Manage 15(2):38K–38L, Feb 1984.

Blume E: 'Tricks' of trade aid kidney transplants, JAMA 249(17):2288–2290, May 6, 1983.

Bohr R: A whispered beginning, Surg Technol 14(6):57–58, Nov–Dec 1982.

Bourbonnais F, Bédard J: Total nursing care for the bone marrow transplant patient, Can Nurse 78(11):17–21, Dec 1982.

Cerilli GJ: Transplantation, Bull Am Coll Surg 67(1):58–61, Jan 1982.

Copeland JG et al: Heart transplantation, JAMA 251 (12):1563–1566, Mar 23/30, 1984.

Cyclosporine approved for kidney, liver and heart transplants, FDA Drug Bull 14(1):6–7, Apr 1984.

Diethelm AG: Transplantation, Bull Am Coll Surg 70(1):57–60, Jan 1985.

Duran F, Lamb J: Cardiac transplantation, Todays OR Nurse 5(2):20–23, 50, Apr 1983.

Fuller BF: Organ graft rejection: The biological process, AORN J 41(4):738–745, Apr 1985.

Fuquay LW: Heart to heart, Surg Technol 15(3):8–14, May–June 1983.

Gimelson P: The artificial heart: A pioneering effort, Todays OR Nurse 5(2):10–13, 50, Apr 1983.

Golden D et al: Understanding the magic of cyclosporine, RN 48(6):53–54, June 1985.

Hardy MA: Transplantation, Bull Am Coll Surg 68(1):57–61, Jan 1983.

Houlihan PJ: When your patient is a transplant recipient, Can Nurse 78(7):40–44, July–Aug 1982.

Jacobs SC, Stoldt L: Replantation for traumatic amputations, AORN J 39(6):956–963, May 1984.

Jamieson SW et al: Heart and lung transplantation for pulmonary hypertension, Am J Surg 147(6):740–742, June 1984.

Kosel K et al: Total pancreatectomy and islet cell autotransplantation, Am J Nurs 82(4):568–572, Apr 1982.

Lahde RE: Heart-lung transplant: A first, AORN J 34(4),627–635, 638–639, Oct 1981.

Maletic-Staschak S: Orthotopic liver transplantation: The surgical procedure, AORN J 39(1):35–39, Jan 1984.

Mallard G et al: Collecting, preserving, and transfusing bone marrow, AORN J 36(3):378–384, Sep 1982.

Mathias JM: Immunosuppression: Postoperative management of heart transplant recipients, AORN J 41(4):748–753, Apr 1985.

Mauldin BC: Harvest of hope: Bone marrow transplant, AORN J 36(3):385–390, Sep 1982.

Nuscher R et al: Bone marrow transplantation, Am J Nurs 84(6):764–772, June 1984.

Parrish BL: Cadaver donor nephrectomy, AORN J 34(2):237–244, Aug 1981.

Patterson P: Replacing a human heart, AORN J 37(2):183–186, 189–194, Feb 1983.

Reitz BA: The current practice of heart transplantation, Bull Am Coll Surg 70(5):11–12, 15, May 1985.

Richard AB et al: Renal transplantation: Nursing management of the recipient, AORN J 41(6):1022–1036, June 1985.

Salinger JH: If your patient gets a bone marrow transplant, RN 47(5):62, 67–68, May 1984.

Salvatierra O Jr: The current status of renal transplantation, Bull Am Coll Surg 70(5):2–7, May 1985.

Schroer K, Hartin P: Cardiac transplants, AORN J 40(2):220–221, 224–225, 228–229, Aug 1984.

Starzl TE: The status of liver transplantation, Bull Am Coll Surg 70(5):8–10, May 1985.

Stuart FP Jr: Transplantation, Bull Am Coll Surg 69(1):54–58, Jan 1984.

West NJ: Liver transplantation: Intraoperative nursing care, AORN J 39(1):40–41, Jan 1984.

CHAPTER 35 ONCOLOGY

Anderson MA et al: The double-lumen Hickman catheter, Am J Nurs 82(2):272–273, Feb 1982.

Balch CM: Cancer surgery, Bull Am Coll Surg 69(1):3–7, Jan 1984.

Bane CL, Rich TA: Intraoperative radiation therapy, AORN J 37(5):835–839, Apr 1983.

Bane CL, Shurkus LM: Caring for intraoperative radiation patients, AORN J 37(5):840–846, Apr 1983.

Beahrs OH: The American Joint Committee on Cancer, Bull Am Coll Surg 69(9):16–17, Sep 1984.

Brozenec SA: Surgical implants: Medication & alimentation devices, AORN J 37(7):1353, 1356, 1358, 1360, 1362, 1364, 1366, 1368, June 1983.

Cozad J: Hyperthermic perfusion for melanoma, AORN J 38(6):974–978, Dec 1983.

Cozad J: Indwelling central venous catheters, Point View 22(3):14–15, Sep 1985.

Gullatte MM, Foltz AT: Hepatic chemotherapy via implantable pump, Am J Nurs 83(12):1674–1676, Dec 1983.

Hushen SC: Dilemmas in practice: Questioning TPN as the answer, Am J Nurs 82(5):852, 854, May 1982.

Jenkins JF et al: Managing intraperitoneal chemotherapy—a new assault on ovarian cancer, Nursing (Horsham) 12(5):76–83, May 1982.

Johnston S, Patt YZ: Caring for the patient on intraarterial chemotherapy . . . Are you ready?, Nursing (Horsham) 11(11):108–112, Nov 1981.

Jones SG: Bilateral adrenalectomy: Post-op dangers to watch for, RN 45(3):66, 68, Mar 1982.

Karrei I: Hickman catheters: Your guide to troublefree use, Can Nurse 78(11):25–27, Dec 1982.

Kelly PP, Tinsley C: Planning care for the patient receiving external radiation, Am J Nurs 81(2):338–342, Feb 1981.

Klopfenstein ML: Hepatic artery cannulation, AORN J 34(5):956, 958, 960, 962, 964, Nov 1981.

Koren ME, Herrmann CS: Cancer immunotherapy: What, why, when, how, Nursing (Horsham) 11(1):34–41, Jan 1981.

Mattia MA, Blake SL: Hospital hazards: Cancer drugs, Am J Nurs 83(5):758–762, May 1983.

McKneally MF: Surgical oncology, Bull Am Coll Surg 70(1):53–55, Jan 1985.

Nonkin R: The Broviac catheter: OR technique, AORN J 35(2):215–217, Feb 1982.

Nursing update: Nursing implications of cancer chemotherapy, Nursing (Horsham) 13(7):56a, July 1983.

Palmer PN: The tunable dye laser: Photoradiation of malignancies, AORN J 39(5):782–786, Apr 1984.

Raaf JH, Callery C: An easy technique for tunneling the Broviac catheter, Surg Gynecol Obstet 157(5):485–486, Nov 1983.

Rosenberg SA: Oncology, Bull Am Coll Surg 68(1):26–29, Jan 1983.

Schulmeister L: Vascular access grafts in cancer chemotherapy, Am J Nurs 82(9):1388–1389, Sep 1982.

Siebel J: Playing it safe around cesium implant, RN 46(10):42–43, Oct 1983.

Steuer K: Liver carcinoma: Treatment with an implantable pump, AORN J 39(5):787–792, Apr 1984.

Varricchio CG: The patient on radiation therapy, Am J Nurs 81(2):334–337, Feb 1981.

Watne AL: Head and neck cancer: The ideal stalking-horse for solid tumors, Am J Surg 146(4):422–424, Oct 1983.

Watson SC: OR nursing care of cancer patients, AORN J 34(2):215–222, Aug 1981.

Wilson RE: Progress in breast-cancer treatment, today and tomorrow, Bull Am Coll Surg 68(9):2–6, Sep 1983.

Wittig P, Semmler-Bertanzi DJ: Pumps and controllers—A nurse's assessment guide, Am J Nurs 83(7):1023–1025, July 1983.

CHAPTER 36
POTENTIAL COMPLICATIONS IN SURGICAL PATIENTS

Aish A, Brown A: How to use risk factors and assessment skills to individualize patient care, Can Nurse 78(11):46–49, Dec 1982.

Allen P: Applying standards to practice, AORN J 31(5):805–813, Apr 1980.

Barrows JJ: Turning the tide against acute pulmonary edema, Nursing (Horsham) 14(3):34–41, Mar 1984.

Becker RC et al: Pulmonary embolism: A review of 200 cases with emphasis on pathophysiology, diagnosis, and treatment, Cleve Clin Q 51(3):519–529, Fall 1984.

Blaisdell FW: Traumatic shock: The search for a toxic factor, Bull Am Coll Surg 68(10):2–10, Oct 1983.

Bobb J: What happens when your patient goes into shock?, RN 47(3):26–29, Mar 1984.

Borchardt AC, Fraulini KE: Hypothermia in the postanesthetic patient, AORN J 36(4):648, 652–653, 656–657, 660–661, 664–665, 668–669, Oct 1982.

Bubela N: Is your client at risk for respiratory complications?, Can Nurse 79(3):46–48, Mar 1983.

Callahan M: COPD: A special postop challenge, RN 47(5):44–47, May 1984.

Darovic G: Ten perils of mechanical ventilation, RN 46(5):36–42, May 1983.

Darovic G: Was this postop death preventable?, RN 46(10):47–48, Oct 1983.

Dossey B, Passons JM: Pulmonary embolism, preventing it, treating it, Nursing (Horsham) 11(3):26–33, Mar 1981.

Drain CB: Managing postoperative pain: It's a matter of sighs, Nursing (Horsham) 14(8):52–55, Aug 1984.

Fahey VA: An in-depth look at deep vein thrombosis, Nursing (Horsham) 14(3):34–41, Mar 1984.

Fernsebner B et al: Surgical prevention of pulmonary emboli, AORN J 39(1):56–64, Jan 1984.

Frace RM: Mechanical ventilation: The patient's viewpoint, Todays OR Nurse 4(6):16–21, Aug 1982.

Fuchs P: Before and after surgery stay right on respiratory care, Nursing (Horsham) 13(5):46–50, May 1983.

Gammon SS: Respiratory acidosis, Nursing (Horsham) 12(8):65, Aug 1982.

Hall KV: Detecting septic shock before it's too late, RN 44(9):28–32, Sep 1981.

Hammond C: Sinus irregularities: From arrhythmias to arrest, RN 46(6):58, June 1983.

Jackson BS, Carlisle PM: How post-op complications can burgeon into crisis, RN 44(1):26–32, Jan 1981.

Lovvorn J: Coronary artery bypass surgery: Helping patients cope with postop problems, Am J Nurs 82(7):1073–1075, July 1982.

Ostrow LS: Air embolism and central venous lines, Am J Nurs 81(11):2036–2038, Nov 1981.

Patras AZ: The operation's over, but the danger's not, Nursing (Horsham) 12(9):50–56, Sep 1982.

Patras AZ, Brozenec SA: Gastrointestinal assessment: Identifying significant problems, AORN J 40(5):726–731, Nov 1984.

Petlin A, Carolan JM: Halt hypovolemic shock, RN 45(5):36–42, May 1982.

Pfister S: Respiratory arrest: Are you prepared?, Nursing (Horsham) 12(9):34–41, Sep 1982.

Platt R et al: Mortality associated with nosocomial urinary-tract infection, N Engl J Med 307(11):637–642, Sep 9, 1982.

RN Master Care Plan: Preventing postop wound infection, RN 47(6):31–32, June 1984.

Shires GT: Shock, metabolism, and organ failure, Bull Am Coll Surg 70(1):48–52, Jan 1985.

Sigg LV, Fallucca LL: Recognizing hypoventilation in the recovery room, AORN J 38(2):270, 272, 274, 276–277, 280, 282, 284–285, Aug 1983.

Skillcheck: Recognizing fluid and electrolyte imbalance, Nursing (Horsham) 12(9):86, 88, 90, Sep 1982.

Stevenson RCK: Take no chances with fat embolism, Nursing (Horsham) 15(6):58–64, June 1985.

Stuhler-Schlag MK: Pre and postoperative fluids and electrolytes: Nursing assessment and intervention, Todays OR Nurse 4(7):10–15, 66–67, Sep 1982.

Sumner SM, Grau PA: To defeat hypovolemic shock anticipate and act swiftly, Nursing (Horsham) 11(10):46–51, Oct 1981.

Taylor AG et al: How effective is TENS for acute pain?, Am J Nurs 83(8):1171–1174, Aug 1983.

Taylor DL: Thrombophlebitis: Physiology, signs, and symptoms, Nursing (Horsham) 13(7):52–53, July 1983.

Treloar DM: When a surgical wound bursts, RN 47(6):26–30, June 1984.

CHAPTER 37
REALITIES OF CLINICAL PRACTICE

AORN ad hoc Committee on Basic Competencies in Operating Room Nursing: *Developing Basic Competencies for Perioperative Nursing,* Denver: Association of Operating Room Nurses, Inc., 1982.

Arnell I: The right to live/The right to die, Todays OR Nurse 6(9):27, 30–31, Sep 1984.

Benner P: From novice to expert, Am J Nurs 82(3):402–407, Mar 1982.

Case BB: Moving your staff toward excellent performance, Nurs Manage 14(12):45–48, Dec 1983.

Clouser KD: Life-support systems: Some moral reflections, Bull Am Coll Surg 68(6):12–17, June 1983.

Creighton H: Law for the nurse manager: Refusing to participate in abortions, Nurs Manage 13(4):27–28, Apr 1982.

Dunlop GR: President's commission offers guidelines on life-support therapy, Bull Am Coll Surg 68(6):8–11, June 1983.

Gaylin W: Modern medicine and the price of success, Bull Am Coll Surg 68(6):4–7, June 1983.

Ghiglieri S et al: Toward a competency-based safe practice, Nurs Manage 14(3):16–19, Mar 1983.

Mittler J: Tell me when you're ready, an open letter to the patient facing death, Can Nurse 78(5):20, 22, May 1982.

Nursing Practice Committee: Guidelines for developing clinical ladders, AORN J 37(6):1216–1217, 1220, May 1983.

O'Neill S et al: A conversation about death and dying, Can Nurse 80(6):25, June 1984.

Opinions: Is there a gap between your ideals and job satisfaction?, AORN J 32(4):661–662, 665, 668, 672, 674, 676, 678, Oct 1980.

Patterson P: Fetal therapy: Issues we face, AORN J 35(4):663–668, Mar 1982.

Prato SA: Ethical decisions in daily practice, Superv Nurs 12(7):18–20, July 1981.

Preston CA et al: Stress and the OR nurse, AORN J 33(4):662–671, Mar 1981.

Regan WA: Legally speaking: Assisting at abortions: Can you really say no?, RN 45(6):71, June 1982.

Regan WA: Legally speaking: She wouldn't play by the rules, RN 44(4):88, 94, Apr 1981.

Richardson JD et al: Ethics and surgery: Bedside teaching and learning, Bull Am Coll Surg 67(7):10–13, July 1982.

Rothrock JC: Reality shock: Some questions and answers, Surg Technol 14(4):8–10, July–Aug 1982.

Rudy EB: Brain death, Dimens Crit Care Nurs 1(3):178–184, May–June 1982.

Schaal PG, Slemenda MB: Nurses' response to transplants, AORN J 39(1):42–45, Jan 1984.

Selye H: A code for coping with stress, AORN J 25(1):35–42, Jan 1977.

Smith SJ, Davis AJ: Ethical dilemmas: Conflicts among rights, duties, and obligations, Am J Nurs 80(8):1463–1466, Aug 1980.

Sredl DR: The head nurse as ethical and legal leader, Nurs Manage 14(11):55–57, Nov 1983.

Thompson JE, Thompson HO: Ethics: Ethical decision making is an integral part of nursing, AORN J 39(2):157–158, 160, Feb 1984.

Uustal DB: Exploring values in nursing, AORN J 31(2):183–187, Feb 1980.

Wolf JS: Ethical ingredients in organ replacement, Bull Am Coll Surg 69(5):12–13, May 1984.

INDEX

ISBN 0-07-002541-X